SURGERY AND ITS ALTERNATIVES

SURGERY AND ITS ALTERNATIVES

HOW TO MAKE THE RIGHT CHOICES FOR YOUR HEALTH

Sandra A. McLanahan, M.D.

David J. McLanahan, M.D.

Preface by Bernie S. Siegel, M.D.

TWIN STREAMS
Kensington Books
http://www.kensingtonbooks.com

We dedicate this book to our parents, C. Jack and
Connie McLanahan; Rev. Swami Satchidananda, Dr.
Gerald and Janey Lemole, Dannion Brinkley, Gail
Tanaka, and Lianne Tanaka McLanahan.

TWIN STREAM BOOKS are published by

Kensington Publishing Corp.
850 Third Avenue
New York, NY 10022

Library of Congress Card Catalogue Number: 2001092972
ISBN 0-7582-0201-6

First Printing: July 2002
10 9 8 7 6 5 4 3 2 1

Printed in the United States of America

CONTENTS

Acknowledgments xiii
Preface xv

INTRODUCTION 1

This Book Is for Everyone 3
Surgery and the New Nonsurgical Choices 5
Educating Yourself 6
Introducing the Authors 7
Making the Best Use of This Book 12

CHAPTER 1. WHAT IS ALTERNATIVE MEDICINE? 13

Why "Alternative" Medicine? 14
Getting in Touch with Your Inner Chocolate 17
Fundamentals of Alternative Medicine 18
The Most Common Alternatives 25
Scientific Research on Alternatives 26
Choosing from Among the Alternatives 26
Protecting Yourself from Unreliable Alternatives 27
Avoiding Blaming the Victim 27
Life Support Considerations 28
Death 28

The Operating Room of the Future 30
Alternative/Complementary/Integrative Health Centers 30

CHAPTER 2. SPECIFIC ALTERNATIVE MEDICINE APPROACHES 33

Designing an Alternative Program: The First Steps 34
Stress Management Techniques 35
Diet 64
Alternative Healing Methods 73
Fasting 83
Quitting Smoking 84
Getting a Good Night's Sleep 86
Alternative Approaches Instead of Surgery: Are They Worth It? 87
Physician, Heal Myself 88
Alternative Approaches in Addition to Surgery 89

CHAPTER 3. HOW TO MAKE A DECISION ABOUT SURGERY 91

Making an Informed Decision 91
Choosing Your Opinions 92
Choosing Your Surgeon 93
The Second Surgical Opinion 94
The Alternative Medicine Third Opinion 94
Other Sources of Information 95
Questions to Ask at Your Initial Doctor Visits 95
Finalizing Your Choice of Surgeon 101
Choosing Your Hospital 101
What Can You Do If You Are Restricted in Your Choice of Doctor or Hospital? 102
The Philosophy of Risk Taking 103
Cure, Quality of Life, and Life Extension 103
The Special Benefits of the Surgical Approach 103
The Special Benefits of the Alternative Medicine Approach 104
Should You Have the Operation? Putting It All Together 104

CHAPTER 4. THE OPERATIVE PERIOD: WHAT TO EXPECT 105

The Preoperative Period 105
The Operative Period 114
Early Postoperative Period 123
Late Postoperative Period 125
Hospital Discharge 136
Alternative Medicine Approaches to Convalescence 137
Adjusting to a New Lifestyle 139

CHAPTER 5. SKIN 141

How Your Skin Works 142
How Skin Disease Is Diagnosed 143
Nonmalignant Growths On and Beneath the Skin 143
Moles 144
Lipomas and Sebaceous Cysts 146
Lymph Gland Enlargement 149
Skin Infections 151
Pilonidal Cysts 155
Skin Cancer 157
Malignant Melanoma 163

CHAPTER 6. BREAST 171

Development, Structure, and Function of Your Breasts 172
Appearance of Your Breasts 174
Breast Enlargement 174
Breast Reduction 179
How Breast Disease Is Diagnosed 181
Fibrocystic Disease and Benign Lumps 190
Breast Cancer 193

CHAPTER 7. LUNG 231

How Your Lungs Work 232
How Lung Disease Is Diagnosed 233
Collapsed Lung 236
Lung Cancer 239

CHAPTER 8. HEART 249

How Your Heart Works 253
Coronary Artery Disease and Atherosclerosis 254

CHAPTER 9. ARTERIES 285

How Your Arteries Work 286
Artery Disease 288
Aneurysms 307
Stroke 311

CHAPTER 10. VEINS 325

How Your Veins Work 326
Varicose Veins 327

CHAPTER 11. ESOPHAGUS 337

How Your Esophagus Works 338
How Esophageal Disease Is Diagnosed 339
Hiatal Hernia and Esophageal Reflux 341
Esophageal Cancer 349

CHAPTER 12. STOMACH 355

How Your Stomach Works 356
How Stomach Disease Is Diagnosed 358
Peptic Ulcer Disease 359

Nonpeptic Stomach Ulcer Disease 372
Stomach Cancer 374

CHAPTER 13. GALLBLADDER 379

How Your Gallbladder Works 380
Gallstones 380
What Happens After Your Gallbladder Is Removed? 391

CHAPTER 14. PANCREAS 393

How Your Pancreas Works 393
How Pancreatic Disease Is Diagnosed 394
Acute Pancreatitis 397
Chronic Pancreatitis 400
Pancreatic Cancer 402

CHAPTER 15. COLON 411

How Your Colon Works 412
Alternative Medicine Approaches to Keeping Your Colon Healthy 414
How Colon Disease Is Diagnosed 415
Screening for Colorectal Cancer 418
Diverticular Disease 419
Inflammatory Colitis (Ulcerative Colitis and Crohn's Disease) 424
Colon Polyps 431
Colorectal Cancer 433
Colon Operations 443

CHAPTER 16. APPENDIX 451

Anatomy of Your Appendix 452
Appendicitis 452
Surgical Approaches to Appendicitis 456

CHAPTER 17. ANUS AND RECTUM 459

How Your Anus Works 460
How Anal Disease Is Diagnosed 461
Hemorrhoids 462
Anal Fissures 472
Anal Warts 476
Anal Infections 478

CHAPTER 18. HERNIA 481

Groin Hernia 482
Umbilical Hernia 489
Ventral and Incisional Hernias 491
Groin Hernias in Children 496
Umbilical Hernias in Children 497

CHAPTER 19. FEMALE REPRODUCTIVE SYSTEM 499

Structure and Function of the Female Reproductive System 501
How Disorders of the Female Reproductive System Are Diagnosed 502
Dysfunctional Uterine Bleeding 507
Endometriosis 515
Adenomyosis of the Uterus 520
Uterine Fibroids 520
Cervical Cancer 527
Uterine Cancer 533
Hysterectomy 536
Ovarian Cysts and Benign Tumors 542
Ovarian Cancer 545
Prevention of Ovarian Cancer 549
Oophorectomy and Salpingectomy Operations 550

CHAPTER 20. MALE REPRODUCTIVE SYSTEM 553

Structure and Function of the Male Reproductive System 554
How Disorders of the Male Reproductive System Are Diagnosed 556

Benign Prostate Enlargement (Hypertrophy) 558
Prostate Cancer 567
Specific Prostate Operations 575
Erectile Dysfunction 579

CHAPTER 21. THYROID 589

How Your Thyroid Gland Works 590
How Thyroid Disease Is Diagnosed 591
Hyperthyroidism 593
Goiter 598
Thyroid Cancer 600
Specific Thyroid Operations 604

CHAPTER 22. BACK, NECK, AND JOINTS 607

The Back 607
How Your Back Works 609
Back Problems 610
The Neck 627
How Your Neck Works 628
The Knee 634
How Your Knee Works 634
Knee Meniscus Injury 636
Knee Ligament Injury 639
Knee Joint Cartilage and Bone Damage 644
The Hip 649
How Your Hip Works 650
Hip Joint Damage 650
The Wrist 658
How Your Wrist Works 659
Carpal Tunnel Syndrome 659

CHAPTER 23. OTHER SURGICAL DISORDERS 665

Excess Body Fat 666

Facial Cosmetic Problems 672

Nasal Disorders 677

Thinning Hair and Baldness 680

Tonsil and Adenoid Disorders 684

Cataracts 690

Kidney Stones 698

CHAPTER 24. AN INTEGRATED APPROACH TO YOUR OPERATION 709

Getting Ready for Surgery: A Program of Diet, Supplements, and Stress Management 710

During Surgery: What Your Surgeon Can Do 713

After Surgery 713

Preventing Future Recurrence 716

Examples of Integrative Surgery 717

Beyond the Scalpel 718

For Further Information 719

Publisher's Resource List 733

Notes 753

Index 797

ACKNOWLEDGMENTS

We are very grateful to acknowledge the diverse group of teachers, coworkers, advisors, and inspirational resources who assisted with this book.

All of our spirited Irish family pitched in: Jack and Connie McLanahan, Michael and Astride McLanahan, Gurnam and Martha McLanahan Bajwa, C. Scott, M.D., and Mary McLanahan; Eileen McLanahan and Gary Livingston.

For their expert advice and assistance, we would especially like to thank our editors Claire Gerus and Elaine Will Sparber; our agent Eric Simonoff; and Bernie S. Siegel, M.D, for kindly agreeing to write our Preface.

We also greatly appreciate the help of artist Liang Wei, who helped work out the illustrations, and Lloyd Birmingham, who finalized them.

Sandra would especially like to thank Reverend Sri Swami Satchidananda; "writing angels" Carole and Bruce Hart; Gerald Lemole, M.D., and his extraordinary wife, Janie, and their entire family: Mehmet Oz, M.D., and Lisa, Daphne, Arabella, Zoë, and Oliver Oz; Laura, Emily, Michael, Samantha, and Christopher Robin; Dean Ornish, M.D., his wife, Molly, and his entire staff: Dr. Jim Billings; Amy Klein Gage, Chip Spann, Heather Amador, Laura Nugent, and Myrna Melling; and all of the Preventive Medicine Research Institute research participants; especially former Top Gun Doug Hawley; Michael Lerner, Ph.D., of Commonweal Cancer Help Retreats; Gloria Steinem; Craig Bradley, M.D.; Ray Haling, M.D.; Robert L. Schwartz; Paul Rosch, M.D.; Jay Neufeld, M.D.; Ernest Shearer, D.O.; Dr. James Duke; Alan Gaby, M.D.; Marty Albert, M.D.; Eugene Schoenfeld, M.D.; Sterling Bunnell, M.D.; Andrew Weil, M.D.; Randy Van Nostrand, M.D.; Richard Prince, M.D.; Dr. Jeffrey Bland; Neal Barnard, M.D.; James Gordon, M.D.; Dr. Ann Gill Taylor; Charlotte McCutchen, M.D.; Robert L. Painter, M.D.; and Jeffrey Mast, M.D.

Sandra also wishes to thank the past and present staff of the Integral Health Center, especially Dwight McKee, M.D.; Alan Dattner, M.D.; Brahman Levy, M.D.; Muktan Michael Sullivan, D.C.; David Harden, D.O.; Divya Heidi Bertoud; Surya Lipscomb; Saraswati Neumann; acupuncturists Lalitha Stone, Sheila Doyle, Jody

Forman, and Dr. Frank Shieh; Hope Mell; Sumati Metro; Mangala Warner; David Douglas; Jacqui Gresham; and architect Kennon Williams; Vernon Sylvest, M.D.; Rolfers Viki Van Wey, Scott Gauthier, Sharon Hancoff, Eva Jo and Frank Wu; medical intuitives Hilda Swiger, Jane Mullan, Carol Keppler, Christine Whitehead, Dale Schear; Poet Coleman Barks; Attorney Sat Nam Singh; Physicist David Okerson; Sam Busch; all of the members of the Integral Yoga Institutes and ashrams: especially all of the Swamis, Rev. Shanti Norris, Peter Max, Arjuna Zurbel, Rishi Schweig, Paramesh and Sadasiva Adie, Prem Anjali, the Metros, Rudra Altman, Lata Altman, Kenneth Shapero, Lila Steinberg, Kalyani Neuman, all of the Rasiahs, artist Ann Sjogren, musicians Radhika Miller and Paul Winter, Cancer researcher and transcendent actor John Jai Fink, hairdressers Luis, and Chrissy; Indians Sri N. Mahalingam, Mr. A.U. Ramaswamy and family, and Jatin and Nalini Bhabhalia; and Hari Barker.

In addition, Sandra thanks Apollo 13 astronaut Dr. Edgar Mitchell, Senator Claiborne Pell, George Vecchio, John Premdas Cinciarelli, Ester Cutler, Ed Brown, Ruth Goerhing, Rene Frank, Elsie Kidd, Sally Todd, Kumar Zelin, Henrietta Near, Arnold Ablon, Gerald and Barbara Hines, Gail and Genard Gross, and Dr. Joe Veltmann. A loving Irish poet, the late Sidney Paul Steed, provided an essential contribution of faith, thoughtfulness, and timely financial assistance.

Finally, Sandra wishes to especially thank Dannion Brinkley, author of *Saved by the Light*, and *At Peace in the Light,* for his essential support and contribution to the spiritual reflections in this book.

David wishes to especially acknowledge his patient wife, Gail Tanaka, and daughter, Lianne Tanaka McLanahan, who gave up some "Daddy Time" for this book.

Also, David would like to thank several of his colleagues who reviewed parts of the manuscript in their area of expertise. While not necessarily agreeing or disagreeing with the final product, their comments were very helpful. Specifically: Drs. Judy Jacobson, Sandy Levy, Tom Preston, Dick Wonderly, Jordan Gottlieb, Piro Kramar, Jim Pritchett, and Jeff Bailett.

PREFACE

BERNIE S. SIEGEL, M.D.

I highly recommend this book. Study it carefully, and share it with your friends, to become aware of the important new choices and changes taking place for both patients and their caregivers. Through this process, we all can become a part of a truly loving, healing community.

Twenty-four years ago, I decided to create a self-portrait. I painted myself totally covered by a surgical cap, mask, and gown. Looking at this picture, you wouldn't recognize me, and it might even frighten you to see the pain in my eyes.

Since then, I have learned how critically important it is to take off such layers, for the health of both surgeons and their patients. We both need to deal with our feelings.

Surgeons are really just tourists, visiting your body and your disease: usually we haven't had the illness, we haven't "been there," so we are not natives. When I talk to large groups of patients, and ask them what is the thing they want most from their doctors, they universally say: "Tell them to treat me like a person!"

Patients want someone to care for them; to listen to their questions, concerns, and fears; to touch and, yes, even to love them. In our "advanced" civilization, we have become less inclined to do this: we have become so mechanistic now we are even surprised when a *person*, rather than a machine, answers the phone. Appliances do our work for us, but they can lead us to a strong sense of disempowerment.

This is especially true in medical care. Modern medicine has trained us to look primarily at variables such as your blood pressure and your organ systems, but not at your lifestyle, what is going on in your life, what you are *feeling*, and what is your story. These factors, which may be the most fundamental to your road back to wellness, are addressed by neither surgery nor drugs.

The *Journal of the American Medical Association* published a study of labor and delivery showing that if a loving labor coach was present, the cesarean section rate and need for anesthesia could be markedly reduced. When such mind-body considerations are included in the practice of medicine, two people are saved: the doctor and the patient. Then the doctor also can become what the word originally meant: "teacher."

Someone remarked to me about a colleague, "He's too closed-minded to be scientific," and I think this summarizes the problem with many surgeons and patients. Open-mindedness includes embracing anything that *works*. You may not know why gravity works, but you can still make use of it. I *like* the word "mystery." Those things we regard as mysterious may someday be explained, but even while they remain mysterious, we can make *use* of them, tell the next person, pass them on. No one should be against success, even if you can't explain it.

Here are the alternative medicine approaches I have found most useful when integrated into my own surgical practice:

Preoperatively, let your surgeon get to know you as an individual. Surgeons need to be aware that there is a *person* there. Before your operation, draw a picture of what you imagine the operating room to look like. If it is a loving supportive scene, your chances of an uncomplicated outcome are better. If it is empty or menacing, you can take action to alter your expectations and degree of support. Practicing the self-hypnosis techniques given in this book, you can "ask" your body to divert blood from the operative site, to help your surgeon, and use other images to help you heal more rapidly.

Give your surgeon a list of suggestions of what he or she can say to you while you are under anesthesia, and have him or her ask the staff to avoid making any negative remarks. Patients under anesthesia are in an altered, trance state, but one in which they *can* register everything said to them. For a while, I suggested to my patients while under anesthesia that they would wake up after their procedures "comfortable, thirsty, and hungry," but I had several complain to me that they *gained* weight after their operation, so I had to modify my suggestion to, "You will awaken feeling comfortable, thirsty, and hungry, but you don't have to finish everything on your plate."

Inform your surgeon about your preferences. Doctors need to be aware of their individual patient's needs, and you can help them by making yours known to them. For instance, having an open mind means that, in some cases, the doctor can write in your chart "patient doesn't *need* pain (or sleep) medication," not "patient *refuses* medication."

During surgery, I have asked patients, while they were under anesthesia, to help change their blood flow and blood pressure, and I then saw the positive results; and the operating room staff also witnessed them. I even challenged this with numbers: "Adjust your heart rate to 68." Then we'd all watch the monitor, and bingo, there it would be at 68. If I noticed a patient with a very fast heartbeat due to subconscious anxiety, I'd say, "Everything is fine. You're doing very well," and see the pulse slowly come down into the normal 80s as the patient relaxed, even while asleep.

People who do best postoperatively are those who see their operation as a source of healing. In my experience, those who look at their operation as a mutilation have more postsurgical pain than those who see it as their choice of therapy or even as a gift. Surround yourself with love. Ask for the help you need. *Express* appropriate sadness or anger, especially if you are not treated properly or with respect.

The pendulum of releasing patients from the hospital may have swung much too far, from previously too-lengthy hospital stays in the 50s to too-short ones now. My father, when close to death, was abruptly sent home by his doctors. My mother was not at all prepared to have him at home, and had no accommodations for such a sick person. When I confronted his doctor, he said, "But I thought you wanted him home." We *had*—but not in *that* condition. He was rushed back to the hospital, where he died a day later. No one was benefited by this disastrous, traumatic attempt at home care that became so uncomfortable for everyone.

Speak up. Let whoever is caring for you professionally know what you need. Say, "Hold it! That's crazy!" if something doesn't feel right to you. Speak up, so that your caregiver gets to know you as a person. One patient, who'd had a laryngectomy and *couldn't* talk, wrote to me, "It's a good thing my wife was here, so she could tell them several times that they were about to give me the medication for the man in the next bed."

The word "patient" comes from "suffer" and "submit." Many studies have now demonstrated, however, that patients who are "feisty fighters," who fight for what they want, actually have higher rates of survival. Communicating your needs and wants is also the most important preventive measure you can take to avoid the postoperative blues. This book can significantly help you avoid postoperative depression by informing you about what to expect from your surgery.

Surgeons need to learn to take care of themselves, too. They can help themselves stay healthy by taking time out for their own daily meditative practices, and other sources of renewal. Even on a busy day, I take fifteen minutes in the hospital chapel, or elsewhere, to meditate, because I know that I treat people better by a small application of my time to this attunement.

I also run. I find it induces a reflective state—it's been shown to shift blood flow to the right brain as well as to increase the body's natural painkillers. On Cape Cod one day last summer, I was amazed to discover I had lost all sense of place and time while I was running—an uplifting experience that encouraged me to continue running as a regular part of my life.

Being a surgeon was a source of great joy to me. Almost every day brought some delight about a patient's progress, and the benefits surgery could bring to them. But I also stored up enormous pain. It was only through keeping a personal journal, then writing books, that I released enough of this pain to even remember the stories of humor and success I had selectively shared with my family at our nightly dinner table. Not sharing my pain made me repress and forget those other, happier parts of my experience.

Where do *doctors* go to express their human emotions? I have seen surgeons crying in the stairwells of hospitals, and in empty classrooms, rather than sharing their grief with the families of their patients.

The current practice of Western medicine and our culture in general is to regard death as a failure. However, everybody *does* die. In our surgical training, we are taught to take care of anatomical parts and diseases, not people. Our entire health-care system is disease-oriented, not people-oriented. But it is *people,* not *organs,* who get sick. And we surgeons are people, too, and when patients do die, we feel it too.

We now understand that sharing the full range of our human emotions, including humor and hope, laughter and love, helps us all to heal. No patients object if their doctor gives them hope and makes them laugh. Once I wheeled a particularly anxious patient into the operating room, and she looked up at me saying, "I'm so glad I have all these wonderful people to take care of me." I leaned over and whispered conspiratorially, "I *know* them. And they are *not* all wonderful people." Everyone laughed, and the tension left the room.

All of us, as humans, are doing the *same work.* We are learning how to love and feel connected and whole in our lives. Were families always a problem, or is this generation having a worse time? What will a generation of children who have been so abused be like as adults? Will those who have never been loved ever learn how to love?

We can't be afraid and laugh at the same time. We must be honest, but when and where can make a significant difference to our subconscious selves. Surgeons giving risk information in the hallway just before surgery had higher cardiac arrest rates in their patients than surgeons who gave the same information the night before, when the patient had time to adjust to it and resist its negative implications. The first group of surgeons was literally "scaring the patients to death."

Health care, our nation's largest business, has not adequately taught us to take responsibility for our own health. We should. Studies have indicated that those who know their options and make their own choices are likely to do better.

"Choice" is the operative mode of this book. Choose the option most suited to *you. Any* operation is your choice and your responsibility. I don't believe there is a *right* or *wrong* choice; I can tell you what *I* would do or what I would suggest to you if you were my child, but ultimately it must be *your choice.* Perhaps you would rather have surgery or chemotherapy than go on a restricted diet. No one can make a choice for you that is as good as the one you make for yourself.

Don't choose a course of action to "not die," and don't choose anything just because someone tells you to. We *are* all going to die anyway. What you choose should enhance the quality of *your* life. Life is a labor pain, but you can say yes or no to the painful choices that ultimately lead to giving birth to yourself.

This book uniquely and completely presents the panorama of possibilities for treatment of your disease. Significantly, you need not be limited by even one choice: if your first preference doesn't work, you can go on to one of the other approaches given here. Nothing is more important, however, than your simply becoming familiar with the full range of your healing choices and subsequently participating in the surgical process as an important member of your own surgical team.

INTRODUCTION

Surgery is one of the most effective ways of influencing the course of disease, but, as is the case with most other treatments, it is a double-edged sword.

George Crile, M.D., surgeon

I think that surgery is an archaic way of treating disease. I do not believe it will be here forever. I see evidence of that even within my own professional lifetime. Many of the diseases for which I performed operations twenty years ago I don't operate upon any more because there are now less brutal, better ways of treating them.

Richard Selzer, M.D., surgeon

June, a 54-year-old clinical social worker, had been overextending herself, commuting to another state to maintain her long-distance marriage, while at the same time experiencing stress caused by her mother's terminal illness. She became increasingly fatigued, then noticed worrisome shortness of breath on exertion, accompanied by chest pain and an irregular heartbeat. A medical examination revealed she was suffering from a degenerative heart condition termed severe progressive cardiomyopathy that had caused congestive heart failure. The only solution her local conventional doctors could offer was an operation: a heart transplant, which has a 35 percent failure rate within five years. Even then, the odds of finding a donor are quite poor: more than 40,000 persons need a heart transplant each year, while only about 2,500 hearts become available. Three other options—a mechanical heart support device, a mechanical heart, or a wrap of her own back muscle around her heart to help it function—were not widely available, and so far had no research showing how they would function after only a short period of time.

June decided instead to embark on a program of lifestyle change to reverse her heart disease, as discussed in Chapter 8 of this book. She switched to a low-fat, vegetarian diet, began walking one hour every other day, and faithfully practiced one and a half hours of yoga every day. She felt better immediately, and her friends began to exclaim at how radiant she looked. An examination six months later showed her heart function so much improved that she no longer needed a transplant, and she was taken off the transplant waiting list.

Douglas, on the other hand, exemplifies the new surgical choices. A 46-year-old nurse, he had been a three-pack-a-day smoker since he was a teenager, though he had finally quit a year previously. After an upper respiratory infection developed that he just couldn't shake, he had a chest X-ray. A small lung nodule was found in the periphery of his right lung. His first surgeon recommended removing a segment, or lobe, of the lung through a standard incision between his ribs.

Douglas investigated his options, getting a second opinion from another surgeon, who suggested his operation could be conducted using a thoracoscope, similar to the laparoscope being used for abdominal procedures. He had the thoracoscopic surgery and his nodule was found to be benign. By choosing to have the operation with this technique, he was left with almost no scar and significantly less postoperative pain, and he went home from the hospital much sooner, two days after his operation.

Marie, a 49-year-old aging baby boomer, thought she might need a hysterectomy. She was experiencing some menopausal symptoms, and had suffered from such marked episodes of bleeding that she had become tired and anemic. In addition, several uterine fibroids were found to be pressing on her bladder. However, instead of simply submitting to an operation, she educated herself about her choices, and discovered, as discussed in Chapter 19 of this book, that the uterus participates in orgasm, exhibiting a series of contractions that contribute to the plea-

surable sensations of the complete experience. Although many women feel better after a hysterectomy, a significant number do not. Marie also learned that after losing her uterus, even if she kept her ovaries, her menopausal symptoms could be worse, and if she chose to take replacement hormone, she would have an increased risk for breast cancer.

Marie decided to try the alternative medicine program given in this book, which includes dietary change, vitamins, herbs, homeopathy, and acupuncture. Her periods quickly reverted to normal, her menopausal problems disappeared, and she felt better than she had in years. She is very grateful to have learned just in time that many hysterectomies are unnecessary, and to have retained an important part of her anatomy.

Bruce Hart, a 60-year-old Emmy award–winning song and screenplay writer, author, and one of the creators of Sesame Street, exemplifies how the conventional and the alternative paths can be combined. He suddenly needed kidney surgery, to remove a small cancerous tumor but, owing to this type of tumor, could not have the surgery done laparoscopically. He utilized an initial draft of this book to design a program integrating traditional surgery with alternative medicine methods. He prepared by making a music tape, practicing hypnosis and yoga, having acupuncture treatments, and following a special diet and supplement program. He also wrote a "script" for his doctor to read aloud during the surgery.

The results were remarkable. During the operation, Bruce's surgeon made suggestions to him. Although he had put aside a quart of his own blood, he needed none during the five-hour procedure. Despite having a rib removed, he experienced no significant postoperative pain.

The surgeon's, residents', and interns' reactions were immediate. They came streaming into Bruce's room afterward, demanding to know more. They had believed it possible to "will" blood to shift from the operative site, since this result of hypnosis has been documented,[1] but because currently so few patients do it, they had never seen it before. They loved the effects of the music, which had transformed a routine operation into a more peaceful, meditative experience for them, too. Bruce's recovery was achieved in record time, and he was soon back crafting his superlative scripts, while continuing to practice daily yoga, to assure his ongoing health and prevent recurrence, though mainly just for the enjoyment of it.

This Book Is for Everyone

The landmark collaboration of doctors of alternative medicine and surgery in this book can help you avoid operations whenever you safely can, and get through them in much better shape when you must endure them.

First, the normal anatomy of each organ will be explained and its tests and evaluations described. Then, the various disorders affecting each organ system will be detailed along with the predisposing lifestyle and other risk factors for each disease. An integrative medicine physician will review and recommend supplements, dietary practices, lifestyle changes, and other alternative measures to replace the operation or assist you through it. An experienced surgeon will tell you what you should know about the surgical options.

Facing the possibility of surgery is generally very difficult. As humans, we want to avoid pain, and often may choose to deny our symptoms up until the last possible minute.

The two authors of this book, having seen how challenging surgical health problems can be, will provide you with readable, accessible information that can help you choose what is best for you.

The remarkable truth is that every three years, you are likely to face a recommendation for surgery for yourself or a family member. Twenty-five million major and multimillions of minor operations are performed in the United States each year. It might be as simple as a hemorrhoid operation or a varicose vein removal, or as complex as a coronary bypass, but in all likelihood, each of us will have to make many decisions about surgery over the course of our lives.

The chances that you will have an operation during your lifetime are 50 percent. How do you decide whether to have surgery once it is suggested to you? Unless your problem is an emergency, you can take some time to consider your options before you make a decision.

This book will help you understand and evaluate a recommendation for an operation. If surgery is necessary, it will tell you what you can do for yourself to help assure a successful outcome. If not, it will inform you about alternative approaches you can pursue, and help you decide when it is safe to avoid the scalpel altogether. You can consult this book whether you are contemplating an operation, faced with an emergency procedure, or recovering from surgery.

The first book ever to bring together specific information from alternative medicine and traditional surgery—two separate disciplines historically not even on speaking terms—it is the result of a unique sister–brother collaboration.

Dr. Sandra McLanahan, M.D., is a family physician specializing in the newly emerging sciences of alternative, complementary, and integrative medicine, nutrition, stress management, and mind-body therapeutics. She will provide the information you need to decide if these newer alternative treatment options may replace your recommended operation. Her expertise will help you make an informed decision on when and how to use alternative and complementary medicine either as a substitute for or as an aid to successful surgery. Should you need surgery, she will help you prepare for it, physically and mentally, with advice about nutrition, vitamin therapies, and stress management techniques to ease postoperative discomfort and speed your recovery. She will also discuss how to improve both the hospital environment and the quality of your relationship with your surgeon and other hospital personnel.

Dr. David McLanahan, M.D., her brother, is an experienced general surgeon. From the world of traditional surgery, he will discuss those aspects of treatment and recovery that many surgeons are too busy, too preoccupied, too protective, or sometimes too patronizing to tell their patients. He will explain the preoperative tests you should have before surgery, lay out the advantages and disadvantages of various anesthetic and surgical options, and provide precise and accessible descriptions of the most common surgical operations.

Of course, you may find an operation is crucial: if you develop acute appendicitis, for example. But you can still use this book to help you choose the type of procedure and those alternative medicine methods that can reduce your risks, prevent complications, minimize your scar, and help get you back on your feet quickly. The underlying cause of the problem in the first place will be addressed. If your illness is not an emergency—say, back pain—you may be able to save yourself from the unneeded dangers and side effects of an operation by using the recommendations given in this book.

Surgery *can* be an enormous blessing to relieve suffering and disfigurement from diseases that cannot be ameliorated with medicines, shifts in lifestyle, or other alternatives. On the other hand, *needless surgery may be responsible for tens of thousands of deaths per year*, according to Rep. John Ross, former U.S. Congressman.[2] Ralph Nader's Public Citizen's Health Research Group has asserted that one-quarter of the money Americans spend each year on surgery is wasted on unnecessary operations.[3] The Department of Health and Human Services surprisingly found that *one-third of surgical recommendations were not confirmed by a second opinion*.[4] Surgery on the tonsils and adenoids is still the most frequently performed operation in children, despite its general abandonment by most major medical centers. Even the American College of Obstetrics and Gynecology admits that one-third of hysterectomies are clearly unneeded.[5] How can you discriminate between appropriate and unnecessary procedures?

To make an informed decision about accepting or rejecting any proposed surgical treatment recommendation, you must understand the important questions to ask: What is the usual course of the disorder without *any* therapy, the probability of cure or progression with or without surgery, and the possible complication and side effect risk of each procedure? What are the costs of each operation or therapy in terms of time, money, and quality of life? Which alternative medicine techniques are well researched and appropriate, and which have not been adequately proven to be successful? You will find the answers to these and other concerns in this book.

Surgery and the New Nonsurgical Choices

On Christmas Day in Kentucky, with the patient on a table in his living room, Dr. Ephraim McDowell, without the aid of anesthesia, successfully removed a seven-pound ovarian tumor from Jane Todd Crawford, who sang hymns to distract herself from the pain. He thus became, in 1846, the first surgeon to perform a successful operation in the United States.

Interestingly, Dr. McDowell was also perhaps the first surgeon to practice the now-emerging field of "integrative surgery," combining alternative with conventional operative techniques. A believer in the healing power of prayer, he had chosen that day for the surgery because he felt the prayers of the congregation at the local church would reach his patient, helping in her operation. He himself kept handwritten prayers in his pocket while he operated.

Some surgical procedures were carried out as early as 5,000 years ago in ancient India; the Egyptians and Greeks also used some operative means for treating disease, although their success rates are unknown. During the following centuries, surgeons were often butchers and barbers who simply extended their services, helping explain why, until the importance of sterile technique became known in the 1850s, less than half of all surgical patients survived. Anesthesia by use of drugs was not developed until 1845, and only in 1937 was a Board of Surgery founded to certify the quality of individual surgeons.

Surgery is now very well defined, with safe, reliable solutions for a wide variety of diseases. Despite some areas of controversy, general agreement exists on which operative options can be recommended, their expected results, and their possible complications. Currently, a major trend has also developed toward "minimally invasive" surgery performed through small incisions, using special instruments such as the laparoscope, and utilizing tiny video cameras that allow the surgeons to watch their manipulations on television monitors. Many common operations have been modified to use these techniques, and others are under investigation to see if they, too, can safely be done this way. Modern technology is allowing today's surgical patient less hospital time, more comfort, and a quicker recovery.

The authors' grandfather, for example, developed an abdominal aneurysm at age 72; this ballooning out of the main blood vessel in the abdomen could result in rupturing. A simple replacement of the faulty area with a Dacron tube allowed him to live healthfully to the very hearty age of 92.

Despite these and other glamorous new medical advances, many people have become suspicious of the traditional medical establishment and its reliance on technology and drugs. Scientists, manufacturers, salespeople, and physicians have their own vested interests in researching, producing, and distributing their costly innovations. Treatments are at times advocated before their effects can be shown to be safe—as seen in the continuing breast implant controversy—or worth the often astonishing expense.

As a result, some people choose simply to delay *any* care because of distrust, monetary costs, or fear of surgery and other conventional treatments, occasionally waiting until advanced disease necessitates less successful treatment at a much higher personal, societal, and economic expense.

Many others look outside the medical establishment for help with their health problems. A 1993 study in the *New England Journal of Medicine* found that in 1990, one in three adult Americans used alternative therapies, making an estimated 425 million visits to providers, more than the number of visits to all U.S. primary care physicians combined. Out-of-pocket expenditure was comparable for alternative and conventional treatments.[6] The trend continued, and by 1997, 42 percent of the population—83 million patients—were choosing alternative medicine, with an increase to 629 million visits. The number of visits to practitioners of alternative therapies in 1997 exceeded the projected number of visits to all U.S. primary care physicians combined in the United States by an estimated 243 million visits.[7]

The potential for alternative medicine to play an important role once it has become integrated into our healthcare system has become more clear within the last few years. Alternative medicine is described by the National Institutes of Health (NIH) as "an unrelated group of nonorthodox therapeutic practices, often with explanatory systems that do not follow conventional biomedical explanations." The techniques range from acupuncture, hypnosis, biofeedback, dance therapy, yoga, and tai chi to comprehensive dietary and lifestyle changes.

A number of these approaches are now well documented as beneficial. Examples are massage and acupuncture, shown to reduce postsurgical pain, and Dr. Dean Ornish's comprehensive program of lifestyle change, proven to reverse heart disease. Many insurance plans now cover such options. In 1992, the NIH opened an Office of Alternative Medicine to coordinate and give grants for research into these therapies, within the context of Western technology; since then, this office has grown into the National Center for Complementary and Alternative Medicine (NCCAM).

An increasing number of surgeons are beginning to embrace alternative medicine, because much of it *works*, often when Western medicine and surgery have nothing more to offer. Surgery may indeed be an area of medicine in which alternatives can be integrated most readily, since the bottom line of results is so easily measured and compared to determine the alternative's contribution.

Alternative medicine's generally simple, natural, noninvasive forms of healing have added an exciting new dimension to surgery. The purpose of this book is to help you sort through the immense amount of new material, both in surgery and in alternative medicine, and choose what may be most beneficial to you. The therapies described in the following chapters may help you avoid an operation if you can, and assure that if you must have surgery, you can act to optimize the whole experience.

Educating Yourself

Many surgeons just don't have the time or inclination to explain the complicated aspects of surgical illness and your legitimate choices. A short description of the proposed anatomical change resulting from the operation is all that you generally now receive. During the high-stress time of a surgical decision, you may not even be able to remember what is said to you. Videotapes taken of briefings by surgeons reveal that only a small percentage of the information is recollected. You should spend whatever time you can educating yourself, at your own pace. The information in this book, and in the other sources listed in its Resources section, is designed to encourage your learning process.

Sometimes an alternative avenue can provide such enormous relief from a disease conventionally treated with surgery that it seems like a miracle. One of Sandra's patients, for example, had experienced chest pain (angina) due to underlying heart disease every day for seventeen years. On only the third day of a yoga and lifestyle retreat, he had his first pain-free day since the onset of his illness!

At other times, using alternative medicine on your own can pose a grave risk. Another of Sandra's patients tried to use alternative medicine on her own and became so emaciated while self-treating her colitis using enemas and an extreme diet that she narrowly escaped death from starvation. Emergency hospital care, with intravenous feedings, helped her survive just in the nick of time.

Therefore, learning how to more safely use the alternatives is one of the key benefits of studying this book. With this knowledge, you will have a starting point for making treatment decisions, with the help of your healthcare providers. Learning about your realistic alternatives may help save your life.

You may wonder if knowing all the details of your proposed operation is necessary, or even a good idea. It is. Several studies have shown that patients who are aware of what to expect and are encouraged to participate have increased surgical survival, faster recovery, lower postoperative blood pressure, and less postoperative pain.[8] Your belief in and understanding of *whatever* therapy you choose may enhance its effectiveness. When you understand your disease and what happens during

surgery, you can work with your body to help it heal. Your personal contribution can make a difference: by guiding your body to respond using the techniques given in this book, you can change your nervous system and body chemistry to optimize your results.

Introducing the Authors

Dr. Sandra McLanahan: The Alternative and Complementary Medicine Approach

My older brother, David, and I grew up in a family steeped in medicine and surgery, in the fifth generation of doctors. My great-great-grandfather was a horse and buggy surgeon in rural Pennsylvania and was followed by my great-grandfather, grandfather, aunt, older brother, twin brother, and brother-in-law, all surgeons. We do have some very interesting family reunions.

As a medical student, I myself found surgery fascinating. The colors, smells, drama, jokes, clothing—here was a true calling, a fairyland with its own strange rituals and gremlins, dragons to slay, and knights in shining sterile waistcoats wielding lances.

From my feminine perspective, I appreciated an operation's beauty: it seemed as if the abdominal organs themselves are color-coded: the liver is purple paisley; underneath it is the bright green gallbladder; next to it is the yellow pancreas; and running through the abdomen are the glistening pink snakes of the intestines.

I liked watching the way the surgeons dealt with their patients: they were generally positive and optimistic within the realm of the limited operative problem. The internal medicine specialists seemed contradictory, vague, and depressed by the seemingly endless and ultimately fatal nature of the illnesses and aging processes they addressed. The surgeons usually were very alert to each patient, and fervently involved with them, perhaps because they had a chance to *do* something, and a strong personal stake in being successful with each one, within the more circumscribed arena of an operation.

However, I also saw that so much of illness has a preventable aspect, a root cause tied to choices in lifestyle: diet, alcohol, cigarettes, exercise, and relaxation habits. Many diseases are related to the effects of how we handle our human emotional stresses. In addition, the main problem with drugs or surgery as a solution is that in their attempts to heal, they both can also hurt the body, creating the challenge of surgical recovery or the unpleasant side effects so common with drugs.

Like most medical students, I received for my graduation a large leather "doctor's bag," donated by a pharmaceutical company. These companies continue to deluge me with samples, magazines, conferences, and other perks, all in a quite compelling and largely effective effort in this country to influence the practice of medical doctors. Surgeons similarly receive this onslaught, as well as devices and products related to their operations, promoted by the very manufacturers with financial interests in them.

Like so many of us who now practice medicine from the new "integrative" perspective, my first encounter with alternative medical approaches came during a search to relieve my *own* suffering. The transcultural journey that was to take me around the world began literally in my own backyard—with my own aching back.

During medical school, I took a giant leap for womankind—and while on vacation, did splits wearing water skis. My lower back started to hurt, and the pain was further aggravated by the long cramped sitting required during school lectures and study. I tried all kinds of remedies—exercises, drugs, traction, physical therapy—but I was still unable to stand or sit comfortably for long. In desperation, I became willing to consider something unorthodox. Someone suggested I try a yoga class. I went, although I expected it to be difficult, or boring—or both.

As I bent over to try to touch my hands to my toes, I was stunned to discover I could barely reach my knees! However, with the teacher's patient assistance, I was able to shed the belief that I would need to tie myself into knots. After a few classes I noticed not only that my back was feeling surprisingly better, but also I myself felt deeply refreshed, both physically and mentally.

I had been a college athlete, but this type of exercise, consisting of placing the body in various positions, then practicing deep breathing, relaxation, meditation, visualization, or chanting, felt different. My energy felt more restored than even after an aerobic workout. In addition to eventually being able to touch my toes once again, I felt stronger on the *inside*.

After some time, I began to reflect on what medicine could do to incorporate such alternate methods, which also can act preventively to protect us from illness rather than just help us once we are sick. I commenced a worldwide study of alternative therapies, many of them, such as acupuncture and ayurveda, rooted in quite different understandings of illness than our Western medicine. The renowned yoga master Rev. Swami Satchidananda, also a naturopath and homeopath, has been my teacher for the last thirty years. Much of what I have discovered about natural approaches to health I have learned from him, while accompanying him on many fact-finding trips to Europe, India, and Asia and residing at his main teaching center, Satchidananda Ashram-Yogaville, in Buckingham, Virginia.

While Director of Stress Management Training for the Preventive Medicine Research Institute for twenty years, I investigated and published research along with Dr. Dean Ornish about these methods when applied to heart disease. In addition, I studied with Dr. Bernie Siegel and worked with Dr. Michael Lerner, looking at alternative methods of health care around the world, especially in reference to cancer patients; and I helped initially with the Commonweal Cancer Help Program.

As Executive Medical Director of the Integral Health Center in Virginia, I have witnessed the success of a wide variety of alternative medicine approaches with my patients over the past two decades. I also now collaborate with Dannion Brinkley, whose organization, Compassion in Action, aims to bring alternative medicine's compatible techniques and spiritual healing centers to hospitals, veterans' organizations, and hospices around the world.

We have often paid more attention to the science of feeding and caring for our animals than to feeding and taking optimum care of ourselves. "Alternative medicine is alive and well in veterinary medicine," states Carville Tiekert, founder and Executive Director of the American Holistic Veterinary Association, with more than 700 members. Over 600 certified veterinary acupuncturists are practicing in the United States. The results of using alternative care with animals include their successful application to a wide variety of disorders in humans, and I will draw on this long history in the context of this book. There is

much to learn by integrating these vets' experience.

Western surgery as a science, when compared with some of the world's more ancient medical systems, *is* very young, and although precociously accomplished at achieving dramatically useful results for a myriad of illnesses, is ready—and I believe needs—to continue to evolve, becoming increasingly inclusive and embracing what works from among the alternative approaches, such as acupuncture.

I, like almost everyone, do perceive surgeons as heroes, the "Sir Galahads" of modern medicine, applying their swordly skills for good causes. However, because they are on average taller, more politically conservative, and usually more powerful within their medical center settings, they can be intimidating. They are more financially important to the hospital and—perhaps reflecting the measurably positive outcomes of so many of their procedures, compared to the rest of medicine—longer-lived.

For all these reasons, they can be unused to being questioned, accepting differences of opinion, or embracing change. Marcia Millman, in her groundbreaking book about the back streets of surgery, *The Unkindest Cut,* quoted an anonymous surgeon: "Oh, she'll have the surgery. I very rarely have a patient refuse me surgery."[9]

Many surgeons themselves are aware of their specialty's weaknesses. One story circulated among them describes how a general practitioner, an internist, and a surgeon go duck hunting together. They agree that whoever shoots the first duck will be treated to dinner by the others. When a group of birds comes along, the GP states: "There's a bird— it looks like a duck," and shoots. The internist says, "There's a bird . . . it looks like a duck . . . well, maybe not . . . well, maybe yes . . . I'm not sure . . . ," and so misses the opportunity to shoot. The surgeon says, "There's a bird," and shoots. As the bird is falling, he says, "I hope it was a duck."

Although I admire surgeons' attitude, I also see the limitations of considering the body merely as a "machine with parts that break down." To operate without an awareness of the mind-body connection is emotionally hard on *both* the surgeon and the patient.

For example, many surgeons routinely relieve their own tension by making negative remarks and jokes about the patient while he or she is under anesthesia. However, evidence has now shown that even while unconscious, patients can subconsciously hear and remember what is said.[10] What just the past two decades of mind-body research has shown us is the astonishing potential of the mind to affect the onset of illness, its course, and recovery.

My opposition to surgery as a routine solution to many health problems takes into account its profound ability to save lives in an emergency, and to "take action" in the alleviation of chronic ailments. Despite these benefits, I feel the physical and financial price is often too high and may frequently be unnecessary. Patients commonly tell me, "I've never been the same since my surgery," and "I didn't expect it to be this bad."

Being told you need an operation is scary. You may even feel stupid questioning a doctor's advice. The more natural, gentle alternative approaches may take longer, but they encourage and help the body to heal itself. This often gives them the additional advantage of helping you improve your experience of life.

I have written this book's "Alternative Medicine Approaches" sections mainly to as-

sist you in sorting through the wide variety of innovative alternative medicine therapies now available. These compatible techniques, also termed "complementary" and "integrative," I have chosen to label "alternative medicine" simply because that is now the most commonly applied title. In the near future, I believe many of these methods will simply become part of the usual practice of medicine and surgery.

Surgery may, in fact, be the best arena to *test* alternatives. The problems are limited, the results easy to measure. Many of the narrow constraints of our medical-surgical centers could be broadened: adding massage and music postsurgically, for example, which has been found beneficial, might lead to massage and music for all hospitalized patients.

Overall, medical research in this country currently creates special problems for alternative approaches because it is largely funded by private drug companies, which choose to investigate only those substances or procedures for which they can obtain a patent. Scientific papers on alternative medicine, therefore, are rarer, or have been less than rigorously composed—although the latter is true of much of conventional medicine as well.

This book's consideration is not exhaustive, and I have included only those alternative medicine tools currently being applied with some scientific indication that they may be useful. Further research is greatly needed, especially to more precisely answer questions such as those about relative effectiveness, safety, and drug-herb interactions.

As noted, these measures may help you avoid surgery, or may be utilized to aid you through an operation should you choose it. Their main advantage is their effect on the *quality* of your life, as well as on the quantity. Many of them just feel good, a particular boon in our exceedingly stressful times. The recent openness to systematic examination of such therapies should continue to clarify our understanding of their exact benefits and limitations in the years to come.

Dr. David McLanahan: The Surgical Approach

As long as I can remember, I wanted to be a surgeon. Working with my hands on various arts, crafts, and building projects gave me great satisfaction, and surgery seemed a natural expression of those interests and enjoyments. While in medical school, I became even more convinced that surgery should be my choice. During my third year, in 1966, I wrote to then-Attorney General Robert Kennedy suggesting he ask the State Department's USAID Division to set up a pilot program for medical students to serve the local population in Vietnam. This led to an incredible, indelible two-month experience at the Danang Civilian Hospital, where I helped take care of civilians with war injuries and assisted with a number of operations. I saw what impressive results surgery could achieve, and became even more certain that this field of practice was right for me.

Over the years, I have also had the opportunity to see the importance of health education. I spent thirteen years in New York City working with the underserved and organizing around community and individual healthcare issues. For the last twenty years, in Seattle, I have been on the staff at Pacific Medical Center, now PacMed Clinics, a nonprofit group practice chartered by the city of Seattle with a specific mandate to provide health care for those without the means to afford it, and to teach other healthcare providers. I work closely with University of Washington and Swedish Medical Center surgical residents and medical students, and hold weekly surgery sessions at the International District Community Health Center and the Country Doctor Community Health Clinic. These are community-controlled neighborhood clinics that cater to patients who might not otherwise have access to first-rate care.

After thirty-three years, I have had plenty of experience with the "emotional roller coaster" that is a surgical career. I can often save a person's leg, cure a dread disease, or relieve years of pain with a simple procedure. Such cases are richly rewarding. Unfortunately, surgery also entails long hours and high pressure, and is often disruptive to family life. There are times when things do not go well, due to underlying disease, unforeseen complications, or inevitably, mistakes. I sometimes lie awake at night, tossing and turning, going over and over an unsuccessful procedure in my mind. When there is nothing further that a surgeon can do, I always find it difficult, especially when a person is suffering. Self-doubt, personal pain, and the desire to retire at an early age follow. On these occasions, I am particularly open to alternatives.

During the course of writing this book, I learned about some of the alternative medicine approaches used in traditionally surgical diseases, and as adjuncts to surgery. Whether or not the current theories of how these things work will be proven sound, some of the experience is quite impressive. I am beginning to apply a few of these techniques in my own practice.

On the other hand, I see people who, for various reasons, avoid the traditional system and place their hopes and lives only in the hands of alternative practitioners. It can be very frustrating if these patients don't follow the advice I give them, especially when it does not seem controversial. Those who temporarily delay necessary surgery, because of fears that usually turn out to be unwarranted, often create more problems for both themselves and their surgeon. Some, who refuse standard treatment altogether, may subsequently lose their chance for cure, or at least a significantly better quality of life.

I welcome this opportunity to present this book with my sister, Sandra. Medicine and surgery are changing, and with the development of both new technology and a greater appreciation of the effect of the mind on the body's physiological resources and defenses, the patient will increasingly be the winner. However, I also feel that the value of an alternative approach should be clearly proven before it is accepted as a true alternative, rather than an adjunct, to the traditional recommendations more solidly grounded in research, experience, and documentation.

I have written the "Surgical Approaches" sections in this book to give you the information you need to understand your conventional surgical choices. I have included comments on which of the alternative methods I consider appropriate options to surgery and which I feel may help you recover from an operation.

Making the Best Use of This Book

This book is intended to help create something new: a dialogue between surgery and al-ternative medicine, and when appropriate, a combination, for the benefit of both sides. It aims to break down the stereotypical lack of patient communication, involvement, and empowerment, presenting you with your best options. It can also protect you from the remnants of such past imbalances.

You can read this book straight through. For optimum results, we recommend you do read all of the chapters, to learn the full range of prevention and treatment options for the most common surgical illnesses you may face.

If you are contemplating a specific surgery, before you skip to the section dealing with your illness, make certain to first read Chapters 1–4 and 24, which together give both a philosophic overview and practical information to be used before deciding about, preparing for, or recovering from an operation.

Once you begin reading the section dealing with your problem, you will find that, after a short description of the disease, Sandra gives "Alternative Medicine Approaches," discussing the newest nonsurgical treatment plans, then David provides "Surgical Approaches," describing the latest surgical options and what to expect should you choose a particular operation.

You can use this book as a springboard for discussion with your doctor during the various decisions you will need to make. It can thereafter serve as a reference source for yourself, your family, and your friends.

WHAT IS ALTERNATIVE MEDICINE?

The doctor of the future will give no medicine, but will interest his patients in the care of the human frame, in diet, and the cause and prevention of disease.
Thomas A. Edison

Dr. *Craig Bradley, a prominent plastic surgeon at the Rush-Presbyterian St. Luke's Medical Center in Chicago, loved his challenging work, especially the art of reconstruction after cancer surgery. However, since he had to spend extended periods bending over the operating table, he began to experience annoying backaches. He decided to seek Shiatsu massage treatments. His back felt so much better, and his energy so renewed, that he wondered if this therapy could help his surgical patients, too.*

In subsequent application, he found that those patients given postsurgical massage healed much more quickly, developed fewer complications, experienced less pain, and had a significantly better adjustment to their operations. He also began prescribing some herbal medicines, which he discovered to be more effective and have fewer side effects than the standard drug regimens. Other surgeons at his hospital soon began using these new additions to rehabilitation with similarly excellent results.

The scene was the typically chaotic yet calm, tense yet focused 911 resuscitation effort. A woman with no previous history of heart disease had suddenly experienced a heart attack, then suffered a cardiac arrest. Two of my physician friends were doing the cardiopulmonary resuscitation (CPR), so I (Sandy) simply began giving the woman's feet and legs a massage.

The woman opened her eyes and smiled. With all the technical wizardry of Western medicine, she recovered fully. But afterward she related that she was especially grateful to have someone massaging her during her ordeal, and she had leaned on it both physically and emotionally to help her recover. One of the physical means by which massage has been found to assist healing is by improving blood and lymph flow; it thereby reduces the amount of work the heart must perform and decreases its need for oxygen. Massage has been found to improve the chance of survival of heart attack victims.[1]

Even in emergency situations, I have found that many alternative techniques can be utilized right alongside more conventional therapies. For example, patients can be given massage in an intensive care unit. Another patient told me, "What I noticed most about my first massage was that afterwards I felt an increased will to live."

My personal and professional experience with a wide range of the new techniques that are included under the umbrella of "alternative medicine" has been heartening. In 1975, I began working with Dr. Dean Ornish and witnessed thousands of patients who were unhealthy and suffering, with significant pain and limitation recover their well-being, improve their heart function by objective testing, and at the same time renew their joy of life. This approach to heart disease is now so firmly established with scientific support that it is often no longer considered alternative, but rather simply another option of conventional medicine.

Alternative methods now offer an increasing variety of therapeutic options. However, the burgeoning choices of therapies and supplements can be bewildering. Just walk into any large health food store—where do you start? In this chapter, I will give you an introduction to the central principles of alternative medicine.

I will then discuss, in Chapter 2, some of the specific alternative techniques, along with scientific studies demonstrating their benefits. After categorizing the techniques and ranking

them according to how useful I have found them to be, then I will give you instructions for their use. I have included only those approaches I myself have found, over the last three decades, to be effective, safe, reliable, easy to apply, and cost-saving.

In subsequent chapters, David and I will help you sort out what is best for your individual problem. Working together as an alternative medicine–surgical team to choose, rate, and integrate what is available, we will show you how to gather all the facts, talk to your healthcare providers, and develop a detailed healing plan for your specific disorder.

You, therefore, will no longer have to abandon conventional medical and surgical care and advice to use alternative medicine, nor will you have to simply submit to whatever is recommended to you by your standard health providers. By educating yourself about both customary treatments and alternatives, you can create a combined program to give you the best of both worlds.

Why "Alternative" Medicine?

In high school, I was not the popular, in-group, cheerleader type. I was the girl in the corner with buck teeth and glasses, her nose buried in a book. A science book. Sputnik had happened, new technical discoveries and worries made the *Detroit News* front page, and the Science Fair was the event of the year for us nerds. Praise, attention, and awards were given to science students, and white-coated wisdom-bearers received more acclaim in advertising and on television than artists or teachers or even clergy. Scientists were the priests of our 1950s generation. The sayings "Better living through chemistry," and "Four out of five doctors recommend" were in our cultural bible.

So I entered the Science Fair, won a trophy taller than I was, and naturally, to continue this sort of success in my isolated and defensive bookish life, chose medicine as a career. Science plus service, I thought: what an idealistic combination.

When I got to college, I began to notice something strange. The premed and science groups of students seemed to lack so much of the fun, freedom, creativity, and general liveliness of the literature, music, and art majors. It wasn't the same feeling of being on the outside of things I'd had in high school, and it certainly wasn't a question of brains. The science group was just so generally serious that something about life and its essence seemed missing.

It wasn't until years later, after college, medical school, residency, lots of medical practice, and many trips around the world, that I began to truly question our Western culture's rush to structure and its view of our world entirely through the necessarily narrow though currently prestigious spectacles of conventional science.

Perhaps the first glimmer came while I was still in medical school and was upbraided for whistling on the stairwell of the hospital. No joy here; this is a *serious* place. Something whistled deep inside me then, some alarm bell that now has become my own personal continuing gong on behalf of sanity.

"Just the facts, ma'am," my teachers emphasized to me. But what about the emotions? Couldn't they be equally, or even more, important to our health? What about stress? We humans are social creatures, and our emotional lives are dependent upon achieving comfortable social connections and intimacy.

These dimensions, along with the spiritual ones, have remained until recently, relatively unexplored for the most part in medical schools and hospitals in relationship to patients' health.

By separating religion from science, and putting the fine arts and creativity into their own boxes, we have made the healing arts so dry that they are almost devoid of life. But it is the *quality* of life that is vitally important. You can have all your body parts and still be dead. It is the flow of energy that gives us life, and this flow is in need of whistles: love, touch, laughter, dance, joy. Right in the hospital too.

Science is, after all, simply a flashlight looking at reality. Its perspective is precocious and dramatic, but it is limited by definition because it uses only one aspect of the human mind: the logical, left-brain, rational, cause-effect function. The right-brain, musical mind is missing. As the mystical poet Rumi stated, "When love first tasted the lips of being human, it started singing."

The term "alternative medicine" in large part derived from the public's search for "alternatives" to drugs and surgery—and attempts to find alternate solutions free of the difficult side effects so often associated with these mainstream modalities. As we shall see, alternatives also often have alternate characteristics, that make them differ from the accepted body of scientific knowledge and usual pathways of such inquiry.

Researchers such as Dr. Dean Ornish and I have been able to show by the rigorous rules of conventional scientific research itself that simple alterations in lifestyle such as a change in diet and the addition of yoga not only improve the quality of our lives, but often increase longevity as well. Many alternatives can now be said to be based soundly in "good science." Continued research is urgently needed, to help sort through and decide which are really the best of the alternatives currently being advocated.

We may also begin to explore more alternatives through "soft science" means—outcomes research, case studies, cross-cultural comparisons—and thus bring a wider therapeutic base into the discussion of the shape and art of medical practice. The recent confirmation that we as humans need social support, and studies showing that joining a support group extended life expectancy for some patients, is just one example of this principle. Interestingly, this research was initiated in an effort to disprove the empirical finding of a mind-body medicine supposition, but ended in helping establish its importance.

In addition to using the current scientific processes to look at alternatives, what I'd like to propose is a real taking down of the Berlin Wall of medicine: the barrier that separates "hard science"—double-blind, randomized prospective trials—from folk wisdoms and techniques—such as relaxation, music, dance, art, caring, love—from around the globe. Of course, one way to assess these approaches is to direct the scientific flashlight at them. Some can be studied by controlled, randomized scientific rigor, such as the interventions in Dr. Ornish's and my research. Although double-blind studies are generally more difficult to design in this context, even touch and caring can to some extent be looked at in a scientific light.

However, as I noted in the previous chapter, since scientific research in this country has been so limited and focused, until recently, almost exclusively on drugs and surgery, alternatives research cannot currently match the volume of that for conventional approaches.

Much is already known from alternative traditions around the world, and it would take years to prove all of these customs in this country by individual scientific projects. Perhaps some of these applications, even though now resting on soft science, can be utilized without waiting for more double-blind studies and can be tested by outcomes research: particularly with such benign approaches as massage, music, relaxation training, yoga, and deep breathing—and especially in the surgical setting.

What I thus envision as most useful for the future of medicine and surgery is a reintegration of the arts, laughter, and spiritual comfort in day-to-day treatment. Alternative medicine at its best for me fundamentally joins together science with the whistling of life, for the benefit of us all.

Even Einstein, the premier scientist of the twentieth century, observed, "Religion without science is dumb, but science without religion is blind." Without interfering with our nation's commitment to freedom of religious choice or nonchoice, we can address our deepest yearnings as humans. With the addition of music to medicine, for example, we can put the "hum" back into "*hum*an."

The word "religion" comes from the root "re-ligio," to "bind back," to feel connected to a larger whole. As the American yoga teacher Ram Das stated, all religions "call us, in one voice, to undertake the journey back to unity." The function of such feelings may be studied in this context as the "physiology of theology": how our spiritual beliefs affect our emotions, for example, which in turn affect our cardiovascular and immune systems.

In the course of my research for this book, I traveled around the world with Dr. Michael Lerner and John Fink to look at the major alternative medicine healing centers. We visited health centers and spas in Mexico, North America, the Bahamas, Europe, and India. John Fink's book about our tour, *Third Opinion*, is a rich resource cataloging what is available in these different centers for the alternative treatment of cancer. Dr. Lerner's book, *Choices in Healing*, discusses in detail these new approaches in the context of preventing and treating cancer. In the next chapter, I will discuss my findings within the context of surgically treated diseases.

Getting in Touch with Your Inner Chocolate

Most alternative medicine methods act to improve your body's own *self-healing* capacities. Even a small amount of practice can make a marked difference: usually within a short time you feel *much* better, so that whatever course you eventually choose to treat your surgical disorder, these approaches may still be worth a try. They can help you through your operation. In addition, they may serve to thwart future recurrence of your disease, as well as prevent other related—and even unrelated—illnesses.

One day, as I was driving home from a long schedule of seeing patients, I felt a dreadfully familiar twang in my midback. Oh no . . . I instantly knew what this meant. I had experienced my first kidney stone two years previously, after a morning of jogging in San Francisco's Marina Green Park. Like 80 percent of all stones, it had eventually passed through, but not until after I had endured a few days of the most exquisite torture imaginable. Now, here I was again, in agony.

But this time I decided to try acupuncture. Almost immediately after the practitioner inserted the needles, I began to relax. By the end

of the session, I was free of all pain. The stone passed on its own with no further distress, and I then followed the program for preventing such stones, as given in Chapter 23 of this book, and have suffered no further recurrences.

How was it that a few needles could solve my problem? The usual treatment includes painkillers and/or lithotripsy; both of which may have significant side effects. Surgery is also sometimes needed. What the acupuncture accomplished was self-healing: it assisted my body in repairing itself, as opposed to just covering the pain with drugs or manipulating relief via an operative intervention. The specific mechanisms by which acupuncture is thought to work are described in the next chapter.

Certainly, my acupuncturist, like many alternative care providers, also had a bedside manner different from many conventional physicians: perhaps because he was implementing such a unique style of therapy, he was very empathetic and reassuring, and spent a significant amount of time selecting and checking the needle points.

Indeed, alternatives may work for various reasons. They do often provide contrasting ways of assisting the body to correct itself, but they also are often delivered in a differing style, one which may itself help elicit a healing placebo response in your body.

One of my patients put it this way: "Recently, I broke off a portion of my tooth. I needed a brave, technically efficient dentist who would be willing to create a tricky filling, so that I could avoid a root canal. I was fortunate to find exactly the right person to attempt this solution, and he completed it perfectly.

"However, like most healthcare practitioners, he treated me as if I were a car with a part that was broken. He was nice enough, but he did not act as if a person were inside, who was having this procedure, with a strong mind-body connection during the operation and afterwards.

"I wanted both. I definitely wanted the latest technical expertise, and a swift and daring dental surgeon to focus on what needed to be done, when I couldn't avoid an operation. However, I wanted the soft, nurturing, and caring comfort that makes my feelings, my emotions, and my spirit *just as important as my material self.*"

Investigating and validating the power of simple interventions that can assist in healing, such as caring, touch, and love, is one of the most important contributions of alternative medicine.

In addition, a willingness to use remedies that are more "natural"—that is, that evolved from nature—without the dramatic intervention of drugs and surgery also creates results that may appear more slowly, but that do not have troublesome side effects. For example, premier herbologist Dr. Jim Duke calls therapy that supports the body in healing itself on many levels an "herbal sling." The "herbal shotgun," he says, is more effective than the "magic bullet." However, as mentioned, you need not be limited to one or the other approach. Alternatives plus conventional techniques simply give you a much broader set of tools from which to choose.

As we shall show in the course of this book, a number of diseases can be ameliorated by changes in lifestyle. But how can you effectively change a damaging lifestyle habit? Eating chocolate, for example, increases the levels of the endorphins and serotonin, the brain's antidepressants. However, since in its initial state chocolate is unpalatably bitter,

deleterious amounts of fat and sugar are usually added. You can raise your levels of these hormones in your brain naturally by the regular practice of alternatives such as yoga, exercise, laughter, and massage. During meditation you can get in touch with your inner chocolate—and avoid the "side" effects of those extra addictive calories—on your sides!

The discovery that our emotions and spirit influence our health may be the most pivotal contribution of alternative medicine. That love is important in healing, that it matters, that it helps us heal, and that spirituality, and our relationship to it, lie at the heart of healing, are the essence of many alternative approaches and the core philosophy of many of its practitioners.

Certainly, many doctors and surgeons have traditionally utilized a warm, encouraging bedside manner, like that of Marcus Welby, M.D., but the value of taking this time during recovery from illness has often gotten swept away from the routine practice of medicine, buried beneath lab test results and prescription pads.

An average doctor visit in this country is scheduled every fifteen minutes. Some HMOs have even encouraged their doctors to keep visits as short as five minutes. How much can you really understand, and especially learn, about your legitimate choices, prevention, and lifestyle from this brief, not very close encounter? Many alternative practitioners choose to spend more time with their patients, even at the cost of lowering their salaries.

Fundamentals of Alternative Medicine

From my personal and professional experiences with alternatives, I have concluded that love, caring, empathy, touch, and spiritual connection are the *most* important elements in healing. Many alternatives and alternative healthcare providers choose to focus on just these dimensions, which, as I mentioned earlier, have somehow been largely lost from our medical care system with the inrush of the technical dazzle of the last century.

You may be experiencing a symptom you find especially frustrating, such as weight gain at menopause. Treating only the symptom is tempting, and drugs or surgical measures may be helpful. However, if you do not address the root of the problem—in this case, subclinical adrenal exhaustion or thyroid dysfunction—a number of other problems down the road may follow.

One unique aspect of alternative medicine, then, is that instead of simply covering up a symptom, the practitioner often looks for the fundamental cause, and chooses a treatment that simply helps your body to self-correct. For example, while antibiotics kill specific bacteria, the herb echinacea increases your white cell numbers and activity, enabling your immune system to get rid of the problem and avoiding the short and long-term dysfunctions and risks associated with antibiotics.

Eighty percent of the earth's population presently uses what we in this country call "alternative" approaches to maintain and restore health, making these techniques "conventional" to the rest of the world. The shift toward alternative, "natural medicine" in the United States is taking place in a way similar to that by which "natural childbirth" came about here: it wasn't the obstetricians who first wanted labor without drugs, fathers in the delivery rooms, bonding with the baby, and a soft entry for a new soul into this earthly life. It was the general public who educated themselves, then informed their doctors. Finally, research was initiated that demonstrated the benefits of these changes. These techniques were also first used in separate centers, then gradually adapted into the hospitals themselves, and are now universally available. A quite similar unfolding seems to be under way for alternatives.

Many people simply try alternatives on their own. However, we strongly recommend you first consult an experienced provider. The majority of alternative medicine users do consult practitioners, utilizing mainly massage, chiropractic, hypnosis, biofeedback, and acupuncture.

A recent study of why patients turn to alternatives found that "the majority of alternative medicine users appear to be doing so not so much as a result of being dissatisfied with conventional medicine but largely because they find these healthcare alternatives to be more congruent with their own values, beliefs, and philosophical orientations toward health and life."[2] Interestingly, alternative medicine use by physicians for their own personal health problems appears to be similar to the rate of use in the general population.[3]

What makes us cleave to unhealthy lifestyle choices in the first place? How can we motivate ourselves to change, and stick to it?

Here are the ten most important principles of alternative medicine, which I think would give you the best possible answers to these pivotal questions. Instituting the following changes, I feel, would also provide the most optimum integration of alternatives into conventional Western medicine and surgery, and could help our entire healthcare system itself become healthier.

1. Shifting from Treatment of Illness to Active Prevention

What we have now in the West is not generally a "healthcare system," but an "illness-care system." It largely acts only once we have become sick, with little intervention at the level of root causes of illness.

As we begin to more clearly understand the links between lifestyle choices and health, mind and body, we can move to act earlier to prevent illness, rather than simply fix Humpty Dumpty once he or she has fallen.

The word doctor means "teacher," and "physician" stems from "of nature." The doctor of the future needs to be a teacher of wellness and natural healing methods, not just a dispenser of drugs or surgery. Diet, exercise, stress management, massage, relaxation training, music and poetry then become the "First Aid," to assist the body in healing itself, leaving the more drastic interventions of drugs and surgery, which hurt the body while contributing their healing effects, as "Second Aid."

2. Rebalancing High Tech with High Touch

As I will discuss more fully in the next chapter, the medical value of traditionally "feminine" healing modalities such as touch, caring, talking, and sharing are now being documented by science itself to be of powerful value, due to their profound ability to reduce stress.

I don't blame the mostly male medical and surgical establishments for the loss of these values and therapies. I don't even blame the mostly male cultural ethic, as some feminists do. I don't think it useful to look at these problems as a power struggle that would further alienate us from the touching, loving values so needed for all of us to heal. I just

simply see it as an evolutionary mistake, like meat eating—a genuine mis-steak, as it were—and circumcision, that it is time for our culture to self-correct.

The sometimes painful process through which this book you are now reading came to fruition is illustrative of this journey. I don't think that my brother and I would have had occasion to speak to each other if we had not been born into the same family; we are just about as far opposite as possible on the spectrum of medical-surgical practice and thinking. And after the struggle of writing this book together, we would not probably still be speaking except that we began as good friends, and we have come to further understand and respect the unique values that each of us holds dear.

During the book's evolution, there were moments when we even shouted at each other on the phone; even called each other names. "You're a dreamer," my brother roared, so labeling my judgment that alternative medicine techniques and traditional surgery could be integrated into a book format. "You're too rigid and unfeeling," I raged back, thinking that I spoke for all womankind, from generations of lack of respect for the feminine voice. Somehow, slowly, we learned from one another. I began to see the artistry in his commitment to thorough documentation of these new pathways, and he began to eat more fruits and vegetables.

Both voices are needed: they create a richness of diversity in our universe that is so "dancy," as the poet Rumi writes. All of nature celebrates diversity; can't we as humans begin this expedition too? My brother and I have started it, a "journey of a thousand miles" (or more, if you count the distance of Venus from Mars), begun with the few small steps of making peace with one another; I look forward to the development of many more unique alternatives and conventional combinations, contributing to an enrichment and broadening of available pathways to health.

3. Moving from Doctor Care to Self-Care

One of the principle aims of this book is to promote self-education and self-care. At present, reliance upon the expertise of doctors leaves you vulnerable from many points of view. You depend upon whatever individual doctors you are able to find. Except for the rare new-thinking alternative insurance company, you have to wait until you are sick to seek assistance covered by insurance. And unless you find one of the few newer alternative doctors, you are left with only the tools of drugs or surgery for the treatment of your illness.

Self-care can be exciting. Personally watching my own patients and the participants in the Dean Ornish Program not only enhance their health, but become glowing and exuberant with a heightened quality of their lives as well, I have seen results that have often seemed nothing short of miraculous.

4. Changing from Individual Care to Group Support

In order to accomplish true preventive health care, the current wisdom of a one-to-one doctor visit as the main form of medical-surgical care may need to change drastically.

We humans are social creatures. To stick to changes in lifestyle, we do best when we can be inspired by and, when needed, can lean on other human buddies swimming up the stream of the generally unhealthy lifestyle current. Weight Watchers, AA, and other groups have proved more beneficial than trying to go it on our own. Research on the relationship between social support and stress substantiates the efficacy of group support. As a pivotal part of the Dean Ornish heart research, support groups help the participants stay on the program. It became clear to us that if this support was not utilized, it was very difficult for participants to stick with the essential lifestyle changes necessary for health.

Surgical care needs to reflect this new understanding. Perhaps surgeons could see their patients in groups, as well as individually. Everyone needs a "functional family"; unfortunately, many of us do not have one. If you do not have access to a support group, you may do best to form one of your own.

5. Integrating a New Paradigm for Medicine and Surgery

When the astronauts went into outer space and photographed the earth from that perspective, it changed us forever. The old identification with human subgroups has to give way to a larger vision of "we humans all in this together."

Likewise, with the advent of biofeedback, and the current exploration of mind-body connections, we have begun to see the human body differently. Particularly for the last two hundred years, the body has been mainly considered by Western medicine materialistically, a mechanism with parts that break down. Generally, even now, if you present yourself to a doctor or an emergency room, for evaluation of disease, that is how you will be treated: as if you were an automobile coming in for repair.

The heady success of the germ theory of disease, and the dramatic changes that surgery can provide, have obscured Western medicine's less-than-perfect result with chronic diseases. Even Pasteur, on his deathbed, referring to his lifelong debate with Claude Bernard, was reported to have said, "You are right, Bernard, it is not the organism, but the soil." Modern immunological theory supports his statement: an individual's resistance is often more primary than the mere presence of an infectious organism.

Within the last ten or fifteen years, with the advent of mind-body research, and the understanding that the mind and its reaction to stress have such an important place in the sequence of events leading to development of symptoms, a move toward seeing the body as "bodymind" has taken place. Since as much as 80 percent of illness may be precipitated by stress, via effects on both the cardiovascular and immune systems, stress management has taken its pivotal place in both prevention and treatment of illness.

However, some persons are not adversely affected by major life changes associated with stress, and do not become ill, while others get sick. Rather than focusing on merely physical causes, or even on mental ones, whether we develop subsequent symptoms when we experience stressful events may depend upon our basic assumptions about life. This "spiritual" aspect, left out of usual Western scientific investigation, may most fundamentally affect health. It is the "meaning" dimension of our lives, how we answer the questions of personal purpose, why we are here on earth, and the importance of our relationships, our family, and our work. As further explored in the next chapter, studies such as those that show people who attend church regularly survive their heart attacks 60 percent more often than those who don't, reflect this significance.

Modern concepts of physics may again be helpful here. It was natural for our culture to view the body as a machine. It was the ma-

chine age, and this was our generational paradigm. The head was seen as independent from the body, each part of the body an individual entity, just as the nucleus was imaged as separate from the circling electrons. All this empty space between.

Newer images of physics envision a different set of rules by which the universe works. An overflowing connection between everything is seen, expressed as a web, as a set of waves by which things constantly and continuously communicate. One saying of contemporary physics summarizes it poetically: "A butterfly can't flap its wings in Delhi without creating a breeze in New York City."

Instead of a picture given to us by science—in this case, physics—of a universe consisting of separate parts that interact against a background of nothingness, this current shift in the basic scientific paradigm suggests that observers affect what they study: if the investigator looks for atomic particles, they can be seen, but a wave looker seeking them at that level will find our atomic universe made up of waves. The characteristics of a wave make it constantly and always connected. The consequences of this change in understanding may be quite far-reaching, in terms such that our own thinking may, in fact, change what happens to us.

Wave theory helps explain more precisely the connection of mind to body, of our emotions and spirit to our health. We are, in origin, beings of light. If you walk into a room and two people have just had an argument, they don't have to say a thing. You can feel it. We emit energy, which can be seen as light or electromagnetism, depending on the recording device. And from another point of view, simply physics at its essence, we are all a part of one huge being of light, the sum total body of energy in the universe.

Healing then means that the process of working on each level—of your body, mind, spiritual self, and community—is interconnected with the others. Anything that affects your emotional self may affect your physical self, and so on. Exercise, yoga stretches, music, the arts, meditation, prayer, and other aspects of spiritual connection take on new importance as therapies, both preventively and within the surgical setting.

6. Applying the Healing Powers of Plants, Pets, Poetry, Laughter, and Love

Whatever makes your spirit sing may prove to assist your healing process, as Norman Cousins and Dr. Patch Adams found with laughter, and Drs. Bernie Siegel and Dean Ornish with love. Scientific research in these specific areas is very promising; it may yet prove to be the most fertile ground for successful avoidance of, or recovery from, surgery. Many of these therapies are so much the opposite of the pain-associated scalpel: they are enriching and often fun, and they help heal our hearts and spirits from the disconnection felt so commonly in our current culture.

It was one of the most moving moments of my medical practice. A number of participants in a Dr. Dean Ornish heart retreat were sitting in a healing circle, as we do during these programs. One participant had not been able to access his true feelings, and share them with the group. At one point another member reached out to him, saying, "I wish I could feel connected to you." He responded by saying, "I want to love, but I just don't know how."

This simple statement was so touching and instructive to me, because we rage at ourselves and others, make ourselves sick with anger, and feel separation from the social support we need to stay healthy, in our search for just this: love. But we are all still learning, and though many of us have very poor models, we begin to learn how to love.

Our cultural myths have limited their focus of love mainly to a male–female sexual context, and thus we have lost the continuous safety and connection that a broader definition of love might give us. The most helpful definition, I think, would act to expand our cultural limitations of sources for obtaining love.

Love would then be "the choice of increasing meditative connection to deepest self, to each moment, person, and thing." Love then becomes a verb, an action we can take, and practice, and we can gradually become more skillful in its application, to stay connected to the web of this new, largest planetary definition of what it means to be most fully human by being fully conscious.

7. Investigating Intuitive Healing, Vibrational Medicine, Magnets, Music, Light, and Color

Many of us have experienced times in which intuition has enriched our perceptions of life: information from a dream, or a sudden "feeling" that turns out to be correct. Now many researchers are applying these concepts within the context of healing. Including simple healing touch and life-review, intuitive mind-body methods can provide a deeper understanding of the emotional and spiritual roots of your specific health problem.

I have found intuitive techniques very useful in assisting my patients in recovering from illness, and in helping them discover the context of their illness within their own unique human story. For example, Dr. Bernie Siegel teaches his patients how to examine their drawings for the subconscious roots and implications of illnesses. You can apply this yourself, by first drawing a picture of yourself and your symptoms, and then of your various choices for therapy, and by next looking for informational clues within the pictures, about what is happening to you emotionally, and about which therapy is optimum for you.

Additional intuitive tools include meditation, muscle or pendulum testing, interpreting dreams, and listening to the tugs of the still small voice of guidance within. Some of these techniques are currently undergoing scientific scrutiny.

Other new approaches may also prove worthwhile. As I will discuss in the next chapter, I have personally witnessed magnets benefiting a variety of problems, and color and music likewise being remarkably effective. For example, a magnet can often eliminate a toothache within a few hours, and sound can treat carpal tunnel syndrome and sciatica. These and other such modalities will be considered in the next chapter.

8. Using Your Illness as a Chance for Transformation

Alternative medicine and mind-body perspectives also give us a different way of looking at illness per se. A disease is seen to give us information about ourselves and our lives. Symptoms can be seen as signposts of disharmony and stress, and when we explore their significance, we can open our eyes to new experiences of meaning. You can thus use your illness as a time to step out of the rat race, gain new insights, and change your life for the better.

You can then see the sword of surgery itself as an opportunity to attain a deeper trans-formation of your experience of the physical, mental, social, and spiritual aspects of yourself. Even something as simple as President Lyndon Johnson lifting his shirt to show off his gallbladder surgical scar exemplifies the ability to be proud of what the school of hard knocks can do.

"I took the cards the way they were dealt," one of my patients told me, relating how he successfully underwent removal of a brain tumor, and against expectation made a complete recovery without recurrence.

Many patients have been able to make peace with the changes in their bodies induced by the scalpel, learning to love what their scars represent in terms of deepening their wisdom. "No pain, no gain" may not be the first choice of ways to learn, but we can take the opportunity to transform the pain that life of necessity gives us, by choosing to learn from it skills of more loving connection with others and our most essential, eternal self.

9. Seeing Everything as a Meditation

"The naked fact of death makes everyone spiritual," someone once observed. The success of Jon Cabot-Zinn's program of mindfulness training for treating chronic pain patients gives us hope that these practices which so enrich the quality of our moments can help heal our physical ailments as well.

Facing surgical illness generates dreadful fear; and then sometimes despite the best surgical care and alternative approaches, you still must experience severe pain and suffering. Practicing daily meditation and yoga increases the natural brain chemicals associated with tranquillity and pain relief, as well as helping you get in touch with the deeper spiritual aspects of your inner self.

10. *Preventing and Treating Disease by Lifestyle Choices*

We all want to be happy and healthy: our country was founded on the essential premise of our right to it. And it turns out, happy people tend to be healthier. Research supports this; those who describe themselves as happy, as a whole, remain healthier; optimists live longer,[4] and altruists likewise have lengthier life spans.[5] Or perhaps it's just optimistic researchers who *think* all this is so.

But nonetheless, how can we stay happy, living in the kind of world that we do? Many of the alternative medicine approaches address prevention by teaching attitudinal skills, to prevent the buildup of stress, which adversely affects both immune and cardiovascular function. Spiritual practice can help us cultivate an interior source of happiness not dependent on exterior events or persons, giving us resilient strength to maintain our health from the inside out.

Massage can be an important part of a stress prevention lifestyle. If you can't afford a massage, you may be able to trade with a friend, or visit a local massage school, where massages are often available free, or at a discount. Yoga postures are also a kind of massage which you can do on your own.

Prevention of surgical illness needs to begin with better education in childhood. "Children exposed to health education showed increased knowledge, healthier attitudes, and better health skills and practices," the Centers for Disease Control reported. For example, their School Health Curriculum Project, which teaches the dangers of smoking, kept the increase in smoking rate to only 2 percent between sixth and seventh grades, while a control group rose 5 percent. They concluded that 146,000 students in the United States could be prevented from smoking each year if every school utilized such an approach.[6]

Educating yourself about your disease, its prevention, and the new alternative approaches to treatment is your first duty. Self-care education has been shown to relieve stress, provide you with the opportunity to transform your illness into a learning experience, and help assure a successful outcome. Each of the general dietary and stress-management approaches in the next chapter has its greatest efficacy when used preventively.

The Most Common Alternatives

The most frequently utilized alternatives can be grouped into four categories: stress management, diet, exercise, and alternative healing methods. Stress management includes processes that provide emotional and spiritual support, such as group support and prayer, as well as practices and therapies that enhance relaxation, such as yoga postures, meditation, massage, and aromatherapy. Alternative healing methods include interventions such as chiropractic and osteopathy, acupuncture, hypnosis, herbs, and homeopathy.

In order to choose an alternative approach or approaches that may replace or supplement your specific surgery, you need to understand both your own problem and how these new methods work. "In college I was taught all about the motions of the planets as carefully as though they were in danger of flying off the track if I did not know how to trace their orbits; but nothing about the organization of my own body," stated Horace Mann.

My brother and I have chosen to provide you with a broad spectrum of information about both alternatives and your conventional surgical choices, so you can make optimum choices for your specific situation.

Scientific Research on Alternatives

Although scientific investigation of alternatives is evolving rapidly, the amount of research for these methods lags far behind that for drugs and surgery.

Three main factors are at the root of this deficiency. The first and foremost, as already mentioned, is the way in which scientific research in this country has been conducted. Much of it is funded by drug companies, medical schools, and the National Institutes of Health, which have generally only considered conducting interventions that fit the traditions of drugs and surgery as the prominent treatments.

The second problem is the difficulty in neatly fitting these modalities into a scientific format for research. For example, a drug is fairly simple to test, and a control can be created to match it. But how do you accurately or adequately measure the healing effects of love, prayer, massage, or emotional support? And how do you control for these interventions? Some studies have now attempted to look at such questions, but many alternatives are more complex than can be easily reduced to the parentheses of prospective, double-blind scientific inquiry.

The third is that many of these therapeutic pathways do not fit our conventional models of Western science: how and why homeopathy works, for example, or traditional Chinese medicine explains disease, can not be easily integrated into present scientific theo-

ries. These modalities can be looked at from "outcome" studies, research to simply assess their results; however, for some conventional scientists, that investigational avenue remains problematic.

Despite these limitations, the field of scientific study and outcome application of alternative medicine is quickly growing. The American Medical Association, in response to the public's increased use of alternatives, has devoted whole issues of its eight established medical journals to publish articles on alternative therapies. Results of the Center for Complementary and Alternative Medicine research work can be found in their on-line data base at www.altmed.od.nih.gov.

When Dr. Dean Ornish and I began our research in Texas, to document the ability of a lifestyle program to reverse heart disease, no one believed that heart disease was even stoppable, to say nothing of using changes such as diet and yoga to accomplish reversal. Down there, of course, beef is still placed in esteem right next to God and mother, as Oprah Winfrey found out. But we were able to persevere, as was Oprah, and now this method of treating heart disease is widely appreciated.

Within the scope of this book—an overview meant simply to begin to bridge surgery to the new alternatives—it isn't possible to cover the research on each alternative in great detail; they are presented in brief, with the hope that future studies will continue to elicit more complete information.

Choosing from Among the Alternatives

With many medical schools having departments of alternative/complementary or integrative medicine, and some actively conducting research and offering patients these therapies within their routine medical and surgical settings, the integration of such approaches into our medical care system is now under way. As you can see in the next chapter and the one relating to your specific illness, when applied to surgical disorders, alternative techniques have many profound physiological, psychological, and spiritual benefits, to help you better come through any operation.

Using an alternative therapy to completely replace an operation is also becoming a realistic option for many illnesses. You most likely want to avoid surgery whenever you can. Yet at the same time, you may feel wary of unproven remedies, those that sound promising but don't really do the job of effectively curing the problem. When you are faced with a surgical illness, delay might lose for you an opportunity for cure, making your choice especially difficult.

In the next chapter, I will explore more fully the various alternatives, either to replace an operation or to help you come through it. If you are familiar with only one type of tool, you can learn about the others' contributions. Through a step-by-step process, you can move toward wholeness: the roots of the words "heal" and "health" mean "whole." We all become enriched when we appropriately include what the various traditions, both conventional and alternative, legitimately have to offer.

Protecting Yourself from Unreliable Alternatives

How can you protect yourself from a "quack" approach, one that is simply "snake oil," taking your time or money without being of any real help to you, and perhaps even inducing harm? This book endeavors to help you with such an important problem, by providing you with the best estimates of effectiveness, and a review of the reliable scientific studies that are presently available. David's careful analysis of what are your best surgical options is especially helpful here, to see what you are missing whenever you choose an alternative route.

Since rigorous full scientific evaluation of these therapies is ongoing, you therefore do often enter less well-charted territory whenever you undertake an alternative pathway. Fortunately, since many of these remedies have been used for centuries, they are time-tested, with side effects and long-term effects even more well known anecdotally than those of the latest drug or surgical innovation. Follow the guidelines in the chapter in this book on making a decision about surgery, and use your local library and the Internet to obtain the latest information. The Resources section, at the back of this book, contains recommended books and further information. Informing yourself is your best protection, and freedom of choice your best guarantee that a worthwhile option will not be missed.

Avoiding Blaming the Victim

Whenever things go wrong, we often very quickly seek to find someone or something to blame. The mind-body connection is a two-sided coin. If on the one hand we accept that various lifestyle choices increase risk for illness, on the other we are likely to experience feelings of guilt or regret.

Of course, we do not consciously wish ourselves sick, nor can we will ourselves well. Once we understand that our emotional and physical habits can contribute to our getting sick, self-recrimination and victimizing the sufferer of a disease are dangers to be avoided.

It has been clearly shown scientifically that since our responses to stress and our lifestyle choices do contribute to our risk of illness, we can take *some* action to do something about getting well, creating ultimately a *more* empowering way of thinking. If you do fail to get well using alternatives, you need not consider yourself a failure; often conventional medicine fails as well. And as noted, since the alternatives generally have the advantage of helping your quality of life, their use alongside conventional medicine can give you the best of both pathways.

Life Support Considerations

Two of the most important and difficult challenges of modern surgical treatment of illness are when to decide against a surgery that cannot offer cure, and when to turn off the machines.

What, after all, is "natural"? Although intensive care is not the same as letting nature take its course in the woods somewhere, isn't it "natural" to want to help those we love to live with us as long as possible? The real problem arises when there is no hope of ultimate cure, and all that can be expected is more suffering.

Perhaps there is a midpoint somewhere between Kathleen Quinlan, who although clinically brain dead was kept alive for years by machines despite her family's wishes, and Jack Kervorkian. All that can be done with expectation of some quality of life can be initiated. But then we can also begin to look at death from an alternative medicine perspective too.

Death

Perhaps we as a Western society can learn from other cultural traditions to make better peace with death. Taking from variations around the world, death itself could be celebrated, in a truly joyous way, rather than the mostly somber, sad, even macabre and devastating rituals we have developed here. It is considered "bad juju" even to speak of death; its inevitability is shoved aside in medical training. We in the West see death as a "defeat." But looking at it squarely may actually enrich our experience of living, and help us remain relaxed when facing an operation.

I was in San Francisco in one of the earthquakes that preceded the big one of 1989. I awoke at 4:30 A.M., and it sounded like a freight train was headed straight through my bedroom window. I dropped to the floor, and became drenched in sweat. Later, I related the incident to my yoga master. "What were you afraid of?" he asked.

"Well, death, I suppose," I answered.

"Death!" he laughed, gesturing with his hands as if it were nothing. "You should be afraid of not living!"

In the Eastern tradition, death is not perceived as the great tragedy we Westerners anguish over: the immortal soul has more chances to evolve. What he was trying to teach me, I felt, was not to let fear of future death keep me from training my mind to enter ever more completely into the "present moment" way of living: living more fully while alive, being-here-now, where the juice is, not missing the opportunity to "make hay while the sun shines."

Even in the United States, 71 percent of the people say they believe in life after death, according to a recent Gallup poll. Sixty percent believe in Hell—but only 4 percent think they will end up there!

As a doctor and person, I don't comprehend, or even know quite how to deal with, even one death. "Rage, rage, at the dying of the light," has always been my attitude. Indeed, there is no quick or sure cure for the sadness we all feel on losing even one treasured person from our lives. But as for what lies ahead, $E = mc^2$ implies that the essence, the amount of energy of our universe, always stays the same, only the forms of it vary. Matter and energy interconvert, with the sum total remaining constant. Since we are also made from this one sum of energy, in that sense we are necessarily immortal, just changing shape. None of us are going anywhere, anyway, so we might as well relax. The light doesn't die, because it can't.

If someone walked up to you and informed you, "I have news for you: you are eternal," perhaps that would be the best stress management tool of all. One form of energy just moves into another form. In a world having lost most of its religious assurance, perhaps we can allow the wisdom of Einstein to provide some sense of comfort derived from science, after all.

My own experiences have convinced me of this truth. When my cousin died unexpectedly, I drove a long way to be at the funeral and console her children. That night, as I lay in my bed, wide awake, thinking about the day, I felt her spirit come and kiss me on the cheek. It wasn't something I would have thought to "make up," and it was so real that I am certain it was not a dream or a hallucination. However, it was just like her to do that, in a gesture of gratitude and farewell.

When a friend of mine died suddenly, his spirit woke me up in the night and asked me to take some dictation. I wrote a note to his wife, containing many personal references about which I could not have known. Some of what he told me included, "The light is much better over here," and "Time doesn't just stand still, it sits still. So much peace!"

Whatever your belief, fear of death can be immobilizing when you are facing a surgical decision. It may cause you to put off any medical care, thus allowing your disease to go beyond a phase at which it can be repaired. As the work of Elisabeth Kübler-Ross and others has shown, facing death and the stages of its unfolding with prior knowledge of what to expect can be enormously helpful. Educating ourselves and our children about these issues may be a fruitful contribution of mind-body, alternative approaches to the functioning of our entire healthcare system.

We are so afraid of death that we abandon the dying. A *New England Journal of Medicine* study found that of 400 patients, 350 on average die alone. Author Dannion Brinkley, incredibly, came through three near-death experiences, then began his work to passionately reassure others that the soul continues after death, and that the love we create in this world we take with us into the next. His books, *Saved by the Light*, and *At Peace in the Light*, tell his dramatic story. He also single-handedly founded a campaign to help promote alternatives within our healthcare system and to prevent people from having to die in unresolved emotional pain, alone. His organization, Compassion in Action, can be reached at www.dannion.com.

Alternative medicine can assist enormously to help the transition to death be less difficult. Especially helpful is hypnosis, which has been shown to relieve pain in the terminally ill.[7] One Denver hypnotist reported that one of his terminal patients "drove her little daughter to the shopping center, picked up some groceries at the Safeway, and then went home and died, alert and feeling like a useful wife and mother to the very end."[8] He concluded that "what we are talking about is a means of helping people die with their boots on, instead of a pair of paper slippers."

Other important adjuncts include aromatherapy and massage, especially with the scent of lavender, which promotes relaxation; homeopathy, especially Arsenicum album, given right before death, as a means of relieving anxiety; acupuncture and yoga, to promote relaxation and assist in pain relief; and group support, love and laughter to help resolve emotional family issues. Hospice care, in the hospital, home, or at a special hospice center, can greatly assist in these areas, since its volunteers are specially trained for this work. See the back of this book for further information on Compassion in Action and hospice care.

The Operating Room of the Future

Both mind-body approaches and nontraditional agents of healing may soon be part of standard operating room procedure. For example, light, sound, electricity, magnetism, and massage may be more a part of the range of equipment for surgery in the near future. Laser scalpels are already common. Electricity is used to assist the union of bone fractures, and has showed initially promising results in Swedish studies utilizing it for the treatment of cancer. Hopefully, further research into the benefits of magnetic and electrical treatments will help set aside the need for the painful kind of healing the scalpel of necessity entails. Perhaps one aspect of the most healthful

future of surgery would include a consult with an alternative medicine specialist whenever nonemergency operations are considered, and even in urgent situations, postsurgical recovery enhanced with the additions of massage, relaxation training, dietary change, nutritional supplements, music, poetry, and art, as discussed in the next chapter.

Alternative/Complementary/ Integrative Health Centers

Since a number of medical centers and hospitals around the United States have now established departments for alternative medicine, some options are increasingly available. The University of Arizona Medical Center, under the guidance of Dr. Andrew Weil, teaches integrative medicine to medical students, and within a fellowship specialty program. In the Planetree Project, a homelike hospital setting is available in a number of hospitals nationwide. This project features whole floors of participating hospitals offering patient-oriented services such as kitchens, libraries, and videos. Integration of such promising mind-body explorations with surgery are exciting, and documentation of their usefulness may lead to making them more widely available. See the Resources section at the back of this book to find a Planetree project hospital near you.

When I first heard an audiotape narrated by Dannion Brinkley, and listened to the pitch of excitement in his voice when he spoke of "The Centers," which the Beings of Light had revealed to him during his near-death experience, I wanted to know more. Specific instructions were given to him about creating exemplary sites to help humans improve our health, understand our emotions, evolve spiritually, learn to be less afraid of death, and help our friends and families through that transition.

These "Centers" are designed to demonstrate the power generated when compatible techniques from diverse and separate disciplines come together to achieve something more comprehensive. The various tools of alternative and complementary medicine are integrated with technological advances directed at relaxation and rejuvenation, for the benefit of patients, caregivers, and their families. A musical bed, for example, provides such significant renewal that, afterward, a new sense of the meaning of life and a deeper ability to heal psychologically and spiritually are the results. The unique eight-step process, described in *At Peace in the Light*, may ultimately best be a routine part of all of our medical institutions, as a part of optimum care for all.

Love, as I noted earlier, I have found to be the most important element in healing, and alternative medicine centers often focus primarily on this dimension. We all want love, and science has begun to appreciate how much a lack of it can affect out health. But how do we make use of this powerful force to prevent disease, or help us when we are sick? The Centers offer a new way of looking at who we are as humans, and a new window on the world: and as the process of this work allows us to first become aware of an ongoing source of love within ourselves, then we learn to see everyone else as a part of the larger body of energy to which we are all connected.

I have come to feel, after my now thirty years of medical practice, that what we get to take with us beyond death are not our technical accomplishments, not so much what we have achieved with our time here on earth, but what we have become as people. What our souls have become. And this includes our feelings and spirit.

In this age of fractured families, such centers can provide space for ongoing support groups, and serve as focal places for community awareness, education, classes, and meetings.

With the current ongoing wider acceptance of integrative medicine, hopefully all hospitals will eventually offer such services. All six major hospitals in New York City have already established alternative/complementary/integrative medicine centers, which provide strategic sites for research alongside treatment.

The word "hospital" originally derived from the root "hospitality." With the Centers project, hope emerges for a transformation of our hospitals back into community resources that really serve us—transforming them from simply sterile "automobile repair shops" into warm, nurturing, caring, empathetic beacons of light and love.

SPECIFIC ALTERNATIVE MEDICINE APPROACHES

Most of us would say, if asked, that we want perfect health. We'd be telling the truth as far as the answer goes, but it doesn't go far enough. What we'd have to add, if we were going to be completely honest, is that we'd like to have perfect health, but only under certain conditions. To achieve it we don't want to give up cigarettes, stop drinking alcohol, and drive under fifty miles an hour. We all want perfect health, but only if we can have it without making too many sacrifices. We want it—but only at our price.

Usually, when the gun is at our head our attitude changes.

William Nolen, M.D., surgeon

Any patient who turns responsibility over to the doctor is giving it to an overworked person.

Norman Cousins

Gerald Lemole, Chief of Surgery, Medical Center of Delaware, one of the foremost heart surgeons in the country, had ventured into the realm of alternatives first with his own family. He treated them with vitamins and other supplements for various ailments, and became convinced of their effectiveness. He began a vitamin program for some of his postoperative patients, and noted improved cardiac function, decreased bleeding, less swelling and pain, and more rapid healing in the patients given this treatment.

He now routinely recommends a specific postsurgical supplement regimen to all his patients, to help them achieve optimum recovery. For congestive heart failure and *peripheral edema, he uses the supplement coenzyme Q_{10} and the herbal remedies mullein tea and watermelon tea. For a number of patients found too sick for surgery, after he placed them on supplements, he discovered their heart function so improved they could then withstand the needed procedure. For several, they were so much better, their tests showed they no longer required the proposed operation.*

Dr. Lemole also uses other alternatives with his patients. He came to appreciate the healing benefits of music, and became so well known for his therapeutic use of it in the operating room, the game Trivial Pursuit created a question in his honor: "Which doctor is known by the nickname "Rock-a-Doc"? In addition, he helped explore the importance of lymph flow's contribution to the prevention, onset, and recovery from illness, and the application of alternative medicine methods such as yoga and massage to harness the lymph's healing potential, summarized in his groundbreaking book, The Healing Diet.

Music, acupuncture, herbs, homeopathy, exercise, yoga—once you consider utilizing one or more alternative approaches to treat your illness, how do you decide which one or ones are best for you? Which should you use as an adjunct alongside an operation, and when can you safely rely on them to help you avoid surgery? Which are most important, and how many should you choose?

In answer to these and other such important questions, in this chapter I have put the alternative medicine techniques into the following three groupings:

1. Stress management techniques
2. Diet
3. Alternative healing methods

According to which I have found most helpful, I have included the various subsets of these distinctions, added a discussion of their scientific rationale, and provided instructions for their use.

Children can also respond to these methods, learn relaxation techniques quickly, and exhibit excellent responses to homeopathy, herbs, hypnosis, and acupuncture. For example, one young person with leukemia learned hypnosis by listening to his favorite stuffed animal being given "instruction."[1] For older children, another method often used is for them to visualize that their brain is typing a message onto an imaginary computer screen.

To maximize results, combining alternatives is generally possible. However, make certain not to overload yourself—to avoid *becoming* stressed by trying to do more than you can comfortably handle during the course of your return to health. In the subsequent chapters of this book, I have indicated which alternatives are especially applicable for your own particular disease, so you should refer to those sections to find which approaches are particularly important for your individual problem.

Natural healing avenues often do require some effort, and you may need to stick to them for some time before you see their full results. Therefore, it is imperative you be carefully monitored by your doctor, to make certain you are making progress.

Designing an Alternative Program: The First Steps

When creating an alternative approach to your specific illness, you first need to carefully analyze the four elements that address your basic lifestyle habits:

1. **Your habitual response to stress**
2. **Your usual daily diet**
3. **Your general exercise pattern**
4. **Specific lifestyle problems, such as cigarette smoking**

Once you have looked at these aspects of your disease, you can then select one or more of the healing techniques included in the self-healing tools section at the end of this chapter, which are intended to stimulate your body to repair itself.

Stress Management Techniques

Use of the word "stress" in the context of medicine first was applied to describe the action and reaction of any change on the human body: whether it is a good event, or a difficult one, change itself invokes a "fight or flight response." Stress management is then a process of learning to choose the most optimum response to the inevitable changes with which we humans are faced.

Stress management techniques can be divided into the following important three categories:

1. **Relaxation techniques:** yoga postures, yoga breathing, meditation, visualization and imagery, tai chi, qi gong, massage, water and other spa therapies such as aromatherapy, and exercise.
2. **Emotional support:** group support, love and intimacy, laughter, plants, and pets.
3. **Innermost or spiritual connection:** reflection, prayer, and spiritual belief and practice.

Since each of these three avenues have differing effects, you should endeavor to choose one or more practices from all three categories. In the following sections, I have included those practices I have personally found most essential and effective.

Stress management training has been found directly helpful in treating many illnesses for which surgery is proposed, including the prevention and treatment of back pain and other forms of acute and chronic pain, cardiovascular diseases such as angina and high blood pressure, digestive disorders, menstrual problems and menopause, sexual dysfunction and urinary diseases, and as an adjunct to cancer treatment.

To describe how you feel after a good deep relaxation taxes the limits of words. The first time I went to a yoga class, this part of the session was a revelation. I felt as if I were floating, not bound by the tightly wrapped muscles I had initially carried into the room. From what I knew about physiology, I felt certain the effects on my physical functioning were significant. Research has now supported this belief, as we shall see. In teaching the technique to my patients, I have witnessed a shift, usually within a very short time, into a deeply restorative state of consciousness which has unique stress-relieving and healing abilities.

Many scientific studies have demonstrated that stress plays a significant role in the onset of as much as 80 to 90 percent of all illnesses. Stress management, therefore, can be pivotal in the prevention and alternative treatment of these disorders, as well as help you more easily and quickly recover from an operation, should you choose one. Although many of the techniques described in this chapter, such as the yoga postures, are not aimed exclusively at stress reduction, this benefit is often a prominent one.

Many of the methods described below are

quite simple, yet they are surprisingly powerful. They are specific tools used in ancient, and now modern, times to relieve stress, prevent disease, and return you to health. Stress reduction, however, can take *any* form that feels comfortable to you—golf, tennis, reading, hiking, swimming, or swinging in a hammock. Work itself can reduce stress in some persons. One study of chief executive officers of corporations found that those who did not take vacations were just as likely to be healthy as those who did. Whatever really gets you to feel most restful is what counts. In order to rest, it is not necessary to rust; but it is critically important to change your physiology to a relaxation mode—and the methods of yoga can be most helpful in achieving this result.

Just moving quickly, originally part of the Type A lifestyle traits felt to increase the risk of heart disease, on further investigation has been shown to not itself be a problem unless it causes you to tense up into the fight-or-flight mode. Something so simple as how fast you talk may reflect your stress, and even affect your risk for heart disease or stroke. Remember the fastest talking person around, who dazzled us in Federal Express commercials with his mile-a-minute speech? His untimely death illustrates the stress effect found in research by Dr. Sue A. Thomas, of Life Care Health Associates, Ellicott City, Maryland. She showed that 111 subjects, asked to read aloud two passages from the Constitution, first fast and then slowly, exhibited increased blood pressure when they read the lines quickly. If you have a habit of speediness associated with stress, you may be raising your blood pressure or heart rate, and once this has become part of your lifestyle, you may set yourself up for disease. The slow, deep breathing of yoga, meditation, and other stress management approaches can help you remember to calm down, and thus lower your risk for a variety of diseases or their recurrence.

Relaxation Techniques

The significant aspects of the mind-body connection can be widely helpful within the setting of surgical illness, a time of obvious anxiety and stress. A variety of relaxation aids and approaches have been shown to be useful.

Especially when your mind is restless, it is difficult to relax. But you can first use body-to-mind pathways to move your body in prescribed ways, which can then assist in establishing calm in your mind.

Following are the most important and promising relaxation techniques for use in the context of a surgical challenge.

Yoga

Janice, a 33-year-old mother of three small children, had a great reluctance to visit a dentist, based on some very unpleasant childhood experiences. Then she read about the use of a yoga program and its success with dental operations, known to be one of the most feared types of surgery. Determined to be a good role model for her kids, she used yoga techniques to help herself undergo the work she needed. She then taught simple yoga techniques to her kids. Now they all have beautiful smiles. In a report entitled "Tension Free Dentistry with Tension Free Patients," the authors report on the success of such a yoga regimen.[2] Another report called "Meditation in Dentistry" confirms these findings.[3]

I have found yoga practices to be the most powerful of all the avenues to achieving relaxation. Yoga is an ancient system for renewing and maintaining health, consisting of techniques addressing the body, mind, and spirit. Although some yoga schools promote certain beliefs, the yoga tradition itself does not have religious dogma associated with it. You may choose to use its methods to enhance your own spiritual path, but it can also be practiced by anyone, of any faith, simply for its many health benefits. Virtually all stress management techniques now utilized in the West were derived from this Eastern root. In the later chapters of this book, aspects of this system with significant physiologic benefits for your particular surgical illness are presented.

Yoga techniques have been studied extensively, with the varying components providing differing benefits. Research indicates its helpfulness for heart disease, cancer, digestive disorders such as ulcers or hemorrhoids, diabetes, as well as for pain control, insomnia, drug addiction, and a multitude of other problems. Dr. Robin Monro, an English molecular biologist, compiled a 1,500-item bibliography of scientific papers, documenting the many medical benefits of yoga.[4]

Numerous studies have now demonstrated the ability of the yoga postures to lower blood pressure. Much heart bypass and vascular surgery today is the result of ongoing long-term effects of high blood pressure on the heart and arteries. Since coronary bypass surgery has become such a common major operation in adult American men, a preventive and therapeutic program that can help "bypass the bypass" takes on great importance.

Stress elevates cholesterol directly, and the yoga postures have, by their antistress effects, been found to lower cholesterol levels independent of dietary change. This is important not only in the prevention of cardiovascular disease, but also in preventing the many types of cancer, such as breast, colon, and prostate, that have been linked to high cholesterol levels.

In my exuberant Irish family, New Year's Eve was always a Big Deal. My father would create a Grand Celebration, with bells and whistles, and banana splits with hot fudge too, spread out for all us six kids and our friends. We then would write New Year's resolutions and predict *where* we would be the next year, since my dad was something of a spiritual Don Quixote, and we moved thirteen times before I graduated from college.

One New Year's Eve early in my studies of yoga, I was on tour with a group of physicians in India. The others went to bed early. I missed the excitement and comfort of my family's traditions and began to feel somewhat lonely and glum. I decided to "celebrate" the incoming year by doing the headstand—it has similar benefits to the simpler shoulder stand—to greet the newborn year from a new angle. So at five minutes to midnight I positioned myself upside down, and held the position until five minutes into the new year.

One of the physiological changes that occurs as a result of the shoulder stand and headstand is a relative shift of blood flow to the brain, along with an equalizing of blood flow to its right and left hemispheres. When I finished the posture, I found that I suddenly had a new "perspective," and felt refreshed and content to be just where I was. In fact, I enjoyed it so much that I have made it my own new tradition, to greet every new year upside down, often in some very interesting locations—including the Golden Gate Bridge! All the yoga practices can be thus used to more clearly observe our emotional reactions, reduce stress, and shift from unhealthy habits of responding to external stressors.

Diabetes is responsible for much of cardiovascular and renal disease. It is also a major factor in peripheral vascular disorders, limb surgery, and eye disease. Studies have been able to show that yoga practice lowers the fasting blood sugar in insulin-dependent diabetics. Many type II diabetics can revert to normal blood sugars with weight loss; a yoga program can thus have a two-pronged effect to lower blood sugar directly and through weight loss. One specific yoga posture, the bow, has been evaluated in relation to both types I and II diabetes, and found to be beneficial to both, working by improvement of blood and lymph circulation to the pancreas itself.

Yoga practice has been found helpful for the functioning of other endocrine glands. Physiological and biochemical studies show normalization of glandular function in the thyroid, adrenals, and pituitary.[5]

In addition, a yoga program has been shown to help greatly in maintenance of correct weight. Yoga is able to achieve success where other programs have failed, because its deep relaxation addresses the eating patterns that result from tension and stress. Studies have been able to document that simply by the regular practice of yoga postures, both overweight and underweight subjects return to their optimum weight.[6]

Although the exact cause or causes of colon cancer remain unproven, chronic constipation has been found by Dr. Denis Burkitt and others to be associated with disorders of the colon such as diverticulosis and cancer. Regular yoga practice has been shown to relieve constipation.[7]

Yoga can help your exercise program. Muscle strains and sprains, and bruises are disorders that are especially benefited by a yoga program. Most athletes know the importance of stretching before active exercise.

Both preventive and therapeutic, these stretches have the added dimension of immediately feeling soothing, relaxing a strained muscle. Research has confirmed their usefulness in this field.

The yoga postures are particularly good for persons who have back problems. When performed daily, they have been shown to help avoid the necessity of back surgery. Especially beneficial are the forward bends, as discussed in the chapter in this book dealing with back surgery.

Dr. Michael Lerner and I conducted a preliminary study of yoga for the treatment of systemic lupus, and found significant lessening of pain within only one week of practice. Similarly, Dr. Ornish and I observed improvement in heart patients within only a few days of practice.

Our research has also shown, in an ongoing study of lifestyle and yoga change in the treatment of prostate cancer, evidence of delay in progression and even reversal of tumors. Improved white cell activity after a period of meditation has been documented. White cells act to defend the body against both infection and cancer, so the addition of a yoga program may act as a preventive and therapeutic agent for the surgical disorders associated with decreased immune activity. One patient with metastatic (spread beyond the breast) cancer of the breast, unresponsive to conventional approaches, achieved remission by the use of a yoga program.[8] Yoga has been demonstrated to reduce the anxiety caused by radiation treatment, so it may also serve as a helpful adjunct to other therapies, as a direct immune enhancer.

Specific yoga postures may feel especially soothing to your individual problem. For example, I recommend more rounds of sun salutation for back and hip problems, and I myself used the child pose to help me pass a kidney stone. The basic principle is to do the full general program, as is comfortable to you, and spend more time in whichever poses give you the most relaxation. Specific postures are emphasized, where appropriate, in the following chapters.

In summary, the yoga program may be able to help prevent and treat surgical diseases of many types.

Yoga Postures Daily Program

The yoga postures are designed to be gentle stretches that anyone can do. They are not really "exercises" at all, but simply a series of postures that have specific beneficial effects. They return flexibility to your spine, and are very relaxing. Taken in series, they squeeze and stretch each separate part of the body in a systematic way. They act more deeply than active exercise, to give a physical and circulatory massage to the internal organs. They can thus be added to a preventive program to keep your body fit, as well as to treat acute and chronic disturbances.

Prepare for your yoga session by wearing loose clothing, such as a jogging suit, or shorts and T-shirt. Use a folded blanket or padded mat. Begin with deep breathing, then slowly assume the positions given below. Go only half as far as you can, and hold the pose only as long as is comfortable.

You can learn the basic yoga routines on your own, though it is helpful to find a qualified teacher if you can. Ask for one who teaches a gentle beginners' class. You can find where to obtain cassette tapes of a beginners' class and nearby certified instructors of a gentle type of yoga in the Resources section at the back of this book or by calling 800-858-yoga.

The combined program of stretching, breathing, deep relaxation, meditation, and visualization is recommended before your surgery. Yoga postures are uniquely suited to help you prepare for and recover from surgery. You are likely to be especially tense and your muscles tight before and after surgery, so you may find the yoga stretches especially soothing during this time. They are nonstressful, and can really help you relax. Someday soon, yoga teachers may routinely come to the surgical bedside and give classes right in the hospital, where such instruction is most acutely needed. At Columbia-Presbyterian Medical Center in New York City, Dr. Mehmet Oz is already pioneering this approach, as described in his book *Healing from the Heart.*

After surgery, the yoga practices can help decrease your need for pain medication and sleeping pills. Yoga's ability to relieve constipation can be especially important as you recover from surgery, since many surgical procedures and pain medications have constipation as a side effect.

Yoga Stretches After Your Operation

After an operation, although you must be quite cautious in returning to the stretching, even a little bit may greatly help your rehabilitation. Concentrate first upon the deep relaxation, breathing, and meditation, then add some very simple stretches in areas away from your incision. The poses should be performed very carefully and under your doctor's supervision, since you will need to avoid any pressure at the site of your incision. The illustrations in Figure 2.1 depict a program that you can begin right in your hospital bed. Choose only those poses that will not affect the operative area, and follow the good general rule to *do just half as much as you think you can*. Slowly increase the time spent.

Recovery from surgery takes time and patient effort on your part. If you have had major surgery, especially with a large incision, wait until six weeks to three months after your surgery to return to or begin the full yoga program.

Yoga Deep Relaxation

This practice is one of the most powerful of all the yoga methods. For example, many of my patients have difficulty sleeping. After I prescribe a deep relaxation tape for them, I have received glowing testimonials about how much relief even a small amount of this particular exercise can give. One of them related to me about how, after his prostate surgery, he was having great difficulty with urination. However, once he began doing the deep relaxation regularly, he was able to quickly resume normal function.

Deep relaxation is also one of the easiest of all the yoga techniques and consists of a directed relaxation to each of the various parts of the body. It is very comfortable and rewarding. This practice alone has been shown

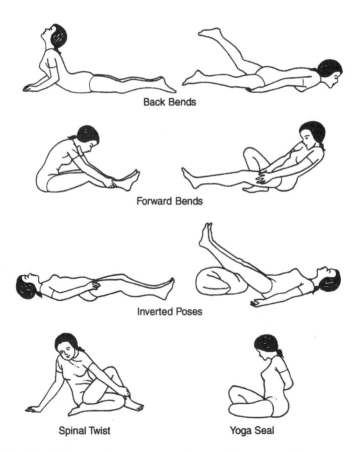

Back Bends

Forward Bends

Inverted Poses

Spinal Twist   Yoga Seal

Fig. 2.1 Eight simple yoga poses that can aid recovery from surgery

to lower blood pressure.[9] *Anyone* can do it, no matter what their physical limitations. Regular practice acts as a direct stress reliever. Now that we understand the relationship of stress to the prevention and treatment of so many diseases, we see how important such a simple step can be. Its use allows imagery to be much more effective, and should precede these sessions, as discussed below.

The time it takes to go through the deep relaxation can vary, depending upon how much time you can spare. You can just quickly scan your body, and then spend a few moments experiencing the resulting relaxed effects. Just before and after surgery, I recommend that you spend additional time in the relaxed state you achieve at the end of the full process, when possible as long as half an hour.

To do the deep relaxation, first tighten the muscles in various groups. Then lie quietly and use your mind to go over the parts of your body, to relax them even further. In addition to its physiological effects, this technique simply allows you to feel *good*. Use this practice daily to enhance your well-being, and particularly to help prevent and treat the surgical diseases now known to be associated with stress: high blood pressure, coronary artery disease, colitis, ulcers, muscle strains and back pain, accidents, and perhaps even some cancers.

You can directly employ the deep relaxation to help you to effectively prepare for and then recover from surgery. Mental influences make a large difference in rates of healing. This area is only just beginning to be explored. Simply follow the instructions given below or use the tape cassettes recommended in the Resources section of this book.

One double-blind study showed that patients undergoing femoral angiography, an X-ray test requiring insertion of a tube into the groin to reach the heart, when taught relaxation via audiotapes, had less pain and anxiety, and required one-third the amount of medication, when compared to patients who listened to blank tapes or even music.[10]

To practice deep relaxation, follow these steps:

1. Lie flat on your back, placing your feet about shoulder-width apart; if lying flat is painful to you, you can practice this in a chair or raised bed. Your hands should be slightly away from the trunk of your body, with the palms turned up. Close your eyes. Gently move your arms, legs, trunk, and neck.

2. Focus on your body part by part. First think of your right leg. Inhale and slowly raise that leg about one inch above the floor or bed. Hold it fully tensed with the breath held. After five seconds, exhale with a gush out the mouth, and relax the muscles of the right leg at the same time, allowing it to fall to the floor on its own, without forcing it; drop it as if it were a puppet that had its string cut, kirplunk. Shake the leg gently from right to left, relaxing it fully, and forget entirely about the existence of this leg. Repeat this same process with your left leg, and then with both arms, one by one. Repeat the process in turn for your buttocks, stomach, chest, and shoulders.

3. Roll your neck from side to side. Squeeze your face muscles tight, open your mouth as wide as you can, stick out your tongue, and roll your eyes back; then release. Once again tighten your face muscles; imagine squeezing all of the tension in your body out the tip of your nose. Take some deep breaths, and feel your whole body relax.

4. Now use your mind to relax each part of your body, beginning with the toes and moving slowly up the body. Feel each part

relax even further, using your mind. Then relax your internal organs. Finally, focus on your breath. Observe it, and keep your concentration there. Then observe your thoughts. See how they come and go, but don't follow them out, just witness them, and stay centered. Then go beneath the waves of changing thoughts, to the peace and stillness that doesn't change, and just feel that peace. Stay there for some time, then deepen your breath, roll your arms and legs, give a good stretch, and sit up, alert yet relaxed.

At first, you may find you have a tendency to fall asleep when you practice this exercise. It is natural, and you still will receive some benefit. However, you should gradually train yourself to stay awake, in which state you can achieve a much deeper relaxation, better concentration training, more pain relief, and more energy after you are finished. Once you master the technique, you can expect to feel wonderfully refreshed after your practice.

Mental influences sometimes contribute to the healing process via the "placebo effect," a name given to the fact that persons who think they will get well have been documented to achieve a higher recovery rate even when given a sugar pill, instead of "real" medicine. Deep relaxation makes use of the positive side of that relationship, using the mind to influence the body directly. By practicing regularly, you can thus consciously harness the placebo effect for your own use.

Yoga Breathing Exercises

Since we have begun to map the relationship of negative emotions to health, the power of yoga techniques to transform our detrimental habits has become more understand-able. The most dramatic and portable of the yoga tools are the breathing exercises.

For example, it is now known that the number of times per day you get angry is a risk factor for heart attacks, as discussed in Chapter 8. But what do you do with your anger, when you feel like stewing in it? Here is where the yoga practices have a twofold effect: they can help your fuse become longer, and also assist you once you have gotten into emotional deep water.

I was at the beach, for some much-needed rest and relaxation. Through a phone call, I found out the man I was dating at the time had lied to me. Small geysers of vapor began pouring out of my ears: I was steamed!

But then I started to reflect upon this, and realized I was only ruining my own vacation! So I decided to take some time for yoga breathing. I set my watch down in front of me, and said to myself, "I am going to do fifteen minutes of alternate nostril breathing."

At the end of the session, I felt so relaxed and calm that I could honestly say, "Well, he was just doing the best that he knew how, trying to be happy—the jerk." (No, that last bit is just a joke.) I truthfully did feel peaceful and forgiving—it didn't make his behavior *right*, but I could understand his fear, and didn't have to sacrifice my own health just because he wasn't willing to be truthful. It's not the event itself that is stressful, but our response to it.

The breathing exercises of yoga can also be particularly helpful in the context of surgery: general anesthesia depresses lung function, and the pain of postoperative recovery can lead you to avoid taking deep breaths, putting you at risk for lung collapse and pneumonia. The yoga breathing exercises increase the depth of your average breath. Usually, we breathe in and out about 500 cubic centimeters of air. After just six weeks of yoga training, the average breath becomes about 700 cubic centimeters, keeping you continuously more relaxed.

Patients suffering from chronic lung disease are at especially increased risk during times of surgery. The breathing exercises of yoga can be particularly beneficial for these persons, improving their lung function before surgery and safeguarding it afterward.

In addition, the breathing exercises are profound relaxers and stress reducers. You may be aware that if you simply take a deep breath, you instantly feel more relaxed. This effect happens too quickly for it to be explained simply by an increase in oxygen. A specific physiologic response, called the Hering-Breuer Reflex, is responsible. Stretch receptors are present in your lungs; and when activated by a deep breath, they transmit messages to your brain, which in turn sends a signal to relax all of your muscles.

Therefore, slowing and deepening your breathing can provide excellent relaxation at any time of day. We normally breathe about twelve times per minute. When we are anxious, our breathing becomes more rapid. When we are concentrating upon something, we almost forget to breathe. By regularly practicing the yoga breathing exercises, you can help alleviate anxiety and calm your whole body and mind merely by calming your breath.

Every cell in your body depends upon oxygen for its function. In medical school, we were taught that oxygen is thus the "currency of the body"; every cell spends it according to its own individual needs. When your breath is deep and slow, your body receives a double physiologic benefit: it is able to receive more oxygen, but at the same time it does not then *need* as much. As the body becomes more relaxed, the need of its tense muscles for oxygen supplies becomes less. When you practice aerobic exercise, the resulting increased intake of oxygen goes mainly to your exercising muscles. Yoga breathing allows you to take in a larger oxygen supply that can then be used by all the regions of your body in whatever way needed for repair and maintenance. You are therefore "putting money in the tank."

As noted, normally we exchange about 500 cubic centimeters with each breath. If we first exhale fully and then deeply inhale, we can take in 3,700 cubic centimeters—more than seven times as much air. Most persons do not take advantage of this free increase in vitality. Especially when we are tense, we breathe mainly using our chest muscles. Singers and athletes know the importance of abdominal, diaphragmatic breathing, emphasized as part of the yoga breathing exercises.

In summary, it is not physiologically as likely you will stay stressed if you make yourself breathe slowly and deeply.

Three basic types of breathing exercises can be practiced. They act together to strengthen the diaphragm, the muscle responsible for 60 percent of the air we bring into our lungs.

All of the breathing exercises are performed with the mouth closed. The exercises are as follows:

1. **Three-part breathing:** Let the abdomen expand, then the lower chest, finally the upper chest, feeling the clavicle rise. Exhale in the reverse order. Count to 10 in and then to 20 out.

2. **Bellows breathing:** Rapidly and forcefully exhale, then have an easy inhala-

tion, for about 20 breaths. Rest and repeat three to ten times.

3. **Alternate nostril breathing:** Breathe in to the count of 10, then out to the count of 20, alternating nostrils, using an index finger to hold the unused nostril closed, and following the sequence: out, in, switch.

The alternate nostril breathing exercise is especially relaxing, and it should be emphasized just before surgery, and afterward. You can practice it in sessions of fifteen minutes to half an hour, making sure to stop if you feel any strain. Sessions can be repeated often, at least three to four times per day to ease pain and keep you calm and relaxed before and after your operation. This exercise has been demonstrated to balance activity in the two hemispheres of the brain, as shown on an EEG (electroencephalograph), which gives you an increased sense of relaxation.[11]

Yoga Meditation

Kidney stone pain is one of the worst types of suffering; if you walk into the emergency room with this problem, they usually just get out the Demerol or morphine. As I noted earlier, I know what this kind of agony is like, since on two occasions I have had to endure it.

Rather than take painkillers, the first time I simply drank lots of fluids, did yoga, and had massages until it passed. The second time, I had acupuncture, with immediate good results; then I went on the preventive program given in this book, and have had no further episodes. However, before the first stone passed, I had an experience that personally proved to me the power of meditation.

I had already been scheduled to teach an individual yoga class to a patient who was staying at the world-famous Pebble Beach Golf Resort. While I was waiting to see if the stone would move through on its own, I drove there from San Francisco, barely able to withstand the pain. I taught the basic set of yoga postures, and then suggested we both sit in meditation together for fifteen minutes or so, in order for him to get a feeling of what that practice was like.

I was amazed to discover that as soon as I relaxed into meditation, my discomfort disappeared, and I was completely pain-free for the first time in two days. However, as soon as the meditation session ended, the pain returned. Until the stone finally was eliminated, I found that I could give myself pain relief simply by placing myself into meditation.

Meditation is the most thoroughly studied of all the yoga techniques. Although it usually is at first the most difficult to master, meditation is also the most directly relaxing yoga practice for the body and mind. Even a small amount of effort can lead to immediate rewards. Dr. Herbert Benson and others have shown that meditation directly lowers blood pressure, heart rate, and breathing rate. Ulcers, heart disease, high blood pressure, colitis, muscle strains, back pain, accidents, and some cancers all may be able to be prevented or more effectively treated by the use of regular meditation.[12] Many studies now support the usefulness of meditation in helping people quit smoking and eliminate the need for drugs or alcohol.

The physiologic effects of meditation are centered on powerful effects on the brain, which then affect the body.[13] Changes in the brain waves, as recorded by an EEG, show that during the meditative state, the brain alters its functioning. As a result, your cells' need for oxygen becomes less, and carbon dioxide and lactic acid are not produced as profusely. Benson has termed this a "hypometabolic" state, a sort of hibernation, yet with the mind remaining awake. This relaxed state has been shown to be reflected in increased levels of the brain hormone *serotonin*, which is associated with a sense of well-being, and the natural painkilling morphine-like substances in the brain, the *endorphins* and *enkephalins*.[14]

Meditation differs from sleep in its physiology, and is even *more* relaxing. During sleep, lactic acid and carbon dioxide accumulate, accounting for the stiffness you may feel in the morning. When you awake from sleep, you also may feel drowsy and tired; tension during the dream state may contribute to this. After a period of meditation, however, you usually feel deeply refreshed and alert, because you are *consciously* relaxing your mind, and through that, your body.

Most everyone has difficulty meditating in the beginning; it took me a full two years before the deeper aspects became apparent. But the first thing I did notice was that although my mind would be racing during the period of practice, afterward it would feel calmer. Even five minutes would make a difference in my day.

Deceptively simple in its technique, meditation is a process that also may take some time for you to learn. With a small amount of practice, however, rewards can usually begin to be *felt*. It is best to commence with fifteen minutes twice daily. Usually the best times to meditate are just after getting up and just before going to bed.

To practice meditation, do the following:

1. Prepare a quiet spot for your meditation. A pillow or folded blanket can be used for a seat. Meditating regularly in the same spot can help your mind to form a habit of relaxing. Sit in a relaxed, cross-legged position, Indian style. If you are not comfortable that way, lean against a wall or sit in a chair. The main idea is to simply be as pain-free in your body as possible, so that you can focus upon your mind without strain.

2. Begin your meditation session by taking some deep breaths. Bring your awareness to the space between your eyebrows or to your heart area. Choose a phrase that is relaxing and uplifting to you, and repeat it as you breathe in, then again as you breathe out. Traditionally, a soft phrase called a "mantra" is used, as sort of a lullaby to your mind. It may not have specific meaning, but rather acts as a type of hum, as if you are humming yourself into restfulness. You may also select a phrase from your own religion, such as "Amen," "Lord Jesus," or "Shalom." The words *Om* and *Om Shanti* ("peace") are traditionally used by the yoga practitioners, without specific religious connotation, just for their peaceful sound. You may simply choose to observe your breath.

3. When your mind starts to drift away from the chosen phrase, gently bring it back to center, repeating the word or words, combining them with your breath. At first, your mind may wander quite a lot. This is natural. The act of catching it and bringing it back gives benefit, even if at first your mind moves its focus repeatedly. Gradually, you may be able to notice an increasing sensation of peace during and after the time you sit to meditate. It is this peacefulness that is the physiologic aim of the practice of meditation.

How can sitting for a few minutes, thinking of one thing, actually help you throughout the day to cope with stress and still remain calm? When you meditate regularly, it has effects that extend far beyond what you might think such a simple practice could do. You begin to respond to the stresses in your life from a more relaxed state: your "fuse" is longer. By increasing your resting levels of serotonin and endorphins, you are more prepared to deal with stress.

The point is not that you must choose between leading a productive, active life that is stressful, or sitting beneath a tree, watching life pass you by. The practice of meditation simply gives you a cushion of relaxation, takes you back to baseline, preventing the buildup of tension within your body and mind to the point where the constant invocation of the fight-or-flight syndrome—our physiologic response to all change—can lead to illness. Interestingly, when your mind is relaxed and your body refreshed, you may in fact be able to accomplish *more*.

Regular meditation may be an especially useful approach in the prevention and treatment of surgical illnesses. For example, frequency of irregular heartbeats was shown to be significantly less after heart patients were trained in meditation, then practiced it for twenty minutes twice daily.[15] If you must have surgery, meditation can help reduce your stress before and after your operation. Once you have trained your mind, you can then make more effective use of imagery and visualization techniques.

Visualization and Imagery

*T*he power of the imagination is a great factor in medicine: it may produce diseases in man and it may cure them.

Paracelsus

*T*hink of your body as a television and your mind as a VCR. You can put anything into it,

and it will show on the screen. If you put in a horror show, it'll show on the body.

Jan Marshall, humor consultant[16]

*D*r. David Bresler, a University of California at Los Angeles researcher, was using visualization with a cancer patient in order to help him reduce his pain. Dr. Bresler asked him what image the pain felt like, and he reported that his lower back "felt like a dog biting him." Dr. Bresler suggested that he "make friends with the dog"; after the patient did so, his pain immediately and significantly diminished.

Visualization is the process of creating mental *imagery* of persons, places, things, activities, or whatever else we choose. In fact, we are visualizing all the time. Unfortunately, these mental pictures are often not positive. If someone suddenly cuts in front of you in traffic, your mind can become quickly focused, but the images are usually not pleasant. Without your specific direction, the images you hold in your mind can be quite destructive to your health. With the process of visualization training, you first become aware of what pictures you are keeping in your mind, and can then begin to change them. Visualization can provide amazing benefits, as you learn the art of how your mind can be harnessed, controlled, and focused in your daily life.

Our inner movies move us. Images may be the "language" of the autonomic nervous system, the relay part of our bodies tied to stress and relaxation. Every time we even think of soothing images, we release different chemicals in our brains than those associated with painful ones. For example, positive mental images act to increase our endorphins and enkephalins, and other natural painkilling substances released by the pituitary. Endorphins give 100 times the pain relief of morphine. Even "thinking of" pain relief can give us actual pain relief.

You can demonstrate the remarkable power of visualization to yourself by performing the following exercise: First, close your eyes. Then, imagine in your mind's eye a table, upon which are sitting a large Ponderosa lemon and a knife. In your mind, see yourself taking the knife, cutting a generous wedge of lemon, bringing it up to your mouth, and taking a big bite. Feel anything? If so, you have illustrated to yourself the significance of the imagery-body connection.

Visualization is well known in its use by athletes to perfect their craft and reduce jitters. Many Olympic athletes have found benefit from these practices. A mental picture of the event is formed in the mind of the athlete, who tries to "see a perfect performance." Gradually the actuality begins to fit this image. As Olympic bobsled driver Bob Said discloses: "I walk up and down the track a lot and visualize myself in every imaginable situation. The last thing I do before I get on a sled is clear my mind and then my mind's eye. I visualize myself driving down that track and I actually see myself the way I want to be and then I get on the sled and I go. The ten minutes before I go each time, I am totally by myself, totally alone, and I just simply program a perfect run down the track." Champion ice skaters Brian Boitano and Tara Lapinsky, and many other athletes, have similarly used visualization successfully before their events.

In many ways, visualization and imagery represent the cutting edge of the new alternative medicine movement, especially appropriate within the surgical setting, where harnessing the power of your imagination for healing takes on such great significance. While meditation can be seen as sharpening the knife of the mind, imagery and visualization can be used to dissect with it. Meditation trains your mind to be focused on one thing. During imagery and visualization, you then apply this focused mind to a specific part of your body to achieve specific therapeutic results.

You can "see" your white cells as more active, and preliminary studies support that your body responds to directions such as this. Norman Cousins studied his own immune system to illustrate this point. Blood was drawn from his right arm, and a number of white cell functions were measured. He then spent five minutes thinking as many positive thoughts as he could: how the Russians and Americans could start talking to one another (this was at the height of the Cold War), better living conditions could be provided for everyone, and so on. Then blood was drawn from his left arm. The immune functions, including T-cell count and NK (natural killer) activity, showed a 20 percent rise in activity.[17] If just five minutes can do this, the potential for such a therapy merits further investigation.

Dr. Carl Simonton and Stephanie Matthews-Simonton pioneered the field of visualization. Several studies by Jeanne Acterberg, performed at the University of Texas, have been able to confirm that patients who were able to imagine their white cells increasing in activity and removing their tumors, had twice the expected survival rate for their cancers.[18]

A fifteen-minute relaxation followed by the instructions to "imagine yourself in a peaceful place in nature" given to breast cancer patients undergoing radiation therapy showed that relaxation was more profound when followed by imagery guidance than simple relaxation alone.[19]

Dr. Pat Norris from the Menninger Clinic reports on one case where a combination of biofeedback, discussed below, and visualization were used. Biofeedback was employed initially to teach the patient how to become relaxed. He was a young boy with an inoperable malignant brain tumor. He made his own visualization tape, "seeing" his white cells as characters from *Star Wars,* which would fly up into his head and zap the tumor with laser guns. After five months of three-times-a-day practice, he came to his parents and announced that he could find no more tumor. His parents told him to go back and try again. Once more he reported that all he could see was a white spot. On re-CAT scan all that showed up was a dot of calcification. The tumor had disappeared completely, and he continues in remission fifteen years later.[20]

Although this is just one case, it still suggests so much. Investigation of the Simonton work supports the powerful possibilities of visualizing. Dr. Bernie Siegel, former surgeon at the Yale–New Haven Hospital, extensively used visualization with his patients. He found that they were able to endure surgery with fewer side effects, and to undergo chemotherapy and radiation with less nausea and hair loss. The summary results of imagery have been striking—lowered but stable heart rates, slower and deeper breathing, much less anesthesia and pain medication needed, and sleep medication unnecessary.

Daniel, a 48-year-old truck driver, and two-pack-a-day smoker, developed a chronic cough that just wouldn't go away. However, since he was in the midst of a very important project, he ignored it. He then began to notice a darkening of his phlegm, even occasional blood. Still, he put off going to the doctor. Finally, he was so weak, his friends insisted he seek help. A chest X-ray revealed lung cancer, and surgery could not remove it all. In addition to his chemotherapy, he decided to practice visualization, imaging his white cells removing any cancer cells in dump trucks. His recovery was astonishing, and five years later he remained cancer-free.

Whatever the surgical problem, visualization can be added to make the therapy more effective, and perhaps even replace a procedure in some instances. It is best to have three to five visualization sessions per day, so that the images become sharper. When conducted right after waking in the morning, after deep relaxation, and just as you fall asleep, this practice is especially powerful.

To practice visualization, do the following:

1. You may benefit from first drawing a picture of your disease, then practice "seeing" the image in your mind, while feeling it in your body.
2. The best time to perform visualization is after deep relaxation. You are then relaxed and calm, and can focus your mind most effectively. Follow the instructions for deep relaxation, given in the previous section.
3. Before you focus on your specific problem, use some general imagery. Many people prefer a general healing image from nature. Fill your mental picture with details. You can imagine you are "breathing in" healing, and "breathing out" pain or disease.
4. Next, choose an image for your visualization treatment process that is appropriate to your specific problem and that encourages recovery. Throughout this book, I have included a sample visualization for each disease: for example, blocked arteries can be seen as opened by a Roto-Rooter, excess body fluid ab-

sorbed by a sponge, your hemorrhoids pushed back inside by a bulldozer and held in place by miracle glue. You can imagine your white cells in any form that appeals to you, such as PAC-men or white knights, and see them gobble up tumor cells or germs. They can carry laser guns or just bring radiant light into the problem area. Choose whatever images seem most positive to you.

5. Finally, use some "open visualization," where you simply allow any image to come up that needs to, by asking your disease area, "What else do you need in order for me to heal?"

6. Draw yourself free of disease.

If you are about to undergo surgery, you can make use of these methods. For example, the Kaiser-Permanente Medical Center in Los Angeles is one of many hospitals that have begun to use visualization tapes with patients. Twenty-minute tapes of soothing images are utilized in order to reduce the need for pain medication, diminish anxiety before surgery, and lesson the side effects of chemotherapy.

"See" yourself coming through the operation in good shape, awakening alert, without pain, feeling hungry and healthy. Patients at Kaiser-Permanente Hospital in Walnut Creek, California, listen to tapes by orthopedist Robert Collins telling them, "Surgery will go well . . . you will block out any negative comments you overhear." Of course, if you can enlist the personnel who work with you, you will not have to block out such comments, but can even have them make positive suggestions to you as well.

Kaiser-Permanente also uses a postoperative tape suggesting, "Your operation is now over and it has been a complete success." The medical and nursing staff report that patients using these tapes need less pain medication, are up and about sooner, and feel generally better. A study of hysterectomy patients reported in *Lancet* found that those patients who had listened to tapes with healing statements, when compared to controls, needed less pain medication and had fewer complications after their surgery.[21] Patients in the tape group also needed less anesthesia and stayed in the hospital an average of one day less.

Tai Chi and Qi Gong

Tai chi, properly called *T'ai Chi Ch'uan* ("great," "ultimate," "fist"), a noncombative martial art form, consists of a series of slow stretching movements and breathing exercises said to have been developed in the thirteenth century by Taoist monks in China. Its dance-like forms have been shown to reduce stress by relaxing the musculature and nervous systems, slowing breathing, and improving balance and posture.

Qi gong means "energy work" and includes a different set of unique movements, breathing, and meditations aimed at allowing the practitioner to first become aware of and then alter the flow of energy—*qi*, pronounced "chee"—through the body. Begun 4,000 years ago along the Yellow River in China as a means to help prevent and treat arthritis, it has become a popular alternative to the practice of tai chi in China and is claimed there to be beneficial for a variety of illnesses. Its movements are generally simple and especially easy for the elderly to learn and practice.

Many of the traditional *tai chi* and *qi gong* movements are similar to yoga, and can be utilized as stress management adjuncts. However, the physiologic benefits of holding the yoga postures have their own unique effects on circulation, so if you choose to practice tai chi or qi gong, you should also do the basic daily yoga poses.

Chi, the Chinese equivalent of yoga's concept of *prana,* is pictured as the "cosmic breath" flowing through us. Once our own energy is flowing healthfully, we can more easily feel connected to the larger flow of energy through everything. When we feel less separate, we feel less stressed. The tai chi and qi gong exercises, similar to yoga postures, are designed to help us feel this flow and connection, and then be able to direct the energy currents to help ourselves, and others, to heal. They deeply relax the body, contributing greatly to stress management.

In his extraordinary book *Saved by the Light,* Dannion Brinkley described how he utilized qi gong methods to help him recover from the paralysis induced by being struck by lightning. After he was resuscitated, he couldn't move at all, except to breathe. Using a copy of *Gray's Anatomy,* he would look at the pictures of his nerves, and then visualize his energy moving down them; finally, he saw his thumb twitch. During this process, he learned to control and send chi to any part of his body that needed healing. This mind-body coordination then helped him come through two more near-death experiences as well.

Massage, Therapeutic Touch, Reflexology, Reiki, Rolfing, Shiatsu, and Alexander Technique

The golden jewel of a moon was rising over the midnight ocean, trailing its light tresses across the waves to our hillside retreat. After sitting for a while in the sulfurous splendor of the hot baths, where time stood still—except for the slow ascent of the moon through the mist—I experienced my first professional massage. The oil, the touch, the letting go of muscular tension, all created an extraordinary feeling of upliftment and renewal. I said to myself, "This seems to be a kind of medicine."

It was 1970, at the Esalen Institute, in Big Sur, California, and I was a maximally stressed medical student from the Midwest, exploring alternatives. Looking at life through eyes so tired they were desperate to find new ways of regaining and maintaining my own health, I had commenced a quest to study, try out, and apply as many healing options from around the world as I could.

I became a massage enthusiast, researching its benefits, introducing all of my friends to its healing capabilities, and recommending it to my patients. When my father had a sudden heart attack at age 80, with no prior history of heart disease, he was placed in the hospital for ten days. I gave him a massage every day, and watched him relax and adjust to this shocking situation with increasing ease. Massage greatly reduces the workload of the heart, aids lymph flow, and changes the physiology to assist with healing. I have similarly witnessed the outstanding restorative powers of body therapies for many types of ailments. In addition to treatment, they also offer a vital form of real preventive medicine.

Touch is a kind of nutrient. Skin-to-skin contact is essential for our health. In a study of institutionalized babies, conducted in the 1930s before this connection was known, 100 percent of the babies who were fed but not touched died. Adults who are not touched may get sick more often, and not heal as well.

Massage is one of the most effective stress-management tools currently available. Premature infants given daily massage have been shown to gain more weight and have shorter hospitalizations than those unmassaged. Both anxiety and depression can be reduced. Pain is diminished, along with blood pressure and heart rate. Skin temperature is increased.

Massage may be especially useful in the surgical setting. Studies have shown beneficial changes in brain chemicals, with decreases in the stress hormones epinephrine and cortisol.[22] Postsurgical recovery is greatly enhanced, with patients found to need less pain medications, have fewer complications, and be able to leave the hospital sooner.[23] Degree of pain and need for hospitalization of colitis patients was shown to be reduced.[24] The Planetree Hospital Program at the Pacific Medical Center in San Francisco has been investigating the benefits of massage for surgical patients since 1985.

Shift from the dominance of our "fight-or-flight" sympathetic nervous system to activity of our "relaxation response" parasympathetic nervous system occurs, so that blood is moved from your arms, legs, and heart, where it must be for fight or flight, to the point of disease, allowing your body to utilize its blood supply more fully for recovery. Since pain is decreased, so is the need for pain medications, which may produce unpleasant side effects and make practicing the self-healing approaches of this chapter more difficult.

Massage can be an adjunct to your personal stress-management program, and its use has been shown to enhance your ability to exercise, as well as leave you less fatigued.[25] Many massage variations exist, including the Alexander Technique, which combines posture training with light touch. Rolfing is a deep tissue technique thought to be able to reverse childhood scoliosis and carpal tunnel syndrome. Therapeutic touch and Reiki practitioners do not touch the body, but attempt to help it heal through energy exchange. Reflexology is based on using pressure points on the sole of the foot to encourage the whole body to heal. Shiatsu is an Oriental approach utilizing pressure points located at various sites on the body.

If you prefer lighter tough, choose therapeutic touch, Reiki, reflexology, or shiatsu. If you can tolerate deeper touch, use Swedish massage or Rolfing. Therapeutic touch, where nurses are taught to concentrate their energies in their hands but do not touch patients, has been shown to effectively increase blood concentrations of red cells, relieving anemia for up to four months.[26] However, other studies have disputed its reputed benefits.

Massage "bars" are now even available in many airports and grocery stores, where, sitting in a specially designed chair, you can receive a fifteen-minute massage for $15 or so. Regularly reducing your stress by massage helps your body to maintain and repair itself internally, thus assisting prevention and reversal of illness.

After a massage, one patient told me, "That was wonderful. I forgot about my surgery and traveled in my mind to Tahiti." Holding such beautiful images in mind can itself help in healing, as discussed in the visualization section.

Touch can help to calm even unconscious patients. Nurses have been found to be more likely to touch patients that are in better health than those who are not—although the latter are the ones who probably need it the most. Depressed, older, and dying patients are less touched. To counteract this tendency, hopefully, all hospitals will soon employ massage therapists as part of the therapeutic team.

Water Therapy, Spa Treatments, Sunlight, and Fresh Air

You float in a horizontal position, totally supported. As images of dolphins and ocean waves are flashed on the walls, the rhythmic music of Enya helps you to drift and stretch gently, letting go earthly gravity into a blissfully therapeutic moment of peace and stress relief.

This is Aqua-traction, invented by Dr. Randy Van Nostrand, whose demonstration pool is located in Tucson, Arizona. His program consists of a simple system of yoga stretches to be performed in the water, and designed for anyone in pain, especially those with back or joint problems. You can do it yourself: Use an air-filled neck collar, a small inner tube under your arms, and small Velcro-fastened weights around your ankles. Pool temperature should be as warm as possible.

Water therapy is an ancient system favored by the Greeks. We humans evolved from the oceans. Our blood is similar in composition to sea water: we are all "walking aquariums." Water settings, and imagery, can profoundly help us relax.

Traditional spas offer various stress-relieving water jets, sprays, and Jacuzzis, along with relaxation devices such as mud-baths, seaweed, and salt applications. Although these simple, nontoxic therapies so far generally lack scientific assessment, their physical and psychological benefits warrant further evaluation.

Steam and sauna treatments increase circulation to the skin, and the cold water applied afterwards increases circulation to the internal organs, creating a restful, stress-relieving effect. Sunlight increases levels of serotonin, one of the brain's natural tranquilizers depleted by stress.

Breathing fresh air, particularly next to water, also acts as a natural tranquilizer.

You can use a daily bath as part of your own stress-management approach. Combine with aromatherapy and music, discussed below. Adding oils to the water will prevent your skin from becoming too dry.

Aromatherapy

Remember Dorothy, in *The Wizard of Oz*, as she ventured into the field of poppies? Ah, just the aroma began to change her consciousness, beckoning her to sleep.

My first experience with the therapeutic power of aroma was at the Greenbriar spa in West Virginia. After soaking an entire sheet in cold water infused with lavender oil, they wrap it around you, then add a metallic "space blanket." Within the cocoon, you slowly warm up, and after an hour, you are floating in a cloudlike wonder of lavender refreshment for body, mind, and spirit.

Inhaling aromas can quickly change our emotions and moods. The nose's olfactory nerves enter into the limbic area of the brain, which registers emotions. Tests utilizing various scents have begun to determine specific effects.

The smell of fresh strawberries has been found to enhance memory, doubling children's test scores, while the scent of cinnamon has proved a significant aphrodisiac. Mint, eucalyptus, and lemon act as stimulants; lavender, chamomile, and rose as calming agents. The French use aromatherapy diffusers in some hospitals, claiming they act as disinfectants; the lavender in the air is felt to kill offending microorganisms.

Eighty percent of taste is smell. We experience only four tastes: sweet, sour, bitter, and salty. All the rest is odor. Complex aromas contain an average of 200 chemicals to which our olfactory nerves respond. One of the reasons coffee is so addictive is that its aroma is composed of 800 to1,000 significantly active aromatic chemicals. Artificial odors can mimic those we recognize, but may not produce the same physical effects.

The complicated, satisfyingly deep fragrance of an old forest may contribute greatly to our moods, and its replacement by concrete may increase the stress of urban dwellers. Changing sidewalks back into plant areas may not only improve air pollution, but act to help us keep our emotional health and sanity.

Aromatherapy has been used in the operative setting to soothe patients following cardiac surgery.[27] Lavender oil has been shown effective in reducing pain following childbirth.[28] This action may be attributed to its ability to sedate nerve function.[29]

You can purchase a small bottle of aroma essence at your local health food store or body shop. You can put some in your bath or use during massage, apply it to your pillow before sleep, or simply place it on your skin like perfume. You can choose the fragrance or fragrances you love best, and use them to help reduce your stress on a regular basis. After you check with your particular hospital, you may also take your personal aromatherapy with you, for use before and after any operation. Inhalers and room diffusers, where the scent is placed on a warm bulb, are also available at larger health food stores. Eucalyptus is especially beneficial for lung congestion, and inhaling it reduces the number of pathogenic organisms in your nasal passages.

Music

The strength of music as a medicine has been generally underappreciated. However, recently, the *Journal of the American Medical Association* (*JAMA*) reported research conducted by the State University of New York at Buffalo showing that when fifty surgeons completed a stress-producing task while listening to their own favorite music, they performed better and felt more relaxed than when working in silence or to music that other persons preferred. Forty-six of the surgeons chose classical instrumental music, two selected jazz, and two Irish folk. The researchers concluded with a quote from Nietzsche, "Without music, life would be a mistake," and went on to add: "Over a century later, our data prompt us to ponder if, without music, surgery would be a mistake."[30]

Both staff and patients can benefit from adding music to their healing regimens, since it is one of the most promising and powerful of alternative medicine techniques.

The patient limped into my office, leaning heavily on a cane. She had been suffering from severe pain in her left hip for six months. The discomfort was getting worse, beginning to radiate down the back of her left leg and give her some weakness in her left foot. Despite physical therapy, her symptoms, typical of classic sciatica, were proving disabling. She was considering surgery.

I decided to try music therapy for her. I placed a speaker right over the hip where the impingement of the nerve was located, and played thirty minutes of calming spiritual music directly into her leg. The sound vibrations themselves can change blood and lymph flow, promoting healing, while the type of music itself induces deep relaxation and taps into the mind-body-spirit healing mechanism, which I will discuss later in this chapter.

I returned to the room to discover she was up and moving easily about, having thrown her cane aside. "I can walk, I can even dance!" she whooped. Her quick and complete recovery amazed even me. I have since seen such music treatment assist patients with a variety of complaints, from carpal tunnel syndrome, aseptic necrosis of the hip, colitis, diverticulitis, and various infections to hemorrhoids.

Music can make us march, and it can bring us to tears; it can relax our muscles, and, on many levels, it can help us to heal.

For my patients, I routinely play music that evokes the relaxation response. Slow, soft, and soothing, it is not "Musak," but rather, like Gregorian chant, its particular rhythm induces slower breathing and heart rate, muscle relaxation, and emotional rescue. Since we now understand the critical relationship of stress to illness, we can begin to consciously utilize the power of music for stress management.

Recent research has shown that listening to soothing forms of music creates "entrainment," a condition in which your brain waves shift toward increased alpha-type waves, associated with an improved state of relaxation. Since so much of illness has now been linked to stress, the regular practice of music-as-therapy may be more than a simple adjunct to your life, but rather be a central tool for maintaining your health. Music may also be used as a powerful adjunct for healing, to help you avoid or come through a specific surgery.

Some relaxation experiments have indicated that if you are very anxious, you may do best to begin with upbeat, active music, and gradually shift to slower, more soothing forms. Such use of a "musical tranquilizer" has been effective in helping break the cycle of addiction. Alcoholics, for example, have been shown to be deficient in alpha waves, and since alcohol increases these waves, addiction

may represent a sort of self-medication that, unfortunately, often carries unhealthy side effects. Both listening to soothing music and meditation increase alpha waves without the negative effects on health associated with using this drug for relaxation.

When you listen to music, you also use a different part of your brain from the portion that speaks and listens to speech. Your brain chemicals change as you listen to the varying forms. A soothing lullaby can help you sleep, and have a rest from pain. A stirring march can move you to get up and exercise. You can thus use music to help you more effectively prepare for and recover from your operation, and to help your body stay relaxed during the procedure itself.

The power of music to "soothe the savage beast" makes it an ideal adjunct to surgical practice. Music has been shown to reduce stress before surgery: measurements of stress hormone levels were lower in patients who listened to music before their orthopedic, gynecology, or urology operations.[31] Some surgeons now work with music therapists, who help patients choose tapes that can be played on portable cassette players while they are under anesthesia. Dr. Bernie Siegel played patients their choice of music over the operating suite's speakers. At first, the other medical personnel at his hospital thought it weird, but now they are also doing it.

What sort of music you choose depends upon your own tastes, and what is elevating to you; you can discuss this with your surgeon and anesthesiologist beforehand, and have it piped into the operating room or played to you only through a portable tape player and headphones. Music tapes can be especially important if you are choosing local or regional anesthesia, to help you relax during the procedure, and reduce your need both for anesthesia and postoperative pain medication. Tapes which include both music and instruction have been found to be most effective.

Promising areas of music research include the ability of certain tones, chants, or music to induce transformative reverie and release of emotional stress. The Australian meditative flute, the digeredoo, may be especially helpful in this context.

Art, Poetry, Beauty, and Color

I walked into the dining room of the hospital and stopped short. Where was I? Here were intimate tables for four and six, set with fresh white tablecloths, beautiful place settings, and fresh flowers; a live string quartet was playing soft classical music. The atmosphere was one of a cherished expensive restaurant, and the effect was uplifting to the soul.

This was an exemplary hospital in Switzerland, where color, art, music, and dance are a routine part of the therapy given every day to every patient. Five such hospitals, inspired by the work of the forward-thinking teacher and author Rudolph Steiner, who also founded the Waldorf Schools around the world, embody an understanding of how important the joy of our spirit really is to our health, especially during recovery from illness.

All of us have been at one time or another inspired by a certain work of art or phrase of poetry. We humans may need another kind of "B" vitamin: a daily requirement for *beauty* in our lives, uplifting us and generating beneficial chemicals in our brains. These modalities can be a conscious part of your personal stress-management program, as well as utilized to help you heal from surgery.

Color itself is a type of therapy. The color red has been found to increase temperature and bodily functions and is psychologically associated with love. Its warming effects may be the reason long flannel underwear is traditionally red. Gazing at the color red was found to significantly increase grip strength, while the color pink diminished it. Rose- or amber-colored glasses decrease the frequency of migraines. Pink reduces anxiety, and has been effectively used to calm schizophrenics and prisoners. Yellow stimulates the mind, aids digestion, relieves constipation, and acts as an antidepressant. Orange increases energy. Green promotes healing and relaxation: salesmen who removed their watches guessed that time had passed more quickly in a green room, whereas those in a red room believed that meetings had taken twice as long as they actually had. Perhaps this is why so many television talk shows have a "green room" for waiting guests: it acts to help reduce their preappearance anxiety and estimation of their waiting time. Blue is calming and cooling and lowers fevers: people in a blue room were found to feel cooler and set the thermostat four degrees higher than those placed in a red room. Violet promotes meditation and sleep.

White, gray, or beige, often the choices for hospitals, have been found to be understimulating, leaving you cranky and restless, and making it difficult for you to concentrate. You may, therefore, help yourself heal while in the hospital by bringing in colored pajamas or jogging outfits, bedclothes, and posters, to create the optimum effects for your individual problems, needs, and preferences. (For a further discussion of this, see Chapter 4.)

I utilize colored lights, shining them directly onto the body, to improve blood and lymph flow, and thus promote healing. I find this type of treatment helpful for a wide array of illnesses, especially chronic infections, digestive and menstrual disorders, menopausal symptoms, fatigue, and obesity. You can also combine mental imagery, discussed above, with color therapy, to achieve these results by "breathing" specific colors into your body and then directing that energy to any problem area.

Exercise

That April morning was the dawning of a classically dark and stormy day. I had driven up to watch a fellow physician run the celebrated Boston Marathon. On a lark, although I had never run more than five miles in my life, I decided just before the beginning of the race to see if I could run with him. The officials let me enter because I was a doctor.

My colleague, who had been training for months, became anxious, nauseated, and almost couldn't finish the distance. As I began to feel my body adjust to the exercise, I used my meditation training to stay relaxed, and "sent my mind" down into my legs to encourage them. The faces of the people along the way looked like beautiful multifarious flowers, a garden of blossoms cheering me on. I breezed past "The Wall," a metaphorical upward stretch of the road two-thirds of the way through, which serves as a point of great fatigue and for which the Boston course is particularly infamous.

Without stopping, I ran the twenty-six miles. About halfway through, it started to rain. Then during the last mile of the race, giant-sized hailstones began tumbling out of the sky, making it seem as if the gods were unloading their ice cube trays. Because of my mind-body training, though, I still had enough energy at the end to actually do a few celebratory cartwheels over the finish line.

Generally speaking, you can expect to add two hours to your life expectancy for every one hour you exercise. Lower rates of heart disease, cancer, diabetes, arthritis, and other chronic ailments have been documented to be associated with regular aerobic exercise. Exercise itself may be an excellent treatment for the anxieties and depression that sometimes cause you to smoke cigarettes, use alcohol, or overeat, placing you at risk for surgical disease.

Active exercise is critical for the success of an alternative medicine program. We are not just "what we eat," but also what we circulate. In addition to assisting us to a level of physical fitness that may prevent many disorders, active exercise changes your brain chemicals to create a buoyant sense of well-being sometimes termed the "runner's high." This vibrant feeling carries over into the rest of the day. It is hard to simply imagine how *much* better you can feel by adding exercise to your lifestyle: it is really worth a try.

Exercise programs first aim to achieve an "aerobic" state, one in which the heart rate is increased and oxygen is used by the body to burn up fats; at least twenty to thirty minutes of very active exercise each day is required. It can be taken in ten minute segments. Slow walking or golf doesn't usually achieve this optimum level. Fast walking, running, bike riding, swimming, tennis, and dancing are excellent forms of aerobic activity. You need to start slowly and gently, then increase until you have reached thirty minutes to one hour each day. Regular exercise has been shown to slow the progress of atherosclerosis, and add to life expectancy, even in smokers with high blood pressure and high cholesterol levels.

Although very active exercise is ideal, less vigorous exercise is still beneficial. Brisk walking for three hours or more per week was found to be equivalent to other more strenuous types of exercises in reducing risk for coronary events (heart attack or death from coronary disease) by 30 to 40 percent in the women in the Harvard nurses' study.[32] A recent study from Hawaii showed that even lower-level activity in seniors is advantageous. Seven hundred nonsmoking men, ages 61 to 81 years, were followed for twelve years. The mortality rate among those who walked less that one mile per day was nearly double of those men who walked more than two miles per day.[33]

Weight training is also necessary. Performed three times per week, it helps maintain muscle mass, prevent and treat osteoporosis, and maintain optimum metabolic rate, preventing obesity. You can start at home with small hand and ankle weights, and graduate to larger heft.

Our research suggests that exercise must be accompanied by dietary change and stress management in order to reverse heart disease. Exercise alone does stimulate the immune system, helps your psychological function, and aids in stress reduction. Since much of surgical disease, such as ulcers, heart attacks, and even infections, may be stress-related, exercise fulfills both preventive and therapeutic roles.

Active exercise specifically may be able to help you avoid surgery for certain problems. Back disorders respond particularly well to regular exercise. Glandular imbalances, menstrual problems, and digestive tract diseases sometimes disappear when a regular exercise program is added to the lifestyle. Lung, blood vessel, and heart malfunctions may also respond.

Even if you can't exercise, particularly before or after surgery, you can almost always chew gum! This simple motion increases brain levels of the naturally tranquilizing hormone serotonin, which is depleted by stress, perhaps explaining why this habit can be so addicting for some people.

You should begin any new exercise routine very gradually, under the guidance of a supportive physician, who will need to monitor your progress to make certain your program is not in itself stressful, and that your surgical disorder is responding to this plan. If you have time, beginning an exercise program before your surgery may help assure its successful outcome and speed your recovery. It adjusts your body to optimum metabolism and circulation, helping you better withstand the rigors of an operation.

After your surgery, how soon you can return to exercising varies with the type of operation; most surgeons favor early walking after surgery, and early return to full activity, since exercise is thought to contribute to the healing process.

Active exercise contrasts with the type of relaxation training in many of its effects, as previously discussed. I recommend *both* be included in your daily regimen.

Emotional Support

The particular stresses of dealing with a surgical illness engage our emotional selves. Fear, anger, sadness, isolation, the stages of grieving all may be invoked. Because of the mind-body physiology, directly examining these emotions may help in your recovery process. Finding support from others dealing with similar issues may be beneficial, especially if you are the kind of person who takes comfort in sharing your experiences. Support groups have been found to work best if you are comfortable with the group interactive format. If you are not, you may wish to try one or more of the other means listed below by which you can help yourself achieve emotional comfort, according to your individual needs.

The following are the most significant emotional support approaches.

Group Support

Even a donkey doesn't go out into the desert alone.

Rumi

Jack McLanahan, the authors' father, a very active 81-year-old, suffered a heart attack while watching a basketball game. An angiogram showed blockage in the arteries of his heart. He decided to use the Dean Ornish program for cardiac disease reversal, to prevent further problems and reverse the ones he had. Since he lived in a rural area of Kentucky, no existing groups were locally available. He and the authors' mother, Connie McLanahan, contacted his cardiologist, asking for referrals of other patients interested in this new and exciting approach to heart disease reversal. The group was so successful that, soon realizing that he also had risk factors that should be addressed, Jack's cardiologist himself joined it.

Having the support of a group to develop and maintain healthier lifestyle choices may be the most important act you can take on behalf of your health. It can help reduce your physical symptoms, such as pain, diminish anxiety and depression, decrease your length of hospital stay, help relieve stress, and even extend your life.

Dr. David Spiegel of Stanford showed that in terminal breast cancer patients, just use of a support group, meeting once a week for one and a half hours, doubled life expectancy,

from 18.9 months in the control group to 36.6 months in the supported group.[34] A group of emphysema, asthma, and bronchitis patients were able to reduce their hospitalizations from 64 percent to 20 percent by attending a support group. Joint pain in those with rheumatoid arthritis decreased after only 10 weeks of being in a support group. Patients undergoing radiation therapy diminished their stress, and demonstrated physical and psychological improvement, after 14 weeks of group support.[35]

Support groups may help to improve health in a number of ways. Simply inspiring participants to improve their diets, exercise habits, and responses to stress, or to sleep more peacefully, may assist healing, and those who commit to a group may be more assertive in seeking out treatments for illness. Benefits extend to quality of life: widows joining a support group were found to have more new friends and activities after one year.

"Psychoneurocardiology," showing links between emotions and the heart, and "psychoneuroimmunology," documenting connections to the immune system, have produced research broadly indicating that mind-body connections directly affect health. Cascades of biochemicals are produced by emotional states, meaning that our emotions can be helpful or harmful to our bodies. Harvard's Steven Locke, M.D., asserts that "solid evidence" has shown biochemical and neurological connections between the nervous system and the immune system. How this translates into any specific disease requires further investigation.

Obviously, you cannot simply "emotion" your disease away, and the complex interplay of emotions and physiology requires much more research. However, enough data indicates that for your own safety, you simply increase your probabilities of health, if you feel comforted by a group setting, by making certain to joining a group meeting once a week, and use this forum to address your emotional issues. It can be associated with your religious affiliation, be an existing organization devoted to your particular disease, or you can start your own group.

In the context of coming through surgery successfully, it is hopeful to note the success of a support program of postsurgical intervention in malignant melanoma patients, a study conducted by Dr. F. Fawzy and others of the University of California at Los Angeles. Depression, fatigue, confusion, and mood disturbance were lower in the patients given support. In addition, changes in the immune system correlated with changes in mood. Dr. Fawzy's study lasted only six weeks, and he concluded, "We showed that it is possible to take someone who is struggling and distressed and change them very quickly" ... they "learned something in the group that reduced their distress, and they applied it to other areas of their lives."[36]

"The evidence is overwhelming that a lot of people get real help from these groups," summarized Dr. Marion Jacobs, of the University of California at Los Angeles Self-Help Center. "Many scientists agree that social isolation increases the risk of poor health. That's why self-help groups are so valuable—they bring together people with common concerns."[37]

The recommended format of these groups is "expressive-supportive," meaning that the sharing of emotions within a positive and supportive atmosphere is encouraged. Such groups are not classical therapy groups *per se*, but patterned on the Alcoholics Anonymous model, where everyone is encouraged and given what support they need to feel con-

nected. Attendance is not optional: to be most effective, you must try, except when you are traveling, to make every meeting. As Dr. Spiegel said of his experience with a group, "They cared about one another deeply. The group's support meant a great deal." Further explanations of what has been learned from this type of group is available from reading *Dr. Ornish's Program for Reversing Heart Disease* and the follow-up book, *Love and Survival*, as well as by contacting Dr. Ornish's organization directly (see the Resources section of this book).

Most people may benefit from this sort of "intimacy group," one that meets at least once a week, although those forced into it may not. If no local support group exists for your specific illness, you can either start your own or join a general one.

Whether emotional change may help you live longer, or even reverse your individual disease, needs further scientific attention. Meanwhile, as Dr. Spiegel summarizes: "What helps patients most is focusing on living better rather than living longer. To focus on psychosocial support as a technique for living longer is missing the point."[38]

Laughter and Play

Life must be lived as play.

Plato

Hah. Hah. HaHaHaHah.

Laughter is like a kind of yoga breathing exercise, and just as powerful. While you may find taking time for the discipline of yoga practice sometimes dauntingly difficult within the context of a hurried life, you can most certainly find time to laugh, and count it as part of your daily yoga practice.

A good laugh affects your whole body.

Scientific appreciation and application of the healing power of laughter is officially termed "gelotology," from the Greek *gelos*, meaning "humor." It was spearheaded by the journalist Norman Cousins, who used the regular application of laughter therapy to help himself recover from ankylosing spondylitis, a debilitating bone disease. Laughter as therapy was further promulgated by Patch Adams and Robin Williams.

We first laugh as early as 29 days old, often as we pass gas, perhaps an important clue to a whole lineage of jokes. By the time we are 16 weeks old, we are laughing once an hour, and by age 4, as often as every 4 minutes! Laughter may represent one way we convert tension to relaxation, making it an adaptive stress response.

One study found that children laugh, on average, 400 times per day, adults as little as 15 times. As Dr. Joan Coggin, Professor of Medicine at Loma Linda University School of Medicine, the laughter researcher who conducted this investigation, put it, "That means somewhere along the way we lose 385 laughs a day. *This has got to stop.*"[39]

Your body's physiology profoundly changes whenever you laugh. Electrical and chemical alterations develop quickly: the speed of a blow-out guffaw of laughter from your mouth can reach seventy miles per hour! The many physical and psychological benefits include lower blood pressure, pulse rates, and muscle tension—though these are all initially increased, they are followed by a fall *below* baseline. Norman Cousins found that ten minutes of belly laughing—he chose videos of the television show *Candid Camera* and Woody Allen movies—could leave him pain-free for two hours. His blood sedimentation rate, reflecting inflammation, was lowered, and this effect held over time.

Cortisol levels decrease and pituitary release of endorphins, the body's euphoric natural painkillers, are increased; adrenaline, initially increased, is then lower than before. All these changes physiologically reflects a diminished sense of stress. Interleukins, an important component of optimum immune system functioning, are increased.

Right brain activity increases, giving you a new perspective on nagging problems. A therapy group in California has participants "sing" their problems into a microphone: it makes you laugh just to think of it. When we sing, we generally use the right brain, which steps outside the time and space constraints of the logical left brain, and can leave us refreshed and more in the "present moment." The mystical Sufis believed that laughter was a significant spiritual tool, since the quality of our attention changes, even as we begin to anticipate listening to a good joke.

Sometimes called "inner jogging," laughter is a kind of "workout," the easiest form of exercise, with its effects felt faster. Heart rate increases within twenty seconds and lasts for three to five minutes, while exercise may take three minutes to exhibit its heart rate effects. It does burn calories, so in addition to being part of your daily yoga, it counts as part of your daily aerobic component as well. Oxygen in the blood is increased, carbon dioxide decreased. Rapid expulsion of the breath clears out the old, stale air in the lungs, making way for fresh, oxygenated air to enter. Jan Marshall stated, "I actually prefer to laugh rather than jog. You save money on shoes, and you smell better. You don't have to be hosed down after you finish."[40]

Laughter, then, really a kind of rapture akin to orgasm, leaves you more relaxed and, by interrupting the panic cycle of pain and disease, can be especially helpful in the setting of surgical illness. As far back as the thirteenth century, the surgeon Henri de Mondeville used laughter to help his patients recover from their operations. Laughter is contagious, as witness the success of canned television laughter. The infamous stress response, the fight-or-flight syndrome, is opposed. Humor therapy programs have been shown to improve the quality of life. Many hospitals, including DeKalb General Hospital in Decatur, Georgia, have effectively utilized a humor room, which they call the "Lively Room," since 1983; some hospitals have a "Humor Cart." St. John's Hospital in Los Angeles has a twenty-four-hour comedy television channel. Some dentists now make use of laughter to decrease the patients' need for pain medication.

"The idea," stated Norman Cousins, "is just to get away from all those reminders that you are sick and to create an environment in which a doctor can do his best . . . We have made the interesting observation that if you can liberate patients from the depression which almost always accompanies serious illness, you get a corresponding increase in circulating interleukins."[41]

Playing is also a lost art. Remember when your mother said to you, "Just go out and play." The rules of this game were that *anything* could be fun, not just celebrating the end goal, as we do in work, and then relaxing. Rather than wait to feel better and then play, we may do best to *first* play, and *consequently* feel better.

Sand tray therapy applies the playfulness of various figurines on a bed of sand to help access subconscious issues, and assist in healing. Hopefully all hospitals will one day provide such tools to kids and adults alike.

Pets and Plants Therapy

I've always known I love having animals . . . what a surprise to find something you love is neither immoral nor fattening but good for you.

Betty White, actress

It is a known scientific fact that the mere sight of a friendly dog induces the body to produce "puptides," chemicals which help the body fight disease and create a general feeling of well-being.

Dog owners have fewer heart attacks. It's a fact. That's because dogs get their people to go for walks instead of watching the 11 o'clock news. Says noted researcher Dr. Hugh Manitarian, "Not only is the walk much-needed exercise, but not watching the news results in 34 percent less stress."

Swami Beyondananda, humorist

Orchids helped me write this book. Whenever I would find myself particularly flagging, I would purchase some large, fragrant cattleya orchids, and place them around my computer screen. The aromatherapy refreshed me, their colors buoyed my spirits, and their oxygen content helped my concentration.

Plants and pets can serve as both stress-relieving preventive medicine and therapeutic inspiration, shifting our physiology to a healing mode. A nursing home project entitled Edencare discovered that when they introduced plants, free-flying birds, and live-in pets to their facilities, their infection rates dropped in half, and their mortality went down by 25 percent.[42]

Pets can help us reduce our stress and get our exercise, both physically and emotionally. Owning pets has been found to be beneficial to health—those who own pets were discovered to be more likely to survive their heart attacks, and getting a pet makes you less likely to have a second one. Looking at fish in tanks, or talking to animals, *lowers* blood pressure, while talking to humans *raises* it. In one study of atherosclerosis in rabbits, the investigators discovered that the rabbits in the lower cages had a diminished rate of plaque accumulation. When this phenomenon was investigated further, it turned out that the lab attendant was taking out the rabbits at night and petting them, but since she could not reach the upper cages, these rabbits did not receive any holding or petting. Repeated in a double-blind fashion, the results of the study were the same.[43]

A University of Pennsylvania research project studied 100 volunteers, placed alone in a room with a fish tank for twenty minutes. For half, the tank contained fish, while for the others, only plants, pebbles, and bubbles. Blood pressure levels became significantly lower in those with the fish to watch, compared to the control group. If you don't want the work and mess of maintaining a fish tank, many videotapes of various aquarium scenes, as well as screen savers for your computer, are now available.

The stress reduction effects of having a pet were elicited by another study, where math problems were given to women whose dogs were present. Their blood pressure and heart rates were better than when they were given the test with a human friend there.

The result of such scientific studies of pets indicates that whether you are the "petter" or the "pettee," touching, petting, playing, and love can have therapeutic and preventive value. Antistress measures can take many different forms, and have turned out to be more important than we have previously realized.

Dolphin swim programs have been used by many people to help them restore health by reducing stress, to come back in touch with the joys of childhood. Pets and animals in general help us remember to play and to stay in the present, essential spiritual values. The therapeutic benefits of their unconditional acceptance provide a great example of the healing power of love. In a culture with rampant family dysfunction, having a pet can help provide the social support essential to health. One survey found that among older Americans who owned pets, 98 percent responded that talking with their animals was the most important social interaction of their day.

Even owning a plant can be beneficial to your health. A Kansas State University study showed that the act of gardening, by its physical and psychological effects, lowers blood pressure and pulse rate. Being surrounded by the green of plants was demonstrated to calm harried Type A personalities and get the couch potato Type B's moving. For more information, contact the American Horticultural Association at 800-634-1603.

Catherine Sneed Marcum developed chronic kidney disease. After reading The Grapes of Wrath, *by John Steinbeck, she thought perhaps working with the soil might help her recover her strength. Gardening became her method of healing, and was so successful, inducing remission, that she went on to found the Farm and Horticultural Program at the San Francisco County Jail, where prisoners learn to be landscape gardeners. Her project, begun with five prisoners, now has a 100-person waiting list. The food they grow goes both to the prison and to the ill, elderly, and homeless, providing a sense of restored community connection, important for health.*

"I use gardening as a metaphor. Because it is an organic garden, I am able to say, 'Well, we could take this chemical here and spray it on this stuff. But what's it going to do to us? What's it going to do to the other plants? It's just like you. When you shoot up heroin or smoke crack, what does it do to you? What does it do to your family? What does it do to society? It's just the same thing... To see people who we as a society have given up on turn on to life again... that's superstrong stuff. I've had these big bad tough guys say to me, 'Oh, Cathy, this is girls' work. I don't want to do nothing with these plants.' And two weeks later the same macho giant with the tattoos and the tracks down his arm is out there saying, 'Hey, don't step on my babies!'"[44]

You can bring your own plants into the hospital, where they provide, in addition to color and beauty, extra oxygen, and also take away carbon dioxide. Early fears that such plants would spread disease have proved unfounded. Eventually, I am hopeful that all hospital rooms will routinely contain plants, perhaps as part of small healing gardens.

Innermost or Spiritual Connection: Prayer and the Power of Spirit

When you go into a hospital, you see a sign with big red letters:"Emergency." That's me, you say. Every test you take seems to measure the explicit rate at which you are dying. The person who is ill should not be confronted with the evidence of illness on all sides. Nothing is more important when you are sick than reassurance.[45]

Norman Cousins, author

A broken spirit makes one sick.

Proverbs, 17:22

No bird ever flew from its nest without first having faith it could fly.

Traditional proverb

John, a 58-year-old orthopedic surgeon, had little faith in alternative medicine. In excellent health, he loved his work, was happily married, and saw no need to pursue any of these new options. He dismissed anyone who even mentioned therapies other than the standard ones he read about in his medical journals, or learned about at conferences, and refused even to treat patients who wished to try alternatives. However, one day during surgery he found himself in a sudden crisis. He had placed a pin in a patient's broken hip, and it had become lodged in such a way it would neither go farther in, nor could he pull it out. He tried and tried. Nothing happened. The pressure was on: he could not keep the patient under anesthesia much longer without risking worsening consequences, and no other solution presented itself. He took a deep breath, backed up from the surgical table, and asked everyone in the room to pray. He had never prayed before, and was known for his atheistic beliefs. After an astonished period of silence, in which everyone joined him in prayer, he stepped forward, tapped the pin, and it moved into place.

This event changed his life. He began to read all he could about spiritual subjects. After his retirement, he began devoting himself to his own meditative practices, and now conducts seminars on the healing power of spirit.

Why spirituality? Contemplating death encourages us all to look at spiritual issues. We are not just cars. We are going somewhere, and how we find the answers of who we are, and where we are going, affects our health.

We *are* all going to have to deal with death. If we don't know what we are doing here, how can we make any sense of this inevitability? Spiritual seeking offers the experience of another, eternal part of ourselves, which helps us understand what we are accomplishing by being alive. A sense of spirituality connects us to something beyond our limited human selves.

Unless we reintegrate emotional truths and spirituality into our healthcare system, we can become like drifting sailboats without a rudder or an anchor or a destination. Life simply makes little sense, and we are subject to the ups and downs of its surf affecting our immune and cardiovascular systems for the worse. We then face death with frantic denial, and make it a disgrace to die.

However, if we can begin the process of healing the rift between science and spirit, between the emotions and the scalpel, we can all begin to heal, from the inside out. We have a chance to benefit from the beautiful gifts conventional and alternative approaches have to bring, to enrich us all.

Writing this book has been a unique opportunity. I have both learned more respect for surgery, and become more passionate to change the way it treats patients as if their emotions were unimportant.

One of my patients put it this way: "I have told my doctor many times that I would like him to be kind, and other than curt, over the phone, as if his business were more important than mine. He gets angry at any disagreement, and hangs up the phone abruptly, as if my feelings just didn't matter. However, they do matter to me. I want my emotions to be important. I want to be treated kindly and caringly just because I am human."

This is the essence of what I think it means to be spiritual: to be kind. To notice how your actions affect another person, your community, and the planet as a whole. To be aware of their emotions and to act to help and support and encourage them, rather than judge and condemn.

A number of studies have documented the benefits of prayer to assist healing, most astonishingly even when the subject does not know he is being prayed for.[46] As author Larry Dossey, M.D., writes, " . . . I believe that if science can demonstrate the potency of prayer, people who pray are likely to feel empowered and validated in their beliefs as a result." In his book, *Healing Words*, Dr. Dossey notes that research has shown the effects of prayer on the rates of growth of laboratory colonies of yeast and bacteria, the activity of enzymes, and the health of mice, chicks, and humans.[47] In the most stringently designed study of coronary care unit patients randomized into groups prayed for by a home prayer group, those prayed for were one-fifth as likely to need antibiotics, one-third as likely to develop fluid in their lungs, and showed lower morbidity and mortality.[48] In another study, a variety of subjects were able to influence the physiology of another subject at a distance by the method of first developing a calming or activating feeling in themselves, then imaging it transferred to the unaware distant subject.[49]

Further studies are needed to investigate the implications of this preliminary research. According to your faith, however, you may want to include prayer in your healing program, and enlist others to pray on your behalf.

Diet

I knew *all* of the secret places underneath the dining room table. Most were already filled, but even then I could often cram a bit more Brussels sprouts or prunes into them. If my mother got distracted away from the table long enough, I could make a run for the garbage can, hide the offending food underneath a few layers, and hope for the best.

In the last decades, the emerging science of human nutrition has shifted and grown by bounds, leaps, and curlicues. The wisdoms of many of my parents' insistences have been set aside, but it looks as if, especially in the case of vegetables, about some things they were right. Though I am still entangled in the long process of making peace with some of the battalions of obnoxious vegetables and fruits of my childhood, as a physician, I see more and more that the Hippocratic injunction, "Let food be your medicine" is leading to new fields—often dark, green, and leafy—of medical research and health maintenance.

Food choices help determine our risks for heart disease, cancer, osteoporosis, migraines, and a smorgasbord of other physical complaints. Some foods are especially detrimental, while others seem to offer protection and even therapeutic benefit once an illness has developed.

The Good News

I am the kind of person who always likes to hear the good news first. Maybe it's because I think it can brace me up for the bad news, or that first impressions tend to last a tad longer. I always did save the yukky foods for last.

The good news in foods is that more and more substitutes are available for detrimental items. Some old favorites like oatmeal have achieved a new status, with increasingly interesting ways emerging to prepare and present dietary items that my mother never knew

about, which place the more painful medicinal aspects in the background.

"We dig our graves with our teeth," goes an old saying. What kind of diet should you be following in order to reduce your chances of having to undergo surgery, or help you recover if you need an operation? In general, I recommend the scientifically well-researched approach of Dr. Dean Ornish. Many researchers have concluded that enough data exist to support his suggestions, as follows.

In general, a high-fiber, low-fat, whole foods vegetarian diet is the diet associated with your least risk for surgical problems, and your best potential for healing. Years of scientific investigation support this conclusion. For example, this diet relieves complaints that often lead to surgery, such as those of hiatal hernia and hemorrhoids, especially if these dietary habits are begun early. Circulatory disorders such as coronary heart disease and varicose veins, as well as kidney disease, have been well documented to be helped simply by this diet. Evidence suggests that one-third to one-half of cancer deaths in the United States are due to dietary factors, and another third due to smoking. If you don't smoke, dietary choices that include a high proportion of plant foods and eliminate meat, full-fat dairy, and other high-fat foods, along with daily exercise, are the most important things you can do to reduce your cancer risk.

If your surgical problem is not an emergency, you may want to pursue a trial of dietary change as an alternative treatment before you sign on for an operation. Specific dietary therapies have been used to treat many individual surgical conditions with much success, each of which is discussed in this book under the heading of your particular disorder. Following are the overall guidelines.

Fiber

Much documentation suggests that a high-fiber diet is essential for the health of the colon, as well as other parts of the body, and may prevent or assist in treatment of the following diseases that commonly require surgery: appendicitis; colitis; diverticulosis and diverticulitis; colon, breast, and prostate cancer; hemorrhoids; varicose veins; gallstones; diabetes; coronary artery disease; benign hypertrophy of the prostate; and hernias. About *20 to 40 grams* of dietary fiber per day are considered optimum. The average American takes in only 5 grams. As a result, we are one of the most constipated countries in the world.

Just adding bran cereal to a diet low in fiber may not provide adequate protection. Count the number of bowel movements you have per day; *two to three movements,* for a total of a pound to a pound and a half of stool per day, are now considered optimum. If you are not in this category, you may not be getting adequate fiber to keep your bowels safe from disease. Eliminate low-fiber foods, such as white bread and refined sugar, and replace them with whole grains and fresh fruits and vegetables. Follow the menus on page 70 to make certain your intake of high-fiber foods is sufficient.

Fats

Fats in the diet, especially those from animal sources, when taken in excess, have now, in many studies, been correlated with both heart disease and cancers of the breast, prostate, colon, rectum, uterus, ovary, skin, pancreas, and liver. Saturated fats and total fat content are most often implicated, but total amount of fat taken in per day is probably the most important consideration.

Most Americans eat from 30 to 50 percent of their calories from fat. The current National Cholesterol Education Project recommends Step I (30%) or Step II (24%) diets, depending on cholesterol levels. However, to prevent and treat disease, Dr. Dean Ornish believes the ideal number to be 10 to 20 percent. You can best achieve this by eliminating red meats and poultry, eliminating or rarely eating seafood or fish, replacing full-fat cheese and butter with small amounts of nonfat dairy, and instead using sources of protein not linked to fats, such as beans, lentils, green beans, green peas, dal (a small, quick-cooking Indian lentil), soy products such as soy cheese (tofu), and bean sprouts, along with whole grains, fruits, and vegetables.

Essential fatty acids consist of two types: omega-3 (from the leaves of plants, seeds, eggs, and cold-water fishes) and omega-6 (found in meat, chicken, dairy, and vegetable oils). We help avert disease when we consume more threes than sixes, which acts to reduce inflammation and promote optimum circulation. You can best obtain what you need of both from low-fat vegetarian sources, such as green leafy vegetables, flaxseeds, seaweed, algae, and soybeans. Since flaxseed oil can quickly become rancid, grinding your own flaxseeds is safest; you can take 2 tablespoons per day.

It is important to note that you do not need to eat fish to obtain an optimum ratio of omega-3 to omega-6 fatty acids. After more than twenty years of research, no lack of these two fatty acids has shown up in those who follow the Dr. Dean Ornish program. The lower intake of omega-6s from a vegetarian diet means that you do not require as large amounts of omega-3s in your diet, since it is the ratio of these that is felt to contribute to the deficiency of omega-3s and to the onset of disease. If you are not able or do not choose to follow a vegetarian diet, however, you can add cold-water fish to your diet, in order to obtain extra omega-3s, in at least three servings per week, to obtain a healthy ratio.

Make certain also to avoid trans-fatty acids, listed as "partially hydrogenated" oils, since these man-made substances have been linked to increased free radical damage, and they raise the "bad cholesterol" LDL levels while lowering "good cholesterol," HDL. Cook only with small amounts of olive oil or canola oil, since these monounsaturated oils do not contribute to such free radical damage.

With some modifications, the type of low-fat diet I am recommending is also ideal post-surgically. In healing from an operation, excess fats in the diet, once they reach the blood, act to interfere with the flow of blood through your capillaries, and slow down your circulation of lymph, as discussed in Dr. Gerald Lemole's book, *The Healing Diet*. You will need extra calories and protein for recovery; use the Superdrinks listed below, and take numerous small meals and snacks of high-protein, low-fat foods, such as lentils and beans, to provide for these special needs. Take Beano to prevent gas formation.

Proteins

Proteins from animal sources have been associated with cancers of the breast, colon, prostate, kidney, pancreas, and uterus. Protein from vegetable sources has not been found to correlate with these cancers. The particular ratio of amino acids in animal foods, compared to that of vegetables, when presented to the glands, such as the breast or prostate, creates altered hormone output, which in turn, is felt to account for the increased cancer rate. An excess intake of protein has also been correlated with chronic kidney disease. In any case, I recommend shifting to a largely vegetable-based diet to avoid these important risk associations. The best nonanimal sources of protein include peas, beans, green beans, and soy products.

While 35 to 50 grams of protein per day are adequate for most people, very active persons and pregnant women may need as much as 100 grams per day. Recovery from surgery also requires extra protein, in order to achieve repair, so for some time after your surgery, eat 100 grams per day. Eat at least five small meals of protein per day for the first six weeks; you can use the recipes for the Superdrinks given below to achieve this.

Nonfat dairy products may be taken in small amounts, a cup per day. If you choose to avoid dairy products altogether, make certain to take a vitamin B_{12} supplement. Frozen yogurt does not give the digestive benefits of acidophilus-containing yogurt, and often contains so much refined or artificial sweetener it can't be considered a health food, as elaborated below.

Refined Sugar

Regular ingestion of refined sugar has been associated with the development of some cancers, as well as with the onset of diabetes. A 60 percent higher refined sugar intake was found in women who developed cancer of the breast.[50] Diabetics have more vascular and circulatory problems requiring surgery. Even as little as one tablespoon of refined sugar has been found to interfere with white cell function, thereby sabotaging the immune surveillance system that protects us against the multiplication of cancer cells.

Vitamins and Minerals

Vitamins A, B, C, and E in the diet are associated with a decreased risk of some cancers.[51] The protection derived from a diet high in fruits and vegetables is due not only to the high-fiber, low-fat, favorable type of protein content, but also to the higher content of vitamins A and C. Diets high in these vitamins have been found to protect populations from some cancers, even if they have other cancer-inducing behaviors such as smoking or alcohol use. Whether taking these vitamins by themselves as pills will prove as protective as eating foods rich in them remains to be seen. Some early studies have shown that taking a tablet a day of beta-carotene (a precursor to vitamin A) does give some benefit, while other research has come to the opposite conclusion. Eating the actual vegetables themselves may give the best protection. Make certain, then, that you eat three to five servings of fresh fruits and vegetables every day for their vitamin content as well as their fiber, low-fat, and optimum protein content.

The antioxidant vitamins, especially C and E, may help reduce your risk of heart disease by inactivating free radicals, the harmful by-products produced when the body breaks down oxygen. Free radicals can interact with some dietary fats to produce compounds that clog arteries and injure the cells that line the heart and arteries.[52]

Areas of the United States with soil and water content low in the mineral selenium have higher levels of leukemia and gastrointestinal, genitourinary, breast, skin, and lung cancers. Whether artificially adding this nutrient to the diet will decrease the cancer incidence is as yet unknown. However, at this point, it seems prudent to add a moderate amount of selenium to your vitamin program, as indicated below.

Whenever specific vitamins have been shown effective in alternative treatment of individual surgical illnesses, I have included that information in the individual chapters of this book.

Phytochemicals

Phytochemicals are natural constituents of plants and fruits that provide particular benefits to your immune system and hormone levels. For example, lycopene, a carotenoid, found in tomatoes, pink grapefruits, and watermelons, is a powerful antioxidant, with proven ability to help prevent prostate cancer. More than a hundred phytochemicals have been differentiated and implicated in helping prevent disease. The best way to assure adequate intake is to frequently include berries, citrus fruits, tomatoes, cruciferous and dark green leafy vegetables, whole grains, seeds, and beans in your diet, along with onions, garlic, and cayenne pepper. Specific phytochemicals will be discussed in the section of this book relating to your particular disease.

Cigarettes, Alcohol, and Caffeine

Out of all the people I knew in medical school, he stands out. Eddie Silver. It's significant, since we spent very little time together; his girlfriend was the roommate of one of my friends. But I had learned how to chain-smoke, as an antidote to the daily stress-press, and from across a smoke-filled room, he was watching me closely. He came over, put his hand on my arm, looked me in the eyes, and said very sincerely, "What's a beautiful person like you doing smoking?"

No one was telling me anything like that. At the most, they would shake their fingers at me, telling me not to smoke, and I would just smoke *more*. I didn't quit right away, but his message—that I was valuable, and it was worth taking care of myself—got through. What most inspires us to change bad habits is love and caring. I quit a month later, never to go back.

Cigarettes, alcohol, and even coffee and tea are all drugs correlated with increased rates of diseases that might necessitate surgery.

Some estimates have found that *from a third to a half of all illness in this country could be prevented if everyone stopped smoking*. Cigarette smoking, of course, causes 85 to 95 percent of all lung cancers, but you may not be aware that it induces many other cancers: stomach, mouth, esophagus, larynx, pancreas, colon, and bladder cancers. If you do smoke, please see the section on quitting, at the end of this chapter.

Alcohol use is particularly associated with cancers of the mouth, esophagus, stomach, and liver, especially when taken in conjunction with cigarettes. Moderate drinking, of a glass of wine or one ounce of alcohol per day, may protect against heart disease, as shown in some studies, perhaps due to changes in fat metabolism or to its relaxation effects, but even a small amount increases womens' risk for breast cancer. Persons who use relaxation techniques and eat a low-fat diet may be able to protect themselves without the potentially dangerous side effects of alcohol use; further research on this point is needed.

Caffeine is a very socially accepted *drug*. Coffee increases insulin secretion, making your blood sugar become elevated, then depressed, and encouraging your body to store calories as fat. Our national coffeehouse fasci-

nation may thus help explain our accelerated obesity levels. In addition, it is associated with elevated amounts of cortisol, which interfere with your immune system functioning. Coffee use, especially if it is in excess of three cups per day, may increase your risk for cancers of the prostate, bladder, kidney, and possibly pancreas, although, since scientific studies are contradictory, the latter remains controversial. Coffee may also predispose a person to ulcers. Black tea and coffee increase the rates of fibrocystic disease of the breast, which in turn may elevate your risk for cancer of the breast three- to fivefold, and also make it more likely you would need a breast biopsy to analyze these lumps for cancer.

Decaffeinated coffee also contains significant amounts of caffeine: a cup of regular coffee or tea has 80 mg of caffeine; decaf may have up to 30 mg. Caffeine use has also been shown to be strongly associated with rectal disease, and a 27 percent increase in infertility has been found in women drinking three or more cups per day. Black tea intake correlates with cancers of the lip, tongue, esophagus, and stomach, as well as that of the bladder; adding milk to tea seems to lower this risk. Our typical soft drinks have several problems: caffeine, phosphates (which cause osteoporosis), and either refined sugar, with its bad effects, or aspartame, which lowers serotonin levels in the brain (the hormone associated with tranquillity).

Green tea intake has been associated with a reduced risk for cancer, though these studies are preliminary, and such reduction may be due to other factors. Green tea does contain high levels of antioxidants, and possible tumor growth–inhibiting factors. However, even the decaffeinated versions contain some caffeine, so you may feel better obtaining your antioxidants from other sources, such as berries. If you do drink green tea, it is best to choose the decaffeinated type.

Your most optimum avenue, in terms of healthy drinks, is probably to try to find an herb tea you can use as a hot-drink substitute. The spicy ones work best; see the substitute list, later in this chapter.

Choosing Whole Foods

So what *is* best to eat and drink? I believe that the answer is really relatively simple, though it may not be easy at first. The way the food appears in nature is the way to eat it; a diet similar to what our closest genetic relatives, the chimps, gorillas, and apes eat. The body doesn't *need* animal protein or fats; a diet based on these foods does not confer any advantages and does not make us stronger—the strongest animal is the elephant, a total vegetarian, and apes are quite healthy and strong on an almost universally vegetarian diet. Some anthropological data supports the finding that the first human beings were not meat-eating hunter-gatherers, but fruit and nut eaters like our chimp and gorilla cousins.[53]

Since 55 percent of Americans are now overweight, everyone is looking for a quick fix. The Atkins and Zone approaches sound good at first, and they may help with short-term weight loss by restriction of calories, but since no long-term studies have shown either efficacy or safety, these methods are un-proven, and most likely dangerous. We do know that a high intake of fats is associated with heart disease and many cancers, so I would recommend you follow the program given in Dr. Ornish's *Eat More, Weigh Less* if you are battling the bulge.

Whether or not you are trying to lose weight, choose the foods you eat each day from these new "four food groups":

1. Whole fresh fruit, three to five servings.
2. Whole fresh vegetables, three to five servings.
3. Whole fresh grains such as brown rice, whole-grain pasta, and potatoes, one to three servings.
4. Peas, beans, lentils, dal, tofu, nonfat dairy products, one to three servings.

These foods can be combined in a variety of ways to create daily menus that are not only healthy, but tasty. Use the following menu as a template:

Breakfast—Fresh whole fruit; whole-grain cereal (without added sugar or honey—use cinnamon instead); whole-grain or Essene bread (made from sprouts); and scrambled tofu.

Lunch—Raw vegetable salad and sprouts and fat-free, sugar-free dressing; fat-free soup such as pea, bean, lentil, or vegetable with tofu; and whole-grain or Essene bread, whole-grain pasta, or potatoes.

Dinner—Three to four steamed fresh vegetables; whole grain such as brown rice; and entrée made from tofu, peas, beans, lentils, hummus, or tempeh.

Snacks—Any fresh fruits or vegetables; whole-grain or soy products; popcorn; rice cakes; or frozen fat-free, sugar-free desserts.

When planning your meals, remember to avoid red meat, poultry, fish, eggs, dairy products, sugar, alcohol, honey, coffee, tea, and soft drinks (except for sodium-free sparkling water). If you wish, try the following substitutes:

Coffee. Use a coffee-like grain beverage, many of which even look like brewed coffee. These products come in several forms, including tea bags and crystals.

Tea. In place of regular tea, try any herbal tea.

Meat. Use textured soy protein, also known as textured vegetable protein (TVP), tofu to make "meat loaf," chili, spaghetti sauce, and other main dishes.

Eggs. Try scrambled tofu, or low-fat yogurt or cottage cheese.

Dairy. Use soy milk to replace cow's milk and tofu to replace cheese. You can also try making a "milk" for cereal or shakes by blending a banana until liquified.

Alcohol. The best substitutes are mineral water with lime and tomato juice. Malt brews and wines are available without alcohol, but should not be used by anyone sensitive to yeast.

Unfortunately, there are no really good substitutes for sugar that are also good for you. Aspartame (NutraSweet, Equal) may be used in moderation, but regular intake can lower brain serotonin levels. You can use fresh well-ripened fruit to satisfy the urge for something sweet, and put fruit into recipes that call for sugar. The sweet spices cinnamon, cardamom, coriander, anise, fennel, and licorice root can be used for cooking and in tea. You *do* get used to this with time, and most people feel much better physically and mentally when they eliminate sugar, and they also reduce their risk for diabetes, heart disease, and cancer.

If you are unable or do not choose to stick to the guidelines given above, the next best thing is to follow an Asian-style or Mediterranean diet, eating lots of fresh organically grown fruits, vegetables, and whole grains, and choosing very limited amounts of organically raised free-range animal products in small portions as part of your meals. Fish has half the saturated fat of red meat, and the cold-water fishes—tuna, mackerel, salmon, and sardines—contain the important omega-3 essential fatty acids, which help protect against the effects of harmful fats in your diet. For this approach, consult the books of Andrew Weil, M.D., for details.

Special Nutritional Formulas

By adding certain foods to the basic good diet described above, you may enhance your intake of nutrients to assure your health. You can take the Superdrinks, described below, every few hours, to build your strength during the two weeks before your surgery, and then afterward to help you recover. If your operation must be performed as an emergency, in addition to the vitamin regimen below, you can drink as much of these formulas as tolerated.

Superdrink I

In a blender, combine 1 to 3 bananas (frozen for thicker consistency), 1 tablespoon whole bran, 1 tablespoon raw wheat germ, 1 tablespoon lecithin powder, 1 tablespoon bee pollen, 1 tablespoon nutritional yeast flakes, 1 tablespoon protein powder, 1 tablespoon flaxseed oil, 1 tablespoon powdered multivitamin-mineral formula, and 1 cup ice cubes. Add your favorite fruits for a fruity flavor or carob powder for a chocolatelike flavor, and process until smooth. Add water if necessary.

Superdrink 2

In a juicer, combine one or all of the following to taste: parsley, carrots, celery, beets, wheat grass, green peppers, sprouts, broccoli, and zucchini. Add 1 tablespoon powdered greens (available in health food stores). If desired, add ginger or garlic.

Vitamin and Mineral Supplements for Your Surgery

Even if you do eat a good diet from the new four-food groups, the depletion of soil nutrients as a result of mass farming techniques reduces your intake of necessary vitamins and minerals. In addition, hospital kitchens may use processed food and devitalizing preparation methods, such as boiling or frying, and your state of illness may contribute to decreased absorption of vital elements.

For all of these reasons, vitamin supplements as a treatment for disease, or adding vitamins to your diet before and after surgery, can provide your body with an assured supply of repair materials.

Vitamin C has been shown to improve wound healing and hasten recovery from surgery, and should be taken in higher doses right before and after the operation.[54] Vitamin C has also been documented to have dramatic results in treating hepatitis, especially chronic and recurrent disease; hepatitis is a risk whenever you receive blood or anesthesia.

The mineral zinc is needed for wound repair, and is reduced in persons who eat a refined diet. Calcium and magnesium are required in higher amounts when bone or tissue is damaged.

Take vitamins and other supplements under the supervision of a physician.

Choose a good multivitamin-mineral formula, and add other supplements to obtain the following doses:

Vitamin A 10,000 units daily of oil-based A

Vitamin B-complex 50 mg once daily

Vitamin C 1,000–2,000 mg of the complex 2–3 times daily (reduce if causes digestive gas or diarrhea)

Vitamin D 400 IU once daily

Vitamin E 400 IU D-alpha type, once daily

Essential fatty acids (EFA) 1–3 capsules 3 times daily or 1 tablespoon flaxseed oil

Selenium	200 mcg once daily
Zinc	50 mg once daily
Calcium citrate	1,000 mg once daily
Magnesium	500 mg once daily
Chromium	200 mcg once daily
Copper	2 mg once daily
Iodine	150 mg once daily
Iron	10 mg once daily
Potassium	99 mg once daily
Manganese	2 mg once daily

This program is a general one for you to take for from two weeks before surgery to two weeks after, added to the diet outlined above, along with the Superdrinks as tolerated. Levels should ideally be individually assessed with your physician or holistic practitioner. Whenever you take vitamins, the color of your urine may change, usually to bright yellow.

Added digestive enzymes, one to two multiple tablets per meal, may be helpful in increasing your ability to utilize the nutrients you ingest, and contribute to the healing process. The following nutrients round out a balanced program:

Betaine HCl	330 mg once daily
Pancreatin	60 mg once daily
Pepsin	30 mg once daily
Papain	30 mg once daily

Alternative Healing Methods

A number of alternative systems that act by assisting the body to heal itself have now been shown by initial scientific research to provide benefits within the context of surgical illnesses. Further research is needed, but seems warranted.

These methods, based on differing traditional understandings of how the human body's resources can be utilized in fighting disorders, diverge from conventional Western science's biochemical model. Some, such as acupuncture and osteopathy, are rapidly becoming mainstream.

Following are the most promising and best documented alternative healing methods that may prove especially useful within the context of surgical disease.

Acupuncture and Chinese Medicine

Elsie, a 68-year-old avid gardener, developed chronic arthritis in one knee. She could no longer tend her lush plants and roses, and so became morose, as well as increasingly obese from lack of exercise. Her physician, after an X-ray, told her, "Your knee is just worn out," and suggested knee-replacement surgery. However, with known heart disease, she was a poor candidate for such a long and difficult operation. Despite deep skepticism, she decided to try acupuncture. The results were immediate, and amazing. Not only was her knee free of pain for the first time in years, but both

of her ankles stopped swelling. She was soon once again walking easily, looking and feeling remarkably younger, and back growing her prize roses.

In Chapter 4, acupuncture is discussed as a useful, promising method of anesthesia. Acupuncture, from the Latin *acus*, meaning "needle," is one of many traditional Chinese medical techniques, including dietary change, herbal preparations, manipulation, and massage, as well as qi gong energy balancing, that may prevent complications and promote healing in surgical patients. Traditional Chinese medicine might even be utilized to treat your underlying surgical disease, to help you avoid an operation.

According to traditional Chinese medical theory, the body's vital energy, termed *qi* or *chi*, circulates through specific channels called meridians. In healthy people, the energy flows smoothly, and its various qualities are in balance. Illness or disease occurs when flow is disrupted and/or the qualities of the qi become unbalanced. The same energy flowing through our bodies permeates the universe as well, making us intimately connected to environmental influences.

A uniquely designed Kirlian photography machine is able to photograph the flow of qi in the body. Researchers in Europe have utilized these pictures to identify illness even before clinical symptoms appear. Although still experimental, these investigators have found that even some cancers can be signaled up to six months before they manifest clinically.[55]

In the ancient China of 2,000 or more years ago, practitioners did not have such technical equipment. They relied on other diagnostic techniques, still in use by the Chinese medicinal specialists of today. An acupuncturist feels the pulses on each of your wrists; examines the shape, color, and coating of your tongue; notices the general state of complexion, and the tone of your voice; then asks you questions somewhat different from those of the usual Western medical examination.

Based on the diagnosis resulting from this evaluation, the acupuncturist may insert extremely thin needles—about the width of two human hairs—into specific points on your body's surface to manipulate the qi and thereby restore its balance. Most patients report either no or only very slight discomfort as the needles are inserted. In addition to this insertion, other Chinese medical therapies include "moxabustion," warming the surface of your skin by burning an herb, usually mugwort (*Artemesia vulgaris*), over the acupuncture points, applying suction cups to tight or painful muscles, or employing electrical stimulation.

Chinese herbal medicine has had a long and venerable reputation in the Orient. Many Western pharmaceutical preparations are derived from the vast store of plants, animals, and minerals that make up the Chinese pharmacopoeia. Ren shen (ginseng) is available in most drugstores to improve general energy. Dong quai can relieve menopausal symptoms. Herbs useful in surgical illnesses are discussed in the section on herbs in this chapter, as well as under the specific illnesses.

Although the general Chinese herbs may be helpful, a person trained in Chinese herbal medicine should formulate a specific prescription based on your unique symptoms. This herbal formula may contain from three to fifteen dried whole herbs, which must be soaked before use. Pulverized herbs combined into a granular formula, which do not require preparation, may also be prescribed.

If your surgery is planned because of chronic pain, a trial of acupuncture may help you avoid the operation.[56] It has been found effective in relief of low back pain,[57] and neck pain.[58] Its use may help you avoid a cesarean section, the most common operation performed on American women.[59] Acupuncture and other Chinese medicine modalities have even been documented to treat gallstones.[60] It has been demonstrated to help in stopping smoking and in treating the acute symptoms of drug and alcohol withdrawal.[61] Though further research is needed, there appears to be a promising future for Chinese medicine and acupuncture in the West.

Should you decide to have surgery, acupuncture can help relieve your postoperative pain, without the side effects of drugs, leaving you more alert to practice the other self-healing techniques given in this chapter and that of your specific disease. Healing of incisions has been found to be accelerated.[62] Vomiting, particularly after chemotherapy, can be reduced.[63] The drop in white cell count after chemotherapy can be reversed.[64] I recommend a session with a Chinese medicine specialist both before and after your operation.

Ayurveda

Eight warm, oiled hands were gliding smoothly across my tired muscles, while the cool, fragrant buttermilk tenderly dripped onto my forehead. Ah, I thought, this is certainly a taste of heaven. Just imagine, and it's good for you too.

This rejuvenation treatment, aimed at body, mind, and soul, has been conducted for centuries in India. Hot medicated oils are massaged into the skin by two practitioners on each side of the body, while above a ban-danna placed over your eyebrows, cool oil or buttermilk is poured steadily onto the third eye region. Sessions last an hour, and may be repeated daily for as long as needed.

The oldest medical system in the world is *ayurveda*. It literally translates as the "science of life," or how to live your life in order to maintain your health. Many of its herbs can be of benefit for surgical illnesses, and within the surgical setting.

The first principle of ayurveda is that each of us has certain tendencies of body and mind, and the aim of its recommendations are to help us lead a balanced life, taking these differences into account.

Three constitutional types are recognized, primarily reflecting your tendency of mind. The wind, *vata*, hummingbird-type is associated with the element air, with a tendency for worry and anxiety, a quick mind, many projects, changeability and irregularity, and aversion to cold. The fire, *pitta*, tiger-type is mentally powerful, enterprising, gets angry easily and has a temper, doesn't like heat, and can't go without eating. The earth, *kapha*, elephant-type is physically powerful, stable, sturdy, reflective, with a tendency to overeat.

Treatment begins with recommendations to balance your mental habits. Various herbs and cleansing techniques enhance this aim. Therapy is optimum when recommended by an experienced practitioner, though some herbal remedies may be generally applicable, as noted under individual diseases in this book.

Its role with surgical disorders warrants further investigation. Research has indicated its possible efficacy in treating arthritis, high blood pressure, stress, digestive disorders, cardiac disease, and certain cancers.[65]

Biofeedback

"Maybe you're not measuring the right thing," the anciently wise-appearing, white-bearded swami commented, with a twinkle in his eye.

Some of my colleagues had decided to test my yoga teacher, Swami Satchidananda, by placing electrodes onto his head, and had connected them to an EEG machine. They were looking for more alpha waves, which are associated with the more relaxed, meditative state. When they couldn't document an increased presence of these undulations, they were starting to feel a bit embarrassed. Here's the big swami, and they can't show anything?

But after the swami's wry comment, they shifted their machine to measure theta waves. These are the very slow peaks found just before deep sleep. The monitor showed a predominance of theta, while the yoga master was sitting with his eyes open and talking, something most persons find impossible to accomplish. His mind was remaining as calm as to be almost sleeping, while he was awake!

Research from the prestigious Menninger Foundation was among the first to experiment with the science of biofeedback. They had heard that certain Indian yogis and mystics were able to control some of their physical functions, such as body temperature and blood pressure, which had previously been felt by Western science to be beyond conscious control. Although biochemical and nervous control of blood pressure do not directly depend upon conscious cortical activity, they may both be connected to activity in other parts of the more primitive brain, and linked to conscious activity.

Both in India and again in their own laboratory, the Menninger researchers were able to demonstrate that conscious control of bodily functions was possible. The next step involved hooking subjects to machines that could give them feedback of their various bodily biologic parameters—thus, this method became termed "biofeedback." Biofeedback devices can measure a variety of elements that reflect virtually every disease. Within a few sessions, you can be taught to lower your blood pressure by thinking calm thoughts, redirect blood flow to your hands, treat headaches, relax specific muscles, and change your brain waves.

Thus far, biofeedback has had its main application in the treatment of high blood pressure, migraine headaches, muscle disorders, chronic pain, and in the psychotherapeutic field. One enterprising psychologist hooked himself up to a feedback device measuring anxiety, via skin resistance, and used this in combination with a videotape to find out when *he* was having emotional reactions that he might not have otherwise noticed while he was treating a patient. Six to ten sessions are generally needed to accomplish the training, and you can usually begin to see the results quite quickly, although sometimes it may take six to twelve weeks for the full effect to become apparent.

The applications of biofeedback are potentially vast. You can combine the use of the yogic deep relaxation, followed by visualization methods, and use a biofeedback machine to let you know how you are progressing. You can choose among machines which measure muscle tension, brain wave activity, skin temperature and resistance, blood pressure, heart rate, or respiratory rate.

Even rats, when given rewards, can be taught to adjust their own blood pressure, blood flow to specific areas of their body, stomach acid, and brain waves.[66] They were able to decrease muscle tension, and elevate their peripheral blood flow with EMG (electromyelogram) (muscle tension) and adjust their temperature feedback. Biochemical and nervous control of the mechanism of biofeedback may thus not depend only upon cortical activity, but may be connected to activity in other parts of the brain.

The specific surgical applications of biofeedback have only been investigated in a preliminary way, and this promising technique may eventually become more widely applied. It may help with back pain, gastrointestinal disorders, elevated blood pressure, and sexual dysfunction, as well as help relieve the side effects of surgery, such as insomnia, headaches, and chronic pain.[67] Since biofeedback can successfully lower blood pressure, it can potentially help you avoid heart and circulation disorders that might require surgery.[68] One study showed that 58 percent of patients taught biofeedback were able to come completely off blood pressure medication, with blood pressure 15 mm Hg below baseline; another 35 percent were able to cut their medication requirements in half; only 7 percent exhibited no improvement.[69] Another study showed how successfully biofeedback could be used to rehabilitate musculoskeletal problems.[70] Biofeedback has been shown to help eliminate low back pain.[71]

If you are having an operation, your goals are to decrease anxiety, decrease postoperative pain, and decrease bleeding. Begin training by using any of a number of small devices now available to purchase; those that measure muscle tension or skin resistance tend to be more reliable than those measuring brain wave activity. A temperature trainer is a small, inexpensive device that you can slip on to your finger. When you are anxious, skin temperature tends to drop; a relaxed state will cause it to rise again. Three to five sessions per day are recommended.

Biofeedback may be especially important for you if you have trouble with guided relaxation or visualization, or have difficulty with self-hypnosis. A professional association of biofeedback practitioners is listed at the back of this book to help you locate someone in your area.

Chiropractic and Osteopathy

The band was Three Dog Night, in a reunion concert, and everyone was dancing. We were under a tent in the cool New Mexican night, outside Santa Fe. The theme was Close Encounters, and many of the revelers were dressed as aliens. The musicians were playing alongside periodic surges of mist, while a giant silver remote-controlled spacecraft balloon was propelled around the domed ceiling. More than three dogs were howling that night.

My friends and I were dancing in a circle, and we decided to play limbo. I was soon to discover that you cannot necessarily do at age 50 what is easy at age 25. I won the contest, but as I came up and resumed dancing, I felt a sudden pain in my hip as if I had been shot.

I had dislocated it. Limping embarrassedly back to my seat, I considered my options. I decided to give alternative treatment a try. After locating a good-hearted chiropractor willing to see me at one o'clock in the morning, I took a taxi to his office, and received an adjustment which gently nudged my hip back in place. My relief was instantaneous, and within a week I was back dancing, although with a lot more moderation.

Andrew Taylor Still, a Virginia country doctor, introduced osteopathy in the midnineteenth century, believing that free flow of nu-

trients to accomplish repair work depended upon releasing tension—from old injuries or stress—to achieve optimum function. Iowa grocer and self-taught healer Daniel David Palmer developed chiropractic in the late nineteenth century. He first used his techniques to restore the hearing of a local janitor, and his system has evolved into a staple of alternative medicine, with 20 million Americans seeking such treatment each year. Multiple adaptations of both treatment techniques have followed.

Both of these therapeutic modalities attempt to assist the body to heal itself by altering posture, thus changing circulation and energy flow. The difference in the two techniques is that the chiropractor focuses mainly on the spine, manipulating its vertebrae, while the osteopath uses osteopathic manipulation therapy (OMT) to adjust the soft tissue, muscles, and ligaments as well. Specific modifications include kinesiology muscle testing, cranial-sacral manipulative adjustment (where the neck and sacrum are gently adjusted to move more freely), electrical muscle stimulation, traction, hot and cold packs, ultrasound applications, as well as gentle and more forceful manipulations.

Osteopaths, called D.O.s, also learn conventional Western medicine, and may simply opt to practice with drugs and surgery; only a small percentage of practicing osteopaths currently even use OMT.

Pressure on nerves by dislocation (termed "subluxations" by chiropractic) as a cause for a wide range of diseases found some support when research showed that even 10 millimeters of mercury (mm Hg) of pressure differential (about the same as a light finger touch) on a nerve root created a 50 percent diminishing of the electrical transmission capability of the associated nerve.[72]

These two therapies may offer relief from surgical disorders, particularly if they are treated by such manipulation early in their course. Most responsive to these methods are back and neck problems, menstrual disorders, high blood pressure, and general pain relief. One study found that immune system activity was increased after thoracic spinal adjustment, when compared to pseudo-manipulation and simple soft-tissue touch.[73] Chronic back pain has been well documented to be relieved by chiropractic, in up to 70 percent of patients.[74] Recently, the Medical Research Council in Great Britain recommended chiropractic as more effective than conventional therapies for chronic or severe lower back pain. Tests included in their evaluation of results were "Changes in the score on a pain-disability questionnaire and in the results of tests of straight-leg raising and lumbar flexion." When followed over two years, manipulation for chronic low back pain was found in one study to be more effective than hospital outpatient care using conventional remedies.[75]

Herbs

Suzannah, a 46-year-old surgeon, had to stand on her feet for hours at a time during her long workdays. She began to notice significantly protruding hemorrhoids, which would occasionally itch and bleed. Over-the-counter remedies didn't solve the problem, so she considered surgery. However, she knew it would mean several weeks of painful recovery, time during which she couldn't work, and it might not prevent the problem returning in the future. She decided to try the alternative medicine program given in the chapter on hemorrhoids of this book: she changed her diet to include more fiber, added yoga stretches, especially emphasizing the shoulder stand, which turns the body upside-down. She applied an herbal remedy, calendula ointment, three times a day, to the area. Within a few days, she was free of pain and bleeding, and her hemorrhoids disappeared after a few weeks. More importantly, she felt other significant benefits, including increased energy and better overall bowel function. Her own relief from pain made her a supporter of alternative approaches, and she began to utilize them with her surgical patients.

I have used herbs for years, preferring them as a first line of treatment for many illnesses, because they often address the root cause of the problem—such as boosting your own immunity, rather than simply getting rid of an infecting organism. Partly because of this, they almost always have fewer side effects than standard drug regimens.

Herbs are simply weeds for which we have found a use. If you have ever grown them yourself, or observed them in a garden, you know how hearty they are. When we eat them, or take them in the form of tinctures or tablets, they transfer some of that vital energy in the service of prevention or treatment.

All foods have some druglike effects on the body: they change our physiology. Herbs do this in a more dramatic way, though not as quickly or specifically as drugs themselves. So the line between food, herb, and drug is a blurred continuum.

Comfrey, one of the most helpful herbs in the surgical setting, can be used for any bruise, break, sprain, or other acute injury. It reduces the amount of bruising, swelling, and pain after surgery. Traditionally called "knitbone," and "the bruise plant," it was found by Native Americans to assist in the mending of broken bones. It can also be used to help heal any chronic skin ulcers. In one trial, one-half of a sprained area was treated with comfrey and the other untreated. The side that got the regular treatment of ice, elevation, and an Ace bandage showed marked swelling and bright bruising. The segment which also received the comfrey compress showed minimal bruising and no swelling.[76]

You can prepare a comfrey pack by boiling the leaves for a few minutes, in enough water to create a compress with the consistency of clay, then placing it onto a washcloth. Where possible, apply the leaves directly to the skin over the bruised, sprained, or broken area. Wrap the area in plastic, then cover by a wet-proof heating pad or hot water bottle for an hour. Repeat three to five times daily, or as needed. Although it may provide some assistance, comfrey salve is not as effective as the fresh leaves.

After an operation, in areas away from the incision where no danger of loosening your stitches exists, you may use the comfrey pack or cream to speed healing and prevent the bruising likely with any surgery. Apply two to three times per day, until healing is assured.

Although regular comfrey should not be taken internally, due to rare liver toxicity, a newly formulated composition, called "alkaloid-free comfrey" with the potentially harmful substances removed, can be taken one to two droppersful, three times daily, to take advantage of comfrey's wound healing ability.

Aloe vera is another substance found in some studies to have success in encouraging wound healing. It may help to soothe minor burns, and prevent scaring at your incision site. When ingested, this naturally laxative gel may help heal ulcers or gastritis. Start with only a half-teaspoon; excess may make stools too loose.

Several substances appear to stimulate your own immune system to fight infection more effectively, and help the body's innate antibiotic and antiviral activity: the herbs echinacea, goldenseal, and garlic can be utilized to increase numbers and activity of white cells. Take them as follows:

Garlic: 2 capsules 3 times daily; since this herb also reduces clotting, stop seven days before and after surgery.

Echinacea: Begin dose at 2 capsules or one dropperful 4 times daily a week before surgery, and increase if needed for infection; take for no longer than 3 weeks.

Goldenseal: 1 capsule or dropperful 4 times daily.

Homeopathy

I was slow to come to believe in homeopathy. For years, I had been hearing about its benefits from my patients, but since its mechanism of action is not well understood, and the choice of remedies can be confusing, I was skeptical.

Then my cat got sick. He was a fighter, and had been through a number of subcutaneous infections, which had required intravenous antibiotics and lengthy stays at the veterinary hospital. When he walked in again with a walnut-sized lump under his cheek, I decided to try homeopathy.

As soon as I gave him the remedy, although he had been very alert, he curled up and fell asleep. Right before my very disbelieving eyes, I watched as the abscess slowly disappeared. By morning, it was gone, and he was feeling his mice once again. I knew it wasn't a placebo effect, and I began to take homeopathy more seriously.

I have since used homeopathic remedies with my patients and witnessed their great success for a variety of ailments. I also discovered that many veterinarians now use homeopathy, and it is especially useful when standard treatments have nothing more to offer.

The term "homeopathy" derives from the Greek words for "similar" and "suffering." In the early 1800s, a German physician named Samuel Hahnemann developed a system of healing based on the idea that "like cures like." He identified several hundred substances from the plant, mineral, and animal kingdoms that caused certain symptoms when taken in minute amounts. These preparations were then used to treat patients who suffered from illnesses associated with similar symptoms.

In the United States in the early 1900s, there were twenty-two homeopathic medical schools and over a hundred homeopathic hospitals, and about one in six physicians in this country was a homeopath. Decline in popularity resulted from advances of surgery and drugs combined with strong political pressure from conventional medicine, infighting among homeopaths, and the cultural climate that valued certain scientific theories over empirical healing practices. Difficulty explaining how such minute amounts of substance could have curative effects also contributed to diminished popularity. With medicines generally, the higher the dose, the larger the effect. With homeopathic treatment, the opposite is true: the smaller the dose, the larger the result. Such a system of medication strains our usual medical reasoning.

However, homeopathic principles may now be more logically explained. Symptoms are not simply random responses of the body, but adaptations of the organism to defend and heal itself. Symptoms are thus not indicative of the disease, but they are the response of the body to the underlying disease. By the homeopath's use of substances that create *similar* symptoms to what the person is experiencing, they mimic the body's wisdom in defending itself, and seek to *aid* rather than *suppress* its attempt at healing itself.

The minute amounts of substances that the homeopaths use are thought to trigger your body's own immune system. Studies conducted at the National Institutes of Health in the immunology section have been able to demonstrate that some white cell functions respond to smaller doses rather than larger ones. Numerous laboratory and clinical studies have shown that the "microdoses" do, in fact, have biological action. More research is needed to further understand how and why the small doses work.

Homeopathy has been described by writer Stewart Brand as "medical *aikido*," meaning that this is a medical science that uses the strength of the force (in this case, the disease) coming at it to defend and heal. You may have seen judo or aikido masters use the force of the person coming at them to turn aside an assault. In a similar way, homeopathy uses the symptoms you already have to choose a remedy that will accelerate and exaggerate these symptoms, to help your body correct its problems. Homeopathy is also uniquely holistic because it takes into account both physical and emotional symptoms.

Homeopathy is undergoing an enormous resurgence in popularity, as many physicians have become disillusioned by the less-than-perfect results of traditional Western medical approaches to many diseases and the troublesome side effects of both drugs and surgery. A national organization of homeopathic physicians exists, and much research is being undertaken to further investigate homeopathy's healing potential.

The royal family of England have been enthusiasts for homeopathy for many years; the Queen credits her record of only two weeks of illness in thirty years to this regimen. According to the *New York Times*, visits to British homeopaths are growing at a rate of 39 percent a year.[77] Homeopathic physicians are located in virtually every country in the world, and this system of treatment is particularly popular in France, Germany, Italy, Brazil, Argentina, Nigeria, Pakistan, and India.

If your disease does not require immediate surgical correction, a trial of homeopathy may be worthwhile. The homeopathic literature is replete with cases of individuals for whom surgery was recommended, though not immediately necessary, and in whom the correct remedy eliminated the need for an operation. A wide range of surgical conditions are included, such as heart disease, ulcers, hemorrhoids, cataracts, cysts, and sports injuries. Success in treatment with homeopathy is dependent upon the seriousness of your disease, the strength of your own defenses, and the competence of your homeopath. Homeopaths may be able to effectively treat some individuals with serious illness, but of course acknowledge that surgery is also sometimes necessary.

Homeopathy can also provide great benefit if you must undergo surgery. Arnica is a common medicine, derived from the mountain daisy, given both before and after surgery to help the body deal with the shock of an operation. Calendula is often very helpful when applied externally to the wound, to speed healing and prevent infection. Hypericum (St. John's wort) is used for surgery where nerve tissue is involved. Staphysagria is appropriate for people who have abdominal surgery. Ignatia is chosen when there are feelings of grief or loss. The Bach Flower Remedies, a form of homeopathic preparation, are sometimes helpful in treating different emotional states before and after surgery. You can refer to books detailing how to use homeopathic therapies, but to find an experienced classical practitioner, contact the national center listed in the Resources section at the back of this book. A general program of homeopathic recommendations for preop and postop is given in Chapter 24.

Hypnosis

I watched as the patient slowly drifted into a state of apparent deep peace. I was using hypnosis to help her battle a 40-year cigarette addiction. "Whew," she told me afterward, "I have never felt so peaceful." After a few sessions, her cravings to smoke were gone.

Beyond a party tool, hypnosis is a little-used medical marvel, similar to visualization and imagery practice, that has exhibited enormous potential for healing. The word "hypnosis" literally means "sleep," but it is not a type of sleep. Rather, a focused state of increased central awareness is attained, combined with decreased peripheral awareness. In sleep, both central and peripheral consciousness are diminished. The brain wave patterns for hypnosis and sleep are quite distinct.

All hypnosis is actually self-hypnosis, a process by which you induce the hypnotic state within yourself. You are taught to center your mind, then can use this focus to assist your body's own ability to heal itself. In several studies with blood flow, differences in healing rates were seen even after only one session.[78] What separates hypnosis from guided imagery and visualization is the use of specific suggestions. These two avenues are also more effective when a trancelike hypnotic state is first obtained, through an instructor or tape.

It is now generally accepted that we have far greater conscious control over our bodily functions than had previously been believed. Hypnosis research has documented that bleeding can be controlled by attaining an altered state of awareness. Thus, even if the psychic surgeon *is* a fake, your body's own placebo mechanism may help you heal; more investigation is needed before any approach is completely discounted.

In Chapter 4, hypnosis is discussed as an effective anesthetic; even major surgery can be performed with hypnosis as the only anesthetic, with fewer side effects than conventional anesthetics. It can also help you come through surgery, by reducing your postoperative pain, nausea and vomiting; preventing infection; and speeding the healing of your incision. It can even help you avoid some operations, such as for removal of anal warts,[79] surgical treatment of skin infections;[80] and may even play a role in the treatment of cardiovascular disease[81] and cancer,[82] especially when applied early in these illnesses. It has been shown to be effective in the relief of pain in terminal cancer patients.[83] It may also lessen the side effects of chemotherapy, such as nausea and vomiting.[84] For such problems, the hypnotist may use instructions such as "Imagine yourself on a wonderful vacation in San Francisco."

Hypnosis gives patients a sense of self-mastery, which is very important during a time of illness, and especially helpful with children. It is especially successful in helping people quit smoking: in one study, one year later 78 percent were still nonsmokers, and their average weight gain was only 3.5 pounds.[85]

How does hypnosis work? Contrary to popular myths, you cannot be hypnotized against your will. In fact, strong-willed subjects tend to be less fearful and able to concentrate their minds in such a way as to achieve better results. Hypnosis seems to act through central mechanisms in the brain. A quick screening test, to see if you can easily be hypnotized, is called the Hypnotic Induction Profile. While keeping your head level, you look up with your eyes. If you can close your eyelids while you are still looking up, you are judged a good candidate; this maneuver is termed the "eyeroll."

The remarkable extent of the body's ability to control all aspects of its function was revealed in a study of hypnosis in a dental setting. The patient was asked, under the influence of hypnosis, to stop bleeding from the socket from which a tooth had been pulled. The bleeding stopped. Then the patient was asked to allow the blood to fill the socket half full. The socket filled halfway.[86] How did the body know that the socket was half filled? We probably have more subtle feedback from various points in our body back to our brain's central control than has previously been imagined. Hypnosis seems to be especially able to affect blood vessels, clotting, and other aspects of wound healing.

You can practice self-hypnosis in its simplest form after you have relaxed via the deep relaxation technique, by consciously suggesting and picturing the desired result to your quieted mind. Persons who have a hard time seeing pictures, as in visualization, can repeat words. You can also find a trained hypnotherapist, through the professional association listed in the Resources section at the back of this book.

Magnet Therapy

The hot flashes were driving me crazy. In jest, they may be called "power surges," but in reality I found that darn uncomfortable. I decided to try taping small magnets to the middle of the bottom of my foot, right where the central small indentation is when you curl up your toes. This is the adrenal point in Chinese medicine; they believe menopausal symptoms are a sign of adrenal insufficiency.

Immediately, I felt relief. No other herb or homeopathic remedy had given such instant help. I then followed the other aspects of treatment for a natural menopause, and felt better than I had beforehand.

We say someone has a "magnetic personality" when they are radiant with good health and vitality. The use of magnets to prevent and treat illness has only recently come under scientific scrutiny, and results are quite promising. Problems such as arthritis and back pain seem to respond especially well. A number of hospitals, especially in the Midwest, have electromagnetic machines for use with patients, and they have been shown to accelerate postsurgical incision healing by two days, improve blood flow, and prevent infection.[87]

Jeffrey H. Lipsky, Vice President of International Medical Electronics, Ltd., reports the successful use of the Magnatherm type of short-wave electromagnetic machine in 71,000 postsurgical patients, to improve surgical outcome and reduce scarring. Some machines have even been placed right in the recovery rooms, and therapy begun there. Magnet therapy has been extensively used for hip replacement and knee surgeries, is especially helpful in treating diabetic ulcers, and has been found to improve joint function in arthritic disease.[88]

Applications of magnets, which presumes inadequate circulation of nutrients as one of the root causes of the body's inability to provide adequate repair, are varied, but research is still in its early stages. Some practitioners suggest simply taping a small magnet over the area of your dysfunction or incision.

Many athletes swear by magnets, to reduce pain and swelling after injury, and to promote optimum muscle function. I have witnessed disorders such as carpal tunnel syndrome and toothache, as well as chronic infections, respond well to their application. Further inquiry seems especially indicated, since the potential range of use is unexplored and the presence of harmful side effects has not yet been disproved.

Fasting

We all watched Oprah Winfrey try to lose weight simply by fasting, then gain it all back again (plus more) when she once again commenced eating. Certainly, fasting does not work for weight control, but it does have other benefits which make it an important preventive and therapeutic tool for everyone to adopt.

Fasting could have gained its name from the fast effect it can have. Indeed, in repeated laboratory experiments, animals that fast regularly live longer, have fewer illnesses, and maintain more competent immune systems.[89]

Animals naturally fast when they are ill. Sometimes we hear the adage, feed a cold starve a fever. Actually, history distorted this phrase; it started out, "*If you feed a cold, then you will have to starve the fever.*" In other words, the ancients knew that if you ate when you were sick with a cold, you would become *so* ill you would develop the complication of a fever, and then you would *have* to fast.

Why is fasting so beneficial? We Westerners have a hard time understanding its merits. It would seem that when you are in trouble, you would be needing extra nutrients. However, the process of digestion itself requires energy and blood supply. If you are eating, some of the blood and bodily resources must be diverted to digestion. If you fast, all of your body's attention can be focused upon the illness.

Liquids such as soup broth can give you the essential nutrients you need to function on a daily basis. Your body usually has two weeks of protein stores in the liver, after which time it starts breaking down its own muscles to obtain nutrients; this is accelerated with chronically ill and postsurgical patients, who break down proteins much sooner. Therefore, though a regular fasting program may be able to prevent or treat surgical disease, all fasting should be undertaken only under your doctor's supervision.

Dr. Roy Walford of University of California at Los Angeles, whose pioneering studies in animals demonstrated the benefits of fasting, suggests one to two days per week of "undereating" if you don't wish to fast completely. On that day you can simply take a large bowl of soup broth, or several glasses of diluted fruit juices or vegetable juices, three or four times per day, supplemented by eight glasses of water.

A fasting soup you can easily make is to take zucchini and green beans: chop them, boil in a large pot of water, blend, and then take as much as you wish during the day, at least three to four servings. Once a month, a three-day fast on this broth helps further stimulate your immune mechanism. Twice a year,

every six months or so, a longer fast of seven to ten days is a useful maintenance plan. Other fasting options include the superdrinks, described above, and watermelon or other fresh fruit.

Arthritis and other autoimmune and allergic diseases respond especially well to supervised fasting, particularly if you are sensitive to foods such as wheat, dairy, or refined sugars. Difficult problems may not respond to simple fasting, and prolonged fasting without obvious results may be harmful. Therefore, close medical supervision is always extremely important.

If your surgery is not an emergency, fasting for a few days several weeks before elective surgery can be undertaken in order to boost your immune function, which is normally depressed by surgery, and may serve to help you avoid surgical complications. A fast boosts immunity for several weeks.[90] Particularly true for infectious and colon problems, such fasting stimulates your immune system so that it will better resist infection. However, as noted, due to the fluid and nutrition demands of surgery, fasting is not recommended right before or after surgery. Protein is very important for wound healing. The especially nutritious drinks outlined earlier in this chapter can help provide those needs before and after an operation, along with extra nutrients available for healing. Blood tests can help monitor your nutrient status.

Quitting Smoking

If you smoke, the most important action you can take to reduce your chances of surgery or improve your outcome should you need an operation is to quit.

Half of all illness in the United States could be eliminated if everyone stopped smoking. Some surgeons now even refuse to operate on smokers, since their outcomes are so much worse. Alternative medicine offers you much help to quit and stay off cigarettes for good. Here are some tricks to help you quit:

- **Decide to Just Do It** The first step in quitting is deciding to do it. Making up your mind to do it *now* is often all it really takes to be successful. Focusing on the bad effects of even one cigarette—which interferes with your circulation enough to lower the skin temperature in your hands and feet by two degrees—may help get you motivated.

- **Practice Daily Yoga** Permanently quitting smoking, like losing weight and keeping it off, is often preceded by many unsuccessful skirmishes. This addiction may have its psychological roots in oral or other nourishment issues, and let's admit it, it's useful as a specific stress-reducing habit. Therefore, you need to have a substitute stress-management program in place, to achieve the relaxation represented by the magic of the cigarette break.

  That's the role of your daily yoga practice. Many studies have documented the remarkable effectiveness of these techniques in helping people permanently stop smoking, and they have the side benefit of improving the quality of your life as well.

- **Practice Visualization** Circling in red the exact date on the calendar I quit seemed to help me. I had learned to be a chainsmoker in medical school, one of many unhealthy habits acquired with that stressful hazing process, and finally I decided I had my health in one hand and my cigarettes in the other—and I couldn't have both. Which, after all, was more important? So I circled a date: February 1, 1970—I didn't quite make my New Year's Resolution—and every time I was tempted to begin smoking *again*, I saw that calendar in my mind, and said to myself, "No. That's It. Never again."

- **Use Massage and Water Therapy** Smokeenders retreats have found relaxation in a bathtub or hot tub to be especially soothing. After such weekends at one spa, one of the staff told me that they found it necessary to drain the Jacuzzi and scrub it down, because it turns yellow from all the nicotine sweated out from the bodies of the smokers!

- **Use Hypnosis and Acupuncture** These modalities have quite high success rates, though you may need more than one or two sessions.

- **Use Chewing Gum and Toothpicks** Smoking is orally satisfying. Gum and flavored toothpicks helped me, and still do.

- **Use Herbal Remedies** The herbs chamomile, valerian, lobelia, and lavender oil can provide soothing relief to the jagged feelings associated with withdrawal.

- **Use Medications** A nicotine patch or nicotine gum may be necessary. The blood pressure drug Clonidine, administered through a patch, binds with receptor sites in the brain that make you crave nicotine, though its use may lower your blood pressure enough to make you feel weak.

Getting a Good Night's Sleep

(O) sleep, O gentle sleep,
Nature's soft nurse . . .

Shakespeare

You plump the pillow. You try a new position. You sigh. You get up for yet another trip to the bathroom. You come back and toss for hours. Once blissfully unconscious at last, you suddenly find yourself wide awake at 3 or 4 A.M., exhausted but unable to go back to sleep.

A good night's sleep when you are faced with the possibility of surgery, and especially if you are in the hospital, can be a daunting challenge. Getting adequate, uninterrupted, and blissful sleep is especially important for healing from any illness, and critically so before and after an operation. However, you may discover "Nature's Nurse" hauntingly impossible to find during this crucial time.

Alternative approaches have much to offer in the realm of a great sleep, with fewer side effects than sleeping pills.

Here is a summary of what you can use at home or in the hospital:

- **Practice Deep Relaxation** This yoga exercise can quickly and very effectively put you into deep sleep. Follow the instructions given earlier in this chapter, and then tell your mind just to drift off into all the sleep you need.
- **Avoid Caffeine, Alcohol, Sugar, and Other Drugs** As little as one cup of coffee or tea, even when decaffeinated, can affect sleep patterns. See above for healthy substitutes.
- **Take a Hot Bath** The Old Wives were right about this one. Drawing your blood supply to the skin carries it away from the brain, making you sleepy. You can add Epsom salts to the bath to provide the relaxation benefits of magnesium, and use aromatherapy oils as well.
- **Take Minerals** Oral calcium-magnesium—1,000 milligrams and 500 milligrams, respectively—encourages muscle relaxation. Even higher levels of an additional magnesium, 250 to 500 milligrams, may be needed to achieve full muscular relaxation.
- **Have Hot Milk and a Banana** Hot milk has been called a "liquid lullaby," and there are biochemical reasons for its place in the hearts of our grandmothers. It contains naturally occurring tryptophan, a precursor to the relaxing hormone serotonin, making it a natural tranquilizer and antidepressant, a natural Prozac. (Prozac acts by increasing serotonin levels in the brain.) It also delivers muscle-relaxing calcium, and increases natural brain opiates via elevation of the hormone cholecystokinin. Its warmth helps your muscles relax, and its ingestion shifts blood supply from the brain to the stomach, making you sleepier. If you prefer, you can use soy milk.

  Bananas contain trace amounts of tryptophan, as well as potassium, a mineral necessary to increase available levels of calcium for muscle relaxation. They also contain high levels of pectin, a type of fiber now shown to reduce cholesterol levels, so you can accomplish two goals at once: lower your cholesterol while you sleep!
- **Use Herbs and Aromatherapy** Chamomile, hops, valerian, lobelia, and catnip all are caffeine-free relaxant teas that can be taken before bed to help you sleep. A

study of chamomile tea, reported in the *Journal of Clinical Pharmacology*, demonstrated "A striking hypnotic (sleep-inducing) action of the tea as noted in ten of twelve patients."

This research was conducted on cardiac catheterization patients, and the investigator concluded that, "It is most unusual for patients undergoing cardiac catheterization to fall asleep. The anxiety produced by this procedure as well as the pain associated with cardiac catheterizations all but preclude sleep. Thus, the fact that ten out of twelve patients fell into a deep slumber shortly after drinking chamomile tea is all the more striking."

You can use these teas in your bath, or choose any other aroma soothing to you. Lavender oil classically helps greatly, and can both be put in your bath, or into a "sleep pillow" under your head.

- **Exercise Regularly and Have a Massage** Exercise increases brain opiates and serotonin, contributing to the feelings of general well-being that make it easier for you to sleep at night. Even a small amount of touch can help you relax enough to sleep better.

- **Use Cotton or Flannel Sheets, and Sheepskin** One hundred percent cotton sheets absorb moisture more effectively and cause you to perspire less than synthetic ones, and flannel sheets in winter can be especially cozy. A study published in the *Medical Journal of Australia*, and another conducted at Ohio State University, showed that even normal subjects have a better night's sleep when sheepskin is placed beneath the sheets. Apparently, the softness of the wool distributes pressure across the skin, helping you to relax more, since the trapped air pockets more effectively absorb your perspiration during sleep. You needn't worry about sacrificing a sheep for a night's sleep counting sheep, though, since mattress pads made from sheared wool are now widely available. Carrying your own sheets into the hospital can be a great source of comfort, though you will have to make certain your particular hospital allows this.

- **Use Music** Music can, of course, "soothe the savage" in us, contributing to the relaxation needed for falling asleep. The most effective way, as noted above, may be to begin with relatively rowdy music, then gradually shift to more slow-paced instrumentals. Research has shown that this conditions the nervous system from higher "wired" feelings to a more relaxed state.

- **Lie on Your Left Side** Yoga texts even recommend the best position in which to sleep. Lying on your left side, with your right knee drawn up, opens the ileo-cecal valve between your small and large intestine, to allow for more ease of digestion. This position also keeps your right nostril open, shown to help you stay warm. If you are too warm, or have a fever, you should lie on your right side.

Alternative Approaches Instead of Surgery: Are They Worth It?

Is it worth it to you to adopt some of the alternative medicine approaches and lifestyle changes outlined in the preceding sections? Does this take too much effort? Isn't it simpler to go to the surgeon, have the operation, and just continue on with your life?

These are all legitimate questions! What argues most favorably for alternative methods is that they also *feel good*, and may prevent recurrence or other future diseases. In addition, many people are choosing to exercise more, eat a higher-fiber diet, avoid fat and sugar, not just to prevent disease in the long haul, but because it helps them feel much better in the short run. Even if you are feeling "fine," you may find that once adopting these programs, you feel "finer." Small, chronic aches and pains disappear, vitality increases, and a general sense of well-being and strength is the usual result of this kind of shift to a healthier lifestyle.

What does it take to achieve this benefit? Twenty minutes of yoga in the morning before work and ten to fifteen at night are probably the minimum daily requirements. In the morning you can meditate, do some stretches, deep breathing, and the deep relaxation. In the evening, you can have a short, deep relaxation and meditation just before bed. You can fit in your active exercise such as fast walking, jogging, swimming, or aerobics either in the morning or evening, three to five times per week.

The diet itself may be an easier transition than you at first might expect. You can begin by eliminating red meats and heavy dairy products such as cheese, butter, and eggs. Eat a high-fiber breakfast, choosing a whole grain cereal without sugar, and switch to whole grain bread. Read labels, and replace sugared foods with fresh fruits, fresh steamed vegetables, and whole grains. A food plan such as that suggested earlier in this chapter, or in one of the widely available whole foods cookbooks, should start you on your way.

Physician, Heal Myself

The moment I grabbed the handle of my suitcase from the baggage belt and began to pull, I knew I was in trouble. "Tucson, we have a problem." I'd flown into that city to give a lecture on stress management. "I never go anywhere without my rock collection," I used to joke to my friends; this time when I tried lifting the overstuffed bag, my back rebelled with such ferocity I couldn't keep from letting out a horrified howl that echoed up into the terminal rafters.

When I tried to walk, the pain centered in my lumbar-sacral junction. I reached behind and felt the area, but rather than my normal curvature and spinal processes, a strange board seemed to have inserted itself into my lower back. It was stone-hard, and any movement on my part produced sensations as if ground glass was being moved about inside my spine. If pain is on a scale of 1–10, this felt like an 11.

In Chapter 22, I discuss alternative medicine therapies for back disorders. Fortunately, I was familiar enough with alternatives by then, and had witnessed their results with my patients, that I chose to try them first. With the help of these techniques, I was not only able to give my talk the next day, but I was free of all pain within ten days.

I created my own combined program for recovery. The first thing I did was take the homeopathic arnica, in a high potency; this remedy has been found to relieve the discomfort of any strain or trauma, and in scientific studies has been found effective in reducing even postsurgical pain. Then I took the herb comfrey, in a nontoxic form designed for internal use; this herb also acts to reduce the swelling and bruising associated with any acute injury.

Next, I assumed a yoga pose called the "child" pose, one which reduces stress on the disks, and allows the muscles in the back to relax. I practiced "breathing to" the area of pain, a method used in both yoga and qi gong; and then added meditation and visualization. I also arranged for chiropractic, osteopathic, and Rolfing manipulations.

Cold packs for the first twenty-four hours helped, followed by hydrotherapy in a bathtub and alternating hot and cold compresses. Tucson is the home base of a remarkable form of water yoga, called Aqua-traction, invented by an enthusiastic alternative medicine specialist, Dr. Randy Van Nostrand. For this type of therapy, you enter an extra-warm pool, with a collar around your neck, a small inner tube under your arms, and ankle weights strapped around your ankles, all of which results in your floating longitudinally upright. Hanging on to side bars, you perform a series of modified yoga positions that Dr. Van Nostrand, having suffered from a back injury himself, developed specifically for bad backs. As soon as I was in the water, I began to feel better.

After a few days, I began to gently do the twelve basic yoga postures, given early in this chapter, as comfortably as I could assume; then, as I began to feel even more improved, I focused on the sun salutation, which gives a range-of-motion workout to all parts of the back. Gradually, full flexibility returned, everything was "back in place," and I felt stronger and better than I had in the first place—though now I definitely do try to travel with less hefty luggage.

How long should you try an alternative plan? I have presented the options I feel are appropriate under your individual condition. Obviously for most surgical illnesses, it is usually *not* safe to simply wait and see; you must be monitored by a physician, so that a poten-

tially surgically *curable* disorder does not progress into one that is beyond help. Self-care *should* have its limits, and you need to take advantage of the experience gathered in alternative medicine thus far.

Alternative Approaches in Addition to Surgery

When the best option *is* an operation, you may choose many of these important adjuncts to help it be successful, to recover quickly, and prevent recurrence. Most hospitals are now open to your utilizing alternatives along with your operation. Chapter 24 gives a handy summary of how you can do this, and recommends the most effective choices. Just make certain to explain what you are doing, and why, to the various personnel involved.

SPECIFIC ALTERNATIVE MEDICINE APPROACHES SUMMARY

Prevention

Lifestyle

• Quit smoking.
• Exercise regularly, 1 hour 3–5 times weekly.
• Practice daily yoga.
• Eat a low-fat, high-fiber diet.

Vitamin and Mineral Supplements

• Vitamin A, 10,000 IU daily.
• Vitamin B complex, 50 mg daily.

- Vitamin C complex, 1,000–2,000 mg, 2–3 times daily.
- Vitamin E, D-alpha, 400 IU daily.
- Zinc, 50 mg daily.
- Selenium, 200 mcg daily.
- Calcium citrate, 1,000 mg daily.
- Magnesium citrate, 500 mg daily.
- Chromium, 200 mcg daily.
- Iodine, 150 mg daily.
- Iron (premenopausal women only), 10 mg daily.
- Potassium, 99 mg daily.
- Maganese, 2 mg daily.
- Boron, 750 mcg daily.

Enzyme Supplements

- Betaine, HCL, 330 mg daily.
- Pancreatin, 60 mg daily.
- Pepsin, 30 mg daily.
- Papain, 30 mg daily.

Superdrink #1.
Superdrink #2.
Maintain proper weight.
Practice stress management.
Laughter, play, pets, plants, music, massage, aromatherapy, art, poetry, beauty, color.
Nature cures: water therapy, spa treatments, sunlight, fresh air.
Group support.
Prayer and spiritual approaches.

Treatment

- Follow the preventive guidelines above.
- Herbal remedies: individualized.
- Additional supplements, individualized.
- Homeopathy, individualized.
- Ayurveda.
- Yoga practices specific to your disease.
- Hypnosis.
- Tai chi and qi gong.
- Chiropractic and osteopathic treatment.
- Massage, Rolfing, Reiki, shaitsu, reflexology, the Alexander Technique.
- Acupuncture.
- Biofeedback.
- Magnets.
- Fasting.
- Seek help for psychological problems, or join a support group.
- Visualization specific to your disease.

CHAPTER 3

How to Make a Decision About Surgery

Remedies are beneficial only through correct applications, but they are harmful when applied wrongly. I assert that there is no science where there is neither a right way nor a wrong way, but science consists in the discrimination between different procedures.

Hippocrates

John, a 60-year-old truck driver, had waged a long battle with hemorrhoids. They became increasingly painful and bothersome, despite repeated applications of a myriad of over-the-counter preparations. Finally, he decided to consider surgery. The first surgeon he visited suggested an operation termed a hemorrhoidectomy, which would leave him unable to drive his truck for several weeks. He decided to seek a second opinion. The second surgeon recommended a rubber-band procedure, which could be done in the office. He chose to follow this advice, and was back at work the next day, without pain.

Making an Informed Decision

When you are faced with a decision for yourself, your family, or your friends about whether or not to have an operation, you must first understand that you do have important input, even in the context of a surgical illness. You can empower yourself by becoming aware of the relationship of lifestyle choices to illness, and the most recently developed options within surgery and alternative medicine.

Do you *really* need the operation? In this chapter and the specific chapter discussing your disease, you will find information needed to help you determine if you must have surgery or what alternative therapy you could choose instead. Making an informed choice may save your life. If you do find an operation is necessary, you will learn what to ask for to increase its chances for success and minimize its discomforts. If the operation can be delayed, you will be advised how to get yourself in the best possible condition beforehand, Of course, in an emergency, you may not have time for gathering more than one opinion and preparing for your surgery, but at least you can discuss the issues with your surgeon, and participate in the thinking about which surgical choices are appropriate.

Each section of this book is meant to help you, step-by-step, in making your choice. You may wish to take it to your doctor's office, and ask about the details of your specific disease. A clear and honest communication process can help ensure your return to health. The more you know about your disease, the more you can assist with your healing.

Knowing what to expect can help you prepare and face the results positively. You can alleviate unreasonable fears and vague apprehension, rather than becoming overwhelmed with what happens. The stress management, relaxation, and visualization techniques discussed in Chapter 2 are designed to help you turn events in a positive direction by reducing tension, fear, and anxiety that can interfere with your healing.

Of course, some people prefer not to know about their illness. They would rather think about something else, and leave the decision making to the surgeon. This *is* a choice you can make. However, if you are well informed, you may be able to help your doctor achieve better results. Whichever path you take, this book can give you some helpful tools to make your choices be most successful.

You can simply add alternatives to conventional approaches on your own. Most Americans hate to go to the dentist; it is the number one medical treatment we dislike. What Sandra has discovered is that the discomfort of the anesthesia injection is worse than the pain of the drill. So she has learned to use the yogic techniques of deep relaxation, given on pages 40–42, to become able to withstand the pain, and thereby avoid a full day stuck with a swollen and numb jaw.

Choosing Your Opinions

Surgeons may be at least subconsciously prejudiced in favor of surgery. A few always seem to recommend an operation, no matter what the indication. You must be wary of simply accepting the recommendation of one doctor only. Seek out a second opinion from another physician or surgeon, unassociated with the first. Finally, find someone to give you a third opinion, one from the new field of alternative medicine, before you agree to *any* operation.

Find doctors who explain things in a way you can understand, and who are willing to answer your questions. Sometimes in the midst of illness, especially a surgical emergency, it may seem that there *are* no choices. However, even then you may be able to gain strength and support from a physician in whom you have confidence and with whom you can talk comfortably.

―――――――――――――――

Here is an interesting, though not typical, example of how a remarkable synchronicity determined one patient's choices. One of the lifestyle heart patients of the Dean Ornish Lifestyle program literally fell into the project. Dr. Ornish had decided to run San Francisco's annual Bay-to-Breakers race, a *seven-mile stretch from the eastern bay down to the ocean. About five miles into the distance, William collapsed right in front of Dr. Ornish, who administered CPR, and helped revive him. That he had collapsed right in front of one of the most prominent heart researchers in the world was not lost on this man, a teacher from Seattle, once he was resuscitated. He then had emergency bypass surgery and was operated on by a student he himself had taught in school. What goes around comes around sometimes in the strangest of circumstances! Two weeks later he chose to come to one of the heart disease reversal retreats, to make certain that his disease would not return. Incidentally, even though Dr. Ornish was not able to finish the race, he was given a commendation and an honorary T-shirt, which contestants receive at the end of the race, by the organizers to express their gratitude for his services.*

Choosing Your Surgeon

Most likely, you will be referred to a particular surgeon by your family doctor or another specialist. Your referring provider will have had previous experience with this surgeon and confidence that you are in good hands. Your provider may, indeed, "know best." However, at times, friendships and economic issues may play a role, and after initial investigation you may find that you would rather have a different surgeon. Most providers will be open to your wishes.

Occasionally, all surgeons make mistakes, or have complications arise. Some are due to their own technical incompetence, and others as a result of the nature of any risky venture. How can you find the best surgeon? You can find surgeons in the telephone book and

through the local county medical society, but you should also ask around. Some surgeons are well recognized in their medical community as practicing a very high standard of care. One way to avoid the rare problematic surgeon who operates too often without adequate reasons, or is otherwise less competent, is to find out who your local doctors and nurses themselves use. Relatives and friends may be able to give glowing recommendations based on their own experiences.

Investigate your potential surgeon's training. Make certain he or she is "Board-Certified," which means he or she has passed written and oral examinations of academic competence, conducted by the American Board of Surgery, a peer organization established in 1937. The American College of Surgery is a professional organization of surgeons established in 1913 "to improve the quality of care for the surgery patient." Surgeons who have passed the board exams and practiced for three years and then passed a review of their skills and personal credentials by the American College may use the initials FACS (Fellow American College of Surgeons) after their name. You can look up your surgeon's credentials in The Official American Board of Medical Specialties *Directory of Board Certified Medical Specialists*, available in your local library, or on their website.

It is usually wise to choose a surgeon who has performed a large number of the procedure that you need. If, for example, you must have a thyroid operation, try to find a surgeon who has a special interest in thyroid surgery, rather than one who only does a few of these per year. Gynecologists usually have more experience than other surgeons in operating on the female pelvis, and so forth.

Make sure that you see your potential surgeon(s) well before the time of your operation. Before you finalize your choice, make certain you are very comfortable with the initial interview and exam, as described later in this chapter, and have full confidence in your surgeon's abilities.

The Second Surgical Opinion

Sandra needed to find a dentist; one of her teeth had broken. The first one told her it was impossible to save the tooth, and recommended root canal and a replacement cap. She persisted, and went to find another opinion. This dentist was able to fix the tooth, and she is happily still enjoying the tooth, without further problems.

A second surgical opinion is best sought in a setting different from that of the first, preferably in another city or at another doctors' group or hospital. Many doctors hesitate to show disagreement with their colleagues, so if you do find *any* difference of opinion, it may be significant.

If the opinions you receive turn out to differ, be certain to ask for details of the alternate plans. You can then go back to the first surgeon, if you choose, and once again discuss your options. Most surgeons are quite agreeable to do all this, but if you find one that is not, do not be discouraged. Getting all the facts gives you the best opportunity to enhance your own health and protect yourself from unnecessary risks. For example, a less disfiguring procedure, or an alternate method of performing it, such as with a laparoscope or endoscope, may be discovered by seeking a second surgical opinion.

As noted earlier, in a study of New York City employees, retirees, and their families who had operations recommended and then obtained second opinions, 30 percent of the surgeries were felt to be unnecessary and were not recommended by the second opinion. This program led to improved physician–patient communication, in the event surgery was decided to be necessary, because the act of asking for another opinion clarified the issues and made dialogue easier.[1]

Voluntary second opinion programs are not as successful as those that are mandatory. States that have such mandatory projects for Medicaid and Medicare patients have saved millions of dollars annually. Although one study did show an increased number of surgeries, most research has demonstrated decreases. Dr. Richard Kusserow, while inspector general at the Department of Health and Human Services, estimated that if a second opinion were required for all Medicare patients, 90 million dollars would be saved annually.[2]

Suppose that the two opinions you obtain *do* differ. How do you know who is right, or if they *both* may be correct? The facts in this book should help you decide. In addition, you may use the third opinion of an alternative medicine practitioner to help you choose between the two.

The Alternative Medicine Third Opinion

Sandra was speaking in Sante Fe, and while attending the final party of the conference, dancing to the live music of Three Dog Night. She was doing the limbo, and somehow at age 50, things sometimes don't work like they do at 25. Her years of yoga had maintained her flexibility, and she won the limbo contest, but afterward, jumping up and down on the stretched-out hip, she dislocated it. She felt as if she had been shot in the hip, and hopped awkwardly back to her room.

Such an injury would conventionally be treated by drugs, manual manipulation, then traction and bed rest, with possible hospitalization. Sandra decided to seek alternative methods, and found a sympathetic and generous chiropractor in the yellow pages. She roused him from bed at 1 A.M. and via chiropractic, he moved the hip back into place without anesthesia. She was free enough from pain to fly back to Virginia, where several follow-up treatments by the chiropractor she works with at Integral Health Center, Dr. Michael Sullivan, solved the problem, and she was grateful for the ease of therapy and avoidance of medications and hospital care created by this effective alternative.

A "third opinion" is one from an alternative medicine, "holistically" oriented perspective. Though used in varying contexts, the word "holistic" comes from the Greek word for "whole" and means the doctor is trained to look at the whole picture, including your lifestyle, habits of body and mind, diet and exercise, and the influence of stress and belief on your health.

He or she should be able to tell you if any alternative medicine, dietary, or other lifestyle alterations may be of benefit to you, to assist you in avoiding surgery or making the best of it. This "third opinion" can be used to create a more balanced view, weighing the newest thoughts from the orthodox with the less traditionally accepted avenues. A list of organizations of these doctors is included in the Resources section at the back of this book.

Other Sources of Information

A number of other resources for decision making are also available. Your local library is a good place to begin. You can look up your disease in the medical references there, and read about further details. Especially helpful is the *Index Medicus*, a source list of recent medical journal articles, providing the very latest information. Ask the librarian to help you do a computer literature search. *Medical Self Care*, *American Health*, *New Age Journal*, and *Natural Health* are magazines published to inform readers about medical options and alternatives. Other useful references are listed at the end of this book.

The Internet is a vast source of information. Hundreds of articles can be found by doing a "search" for your disease. If you are not computer-literate, find someone to help you. Many organizations' web addresses are listed in the Resources section at the back of this book.

Questions to Ask at Your Initial Doctor Visits

Interview your first, second, and third opinion doctors systematically during the course of the initial visits. Take the following list along with your own questions, and gather all the facts and answers, before you make your decisions. Take with you a record of all your symptoms, in chronological order. Most doctors welcome a chance for orderly dialogue. Take notes or make a tape recording, so that you don't lose any information you may not have heard or understood during these appointments. It may be useful to keep a journal or a file, with different options, opinions, records of your conversations, and anything else relevant to your condition.

QUESTIONS TO ASK YOUR DOCTOR

1. What is your experience with my disease?
2. Can you explain my disease to me?
3. What is the usual course of my disease without any treatment?
4. Are there any surgical, conventional, or alternative medicine approaches?
5. Exactly what does the proposed surgery involve?
6. What are the possible side effects and risks of surgery and other treatments?
7. What is my prognosis?
8. What can I expect during the recovery period?
9. Will there be any changes in my lifestyle after surgery?
10. What are the anesthesia options, their risks and side effects?
11. Can the operation be done in ambulatory surgery or is hospitalization necessary?
12. What is the best timing for surgery?
13. What are your fees and payment schedule?

I. What Is Your Experience with My Disease?

Ask about your surgeon's experience with your specific disease. Ask how many of the operations that he or she has done, and what the results have been, if known.

2. Can You Explain My Disease to Me?

Begin by asking for an explanation of your disease. How common is it? What caused it? Is there anything you could have done to avoid it, or do now to prevent it from happening again? Have your physician draw a picture of what you have, and what the operation would entail. Make certain you ask for interpretations of any words or procedures you do not understand.

In the case of back pain, for example, just having a positive X-ray showing disk degeneration ("slipped disk") does not necessarily mean you need an operation. One study, discussed in the chapter of this book dealing with back disorders, was conducted in a mall. Two hundred persons were X-rayed at random. Many showed disk degeneration without any back pain at all, while many had back pain with no evidence of disease on an X-ray.

3. What Is the Usual Course of My Disease Without Any Treatment?

Ask for an explanation of the usual course of your disease without any treatment. Is it possible your body will heal itself or symptoms will decrease over time? Does doing nothing now increase your risk for later complications or cancer? See if you can acquire a good understanding of your problem. You can read about the usual course of your disorder in this book, as well as go to the library for further details.

Sandra's own experiences with kidney stones exemplifies how watchful waiting can sometimes help you avoid a procedure that includes side effects and risks. Eighty percent of kidney stones pass on their own eventually, and in her case the addition of acupuncture assisted this process and relieved the pain.

4. Are There any Surgical, Conventional, or Alternative Medicine Approaches?

You will need to know what different types of surgical procedures are possible and available to you. Could a laparoscope or an endoscope—newer tools for operating that minimize scars, postoperative discomfort, and convalescence—be used for this procedure? Are alternatives to the surgery available, either in the form of conventional medical treatment or the newer lifestyle, dietary, and alternative medicine techniques given in this book? Since conventional surgeons and medical doctors are often unfamiliar with all of these options, obtain what information you can from the doctors you interview, then seek out answers to the other questions with your third opinion consultant.

One of Sandra's patients, who had developed breast cancer, was told that her tumor was too large, and her breast too small, for her to qualify for lumpectomy and radiation. She did not seek a second opinion, but underwent a mastectomy. Her doctor also did not explain to her what reconstruction options were available, and she thought that having reconstruction at the time of surgery would somehow make future cancer less easy to detect, which is not true. It was only much later that she discovered she might have avoided disfigurement and a second operation by choosing reconstruction at the time of her breast removal.

Our sister Martha needed an operation to repair an abdominal hernia. She simply opted to do what her local surgeon recommended, without exploring her options, which would have included the use of a laparoscope, which significantly reduces the size of the scar and time it takes to recover. However, it was only after her procedure that she realized another avenue was available to her.

5. Exactly What Does the Proposed Surgery Involve?

Ask about what will be done during the operation. What organs, or parts of them, will be removed or rearranged? Exactly what kind of incision is planned, and what kind of scar can you expect? Ask for pictures or a diagram. How long will the operation take? Will you need tubes to drain your stomach, bladder, or wound discharge postoperatively? When will your family be able to see you after surgery? How long before you can eat, and how long will you be hospitalized?

6. What Are the Possible Side Effects and Risks of Surgery and Other Treatments?

Make certain to ask exactly what you might be feeling after your surgery. In addition to the general malaise and bruising associated with the body's reaction to being cut, each operation is accompanied by a certain mortality risk, or possible complications ("morbidity") and side effects. Ask about these for your operation, as well as for the medical or alternative medicine treatment programs. Ask about side effects of any drugs recommended.

Morbidity and mortality rates for each operation are generally known. Most surgeons are able to tell you quite fully what could go wrong during your surgery and what you may experience afterward. We have included a discussion of these for each operation in this book.

Effects of the alternative lifestyle therapies are not as extensively documented, but within the last few years, much research on modalities such as diet, exercise, and stress management has been conducted, and can be found in the medical literature.

One of Sandra's patients called frantically, late at night, to complain about a red ridge at the site of his hernia repair. He was afraid that infection had set in, which would disturb the results. His doctor had not explained to him that such a swelling is common after this procedure, and is called a healing ridge. Make certain you take time to listen to all the details of what to expect, and note them down.

Dwayne, a 45-year-old graphic artist, finally decided to have his small inguinal hernia repaired. However, he was not prepared for the numbness that followed the procedure. Small skin nerves had been cut, and the area below his incision had no feeling, a condition he had to learn to live with for a few months, until the nerves had time to regrow.

7. What Is My Prognosis?

"What's my prognosis, Doc?" This means, "What is the change in life expectancy and quality of life that can be expected with or without surgery, or with other possible forms of treatment?" Prognosis varies significantly with combinations of therapies, and is constantly subject to updates. Make certain you have the latest information.

8. What Can I Expect During the Recovery Period?

Ask about what to expect after the operation. You will need to know about any discomfort as you recover and any necessary restrictions in diet and activity. How long before you will be "back to your old self"?

When will you be able to drive a car and return to work? It is extremely important you know what to expect for the period after your surgery, so that you can prepare for this ahead of time. You can make arrangements with friends, and use the stress management, dietary, and other recommendations discussed in Chapters 2, 4, and 24 to assist you before, during, and after surgery, to reduce pain and encourage your body to heal.

9. Will There Be Any Changes in My Lifestyle After Surgery?

You need to inquire about permanent changes in lifestyle that may be necessary after surgery. Some operations such as breast removal and ostomy procedures, where colon contents or urine are diverted externally, create marked alterations in your body, as well as your feelings about yourself. Ask about supportive organizations that can help you during the recovery period; these can make an enormous difference. Many are listed at the back of this book.

10. What Are the Anesthesia Options, Their Risks, and Side Effects?

The anesthetic agent itself carries a risk. It may, in fact, be the *most* dangerous part of your operation, especially if you are elderly. Anesthetics can damage your brain, heart, liver, or kidneys. Be certain you ask about the specific side effects of the anesthetics being considered. Special care should be taken if you or any members of your family have any history of reaction to anesthesia. These issues are discussed more fully in the following chapter.

For most operations, you may choose from various anesthetic options. Ask your first, second, and third opinion sources which anesthesia they would recommend and why, and if they would be comfortable if you choose a different type. A few hospitals offer hypnosis or acupuncture as alternatives. Request the least amount of anesthesia that will still keep you comfortable.

Many persons, for example, do not know that they can choose not to have anesthesia for dental work. Sandra, as she described earlier, much prefers to submit to the temporary pain of the drill than the several hours of numbness and swelling of the anesthetic.

11. Can the Operation Be Done in Ambulatory Surgery or Is Hospitalization Necessary?

Should you have your operation in your doctor's office, in a special surgical clinic, as an outpatient at a hospital, or as a hospital in-patient? Dr. Carson Lewis, a plastic surgeon from San Diego, is president of the Society for Office-Based Surgery. He asserts that billions of dollars could be saved by moving many surgeries right into doctors' offices, where costs for supplies and overhead are lower. A $1,000 hospital operation may cost only $400 in the office. If your lipoma is removed in your doctor's office, for example, the hospital fee is avoided. In addition, errors such as administration of the wrong anesthetic or medication, sometimes attributed to the large size of hospitals, might be avoided.

Blue Shield of California has recommended 700 surgical procedures that could be best performed on an outpatient basis, including hernia repair; vasectomies; plastic surgical repairs; eye operations; gynecological interventions including D&Cs (dilation and curettages), tubal ligation, and diagnostic laparoscopy; tonsillectomy; endoscopy; tooth extraction; arthroscopy; and thyroid and breast biopsies.

Even laparoscopic gallbladder removals are routinely done this way. At outpatient surgical centers, special sites for one-day surgery, several studies have shown that patients receive less anesthesia and sedation than comparable hospital patients having the same operation. They are, therefore, more awake, can go home sooner, and decrease their risk for anesthetic side effects.[3]

At one such center, perhaps because outpatient operations are less intimidating, patients needed to be given less premedication and less anesthesia, reducing costs and complications.[4] Reclining chairs are used in the recovery room; gradually, these chairs are elevated to a sitting position following your procedure. Emotional influences have been found to affect surgical recovery, and by creating a homey atmosphere, with lots of personal attention, these centers harness the mind-body connection for help in healing.

However, even though more than 1,000 such clinics are now available, most outpatient surgery is still undertaken in an operating room connected to a hospital. Whether in a doctor's office, freestanding surgery center, or hospital, about 60 percent of surgery is outpatient—performed without you remaining overnight.

Outpatient surgery has the advantages of lower cost, less anesthesia, lower infection rates, easier mobilization afterward, and reduced psychological stress. Hospitalization is needed for very complex operations, but more and more procedures now qualify for day surgery. Investigate your community for one-day surgical options.

Some *disadvantages* of outpatient surgery are less time for preparation and discharge, and the occasional complication that necessitates hospitalization. If you have a low pain tolerance, hospitalization may be better for you. Discomfort is almost always present after any operation. On the other hand, you may be more relaxed, and recover more easily, in the familiarity of your own home.

If you are to be hospitalized, ask your doctor about your expected length of stay. Although the average time spent in the hospital has been decreasing overall during the last ten years, a large difference still exists in how long patients are kept in various geographical sections of the country—patients tend to be kept longer in the Western United States. Using relaxation techniques and biofeedback may help shorten your stay.

Have a look at the potential hospital and outpatient sites, compare them, and assess what they do to reduce stress. Sandra prefers to visit a dentist who has an M. C. Esher print on his ceiling, soft colors, and relaxing music.

12. What Is the Best Timing for Surgery?

We all know the adage, "The operation was a success, but the patient died." Studies have shown an intriguing relationship of the mind to surgical outcome. Patients who state beforehand they "have a strong feeling they are going to die from their operation," and tell their doctor or family, actually end up having a higher mortality rate. Thus, if you do have feelings of distinct dread before an operation, you may request to delay the operation, discuss your feelings further with your surgeon or another doctor, or use some alternative to a surgical solution.

Some evidence suggests that bleeding and mortality are increased slightly during the phase when the moon is full.[5] In a study of over 1,000 tonsillectomy patients, increased postsurgical bleeding was found to be present at the time of the full moon.[6] Neurosurgeon Dr. Norman Shealy, while at the Pain and Health Rehabilitation Center in Green Bay, Wisconsin, "checked with blood banks all over the country and found that 'the demand for blood transfusions is always highest at the time of the full moon and the two days following.'"[7] If you have a choice, you may wish to schedule elective (nonemergency) surgery at times away from the full or new moon.

Often, the surgery can be safely delayed, and a trial of alternative medicine begun. If these gentler methods do not then work, the proposed repair can be initiated. For example, Sandra has witnessed thousands of patients with heart disease able to bypass the bypass and angioplasty utilizing the Dean Ornish program.

If you are still having menstrual periods and you need a breast operation to diagnose or treat breast cancer, schedule it in the middle part of your cycle, in the week following ovulation. Although retrospective and difficult to interpret with confidence, several studies have found recurrence rates much lower when surgeries were scheduled during this part of the cycle, when a high progesterone to estrogen concentration ratio prevails, which may inhibit tumor cell dissemination.[8]

13. What Are Your Fees and Payment Schedule?

A wide variation exists in what surgeons charge for the same operation, so this is a good item to check. If you have financial problems, don't have insurance, or carry inadequate coverage, most doctors will allow you to pay over time rather than delay necessary surgery. Most hospitals likewise have such a plan for their fees. However, like in all things, to some extent you get what you pay for.

Sandra's dental experience has led her to conclude that seeking a sometimes more expensive second opinion has been worth it.

Finalizing Your Choice of Surgeon

After you have had your first, second, and third opinion interviews and examinations as just described, you need to evaluate each experience. Were your symptoms taken seriously? Did the doctor listen carefully? Did he or she take a detailed history and do a careful physical examination? Did you feel respected while you were asking your questions and being examined? Were you given enough time to discuss *all* of your questions and concerns? Did the doctor seemed rushed, or distracted? Importantly, did you feel a sense of trust and confidence in this doctor such that you would be comfortable putting your life in his or her hands?

Sandra's ideal surgeon is exemplified by Dr. Robert L. Painter. During her first years in medical practice, Sandra observed this remarkable and beloved Connecticut surgeon. His caring and compassionate yet humorous way with his patients, it seemed obvious, made a difference in their mind-body connections, and his career was characterized by such outstanding successes that he was coaxed out of retirement by the local teaching hospital to share his skills with future generations of surgeons.

If you feel uncomfortable about making a decision, you can ask for more time to think about it and do more investigation. Follow-up visits for more discussion should be encouraged until you are very comfortable with the surgeon you choose.

Choosing Your Hospital

Your surgeon will want to admit you to a hospital where he or she has privileges and where your insurance covers the expenses. Most surgeons are affiliated with more than one hospital, and will give you a choice if you ask for it. All hospitals do not have the same track record, particularly with more complicated procedures. Mortality rates for risky procedures are usually lower at larger centers, where increased volume gives the doctors and nurses more experience. For example, a large study of Medicare patients found operative mortality for removal of the esophagus for cancer rose to 17.3 percent in low-volume hospitals compared with only 3.5 percent in high-volume hospitals.[9] A 2000 study reported in *JAMA* found mortality rates significantly higher in low-volume hospitals for abdominal aortic aneurysm repair, carotid endarterectomy, leg bypass, heart artery bypass, heart artery balloon angioplasty, heart transplant, pediatric heart surgery, pancreas cancer surgery, esophagus cancer surgery, and brain aneurysm surgery.[10, 11]

A "teaching" hospital" affiliated with a medical school, with a "house staff" of medical students and residents, provides top-flight, round-the-clock care, which could prove critical should you have an emergency during off hours. On the other hand, several visits and exams a day by different house staff members, often discussing you as an example of an illness, is the necessary trade-off, and may be irritating to you. If you have a common low-risk problem, the quieter, more personalized attention at a smaller center has its own advantages.

You can find out about a particular hospital's healthcare record by contacting the Joint

Commission on Accreditation of Healthcare Organizations, listed in the Resources section of this book. They can send you a report on the hospital's results compared with other hospitals in your area and the national average. With the rapid increase in the popularity and ease of Internet searching, this sort of information is becoming readily available. For example, since 1992, the state of Pennsylvania has published its *Consumer's Guide to Coronary Artery Bypass Graft Surgery* showing mortality rates for all cardiac surgeons and hospitals in the state on its website at www.phc4.org.

Visit the hospitals that you can choose from ahead of time. Ask friends about their experiences. Choose the hospital where you think you will be most confident and comfortable. Check to see if it will be open to any alternative medicine therapies you want to include in your care. See if a Planetree project unit, known for its compassionate care facilities and discussed in the next chapter, is available near you. Their number is listed in the Resources section of this book.

What Can You Do if You Are Restricted in Your Choice of Doctor or Hospital?

Of course, managed care is a growing factor in determining the choice of healthcare providers in the United States, as it already is in most other countries. The type of HMO you have may have a bearing on the quality of care you receive. After you have an illness that needs to be treated may be too late to make changes, but if you have a choice of HMO plans, choose one that is "not-for-profit." Owing to the need to earn a profit to

pay high administrative salaries and satisfy investors, the healthcare related expenses of a for-profit HMO may be cut. A 1999 study reported in *JAMA* comparing 248 investor-owned plans to 81 not-for-profit plans and representing 56 percent of total HMO enrollment in the United States found that the investor-owned plans had lower ratings for all fourteen quality-of-care indicators tested.[12]

If it does not already, your health insurance plan may eventually place restrictions on whom you can choose as your surgeon and where you can be hospitalized. Your primary care provider will have to refer you to a specialist affiliated with your health plan. If you choose a surgeon or an alternative practitioner outside of it, you will most likely have to pay for a higher portion or all of your bill.

Does this make all the information given in this book about choosing a doctor worthless? Absolutely not! If you do not have full confidence in your first surgeon, express this to your primary care doctor or, if necessary, to the health plan administrator. Despite some restrictions, you may ask your primary care doctor to refer you to someone else. All plans have avenues for alternate referrals. Just make sure you know exactly what your healthcare plan will and won't pay for.

Most health plans pay for chiropractic care, and now some even cover Rolfing, the structural work especially suited for certain back disorders such as scoliosis. As alternatives become more popular, more companies are finding they may save money including these options. Fifty insurers cover the Dean Ornish Heart Disease Reversal Program as described in Chapter 8, and Medicare has agreed to reimburse for an initial pilot study as well.

The Philosophy of Risk Taking

Risks are inherent in any decision-making situation. As discussed above, before you make your final decision, you need to know and compare all the risks of the surgery, of medical therapy alone, and those of an alternative medicine program.

What risk *should* you choose to take? Unless your mental status is compromised, no one can make this choice for you better than you can. Delay in deciding may itself increase the possibility of a less successful outcome, but usually there is time for you to gather information and make a considered decision. Then you can choose the option *you* feel will work for you.

Don't take a risk you do not *have* to take. On the other hand, even though any operation carries some danger, you *should* opt for surgery when you find you will be greatly benefited, as when your disease is clearly life-threatening, or when the operation is likely to bring an enormous boon to your daily functioning.

At times the choice can be especially difficult, such as when a dangerous operation offers the *only* hope for cure, but the likelihood of such an outcome is small. Radical surgery for some types of cancer, for example, may only offer a 5 to 20 percent chance of cure, and the mortality rate of the operation itself may approach these figures. A failed operation *can* bring with it a shortened and less comfortable remaining time with family and friends, and even a successful, life-prolonging operation may lead to drastic changes in quality of life. Facing this type of decision, it is obvious you need to take time to gather and understand as much of the latest information as is available, then make your choice based on consultation with physicians, family, and friends.

Cure, Quality of Life, and Life Extension

Especially in the case of malignant disease, surgery that aims to cure the problem is not always possible. However, that does not mean you have to forsake a potentially beneficial operation. Many procedures can vastly improve your quality of life, even if they do not lengthen your life expectancy. This is often true of "palliative" surgery, which does not aim to cure the disease, but can, for example, bypass a liver bile duct blocked by cancer to relieve jaundice, or provide other temporary relief. The risk of such a procedure may be worth taking.

Many of the operations discussed in this book clearly add to life expectancy. However, even these may at the same time have such unpleasant effects upon your life quality that you may not find them worth it for you. These choices are especially difficult.

The Special Benefits of the Surgical Approach

A clear benefit of surgery is that it often provides rapid relief of symptoms. Alternative medicine remedies, in general, though not always, may take longer.

If you are a person who tends to worry, living with your disease without acting upon it dramatically, as by having an operation, may not be tolerable. Since we have begun to understand the important effects of the emotions on health, we now appreciate the contribution it makes to your recovery when you honor your own feelings about the different choices.

The Special Benefits of the Alternative Medicine Approach

In addition to helping you avoid an operation, choosing to use an alternative medicine program gives its own real advantages. Changes in diet, exercise, and stress management act to help you feel much fitter in the short run, as well as assist in preventing other medical and surgical diseases later in life. You will most likely need to make these changes *anyway,* to prevent recurrence of your original surgical illness. An experience of mastery over your health also often follows, which can help you feel an improved quality of life in its own right.

Should You Have the Operation? Putting It All Together

Before you decide whether you can avoid surgery, or can't live as well without it, make certain you have addressed as cautiously and thoroughly as possible all the issues considered in this chapter, as well as in the section dealing with your specific disease. A final guideline to your best approach when facing the knife: *Take time to make your decision.* Even though everyone is apprehensive about having an operation, you should be very comfortable you are making an appropriate decision. Once you have decided upon a course of treatment, let your "three opinion" doctors know what you are doing, and give them complete follow-up on your results.

THE OPERATIVE PERIOD: WHAT TO EXPECT

But not once, in the three days I was there, did any one doctor sit down and talk, personally, one on one, with me. Five doctors made rounds on me every day—always in clumps. Great scientific medicine—but impersonal as hell.

William Nolen, M.D., surgeon,
describing his own surgery
in *A Surgeon Under the Knife*[1]

The Preoperative Period

Suppose you have consulted the previous chapters, met with your prospective surgeon, obtained the second and third opinions as outlined in the preceding chapter, and read the section in this book dealing with your disease. If you decide in favor of surgery, this chapter's information can help you know what to expect and what to request before, during, and after your operation.

We have included information in this chapter about how alternative medicine's effective techniques, such as relaxation training and acupuncture, can help you have a successful hospital course. Specific applications are given in the section relating to your individual disorder.

If possible, to fully prepare yourself for any elective major surgery, spend several weeks following the guidelines for diet, exercise, and relaxation training given in Chapter 2. Even in an emergency, however, you can make use of the information there in conjunction with the following guidelines, to help you through your surgical experience.

An important first step is to choose one or more loving friends or family members to be with you before and after your operation. They can give you a massage, hold your hand, and perform many other small services that the doctors and nurses may be just too busy to carry out.

Each surgeon usually has a standard set of preoperative orders and routines for the specific surgery. In the past, activities were restricted before operations. Now it is known that keeping you inactive beforehand can *increase* your risk of lung problems, circulation disorders, and muscle weakness. Being up and about until the time of your operation is to be encouraged, within your capacity; just make certain to be well rested.

Preoperative Testing

If you are having your operation performed in your doctor's office, you probably will not need preoperative testing, but for many procedures a series of routine tests may be ordered before your surgery. You can avoid unneeded procedures by educating yourself before surgery about what is appropriate.

Blood Tests

Most likely, some blood will need to be taken for testing before your operation. A tube or tubes are drawn from a vein in your arm with a simple needle stick. If you are otherwise healthy, you may need only the *CBC (complete blood count)*. A CBC makes certain you have enough red and white blood cells, and platelets, to withstand the rigors of surgery. African-American patients may be screened for sickle cell anemia or trait. Other tests may be needed, depending on your age, the medication you are taking, or if you have a history of or risk for certain underlying diseases.

Serum electrolytes measure the amounts of sodium, potassium, chloride, and bicarbonate that give your blood its degree of minerality. This screens for underlying medical disease, and may determine the type of intravenous fluids you receive. *BUN (blood urea nitrogen)* and *creatinine* reflect kidney function, and makes certain you are not dehydrated.

Glucose levels are particularly important, since all cells depend upon an appropriate amount of this sugar, and high levels may indicate unsuspected diabetes, which in turn increases the possibilities of infection, heart disease, and other circulation disorders. *Calcium* levels that are high or low can indicate hormone imbalance. *Magnesium* is another important mineral necessary for proper muscle relaxation and regularity of heartbeat. Proteins—measured by the *total protein, albumen, globulin,* and *albumen/globulin ratio*—are essential for the healing process and immune function. *LDH (lactate dehydrogenase), SGOT (serum glutamine oxalate transferase), SGPT (serum glutamine pyruvate transferase),* and *alkaline phosphatase* are used to look for liver disease, important knowledge for your anesthesiologist, especially if you have a history of liver problems. *PT (prothrombin time)* and *PTT (partial thromboplastin time)* are tests of your blood's clotting ability, only necessary if a disease affecting this ability is suspected.

Blood gases (levels of oxygen, carbon dioxide, bicarbonate, and acid-base balance) are drawn from an artery at your wrist. These are only needed preoperatively if you have severe lung disease or are very, very ill.

Heart and Lung Tests

An *electrocardiogram* (*EKG* or *ECG*) and a *stress exercise test* (see Chapter 8) are unnecessary if you are young and healthy with no cardiac risk factors, but may be requested to screen for heart disease if you are an older individual or have a history of heart problems. *Lung function tests* (see Chapter 7) may need to be performed if you have a long history of heavy cigarette use, emphysema, asthma, or other lung problems.

Chest X-Ray

If you are healthy and not at increased risk for lung or heart disease, you do not need this test, and thus can avoid its extra costs and X-ray exposure. Some hospitals *still* require a *chest X-ray* at the time of admission for all surgical patients. You can request this not be done, although you may need to sign a special waiver form.

In order to protect themselves from missing something, and thus later being charged with malpractice, some doctors currently order an excess of laboratory tests, increasing costs of health care. Dr. William Nolen, in his book, *A Surgeon Under the Knife,* describes how lab tests were incorrectly ordered for him, despite the preferential treatment usually given to physicians when they are patients. To protect yourself, we suggest you ask for an explanation for each test ordered, and find out how this information applies to your specific case.

Checking into the Hospital

Alice, *a 69-year-old retired secretary, never thought it could happen to her—she had never been in a hospital in her life. However,* one night she developed such severe abdominal pain she had to go to the emergency room. *Unfortunately, she was by herself, and did not give the doctor a complete description of the timing and characteristics of her pain, as she sometimes experienced short-term memory deficiencies when she was nervous. Tests initially revealed a urinary tract infection, for which she was treated, but during the subsequent delay, her swollen appendix ruptured, necessitating a much riskier operation and longer recovery time. She might have avoided these problems had she taken a friend with her, to give the doctor more information about her pain and its sequence of onset.*

You need to know what to bring with you when you check into the hospital. If you are staying overnight, you need your toiletries, magazines, books, a personal cassette player with earphones, hobby supplies, stationery, and anything else that may make your stay more pleasant. Some hospitals will let you wear your own pajamas, bathrobe, and slippers. Bring a warm-up suit if you like. Photos of family, friends, and yourself during happy times can help cheer you up. Don't forget a list of your medications, and the phone numbers of relatives or friends for your surgeon to contact after your operation or about changes in your condition. You should not bring much money or valuables.

Walking through the doors of a hospital for the first time as a patient can be a daunting experience. Your fears and sense of vulnerability can suddenly be overwhelming. Take some deep breaths to calm yourself, and practice the other relaxation techniques given in Chapter 2.

The first step is to check in with Admitting, where you will be asked for your name, address, phone number, employer, date of birth, religion, Social Security number, closest family member or friend, and insurance information.

Most hospitals now ask you to sign an *Advance Directive,* which details how you want to be treated if an unforeseen complication arises in the hospital and you are not able to make a decision for yourself. You should not sign this until your doctor explains it to you. For example, if you were to have a cardiac arrest, would you want a "full code," meaning that all resuscitative measures would be used to try to bring you back, including external heart massage, cardiac electric shock, drugs, and a breathing machine? If your condition was judged to be terminal or you were unlikely to have any meaningful recovery, would you still want to be kept alive by drugs, feeding tubes, and mechanical devices? This is not an easy decision if you are seriously ill or have a terminal illness, and should be made after consultation with your doctor and family.

If you are having day surgery, you then proceed to the changing room, where you slip on a gown. If you are being admitted before your operation, you are assigned a hospital room with a closet for your clothes and personal effects.

One of the most important things you can do to improve your hospital experience—and even save your life—is to get to know all of your hospital staff personally. Even though they change shifts every eight hours or so, you should try to become a person to them, and make friends. They commonly have even more experience with certain problems than the doctors do. For example, constipation can often follow surgery, and they can help you know what to expect and how to best treat it. Medical students and residents are able to

spend more time with you, often seeing you several times a day, and may be more open to helping you with alternatives. Many hospitals use such a "house staff" to help their surgeons, who are likely to be tied up in the operating room or in their offices.

You may have a choice between a private or a shared room, usually with one other person. If you can afford it, you may wish to ask for a private room, so that you can focus on your alternative medicine approaches. If you cannot budget for this, you can try to create a sense of privacy by the use of special pictures and photos. On the other hand, especially if you are a gregarious person, you may do better with a roommate who has already been through surgery, as discussed below. Hospital noise is often a significant problem, so your personal tape player can help you relax. Earplugs, either foam or wax, are available at local drugstores, and are a wise addition to your toiletries.

Hospital History and Physical Examination

After you are settled in the outpatient surgery waiting room or your hospital room, your nurse asks a series of routine questions about your health, medications, and allergies. In larger teaching hospitals, be sure this information stays with you, so that medical students and residents do not have to repeat the same questions for their reports—unless you want to allow them to, since they do need the practice. The nurse takes your weight, temperature, pulse rate, and blood pressure.

You will likely have already had a medical history and physical exam and necessary tests before you enter the hospital. If not, your doctor or a medical student and/or resident then asks more detailed "history" questions.

The standard history form has headings concerning your:

- Chief Complaint—what your symptoms are.
- History of Present Illness—the history of your symptoms.
- Past Medical History—significant medical problems.
- Review of Symptoms—general questions about your body systems.
- Medications.
- Allergies—to medications, foods, bee stings, or others.
- Smoking—in packs/years.
- Previous Surgery.
- Family History—of medical problems.
- Social History—your family, job, present living situation, hobbies.

After your history is taken, you next have a physical examination. A routine exam includes checking your eyes, ears, mouth, neck, lungs, heart, abdomen, rectum, external genitalia, lymph nodes, pulses, nerve reflexes, and muscle strength. A pelvic examination or other more detailed exams, based on your specific illness, may be included. If you are generally healthy, a quick exam limited to the heart and lungs may be all that is done. You can decline any part of the exam, especially if it has been performed recently.

The *history and physical exam (H&P)* can take anywhere from a few minutes to an hour. The result of all this is a report, written or dictated, that is placed into your hospital chart.

Immediate Preoperative Tests and Preparations

It may be necessary to repeat some of the blood tests or other tests, described above,

immediately prior to your operation. If so, you may be visited by the phlebotomist, a member of the blood-drawing team, and the EKG technician. As you must not eat anything for at least eight hours before anesthesia, an intravenous line may be necessary, especially if you are dehydrated or need to wait more than a few hours before your operation. Antibiotics or other preoperative intravenous medications may be given.

If you are having bowel surgery, you may need to have a "bowel prep" to flush your intestines. This includes drinking the nonabsorbable mineral solution "Go Lightly," citrate of magnesia, or other laxative solutions, perhaps followed by an enema.

Consultations from Specialists

Your doctor may ask for one or more specialists to help with your hospitalization and visit you before your operation. For example, a cardiologist may be asked to evaluate your heart and help with postoperative management. Usually, the consultant will see you before hospital admission, although there may not be time if your problem is urgent. If consultation is necessary, your doctor should explain this to you beforehand.

Reading Your Chart

*J*ordan, *a 49-year-old artist, experienced severe chest pain and shortness of breath soon after an angry phone call from his ex-wife. Diagnosed as having a heart attack, his initial hospital recovery was prolonged. He decided to read his chart, to create artistic impressions for himself of the problems cited there by the doctors, and use them to practice visualizing his heart function improving. In a short time, his tests were much improved, and he was* *able to leave the hospital. He then entered a lifestyle-oriented heart disease recovery program, based on the research of Dr. Dean Ornish, as discussed in Chapter 8 of this book.*

———————

You may want to obtain permission to read your chart, so you can keep up on your progress and gain insight into your physician's planning and the nurses' evaluations. You have the legal right to do this. The more informed you are, the more you can focus your relaxation and visualization therapies to assist your healing. Though many physicians and nurses may not yet be familiar with this practice, it can be quite helpful; it is now a part of the Planetree Hospital Program, utilized at a number of medical centers; to contact Planetree, see the Resources section at the end of this book. Make certain you discuss the advantages of personal chart-reading with your doctor first, and have him or her inform the entire staff that you will be reading their notes.

Surgical Consent Forms

Surgical consent forms list your problem or illness, what the proposed operation will be, and the name of your surgeon. You are asked to sign your name, indicating you understand what will be done; that the risks, possible complications, and alternatives have been explained to you; that you have had an opportunity to have all of your questions answered; and have read the form. Also, the form probably will contain a clause indicating that you give permission for your doctor to use his or her judgment should unforeseen circumstances arise during your operation. For example, if you have signed consent for an appendectomy and a colon tumor is found, your doctor has your permission to remove it.

Trying to understand the consent form at a time of illness and apprehension is especially problematic. A study of Pittsburgh Hospitals conducted by Carnegie-Mellon University found that twenty-one years of education were needed to understand surgical consent forms, while most Americans can read only at or below the eleventh grade level.[2] We suggest you have a family member or friend help you completely comprehend these forms before you sign, and if you can't understand them, ask your doctor for more information.

The information given on consent forms can be very scary. In order to protect themselves from lawsuits, surgeons and hospitals often present the worst possible circumstances either verbally or on the printed form. To counteract this, you can affirm in your mind you will *not* have complications, and will come through the operation without incident. Such mind-body practices, and the research that supports them, are discussed further in Chapter 2.

The Patient Advocate or Ombudsman

Most hospitals give you a Patient Bill of Rights when you are admitted. It outlines your rights regarding refusal or acceptance of tests and treatments, and what you can do if you feel you are not getting the best of care, or have disagreements with your doctors, nurses, or other hospital staff. Most hospitals have a patient advocate or ombudsman who can act as your intermediary to help resolve dissatisfactions. If you meet resistance, he or she can also help you implement your integrated alternative medicine program, as described in Chapter 24.

Hospital Environment: Conventional and Alternative Possibilities

It is interesting to contemplate the invention of hospital gowns. Were the ties placed in back in order to prevent patients from getting out of them? Were the materials and shapes a matter of expedience? Or were there other considerations that justified these embarrassing outfits? The rationale appears to have been lost over time.

Since mind-body research now indicates that the state of your mind influences the competence of your immune system, then how you are feeling about yourself can be important to your recovery. In whatever ways your stress can be reduced, your immune system can function more effectively.

You may, therefore, want to avoid the standard hospital gowns, and instead choose very comfortable and enjoyable outfits for your hospital stay. They need not even be restricted to pajamas; it might help your identification with health if you wear pajamas only for sleep. Getting up and dressed can give you a lift in itself. Most hospitals now allow you to do this.

In an experiment called the "Pritikin Hospital Plan," patients were issued jogging suits upon admission to a special section of a New Orleans hospital. They ate their meals together in a common dining room, and took exercise classes together each day. Exercise suits would seem a good choice for both before and after surgery, to make you feel healthy, and remind you of the benefits exercise can have for a return to health.

The Planetree Hospital Program exemplifies such principles. The "planetree" is the tree under which Hippocrates, the father of modern medicine, taught his students on the Greek island of Cos. Started in 1985 by Angelica Thierot after she had witnessed several of her family members suffering in the usual hospital environment, this program consists of patient-oriented architecture and facilities, where patients are encouraged to participate in their care. A kitchen is provided, so that family members can prepare meals. Patients can write in their own charts, take their own medications at bedside, and take advantage of many other features of a homelike setting. The Planetree Program is now available in a number of hospitals around the country.

At least twelve California hospitals have "surgery hotels," located next to the conventional hospital. For example, the Fresno Recovery Care Center, and the Sharp Recovery Center in San Diego offer hotel room–like suites, with gourmet meals, a snack-filled refrigerator, a VCR, and a sofa bed for guests. At a cost only slightly above a conventional room, they are covered by most private insurance plans, though not yet by Medicare or Medicaid. As further mind-body research documents the healthcare savings from attention to these elements, translated into quicker recovery, with less medication and shorter hospital stays, the transformation of hospitals to becoming truly hospitable may become more universal.

Noise, color, aromas, and our visual and architectural environment affect our stress levels. The simple presence of windows in an intensive care unit has been shown to reduce the number of episodes of delirium in patients by 50 percent, compared to patients in a unit without windows.[3] The arrangement of chairs into a homey distribution was found to increase appropriate interaction[4] and eating behavior of mental hospital patients.[5] Piped-in rock and rap music increased the number of inappropriate behaviors, when compared to easy-listening and classical music,[6] reflecting this mind-body connection.

When exposed to noisy circumstances, our hearts beat faster and our blood pressure increases; even normal sound levels of talking or television elicit this stress response.[7] Conversation within a room elicits higher stress response than that outside the room. "Shh . . . Hospital Zone" was the early wisdom, which may have been grounded in the ability of silence to assist our needed healing rest. You can modify your environmental noise level by using earplugs or headphones.

What sorts of sounds you choose for your tape player may help you or interfere with your healing. Studies in plants have shown that rock and roll decreases plant growth, while classical music increases it. The same has been found to be true for milk production in cows. Please see Chapter 2 for further discussion of music as therapy.

Several studies have indicated that patients who are "feisty," ask many questions, and generally get involved in their treatment, recover more quickly. Perhaps their immune systems are positively affected by a sense of control, and hopefulness—feelings of *control* have been tied to the activity of white cells.[8] The more you can control the atmosphere of your hospital stay, by bringing in photographs of family and friends, clothes you like to wear, music and art that you enjoy, the more you boost your body's innate healing forces. You can choose the colors, aromas, and music that most help you relax; these and other such factors are discussed more fully in Chapter 2.

Beauty affects us. In one example of the importance of such emotional factors in recovery from illness, patients assigned to rooms with a view of trees outdoors needed less pain medicine, had fewer complications, fewer negative evaluations from the nurses, shorter recovery periods, and left the hospital sooner, when compared to patients placed in rooms whose windows looked out on a wall.[9] In another study, persons placed in a room with a photograph of a nature scene on the wall needed less pain medication, and experienced less anxiety when compared to those facing an abstract painting or a blank wall. Alpha waves, the brain waves associated with relaxation, were shown to be increased in those exposed to the nature scenes.[10]

If you can't get a room with a view, perhaps you can have someone bring in pictures of beautiful landscapes or other uplifting images to keep you company. As noted, the Planetree Hospital Program, gradually being introduced into hospitals nationwide, includes many of these mind-body elements.

You may wish to request a roommate who has already completed surgery. An intriguing study compared two groups of patients awaiting surgery. The first group was given roommates who had already had their operations performed and were recovering. The second group had roommates who also had not yet had surgery. The first group exhibited less anxiety, were more active after their own operations, and left the hospital one to four days sooner.[11]

Preoperative Preparation

Conventional Approaches

Up until the time of any preoperative dietary restrictions, you can continue to follow the diet and take the vitamins and supplements outlined in Chapter 2. Because they are not stored in the body, vitamins B and C are especially important; these vitamins can be added to your IV (intravenous) bottle. We suggest that if you will not be able to eat regular food or take vitamin supplements for more than a day or two after your operation, that you discuss the guidelines in Chapter 2 with your surgeon.

A regular diet is usually prescribed until the night before surgery, at which time, if you are to have regional or general anesthesia, you are asked to be *NPO* (short for Latin *non par oris*), meaning nothing is to be taken by mouth, not even water. If you were to have anything in your stomach as you underwent or came out of anesthesia, during the unconscious or drowsy state, you might vomit and subsequently inhale this material into your lungs. Since vomiting may be triggered by medications or nervous reflexes, this advice may also be true even for procedures done under local anesthesia, with or without sedation. Oral medications can usually be taken with a sip or two of water a few hours before your surgery.

Recent information suggests that the standard advice not to eat or drink anything for eight hours before your surgery may be unnecessarily restrictive. A glass of clear liquid has been found to be safe four hours before surgery. Check with your doctor to see if you can have a cup of black coffee or herb tea to help you get out of bed at 4 A.M. for your 8 A.M. surgery.

Operations involving the colon must have specific preparation to cleanse and clear it of roughage and bacteria. This may include liquids-only for two days preop, laxatives, oral antibiotics, and enemas. Take a bath or shower using antiseptic soap to keep skin bacteria to a minimum, and diminish your risk of incision infection.

If you are undergoing major abdominal surgery under general anesthesia, a tube, called a nasogastric (NG) tube, may be placed down your nose in order to empty the stomach of its contents by suction. If not required preoperatively, this is done after you are asleep. Once you are under anesthesia, a *Foley catheter* may also be inserted into your bladder, to drain and monitor your urine output.

Alternative Approaches

The shaving of your body hair is a common practice now known not only to be unnecessary for most operations, but also to increase your risk of infection. Any level of shaving, even looking grossly normal to the eye, causes small cuts and scratches in the skin's epidermal barrier, allowing bacteria to enter and cause infection. Hair removing creams are associated with a much lower rate of incision infection compared to using a razor. However, hair removal creams themselves can cause skin reactions and discomfort. If you have tried depilatories in the past without a problem, perhaps this is the very best option to remove hair when necessary. If you know you have such a reaction, and your surgeon insists on hair removal, you should request hair *clipping*, that is much less traumatic than shaving.

If hair is clipped or shaved in the operating room, rather than the night before, it decreases time for bacteria to become established beneath skin cuts. Don't shave yourself thinking you are doing your surgeon a favor. Although this information is not new, some hospitals, especially in rural areas, may be continuing to shave long before you are actually in the operating room.

It is interesting that only with the advent of the women's movement was routine shaving questioned, and the discovery made that such shaving *increased* infection risk. For most operations and deliveries, preparatory shaving can be entirely eliminated. Even in most cases of extreme hairiness in the incision area, including scalp surgery, requests to keep shaving to a minimum are supportable. Resist any shaving outside of the operating room and ask your doctor if you can avoid being shaved altogether.

Here's a piece of advice: If you are having surgery on one side of your body—your knee, for example—to help protect yourself, take an indelible magic marker and write on the other knee: WRONG KNEE (or hip, or leg or whatever) in large letters. Although it is exceedingly rare, operations are sometimes mistakenly performed on the opposite side of the disorder, so such labeling helps assure that it won't by any chance happen to you.

The Operative Period

After you are prepared for surgery, you are taken to the operating room holding area by stretcher or wheelchair, or may walk there if you are having day surgery. The choice for anesthesia usually will already have been made for major surgery or you will now discuss your choices with your surgeon and anesthesiologist if you won't necessarily have to be asleep.

Nurses will interview you one last time to ensure that you haven't taken anything by mouth in the last few hours, record drug allergies, and confirm you understand what's going to be done. An IV will be started. You then are taken to your specific operating room.

Anesthesia

We can look as far back as the Bible to find the first reference to anesthesia, when God caused a "deep sleep" to be visited upon Adam, during which his rib was removed to create Eve. Anesthesia using ether and chloroform began only in the mid-1800s. These chemicals have been replaced by safer, nonexplosive agents, used singly or in combination.

The word "anesthetic" itself means "not perceptive"; a general anesthetic puts you to sleep. However, being made to sleep carries with it the problem of how to get you *back* from "down under." Such a process requires specialized training. Medical doctors, called anesthesiologists, take several extra years of residency to become specialists in anesthesiology, while nurses can also acquire special training to become "nurse-anesthetists."

Nurse-anesthetists give more than half the anesthesia in the United States. For the most part, they are supervised by the anesthesiologists who examine you, take your anesthetic-related history, and oversee the application of the selected drug, and then are available for emergencies. For prolonged or difficult operations, you should request an anesthesiologist be present, because they have more training with nonroutine problems. You can discuss this with your surgeon.

A preoperative visit to discuss anesthesia is usually conducted by your anesthesiologist, nurse-anesthetist, or an anesthesiology resident prior to your surgery, and preoperative choices of anesthesia are made at that time.

Warning: If you are taking any medications, including herbal supplements or vitamins, you must inform your anesthesiologist and surgeon before your operation. See Chapter 24 for a complete list of supplements which may influence your surgery. For example, some herbs and vitamins may alter the effects of anesthesia, or cause blood pressure or bleeding changes. If you are having elective surgery, you should stop vitamin E, which can slow the clotting of your blood, for two days before and two days after your operation. Likewise, garlic should be stopped seven days before surgery and can be resumed two days after. Ephedra should never be taken; check for it mixed with other herbs. Herbs such as ginkgo biloba, St. John's wort, feverfew, and ginseng should be discontinued for two weeks before and not resumed until two weeks after the operation. Immune-enhancing herbs such as echinacea, and the other supplements discussed in Chapter 2, can be continued, but you must still notify both your anesthesiologist and your surgeon beforehand.

The presurgical visit to discuss anesthesia is much more important than might casually be thought. One study showed that a meaningful, communicative visit to a patient by the anesthesiologist preoperatively resulted in a decrease in mortality and a shorter hospital stay.[12] The anesthesiologist is the person responsible for coaxing you while you drift off to sleep, then bringing you back again. Knowing him or her beforehand may allow you to assist this process, even when you are unconscious.

Sleeping pills are often given the night before surgery, in order to help you rest in the strange hospital environment, and to leave you drowsy the morning of the surgery. You may choose the more natural approaches to a good night's sleep, given in Chapter 2, but if they don't work, you should opt for medication, so that you are well rested. Preanesthetic sedatives may be given an hour or so before your operation. They relieve anxiety and allow for a lower level of anesthetic.

Anesthetic Choice Considerations

Many of the factors in choosing your anesthetic involve your own personal and family history and your specific operation. You can go over the following considerations with your surgeon and anesthesiologist at the preoperative visit.

If you have a history of allergies or reactions to medications or anesthetics that might be used during the operation, your anesthesiologist needs to be told. The anesthesiologist also needs to be aware of any medications you may be taking that may interfere with or affect the strength of your anesthetic.

Very rarely, patients experience a severe reaction to anesthesia that may have a genetic basis, so be sure to report any problems with anesthesia experienced by family members.

For patients with heart, lung, liver, or kidney problems, local or regional anesthesia is usually preferred.

The time of your last meal may have a bearing on the anesthetic chosen if your operation must be performed as an emergency. General anesthesia, which eliminates the gag reflex and increases the possibility of vomiting stomach contents into the lungs, should be avoided if possible.

Your diagnosis, the extent and location of your disease, your position on the operating table, and the location of the incision are likely to be determining factors in what types of anesthetics are reasonable. For example, if you need part of your stomach removed, local or regional anesthesia would likely be ineffective by not providing sufficient relaxation of your abdominal muscles for the exposure your surgeon needs.

Your surgeon's and anesthesiologist's recommendation for your operation is likely based on experience with hundreds of patients with similar diagnoses. However, if you have a strong preference, be sure to express it and determine if it is a sensible choice for you.[13]

Anesthetic Choices

The traditional anesthesia choices are local, regional, and general. The alternative technique of acupuncture or hypnosis can be substituted for or added to the traditional method in many cases.

Local Anesthesia

This is the type of anesthesia given for minor procedures in your doctor's office, such as skin biopsies, removal of small "lumps and bumps," and drainage of small infections. It can also be used for more extensive procedures, as described throughout the book. Local anesthesia relieves pain by the use of nerve-deadening solutions injected directly into the area where the surgery will be performed. Such medications are usually given by your surgeon or doctor, rather than an anesthesiologist. Novocain, Xylocaine, and Marcaine are examples of anesthetics used for this technique. They take a few seconds to a minute or two to inject, and the effect is almost immediate. The duration of numbness is anywhere from thirty minutes to two hours or more, depending on the drug used. You remain wide awake.

You may ask your doctor to use the smallest possible needle, add some bicarbonate to counteract the acidity of the anesthetic, warm the solution, and inject slowly. These measures will lessen the "sting" and pain you feel. Most patients are surprised that they then don't feel a thing while the operation is being performed.

Local anesthetics have the advantage of avoiding the problems associated with general anesthetics, as described below. However, if too much local anesthetic is used, or if it is inadvertently injected into a blood vessel or tissue with a large blood supply, enough can be rapidly absorbed to cause potentially toxic effects. In addition, very rare fatal allergic reactions have occurred.

If you have severe anxiety, a low pain threshold, or are likely to have a procedure lasting much longer than forty-five to sixty minutes, you are not a good candidate for an operation under strictly local anesthesia. To avoid more widely active agents, you may be able to have a local combined with intravenous (IV) sedation ("conscious sedation"). Prior to your operation, an intravenous line is started and you are given a sedative such as Versed and painkillers such as Demerol or morphine. You are thus made slightly "groggy," placed in the "twilight zone," or drifted off to a light sleep. With these intravenous medications, you must be well monitored with a cardiac monitor and watched closely, with oxygen and a breathing tube available, since an overdose would cause you to stop breathing. With deeper sedation, it is safer to have the procedure performed in an operating room setting, rather than a doctor's office. Examples of operations where local anesthetics are commonly combined with IV medications include breast biopsy, hernia, and dilation and curettage (D&C), the procedure used for clearing the uterine lining.

Some operations obviously require general anesthetics, but surprisingly, many traditional major surgeries can be carried out with local or other lesser means of anesthesia. Check further in this book, under each operation, for your best options.

Excretion of the hormone adrenaline, which speeds up your heart and makes you ready to "fight," is an indication of how much stress you are experiencing. These levels are higher in patients who have local anesthetics compared with general anesthetics. General anesthesia has the advantage of full pain and anxiety control, and also produces the full muscular relaxation essential for some procedures. However, more surgeons and anesthesiologists are now giving their patients options, and if you can successfully use the relaxation techniques in Chapter 2 to offset your anxiety, you can obtain the most rapid recovery by opting for local anesthesia.

If you prefer, you may choose to do without any anesthetic for very minor operations. Stitches can be placed and even root canal surgery performed without anesthetic, by use of the mind-body techniques discussed in Chapter 2. You thereby opt for only a few moments of pain, and are able to avoid the postoperative discomfort associated with the local anesthetic injection.

Regional Anesthesia

This technique acts upon a preselected part of the body to provide full anesthesia to that region. The drugs used are similar to those employed in local anesthesia, but are aimed at deadening the larger nerves, which provide sensation to a much wider area. These blocks typically take a few minutes longer to perform and are a bit more uncomfortable to inject, since the nerves are deeper. Typically, it takes longer for the drugs to numb the nerves, but once this is achieved, the duration of numbness is much longer than with local anesthesia, and pain relief more reliable.

Spinal (midback), *epidural* (upper tailbone), and *caudal* (lower tailbone) anesthesia is given by injecting long-acting anesthetics into the space surrounding the spinal cord nerves in the mid or lower back. You sit or lie on your side, with your back arched, so that a thin needle can be guided through the space between your backbone vertebrae. These blocks are very commonly used in orthopedic,

vascular, urologic, and gynecologic surgery. *Paracervical block* is given by numbing nerves on each side of the cervix, accomplished with anesthetics injected by a needle introduced through the vagina. This method is often chosen for gynecologic surgery such as a D&C. *Arm block* numbs part of or the entire arm. Anesthetic is injected around the large nerves between the neck and shoulder, in the armpit, or at various locations in the arm itself. This type of block is used for orthopedic, vascular, and plastic surgery. *Tourniquet/intravenous Bier block* injects anesthetic into your veins below a tourniquet and can be used to anesthetize the arm and hand. The anesthesia rapidly disappears after the tourniquet is released. This technique is usually used for orthopedic and plastic surgery procedures where a tourniquet is desirable. *Intercostal nerve block* can be given for some chest and abdominal procedures. The anesthetic is injected in the back between several ribs. *Regional neck nerve block*, by injecting anesthetic next to nerves in the neck, may even be preferred for thyroid gland and carotid artery surgery.

Usually, regional anesthetics are combined with sedation, because the procedures may take an hour or more, and the position required may be uncomfortable. They are most often given by an anesthesiologist and are rarely performed outside of a monitored operating room.

One drawback to spinal anesthesia is that the initial entry of the needle into the spinal canal can occasionally be difficult, particularly in older patients. After spinal anesthesia, some people experience headaches, neckaches, or backaches lasting for several days or, rarely, even longer. One English study of 11,000 women showed that those with back pain affecting their lifestyle had a higher rate of previous epidural anesthesia.[14] The pain was felt due not to the needle stick or anesthetic itself, but to inadvertent back strain occurring during the time they were unable to feel pain, while under the influence of the anesthetic. Newly triggered chronic migraine headaches were found in 2.9 percent of the women who had received an epidural during the previous year, in comparison to a 1.1 percent rate in those who had not. Choosing an epidural for labor pain may increase your risk for cesarean section: a number of studies have shown as much as a two-and-a-half times increased risk, when patients who chose an epidural were compared with those who did not, although one recent review did not find such association. The mechanism appears to be a marked slowing of the second stage of labor.

If you must have a cesarean section, regional anesthesia is then a particularly appropriate choice, so that you can see your baby immediately, and avoid the risks of general anesthesia. Maternal deaths during labor and delivery are most commonly due to general anesthesia.[15]

General Anesthesia

At present, most major operations are still performed under general anesthesia. Usually, you are wheeled on a stretcher to the operating room. After being transferred to the operating table, your IV lines and monitoring devices are set up. You are asked to breathe pure oxygen through a mask. If you have had premedication, either the night before or just before surgery, you may feel groggy even before the general anesthetic is delivered.

The induction into sleep is accomplished by an intravenous injection. You drift off in a matter of seconds. Once you are asleep, you may be *intubated*, a procedure in which an *endotracheal tube* is placed directly through your mouth into your trachea, the pipelike breathing structure leading to your lungs. Not all operations under general anesthesia require this tube, but most major procedures do. You are then kept asleep with vaporized anesthesia gases, which can be quickly eliminated when the operation is over. General anesthetic agents are often used in combination with muscle relaxants, in order to produce the desired effects quickly and fully.

A new general anesthetic technique employs a *laryngeal mask airway (LMA)*, a floppy, flat, soft plastic device that fits over the opening to the windpipe at the back of your mouth. While delivering the anesthetic gasses to the lungs, it protects against saliva and stomach secretions being sucked into your windpipe. Much less irritation to the vocal cords and trachea occurs than with an endotracheal tube, but it can still give you a sore throat. LMA can be used for shorter operations under "lighter" levels of general anesthesia, whenever muscle relaxation is not required.

Only since the mid-1930s has complete anesthesia during an operation been really safe, though it still carries a risk and may be the most hazardous part of your operation. Damage to the liver and kidneys, heart failure, fluctuations in blood pressure, irregular heart rhythms, and allergic reactions are the main problems. Also, you are more likely to have nausea, vomiting, or disorientation upon awakening, although this has been greatly reduced with the use of the newest anesthetics. As noted, the endotracheal tube may give you a sore throat and a raspy voice for a few days postoperatively.

In 1992 Dr. Ellison Pierce at Harvard estimated the mortality rate caused by anesthesia to be 1 or 2 per 100,000 or 200,000.[16] In 1987, the number of deaths per year due to anesthesia was estimated to be 2,000, and half were felt to be a result of mistakes, according to University of California at Los Angeles's Dr. Ronald Katz.[17]

Which is your better choice for major surgery—regional block or general anesthesia? It may help to answer this question by noting that in one study, 68 percent of the anesthesiologists stated that they would choose regional routes for themselves and their families.[18] Why this preference? The likeliest reason is *safety*. The liver, kidneys, and entire metabolism are less burdened. You also remain more alert and more able to practice the mind-body techniques detailed in Chapter 2.

Alternative Anesthesia: Acupuncture

Although more than 4,500 years old, the practice of acupuncture is still relatively untried in the West. Despite research supporting its usefulness, only a few centers, such as the University of Pennsylvania Medical Center, offer acupuncture as an alternative form of anesthesia. When correspondent James Reston of the *New York Times* needed an emergency appendectomy while on assignment in China, he received acupuncture anesthesia with good results. Through his reporting, he first made Westerners aware of this strange-appearing procedure. Astonishing films of Chinese patients sipping tea and talking while having major abdominal, thoracic, and even brain surgery, have focused attention on the possibilities of this type of anesthesia.

Allen, *a 59-year-old attorney, required knee surgery, to repair a ruptured cartilage, and needed to make a choice about anesthesia. He considered conventional regional methods, but decided to investigate acupuncture. He found a hospital, the University of Pennsylvania Hospital in Philadelphia, that allowed him to choose this approach. He was able to avoid the side effects of a spinal injection, and felt that his recovery from the operation was also enhanced by the acupuncture.*

How does this system really work? Newer research points to specific nervous and hormonal mechanisms, as discussed in Chapter 2. Acupuncture appears to exert its effects through established nerve networks: the insertion of a needle stimulates the nearby nerves, and also affects pain-sensing nerves in other areas of the body and/or the brain's interpretation of pain signals. In addition, secretion of local and central endorphins and serotonin, the body's natural painkillers and hormones of tranquillity, is increased. Acupuncture anesthesia even works in animals, and a number of veterinarians now successfully use this modality.

Acupuncture is effective, but not always totally pain-free. The acupuncture needles can sometimes cause discomfort during or after insertion, even though they are much smaller than the standard needles used to give injections. Usually stainless steel, though occasionally silver, the needles are inserted at depths ranging from one-half to a full inch. Continuous twirling has, for the most part, been replaced by continuous electrical stimulation. A small electrical device is connected to the needles by wires, to provide minute tingling impulses.

The main advantage of acupuncture for surgical anesthesia is that it is markedly free of side effects. General anesthetics, as noted, can impair body organ function and cause allergic reactions. Acupuncture anesthesia causes minimal local discomfort, no adverse effect on organ function, no change in mental awareness, and recovery is immediate. It is especially useful in obstetrics, where it has been documented to shorten labor and even induce delayed labor.[19] Acupuncture anesthesia allows cesarean section patients to remain alert while their babies are born, and avoids the postop restrictions necessitated by spinal anesthetics.

Neurosurgery, thyroidectomy, thoracic surgery, including lung resection and heart operations, breast removal, gastrectomy—the list of operations successfully performed with acupuncture anesthesia is virtually endless. The Chinese have found a 90 percent success rate when acupuncture is chosen for anesthesia, but they allow only 20 percent of surgical patients to opt for this method, since conventional anesthesia is more uniformly simple and effective. The future may find more such services available in Western hospitals—acupuncture is now an elective for medical students at a number of American medical schools, and many states now license non-M.D.s to practice this therapy.

You may think you would prefer to be totally "out of it" while your operation is performed. However, in an encouraging and supportive atmosphere, your chances of a good outcome may be greatly enhanced with the conscious participation made possible by this anesthesia method.

Alternative Anesthesia: Hypnosis

Perhaps it was hypnosis that God used to make Adam fall into a "deep sleep" while his rib was removed. Used by the ancient Egyptians and the American Indians, hypnosis has recently been studied in the Western setting, both as anesthesia and as an adjunct to treatment, with very promising results. Hypnosis was approved by the American Medical Association as a "valuable medical tool" in 1967. An official American Society of Clinical Hypnosis conducts classes to train physicians to become hypnotists. Possibilities for therapeutic applications before and after surgery are very encouraging, and its use as anesthesia quite intriguing.

Risk-free, and without side effects, it can be employed on its own, or as a adjunct to local or regional block. For example, Dr. Bari Bett, a physician in Arlington, Virginia, had been using hypnosis for her patients, and decided to choose it herself, as anesthesia for her own operation. She had a laparoscopic tubal ligation using hypnoanesthesia and an anesthetic injected around her belly button prior to the incision.[20] A 2000 study in *Lancet* documented self-hypnotized patients undergoing uncomfortable invasive medical procedures had less need for pain medication, more stable blood pressure, fewer heart problems, less anxiety, and shorter operative times than patients receiving standard medication or structured attention distraction methods.[21]

The word "hypnosis," meaning "to put to sleep," was coined by James Braid in 1842, before he realized that this was not a form of sleep. You may think that it requires a "weaker" person in order to be hypnotized, but quite the contrary is true. More intelligent, active people do better with hypnosis. A new test to tell whether you can be successfully hypnotized measures the level of homovanillic acid in your cerebrospinal fluid.[22] When applied as anesthesia, hypnosis can be remarkably effective. In one demonstration film, a patient is shown singing while having abdominal surgery!

J*an, a 28-year-old mother, disliked the side effects of the drugs given for pain relief during her previous difficult labor. She noticed an advertisement from an obstetrician who utilized hypnosis. She chose this form of anesthesia for her second child, and loved the experience, sailing through her labor and delivery without difficulty, staying relaxed enough even to laugh through her contractions.*

Much of the experience with hypnosis as anesthesia has been derived from obstetrics. You can be trained in hypnosis during early pregnancy, and be carried quite successfully through labor and even cesarean section solely with this technique. You can learn to use certain fingers as yes and no signals, so your hypnosis can even be conducted over the phone. Your hypnotist asks you to raise your finger when you are fully under hypnosis, and your surgeon reports over the phone when you do so. Your hypnotist then informs your surgeon to start the procedure.

How does hypnosis relieve pain? One proposed pathway suggests that hypnosis lowers the rate of release of the neurokinin hormones in the area of the incision that are necessary for pain nerve impulse transmission to the brain. This effect, in combination with central blocking mechanisms within the brain's pain perception centers, interfere with pain recognition. In the book *One Surgeon's Experience with Hypnosis*,[23] Dr. Ernest Werbel discusses his success using hypnosis for analgesia and anesthesia even in emergency situations. Another book, *Hypnosis in Obstetrics*,[24] documents the use of hypnosis in 1,000 deliveries. Patients were taught the technique in small groups. The resulting cesarean section rate of 2.2 percent was thought to be due to the increased relaxation combined with the absence of the labor-slowing side effects of pain-relieving drugs.[25] In contrast, at many hospitals, the C-section rate is now 25 to 30 percent.

Is there anything to fear from hypnosis? Some myths still continue. It is not possible to get a hypnotized subject to reveal anything that they do not wish to reveal. You *cannot* be hypnotized against your will.

Hypnosis can also be utilized to help your own body's resources aid the healing process. As discussed more fully in Chapter 2, it may help you come through surgery successfully, and assist your incision to heal.

Self-hypnosis methods are discussed in Chapter 2; you can utilize these as adjuncts to your anesthesia. Hopefully, all anesthesiologists will soon be taught this advantageous nontoxic anesthetic method, along with acupuncture, as a routine part of their training.

The Operating Room

Most operating rooms are not friendly, inviting environments. The furniture includes the adjustable operating table, a table or two for instruments, two or three stools, the gas machine for anesthesia, and perhaps other special equipment, such as a heart-lung machine. Large, adjustable lights are suspended from the ceiling. Walls and ceiling are usually white or light pastel tiles. Personnel wear masks, caps, green or blue "scrub" shirts, pants, wraparound gowns, and booties. Gloves are worn whenever there may be contact with blood or any body secretions. There are no distracting decorations. Such simplicity is felt to help concentration upon the work at hand, maximize cleanliness, and make for easy and rapid room cleaning between cases. Operating rooms are quite chilly, kept that way so the bright, hot lights and thick gowns won't overheat the staff. The overall effect is intimidating, high-tech, and sterile.

Is this really the best environment for the healing of a needy body, and the relaxation of the personnel? In a moving passage, Yale surgeon and writer Richard Selzer describes the need for more "life" in the OR:

Not long ago, operating rooms had windows. It was a boon and a blessing in spite of the occasional fly that managed to strain through the screens and threaten our very sterility. For the adventurous insect drawn to such a ravishing spectacle, a quick swat and presto, the door to the next world sprang open. But for us who battled on, there was the benediction of the sky, the applause and reproach of thunder. A divine consultation crackled in on the lightning and at night in an emergency there was the pomp, the longevity of the stars to deflate a surgeon's ego.

It did no patient a disservice to have heaven looking over his doctor's shoulder. I very much fear that having bricked up our windows we have severed a celestial connection. To work in windowless rooms is to live in a jungle where you cannot see the sky. Because there is no sky to see, there is no grand vision of God. Instead there are the numberless fragmented spirits that lurk behind leaves, beneath streams; the one is no better than the other, no worse. Still a man is entitled to the temple of his preference. Mine lies out on a prairie, wondering up at heaven or in a many windowed operating room where just outside the panes of glass, cows graze and the stars shine down upon my carpentry.[26]

Ask your surgeon and anesthesiologist to keep you warm. Even in this chilly environment it is possible to keep you covered as much as possible, and to use external warming devices such as the Bair Hugger, which circulates warm air through a thin plastic membrane pressed against your body. Patients maintaining normal temperature have been shown to have decreased risk of major heart complications.[27] In a 2001 *Lancet* report, Dr. Andrew Melling reported a study of 421 patients randomized to receive local warming to the area of the incision, whole body warming, or no warming beginning at least thirty minutes prior to surgery. A variety of operations were studied. They found that the wound infection rate was three times higher (14 percent versus 5 percent) in the group that was not warmed.[28]

One simple way in which to bring more "life" into the operating room is to introduce music. Many ORs are equipped for this, and the choices can add to a harmonious experience. Recent evidence suggests that when your surgeon chooses the music to play during the operation, his or her stress may be decreased and performance improved.[29] If your taste is different from that of your surgeon, you may use a small portable tape player with headphones, choosing the music best suited for you. Even when you are unconscious, you can still register the music in your subconscious. You may need less pain medication.[30]

What goes on within the operating room while you are having the operation is far more important than was originally thought. Humorous exchanges and negative remarks are often the rule. However, as mentioned earlier, several studies have shown you can hear and subconsciously remember what is said even while under anesthesia.[31] An intriguingly designed study compared patients to whom the sentence "Friday is Robinson Crusoe's apprentice" was repeated while they were under anesthesia with a control group not given this sentence. When asked postsurgically, "What is Friday?" the first group responded it was Robinson Crusoe's apprentice 60 percent of the time, while the control group only named it as a day of the week, with no one mentioning its connection to Robinson Crusoe.[32]

Some patients have said that negative remarks have continued to haunt them for years. On the other hand, positive suggestions may have markedly beneficial effects, which can likewise register for long periods of time.

Even sympathetic surgeons may have a hard time accepting the idea that their negative remarks and/or positive suggestions can make a profound difference. Much scientific research from biofeedback, hypnosis, and mind-body investigations, however, indicate that the body *does* respond to suggestions. You can enlist the aid of your surgeon and anesthesiologist to monitor remarks in the operating room, give you specific positive suggestions, and tell you what you yourself can do to contribute to the success of your operation.

Dr. Bernie Siegel pioneered this approach, and his staff testified to the difference it made in the patients. At the very least, it may be worth a try. Special tapes with positive suggestions are available, listed at the back of this book. The most effective approach seems to be music, combined with suggestions. If your surgeon or anesthesiologist needs to make a specific positive suggestion to you, such as "Help us out, don't bleed so much," your headphones can be removed for a moment. Chapters 2 and 24 discuss more fully how your unconscious self may register sug-

gestions and your body respond in ways similar to hypnosis, and summarize the specific requests to make of your surgeon and anesthesiologist.

Early Postoperative Period

The early postoperative period is when you are waking up from anesthesia in the recovery room and, possibly, during an initial stay in the intensive care unit until your blood pressure and heart, lung, and kidney functions are stabilized. Usually patients are in the recovery room for an hour or so. If an ICU (intensive care unit) stay is necessary, it usually lasts at least overnight.

The Recovery Room

After the operation is complete, you are moved to the recovery room for close observation during the next hour or so. If you were given general anesthesia, the endotracheal tube is usually removed in the operating room, and you will probably be first again aware of your surroundings in the recovery room.

The recovery room contains anywhere from one to eight or more patients in various stages of waking up. The nurses constantly hover around you, checking your "vital signs"—blood pressure, heart rate and rhythm, breathing efficiency, and urine output if you have a bladder catheter. You are hooked up to intravenous lines and monitoring wires. Be prepared for the groans and cries of other patients, as they wake up with discomfort and disorientation. Recovery from minor operations, especially with local or regional anesthesia, is much more pleasant. Outpatient surgery recovery rooms are quieter, better decorated, and less hectic overall.

Postoperative recovery is a critical time. Especially in longer operations, the amount of anesthetic that must be given puts you in a vulnerable position. Nausea is common, and if vomiting were to develop, some of it could be sucked into your lungs, causing pneumonia. Rapid shifts in blood pressure are also frequent. Low blood pressure is treated with extra fluids or blood, combined with elevation of the legs. High blood pressure is treated with medication. You are watched for bleeding. Rarely, a return to the operating room may be needed to open up the incision and tie off bleeding vessels. Your blood oxygen level is monitored by a device which fits on your finger. If you are unable to maintain safe levels, the breathing tube may have to be reinserted.

Here is a helpful hint. *Be prepared:* Nausea, vomiting, and pain are commonly experienced postoperatively. Intravenous morphine or Demerol are often given for pain relief, and these drugs may produce nausea. You may be cold and shivering. Most recovery rooms, therefore, provide warmed blankets and heating devices, to offset the air-conditioning of the OR and the chilliness induced by exposure during the operation and by low blood pressure.

Your throat is likely to be sore from the breathing tube. Ice chips and a hot washcloth on the throat can help. Chloraseptic is one throat spray documented to alleviate sore throats.

Positive suggestions can be very useful here, and can be given by your surgeon, anesthesiologist, nurses, and bedside friend or relative. You may also continue to listen to your portable tape player, using relaxation and visualization tapes, via headphones.

Disorientation is frequent as you emerge from anesthesia. You may have experienced something similar while you were traveling, when you awakened in a different bed, and had a moment before you realized where you were. The tubes, paraphernalia, and starkness of most recovery rooms contribute to this effect, especially in older individuals. Hallucinations may even follow, as a side effect of the drugs you have been given.

Some of the newer drugs used by anesthesiologists reduce nausea (ondansetron, metaclopramide, propofol) and produce a sense of well-being (propofol), thus counteracting these problems to some extent.

Hospitals allow interpreters in the recovery room. Some also now allow relatives to be with you there. An excellent addition from several points of view, they can help orient you, give you positive suggestions and encouragement, and watch you for complications more closely than an overburdened nursing staff can. That this is an important time for close vigilance can't be overemphasized: our cousin died of an allergic reaction that went unnoticed while she was in a recovery room.

One Utah center uses special chair-beds: they start out as beds, but can be raised into chairs as you become more alert, allowing you to reorient more easily, and go home sooner.

Studies need to be conducted of the optimum environment for recovery—if recovery rooms were not so barren-looking, would the process of awakening from anesthesia be easier? The fruits of mind-body research may yet influence recovery room design. Colors and windows might help both the patients and the healthcare workers.

The Intensive Care Unit

After emerging from the anesthetic in the recovery room, especially if you have had a long or difficult operation or have severe medical problems, you may be moved to the ICU. Being monitored here could prove lifesaving, should postoperative bleeding, irregular heartbeat, heart failure, breathing difficulties, or other complications develop.

Time spent in the ICU is variable, from a few hours to a few days. Monitor disks are placed on your chest, so that your heart's activity can be watched on a television monitor in your room and at the nurses' station. Hourly or even more frequent readings are obtained of your blood pressure, fluid intake, urine output, and body temperature.

Some hospitals are making efforts to humanize these special rooms too, but most medical centers still have very unpleasant-looking ICUs, oriented for technical function but with little that inspires your body's natural antipain mechanisms, the endorphins and other hormones of healing.

Just like the recovery room, the ICU can be quite disorienting and uncomfortable. Visitors are often limited to the immediate family and even they are only allowed for short periods. Here again, use of the music tapes, visualization, and nice pictures could be helpful. If possible, you might prepare someone beforehand to give you assistance at this time, using the methods from Chapter 2, to lessen the dehumanizing aspects of the life-amidst-machines of the usual ICU.

Alternative Methods of Nausea and Vomiting Relief

Nausea following surgery may directly result from the operation itself or be a side effect of the anesthesia or postsurgical pain medication. Trying an alternative anesthetic or using alternative approaches to diminish

your need for pain-relieving drugs may help prevent or limit your experience of such common postsurgical nausea.

Acupressure massage stimulation given just below the inner aspect of your wrist, on the side of your thumb—the acupuncture site called Pericardium 6—has been reported to help relieve nausea associated with anesthesia.[33]

If you are unable to take anything by mouth, you can still obtain the benefits of the herbs ginger, cinnamon, peppermint, and chamomile via aromatherapy: sniffing the vapors of fresh-brewed teas or using aromatherapy extracts of these herbs, obtainable from most health food stores.

Once you can take liquids, the powerful ability of the herb ginger to curb nausea, no matter what the cause, can be tapped by grating the fresh root into a tea, using the powder as a tea or capsule, or finding a sugar-free ginger ale that actually contains the root or its extract. Cinnamon, peppermint, or chamomile tea may also prove useful.

Late Postoperative Period

The late postoperative period includes the time necessary for return of your usual body functions and basic activities of daily living prior to hospital discharge. Depending on your operation, it may be a matter of hours or many days.

Postoperative Pain Control

Most surgery leads to pain and discomfort. Even with minor operations, the body is being asked to adjust to quite significant changes, including fluid loss, bruising, swelling, infectious organisms, and associated phenomena.

You can act to help yourself heal by adding alternative medicine approaches.

Types of Pain Medication

Postoperative pain can be controlled by several classes of drugs. As noted, opioid-based medications, or *narcotics,* are most commonly given initially. Morphine, hydromorphone, codeine, and meperidene are the generic forms, with common trade names such as Dilaudid, Demerol, Tylenol #3, Percocet, Vicodin, and Roxicet. These drugs are very effective in alleviating pain. However, they can cause you to feel unpleasantly "high" or nauseated. They also have addictive potential if used for many weeks.

The antiinflammatory medications include the nonsteroidal antiinflammatory drugs (NSAIDs) such as ketorolac (Torudol), ibuprofen (Motrin, Advil, Nuprin), and naproxen (Naprosen, Aleve). They can be very effective and have little effect on mental status, but rarely, cause ulcers and bleeding tendency, and can affect kidney function.

Aspirin (Ecotrin, Emperin) and acetaminophen (Tylenol) are the common over-the-counter antiinflammatory drugs. Aspirin has few side effects if taken in prescribed dosages, but can prolong bleeding, irritate the stomach, and cause ulcers. Acetaminophen in excessive dosage can cause liver failure. Other types of pain relievers with mild addictive potential include propoxyphene (Darvon), and pentazocine (Talwin).

Methods of Pain Control Administration

Pain relievers can be delivered by several different methods, depending on the area of the body affected and your expected intensity and duration of pain.

Epidural Catheters

The "Cadillac" of postoperative pain control is the *epidural catheter.* This method is commonly used in major abdominal surgery on the colon, stomach, and blood vessels, and can also be chosen for chest surgery and procedures on the legs. A tiny catheter (tube) is inserted just before your operation, in a manner similar to administering a spinal anesthetic. The catheter is threaded through a small needle introduced into the epidural space next to the spinal cord and pain nerves are then "blocked" (numbed) with intermittent or continuous injections of anesthetic or narcotic-based drugs. The catheter is usually used for a few days after the surgery, and then removed as you are switched to another form of pain control. The advantage of this method is excellent pain relief, allowing you early postoperative exercise, deep breathing, and coughing, with little effect on your mental status. Disadvantages include expense, difficulty urinating in some patients, and possibility of an overdose, which could cause you to stop breathing.

Intravenous Medication

Pain can be relieved most quickly and effectively by intravenous injection of narcotics. This method is commonly employed after major surgery, when discomfort is expected to be significant, especially if you are unable to eat, drink, or take pain pills immediately after your operation.

Patient-controlled anesthesia, or *PCA,* can be chosen whenever an intravenous route is expected to be used for a few days. In this method, when you start to feel pain, you can punch a button to add a pump-delivered prescribed dose of painkiller through your IV line. Your doctor programs your PCA machine, so that you cannot give yourself too much or too frequent amounts of medication.

Intramuscular Injection

This method provides pain relief similar to that of the intravenous route, but the effect is more gradual and longer lasting. Of course, intramuscular needle sticks are more uncomfortable than IV line injections. This route is usually preferred immediately postoperatively when you are not expected to have severe pain, and are likely to be soon discharged home. Narcotics such as Demerol and morphine, or antiinflammatories such as Torudol, are the usual drugs given.

Pain Pills

Once you are successfully taking fluids, you can be switched to oral medications. Most likely, when you are discharged from the hospital or outpatient surgery, you are given a supply to take home with you. By far the most common prescriptions are codeine variations with trades names such as Tylenol #3, Vicodin, Percocet, and Roxicet. Stronger members of the opium derivative family such as morphine and Dilaudid are rarely prescribed. These pills are usually taken every four to six hours as necessary. OxyContin, MsContin, and Kadian are examples of controlled-release opioid-based formulations that are designed to eliminate the peaks and troughs of pain intensity commonly experienced with the regular preparations. They can be taken every eight to twenty-four hours as directed and can be adjusted as necessary to keep you comfortable.

The more potent the drug, the better the pain relief, but also, the stronger the side effects such as nausea, constipation, mental status alteration (drowsiness, disorientation, mood changes), and addictive potential. Use them only as needed, and for as limited a time as possible. You should not drive a car, operate machinery, or do anything requiring close attention while you are taking these medications. You can switch to nonnarcotics as soon as possible.

Antiinflammatories such as ibuprofen (Motrin, Advil) can be prescribed if you are sensitive to opium-based drugs. Darvon is a different type of pain reliever, with less addictive potential, and can be tried if the other drugs are undesirable.

Local Measures

Ice packs can be applied over the dressing of a fresh wound. This will often decrease pain and swelling in the first twenty-four to forty-eight hours. After this period, a heating pad may be helpful. In general, and especially if you have had anal surgery, sitting in a warm tub may be the most effective thing you can do. Elevation of the operated area, if possible, will decrease pain, throbbing, and swelling. Make sure your doctor agrees with these methods before trying them.

Alternative Medicine Methods of Pain Relief

Pain increases your level of stress, inhibiting your body's ability to heal, as discussed in Chapter 2. As you shall see, the alternative medical techniques of homeopathy, acupuncture, massage, yoga practice, meditation, hypnosis, music, and certain herbal remedies have all been scientifically validated as useful for postsurgical pain relief. Other promising options include visualization, biofeedback, magnetic devices, laughter, and aromatherapy. Application of these techniques can reduce your need for pain medication, helping you avoid the side effects of drugs. Review Chapter 2, and choose the approaches most suitable to you. Prepare yourself by having pictures, and arranging for music, massage, and supportive family and friends.

A very promising first step for achieving pain relief after your operation is to take the homeopathic remedies arnica and hypericum, in doses of four 30C to 200C pellets under the tongue, every fifteen minutes until the pain improves, and then four times daily until it is gone. Double-blind research has shown diminished pain from this regimen after dental surgery.[34]

Several studies have demonstrated the ability of acupuncture to reduce postoperative pain. Acupuncture was found even better at pain relief than the commonly used painkiller Demerol.[35] Another study showed that acupuncture-treated patients experienced significantly less postoperative pain after oral surgery than a placebo "sham acupuncture" group.[36]

In research conducted at the University of Virginia Medical Center, patients given a forty-five-minute massage before and after their surgery needed less pain medication, developed fewer complications, and were able to go home from one to four days sooner than patients who did not receive massage.[37]

Yoga practice has been found to be very helpful in pain relief. Subjects taught to meditate were shown to be able to tolerate increased levels of experimentally induced pain.[38] Especially recommended are the yoga breathing exercises, particularly alternate nostril breathing, as described in Chapter 2. Start very gently, and be careful not to strain. You can use yoga, meditation and relaxation tapes, as listed at the back of this book.

Hypnosis can markedly reduce or eliminate pain.[39] Patients who listened to hypnotic relaxation tapes, with guided therapeutic suggestions and music, were found to have less pain and took fewer narcotics.[40] Simply listening to music has been shown to decrease postoperative pain,[41] and patients who listened to music they chose reported less pain while stitches were placed.[42] Anxiety levels have also been shown to be reduced through the use of music.[43] Easy listening or classical music may provide more pain relief than rock music.[44] Ocean sounds have been shown to help postsurgical patients sleep better and wake less.[45]

The amino acid tryptophan has been shown to allow patients to endure higher levels of experimentally induced pain, when compared to placebo.[46] This amino acid was taken out of health food stores when some was contaminated, but is now available again in its precursor forms of dehydroepiandrosterone (DHEA) and 5-hydroxy-L-tryptophan (5-HTP). You can take one tablet every four to six hours, as needed. Creams containing topical arnica, termed "the bruise plant" in Native American medicine traditions, or capsaicin, the main hot ingredient of red peppers, can be rubbed on sore muscles to help them relax, or around (but not on) your incision.

Electrical stimulation utilizes electrodes to control pain, and many hospitals now offer it as an option to painkilling drugs. Twenty minutes or so of therapy twice a day may be all that is needed. As noted, and as your mobility and healing allow, a hot bath or shower is another simple measure you can take to reduce pain. Just make certain not to allow your incision site to get wet in the first forty-eight hours. Sleep is also a great boon to pain relief, and helps speed your recovery. See Chapter 2 for alternative methods to help you obtain optimum sleep.

Intravenous Lines

After any major operation, you will very likely have an intravenous line for at least a few days. It may give you fluids if you cannot drink, salt solutions to adjust your body's chemistry, medications, antibiotics, and/or nutritional formulations, and be used to draw blood samples for lab analysis. One of several different types of IVs is chosen, depending on how long it is expected to be necessary, what must be given through the line, and the size of your veins.

Peripheral IVs

The simplest IV is a *peripheral line*, usually a short plastic catheter or "butterfly" needle placed into a vein of your hand or arm. It can be inserted with or without a small injection of skin anesthetic. These usually can be used for a day or two, after which they cause vein irritation, and must be changed to another location. If your IV solutions begin to create reddening or local pain, or leak into the surrounding tissues producing puffiness, a change in IV site becomes necessary.

A *heparin-lock IV*, or "hep-lock," is a short tubing connected to the IV catheter, kept filled with a small amount of heparin solution to prevent blood clotting, and capped off. It is not connected to an IV bottle. When you don't need continuous IV fluids but still must have injected medications, you can avoid the agony of repeated needle sticks via this device.

An *enterocoel IV*, or peripherally inserted central catheter (PICC) line, is a cross between a peripheral and a central IV. The long plastic catheter is passed from a vein in the middle part of your arm all the way up to a large vein in your chest. It can be used until it causes local irritation or becomes plugged, and is inserted at your bedside or in the X-ray department, after you are given a small amount of local anesthetic.

Central IVs

There are several different kinds of *central lines*. These IVs consist of a long tiny catheter threaded into one of your large, high-flow veins—usually the superior vena cava, the vein that connects with the right side of your heart.

A *subclavian* line is passed into the large vein under your collarbone, then manipulated to the vena cava. Likewise, an *IJ*, or *internal jugular* line, is passed through a large vein in your neck to reach the vena cava. Since these veins are large and blood flow is rapid, they are less likely to become plugged or allow medications and solutions to irritate your vessels.

These catheters are usually placed during your operation or at your bedside, using local anesthesia. Since deeper veins can't be seen or felt, your bed is cranked to a head-down position to distend them, making them easier to find. After skin preparation with an iodine solution, adjacent areas are covered with sterile drapes, and you are given local anesthesia. Your doctor finds the vein based on bony and muscle "landmarks." A needle is placed into it, and the catheter passed through the needle. A stitch or two holds the external part of the catheter securely to the skin and then it is covered with a small dressing. This process can be uncomfortable if it is hard to find your vein, not uncommon if your neck and shoulders are thick or muscular.

If central lines are expected to be necessary for more than a few weeks, a more permanent line, called a *Hickman* or *Groshong* catheter, can be inserted, usually in the operating room or X-ray department. After gaining access to a large vein as just described, the tip of the line is guided to the correct position using fluoroscopic X-ray. The catheter is then "tunneled" under the skin and brought out through a separate tiny incision. The external part of the tubing is covered with a dressing to prevent infection. These catheters have a small plastic cuff that remains under the skin in the tunnel, helping to prevent infection and keep them securely in place. The catheters come with one or two intravenous channels, and are easily removed at your bedside or in your doctor's office.

A *Portacath* is similar to other central lines except that a plastic or metal "port" is placed completely under the skin in a pocket usually two or three inches below your collarbone. A similar device, the PassPort, is placed in your inner upper arm beneath the skin. To access the port, the needle is passed directly through the skin, through a silicone sealing-disk, and on into the fluid chamber connected to the catheter. A port is usually chosen whenever need for intravenous access is regular but infrequent, commonly for chemotherapy doses given every three or four weeks. It is placed in an operating room or X-ray department using X-ray guidance, and has the advantage of no external parts to keep clean or cover with a dressing. The disadvantage is that you must endure a needle stick each time it is used, and a minor operation is necessary to have it removed.

The most common immediate complication of placing a central IV is the puncture of a lung, causing its collapse. This only happens in 1 percent of all cases, but you might require a chest tube for a few days. Bleeding from inadvertent puncture of a large artery or vein is very uncommon. You may have some swelling, bruising, and soreness for a few days. Often, a central IV is less bother than an arm IV.

Problems with IVs

You may hear an alarm on the IV pump beep if fluid flow becomes blocked in your catheter. Don't panic; it is extremely unlikely you are in any danger. Usually the source is a kink in the IV tubing. Call a nurse to investigate the problem.

All types of IVs eventually need to be removed or replaced, since they leak, become plugged, or cause a local vein irritation, vein blockage, or infection. Sometimes, if the catheter is simply plugged with a blood clot, it can be opened by injecting clot-dissolving medication into it. Arm IVs need to be changed frequently, but central lines can be used for more extended periods. The Portacath, Hickman, and Groshong catheters can be maintained for months.

The vein in your arm or hand may be irritated for several weeks after your IV is removed. It may develop a tender, slightly reddened, firm cord. Moist heat is soothing, and should resolve the problem.

Central catheters can cause a narrowing or complete blockage of a larger vein, leading to arm or neck swelling. You then might need the catheter removed, followed by temporary blood-thinning medication.

Postoperative Nutrition

If your surgery was relatively minor, and you can at least take fluids immediately after the operation, follow the nutrition guidelines given in Chapter 2. You can begin with the Superdrinks, then continue to follow the low-fat, high-fiber program, for your optimum return to health.

After most operations, you are given regular food on the evening of your surgery, or the next day. If you have had an abdominal operation, your intestinal function is tested cautiously, starting oral intake with your doctor's order for "clear liquids only." This is a specific diet consisting of water, black coffee (although Sandra recommends herbal teas only, especially chamomile), broth, and some juices. Clear liquids are chosen because if you were to vomit and these liquids got into your lungs, they would be less dangerous than solid food from more advanced diets. After you have been successful with this intake, with no signs of nausea, vomiting, or abdominal distention, your doctor may order "advance as tolerated."

The next step up is full liquids, which adds milk, custard, and some soups. A soft or regular diet follows, depending on your ability to chew. Special diets such as low-residue, post-gastrectomy (more frequent, smaller feedings), diabetic, or low-sodium, may be given, depending on your operation and underlying medical problems.

Your body, in order to repair itself, needs lots of supplemental calories and proteins after surgery. Otherwise, you would break down your own tissues to simply supply your energy needs, with little left for your healing. This is especially true if your illness caused you to lose weight before your operation. A hospital dietitian may visit with you to assess your nutritional state and make dietary recommendations to you and your doctors. "Calorie counts," which measure and record your actual calorie and protein intake, may be useful, to keep track of your progress.

It is very common to lose your appetite after any type of operation, especially if you have been ill for a prolonged period. Anesthesia gases, drugs, and pain medications can cause nausea and vomiting. Hiccups can be distressing. The passage of time, and becoming as active as possible, helps restore your desire for food. Meanwhile, you can supplement your meals with nutritional preparations such as the Superdrink 1 or 2 (Sandra's preferred choice) or a liquid meal replacement. Nausea can be controlled by medication.

If you have had surgery involving your gastrointestinal tract, your doctor may not want you to take anything by mouth for several days after the operation. You may not be able to fulfill your nutrient requirements orally for a few days or even much longer after major surgery. If you have a complication, it may be several weeks or more before you are eating normally again.

Over the last thirty years, surgeons have done much outstanding research on nutrition and have developed many strategies to provide whatever you need. If you are not allowed to eat or drink anything, or can't force yourself to do so, sugars given intravenously will provide enough energy to protect you for a few days, assuming you were in reasonably good nutritional status before the operation. If you are unable to resume eating for a more extended period, you may require a feeding tube or a high-powered IV nutritional program, as described below.

Feeding tubes are usually small-diameter tubes passed through the nose and on into the stomach or first part of the small intestine. They are much less irritating than the larger, stiffer NG tubes used to suction out the stomach. Surprisingly, those placed in the small intestine can be used almost immediately after your operation, since function here returns much sooner than in the stomach and colon. Research suggests that this method of nutrition is superior to intravenous feeding. When it may not be safe for you to eat for an extended period, these tubes can be placed directly into the small intestine at the time of surgery and brought out through your abdominal wall, thereby avoiding the discomfort of a nose tube. When they are no longer needed, they can be simply removed in your doctor's office.

If a feeding tube is needed for many weeks, months, or even permanently, a *percutaneous endoscopic gastrostomy*, or *PEG tube*, can be chosen. This tube is inserted directly into your stomach and brought out through the abdominal wall without "opening" your abdomen. The placement procedure is performed using sedation and local anesthesia. You lie on your back while your doctor passes a long, flexible gastroscope through your mouth, then on into your stomach. The light on the tip of the scope is maneuvered to push the front wall of your stomach up against your abdominal wall. Local anesthetic is injected at that point and a small incision made. The tube is then passed through the abdominal and stomach walls, and the tip of the tube positioned in the stomach or passed into the small intestine by the scope. A plastic flange on the inner wall of the stomach and another on the skin hold the tube tightly in place. Afterward, you may have mild discomfort at the incision site. Complications include bleeding and dislocation of the tube. If it is inadvertently pulled out before your stomach has healed against the inside of the abdominal wall, a leak may occur, requiring a surgical operation for repair. After a few weeks, the tube can be safely removed or changed.

Feeding tubes can be used continuously or intermittently, and can supply all of your nutritional needs, or supplement your oral intake, if it is not sufficient. The feedings are run in by a pump or by gravity.

If your intestinal tract cannot function whatsoever, all of your nutritional needs must be given intravenously. This may be the case if you have an intestinal blockage or fistula (leakage of bowel contents onto the skin), a disorder such as Crohn's disease interfering with the bowel's absorption function, severe pancreatitis, or have had a large amount of intestine removed. This method, called *total parenteral nutrition (TPN)*, or *hyperalimentation*, can be utilized for prolonged periods of time, even permanently, given by one of the central line catheters described above. It can also be given continuously or intermittently. Complications include problems with the IV line and body chemistry imbalance, so frequent blood tests may be necessary.

If you are otherwise able to leave the hospital, you can set up the tube-feeding or TPN program at home. Nursing services are available to provide the tube feedings or IV bottles, troubleshoot any problems, and monitor your progress.

Return of Bowel and Bladder Function

When the body is subjected to anesthesia and major surgery, both the bowels and bladder can be affected. Swallowed air and decreased or uncoordinated intestinal activity can cause bloating, cramping, and hiccups. Pain medications also typically slow intestinal movement. In addition, being in a strange environment, combined with disturbance of your usual dietary habits, contributes to disruption of your accustomed patterns. It may take a week or longer before your bowels work normally again, particularly after an abdominal operation.

A stool softener, bulking agent, laxative, enema, or suppository may be helpful.

Men with a history of prostate symptoms may discover that their difficulties with urination have worsened after surgery, and may take some time to improve. A bladder tube or catheter may be necessary for a few days. However, whenever possible, bladder tubes should not be left in place, since this can induce infection; it is better to be intermittently catheterized, which significantly decreases your chances of infection.

Most of all, early mobilization helps to hasten return of normal bowel and bladder function: patients who are up and walking about do much better.

You can also apply the skills given in Chapter 2 to assist your bladder and bowel function. Follow the directions for guided deep relaxation and visualization. For example, you may imagine your bowel as a gentle freight train, whistling through the countryside, and feel this happening within your digestive tract. Repeat three to five times daily, for five to fifteen minutes.

Postoperative Activity

Immobilization is responsible for many of the complications of surgery. You lose 1 percent of remaining muscle strength for each day you remain in bed. Movement helps to minimize the potential for blood clots forming in the veins of your legs while you are lying horizontal in bed, and decreases amount of lung collapse. You are more mentally alert and feel better. Such advice for early mobilization is the opposite of previous recommendations, which suggested you stay inactive during the first few days after your operation.

Postsurgical Problems

The postoperative period is usually uncomfortable and the possibilities of complications developing adds to the ordinary anxiety. Knowing what to expect, what is common, and what to look out for can relieve a lot of your tension and worries.

Postoperative Fever

It is very common and natural to run a fever in the 100-degree range for several days after your operation. This reflects your body's reparative processes at work. Higher temperatures or any shaking chills may indicate an infection, and should be reported to your doctor.

Incision Problems

The normal healing process involves some pinking, mild swelling, and tenderness around your incision. After the first few days, you may feel a *healing ridge*, a linear, firm area underneath your incision. It is also common for the incision edges to be slightly separated, and a small amount of thin fluid to seep out.

A *hematoma* is a collection of blood clots in your incision. It is not dangerous, though it can predispose you to infection and delay incision healing. Small clots are reabsorbed over a period of days or weeks, but larger ones must be removed and your incision reclosed.

A *seroma* is a collection of thin fluid beneath the incision, often found where the operation lifted up a flap of skin, or in the space where a mass was removed. Smaller collections can be left alone, although larger ones should be removed with a needle and syringe.

Incision infection occurs in 2 to 10 percent of all operations, depending on whether the passage was clean or contaminated. When a surgical incision develops increasing swelling and pain, acquires a fiery redness, or exudes a cloudy, smelly fluid, it is probably infected. Some infected incisions can be treated with antibiotics, but if it contains pus, it needs to be opened fully, drained, and left open for dressing changes. Depending on its size, it will usually close spontaneously over days to weeks.

To help prevent an infection from developing, you may follow the nutrition and lifestyle guidelines given in Chapter 2. If you do develop an incision infection, please refer to the section on surgical and alternative medicine methods of treating skin infections, located in Chapter 5: "Skin."

Lung Problems

Lung problems are seen after 5 to 10 percent of all operations. The frequency is 5 percent in lower abdominal surgery (appendix, uterus, and prostate) and increases to 50 percent in upper abdominal surgery (gallbladder, stomach, pancreas, and spleen). Smokers have three times the risk of this problem. Lung complications are responsible for death in 25 percent of the patients who do not survive surgery, and are a significant contributing cause in another 25 percent.

Several factors may play a role in these postoperative complications. Anesthesia temporarily eliminates your cough reflex and your drive to breathe. If you inhale your secretions or stomach contents into your lungs, it can cause severe pneumonia. In the vulnerable early postoperative period, these effects linger for several hours. Your breathing efforts may be insufficient, leading your lungs to partially collapse, and you to become deficient in oxygen. You must be closely watched and supported, if necessary.

Postoperative pain also tends to limit your deep breathing and coughing efforts. Pain medication, especially narcotics such as morphine and Demerol, decrease respiratory drive and reflexes. Abdominal distention, common after abdominal surgery, limits your diaphragm motion, preventing full lung expansion. Nasogastric tubes, although necessary to remove stomach air and fluid accumulation, also decrease the cough reflex, and can create the conditions for the breathing of secretions into the lungs.

For all these reasons, collapse of small areas of your lung tissue, termed *atelectasis*, is very common after surgery, and is the most common cause of early postoperative fever. Findings of atelectasis on physical exam or chest X-ray develop in more than 50 percent of postoperative patients. Usually, as you become more active and breathe more normally, these changes clear up in a few days. If these airways are not reopened, pneumonia can result from the overgrowth of organisms behind the block. Even though you won't feel like it, you can help prevent these complications by breathing and coughing as deeply as you can immediately after your operation.

Surgery produces a temporary increase in your blood's tendency to clot. Bed rest and decreased activity are associated with sluggish blood flow in your pelvis and legs. Blood clots may form, which can then break loose and migrate to your lungs (*pulmonary embolus*), where they can cause severe breathing and heart problems, or even sudden death.

You can act to reduce your risk of lung problems after surgery by both preoperative and postoperative preventive measures. Cigarette smoke causes irritation and inflammation of your airway lining cells, along with increased secretions. Since the tiny *cilia*, the hairs that "beat" secretions and debris up and out of your lungs, become paralyzed, your ability to mobilize and cough out your secretions is decreased. Stopping smoking a few weeks before your operation will allow time for these harmful effects of smoking to be reversed. See Chapter 2 for help in quitting.

Diet can also play a significant role in the development of lung diseases. A diet rich in fats, especially dairy products, makes your mucus thicker and more difficult for your body to remove. Spices such as garlic, ginger, and cayenne pepper have been shown to loosen secretions and help in lung infections. Garlic in the diet serves as a natural antiseptic, with both antibacterial, antiviral, and antifungal activity.[47] Follow the dietary recommendations given in Chapter 2.

You can maximize your cough's efficiency by pressing against your incision as you try to breath deeply, then cough. Breathing into an *incentive spirometer*, a small plastic device that contains Ping-Pong–like balls you try to elevate, helps expand the small air sacs in your lungs. Preoperative practice will make your postoperative efforts more effective.

Percussion, where a healthcare worker pounds on your back, loosens secretions and increases circulation to your lungs, helping prevent infection. A friend or family member can be trained to assist you with this therapy.

Preoperatively and postoperatively, the various breathing exercises of yoga can directly strengthen your chest muscles, while the relaxation techniques can help calm your breathing and diminish all your cells' need for oxygen.

When you are having difficulty breathing, feelings of intense anxiety can worsen the problem. Visualization and meditation can assist in calming your breathing patterns, making them more efficient. The yoga practices serve as excellent, established methods of directly preventing and relieving lung problems. Follow the guidelines given in Chapter 2.

Walking is almost always possible the day of or the day after any surgery. A graduated exercise program can increase your lung function capability. After your operation, you should be up and walking as early as possible, thereby increasing your lung volume and breathing efficiency, as well as preventing dependent fluid collection in the lungs and sluggish blood flow in leg and pelvic veins. Even during bed rest, you should change position and move your feet and legs frequently.

Cardiac Problems

Rhythm disturbances, heart failure, and heart attack can occur after major operations. If you have a history of heart problems, you must be closely monitored. Report any chest pain or shortness of breath.

Blood Clots in the Veins

Surgery, bed rest, and decreased activity are associated with sluggish blood flow in the veins of the pelvis and legs, increasing risk for blood clots that can break loose and migrate to your lungs. Clots are present to some degree in almost all patients after major surgery. If you are debilitated, over 40 years old, have cancer, or overweight, your danger is greater. Small clots may not cause any symptoms, while larger ones can cause leg pain and swelling. If they reach the lungs, they can cause shortness of breath, chest pain, coughing up blood, and even sudden death.

Several measures are taken to prevent blood clot formation. For most major operations special automatic compression stockings

(ACSs) are put on your legs right in the operating room and left on until you are up and around. They intermittently squeeze your legs, acting to promote blood flow in veins, thus helping prevent clot formation. Also, you may be given aspirin or subcutaneous heparin, fragmin, or lovenox, blood thinners injected under the skin to discourage clot development. These have been proven to be very effective in preventing blood clots in the legs and pelvis that could migrate to you lungs. They are standard preventive treatment for many operations, especially orthopedic surgery. These injections may cause some skin bruising.

The most important measure you can take is to keep your legs moving. If confined to bed, rock your feet up and down, and contract your calf muscles, several times a minute. If possible, get up and walk around the halls as often as you can.

The "Postop Blues"

Depression is so common after surgery, it is called the "postop blues." Following the guidelines given in Chapter 2 can make a significant difference in your attitude, owing to the influence of good nutrition and the other gentle techniques discussed there. The herb hypericum (St. John's wort) has been found to be an effective natural antidepressant alternative to drug therapy, with fewer side effects, although further research is needed to completely compare its effects. You can begin with two capsules, three times daily. Passionflower and valerian are other beneficial herbs, taken in doses of one to two capsules three times daily. Meditation has been found to increase serotonin levels, the way Prozac works. Begin with fifteen minutes, three times daily.

After an operation, you need time to recover, both physically and psychologically.

Initially, your body is using much of its resources to recover from the illness and repair any surgical incisions. It can take a month or longer before there is nutritional reserve to rebuild your muscle strength to the point where you start to feel energetic again. Meanwhile, expect to tire easily, sleep a lot, be tearful, and feel emotionally drained and depressed. All this is normal. Ask for help when you don't feel up to doing certain things just yet.

You may have new scars and tender areas, look different, and have lost a part or two. Give yourself time to adjust to these changes. Consider that such changes are simply necessary to get you back to optimum health. This is a time to be with family and friends, catch up on old hobbies, or develop new ones. A support group or counseling may be very beneficial, and is strongly recommended.

Hospital Discharge

The decision for date of discharge has undergone much change within the last few years. Long recovery periods were the usual surgical approach in the past, but have been largely replaced with a move toward early release. Studies have indicated that patients get well faster when they can be at home in a familiar and loving environment. Hospitals and physicians alike are under great pressure from insurance plans and regulatory agencies to move patients out sooner in order to cut costs. In order to limit their costs, Medicare and insurance carriers now reimburse for only a certain number of hospital days. "Peer review" is an overview of surgeons by other surgeons that checks for those who keep patients in the hospital unjustifiably.

Both advantages and problems stem from these changes. Some patients are now being sent home who are not physically or psychologically ready. Some may not have a reasonable environment at home to enable them to get well. A hospital can be very helpful for such persons, and time of discharge should be determined individually for all surgical patients. A week or two in a less expensive "skilled nursing facility" can provide an alternative for patients who do not need intensive nursing care but are not yet able to manage at home.

Patient care and discharge coordinators are new hospital specialists who will most likely be involved in your discharge planning. They can make arrangements for visiting nurses, physical therapists, chore workers, or whoever else you need to visit you at home to help ensure you are making the safest and quickest recovery.

When possible, have your spouse or a friend with you both just before and when you leave the hospital, so he or she can listen to the instructions with you, and give you appropriate physical and emotional support during the time of readjustment at home. Make certain you receive written discharge instructions, and a list of things of importance to look for. You need to watch for signs of infection or other complications that might require immediate attention, and you may need to take new medications. Make sure you know of possible side effects for which to be alert. If you need to follow a special diet or take extra supplements, have a discussion with the hospital dietitian.

Alternative Medicine Approaches to Convalescence

When you have no restrictions on your diet, make sure to select wholesome menu items. When our father was in the hospital following his heart attack, angioplasty, and pacemaker placement, he wanted to begin the Dean Ornish lifestyle program, to begin to reverse his disease and prevent future problems. Despite his indicating on his diet request sheet exactly what he wanted, every day high-fat items such as meat would be sent to his room. So you will need to be vigilant about such matters during your hospital stay, and recruit family or friends to help you.

Randy, a 50-year-old physician, needed surgical repair of a hydrocele, a benign swelling of the testicle. Despite being a doctor himself, he did not anticipate the challenge of postsurgical recovery. "For the first week, my entire life's experience consisted of lying on the couch during the daylight hours and lying in bed during the dark hours. I was very cold no matter what the room temperature; it was as if my body's thermostat was not working. I wore scrubs over a long-sleeved T-shirt, and had a sweat suit on top of them. I had to lie under a heavy blanket dressed like this to prevent shivering, even in a warm room. With great effort and discomfort, I managed to walk the ten feet from the couch to the bathroom or to the kitchen. I wore the same clothing for five days, because it was too much of an effort to change them. The surgical site was too tender to support the tissue and too heavy to support its own weight. Only by lying down could I have some measure of lessened pain. Finally, I consulted an alternative medicine doctor for some advice. I added homeopathy, a comfrey compress, flower essences, the herb echinacea, and a massage to the rest of my body. Immediately, I felt better in both my spirit and body, as if a lightbulb had been turned back on inside of me, and [I] began to heal."

If you can, being well prepared ahead of time for the effort required during the recovery period is optimum. Just like a mother-to-be benefits from prepared childbirth classes, a surgical patient can become equipped preoperatively to allow body and mind to be mobilized for healing during this critical time. Many of the techniques given in Chapter 2 are simple to learn beforehand. Even if you have not had the time to do this, you can learn them during the recovery period. A small amount of application goes a long way, so whatever you can do, starting with the simplest practices, may have some benefit.

As noted above, deep breathing is often quite difficult after major surgery, because the movement of breathing precipitates pain. The lungs therefore tend to collapse, filling with life-threatening amounts of fluid and predisposing a patient to pneumonia. The deep breathing exercises discussed in Chapter 2 can be especially beneficial. Alternate nostril breathing is especially useful for pain relief and induces profound relaxation.

Postsurgical swelling due to lymph congestion is common. Here the yoga stretches can have an extremely beneficial effect to get the lymph flowing again, diminishing pain and distention. The gentle yoga stretches are also ideal for getting you back in motion. You can perform them in bed at first, as pictured in Chapter 2. It is extremely important that you do not strain, especially, of course, at the point of your incision. At first, you may do best to have someone there to assist you in the stretches. The main point is never to strain beyond what feels perfectly comfortable, even in the name of getting well faster.

Walking soon after surgery, so important to good recovery, is not usually fun, requires effort, and calls for an ability to tolerate pain when you already feel pretty wiped out. Here

again you can use the training described in Chapter 2 to help visualize yourself alert and healthy, and enjoying each step.

For the first few days after surgery, a liquid diet of high nutrient value may be the best plan, using the Superdrinks and supplemental vitamins and minerals given in Chapter 2. Such a liquid diet's main benefit is to allow your body to focus all its energies upon fixing the incision, rather than using this energy to digest and process food.

Later, a good regular diet and vitamin program can be a source of strength for recovery. Most hospital food could not and would never be used to nurse a veterinary patient back to health. Coffee, sugary drinks, sugar-filled Jell-O and sugary, fat-filled ice cream are the standard routine for postop patients. Such foods are devastating to the immune system, as discussed in Chapter 2. If possible, locate a friend or relative who can bring you the drinks and foods suggested in that section, or see if the hospital can secure some of them. Most physicians and hospitals will be receptive to your requests and, perhaps in the future, routinely provide more nutritious and vital foods.

Try to limit your pain medication to the least amount with which you can stay relaxed. Pain medicines affect the kidneys and liver, already burdened with the anesthetic and the underlying disease. You can increase your own body's production of natural painkillers by the relaxation and meditation processes. The idea is to "meditate rather than medicate," which can provide pain relief and add the benefit of stimulating your body to its quickest possible healing. In avoiding medication, you keep yourself alert to assemble your body's own resources toward recovery.

However, if the natural techniques given in Chapter 2 are not working for you, you should not be a martyr. Chronic pain can set an "imprint" on the nervous system, in which the nerves continue to relay pain despite healing. Such a pattern becomes more difficult to erase, the longer you have pain. Take the amount of pain medication you need to feel comfortable.

The best approach is to keep the time of convalescence as enjoyable as possible, making it as interesting as you can. You can rent humorous or uplifting videotapes, listen to inspiring music, look at picture books, receive daily massages, and practice other stress-management approaches.

The techniques and dietary advice given in Chapter 2 can help reduce your distress during convalescence. It may be helpful to find a full-time person to provide your care during this time. He or she can prepare the nutritious drinks and give you the vitamins, provide massage and music, or just be there to give you caring support. If you have not already learned relaxation, breathing, and visualization techniques, you can try them now. They can help speed your healing and ease your aches.

An example from Hippocrates, the father of Western medicine, may illustrate a healthful approach to recovery. It is reported that he began perhaps one of the first Western "holistic" medical centers, on the island of Cos in Greece. Patients would be given a liquid diet and encouraged to sleep as much as possible during the first two weeks. Then for the next two weeks, they would receive massages and undertake gentle stretching exercises. For the final two weeks, he would train them like Spartan athletes! You may need to vary the amount of time in each phase, but generally the time from operation to athletic training is three to six months after major surgery.

Adjusting to a New Lifestyle

While many surgeries leave only an incision scar as a reminder of the experience, some operations leave your body obviously and permanently changed. Removal or rearrangement of part of the intestinal tract may require a restricted diet or a need to never venture very far from a rest room. Previously cherished activities such as golfing, hiking, or other sports may have to be eliminated or severely restricted, drastically changing your lifestyle habits. Various "appliances" (postop devices) and medications with their inevitable side effects may prove a nuisance or give you real pain. Your body's appearance may be altered markedly, by loss of a part or significant surgical scars.

Despite these difficulties, adjustments can be made to overcome or accept limitations, so you can move on to a full and satisfying lifestyle. One of the most helpful things to do during this time of change is to join one of the organizations for persons with similar disabilities, such as "Reach-to-Recovery" if you have had breast cancer or an "Ostomy Club" if part of your bowel or bladder has been removed. These groups can make a remarkable difference in your ability to develop positive attitudes and skills. Their members are people who have confronted similar difficulties, and their collective wisdom is far beyond that of a surgeon or other type of doctor or nurse lacking the personal experience of dealing with the day-to-day challenges of your specific problem. Please see the back of this book for a list of resources.

5

SKIN

Randy Van Nostrand, an adventurous 53-year-old ER doctor, had traveled to the outer regions of Mongolia and spent time living with a family there. The conditions were rustic, and he developed a small but deep skin infection on his back. The doctors he sought out were mystified, and despite several courses of antibiotics, the condition continued. Once he began an alternative medicine regimen which included the herbs garlic, goldenseal, and echinacea, along with the vitamin inositol, all taken orally, his wound began to heal, and he was able to once again continue his own personal "fantastic voyaging."

While most skin problems are minor, occasionally they can be very serious. Severe skin infections, moles, cysts, other "lumps and bumps," and skin cancer may need surgical evaluation.

"You have cancer." We dread these words so much we often practice active denial about our risks for it. *However, skin cancer is the most common malignancy found in humans.* More than a million people are newly diagnosed with it in the United States each year. Although most cases can be cured, especially if detected early, 10,000 people die each year from this disease. With the increasing loss of the ozone layer, skin cancer rates are escalating around the world. You can take action to help prevent this prevalent cancer.

President Reagan, while in office, developed a skin cancer on his nose, but thought the problem was only a pimple, until his doctor noticed it. If you detect any unusual change in your skin or an area which does not heal, you should consult a doctor immediately.

The good news is that alternative medicine approaches offer guidelines so you can act preventively, to adopt optimum dietary and other lifestyle habits to help you avoid this and other potentially dangerous skin problems. In addition, they offer new hope when used as adjuncts along with conventional methods of treatment.

In this chapter, we will discuss the most common surgical skin disorders and your varying treatment options, including new alternative medicine therapies for infections you can use at home to help you avoid the surgeon's knife. We will help you learn to recognize skin cancer, and what steps you can take to help in its prevention.

In addition, we advise you on alternative ways you can care for and help speed the healing of a surgical incision.

How Your Skin Works

Your skin, the largest organ in your body, acts as your external "brain," to connect you in the most immediate way to your environ-

ment. If you stretched all of your skin out, it would cover 20 square feet, with each square inch containing, on average, 10 million cells, 100 oil glands, 65 hairs, 650 sweat glands, plus yards of blood vessels and nerves.

Skin provides *protection*—it keeps what is inside your body inside, and what is in the environment outside—and helps your body regulate its temperature, by using sweat glands and blood vessels to retain or release body heat. When necessary, your skin can produce several *quarts* of sweat per day! Your skin's sense of pain, touch, heat, and cold helps you avoid injury, while at the same time giving you the experience of sensation.

Your skin has two layers: a tissue-paper thin but tough outer layer, the *epidermis*, which is completely shed and replaced every three to four weeks; and an inner layer, the *dermis*. (See Figure 5.1.) *Melanocytes* are cells that lie between the epidermis and dermis, manufacturing pigment that protects you

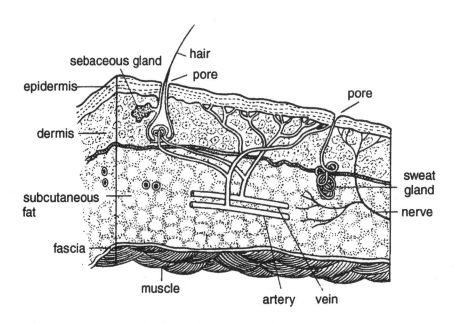

Fig. 5.1 The anatomy of the skin

from ultraviolet radiation. The amount of this pigment determines your skin color.

Your hair, nails, sweat glands, and oil-producing sebaceous glands, located in the dermis, are actually specialized epidermal cells. Your nails protect the sensitive tips of your fingers, and improve your grasp. Your sebaceous glands produce oil to keep your skin soft and pliant. Sweat glands help with heat regulation. Both sebaceous and sweat glands are coiled tubular structures, with ducts going up to your skin surface where they empty through small pores. Elastic fibers keep the skin supple, while collagen fibers give it strength.

You can take care of your skin by avoiding harsh soaps and sunburn, and remoisturizing it to keep it elastic. Maintaining your general health and providing proper nutrition for skin repair also help your skin stay healthy. Aging weakens the elastic fibers and decreases fat beneath the skin. Your glands also secrete less oil and sweat; as a result, older skin appears more creased, dry, and flaky. You can help prevent and reverse this process by following the guidelines given in the alternative medicine sections, below. Cigarette smoking destroys the skin's collagen and elastic fibers, leading to premature aging changes, and especially obvious wrinkling.

How Skin Disease Is Diagnosed

Skin growths and lumps under your skin are diagnosed by a review of your symptoms, an assessment of their distribution and appearance, and if necessary, microscopic examination of a sample of tissue—a *biopsy*. Whether the biopsy removes all of the abnormality depends upon its size and what conditions are being considered.

Four kinds of biopsy can be performed on skin surface abnormalities: a *shave biopsy* uses a sharp instrument to shave cells from the surface of the abnormal area, a *punch biopsy* punches out a small piece of the tissue with a cookie cutter–like instrument, an *incisional biopsy* also cuts out a small piece using a scalpel, and an *excisional biopsy* removes the whole thing. For abnormalities under the skin surface you may have a *fine needle aspiration biopsy* that sucks individual cells out through a small needle, a *core needle biopsy* that removes a piece of the abnormality through a special larger needle with a cutting sleeve, or an incisional or excisional biopsy.

These biopsies are performed using local anesthetic, usually in your doctor's office. Acupuncture or hypnosis, discussed more fully in Chapter 2, are also useful anesthesia options. The incision, if any, may be closed with stitches or skin tape. Discomfort is minimal and pain pills rarely necessary. The biopsy result may be available immediately or within a few days.

Nonmalignant Growths On and Beneath the Skin

Most of us have some skin abnormalities that are usually not a health threat. However, the giant cosmetic industry pushes us to great worry and expense about such "abnormalities" that are so common they may, in fact, be normal. These *can* be treated with surgery or other means, as we will discuss. However, a trade-off always exists between costs and benefits, and it is up to you to weigh these carefully. On the benefit side, the relief of removing an offending problem may be great; but on the cost side are scarring, surgical discomfort, and expense.

A surgical scar is a natural healing phenomenon which can never be entirely avoided, though your incision can be placed to minimize and hide the scar within a natural skin or wrinkle line and the alternative medicine approaches discussed in Chapter 24 can diminish postoperative scarring. Some areas of your body, however, especially at stretch and tension points such as the shoulder, chin, and between the breasts, are notorious for producing wide, thick scars which may become much larger than the original abnormality. Keep this in mind in your decision about any optional skin surgery.

When *should* a skin abnormality be removed? You need to have it removed whenever malignancy or "premalignancy" is suspected, or if future complications are likely. Although not themselves diagnostic of cancer, rapid increase in size, change in consistency or color, symptoms of pain, tenderness, itching, or an ulcerated or bleeding surface are all cause for special concern. Don't attempt to make the critical determination about whether your problem is benign or malignant on your own; have any questionable area examined by an expert.

Other reasons for removal of a lump or bump are to relieve any associated discomfort or irritation, or improve your appearance. Such considerations are quite subjective. Cost may be prohibitive: you may prefer to just put up with minor symptoms. Many people do tell us that if they had known it would be so easy, they would have chosen to spend the money on an operation years before; others come to the opposite conclusion.

If you are diagnosed with a benign problem, ask your surgeon if it will enlarge, cause discomfort or disfigurement, and therefore, should be removed *now*, or will it likely remain stable or even get smaller? What are the possible complications, and what is involved in removing it?

Moles

Mole is a term often misused to describe all sorts of skin problems. *Nevus* is the medical term for mole—a benign growth of brown pigment cells (melanocytes) that forms a flat or slightly raised dark spot.

Most moles are smooth and rounded, with sharp borders; they may contain hair and vary in color from tan to brown, gray or black. Moles may be present at birth or appear at any time, and generally don't produce symptoms or have any significance unless they bother you cosmetically. You need not have your mole removed unless it undergoes a significant change in appearance or is in a position where it is constantly irritated, such as at your bra, collar, or belt line.

However, any change in appearance or enlargement of a mole may indicate the rare transformation into cancer of the melanoma type, the most dangerous form of skin cancer. Although about one-third of all melanomas arise from preexisting moles, the chance of any one of your moles becoming cancerous is less than one in a million.

Specific signals that suggests a mole might be transforming into a malignancy are:

- Increase in size
- Change in consistency (softening or hardening)
- Change in pigmentation (especially if the mole becomes variegated in color)
- Change from symmetrical with clear boundaries to asymmetrical and with poorly defined boundaries
- Loss of previous hair

- New itching or soreness
- Ulceration or bleeding

Change does not necessarily mean malignancy, but does indicate the need for surgical removal, to determine if abnormal cells are present.

Alternative Medicine Approaches to Moles

Some friends and I (Sandy) were horsing around a magnificently blazing campfire, set on the high banks above the Delaware Water Gap in Pennsylvania, celebrating my friend's birthday out in the fragrant fall evening. All of us were college students on a break in the mid-1960s, and we were wearing bell-bottoms. I made a particularly dramatic turn too close to the flames, and my wide pant leg was suddenly ablaze. We quickly doused it with water, but not before I had sustained a significant and very painful burn to my lower leg. One of my companions had to carry me piggy-back to search for the nearest ice.

The area remained red and sore for several weeks. I witnessed a small, flat black circular spot begin to form, and I now have a small mole at the burn site. Since then, I have observed that the best treatment for sunburn or any skin burn is applying lavender oil, which can quickly decrease pain, prevent scarring, and even keep a first- or second-degree burn from accelerating into second or third degree, respectively, as discussed in the section on skin infections, below. This may be one way of helping prevent posttraumatic mole formation.

I watch this particular mole especially closely, since it is this type of burn or sunburn origin that can generate the conditions for a mole to change into the skin cancer melanoma. It's been there now for thirty years without any modification, and I wouldn't want it removed, unless it were to change: I have come to rather like it, since it represents a kind of wisdom, reminding me of both the joys and dangers of playing with fire.

The skin is a reflection of the general health of your body. Where and when you form a mole can be an indicator for this. You should take the time to be fully evaluated, both by a conventional practitioner and one who practices alternative approaches.

When should you even bother to try to make a mole disappear by alternative methods? All moles that show change, as discussed above, must be surgically removed. But if your mole is simply cosmetically located in an inconvenient spot, or one where it becomes irritated, or if the long-term prevention of malignant change causes you to worry, you might choose alternative approaches to try to eliminate it. Otherwise, it is fine to simply leave a mole alone.

However, since the formation of a new mole can indicate a weakness in your body's repair mechanisms, I have observed that noting where your mole is situated may give a clue about a problem in this portion of your body, related to an acupuncture meridian or underlying organ. Act preventively, to assist in optimum circulation to and health of this region, by following the dietary, exercise, stretching, and relaxation guidelines given in Chapter 2.

Following are the most promising alternative medicine approaches for mole removal.

Use Natural Topicals

Rubbing castor oil or liquid vitamin A into the mole, three times a day, has been reported to cause moles to disappear in some people.[1] Retinoic acid, as found in Retin-A, initially may cause a mole to disappear, but it is likely to return within a year.[2]

Change Your Diet; Take Supplements

Switching to a low-fat vegetarian diet provides increased nutrients for optimum skin maintenance, eliminating excess fats—which interfere with circulation to your skin, and give you increased amounts of damaging free radicals. Vitamin A functions to help maintain the skin, and is now felt to be a promising agent to prevent skin cancer.[3] Vitamin C may also give protection.[4] Taking these two vitamins may provide your moles with protection against malignant change. Recommended oral doses are 5,000 to 10,000 IU of vitamin A daily, and 1,000 mg of vitamin C a day.

Practice Hypnosis and Visualization

These techniques have been reported to be effective in removing moles in some people.[5] For example, you can say to yourself, "My skin is perfectly healthy," and "My skin is free from any spots," or image the mole in your mind's eye as "melting like an ice cube." Further instructions for the practice of these techniques is given in Chapter 2.

Surgical Approach to Moles

The only acceptable method of biopsy of a mole is surgical excision, removing the *entire* mole so that all of it can be examined under the microscope.

After preparing your skin with an iodine solution to kill harmful bacteria, your doctor injects a local anesthetic such as Xylocaine to numb the area around the mole, which is then removed, along with a small ellipse of surrounding skin. Your incision is closed with stitches, and/or skin tapes, and your soreness

should be minimal. The incision should be left covered, and kept dry, for twenty-four to forty-eight hours. You should see your doctor for a follow-up visit to discuss the biopsy findings, to make certain you do not have an incision complication, and to have any stitches removed. If your stitches are placed beneath the skin they will dissolve; those that you can see, if any, need to be removed after three to ten days, depending on location. The scar following this procedure is usually small.

Lipomas and Sebaceous Cysts

Ludmilla was a 23-year-old Russian immigrant who lived within 30 miles of Chernobyl, site of the nuclear explosion and radioactive fallout. One of her daily chores was to hang out laundry. Five years after the explosion, she began developing lumps under the skin of her arms and thighs. Understandably concerned about these growths, Ludmilla had three of them removed. Analysis showed them to be typical lipomas without malignant potential, and her anxiety was greatly relieved.

Lipoma, the most common benign tumor underneath the skin, is a proliferation of fat cells of unknown cause, tending to occur more frequently around the neck and shoulder, lower back, and flank. A genetic predisposition is present in some people, who usually develop multiple lipomas on the arms and legs. Usually small, soft, freely movable, and causing no symptoms, lipomas can, however, sometimes assume huge proportions. You may develop symptoms if your lipoma irritates a nerve or pressure is transmitted to underlying tissues. Lipomas do not become cancerous.

Sebaceous cysts are extremely common

skin lumps that also have no malignant potential. In their simplest form they are "whiteheads," most often seen on your face and back. The duct of a sebaceous gland, which empties into a hair pore, becomes blocked. Pressure over the whitehead can generally empty its sebaceous secretion. However, if the duct remains blocked, a cheesy mixture of this oily secretion and dead cell debris accumulates.

Such a cyst usually slowly enlarges, until internal pressure prevents further cell activity, and a stable size is reached. You may notice a foul-smelling discharge. Since bacteria are present on your skin surface and can gain entry through hair pores, these cysts have a tendency to become infected. Those on your back have especially high infection rates due to the poorer blood supply there. If you do develop infection, the affected area becomes swollen, tender, and reddened. The cyst has now become an abscess, which may have to be surgically drained.

Alternative Medicine Approaches to Lipomas and Sebaceous Cysts

Both of these skin problems have potentially important meanings. They serve as small warning flags, indicating dysfunction on a minor level that may reflect underlying dietary and/or immune concerns. Although lipomas can just be a nuisance, a cause for cosmetic concern, and can get in the way of your clothing, creating discomfort, they signal a disorder of fat and sugar metabolism that may be linked to heart disease or diabetes. Sebaceous cysts likewise form more often when excess fats and sugars in the diet combine with local factors to precipitate such a cyst.

One of my patients, for example, devel-oped a troublesome sebaceous cyst on his back, right at his waistline. It became so inflamed that it required not only surgical excision, but also a drain for a week, to give the massive associated infection an avenue for removal. I was interested in what might be done for prevention of future such problems.

As we assessed his lifestyle, two important clues emerged: he was drinking lots of alcohol every day, and holding his guitar strap right at the site of the problem. The wine and beer, acting as a sugar in the body, were affecting his immune system's ability to fight infection, and the strap was providing enough irritation so that bacteria could enter across his skin barrier. Once these two initiating causes were addressed—he switched to various interesting varieties of sparkling mineral water and changed his guitar strap to an over-the-neck type—his skin cleared up nicely, and he was happy to report that both his music and his moods improved too.

Following are the most promising methods for alternative regression of lipomas and sebaceous cysts.

Change Your Diet; Take Supplements

Lipoma growth is felt by some researchers to be directly related to diet. Ludmilla's story, above, may have reflected an increased fat and refined sugar diet, associated with coming to the United States from the relatively food-restricted Soviet Union. Since lipomas are so benign, a trial of a low-fat diet, and avoiding refined sugar, may be undertaken, to aim for their disappearance.

Diet may also play a role in the development of sebaceous cysts, especially a diet that is high in fats, fried foods, and refined sugar.[6] A low-fat, high-fiber diet may cause these cysts to disappear.[7] Oral zinc and vitamin C may also be helpful. Begin with 50 mg of zinc, and 1,000 to 2,000 mg of vitamin C daily. The antioxidants selenium and vitamin E should be taken orally: 200 mcg of selenium, and 400 to 800 IU of vitamin E. The omega-3 and omega-6 fatty acids, as found in sunflower seeds and flaxseed oil respectively, help in skin repair. Take a tablespoon of flaxseed oil and a handful of sunflower seeds with your food daily; the effect may take one to two months to be apparent. Follow the complete vitamin and supplement program given in Chapter 2.

Use Natural Topicals

Daily application of topical vitamin E or topical castor oil have been anecdotally reported to be effective for sebaceous cysts.[8] Apply three times daily; results may take six to eight weeks to become apparent.

Use Immune-Enhancing Herbals

The immune-enhancing herbals given in Chapters 2 and 24 may be helpful, especially important because they increase the ability of your immune system to stave off infection. Particularly effective are garlic and echinacea. Dosages are explained in Chapter 2.

Use Homeopathy

The most common remedies chosen are calendula, silicea, belladonna, and hepar sulph. See Chapter 2 for details. You may need the assistance of an experienced homeopathic practitioner.

Practice Hypnosis and Visualization

These approaches have been anecdotally reported to be successful for this problem. Follow the guidelines given for deep relax-ation and visualization in Chapter 2. Then, for example, imagine your lipoma or sebaceous cyst as a small rain cloud. Picture the sun coming out, and the cloud evaporating. Hold this image in your mind, while you feel it happening within your body. Repeat the process three to five times daily, for five to fifteen minutes. Full results may take three to six weeks.

Surgical Approaches to Lipomas and Sebaceous Cysts

A common role for the surgeon is simply to relieve uncertainty and anxiety about lumps underneath your skin, which can of course sometimes be a sign of cancer. If you have a lump that is noticeable, family or friends may nag you to have it "taken care of." Even when you have no symptoms and your doctor finds your lump need not be removed for medical reasons, you may well just want to be rid of it.

A lipoma is usually innocuous, and can be left alone. It may enlarge slowly, then remain stable after reaching a certain size, but rarely does it spontaneously regress in measurement. If it causes symptoms or changes in consistency, if you don't like the way it looks, or if it otherwise makes you worry, you may want to have an operation to remove it.

Most patients who come to a surgeon for sebaceous cyst removal have had their cyst for a number of years, and have finally decided to have it removed because of mild local discomfort, a foul-smelling discharge, a developing infection, cosmetic reasons, or pressure from family or friends worried that the lump could be cancer. If a sebaceous cyst is no bother to you, once the possibility of infection has been explained and you have chosen to take your chances, you may leave it alone. Once your cyst develops an infection, however, since recurrent infections are likely, it should be removed.

If you need to or choose to have surgical treatment for your sebaceous cyst or lipoma, the following techniques are available, depending on the diagnosis and whether or not an infection is present.

Incision and Drainage

If your sebaceous cyst is infected, it must be first drained and treated as an abscess, as described for "Skin Infections" on page 151. After the infection subsides, usually in three to four weeks, the lining can be surgically removed and the skin closed with stitches. A noninfected cyst is easily excised surgically. All of it must be shelled out, since a recurrent cyst is likely to develop if any lining cells are left behind to continue to form sebaceous material.

Surgical Excision

If you have a sebaceous cyst or a small lipoma, it can usually be surgically removed under local anesthesia, on an outpatient basis. Very large lipomas may have to be operated on under general or spinal anesthesia, since the amount of local anesthesia needed, and associated discomfort, would make this the better choice. After preparing your skin with an iodine solution to kill harmful skin bacteria, your doctor injects a local anesthetic such as Xylocaine to numb the area around the lump. A straight incision may be used in small lumps, but if your skin has been stretched by a larger lipoma, an ellipse of skin is removed over the lump, so that your skin will lie flat once the edges are brought together.

Your incision is closed with stitches or skin tapes. Occasionally, in very large lipomas, a soft plastic drain is used to prevent tissue fluid accumulation under the skin closure. Depending on the size of your lump, the procedure takes fifteen to sixty minutes to complete. Postoperative discomfort depends on the size and site of your procedure, but should not be significant, and most likely, you will not require pain pills. You should keep your incision dry for forty-eight hours. You need to see a doctor again after three to ten days, for removal of stitches, if any, and to be checked for bleeding, infection, and fluid accumulation (which can be evacuated by a needle passed through your skin). You will likely have a small scar.

Liposuction

For lipomas, another surgical choice is liposuction, which uses a high suction device connected to a small tube, passed through a skin incision, to suck out the fatty tissue. This method is often chosen by plastic surgeons and described in chapter 23 (see pages 668–70).

Lymph Gland Enlargement

Your lymph glands contain collections of "lymphocytes," a type of white blood cell very important in your immune defense. Lymphatic channels drain lymph fluid into these glands; outgoing channels eventually connect into the venous system.

Your lymph glands, also called lymph nodes, can cause painful groin, armpit, or neck lumps whenever they perform their important roles of resisting infection. Once the infection clears, your pain goes away and swelling decreases, but the gland may never fully return to its previous size. Occasionally, if an infection overcomes your gland's defense, an abscess can form.

Alternative Medicine Approaches to Lymph Gland Enlargement

If you suddenly find a swelling in one of your lymph glands, it can be quite disconcerting. One of my patients noticed some small tender lumps in her armpit. Having previously had a lung cancer removed via surgery, she was especially alarmed.

However, the glands were quite tender, not usual with cancer. Upon further questioning, I discovered that she had been playing with a new cat the previous week, and still had a few of the scratches on her arm. After testing for the infection known as cat-scratch fever proved negative, her problem was concluded to simply be a small infection that had traveled to her local lymph nodes, and hot soaks combined with the herb echinacea quickly resolved it.

Any gland where cancer could be the cause of enlargement should be biopsied. Infected lymph glands, however, often respond to alternative approaches, and you can thus avoid surgery. These therapies must be carefully supervised by your doctor, but may also be used as adjuncts to surgical treatment if that becomes necessary.

Following are the most promising alternative medicine approaches.

Use Local Measures

Hot wet packs often help in alleviating an infected lymph node, and may be all that is needed for its resolution. The local heat causes an increased blood supply to come to the area, bringing more white cells, enhancing circulation of nutrients and removal of waste products. Use a hot wet washcloth, kept warm with a wet-proof heating pad or hot water bottle, for one-half hour at a time, four to six times daily.

Change Your Diet; Take Supplements

Lymph glands may be responsive to changes in diet. In 1982, a study conducted by Dr. P. Chandra reported that nutritional supplementation could improve white cell function.[9] Other investigators have subsequently found that vitamins A, B, C, E and the minerals zinc and selenium all play a necessary role in immune system function; see Chapters 2 and 24. If you do not observe a response within a week or so, you may require antibiotics; if they, too, fail to relieve your symptoms, you may need surgery.

Use Immune-Enhancing Herbals

Several traditional home remedies have recently been documented to act through stimulation of immune activity. Garlic affects fat metabolism by promoting its excretion via the liver, and may therefore make your lymph less fatty and able to flow more easily, allowing your white cells to more quickly reach the site of infection with increased effectiveness. You can add fresh garlic to your diet, the most effective form, or use deodorized garlic tablets if you have social constraints. Take two cloves or capsules three times daily. Echinacea is an important immune-stimulating herb. Take two capsules or droppersful three times daily. If you do not see results in a week or so, you may need to turn to antibiotics or surgery.

Conventional Medicine Approach to Lymph Gland Enlargement

In addition to the local measures just described, there is a conventional medicine approach you can try. Antibiotic therapy may help you avoid surgery. Your doctor will need to determine which drug is best for your particular infection and how long to take it.

Make certain to take acidophilus at the same time as your antibiotic, two capsules, three times daily, to prevent a subsequent yeast infection.

Surgical Approach to Lymph Gland Enlargement

An enlarged lymph gland is not usually a cause for alarm if you have had an infection in its drainage area. However, three conditions indicate you should have surgical assessment. If the node becomes abscessed, it may need to be drained or removed. If infection persists, a specimen may be necessary to determine the organism present so that treatment can be optimized. If there is a possibility of cancer, analysis of the node can determine type and stage of malignancy, so that the best treatment can be chosen. Although you might fear a swollen lymph gland could be cancer, this is rarely the case. However, any gland suspected of containing cancer must be biopsied to obtain a diagnosis.

Most lymph glands are easily removed in outpatient surgery under local anesthesia. Glands high in your armpit or deep in your neck may best be taken out under general anesthesia.

After preparing your skin with an iodine solution to kill harmful bacteria, your doctor injects a local anesthetic such as Xylocaine, to numb the area around the gland. After the gland is removed, stitches or skin tapes close your incision, unless infection demands it be left open to drain (also see "Skin Infections," on pages 151–52). Your soreness should be minimal, and your incision left covered and dry for twenty-four to forty-eight hours.

You should see your doctor for a follow-up visit to discuss the biopsy findings, to make certain you do not have an infection, and to have any external stitches removed. Stitches under your skin dissolve, so do not need to be taken out; those that you can see can be removed after three to ten days, depending on location. The scar will likely be small.

Skin Infections

Your skin is normally covered by many different kinds of bacteria, some of which can cause infections. It is a tribute to your skin defenses and immune system that you are not one big sore!

The bacteria concentrate in moist areas, and when your skin is wet, it is much more susceptible to invasion by disease-causing bacteria. Excessive dampness can occur if you sweat too much, your oil glands are extra oily, you are overweight and skin folds prevent normal evaporation and skin drying, or you wear clothes that are too tight, especially synthetic undergarments.

A skin infection usually starts when bacteria gain entrance into or through the skin's surface by way of a hair follicle, sweat gland, cut or scrape, or surgical incision. Your immune defense begins with an inflammatory response, which brings increased blood flow to the involved area. Your white blood cells arrive to engulf the bacteria, while your circulating antibodies kill them directly. The classic signs of infection—redness, warmth, swelling, and tenderness—develop during the time the invading bacteria are being battled. Usually few, if any, bacteria are able to gain access to the rest of your body as this inflammatory reaction isolates the infected area from neighboring uninfected tissue, blood vessels, and lymph channels.

Your body's defenses can be overwhelmed by particularly virulent types of organisms.

You are at increased risk if you have poor blood supply, dead tissue, or foreign material in a wound or incision, or if you are diabetic, have a chronic disease, are nutritionally deficient, or immune-suppressed. Signs of possibly life-threatening infections, which appear if bacteria gain access to your bloodstream, are malaise, fatigue, fever, and especially chills.

Staphylococcus, the most common bacterial invader, is normally present on your skin's surface, and is involved in pus-producing "staph" infections. Pus is a combination of bacteria, white blood cells, plasma, and tissue breakdown products. An abscess or boil is formed when pus is trapped beneath your skin. Such a boil may drain spontaneously by "coming to a head" and rupturing through the skin surface, as is the case of the common pimple, itself a small abscess. On the other hand, it may continue to enlarge without draining spontaneously.

Once an abscess forms, your body's defenses and even antibiotics are not as effective. Your circulation cannot get to the area that is "walled off" by the reaction around the abscess space. You may, therefore, require surgical drainage.

Streptococcus bacteria—"strep"—skin infections tend to spread without forming pus. Antibiotics, especially if given early, are usually rapidly effective. No barrier is present to prevent the white cells and antibiotic from reaching the area of infecting bacteria. However, if you put off treatment too long, the infected tissue may die, and then must be surgically removed.

Alternative Medicine Approaches to Skin Infections

Most small skin infections simply resolve themselves, with little or no local care. How-

ever, they can pose significant problems, especially after an operation. Or if you are in a foreign country.

What allows bacteria to enter, then survive and multiply once they get through your skin, via a hair follicle, sweat gland, or small crack? Your skin should be able to prevent such breaches, and your immune system, under conditions of good health, able to fight off even these invaders. Alternative medicine approaches analyze nutritional and immune aspects of skin problems, to address the root of the disorder. Just make certain to have any alternative treatments supervised by a doctor.

Following are the alternative medicine approaches that may help you avoid the surgeon's knife as a solution to your skin infection.

Practice Preventive Maintenance

All "soap" has lye in it, which can reduce your skin's natural lubricating oils, predisposing it to cracking and thereby providing entry points for harmful bacteria. Keeping your soap use to a minimum can thus actually help *prevent* infection; use one of the newer lye-free "nonsoaps" available at health food stores. Whenever you suffer scratches or abrasions, you can use soap just at that point, to reduce the number of organisms that might enter the break. Another preventive measure is to keep your immune system in good shape by following the dietary and supplement information given in Chapter 2.

Use Warm Soaks

Warm moist soaks are enormously helpful to the healing of skin infections. They bring increased blood supply and white cells to the infected area and accelerate the speed of your body's immune reactions. Your immune system can thus localize an infection, prevent it from entering your bloodstream, and "bring it to a head," which will then often drain spontaneously. Repeated warm soaks may be all you need to fully recover.

Soaking your whole body won't have this local effect, so just submerge or apply compresses to the affected area. Make a salt solution using one tablespoon of table salt to one quart of warm water, or follow the package directions for mixing Epsom salts; salt solutions prevent your skin from the wrinkling and drying caused by regular water. If you cannot soak the infected part, dip a towel or washcloth, and apply it to the infection, then place an insulated heating pad, hot water bottle, or aluminum foil on top. Repeat three or four times per day, for twenty to thirty minutes each time.

Change Your Diet

Both alcohol and refined sugar act to decrease activity of the white cells of your immune system, as discussed in Chapter 2. See that chapter for optimum dietary instructions.

Use Immune Stimulators

If you utilize immune stimulators early, whenever you have a cut or incision, you may prevent complications that require surgical intervention. Most surgeons are quick to lance an area that may resolve on its own, but whenever a scalpel is used, a scar will be left.

The vitamins and minerals that are particularly useful in skin infections are vitamins A, 10,000 IU daily, and C, 1,000 mg three times daily, and zinc, 50 mg daily. Echinacea is an herb that functions as a reliable immune stimulator when taken as capsules or tincture, 2 capsules or droppersful, three times daily.

Garlic may also be helpful; see Chapter 2 for details.

Surgery *itself* lowers your white cell function, thereby predisposing you to postoperative infections at your incision site. Some components of your white cell activity take as long as three weeks to return to normal. After your operation, follow the guidelines given in Chapters 2 and 24.

Practice Hypnosis

This approach is very effective in modifying your skin resistance. Hypnosis may be an especially helpful adjunct to help resolve chronic infections.[10] See Chapter 2 for details.

Use Homeopathy

The most commonly chosen remedies are cinchona officinalis, sulfur, and hepar sulfuris, 30C, four times daily, until the infection is healed. You may need the help of an experienced homeopath.

Use Magnets

Magnets, when applied to the skin, act to increase capillary and lymph flow, bringing more white cells to the site of infection. Further research on their precise effectiveness is needed, as discussed in Chapter 2. The Magnatherm electromagnet machine has been found to diminish the risk of infection postsurgically.

Practice Stress Management

Your immune system is highly influenced by factors of stress. Even a small amount of stress can cause your white cells to be less active. Meditation has been shown to improve white cell activity. Follow the guidelines for stress management and visualization given in Chapter 2.

After doing deep relaxation, you can, for example, imagine your white cells growing in number and activity, and streaming into the site of your infection, "removing debris with garbage trucks" or "zapping invading bacteria with laser guns," or whatever other images feel strong and healing to you.

Conventional Medicine Approach to Skin Infections

If your infection doesn't respond within a day or two to the measures given above, or if you have any associated fever or malaise, you can try antibiotic therapy. Your doctor chooses the antibiotic on the basis of the most probable causative organisms, the presence of which can be confirmed by laboratory cultures of pus from your infected area.

Although many doctors and patients think so, antibiotics are *not* a panacea. They have side effects, can cause allergic reactions, and may be harmful to your kidneys, liver, or hearing. They kill only sensitive organisms, allowing for the development of new, more resistant and dangerous strains, which can then multiply without competition. In addition, antibiotics create the conditions for acute and chronic yeast infections in the vagina and bowel. Antibiotics tend to be misused and overused, and can't be expected to take the place of surgical attention when you have a significant infection. If your infection does not resolve within a few days with the above measures, seek your doctor's further advice.

Surgical Approach to Skin Infections

Hubert was a 65-year-old diabetic who developed a skin infection on the back of his short, bull neck. The infection rapidly progressed from a "boil" to a large, deep, spreading abscess. His diabetes went out of control and he developed shaking chills and a fever of 104 degrees. Under general anesthesia, I removed a large area of dead tissue. His incision measured three by six inches, by three inches deep. However, "all's well that ends well." He was discharged after three days in the hospital, and managed his own care of the incision, with the help of his wife, obtaining complete healing six weeks later.

The vast majority of skin infections can be handled by your immune system without antibiotics or surgery. It's a scary thing to imagine needing a surgeon to help with a skin infection. Most people who eventually seek a surgeon's attention have delayed their treatment due to fear of the scalpel, so their problems are much worse than they might have been if treated earlier.

You need a surgical evaluation whenever your infection has not resolved after a short trial of the alternative and conventional methods given above. Infections can spread very rapidly, leading to the necessity of much more involved treatments and subsequent discomfort, scarring, disability, and expense.

If spontaneous drainage or resolution of your infection is inadequate, you may need an *incision and drainage* ("I and D"). Most I and Ds can be performed with local anesthesia, but larger infections may require general anesthesia and hospitalization for incision care.

The goal of an I and D is to drain all collected pus, and remove any dead tissue. After preparing your skin with an iodine solution, your doctor injects a local anesthetic such as Xylocaine to numb the area around the infection. Your surgeon makes an incision over the site where the infection is closest to the surface, and may remove an ellipse of skin, so that the area will continue to drain freely. The incision is irrigated to flush out pus and any debris. The whole procedure takes only five to ten minutes. You should feel much better immediately. For larger infections, you may need pain pills for a few days.

After your infection is surgically drained, the incision is left open to heal from the inside out; closing it would just recreate your abscess. You can use warm salt water soaks, or allow water from a shower or Waterpik to flow through your incision two or three times per day, keeping the area clean with a mild soap such as Dial or Ivory.

If you have a deeper incision, it may need to be packed with gauze, which must be changed at least twice a day. A soft rubber drain may be inserted, to continue to drain any pus, and prevent it from accumulating again. You may need the help of family, friends, or a visiting nurse if you have a larger, complicated operative site.

While thin plastic nonadherent dressings, such as Telfa, may seem like a good idea, since they cause less discomfort when your dressing is changed, they also prevent effective cleaning of your incision surface. Use the "wet-to-moist" dressing method, where a salt solution is used to dampen each new gauze dressing. You can get the "saline" salt solution at a pharmacy or make it yourself by adding one teaspoon of table salt to one quart of boiling water. This method keeps bacteria counts to a minimum, loosens crusts, and removes pus and other secretions by their adherence to the dressing. You can reduce the pain of removal by wetting the gauze just beforehand.

You should not use peroxide, alcohol, or other common skin antiseptics such as Merthiolate or tincture of iodine directly on an open wound as these agents are harmful to your tissues, which are trying to regenerate themselves. You may use the topical over-the-counter antibiotic ointment bacitracin, or the prescription cream Silvadene, but only if so advised by your doctor.

Depending on its size, blood supply, and type of infection, an infected incision should heal in a few days or weeks. However, the resulting scar will probably be wider and more irregular than that of a clean surgical incision. If you choose, such scars can be revised later using plastic surgery techniques.

Pilonidal Cysts

A *pilonidal cyst* is a *very* common infection, seen in 5 percent of the population, most often in young men, especially those with increased body hair. This cyst develops when a hair breaks the surface of your skin and then grows inward, becoming a source of chronic irritation. Multiple long hairs may form a surprisingly large "hair ball" beneath the skin. Bacterial contamination follows, and an abscess develops. The ingrown hair acts as a foreign body, diminishing the effectiveness of your body's natural defenses.

Although such cysts can be found anywhere that hair grows, they are most often located in the cleft between your buttocks, over the sacral bone. You first notice a tender lump or thickening in the midline or middle side of your "cheek." You can usually see one or more midline pores, which are the sites where hair entered and where spontaneous drainage may have occurred. Extensive, infected tracks beneath the skin can develop.

Without treatment, you may be subject to repeated episodes of tenderness, swelling, and spontaneous drainage. If it does not drain on its own early and effectively, you may develop a very painful abscess that then will need surgical drainage.

Alternative Medicine Approaches to Pilonidal Cysts

When I saw the scar running diagonally across and around the buttocks, it looked like the California coastal highway. This patient very much disliked the physical annoyance of the scar itself, and found it socially embarrassing. If he had it to do again, he told me, he would never have submitted to the surgery.

Pilonidal cysts may respond to alternative therapies, thus helping you avoid a dramatic scar and the other possible complications resulting from such operative procedures.

Following are the most promising alternative and nonsurgical approaches.

Treat Infection

See the instructions given above for alternative treatment of skin infections. Keep your lower back and buttocks clean and dry.

Change Your Diet; Take Supplements

The low-fat, high-fiber diet and supplement program given in Chapter 2 is essential, to assure proper bowel and immune function. Oral zinc, 50 mg three times daily, may be an effective remedy, since it has been shown to boost the immune system's ability to fight infection, by improving white cell (T-cell) function.[11]

Practice Yoga

The gentle yoga stretches given in Chapter 2 also help make certain that increased circulation reaches the area, so that the body's immune system can keep this area clear of infection. Deep relaxation and visualization can be used as well.

Practice Visualization

Follow the guidelines for deep relaxation and visualization given in Chapter 2. First, do the deep relaxation. Then, for example, imagine your cyst as a small balloon. See it deflating, and then disappearing. Hold this image in your mind's eye, while feeling it happen within your body.

Surgical Approaches to Pilonidal Cysts

Surgery may be necessary for permanent cure of this problem. If an abscess develops, it must first be drained, then you must wait two to three weeks to allow inflammation to subside before anything can be done to prevent recurrence. If your problem is chronic but without an abscess, your operation can be carried out without preliminary drainage. If you procrastinate, allowing infection to progress, you may need a much more extensive operation. You can have this done as an outpatient usually using local anesthesia, but spinal or general anesthesia may be preferable in some cases. One of three surgical techniques can be chosen.

No matter which surgical technique you choose, in the postoperative period, you need to see your doctor on a weekly basis, until your healing is assured. After your incision has fully come together, shave or use a depilatory to keep the affected area hair-free for at least six months, to prevent recurrence.

Excision and Closure of the Skin

If no active infection is present, your cyst and any side tracts can be removed with total excision and closure of the skin, using stitches. This operation takes twenty to forty-five minutes, and heals in ten to fourteen days, during which time no direct pressure should be placed on this area, including sitting. You may need pain pills for a few days. Excision and closure has the advantage that the incision is closed immediately, without the need for dressing changes and open incision care, but carries the disadvantages of increased incision infection rates and a 20 percent recurrence rate. Therefore, I recommended it only if you have minimal disease.

Excision Without Skin Closure

Excision without skin closure is a second surgical option, usually used if you have extensive disease. In this procedure, requiring ten to twenty minutes to complete, all infected tissue is removed, and your incision left open under a gauze dressing, without stitches. After a few days, when your soreness has become minimal, you can resume full and unrestricted activity. Your incision heals slowly, over four to six weeks; during this period, you must keep it clean with showers or a pulsating water spray, such as from a Waterpik. You will also need to change your dressings frequently, to minimize dampness—sanitary pads make an ideal dressing. I find this approach very rarely necessary.

Marsupialization

Midway between the two above options is *marsupialization*, which excises most of the cyst and side tracts, but leaves the fibrous base, which is then sewn to the skin edges. This procedure takes twenty to forty-five minutes, produces an incision smaller than that of excision alone, heals within three to five weeks, and carries a recurrence rate of 5 percent, the lowest of all three procedures. Incision care is similar to that described above. You might need pain pills for a few days, after which time you should be able to resume normal activities. This is the technique I most often use.

Skin Cancer

Skin cancer is the most common type of cancer in the United States, and accounts for one-third of all cancer cases. Since spread to other areas of the body is rare, this cancer is usually very easily treated, and more than 90 percent of the time completely cured by simple surgical excision. However, if you avoid or delay treatment, the results can be devastating. Local invasion can extend widely, and if you leave your skin cancer untreated, it can be fatal.

Prolonged exposure to the sun's rays is well known to be the major cause of skin cancer, and light-skinned, redheaded, blue-eyed individuals are most susceptible. The highest rate in the United States is on the Hawaiian island of Kauai; if you spent your life on Kauai, your chances of having this disease by age 80 would be 50 percent, whereas if you spent it in less sunny Minnesota, it would be 17 percent. Skin cancer is quite rare in blacks, since their increased melanin pigmentation protects their skin by screening out harmful rays.

Men are at greater risk than women, probably because men's clothing is less protective and their occupational exposure is higher. If your occupation or recreational preferences lead to prolonged time in the sun, you are at especially high risk. In Australia, women who wear bikinis when they sunbathe have thirteen times the rates of skin cancer than those who wear one-piece swimsuits. Women who choose low-backed swimsuits are four times more likely to develop these cancers.[12]

Skin cancer has also been associated with large amounts of diagnostic and therapeutic X-rays, and with nuclear blast exposure. Chemical carcinogens in petroleum by-products, as well as arsenic, are also known to cause it. Additionally, it may arise in areas of chronic irritation, such as long-standing skin ulcers, infections, and scars.

Ninety-five percent of skin cancer develops on the most sun-exposed areas: face, neck, and hands. *Most skin cancers could be prevented by avoiding prolonged sun exposure*, especially during the midday period, between 10 A.M. and 3 P.M. Garments and sunscreen should be used to filter out the harmful ultraviolet rays. The B vitamin PABA, used topically, is an effective sunscreen, although some persons exhibit allergic reactions. In our culture, the pleasures derived from "basking in the sun," the stature awarded a natural suntan, the restriction of staying inside, and the annoyance of applying sunscreen make a significant reduction in incidence of skin cancer by preventive measures difficult. *You should always wear a sunscreen, especially if you are fair-skinned, redheaded, or blue-eyed.*

Basal Cell Skin Cancer

The *basal cell* type of skin cancer is the most common type. This cancer usually grows very slowly, and may have been present for many years before you bother to ask your physician about it. Ninety-five percent of basal cell cancers develop on the head and neck. Distant spread is extremely rare; however, these tumors can be very locally destructive.

A basal cell cancer appears as a small scaly or scabbed area of skin, and can easily be con-fused with other skin problems, such as acne or eczema. If you allow it to grow large, it may then be quite difficult to remove and still leave you with a satisfactory cosmetic result.

Of the three types of basal cell cancers, the most common is *nodular*, a firm and pearly gray area, with raised borders, very tiny surface blood vessels, and a central depression containing a crust or ulcer that may bleed. *Superficial* basal cell cancers, tending to grow on your trunk, are reddened and thin, with edges blending into normal adjacent skin. Quite hard to distinguish from benign problems, they tend to be multiple. *Pigmented* basal cancers, with color varying from brown to black, may appear quite similar to the more dangerous malignant melanoma. You need an expert, and most likely a biopsy, to distinguish among these cancers.

Squamous Cell Skin Cancer

Squamous cell skin cancer exhibits a different microscopic pattern than basal cell cancer, and is more worrisome, since it can spread—though rarely—through your lymphatic system, to distant sites. It often appears first as an ulcerated area or wart that crusts, bleeds easily, and never quite heals. Seventy-five percent of these cancers grow on the head and fifteen percent on the hands.

The first thing you must do if you suspect a basal or squamous skin cancer is have a biopsy to determine its exact nature.

Alternative Medicine Approaches to Basal and Squamous Cell Skin Cancers

Alternative medicine approaches offer great hope in the treatment of resistant skin cancer, especially when it is unresponsive to conventional approaches. When added as adjuncts to therapy for the most dangerous type of skin cancer, melanoma, alternative approaches may improve survival rates.

No self-treatment of cancer should be used without your doctor's supervision. The alternative medicine approaches given here may best be used as adjuncts to conventional therapies.

One of my patients, a weekend golfer, was blissfully spending his retirement enhancing his game by going to the golf course every day, and rewarding himself with several glasses of wine, along with chicken and steak, in the evening. He noticed a small, scaly growth on the side of his forehead that just didn't seem to heal. Biopsy showed it to be a squamous cell cancer.

Preventing these cancers is another great reason to consider becoming a vegetarian and replacing your alcohol with Perrier. The sun's ultraviolet radiation damages the ability of the skin cell to maintain its appropriate genetic structure and is at the core of this problem. What alternative medicine can offer is a recommendation of nutrients to help prevent this damage, so that your skin can repair itself, or once cancer has developed, prevent its return after treatment.

Successful treatment of basal and squamous cell skin cancers with alternative medicine has now been documented, and these approaches offer the advantages of diminished scarring and pain, as well as helping prevent future cancers.

Since basal and squamous cell cancers tend to be slow-growing, you can try alternatives, though only once your doctor makes certain your disease has not reached the point of danger. Do not then delay in surgical removal if your cancer has not begun to respond within a few weeks. *All skin cancer therapy must be monitored by your physician.*

Following are the most promising alternative medicine remedies for prevention and treatment of basal and squamous cell skin cancers.

Practice Prevention

Limit your sun exposure, and when you do go in the sun, use sunscreen. You *need* some sun exposure to maintain good health, assure mineral absorption, and *prevent* cancer, most notably cancers of the breast and colon. Vitamin D, activated by sunlight on the skin, may be systemically anticarcinogenic, and responsible for the lower rates of these two cancers in areas of the country getting the most sun.

What is most associated with skin cancers is *burn*. You should monitor your sun dosage, especially if you tend to burn easily, and stay out of the sun during the most intense hours of sunshine, between 10 A.M. and 3 P.M. Wear PABA, the most effective sunscreen, of at least 15 SPF potency, even on cloudy days, when 80 percent of the sun's rays still penetrate the clouds. If you are sensitive to PABA, you can opt for PABA-free sunscreens.

In addition, enjoy frequent steam baths or saunas. Steam baths and saunas help the skin stay healthy by drawing nutrition to it. You can take one every day, or at least once a week. Then apply aloe, topical vitamin E, comfrey, calendula, castor oil, or cocoa butter to any problem areas, to help maintain skin wellness. Check your skin regularly for any abnormal areas, and seek advice if you spot anything.

Change Your Diet; Take Supplements

A high-fat diet has been found to be associated with an increased incidence of skin cancer.[13] Consumption of vitamin A–rich foods may be protective and may partly account for the higher rate of this tumor in men, who usually do not eat as many vegetables as do women. A diet low in fat and high in vitamin A–rich foods such as dark green and dark yellow vegetables, should be instituted. Once skin cancer has developed, vitamin A, in various formulations, is also now being utilized as a therapeutic agent. Specific dietary directions are contained in Chapter 2.

Alcohol and sugar, by lowering the activity of the white cells, as noted in Chapter 2, can interfere with your body's ability to remove abnormal skin cells. Nutrients needed for optimum skin cell maintenance are: primrose, borage, or flaxseed oil, two capsules or one teaspoon daily; multi-B complex, 100 mg; kelp capsules as a source of minerals, one to three daily; vitamin E for its antioxidant effects, 400 IU three times daily.

Vitamin A supplements in animal studies has been found to delay skin tumor appearance, slow tumor growth, and may even cause tumors to diminish in size or disappear. Vitamin A and its derivatives may have a prophylactic and a therapeutic role in human skin cancers.[14] The usual dose is 10,000 IU orally one to three times daily, in addition to topical application of vitamin A. WARNING: Vitamin A in doses of more than 10,000 IU daily must be taken only under the supervision of your doctor.

Beta-carotene, a precursor to vitamin A, has been shown to have an antitumor effect in animals exposed to sunlight. Eat foods rich in mixed carotenoids, such as carrots, cantaloupes, sweet potatoes, spinach, and other dark green leafy vegetables. Mixed carotenoids can also be taken in doses of 25,000 to 30,000 IU daily, as directed by your doctor. *Genistein*, an isoflavone occurring in soy products, is felt to contribute to protection against skin cancer.[15] Take soy milk, one to three cups daily, or tofu, one-quarter cup daily.

Garlic oil and onion oil were found to be effective in reducing the number of skin cancers, when given in doses of 1 mg per kg and 10 mg per kg of body weight, respectively.[16] Adding these elements, by eating fresh raw garlic and onions liberally, may give additional protection.

Practice Hypnosis

Hypnosis, described in Chapter 2, has been shown to be very effective for skin health.[17] Find an experienced hypnotherapist. Since your body may take time to respond, repeated sessions may be needed.

Use Homeopathy

Specific homeopathic remedies for the treatment of skin cancer should be individually prescribed by a trained homeopath. The usually effective choices are thuja, natrum muriaticum, and sulfur. In addition to your homeopath, you should be monitored by a doctor who is a specialist in skin cancer.

Use Natural Topicals

Anecdotally, topical castor oil therapy has been found to be successful in treatment of early basal cell skin cancers.[18] Six to eight weeks are usually necessary to see the full effects, with application three times daily. Topical vitamin A, in the form of tretinoin (Retin-A), has been shown to prevent premalignant skin lesions, such as actinic keratoses, from developing into skin cancer.[19] This treatment was shown effective in eliminating skin cancer in 90 percent of 300 patients with this disease.[20]

Carrot oil and alfalfa oil also contain vitamin A, in a form that avoids the side effects of burning or sun sensitivity, seen with Retin-A. These oils are available in health food store skin-care products, but have not yet been studied in the context of cancer prevention or reversal.

Practice Stress Management

Stress has been linked to skin cancer.[21] When and where any cancer develops may have psychosocial meaning, reflecting the interaction of stress and the immune system. Cancer researcher Dr. Carl Simonton first became interested in the relationship of mind and cancer when he himself developed a skin cancer on his nose during a period of high stress.[22]

Use Acupuncture; Practice Qi Gong and Yoga

These modalities act to address the underlying flow of energy and nutrients that may have influenced the inability of the body to maintain the skin cells. Further research is needed to determine their specific effects. See Chapter 2 for more information on these approaches.

Practice Visualization

Visualization has been extensively explored as an adjunct to cancer therapy, and is described in Chapter 2, along with other stress-management techniques. For example, imagine your skin is a sandy beach, with a small clay balloon sitting on it. Take a hammer, puncture the balloon, and wash it clean with the water. Hold this picture in your mind, while you feel it happening in your body.

Conventional Medicine Approaches to Basal and Squamous Cell Skin Cancer

Nonsurgical approaches seek to avoid the discomfort and scarring associated with surgery. The following are the approaches that may be effective.

Immunotherapy

In research conducted by Dr. Hubert Greenway, at Scripps Medical Center, La Jolla, California, 81 percent of patients were free of basal cell cancer one year following the injection of a gel of interferon alfa-2b (AccuSite) three times a week, for three weeks.[23] The advantage of this approach is avoiding the sometimes large scar caused by surgical removal, especially a problem for cancers on the face.

Radiotherapy

Radiation treatment of skin cancer is not often used unless tissue preservation is very important, such as with the tip of your nose or your eyelids; reconstruction after excision here would be a major undertaking. Advantages of radiation are that treatment is relatively painless, hospitalization isn't required, surgical expertise is unnecessary, and tumor extensions that might not otherwise be detected are destroyed.

Disadvantages include possibility of poor healing, with a resulting ulcer taking months, or longer, to heal completely. The scar itself may be thin and fragile, and permanent hair loss and changes in skin pigmentation often develop. The carcinogenic potential of the treatment itself must be kept in mind, especially if your further life expectancy is greater than twenty years.

Drug Treatment

Anticancer medications can be used locally, and are often successful in treating small cancers. Five-fluorouracil, 5-FU, is a commonly used anticancer drug that can be injected into your tumor, or applied as a cream. As noted above, some dermatologists are experimenting with derivatives of vitamin A applied topically combined with surgical curettage.

Surgical Approaches to Basal and Squamous Cell Skin Cancer

Surgical treatment options for basal and squamous cell cancers are the same. Several different methods of treatment provide essentially the same success—about 95 percent cure—with the first treatment attempt. The therapy recommended depends on your specific tumor's size, thickness, and location. You must consider discomfort, time, and expense of the various treatments, along with their cosmetic results and the possibility of scarring that might limit your movements. Following are the two basic surgical options.

Electrodessication and Curettage

The simplest form of surgical treatment is *electrodessication and curettage,* suitable for small tumors. After skin preparation with an iodine solution, to decrease presence of skin bacteria, your doctor numbs the tumor and surrounding skin with a local anesthetic such as Xylocaine. The cancer is first "desiccated" (burst into pieces) by an electric needle (or laser) that generates localized heat, destroying the tumor cells, that are then scraped away with a sharp curette scraper or scalpel. The raw area is sore for a few days, but should heal in a week or two. If all the tumor is not

removed with the first treatment, a second "cycle" of destruction and scraping will be necessary, perhaps followed by a third.

The major advantages of this technique are that it is quick and easy, and several tumors can be treated at the same time. Stitches are not required, less normal tissue is removed than with surgical excision, and the resulting scar is usually smaller, though it may be wider than with surgical excision. The major disadvantages are that it is not suitable for large, deep, or recurrent tumors, and pockets of malignant cells can be easily missed. Healing takes much longer than with surgical removal followed by stitches, and the resulting scar may be deforming. Complications of this form of treatment can include excessive scar thickening, deformity, incision infection, and recurrence of tumor.

Surgical Excision

Complete removal by surgical excision is usually the best method for treating large and invading cancers. Because cells have not been destroyed, as with the other methods of treatment, it provides the best biopsy specimen for microscopic analysis. If this analysis shows that tumor has been left behind, more tissue can be taken, either during your original surgery (if immediate testing is available) or at a later date.

Most skin cancer operations can be performed under simple local anesthesia with you as an outpatient. More complicated reconstructions, such as on your face or scalp requiring skin rearrangement or grafting, may be undertaken using a local anesthetic with sedation, or general anesthesia.

After administration of the anesthetic, your surgeon removes the tumor, along with an ellipse of skin, carefully trying to avoid damage to adjacent nerves and blood vessels. This approach must remove more normal tissue than with curettage, so that the closure can lie flat, rather than form the "dog ears" of a circular incision. Usually, your scar can be arranged to follow your skin wrinkle lines. The incision is closed either with stitches beneath your skin, which will dissolve, along with skin tapes to hold the upper skin edges together, or with external stitches. Your incision should be covered and kept dry for forty-eight hours. A week following surgery, your doctor should check it, remove stitches, if any, and discuss your pathologic report, ensuring that the tumor was completely removed.

Although you might need pain pills for a few days, healing should be rapid and relatively painless. Cosmetic results are generally good: The fine thin surgical scar compares favorably with the wider, thicker scar that often results from the other forms of treatment. Hair loss and pigmentation changes can be minimized. Disadvantages of surgery are that surgical expertise varies, it can be relatively expensive, and occasionally complications can develop, such as bleeding, incision infection, and excessive scar formation.

Malignant Melanoma

Charles, a 56-year-old, had a dark mole which had been present for five years on his right forearm. He didn't pay much attention to it until it started bleeding. When removed, it was found to be a two-millimeter-thick malignant melanoma. He then underwent a wider skin excision in the area where the melanoma had been, followed by armpit lymph gland removal, which revealed two tiny areas of melanoma spread. After his surgery, he chose to participate in an experimental study using interleukin II, an immune stimulator, now known to be helpful in patients with advanced melanoma. Three years later, he still had no evidence of melanoma recurrence.

A *melanoma*, also termed *malignant melanoma* due to its tendency to spread, is a cancerous transformation in your skin's dark pigment cells (the melanocytes). Unlike other forms of skin cancer, it tends to spread through lymph and blood vessels to distant areas of the body and is therefore quite dangerous.

Most melanomas begin microscopically, gradually enlarging until they are visible to the naked eye, although one-third develop from a previously benign mole. Early melanomas are usually flat and superficial. At this stage, they are 100 percent curable by simple surgery. As they grow, they invade the underlying skin's dermis and fat, where they come into contact with lymph channels and blood vessels. Clumps of tumor cells may then invade these channels and migrate, establishing new tumor sites in other areas of your body.

In the last decade, the incidence of malignant melanoma in the United States has been increasing at a rate of 4 percent per year, faster than any other cancer. In 2002 an estimated 58,300 new cases will be diagnosed and 7,400 people will die of this disease.[24] If you are a man, your chances of developing melanoma in your lifetime is 1.42 percent. If you are a woman, it is 1.08 percent. Your chance of dying from melanoma is 0.31 percent or 0.20 percent, respectively.

Like other forms of skin cancer, melanoma is at least partially caused by ionizing radiation from the sun. You are at higher risk if you have a history of excessive sun exposure and severe sunburn in childhood, have lots of moles or freckles, are fair-skinned with blue eyes and light hair, or have an inability to tan without burning. White-collar working men, with higher education, are at high risk, most likely due to episodic weekend exposure to the sun, making them very subject to sunburn. Melanoma has been found to be increased in patients who have received ultraviolet light treatment for severe psoriasis (PUVA).[25] Melanomas are ten times higher in white than nonwhite populations. They are rare in African-Americans and Asians, where they tend to appear only on the palms and soles. Some families are melanoma-prone, so if you have a family member who develops a melanoma, you should be especially careful to examine your entire skin surface at regular intervals and meticulously avoid sun exposure.

Women most often develop melanomas on their arms and legs, while in men they are more common on the chest, back, and scalp. Arm and leg tumors have the best prognosis, followed by those on the scalp, head, and neck; the trunk carries a more difficult prognosis, while location in the mouth, anus, and genitals has the worst outlook. Peak incidence is in the 30-to-60-year age range, with prognosis worse in older individuals.

The average Caucasian has more than 100 brown spots and about 15 moles. The chance that one of these will change to become malignant is extremely unlikely: less than one in a million for each mole. Most melanomas have been present for a few years before being seen by a doctor. They need to be recognized early, when simple surgical removal is 100 percent curable. Appearing asymmetric, with poorly marked borders, these tumors usually have variable pigmentation of brown, black, gray, pink, or flesh-colored areas, within the same tumor.

The problem is to pick out a melanoma from within the landscape of pigment collections and moles that all of us have. Look for the ABCDs of melanoma appearance:

A = Asymmetry: growth is not round or oval; one half does not match the other.
B = Border: irregular, scalloped, or blurred.
C = Color: variable with multiple color shades.
D = Diameter: usually greater than 6 millimeters.

Melanomas can appear as a flat pigment "stain," slightly raised, or "nodular," the thickest type, with the worst prognosis. One type of melanoma may change to another as it grows. If ulceration is present, your prognosis worsens. Examination of the biopsy specimen, especially its thickness, establishes the probability of your tumor's metastasis, its prognosis, and your optimum form of treatment.

It is helpful if you take Polaroid photos of your moles and brown spots for future comparison. Removal of a normal mole is unnecessary unless it is in an area of constant irritation, such as the bra, belt, or collar line. *However, whenever a mole changes in size, consistency, or coloration; bleeds, crusts, or ulcerates; becomes painful; or itches, it should be removed.*

If you develop a melanoma, your chance for cure depends on the thickness of the tumor and, more important, whether or not spread has occurred to lymph nodes or beyond. If your tumor is less than 1 millimeter thick, your chance for cure is 98 percent. If your tumor is more than 1 but less than 4 millimeters thick, you should probably have your sentinel node checked, as described on page

168. Overall, about 80 percent of melanomas are found at an early localized stage. Table 5.1 shows prognosis for living five years after diagnosis and treatment by stage of spread.

If you develop one melanoma, you have a 3 percent chance of developing another one within three years; you should, therefore, have close follow-up by your doctor.

Alternative Medicine Approaches to Malignant Melanoma

Your doctor should supervise any alternative or complementary therapies for malignant melanoma. Promising alternative medicine treatments center on your immune system. Conventional research into the effects of vitamin A and its derivatives, interferon and interleukin-2, natural immune modulators, and BCG, a vaccine derived from an organism similar to the one that causes tuberculosis, may be supplemented by the following approaches, particularly group therapy. Although these new treatments, used singly or in combination, may be utilized for disseminated melanoma, they are *not* yet recommended as the primary treatment for early disease, since simple surgical removal is so often all that is needed then for cure.

Change Your Diet, Take Supplements

All skin cancers have been found to be less common in vegetarians. This may in part be due to the higher vitamin A levels in this diet. Follow the guidelines given in Chapter 2.

A number of studies in animals have now specifically linked low vitamin A levels to the development of a variety of cancers, and research in humans has shown similar results. In one study, investigators found that patients administered oral vitamin A along with the immune stimulator BCG (made from modified tuberculosis organisms) had fewer relapses than patients who received BCG alone. Both of these agents act to stimulate the immune system in ways not yet fully understood. Dosage of vitamin A is 30,000 IU daily, but must be monitored by your doctor.

One team of researchers reported that topical vitamin B_6 was able to induce regression of metastatic melanoma in two patients.[27] B_6 has been used successfully to treat bladder tumors, a cell type similarly originating from the epithelial tissues that cover the body's surfaces and line its cavities. Dosage of vitamin B_6 begins at 50 to 500 mg daily, but must be monitored by your doctor. Both vitamins C and E have shown antimelanoma cell activity

TABLE 5.1
Prognosis of Malignant Melanoma

	Percent of Patients Surviving 5 Years	Percent of Patients in This Stage
All Patients	88.8%	
Not Staged	73.7%	6%
By Stage		
Localized to skin	96.0%	82%
Lymph node spread	60.5%	9%
Distant spread	16%	4%

in the laboratory.[28] Follow the complete supplement program given in Chapter 2.

Melatonin, an antioxidant hormone normally secreted by the pineal gland, when taken at a dosage of 500 to 700 mg twice a day, has initially shown promise with this disease, though further research is needed.[29]

Use Natural Topicals and Herbs

Echinacea and garlic both have been documented to enhance white cell activity, thought by some researchers to assist in fighting cancer. Freshly crushed garlic applied to the tumor has been historically reported to be able to eliminate melanoma, though research remains to be carried out. Melanoma is a cancer reportedly found responsive to some of the current complementary cancer therapy programs, such as the Gerson program, the Hoxey herb treatment, and a drawing salve made of a combination of herbs including sanguinaria, bittersweet, ginger, galanga, chaparral, and capsicum; whether this is an effect of large doses of vitamin A in the diets and herbs used or by a placebo mechanism is not yet known. Germanium, astragalus, chaparral, coenzme Q10, essiac, and many other herbs are claimed to be of benefit.[30] For further consideration of alternative medicine cancer treatment approaches, see Dr. Michael Lerner's book, *Choices in Healing*, and Patrick Quillin's *Beating Cancer with Nutrition*, referenced in the Resources section of this book.

Practice Stress Management

Positive attitude and strategies to cope with stress affect your immune system, and your resistance to melanoma may be influenced by the stress-management approaches presented in Chapter 2. An assessment was made of melanoma patients' adjustment to their illness, and a high score (good adjustment) was associated with a good one-year outcome; this test was a better predictor of one-year survival than extent of disease, suggesting that psychological variables do play a significant role in this cancer.[31]

Since melanomas are unpredictable cancers, visualization may be an especially important adjunct to your treatment. Some melanomas seem to disappear spontaneously on their own, while others recur after thirty or more years. Psychoimmunotherapy may play an important role in the future, as we learn how to enlist the brain's resources. Follow the guidelines for alternative medicine treatment of basal and squamous cell cancers, given above.

Join a Support Group

As discussed in Chapter 2, research has shown an improved survival in melanoma patients who joined a support group that met once a week for six weeks.[32] You may use the Internet and the Resources section of this book to find a group.

Use Acupuncture; Practice Qi Gong and Yoga

In China, many investigators claim benefits for acupuncture, Chinese herbs, and the energy discipline of qi gong as healing aids to cancer. In the parks, as part of their qi gong practice, you can see cancer patients hugging trees for twenty minutes to an hour, establishing a revitalized energy field to fight their disease. In the same way, yoga stretches and meditation are felt to help rearrange the energy and circulation patterns in the body, thereby affecting immune function. Further research is needed to determine specific effects.

Practice Visualization

Visualization has shown promise when used as an adjunct to cancer treatment.[33] First, do the deep relaxation, as given in Chapter 2. Then, for example, imagine your melanoma as a small spot of mud on a clear cloth. See your white cells as spot remover, and see the cloth bright and clean. See this happening in your mind's eye, while you feel it within your body. Repeat three to five times daily. See Chapter 2 for details.

Conventional Medicine Approaches to High Risk and Advanced Malignant Melanoma

If you have a melanoma with a poor prognosis, or have found to have spread to your lymph nodes or beyond, seek out the latest information about combining chemotherapy, immunotherapy, vaccines, and gene therapy.

Immunotherapy

The Federal Drug Administration has endorsed *interferon alfa-2b* as the first approved agent for use in high-risk melanoma patients without known spread. A 1996 study found that inteferon increased chances for five-year disease-free survival by 42 percent in high-risk surgically treated melanoma patients.[34] However, another preliminary report of a larger group of patients found no survival advantage at 4.3 years.[35] Trials are ongoing.

Experimental Trials

If you have known tumor spread that can't be treated surgically, you may want to enter into one of the ongoing experimental trials, under the supervision of a melanoma cancer specialist.

Monoclonal antibodies have been created in the laboratory and used to attack the melanoma cells. A genetic research technique extracts your own immune cells, changes them in the laboratory to better target the melanoma cells, then reinjects them. Another approach removes some cancer cells, alters them, then reinjects them as a vaccine to get an improved natural immune response from your own body. An antigen to melanoma, called tyrosinase, can be added to your T-cells to help them target the melanoma. Other agents, such as colony stimulating factor and virulixin, which activate white cell activity, and tumor necrosis factor, which assists in tumor breakdown, may also be added. Betulinic acid, a substance derived from the white birch tree, has been found to be selectively toxic to melanoma cells when tested in animals, and will hopefully prove effective in clinical trials, yet to be conducted.

The "Dartmouth protocol" uses a combination of chemotherapeutic agents along with immunotherapy and vaccine treatment. The antiparasitic agents levamisol and suramin have shown promise, as well as the addition of tamoxifen. Although there is no proven benefit as yet, initial results are encouraging.

Surgical Approach to Malignant Melanoma

Any growth suspected of being a melanoma should be completely removed during biopsy, easily performed under local anesthesia while you are an outpatient. If the lesion is large, or in an area where complete removal would be complicated, a piece can first be taken for microscopic evaluation.

The surgical procedure for removal of a melanoma is the same as described above for the other skin cancers, except that, depending on the depth of invasion of your tumor, a 0.5- to 2-centimeter margin of adjacent normal skin must also be removed, to prevent local recurrence.

This procedure is termed a "wide local excision." The defect is usually closed with stitches or skin tapes. If the melanoma is large, or in an area without loose skin, a skin graft or a plastic surgical "flap" may be required to close the incision. You may need pain pills for a few days, but your healing should be complete in a week or so. You need to go over the final pathologic evaluation with your doctor.

The need for, or desirability of, a surgical procedure to biopsy the lymph glands draining the area of your melanoma, to check for and remove possible cancer cells there, is controversial. Evidence regarding its benefits is conflicting. Surgeons and other cancer specialists agree that your glands should be removed if they are enlarged and appear to contain tumor spread. Also, some older studies show that if you have a tumor extending deeper than 1.5 millimeters, but less than 4 millimeters, and have your local glands removed even when they are not enlarged, you have a better chance for cure than if you do not. This advantage is more likely if you have an arm or leg tumor than one on your trunk or at some other site.

Recently, new low-risk, less-invasive techniques have been developed to check for tumor cells in the "sentinel" lymph node. This node is the first node that cells reach when they begin to spread through the lymph channels. If a surgical biopsy of this node does not show tumor cells, you can avoid the discomfort and possible complications of a full lymph node operation.

Prior to this biopsy, the sentinel node is located by the injection of a liquid radioactive isotope tracer into the skin around the melanoma. As the tracer is picked up by and moves through the tumor's lymph drainage channels, it is followed by an isotope camera, which will localize the "hot spot" of the sentinel node where the tracer first accumulates. The spot is marked on the skin with indelible ink.

In the operating room, your surgeon, after first injecting blue dye around the melanoma. makes an incision over the marked area. The sentinel node will pick up the blue dye and can be visually identified. Also, the sentinel node containing the radioactive isotope tracer is found by using a handheld probe and Geiger counter technique. The node specimen is then microscopically examined for tumor cells. If any are found, you should then have the full lymph node operation.

Using these techniques, usually requiring only local anesthesia, it can be determined if you have nodal spread with 96 percent accuracy. Aside from removing tumor in the nodes and improving your prognosis, another reason to have your nodes checked is that if you are found to have microscopic spread to lymph glands, recent studies show that your prognosis can be further improved with interferon alpha-2b treatment, as described in the next section. Ask your surgeon about the latest information on these techniques, since sentinel node biopsy is now the state of the art. However, in the near future, the PET scan may replace sentinel node biopsy as a noninvasive way to determine lymph node status.[36]

Full lymph gland operations are performed under general or regional anesthesia in a hospital operating room. Your surgeon makes a two-to-three-inch incision in your armpit, base of your neck, or groin, depending on the location of your melanoma. The glands and surrounding tissue draining the area of your tumor are removed, and the incision closed with stitches. A soft plastic drain may be left in place for a few days to collect fluid, until your lymph channels seal.

You are taught simple drain and incision management at discharge. You usually stay in the hospital for a day or two, and may need pain pills for several days. If your melanoma was on your arm or leg, you should keep this limb elevated to prevent swelling. You should see your doctor after a few days, to be checked for incision complications, have your drains or stitches removed, and discuss the final pathology report. Complications after armpit and groin lymph node removal may include infection, fluid collections, or troublesome arm or leg swelling.

SKIN CANCER AND MALIGNANT MELANOMA SUMMARY

Prevention

Diet and Supplements

- Follow a low-fat, vegetarian diet, especially dark green, red, and yellow vegetables.
- Eat garlic and onions daily.
- Vitamin A, 10,000 IU daily.
- Mixed carotenoids, 25,000–30,000 IU daily.
- Borage, flaxseed, or primrose oil, 300 mg, 2 times daily.
- Multi-B complex, 50 mg daily.
- Kelp, 500 mg daily.
- Soy milk or powder, 1/4 cup daily.

Lifestyle

- Limit sun exposure. Use sunscreen.
- Take steam baths or saunas.
- Check your skin regularly.
- Practice yoga and qi gong.
- Practice stress management.

Alternative Medicine Approaches

- Follow preventive program, above.
- Topical castor oil, Retin-A, carrot or alfalfa oil under supervision.
- Vitamin A, 10,000 IU, 1–3 times daily under supervision.
- Mixed carotenoids, 25,000–300,000 daily under supervision.
- Hypnosis.
- Homeopathy.
- Acupuncture.
- Visualization.

Conventional Medicine Approaches

Basal and Squamous Cell
- Immunotherapy—interferon alpha-2b.
- Radiotherapy.
- Medications—5-FU.

Melanoma
- Immunotherapy—interferon alpha-2b.

Surgical Approaches

Basal and Squamous Cell
- Electrodessication and curettage.
- Surgical excision.

Melanoma
- Wide local excision.
- Sentinel node biopsy.
- Full lymph node removal.

CHAPTER 6

BREAST

Joyce, a 53-year-old actress, had been experiencing the stress of constantly trying out for parts for which she was not chosen. She comforted herself by drinking lots of coffee lattes at the local café. She had divorced two years previously, and was single-handedly raising the 12-year-old child she had given birth to late in life, at age 41, after several miscarriages. While taking a shower, she noticed a small lump in her breast that had not been there previously. Biopsy showed it to be an early cancer.

She chose breast conservation therapy (lumpectomy) with follow-up radiation, as described in this chapter, but also began a series of lifestyle changes including a low-fat diet, quitting caffeine, daily yoga and exercise, and joining a support group. She remained free of disease at follow-up, five years later, and used her breast cancer as a positive turning point toward a richer experience of life.

You may worry about your breasts, be concerned about their shape and size, or afraid they might develop cancer. What should you do? Can you avoid the scalpel? An integrative approach offers new hope: combining what alternative medicine has to contribute while also giving you the newest choices of surgical techniques, when they are appropriate—for cosmetic concerns, and the prevention and treatment of breast cancer.

The breasts have come to epitomize femininity, in terms of their appearance as well as function. Usually a source of pleasure and human satisfaction, they can also become a cause for severe recurrent anxiety and physical pain. Many women contemplate changing them through surgery, are confused about when they should begin having mammograms and how frequently, and too often, avoid even examining themselves for fear of what they might find.

In this chapter, we present comprehensive information for both prevention and treatment of a variety of breast disorders. The latest research indicates that you can take steps yourself which may help prevent fibrocystic disease and cancer in your breasts. In addition, should you develop cancer, we present your best surgical options for effective treatment, along with alternative medicine approaches that can speed your recovery and improve your chances for survival.

One in eight American women who live to age 85 now develops breast cancer—an alarming rate of increase, making the number of cases of this cancer almost double that of twenty years ago. What is generally referred to as "prevention of cancer" is actually only "secondary prevention," meaning it is simply screening to find problems early; such measures do not act to prevent the onset of disease. We will discuss the latest evidence for "primary prevention," what you yourself can do to prevent cancer from developing in the first place, through preventive lifestyle change.

Even if you do develop cancer, newer surgical techniques can spare your breast, or if it does happen that one or both of your breasts must be removed, reconstructive surgery has been refined to give highly satisfying results. Alternative medicine also has added new solutions for concerns about the size and/or shape of your breasts.

The dictionary defines the breast as "the outer part of the chest," but also as "the bosom conceived of as the center of thoughts and feelings." Your body image, your sense of self and sexuality, and your emotions may be strongly tied to your feelings about your breasts. In addition to their symptoms, your attitudes about them may reflect and express messages from your subconscious self. Once you are aware of such signals, you can choose your own personal path to a healthier and more fulfilling experience both of your body and your life.

Development, Structure, and Function of Your Breasts

In attempting to understand surgical problems of the breasts, it is helpful to know of what they are composed and what factors affect them.

Your breasts consist of glandular and supporting fibrous tissues, with fat interspersed between. The glandular tissue includes twelve to twenty mammary glands or lobes, which make milk during breast-feeding. (See Figure 6.1.) Ducts, positioned to carry this milk up to your nipple, exit through tiny pores. As you age, the ratio of "firm" glandular tissue to "soft" fat tissue changes. When you are young, you have more glandular tissue and stronger supporting fibrous tissue bands creating, therefore, firmer breasts. These glands are gradually replaced by fat and the fibrous tissue weakens, so that a softer, more pendulous breast is normal in older women.

Oil-forming glands appear as tiny "BBs" just under the surface of your areola, the dark tissue surrounding your nipple. Having hair surrounding the nipple is common and also completely normal.

If you divide your breast into four parts, the upper outer quarter extends up toward your armpit and contains the most tissue. About 80 percent of breast cancers develop in this area. Your breast's lymphatic channels, the body's system for draining fluids that accumulate in your tissues, travel mostly to and through lymph nodes in your armpit, with some also leading to nodes underneath your breastbone.

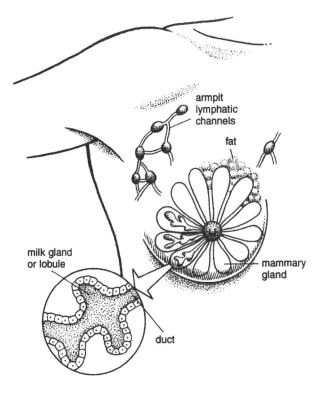

armpit
lymphatic
channels

fat

milk gland
or lobule

mammary
gland

duct

Fig. 6.1 The anatomy of the breast

Breast development and function are controlled by hormones. The immature breast consists principally of ducts. At puberty, estrogen and progesterone, the primary female hormones influencing breast tissue, begin to be produced by the ovaries. These, as well as hormones from the pituitary gland, act to stimulate budding of the terminal ducts, to form the alveolar or acini cells, which may eventually secrete milk. The mature breast is continuously stimulated by fluctuating levels of these two hormones during monthly hormonal cycles that increase and decrease the size and sensitivity of your breasts.

Estrogen remains at fairly uniform levels throughout most of the menstrual cycle, and its cumulative effect is a proliferation of the ductal system, increase in volume and elasticity of fibrous tissue, increased vascularity, and fat deposition, resulting in enlarging breast size. Progesterone primarily affects the breast in the two weeks before menstruation. Along with estrogen, it also increases breast size, by stimulating the alveolar cells to proliferate, enlarge, become more active, take on water, and become secretory.

Therefore both hormones, acting together, explain why your breasts are at their largest and most sensitive just prior to your period. Premenstrual syndrome (PMS) occurs whenever the effects of such hormone fluctuations are extreme.

After menstruation, the two hormone levels drop, the stimulation decreases, and the breasts shrink in size. The result of this proliferation and regression may not be uniform throughout the breast, so that areas of nodularity may develop. The resulting lumpy regions, however, usually disappear after a few cycles, although some may remain, and prompt you to seek evaluation.

During pregnancy, as the breast enlarges and makes itself ready for milk production, estrogen and progesterone levels remain high. After delivery, the levels of these hormones suddenly drop, and the pituitary hormone prolactin causes onset of milk flow from the actively secreting alveolar cells. After pregnancy and milk production are finished, the breasts diminish in size once again, although they often retain some of their increased size. With menopause, as ovarian function decreases, hormone levels fall, and the alveolar cells largely disappear. The breast becomes smaller, consisting mostly of ducts, fibrous tissue, and fat.

Both oral contraceptives and estrogen hormone replacement therapy act to increase the breasts' exposure to estrogen. Some studies have suggested an increased risk for breast cancer in women who began taking birth control pills as teenagers, and a clear association has been found between estrogen replacement therapy and increased risk of breast cancer. These issues are discussed below, in the section considering breast cancer.

Certain chemicals, drugs such as coffee and other caffeinated beverages, and pollutants have hormonelike effects on breast tissue. The breasts can absorb some medications from your bloodstream, and then concentrate them; if you breast-feed, they may be secreted in your breast milk. Alcohol can affect your baby's behavior.[1] Smoking gives a nicotine smell and taste to breast milk and increases the likelihood of this addiction for the baby later in life.[2]

Appearance of Your Breasts

Especially in the Western world, a woman's breasts are symbols of sexuality and attractiveness. "Beautiful" breasts are prominently displayed by glamorous people, and used in advertising to help peddle totally unrelated products. Our culture's notion of what is appealing, based on the Barbie Doll or Playboy image, makes a certain size, shape, or orientation "ideal."

However, *most* women's breasts do not fit these imaginary icons, and though lumpy, sagging, or unmatched in shape or size, they still can provide perfectly graceful sexual response. Your breasts are *unique*, and no two bodies are exactly alike.

Deborah told this story: *"I grew up thinking 'perky' breasts were much more attractive, and really hated my 'pendulous'-shaped ones. They reminded me of torpedoes. One day, my sister and I were sitting in the sauna, and finally started talking frankly about breast shape. She told me she had always admired my breast type, instead of her own smaller, firmer ones. She thought mine must be more appealing, because they were softer. We both had a good laugh, and vowed to feel better about our bodies despite our society's hang-ups."*

Breast Enlargement

Many women, for their physical comfort or to change their appearance, consider having breast surgery to alter the size or shape of their breasts. Currently, thousands of women have breast implants placed into their bodies each year, most of them young, married mothers.

Breasts that are "too" small may genuinely be a source of ongoing embarrassment, and a factor in chronic anxiety or depression. Some women who undergo cosmetic surgery do achieve a much better self-image. However, others are disappointed that the "beautiful" breasts make little difference in their adjustment or happiness or how others act toward them—and occasionally, the results of surgery may be felt to be worse than the original appearance.

Alternative Medicine Approaches to Breast Enlargement

As Shakespeare noted, "From the fairest creatures we desire increase, that thereby beauty's rose might never die." Simply changing the size of your breasts, whether by surgical *or* natural means, may not give you the increased sense of well-being you might expect. Also, many patients experience breasts that became abnormally hard after the operation: as many as one-third of breast augmentation patients suffer from this uncomfortable problem, the result of excessive scarring. You may well find yourself with less appealing and comfortable breasts than those with which you started out.

Another point to ponder: Studies have found that small-breasted women are perceived as more intelligent and moral than large-breasted ones. On psychological tests, both men and women make this judgment, subconsciously. One study compared reactions to the same women, with various-sized breasts created by stuffing cotton in their bras. Photos were shown to students at five colleges around the country, and judgments made of their assumed characteristics. Dr. Chris Kleinke, the psychologist who performed the study, said, "As they stuffed themselves larger and larger, they "became" relatively less intelligent, competent, and modest."[3] You may just decide to keep your breasts the way they are, and rest on your (perceived) laurels!

However, if you still want to try to enhance your breast size, following are the most promising alternative medicine breast enlargement options that are currently available.

Practice Hypnosis

Your mind can be employed to influence the size and shape of your breasts. Since all parts of your body are influenced by the brain via hormonal messengers, this connection can be utilized, by hypnotic suggestion, to change your breasts. Several studies have shown that hypnosis allowed women to adjust the size of their breasts without surgery, usually only with a few months of treatment. For example, in one such experiment, participants' breasts were measured beforehand, then the women were hypnotized, with suggestions that they could feel warm water running over their breasts until they pulsated, or if they preferred, imagine a heat lamp shining upon them. They were given self-hypnosis tapes to use every day at home, and remeasured after twelve weeks. Eight-five percent had some enlargement, at an average of two-thirds of an inch vertically, an inch horizontally, and 1.37 inches in circumference. Forty-six percent needed to buy a larger bra; on average, by two cup sizes.[4]

You may need to have a number of sessions, over a few months, with a skilled hypnotherapist. The Resources section at the back of this book contains information about where to find one near you.

Practice Visualization

This is a form of self-hypnosis. Images held in the mind affect the circulatory, nervous system, and hormonal systems of the body. Visualization practice itself has been shown to markedly affect other areas of the body, within a few sessions.

Follow the guidelines for deep relaxation and visualization practice given in Chapter 2. You may wish to use visualization images such as those above: "warm water running over my breasts"; or affirmations of "my breasts are becoming just the right size for myself and others." Repeat this mental practice three to five times daily for five to fifteen minutes, while feeling it happen within your body. Results may take from one to two months to become apparent.

Use Other Alternatives

No medicine or herb has yet been scientifically shown to enhance breast size. Exercise of your pectoral muscles can help your breasts appear larger and firmer, as well as contributing to their health by improving their circulation. You can use hand weights, or a thigh-master device; simply raise your arms to midchest height, with the elbows bent, and squeeze the lower arms in and out. Massage of your breasts also may help you and others feel happily connected to this area of your body. You may choose to wear a "Wonderbra," to emphasize what you do have, but make certain only to wear it for short periods of time, not all day long, since this may increase your risk for breast cancer, as discussed below in the section on alternative prevention and treatment of that disease.

Surgical Approach to Breast Enlargement

Sally, a 25-year-old who came from a long line of flat-chested women, had always been uncomfortable with her figure. In high school, the boys teased her about having "two fried eggs," and she wore bulky clothes to hide her profile. After completing nursing school, she took a job in the office of a plastic surgeon, and was very impressed with the results she observed in the patients who had breast enhancement. Sally finally decided to take action for herself: she had her breasts surgically enlarged, from size 30A to size 34B, and is quite proud and happy with the results, though they do feel slightly firmer in texture than her original ones.

Your breasts can be surgically enlarged by placing implants, of varying size and shape, in "pockets" created underneath your breast tissue or chest wall muscles. (See Figure 6.2.) Currently, the type used for augmentation surgery is a "saline (meaning 'saltwater') implant." This device has an outer shell or cover of silastic, which is a rubbery form of silicone. The shell is put in place while empty, and then inflated with saltwater during your surgery.

Before your operation, you need to discuss with your surgeon which techniques are most appropriate for the size and shape of your breasts. Your own desires and expectations play an important role. Many plastic surgeons have photographs or diagrams, and even computer simulations, to help both of you arrive at a clear understanding of the desired results.

Smoking slows healing and encourages growth of scar tissue. Therefore, if you are a smoker, you should make every effort to stop completely before you have this surgery.

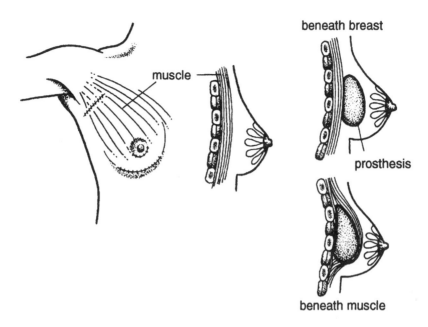

muscle

beneath breast

prosthesis

beneath muscle

Fig. 6.2   Placement of prosthesis in breast enlargement

The enlargement operation, which is called *augmentation mammoplasty,* is a one-stage procedure, performed in your surgeon's office, an independent surgical center, or hospital operating room. It requires one to two hours, and has few complications. Most women choose general anesthesia, though you can opt for local anesthesia with sedation. Your plastic surgeon makes a 1.5-inch inconspicuous incision in the skin fold beneath your breast, at the edge of the dark part of your nipple areola, or in the armpit, where a scar will show the least. Through the incision, your surgeon creates the pocket under the muscle behind your natural breast, inserts the implant and centers it behind the nipple, inflates it, then closes the skin with internal stitches and skin tape, or external stitches.

You can usually be discharged home right after your operation, with pain pills and advice to restrict your activities. Drainage tubes may have been placed under the skin during the surgery to prevent the buildup of fluids. If so, they can be removed after a few days, and you will then be able to wear a surgical bra. Any external stitches can be removed in five to ten days. The change in appearance is immediate, although bruising, swelling, and soreness may last a few weeks. The final effect of the operation will be evident after four to six weeks.

The sensation in your breasts usually returns to normal, and you can nurse after having had augmentation. Possible complications of this operation include excessive bleeding, blood clot formation, wound infection, and extrusion or rupture of the implant. If you have any question about the healing of your breasts, you need to see your doctor immediately. The tissue surrounding an implant can react abnormally, creating a rippled look with unsatisfactorily firm consistency. This is termed "capsular contracture" and may cause substantial pain and discomfort. It can be treated by an operation that breaks up or removes the fibrous capsule. The implant may have to be removed or exchanged. Overall, the risk of a complication requiring surgical correction is 12 percent at five years.[5]

Implant manufacturers did not originally conduct extensive research about possible hazards of implants before bringing their products to the market. Over the past thirty years, as many as two million American and Canadian women have had implants placed for augmentation or reconstruction after mastectomy. Concerns have surfaced that silicone, a material thought to be very nonreactive and inert when implanted into the body, may not be as safe as first supposed. Some studies have suggested that persons with these implants—especially those whose devices have leaked gel—were at increased risk for disorders of the immune system, such as rheumatoid arthritis, lupus, scleroderma, and fibromyalgia.

However, a recent analysis of eighty-eight reports, involving thousands of women, did not show any greater incidence of these disorders in women with silicone gel implants than in the general population.[6] A meta-analysis of all scientific studies published in the medical literature looking at this question was reported in the *New England Journal of Medicine* in 2000 and found no evidence of an association between silicone gel filled breast implants and connective tissue disorders, rheumatic conditions, or other autoimmune diseases.[7] A study from the Nurses' Health Study of 1,183 women with implants also did not find an association.[8] The American Academy of Neurology Practice Committee reviewed the medical literature and found no association between silicone implants and neurologic disorders.[9]

In 1999, the Institute of Medicine, part of the National Academy of Sciences, concluded that no evidence supports the theory that silicone is toxic to humans or has harmful effects on the immune system, or that silicone implants are associated with any disease syndrome. No increased risk for breast cancer has been found in women with silicone gel implants. Although breast cancer may be more difficult to detect by mammograms, no evidence suggests a higher mortality in women who have had implants.

Since 1992, the U.S. Food and Drug Administration has restricted silicone gel–filled implants to women having postmastectomy reconstruction, those who have previously had a gel implant and need to have it exchanged, or those participating in special studies. "Saline," saltwater-filled implants, which also have solid silicone making up their outer covering, continue to be available for everyone. Theoretically, silicone from the solid silicone covering of the saline implant is unlikely to be absorbed, and if the implant leaks, the harmless saltwater is absorbed rather than silicone gel. The disadvantage of the saline implant is that its consistency is less similar to breast tissue than the silicone gel–filled implant. Since all safety questions have not yet been fully answered, you need to ask your doctor about the latest information.

It you have an implant, be certain to have regular examinations and follow screening recommendations. If you believe you are having problems with your implant, you should seek consultation with a board-certified plastic surgeon who specializes in this area. Breast reconstruction using rearrangement of your own tissues, as discussed later in this chapter, is also a possible way to achieve larger breasts. However, it is infrequently used for augmentation because of the magnitude of the surgery.

Breast Reduction

Breasts can be "too" large, assuming dimensions way out of balance to the rest of the body, resulting in back, neck, and shoulder pain; skin problems; and social embarrassment. Juvenile or "virginal" hypertrophy, a condition in which the breasts respond inordinately to the increased levels of hormones during puberty, can be especially difficult if you are a teenager. You may consider surgery to reduce the size and weight of your breasts if you find them psychologically distressing, or simply physically uncomfortable.

Alternative Medicine Approaches to Breast Reduction

As with breast augmentation, you can find yourself with less appealing breasts after your operation than those with which you began. Up to one in five patients loses sensation in one breast, and one in ten loses it in both breasts. Excessive scarring can result in abnormally hardened breasts. Before turning to surgery, try one of the following alternative approaches.

Practice Hypnosis and Visualization

Hypnosis and visualization have not yet been tested as therapies for breast reduction, but since they work for enlargement, a trial seems to be warranted. See above, under "Breast Enlargement," and Chapter 2, for further information on these techniques.

Change Your Diet; Take Supplements

A good nutrition program can eliminate PMS, often a source of excessive discomfort in larger breasts. Follow the alternative guidelines for fibrocystic disease of the breast, below. If you are overweight, simply losing weight may help your breasts become smaller. Excess upper body weight has been linked to a higher risk for diabetes. Follow the guidelines given in Chapter 2 to attain and maintain your optimum weight, and achieve optimum nutrition.

Surgical Approach to Breast Reduction

Juanita was a 15-year-old who developed breasts way out of proportion to her small frame. Her bra straps dug grooves into her shoulders, and the skin under her breasts was always moist and raw. Support bras did little to relieve the constant aching, and the pain, especially during her periods, made it difficult for her to navigate the high school stairs. Gym classes were torture, both because of the running and jumping required and because of having to shower with the other girls. She even considered dropping out of school altogether in order to avoid the stares and snickers of her classmates. Finally, during summer vacation, she had surgical breast reduction, in which two-thirds of her breast tissue was removed, from size 38DD to 36C. Juanita has recovered completely, feels great about her decision, and is now on the tennis team. Because of the painful consequences of her oversized breasts, her family's health insurance even paid most of the cost of the surgery.

As with augmentation mammoplasty, it is very important to begin the process by having a frank discussion with your plastic surgeon about your desires and expectations. Ask to see photographs of some of your surgeon's previous patients to help you reach a mutual understanding about the appearance you wish to achieve. Your surgeon may ask you to have a mammogram to ensure you have no undetected breast disease. If you are a smoker, you should stop smoking, to aid your healing and help you avoid excessive scarring.

The breast reduction operation, termed *reduction mammoplasty,* decreases your breast size by removing excess glandular tissue, fat, and skin. It is a more complicated operation than breast enlargement, and may take three or four hours under general anesthesia in a surgical center or hospital operating room. You can have it done as an outpatient if you are having a moderate reduction. If a large amount of tissue needs to be removed, you may need to spend two or three days in the hospital.

Before you are anesthetized, your surgeon carefully measures and marks your breast with an indelible pen, to serve as a guideline for the incisions and the amount of glandular tissue and skin to be removed. After this tissue is removed, the remaining glandular tissue and overlying skin is brought together with stitches, and your nipple repositioned on the newly shaped breast. *Liposuction* is sometimes used in combination with this surgery to improve the contour of the breast. You wake up with bandages compressing your breasts and drains under your skin, to prevent fluid from collecting. Your soreness and bruising are likely to be significant for a week or two, but can be relieved with pain medication.

If you are discharged before your drains are removed, you can easily attend to them yourself. The visible part of the drain consists of flexible tubing with a small collection bulb at the end of it. You simply empty the collection bulb when it fills, and then squeeze the air out of it to create suction. Your surgeon should see you at least weekly until healing is apparent. The drains are removed after a few days and stitches, if any, can come out a few days later. You should wear a support bra and restrict your activities for several weeks.

Because of the extent of this surgery, scar tissue may cause your breasts' consistency to be more irregular and lumpy than before the operation. Since scarring is often variable, the appearance of one breast may be slightly different from the other. Scars from this operation are noticeable, though they can be hidden under your bra.

Healing problems include bleeding, infection, fluid collection under your skin, and loss of skin along with all or part of your nipple. Your nipple's sensitivity may be decreased to some degree. Since this operation cuts some of the milk ducts, although lactation may still be possible, if you wish to breast-feed, you may want to postpone the surgery until after you have had children.

Other Cosmetic Breast Problems

Asymmetry of the two breasts is actually quite common, though in rare cases it can be extreme enough to make you uncomfortable. Sometimes one breast is completely undeveloped. In these situations, surgery can be performed on one or both breasts to achieve similarity, utilizing the previously mentioned augmentation or reduction techniques. You can also choose liposuction, in which some of your breasts' fat is removed, with the use of a high-power suction device attached to narrow probes passed through small skin incisions into the area to be remodeled. Visualization and hypnosis might be tried in these situations, too.

Other cosmetic surgical operations can be performed to lift sagging breasts, create or restore nipple shape, or remove unwanted hair, all with reliable results.

With or without implants, or whether or not you have had reduction or other modifications to your breasts, a healthy lifestyle is a vital part of improving your body image.

How Breast Disease Is Diagnosed

Breast cancer can threaten not only your breasts, but your life as well. Taking steps to reduce its risks, along with those that improve the chances for early detection of disease, are part of your responsibility to yourself. Besides diet, exercise, and stress reduction, and a generally healthier lifestyle, discussed in detail below, in the sections on alternative approaches to prevention and treatment of fibrocystic disease and cancer, you need to include breast self-examination and mammography as part of your wellness routine.

The importance of your breasts is probably never more apparent than when their loss is seemingly imminent. Accompanying the dread of diminished femininity, sexuality, and body image is the terror of the possibility of death. A newly discovered lump can therefore cause crippling panic. If you are immobilized by your anxieties and avoid seeking medical care, as many women do, and if the mass is cancer, you may lose your chance for cure. Much of the time, such preconceived fears turn out to be much worse than the reality of what you must do to complete treatment and return to health.

Breast Self-Examination

Most women have "lumpy" breasts; it is normal for the breasts to range in consistency because of variations in their underlying glandular tissue and fat. *Breast self-examination* *(BSE)* allows you to "get to know" your breasts, so you can detect a lump that seems different from your "usual" lumps, or has changed since the previous exam. You cannot even totally rely on a mammogram to find a cancer; some tumors can be felt, but not seen, by this study. If you examine your breasts regularly, it will be easier for you to detect early, subtle changes.

Most breast lumps are not cancer, but it is very important that all *new* lumps be found and evaluated as early as possible. This provides a much better chance for cure should cancer be found. Most breast tumors that can be felt are found by women themselves; therefore, the key to the earliest diagnosis is for you to practice BSE.

The average cancerous breast lump has been present for more than five years before it grows to over an inch, when it can be easily felt. If you are very familiar with your own breasts from monthly BSE, you may be able to notice a lump much earlier, when it is as small as one-quarter to one-half inch. It has been shown that women who examine their breasts *regularly* go to their doctors earlier, when it is less likely their cancer has spread, with a mortality rate half that of women who do not do BSE.[10] Cancers found early require less radical surgery.

However, in spite of widespread educational campaigns to encourage women to do BSE, studies report that only 20 to 25 percent of all women now practice it. BSE requires only five minutes a month, and is something special you can do for yourself—because you are worth it! For complete instructions, see "How to Examine Your Breasts" on page 182. Ask your doctor to critique your technique. You can develop confidence by first trying it on a manufactured silicone breast model, available in most doctors' offices.

How to Examine Your Breasts

Breast self-examination (BSE) allows you to "get to know" your breasts. BSE should be done each month, about five days after your period has ended, when the breasts are smaller, less tender, and softer. New lumps are most easily found during this time. If you are postmenopausal, you can do BSE the same day each month. The most effective examination process includes both visual inspection and touch.

1. Face a mirror, preferably one with a light source from the side. Hold your arms above your head, then put your hands on your waist with the elbows bent. Lean forward slightly and look for any subtle difference between your two breasts: a difference in the direction a nipple points, a slight bulge or dimpling, or a minor difference in the prominence of the veins. Any changes in the nipple, such as a sinking or skin irritation, should be noted.

2. Next, while sitting and lying down, feel your breasts and armpits. If you can, lubricate your skin with soapy water, oil, or lotion. Divide your breast into wedge-shaped areas corresponding to the hours on the face of a clock. Feel your breast tissue with three or four fingers of the opposite hand, as your fingers "walk" from the outside edges to the nipple. Examine each area in turn, varying the pressure from light to moderate. Squeeze the nipple gently and note any nipple discharge. A clear, greenish, or milky discharge noticed only with squeezing is normal. A pinkish, bloody, or clear spontaneous discharge should be reported to your doctor. The armpit is best examined while the elbow of that arm is at your side. You should note areas of tenderness, thickening, or lumpiness.

3. If you have breasts with lumps or thickened areas, try mapping them as a way of remembering from month to month where all the irregularities are located. Just draw a simple diagram of each breast, with all the spots indicated. Again, dividing the breast into areas as though it were a clock face is a helpful way to gauge the locations.

Don't be intimidated by these recommendations. Just practice "getting to know" your breasts in the shower, with soap and water on your hands. Most women have "lumpy" breasts; this is a normal consequence of variations in the structure of the breast and the response to hormone fluctuations. The range of "normal" consistencies is quite broad, so the goal of BSE is to detect a lump that seems different from your usual lumps or changes from the previous examination. If you examine your breasts regularly, you will know your breasts more completely, and it will be easier for you to detect subtle changes.

All women, starting in their teens, should perform BSE monthly. If you find any lumps, areas of hardness or thickening, tenderness, nipple discharge, or change in appearance, have them double-checked by your doctor. Your partner can also play a role and may be the first one to notice a change.

Breast Specialist Evaluation

A consultation between you, the one who is "experienced" with the way your breasts feel, and your doctor, who has examined thousands of breasts, is the best possible way to ensure early diagnosis and treatment of breast disease. Your regular primary doctor or gynecologist is likely to be familiar with your breasts and should do a screening exam routinely, at least once a year. If there is a cause for concern, you may be referred to a breast specialist for another opinion.

The breast specialist is usually a surgeon. He or she will first ask a series of questions about any changes or symptoms you may have noticed, how long they have been present, what may have caused them, if they change with your cycle, if you have had any past problems, et cetera. Then you will be asked questions about your menstrual history, pregnancies—if any—breast-feeding, hormone medications, family history, and other information concerning risk factors for breast cancer as outlined on page 196.

You need to undress above the waist, then put on a gown with the opening in the front. If you are uncomfortable, take along your partner or a friend, or ask a female nurse to be present during the exam. Usually you are examined both sitting and lying down, with your arms first raised above your head. Your doctor systematically examines your breast tissue using several fingers of both hands. You may be asked to gently squeeze your nipples to check for discharge. Also, your armpit and neck regions are checked for enlarged glands.

If you have had a mammogram or ultrasound, any findings can be reviewed with you. If suspicious areas are found on exam, your doctor may suggest a needle biopsy on the initial visit. Please see pages 187–88.

At the end of your visit, your doctor makes recommendations based on your history, risk factors for cancer, exam, and any tests that may already have been done. You may need further evaluation via a biopsy or the tests described below. You may just be asked to return in a few months for another exam. If your doctor feels your findings are not suspicious, you need only follow the usual screening guidelines with your primary doctor. Be certain you express any discomfort you have with the recommendations.

The results of a physical exam alone are only 60 to 85 percent accurate. Even the most experienced "expert" examiner can only reliably find tumors that have reached one-half to one inch in size, by which time *20 to 50 percent have already spread*. Therefore, in addition to BSE and regular physical examinations by a doctor, the screening mammogram is used to help discover an early malignancy.

Mammography

Mammography is a low-dose X-ray technique that can find cancers as small as one-quarter inch, before most of them have spread. It is more reliable for finding cancers than BSE or a doctor's physical exam. A tumor too small to feel or cause symptoms, but found on mammogram, has *half* the likelihood of spread and is *40 percent more curable*. Seven randomized studies have shown that regular screening mammograms decrease the risk of death from breast cancer by 25 to 30 percent.[11] Despite this advantage and campaigns to publicize these facts in the mass media, a study by the National Center for Health Statistics found that in 1993 only 60 percent of all women in the high-risk group, over aged 50, reported following recommended screening guidelines by receiving a mammogram within the past two years.[12] This was due to lack of information and awareness, failure of their doctors to make the recommendation, inability to afford the cost, unfounded belief in the harm of this minute amount of radiation, or just plain fear that something might be found.

Chris was a health-conscious mother of four who had her first screening mammogram at age 40. She was shocked to receive a call from her doctor and learn that a tiny area of "suspicious" calcifications was found in one of her breasts. A biopsy showed a one-quarter-inch area of cancer still confined within the milk ducts. Removal of the tumor and follow-up radiation therapy have given Chris a nearly 100 percent probability of cure. Without the mammogram, it is unlikely her malignancy would have been discovered before it broke through the duct and moved into the less curable "invasive" stage.

Mammography requires no special preparation other than avoiding lotions, oils, or deodorants on the breasts or underarm areas on the day of the test, since many contain aluminum or other particles that can interfere with interpretation. After disrobing from the waist up, you place one breast at a time between the X-ray tube and film plates. The compression necessary to thin and spread out the breast's tissue *can* be uncomfortable, and the pain may even last a few days. Scheduling your mammogram for about five days after your period ends will minimize the discomfort, because this is when the breasts are least likely to be tender from fluid retention. Routine mammography consists of a top and side view of each breast; further evaluation of a questionable area may need "tangential," "spot," to "magnification" views.

Breast cancer produces characteristic mammogram changes in density and architecture, skin thickening and/or an increase in blood vessels that show up against the normal background of fat and glandular tissue. A white "mass" with irregular, fingerlike borders, is classic. "Microcalcifications," a frequent cause of concern, are small white specks commonly seen on mammograms, but not picked up on any other type of exam. Rounded ones are benign and associated with blood vessels. Tiny linear microcalcifications can be seen in cancer, though also commonly in other types of breast changes as well. Two out of three breast biopsies done for suspicious calcifications turn out to be benign.

Mammograms are difficult X-rays to read. Mammography is only 85 percent accurate in finding breast cancers; 10 to 15 percent are missed. Small tumors can look quite similar to normal patterns. The error rate is even higher if you are under age 50, when denser breasts tend to hide small changes. Density varies among individuals; is not related to size, shape, consistency, or lumpiness; and is determined by the amount of fat and glandular and fibrous tissue in your particular breasts. In general, more than half of all premenopausal women—and those postmenopausal women taking hormone replacement—have dense breasts, meaning their mammograms must be interpreted with special care. Using a computer to double-check screening mammograms and mark subtle suspicious areas for the radiologist to take another look at is a promising new approach that may make routine screening more accurate. One study using a computer-assisted method in 12,800 women found a 20 percent increase in the detection of early cancers.[13] However, this technology adds extra expense and the $200,000 ImageChecker system is not widely available.

Screening mammograms can also falsely report normal areas as "suspicious," engendering a lot of needless worry and follow-up expense. Elmore and colleagues reported a study of 2,400 women screened for ten years by mammograms. They estimated that after ten mammograms the probability of having a false positive mammogram is 56.2 percent; further special-view mammograms, ultrasounds, or other tests are then required. Nineteen percent of patients would eventually undergo a negative biopsy for something suspicious on a mammogram.[14]

Ten to thirty percent of abnormalities reported on mammograms do prove to be cancer. Most surgeons feel it is "better to be safe than sorry," and recommend you have a biopsy of any suspicious area, since the chance for cure of a small, early cancer outweighs the expense, discomfort, and scar of a negative biopsy.

You may say to yourself, "Well, I have lumpy breasts. They might find something on a mammogram, and then I'd have to have it biopsied. Since most of these biopsies are negative, why have this X-ray in the first place?" Recent evidence indicates that *routine yearly mammograms* are effective in increasing survival in women over the age of 50—and that if all women received yearly mammograms after age 50, breast cancer deaths could be decreased by one-third.[15]

Whether routine mammography is desirable for women under age 50 has been hotly debated for the past several years. Some evidence has suggested that there is no survival benefit, probably because tumors are harder to see in denser breasts and have a worse prognosis, despite early therapy for women in this age group. The biggest objection to routine mammograms for everyone between the ages of 35 to 50 is that they are not cost-effective. This means that although the benefit to the individual may be great, the large expense to society to screen every woman in this age group to find a rare early tumor capable of being cured may not be justified. The argument goes that since most "suspicious" areas seen on mammogram are not cancer on follow-up biopsy, the expense and discomfort generated would not be worth the effort. This controversy is not yet settled, but the introduction of newer less-expensive minimally invasive biopsy techniques is tipping the balance to more frequent screening.

Another concern you may have is that large doses of radiation can *cause* cancer, but this is the case only very rarely. It is estimated that with the low-dose equipment now in use, you would have to have 26 to 40 mammograms to increase your risk of cancer by even 1 percent.

Analysis of the results of eight studies of mammograms done between the ages of 40 to 49 suggests that routine exams could reduce deaths by 14 to 23 percent.[16] The American Cancer Society (ACS), the American Medical Association, and the American College of Surgeons therefore now recommend mammograms every year after age 40 for all women of average risk. The government's National Cancer Advisory Board of the National Cancer Institute (NCI) has recently changed from recommending against routine mammograms between ages 40 and 49 to advising them every one or two years, and that you yourself should decide how often to have them during this period, after consulting with your doctor. The American College of Obstetricians and Gynecologists also say that every one to two years is adequate. Both the NCI and the ACS now advise that after age 50, mammograms should be carried out every year. A mammogram should be done, at any age, to help evaluate suspicious changes. If you have had a previous breast cancer, you should schedule a mammogram every year.

Ultrasound Scan

This technique employs sound waves to take a picture, and is recommended for examining lumps in younger women whose breasts are dense and difficult to read on mammograms. It is also useful in older women with dense breasts, or when something abnormal can be felt but is not seen on a mammogram. Ultrasound, but not a mammogram, can determine whether a lump that can be felt or is seen on a mammogram is "cystic" (contains fluid) or solid (no fluid). The very common fluid cyst contains fluid that can be sucked out ("aspirated") with a needle; if it then disappears, you can avoid a biopsy. Microscopic calcifications seen on a mammogram, often associated with cancer, cannot be seen on an ultrasound, but the ultrasound may reveal an associated mass missed by a mammogram.

CAT, MRI, and PET Scans

These scans are now under investigation in assisting breast cancer diagnosis, and are not appropriate for routine screening. Although expensive, they may help in diagnosis of suspicious areas found by physical exam, ultrasound, or mammography, especially if you have a breast implant or enlarged lymph nodes in your armpit. MRI may be recommended for women with dense breasts and a strong family history of breast cancer and those with BRCA genetic predisposition. Also, in patients with known breast cancer, MRI has been very useful in characterizing its extent when the mammogram and ultrasound do not give enough information for certain treatment decisions.

Breast Biopsy

The most accurate test to evaluate any new questionable lump, bloody discharge, discharge associated with a lump, or change on a mammogram or an ultrasound classified as having a "moderate" or "high" level of suspicion is the breast biopsy. At times, it can be difficult to make a decision about having a biopsy when you have no symptoms, your physical exam is normal, and the only concern is a change on a mammogram that is classified as being "probably benign" (an actual classification recognized by the American College of Radiology). Depending on your risk factors, your doctor's advice, and your peace of mind, if you have a finding with a "low" level of suspicion, you can make a decision to have an immediate biopsy or to just repeat the mammogram in four to six months to look for stability or further suspicious changes. Edward Sickles of the University of California followed 3,184 of these abnormalities and reported that repeating the mammogram in four to six months is a safe, cost-saving approach. Less than 2 percent of findings with a low level of suspicion prove to be caused by early cancers. Studies have shown that in this situation, even if you have a cancer, delaying your biopsy is unlikely to change your prognosis, as long as you are followed closely.[17]

Breast biopsies formerly included a hospital stay and your signing of a consent form permitting the surgeon to perform a mastectomy, should cancer be found. You were put to sleep with general anesthesia not knowing whether you would wake up missing a breast. *Since four out of five biopsies are negative,* many women needlessly went through this terrifying sequence of events. Fortunately, you can now choose to have a biopsy, under local anesthesia, in your doctor's office, a diagnostic imaging center, or an outpatient surgery facility. Should a malignancy be found, you then have several weeks to adjust to the news and consider your treatment alternatives. Several different kinds of biopsy are available.

Needle Breast Biopsy

Needle biopsy of a lump that *your surgeon can feel* requires no preparation and is usually performed on your first office visit. You lie on the examining table, and your skin is cleansed with an iodine or alcohol solution. Local skin anesthetic may or may not be used. The doctor passes the needle directly through the skin into the suspicious area, a procedure usually only minimally uncomfortable and which takes less than a minute. Afterward you may experience some bruising or soreness, lasting for a few days, and you may have a pinpoint scar. Significant complications are extremely rare, and you can resume your activities immediately.

Needle aspiration of a lump (in which the physician attempts to extract fluid) may show it to be a fluid-filled cyst that disappears completely after the fluid is removed through the needle. Need for an "open" surgical biopsy, one requiring an incision, is thus avoided, and your anxiety can be immediately relieved.

If your lump is solid, some cells can be sucked out by *fine needle aspiration biopsy (FNA)* that uses high suction through a fine needle to remove cells from the suspicious area. The pathologist then examines these cells for malignancy under the microscope, in a manner similar to a Pap smear. This technique is becoming less popular because up to 50 percent of samples are insufficient for accurate analysis. FNA will not determine whether a cancer is "invasive" or "noninvasive." (See explanation on page 197.)

Solid core needle biopsy is performed with a special needle that cuts out a one-sixteenth-inch solid core of tissue. It leaves only a tiny scar, is minimally painful, and is often used on very suspicious lumps. Since the needle itself is relatively large and several attempts may be necessary to obtain sufficient tissue, this test does require local anesthetic, which feels similar to dental anesthesia. If your lump is cancerous, more information about the nature and degree of invasion is obtained than with the FNA.

If you have a suspicious area seen on a mammogram or an ultrasound exam that *your surgeon cannot feel* because it is small, deep, or you have firm breasts, you need a specially guided needle biopsy or a surgical "open" biopsy. Five hundred thousand such biopsies of suspicious areas that cannot be felt are done each year in the United States. Twenty to thirty-five percent turn out to be malignant.

Recently, a very strong trend has developed to perform these biopsies using *image-guided* needle techniques, rather than the traditional *open biopsy,* described on page 189. Mammography or ultrasound provides the picture of the target area. These procedures take thirty to sixty minutes, and are otherwise quite similar to the needle biopsy available in your doctor's office, using local anesthesia.

The *"stereotactic" needle biopsy* uses mammography and a device to mechanically guide the needle to the localized area as you lie on a special table with your breast hanging down through an opening in it, compressed between two paddles. Most of the equipment necessary is quite expensive, so you will probably be referred to a radiologist's office or a diagnostic imaging center for this type of biopsy.

All these techniques use local anesthesia. Several types of biopsy devices are available, which employ different size core needles. Generally, five to ten samples are taken. The Advanced Breast Biopsy Instrument actually attempts to remove all of the suspicious area in one specimen. It uses a 10- to 20-millimeter cylindrical "cookie cutter" with a circular oscillating knife that is advanced to the target area. An electrocautery snare cuts through the base of the specimen. A larger 10- to 25-millimeter skin incision must be performed, so you will have a small scar. If successful and no suspicious cells are found, follow-up mammograms may not be necessary. If malignant and all the suspicious area is removed and surrounded by normal tissue ("negative margin"), follow-up surgery might not be needed, unlike with the core needle techniques.

An *ultrasound-guided needle biopsy* uses sound-wave technology to guide the needle into a suspicious area. The breast does not need to be compressed, and an X-ray is unnecessary, but this technique cannot be used to biopsy an area with suspicious calcifications. The equipment is much cheaper than that necessary for the stereotactic biopsy, so some surgeons are acquiring it for their own offices.

Current studies indicate that the image-guided solid core biopsy needle can be precisely placed into an area in question and tissue successfully removed, with a technical success and overall accuracy rate of 95 to 99 percent, similar to open surgical biopsy. However, rebiopsy by needle or open technique may be necessary in 2 to 25 percent of biopsies, if after microscopic study, what is found in the tissue removed doesn't seem to correspond with the mammogram or ultrasound picture ("discordant result").[18] Open biopsy follow-up is also necessary if *atypical ductal hyperplasia* is found, since it is often associated with malignancy.

The advantages of a core needle biopsy are that it is less time-consuming, one-quarter to one-half as expensive, and more comfortable than open biopsy. It has the psychological benefits that less tissue needs to be removed, no deformity is created, and you have only a pinpoint scar. Another value is that when cancer is diagnosed by this method, fewer surgical procedures are likely to be needed to achieve "clear margins" if you choose breast conservation (see pages 217–18).[19] Its major disadvantage is that most of the suspicious area still remains, so that if the biopsy is negative for cancer, it must still be observed on follow-up mammograms, to check for the rare case in which the malignant area was not sampled by the needle. In a 1994, twenty-center study, the missed cancer detection rate was only 1.3 percent.[20]

After any type of needle biopsy, you may experience some bruising and soreness. Usually, any discomfort disappears in a few days. The complication rate is only 0.2 percent. Rarely, a blood clot develops when the needle cuts a small artery. Incision infection is very unusual.

A needle biopsy is useful, when *positive* for cancer, because it gives you a quick and inexpensive cancer diagnosis. If your needle aspiration or needle biopsy is *negative* for suspicious cells, your doctor should recommend a plan for follow-up exams. However, if your lump is still considered very suspicious for cancer, you may be advised to have an open biopsy, since the needle may have missed the cancerous cells.

Open Breast Biopsy

This type of biopsy is usually performed in an operating room, since excess bleeding may be encountered and the specimen must be carefully handled by the pathologist. However, most are performed in outpatient surgery. You can come directly to the hospital or an outpatient surgery center immediately before the procedure, and can go home right afterward.

If your suspicious area was found by mammography and can't be felt, you need a *wire-guided open breast biopsy*. Prior to arriving in the operating room, you go to the mammography suite. The radiologist injects local anesthetic to numb your skin and, using mammography to determine the direction, subsequently steers a thin needle into or next to the area in question. A tiny wire with a hook to keep it from moving is then passed through the needle. The needle is removed, after which you go directly to the operating room for the biopsy, where your surgeon can follow the wire down to the right spot. In this way, a more precise biopsy can be performed through a smaller incision, and less normal breast tissue is removed. The specimen may be X-rayed, to ensure the suspicious problem was in fact removed.

The most common type of open biopsy is an *excisional biopsy,* the goal of which is to remove *all* of the suspicious area with a surrounding rim of normal tissue. This is also sometimes termed a *lumpectomy.* If your tumor is large and very suspicious for cancer, an *incisional biopsy* may be performed: with this method, only a small sample of the tumor is taken. The rest is removed later, after you have chosen your cancer treatment option. Open breast biopsies usually take from twenty to sixty minutes. You lie on the operating table with your arm at your side or above your head. Most likely a screen prevents you from seeing what is happening. You can ask to be told what is going on, or you can listen to music on a portable tape player. If you wish, you can have intravenous sedation to keep you drowsy. You can feel the initial needle as the local anesthetic is injected, but after a few minutes, the biopsy area becomes numb. If your lump is large or deep, if you need multiple biopsies, or if you would *rather* be totally asleep, you may choose general anesthesia.

If your lump is close to or at the edge of your areola, the dark part around the nipple, ask your surgeon to put your incision there, where the scar will be less conspicuous. During the procedure, you may hear sucking sounds from the suction device, and buzzing from the cautery that closes the ends of cut blood vessels with an electrical current. You may feel tugging and pressure, but you should not feel any significant pain. If you do, you should ask for more anesthetic. If the lump appears suspicious, your surgeon may place tiny metallic clips in the biopsy cavity to help the radiotherapist guide radiation treatments, should you choose this option. Once the procedure is complete, the skin is closed with stitches or skin tape.

You may have some postoperative bruising, swelling, and firmness; if necessary, your soreness can be controlled with pain pills for a few days. Uncommon complications such as a blood clot or excessive bleeding may require repeat surgery, or rarely, infection may require drainage. You should watch for signs of these, which are indicated by excessive swelling, tenderness, warmth, and redness. If many breast ducts are removed in your biopsy, nursing from that breast may not be possible. Occasionally, sensation is affected, though this most often eventually returns to normal.

For immediate biopsy results, a *frozen section* report can be obtained on larger specimens. A part of your tissue is quick-frozen, sliced into ultrathin layers, placed on slides, then stained to bring out the details of the cells. However, some cell distortion occurs when frozen cells are cut, and only small areas of the biopsy can be evaluated. Most of the tissue removed in a biopsy is saved for the more reliable and informative *permanent section* analysis, which takes a day or two to complete. The tissue is "fixed" in a chemical called formalin before cutting and staining takes place, which produces finer microscopic detail. Also, the pathologist has more time to evaluate samples from all areas of a "fixed" specimen than he or she does from a frozen section.

If your biopsy is positive for cancer, you need not make an immediate decision about treatment. Postponing therapy for a few weeks after the biopsy allows you to adjust to your diagnosis and investigate and consider your alternatives. No increase in risk of further cancer spread has been found to be caused by this short delay.

Fibrocystic Disease and Benign Lumps

Most women have "lumpy" breasts. That is, most *normal* breasts have variations in consistency, with firm and soft areas, ridges and valleys, lumps from the size of a BB or pea to ones the size of large grapes or grape bunches. Many women are told they have *fibrocystic disease,* when the unevenness is ac-

tually a consequence of the physiologic hormone fluctuations of monthly menstrual cycles. Increased lumpiness and cyclic tenderness may be particularly evident in one or more areas of one or both breasts that are more responsive to these hormone changes than neighboring tissue. Unfortunately, you may feel worry and confusion, given that breast cancer also presents as a lump.

Most breast lump biopsies in the 25 to 45 age group are labeled "fibrocystic disease" by pathologists, but few of the many kinds of changes in cells seen under the microscope are associated with an increased risk of malignancy. The word "disease," therefore, is a misnomer with unnecessarily alarming overtones. The term "fibrocystic disease" should be applied only if you have fluid-filled cysts or if your biopsy is benign but shows the specific "proliferative" microscopic patterns known to indicate your breast has a higher risk for developing cancer.

The fluid-filled breast cysts of fibrocystic disease may contain from a fraction of a cc (cubic centimeter) to several cc's of thin fluid. Such cysts may feel stony hard, making it very difficult to distinguish them from malignant tumors.

The most common noncystic lump in women aged 15 to 35 is the *fibroadenoma,* a solid mass of fibrous and glandular tissue. Very little variation in size or sensitivity is noticeable during the menstrual cycle. Growth is slow, with the lump usually reaching the size of an olive before being brought to the attention of a doctor. After that size is reached, growth tends to stop, though infrequently these adenomas continue to grow quite large. Occasionally, a fibroadenoma will grow rapidly, under the effects of high levels of estrogen during pregnancy and lactation, use of birth control pills, or estrogen replacement therapy. Fibroadenomas are the easiest breast lumps to recognize. Typically, they are firm to rubbery in texture, slip and slide in relation to your skin and adjacent tissue, and are minimally tender or not tender at all.

Alternative Medicine Approaches to Fibrocystic Disease and Benign Lumps

Some studies indicate that breasts which develop fluid cysts and the "fibrocystic" changes discussed above have a two to four times higher risk to develop cancer, and therefore should be watched more closely. You should especially avoid the known risk factors for breast cancer, such as a high-fat diet, alcohol, and obesity. Follow the recommendations in the next section, on alternative medicine approaches, to prevent and treat breast cancer.

Since "fibrocystic disease," fibroadenomas, and painful mastitis are benign, a trial of the following methods may be undertaken to see if you can achieve regression.

Quit Smoking

Cigarette smoking increases your risk for breast problems. Studies have shown a strong association between smoking and periductal mastitis, an inflammation around the milk ducts that causes swelling, pain, and abscess formation.[21] Use the guidelines given in Chapter 2 to help you quit for good.

Avoid Caffeine and Other Methylxanthines

You may find relief from breast cyst formation, tender lumps, and discomfort by avoiding members of the methlyxanthine family of chemicals—including coffee, tea, cola, sodas with caffeine, and chocolate. They are known to increase your body's circulating adrenaline, which stimulates the cell proliferation seen in lumpy, tender breasts.

One study looked at women with a history, physical exam, and mammograms consistent with fibrocystic disease who consumed methylxanthines in average amounts equivalent to four cups of coffee per day. Eighty-two percent of those women who were able to completely abstain experienced total disappearance of their pain and lumps, and another 15 percent improved. Many of those who were unable to give up methylxanthines completely, but lowered their intake, still improved, though to a lesser degree.[22]

Change Your Diet; Add Soybean Products

A high intake of fat in the diet creates excessive estrogen production that stimulates breast tissue to form cysts. "Phytochemicals," such as soybeans, bind at estrogen sites to prevent overabundant activity of this hormone. For a more complete discussion of this subject, see page 203. Cyclical breast pain has been reported to improve with a switch to a low-fat diet.[23]

Take Supplements

By acting to return hormone levels to normal, supplements may help in the treatment of this disorder. In one study, subjects with fibrocystic disease were found to have elevated levels of the adrenal hormone DHEA, which returned to normal after therapy with vitamin E. Eighty-five percent showed disappearance of both pain and nodularity.[24] Several other studies have shown that supplemental vitamin E lessens fibrocystic disease.[25] Recommended oral dosage is 600 to 800 IU of the D-alpha form of vitamin E daily.

Vitamin B_6, a coenzyme in hormonal function, may assist in reversing this disorder, especially if it is related to PMS.[26] Begin with 50 mg daily; take more only with a doctor's supervision.

Take Evening Primrose Oil

A fatty acid deficiency has been suggested to be associated with cyclical breast pain. Evening primrose oil is one of the richest known sources of essential fatty acids. Several trials have shown it to be effective in mild to moderate cyclical pain, with minimal side effects.[27] Take six capsules per day.

Avoid Estrogen Replacement Therapy

Birth control pills and estrogen replacement therapy can cause breast tenderness and fluid cysts. A Boston study showed that twice as many women taking estrogen replacement therapy have to have surgery for significant lumps in their breasts.[28] The longer the estrogen use, the more the fibrocystic disease developed. Follow the guidelines given in Chapter 19 for alternatives to birth control pills or taking estrogen.

Practice Stress Management

Similar to methylxanthines, emotional stress increases blood levels of the catecholamine or "stress hormones." These have been linked to onset of fibrocystic lumpiness and pain. See Chapter 2 for ways to reduce the stress in your life.

Practice Visualization

Follow the guidelines given in Chapter 2. For specific visualization, you can image your breasts and hormones as normal, draw pictures of your breasts with normal internal tissues, and repeat phrases such as, "My hor-

mones and breasts are now returning to normal." Problem areas can be targeted by imaging your cells as "PAC-men (or PAC-women)," or as carrying white light lasers, to shift abnormal cells back to normal.

Conventional Medicine Approach to Fibrocystic Disease and Benign Lumps

If your lump has no suspicious characteristics on exam or imaging studies, you can choose to continue to observe the lump closely instead of having it removed. If you choose this course, you should follow up with your doctor in two or three months. If you have a needle biopsy with a "negative" pathology report, you may be more reassured.

Surgical Approaches to Fibrocystic Disease and Benign Lumps

If your mass has some suspicious characteristics or you would be worried about the observation approach, one of the following surgical approaches can be chosen.

Needle Biopsy

Easily drained with a needle, most cysts then completely disappear, to the immediate relief of both you and your doctor. Ninety-five percent of the time, the cysts do not recur, though more than one aspiration may be necessary. If your cyst does not completely vanish, reappears after two or three aspirations, or is found to contain bloody fluid, surgical removal may then be necessary to biopsy the wall of the cyst. Solid masses can be easily evaluated in your doctor's office by the core biopsy technique. However, you will still likely have an evident lump.

Surgical Removal

Fibroadenomas are usually removed because they don't disappear spontaneously and cannot be 100 percent accurately diagnosed until they are seen under a microscope. Most can be removed on an outpatient basis, through a small, inconspicuous incision along the border of your areola.

Fibroadenomas are a marker for increased risk of malignancy. Although they don't become malignant themselves, women who develop them are at two to four times the baseline risk for developing a breast cancer in the future.

Fibrocystic Disease and Benign Lumps Summary

Prevention

Diet and Supplements

- Follow a low-fat, vegetarian diet.
- Avoid coffee, tea, chocolate, and other caffeine-containing foods, medicines, or beverages.
- Add soy to your diet.
- Take vitamin E, D-alpha form, 600–800 IU daily.

Lifestyle

- Don't smoke.
- Choose a diaphragm or condoms instead of birth control pills.
- Choose supplements instead of hormone replacement therapy.
- Practice stress reduction, using yoga, tai chi, etc.

Alternative Medicine Approaches

- Follow preventative measures, above.
- Vitamin E, 600–800 IU daily.
- Vitamin B_6, 50 mg daily.
- Evening primrose oil, 6 capsules daily.
- Visualization.
- Hypnosis.

Conventional Medicine Approach

- Observation.

Surgical Approaches

- Aspiration of cyst.
- Needle biopsy and observation of solid lump.
- Surgical removal.

Breast Cancer

8 A.M.— less than 48 hours since surgery to remove my left breast. My chest is wrapped in an elastic bandage, and two drainage tubes emerge from small incisions near my lower ribs to siphon fluid from the mastectomy site . . . as the bandage fell away, I snuck glances down, waiting to be shocked by some unimaginable horror—a vision of my body—raw, wounded and bloody. Instead, I saw clean, healthy skin and a thin band of steri-strips covering a neat incision. It was nothing. And it was everything. I looked for what seemed like a long time and felt myself begin to breathe again.

"My Turn," *Newsweek*, March 21, 1994[29]

The threat of death and disfigurement makes breast cancer one of the most terrifying plagues of women, and the battle against it one of the most controversial areas of surgery. In the last two decades, treatment options have grown to include radical and conservative surgery, radiation, chemotherapy, hormonal therapies, and combinations of these. Despite modern therapy, the number of deaths of women in the prime of their lives from breast cancer is still staggering.

Breast cancer is the second most common cause of cancer death for women in the United States; lung cancer is now number one. Twelve percent of all women (one in eight) who live to age 85 develop this disease and 3.5 percent (1 in 28) die from it. In 2002 there will be 205,700 new cases and 40,000 deaths.[30] Although the number of women who must deal with this disease continues to increase, improved public awareness, earlier detection of smaller cancers, and more effective treatment have recently led to better survival rates and cure. For the first time in forty years, the U.S. Department of Health and Human Services reported a decline of about 5 percent in the breast cancer death rate for the period from 1989 to 1992, most significantly for Caucasians and younger women,[31] and the trend continues.

New information on the relationship of breast cancer to diet, exercise, and stress offers hope that changing your lifestyle may help prevent this disease or aid in its treatment; the picture is much brighter than even a few years ago. Breast cancer is far less frequent in countries with diets low in fat and high in fiber, as discussed below, and some indication exists that those who do develop the disease and change to this diet live longer.[32]

The exact cause, or causes, of breast cancer is still obscure, although complex interactions of genetics, hormones, environment, dietary factors, and possibly viruses are suspected. A number of "risk factors" have been identified that increase your chances for developing it.

The biggest risk factor, of course, is gender itself. Female breast cancer outnumbers male breast cancer by 110 to 1. The next most important risk factor is your age: only 3 percent of all breast cancers occur before the age of 30. After 40, the incidence rises fairly sharply, with the average age at first diagnosis being in the early 50s. After age 45, half of all new breast lumps are malignant.

Hormones play a key role in the cause of breast cancer, and increased risk is associated with prolonged, uninterrupted exposure of your breasts to your body's female hormones, especially when estrogen is unopposed by progesterone. Estrogen and progesterone cause breast cells to divide and proliferate, at which time they are more subject to carcinogens and errors of gene division. Early onset of menstruation, late menopause, and lack of pregnancy cause the breasts to be "bombarded" with these hormones for a longer period of time. Early pregnancy, which interrupts this continuous exposure, decreases your risk. Nuns, and other childless women, have five times the risk for this disease. Prolonged use of hormone replacement therapy (HRT) after menopause increases your risk. You may have a slightly higher risk for breast cancer if you take oral contraceptives before age 35.[33]

Your genetic background may increase your risk. If your sister, mother, aunt, or grandmother has had breast cancer, your risk is two to three times greater than the average baseline rate of one in eight women. If your relative developed the disease before menopause or had cancer in both breasts, your risk increases to three to five times the baseline. New research has located a genetic defect in about 5 percent of women with breast cancer, genes called BRCA 1 and BRCA 2, which in the future may lead to earlier diagnosis and preventive treatment. If you are from a high-risk family (four or more family members with breast cancer and/or both breast and ovarian cancers), you can be tested for the presence of this gene. If present, you have a 50 to 87 percent chance of developing breast cancer.[34] If you are found positive, be especially certain to follow the preventive advice given in the alternative medicine approaches section, practice careful breast self-examination, and have regular screenings beginning at an early age. If you desire children, you can consider prophylactic mastectomy afterward. Most women choosing this course report long-term satisfaction, decreased worry about breast cancer, and generally favorable psychological and social outcomes.[35]

Environmental factors—carcinogens in the diet, water, and atmosphere—and their role in the cause of breast cancer may be pinpointed through future research. A study in Long Island, New York, found a 60 percent higher rate of breast cancer in postmenopausal women living close to industrial plants compared with those who lived farther away. Risk increased as the number of nearby industrial facilities increased from one to two or more. Air pollution from the local chemical, rubber, and plastics plants was implicated as the cause.[36] Breast cancer incidence is higher in the U.S. "radon belt," the states with higher radon levels, and a link between radon and breast cancer is now being investigated.[37]

Your chances for developing breast cancer would change if you were living in a culture with a different diet. *Rates of breast cancer are more than five times higher in the United States than in countries eating a low-fat diet.*[38] The excess consumption of proteins in the American diet may also play a role: this leads to early onset of menstruation, known to increase risk by prolonging the breasts' exposure to estrogen.

Recently, the National Cancer Institute developed a computer program that uses a complex formula (Gale model) to determine an individual woman's risk for breast cancer over the next five years. It considers age, race, family history of breast cancer, age at first menstruation and first childbirth, and history of breast abnormalities and biopsies. The NCI sent the software to thousands of doctors. You may ask your doctor to calculate just what your risk is by this formula, and it may help you make decisions about screening frequency and whether to participate in prevention trials. (For a quick list of risk factors and the amount they increase the baseline risk for breast cancer, see Table 6.1.)

A majority of women have at least one risk factor for breast cancer. Even if you aren't at identified increased risk, you still have a 6 percent chance of developing this disease. Some of the risk factors, such as those determined by sex or genetics, are beyond your control. However, *you can take some measures to decrease your risk,* by making lifestyle changes. All women, therefore, regardless of their level of known risk, need to follow the alternative medicine approaches lifestyle advice below, and practice careful breast self-examination and screening.

Breast Cancer: First Steps

If you are diagnosed with breast cancer, before you make decisions about treatment, you first need to gather information about your tumor and the extent to which it has spread. Following are ten questions to ask your surgeon.

1. What Is the Extent of Invasion?

Cancer is a disorganized growth of abnormal cells that can erode or invade into neighboring tissues, then spread by the lymph or blood circulation to distant sites.

Lobular carcinoma in situ (LCIS) is a condition in which the group of abnormal cells stays confined within the breast lobules, microscopic milk-producing sacs. (See Figure 6.3.) This used to be considered a cancer—thus its name. Now, it is not felt to be a true cancer, since it does not invade other tissue. However, it is a "marker," an indicator you have an increased risk of breast cancer in both breasts (ten times the baseline risk, or approximately 1 percent per year for 25 years).

TABLE 6.1.
Risk Factors for Breast Cancer

Risk Factor	Increased Risk (Times Baseline Risk)
Family history—Mother, sister, daughter had breast cancer when:	
Postmenopausal	1.5
Premenopausal	3.0
Both breasts	5.4
Mother and sister*	4.7
Never pregnant or later than age 35	2.3
Early first period (before age 12)	1.2
More than 30 years of periods	1.4
More than 5 years on estrogen replacement therapy	1.4
Oral contraceptives before age 35	1.4
Benign breast disease—fibroadenoma or "proliferative" changes found on biopsy	1.5–2.0
Atypical hyperplasia	1.4–4.5
Obese and over 50	1.2
Alcohol consumption	1–2
Cigarette smoking	1.5
Environmental factors—diet	1.4–2.0

*30% risk of developing breast cancer during ages 20–29.

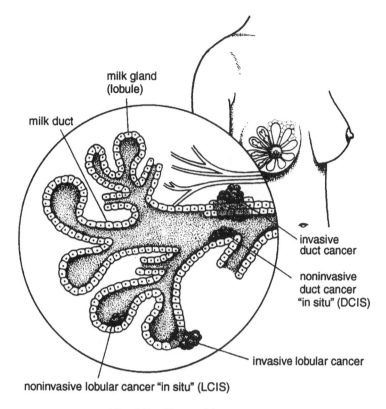

milk gland (lobule)

milk duct

invasive duct cancer

noninvasive duct cancer "in situ" (DCIS)

invasive lobular cancer

noninvasive lobular cancer "in situ" (LCIS)

Fig. 6.3 Types of breast cancer

Treatment is unnecessary, though you should carefully follow the screening guidelines, above.

Breast cancer can be found in a *noninvasive* or *invasive* stage. Currently, thanks to widespread use of screening mammograms, noninvasive breast cancer, or *ductal carcinoma in situ (DCIS)*, is the type found in 15 to 30 percent of breast cancer patients. In this early form of cancer, the cancer cells have not yet invaded through the wall of your milk duct, and are not yet in contact with the lymph or blood vessels in the breast. Therefore, they are very unlikely to have spread to the lymph nodes or elsewhere. This type of pattern is highly curable. However, it has the potential to become invasive, especially the *comedo* type of DCIS. DCIS with *microinvasion*, more commonly seen with bigger tumors, indicates a slight chance for spread. Therefore, unlike LCIS, DCIS must be treated.

If your biopsy shows an invasive tumor, found in 70 to 85 percent of all cases, the cells have already broken through the wall of a duct or lobule. This means there is a chance the cancer may have reached and spread through the lymph or blood systems.

2. What Is My Tumor Cell Type and Pattern?

Invasive or infiltrating breast cancer originates in the cells of the milk ducts or the lobules. Although *lobular cancers* are more difficult to see on mammograms, tend to be larger than first appreciated, may have a higher rate of local recurrence, and more often require more radical treatment, no difference in prognosis has been found, as compared with the more common invasive *ductal cancers*.

A number of specific cell patterns can be identified in tumors. The ones called *medullary, mucinous, colloid, papillary*, and *tubular* have a better prognosis because they are much less likely to spread.

Some invasive cancers have associated DCIS. If a large amount is present, it has an *extensive intraductal component* or *EIC*. This indicates it is harder to remove it all locally, and has more potential for a local recurrence, if you choose breast conservation therapy.

3. What Is My Tumor Size?

The larger your tumor, the greater the chance it has spread through the lymph or blood systems. A study correlating tumor size with lymph node spread found that if the tumor was less than 0.5 cm, there was only a 9 percent chance for spread. The risk increased to 19 percent if the tumor was 0.5–0.9 cm; 32.8 percent if 1.0–1.9 cms; 40.8 percent if 2.0–5.0 cms; and 75 percent if greater than 5.0 cms.[39,40] If your tumor has invaded your skin or underlying muscle, treatment of it is considered to be much more difficult, with a worse prognosis.

4. What Is My Hormone Receptor Status?

Your tumor will be tested to see if it contains estrogen and progesterone receptors, which are sites on the tumor cell wall to which these hormones attach. If receptors are found, you have a better prognosis. Also, tumors with hormone receptors are more likely to respond to tamoxifen, a medication that blocks these receptors and thereby prevents tumor growth and spread. Such receptors are more commonly present on tumor cells in older women.

5. What Are My Nuclear and Cytologic Grade, Cell Turnover Rate, Chromosome Number, and Gene Abnormality Expression?

These tests of "tumor biology" reflect how aggressively your tumor is likely to act. *Nuclear* and *cytologic grade* is determined microscopically, by size, shape, cell division activity, and degree of abnormality of cell components. The more abnormal these characteristics, the worse the prognosis. Your tumor *DNA index* can show a normal or abnormal *number of chromosomes*, with abnormal numbers having a worse prognosis. *Flow cytometry*, or *S-phase percentage*, measures the percentage of cells in your tumor that are dividing and multiplying. A high S-phase percentage, greater than 7 percent, indicates a slightly worse prognosis.

You may also see reference to *oncogene erb-2* and *HER 2/neu expression, p53 tumor suppresser gene mutation*, and *cathepsin D expression*, which reflect gene abnormalities which may correlate with a worse prognosis. These tests are investigational at this time but may have a bearing on the type of treatment recommended.

6. What Is the Status of the Edge of My Biopsy?

If you have an "open" biopsy, your surgeon will attempt to remove your tumor completely, along with a margin of normal tissue surrounding it. This may be difficult, because the tumor cells on the outside edge may not be visible to the naked eye and your surgeon does not want to remove too much tissue, thereby producing a poor cosmetic result. Microscopic examination may show tumor cells at, or very near, the edge of the specimen, a situation referred to as "positive" or "dirty" margins. A 10-millimeter negative margin is considered optimal. Inadequate margins, generally considered when DCIS or invasive cancer cells are within 1 millimeter from the edge of the biopsy specimen, occur in 20 to 40 percent of open biopsies. Further surgery, either local removal of more tissue or removing the whole breast may be necessary to "get it all." Also, a postbiopsy mammogram may be recommended to look for evidence of tumor left behind.

7. What Is the Evidence of Spread?

Because breast cancer tends to spread along the lymph drainage system, you may be advised to have your armpit lymph nodes on the side of the tumor biopsied to look for cancer. (The pathology report will indicate that the nodes are either "negative" or "positive" for cancer.) Removing cancerous nodes may not affect overall cure rates, but the presence or absence of positive lymph nodes—and how many of them contain cancer cells—is, by far, the most important factor in determining your prognosis and treatment. Even though cancer cells may spread elsewhere before appearing in the lymph glands, if cancer is found here it is more likely cancer cells have also spread elsewhere in your body by your bloodstream. Chemotherapy and/or hormonal therapy is then strongly recommended, to treat your whole body for any stray cancer cells. A chest X-ray, blood tests, bone scan, liver scan, and other tests may be conducted to look for possible distant spread.

8. What Is My Stage?

Women with breast cancer can be divided into groups based on the extent of their disease. This is very important in determining prognosis and treatment recommendations; it is also the basis for research comparing the results of different treatments, which is the way doctors are able to continually improve cancer survival. Your *stage* is based on three characteristics of the tumor: how big it is, whether or not it has spread to lymph nodes, and whether it has been spread by your bloodstream. To determine the stage of your disease, see Tables 6.2 and 6.3.

9. What Is My Prognosis?

Once your final stage is known, a *prognosis* is possible. This gives you a general idea about your chances for cure and life expectancy. Such information is derived from the experience of thousands of women who have undergone various forms of treatment. As examples, after appropriate treatment:

- If you have DCIS only, your chance for cure is 97 to 99 percent.
- If your invasive tumor is smaller than 1 centimeter, you have more than a 90 percent chance you will survive for five years or more, and greater than 95 percent if your armpit nodes are negative. If it is 1 to 2 centimeters, your chance is 85 percent; 2 to 5 centimeters, 75 percent; and if larger than 5 centimeters, it drops to less than 50 percent.
- If you have positive armpit nodes, you have a 75 percent chance of living five years and 65 to 80 percent to live ten years. If you have one to three positive nodes, your chance of living ten years is 35 to 65 percent; four to nine nodes, 30

TABLE 6.2.
Information Necessary for Breast Cancer Staging

T = Original Tumor	N = Armpit Lymph Nodes	M = Distant Metastasis (Spread)
Tis—DCIS	N0—no lymph node spread	M0—none
T1—Tumor 2 cm or less	N1—Spread to movable armpit nodes	M1—distant spread beyond armpit lymph glands
T1a—0.5 cm or less	N2—Spread to armpit nodes that are attached to one another, chest wall, or other armpit structures	
T1b—more than 0.5 cm but not more than 1 cm	N3—Spread to lymph nodes under the breastbone	
T1c—more than 1 cm but not more than 2 cm		
T2—tumor more than 2 cm but less than 5 cm		
T3—Tumor more than 5 cm		
T4—Tumor of any size with direct attachment to chest wall or skin		

TABLE 6.3.
Breast Cancer Stages

Stage 1	Stage 2 A	Stage 2 B	Stage 3 A	Stage 3 B	Stage 4
T1, N0, M0	T1, N1, M0 T2, N0, M0	T2,N1,M0 T3,N0,M0	T1,N2, M0, T2, N2, Mo T3, N1, M0 T3, N2, M0	T4, any N, M0 any T, N3, M0	Any T, any N, M1

to 40 percent; and more than nine nodes, 15 to 30 percent.

- If you have positive receptors, you have an 8 to 10 percent better chance for cure than if they are negative.
- If you have spread beyond your armpit, your chance for living five years is about 20 percent.

For the five-year survival rate of the patients in the National Cancer Institute's database, see Table 6.4.

Alternative Medicine Approaches to Breast Cancer

L*inda developed breast cancer at age 45. She underwent a mastectomy followed by reconstruction, but after the operation her husband refused to look at her scar or sleep in the same bed with her. Two years later, she was found to have metastatic (distant spread) cancer. At that time, she sought alternative medicine help. She chose to undergo chemotherapy, but at the same time changed her diet and practiced visualization, self-hypnosis, and the other approaches listed below for alternative treatment of breast cancer. She took meditation tapes and a portable tape player with her to the hospital, to listen to as the medication was being administered. Her doctor told her he had never seen anyone tolerate chemotherapy so easily. She obtained a divorce and began a new career: counseling other women going through difficult times. Fifteen years later, she remains disease-free, and is now considered cured.*

In the United States, breast cancer is a national epidemic. Its incidence has doubled in the last twenty years. It is much rarer in the rest of the world. This should give our entire country pause, and make it seek more definitive action. We can act to prevent this continued plague, if we as a culture make the necessary changes. In addition, alternative medicine approaches offer help for treatment of this disease, and can assist in preventing its recurrence.

Only 5 to 10 percent of breast cancer is "genetic," something you inherit. Even then, whether your tendency is expressed depends upon your lifestyle choices. You may inherit, more significantly than your genes, your lifestyle.

TABLE 6.4.
Prognosis of Invasive Breast Cancer[41]

	Percent of Patients Surviving 5 Years	Percent of Patients in This Stage
All Patients	85.5%	
Not Staged	54.3%	3%
By Stage		
Localized to breast	96.4%	63%
Lymph node spread	77.7%	28%
Distant spread	21.1%	6%

For your own sake, and to assist your family and friends to also prevent this disease, educate yourself as completely as possible about its causes and treatments. Act preventively, especially if you are at risk. If you already have this cancer, construct a support team, from traditional and alternative medicine resources, to help you apply the recommendations given below, and in Chapter 2. The good news is that the deaths from breast cancer have decreased, perhaps due to earlier detection and treatment.

Generally, even alternative medicine practitioners recommend that if you do develop breast cancer, you first have your tumor removed through surgery. The reason for this is that local growth of the cancer can be quite uncomfortable, and metastatic spread is made more likely if the primary tumor is not taken out.

The essential cornerstone of a preventive and therapeutic program for the breast is a high-fiber, low-fat vegetarian diet that avoids sugar, refined foods such as white flour, alcohol, and caffeinated beverages. Such a change in diet may help you prevent, or treat, not only breast cancer, but heart disease and other fat intake–related cancers, such as those of the colon, stomach, esophagus, uterus, skin, ovaries, and prostate. See Chapter 2 for a more lengthy discussion of the beneficial effects of a high-fiber, low-fat diet on the functioning of the immune system. Following are the specific dietary and other alternative medicine modalities most promising in the prevention and treatment of breast cancer.

Change Your Diet

If you eat a lot of dietary fat, your body fat percentage increases, which then creates higher levels of estrogen in your body. Excess estrogen's overstimulation of the breast for prolonged periods is widely thought to be the *major* contributing factor to the onset of breast cancer. Changing to a low-fat diet has been shown to lower the level of circulating estrogen.

Although a study by David Hunter and others published in the *New England Journal of Medicine*,[42] and a few other studies, have *not* found a fat-breast cancer association, their conclusions must be questioned, since virtually all of these subjects still ate too much fat for adequate comparison to a low-fat diet: there were very few patients who took less than 10 percent fat, and a diet below 10 percent is needed to show the correlation, which becomes very apparent in cross-cultural research. "Tell me what a culture eats and I'll tell you its breast cancer risk," asserts Dr. Steven Austin.[43] Studies across cultures indicate that high fat consumption is very directly related to an increased risk of breast cancer. For example, one review of international epidemiological studies looked at fat intake and the incidence of breast cancer, and found that the Asian diet was the most protective, a Mediterranean diet posed an intermediate level of risk, and the typical Western diet was the worst: the more fat eaten, the higher the risk.[44]

A Canadian study showed increased risk with greater intake of beef, pork, and sweet desserts.[45] The Canadian National Breast Screening Study found a 35 percent increased risk with 77 grams of total fat intake per day, and evidence of a dose-response relationship.[46] An analysis of twelve studies showed up to a 46 percent increased risk for breast cancer with increasing saturated fat intake in postmenopausal women.[47] The most frequently named fatty "culprits" from dietary studies are the red meats, especially beef and pork, and high-fat dairy products such as cheese. *Your amount of beef intake can directly predict your breast cancer risk.*

Among Seventh-Day Adventists studied in this country, those who were vegetarian had one-third to one-half the amount of breast cancer, compared to other Adventist women eating the standard high-fat, low-fiber American diet. Even among the vegetarians, those who ate more fried potatoes and other fried foods, hard fats like butter or margarine, and dairy products had a higher risk than those who did not eat these items.[48]

If you already have breast cancer, changes in your diet may increase your longevity, by directly lowering estrogen production. Comparisons of both epidemiologic and experimental studies have shown increased survival after mastectomy of women eating a lower-fat diet.[49] One investigation found that in breast cancer patients the risk of death at any one point in time increased by 40 percent for each 1,000 grams of monthly fat in the diet.[50] A study of breast cancer patients showed favorable changes in immune function after only twenty-eight days on a low-fat diet supplemented with omega-3 fatty acids (as found in flaxseed oil).[51]

Aim for a diet that consists of 10 percent or fewer calories from fat; when fat provides 30 percent of calories, the upper limit recommended by most dietitians and the American Heart Association, you are in the high-risk group for breast cancer. Therefore, simply switching from meat to chicken or fish is not enough to provide protection.

The problem of fat consumption may also be one of its excessive calories or energy intake. Fat provides twice as many calories per ounce as do carbohydrate and protein. Animals fed lower-calorie diets do not develop cancer at nearly the rates of those fed standard diets. Some researchers suggest you adopt periodic "undernutrition"—accomplished by fasting one day a week—to give your body a rest from excess calories. Further investigation of these factors is needed.

Eat a High-Fiber Diet

Since excessive estrogen stimulation of the breast is thought to contribute to this cancer, any dietary substance that lowers excess estrogen levels may help provide protection. By inactivating an enzyme in your digestive tract that promotes estrogen reabsorption, and perhaps also by simply soaking up estrogen, adequate fiber in your diet lowers your estrogen level, and has been shown to decrease risk for breast cancer by up to 30 percent.[52] In one study, simply adding oat, corn, or wheat bran muffins, to increase daily bran intake from 15 to 30 grams, lowered estrogen levels by 20 percent.[53] Add bran to your meals, or make certain your muffins are fat- and sugar-free.

Add Certain Protective Foods to Your Diet, Especially Soybean Products

Cruciferous vegetables—broccoli, cabbage, cauliflower, and Brussels sprouts—contain a substance called indole-3-carbinol, that increases estrogen deactivation and breakdown, thus reducing estrogen stimulation. Broccoli has an additional substance shown to prevent breast cancer in mice.

Women who eat soybean products daily, such as soy milk and tofu, have a significantly lower risk for breast cancer.[54] Eating soybeans seems to provide protection in several ways. They contain *phytoestrogens*, substances that block the effects of estrogen, in a similar manner to the anticancer drug tamoxifen, but without its side effects. They also contain an ingredient called geneistene, an antioxidant that also hinders the formation of new blood vessels. Soybeans have other antioxidant isoflavones, and a substance called the Bowman-Birk protease inhibitor, shown to reduce cancer risk in animals.[55] A 1990 study from the University of Alabama found that rats fed a soybean protein diet developed 70 percent fewer breast tumors than rats getting their protein from other sources. The effects of these substances may help explain the lowered incidence of breast cancer in Oriental populations that traditionally consume large amounts of soybean products. Japanese women eating a high-soy diet excrete 1,000 times more geneistene than Americans.[56] Tofu, soy milk, and soybeans are the best sources; soy powder and soy sauce have lost their phytoestrogens in processing. Beans of all kinds contain phytoestrogens.

A combined analysis of twelve studies found that a diet high in fruits and fresh vegetables and vitamin C was associated with a 30 percent decreased risk for breast cancer. The authors estimated that, along with saturated fat reduction, dietary modification could prevent 24 percent of the breast cancers in postmenopausal women and 16 percent in premenopausal women in North America.[57] This effect may be related to the anticancer activity of *antioxidants*, dietary elements that may help prevent cancer. Antioxidants have "scavenging" ability against toxic-free oxygen radicals, which interfere with immune function.

A study by David Hunter of Harvard Medical School found a modest inverse association between intake of vitamin A and breast cancer.[58] Beta-carotene, a form of vitamin A, is one of the most frequently mentioned of the antioxidants, although research now indicates taking mixed carotenes, especially from foods, may be the most beneficial. Tomatoes have recently been shown to contain lycopene, an antioxidant even more powerful than beta-carotene. Selenium may play a role. For further discussion, see Chapter 2.

Avoid Grilled and Fried Foods

Whenever meat or fish is grilled or fried, at least ten different cancer-causing substances are created, including *heterocyclic amines*, also found in cigarette smoke. When these chemicals are taken up by breast tissue, they may encourage cell mutation.

Avoid Eggs

Another suspect food is eggs; they contain the fowl leukosis virus, known to cause cancer in chickens. Among the Navahos, who do not eat any eggs, breast cancer is rare.[59] Further investigation is needed to clarify the role of this agent. Recently, research found that women who as children were given the Salk polio vaccine, grown on eggs, had a higher incidence of subsequent breast cancer.[60] Such an association may find its origin from the injection of this virus. Whether this virus is killed when eggs are cooked is unclear.

Avoid Alcohol, Caffeine, Sugar, and Refined Foods

The link between alcohol consumption and breast cancer incidence is strong enough to advise total abstinence. Your chances increase with any increasing amounts of alcohol you consume. An analysis of thirty-eight studies found that compared with a nondrinker, *even one drink a day increases your risk by 17 percent; two drinks by 25 percent; and three drinks by 37 percent.*[61] The Canadian National Breast Screening Study found that the risk is even greater if you are premenopausal, up to 86 percent higher with more than 30 grams per day (a jigger of hard liquor, a bottle of beer, and a 6-ounce glass of wine each equals approximately 15 grams of pure alcohol).[62]

You especially should consider giving up alcohol if you are already at increased risk for this disease. "Women who are at higher than average risk for breast cancer should definitely consider abstaining from alcohol consumption. I think the available evidence is compelling enough to support this," stated Dr. Tim Byers, of the Centers for Disease Control and Prevention, Nutrition Division.[63] Alcohol suppresses immune function and raises estrogen levels. Although it may help prevent heart disease, the increase in breast cancer risk is too high a price to pay—and you can act to prevent heart disease by following the guidelines given in Chapter 8. (Eating red grapes may also take the place of the benefits of red wine.)

Likewise, consumption of even 1 teaspoon of sugar has been shown to decrease activity of your white cells, and thus the competence of your immune system, as discussed more fully in Chapter 2. Regular intake of sweet desserts has been correlated with breast cancer risk.[64] Refined foods, such as white flour products, which are low in fiber and other nutrients essential for a vigorous immune system, should also be avoided.

The correlation between caffeine consumption and breast cancer is as yet unclear, although by increasing the rate of fibrocystic disease, some types of which carry a two to five times increased breast cancer risk, a possible association deserves further investigation.

Eat Organically; Avoid Pesticides and Industrial Pollution

Exposure to pesticides and insecticides may increase breast cancer risk, with these carcinogenic substances concentrating in breast fat, as well as fat elsewhere. Due to inefficient metabolism, they may be sequestered there lifelong. Some of these chemicals have estrogenlike effects; DDT is known to act that way. In a study by M. S. Wolff on women in New York City, the group with the highest blood levels of DDT had four times the risk for breast cancer compared to those with the lowest levels. Those in the increased risk group had ten times the level of DDT of those in the lowest risk group.[65] And despite the 15-year ban on its use, DDT is still present in our foods, because of environmental contamination and residual amounts in the soil, and the importation of foods from third world countries to which we still ship DDT. Exposure as an infant or child may have long-term effects.[66]

The 1996 Long Island study, following women in larger numbers than ever before over a 20-year period, found a direct association between increased exposure to chemical pollutants (from living near a chemical treatment plant) and increased breast cancer risk.[67]

Many toxic substances are stored in fatty tissue, another reason to avoid animal products. Avoid using pesticides in your home and on your lawn and garden. The more we *all* buy organically grown foods, the more the marketplace will be encouraged to provide them.

Take Supplements

Because they affect immune activity, vitamins A, B_6, C, E, selenium, zinc, and magnesium supplements may be preventive as well as therapeutic.

Women who have a higher dietary intake of vitamin A and carotenoids, of which beta-carotene is only one, have been found to have a significantly lower risk of breast cancer.[68] Taking vitamin A or beta-carotene as supplements in pill form may not be enough to provide this protection; you may need to eat them in the vegetables themselves. In any case, taking beta-carotene supplements alone has not been shown to provide protection; it should be taken in the *mixed*-carotenoid form, 25,000 IU daily. Vitamin A should be limited to 10,000 IU per day. Once breast cancer has developed, vitamin A may stop tumor growth, as it has been demonstrated to do so in animal tests.[69] Selenium has been shown to prevent breast cancer in animals, and Dutch research has demonstrated that women eating more selenium-rich foods have decreased risk.[70] Follow the vitamin supplement guidelines given in Chapter 2.

Use Herbs and Other Immune Modulators

A number of herbs have shown some ability to assist the immune system in fighting breast cancer. Since studies in this country are funded only for patentable formulas, significant research on their effectiveness is lacking. However, anecdotal benefit has been reported for oral ingestion of the Hoxey Formula, Essiac, shark cartilage, chaparral, astragalus, echinacea, and garlic. Volunteers eating two bulbs of raw garlic daily exhibited an increased NK white cell killer activity, 140 percent more than controls; deodorized garlic showed even more, a 156 percent increase.[71] Research has also shown that garlic can inhibit breast cancer cells.[72]

One study showed that animals fed lavender oil had 60 to 80 percent shrinkage of their breast tumors, while orange peel oil had a similar effect.[73] For in-depth consideration of these adjuncts, see Dr. Michael Lerner's book *Choices in Healing* and Patrick Quillin's book *Beating Cancer with Nutrition*, which are listed in the Resources section at the back of this book.

Quit Smoking

Smoking inhibits wound healing through a great many mechanisms. Smokers undergoing breast surgery have a 30 to 50 percent higher rate of incision complications than do non-smokers.[74] Therefore, if you smoke, and you need surgery to help treat your cancer, you should stop before your operation, and never resume.

Practice Stress Management, Meditation, and Visualization

Of all the things you can do to help prevent and treat cancer, the most important may be to reduce your stress. Several studies have shown that stress-management training can increase survival in breast cancer patients.[75] Anecdotal reversal of metastatic breast cancer by the use of meditation has also been reported.[76]

Connections between the emotions and activity of the immune system may explain the relationship of stress to cancer. This new field of research, called psychoneuroimmunology, documents how your mind affects your ability to resist disease. Several studies have shown a strong link between stress and cancer, demonstrating rapid tumor growth in animals subjected to stress.[77] Women who express an inability to cope have an increased incidence of breast cancer.[78] The strength of "NK (natural killer) activity"—a measure of the ability of your immune system's white cells to eliminate abnormal cells from your body—is felt to be one predictor of outcome for some cancers.[79] Depression and lack of social support have been correlated with reduced NK activity.[80]

Training the mind with visualization techniques, hypnosis, and biofeedback can be used as important supplements to traditional therapy. Dr. Jean Acterberg, while at the University of Texas Medical Center, showed a doubling of the expected life span of terminally ill cancer patients who used visualization techniques three times daily.[81]

In addition, training in stress management and visualization helps you feel *physically* better. As you undergo breast conservation treatment or mastectomy, meditation, deep relaxation, and visualization may assist your body processes to speed healing and recovery. Dr. Bernie Siegel and others have reported that these tools can also be used to reduce the side effects of surgery, radiation, and chemotherapy. Visualize the X-ray or chemotherapy as going straight to your cancer cells without affecting the rest of your body. Follow the guidelines given in Chapter 2.

Seek Support from Family, Friends, and a Support Group

Much evidence now links solid social support to lower cancer risk, and improved outlook for those who do have cancer. Along with your diagnosis of breast cancer you can expect to experience shock, anger, grief, and intense fear. With help, you can also expect to work these through, and need not experience long-term emotional disturbance. Many studies have concluded that the quality of support from partner, family, friends, and healthcare providers may be as important for survival as well as psychological adjustment.

One of the most helpful steps you can take is to join a support group. Stanford researcher Dr. David Spiegel, originally a mind-body skeptic, set out to show that suggestions that the mind could affect cancer were ludicrous. He led a randomized study of eighty-six women with breast cancer that had already spread to distant areas. Half of the women attended a professionally led breast cancer support group, which met once a week, for an hour and a half, for twelve months. Women in the group were encouraged to form strong bonds of support within their group, express their feelings about their cancer, share their fears about death, improve their relationships with family and friends, and communicate more successfully with their physicians and nurses. They were also taught self-hypnosis for pain control. As expected, he found that the women in the support group had less stress and coped better. To his surprise, he documented that these terminally ill breast cancer patients doubled their survival times.[82] In his report, published in the *Journal of the American Cancer Society* in 1997, he showed that there were no differences in the medical treatment the patients received after their group therapy experience which might have accounted for the improved survival.[83] He is now searching for differences in immune function and other mechanisms that will explain this benefit.

Develop a "Fighting Spirit"

A study conducted in England showed that women with breast cancer who were taught to express their emotions had increased survival time. Those who refused to let their cancer diagnosis change their lives, responding with a "fighting spirit," denial, and hostile attitudes toward their physicians (which, in this case, meant resisting the prognosis of failure given to them) did better than those who stoically accepted their diagnosis. British scientist Steven Greer concluded that "the way a patient chooses to psychologically respond to her breast cancer diagnosis determines the outcome more than any other single factor, including initial staging."[84] Suggestions for finding a support group are listed in the Resources section at the back of this book.

Practice Daily Yoga Stretches and Breathing Exercises

Yoga stretches promote circulation of both your blood, which carries your protective white cells, and your lymph system, where your white cell reserves are located. By keeping your lymph channels flowing clearly, the yoga stretches systematically safeguard your immune system, allowing your white cells free access to find and destroy malignant cells before they multiply. Deep breathing also enhances blood and lymph circulation.

See Chapter 2 for details on yoga exercises. The gentle stretches of yoga are especially recommended postmastectomy, to improve your arm and shoulder mobility and decrease swelling. They also may help prevent recurrence of your disease by increasing local blood and lymph flow.

Use Acupuncture; Practice Qi Gong

Acupuncture has been demonstrated to be even more effective than narcotics at relieving pain in metastatic breast cancer patients. Qi gong, a type of tai chi movement therapy, is a way of becoming aware of your own healing ability, and changing your circulation to help you heal. In China, people practicing qi gong use rhythmic movements, and even hug trees for twenty minutes or so at a time. Since flow

of nutrients to all parts of the body can help the immune system function more effectively, these practices may have benefit as adjunctive therapy.

Exercise Regularly

Some studies have found evidence that exercise has a protective effect against breast cancer. Like yoga stretches and deep breathing, it increases blood circulation and lymph flow in the breast, as well as helping to alter breast metabolism and hormone production to prevent disease. Regular exercise can also help you achieve and stay at your optimum weight, thereby maintaining healthful amounts of circulating estrogen.

The U.S. Surgeon General's report *Physical Activity and Health,* 1996, found no consistent relationship between exercise and breast cancer incidence. It cited a few studies that lent "limited support to the hypothesis that physical activity during adolescence and young adulthood may be protective against later development of breast cancer." Their conclusion was that data regarding a relationship between physical activity and breast cancer were too limited to reach a conclusion. However, they also stated that: "The suggestion that physical activity in adolescence and early adulthood may protect against later development of breast cancer clearly deserves further study."[85] Conversely, several studies have found a relationship. A Harvard report indicated that those who exercise regularly had *half the breast cancer rates* of those who did not.[86] Another University of Southern California study showed that as little as four hours of exercise per week is enough to cut your risk by 60 percent.[87] A study from Norway published in the *New England Journal of Medicine* in 1997, involving

25,624 women who reported their level of physical activity during work and leisure time over an average of thirteen plus years, found the breast cancer risk reduced by one-third in regularly exercising women compared with the sedentary group. This effect was more prominent for premenopausal women, those less than 45 years of age, and for increasing levels of activity.[88]

In general, regular exercise is to be greatly encouraged, especially if you are overweight or have large breasts. See Chapter 2 for more information about starting and maintaining an exercise program.

Maintain Your Optimum Weight; Monitor Your Shape

Since your body's fat cells produce estrogen, if you are overweight, you are producing excess estrogen. And as previously indicated, these higher levels of estrogen harmfully overstimulate your breasts and you are therefore at higher risk for breast cancer, particularly after menopause. Studies have also suggested that recurrence rates after mastectomy are higher and survival rates lower in overweight women.[89]

Most studies have found the incidence of breast cancer to be higher in overweight women after menopause, although some have not supported this conclusion.[90] Particularly, postmenopausal women with a high ratio of central body fat to that in their extremities are at a higher risk. Such a distribution may reflect an inability of the liver to store more fat, so it begins to accumulate in the omentum, a thick fatty layer that hangs off the colon. Further investigation of the "apple" shape, already established as a risk factor for heart disease, is needed. Meanwhile, if you have an apple shape, you should make a special effort to change to the low-fat, high-fiber diet given in Chapter 2, and add at least four hours of active exercise each week.

Breast-Feed

Breast-feeding has been found to be strongly protective against the development of breast cancer in premenopausal women. Increased protection is associated with lactation before age 20 and nursing for more than six months. In other words, the earlier and longer you breast-feed, the greater your protection. The protection from having breast-fed a child lasts the woman's entire lifetime.

The mechanism for this risk decrease is unclear, but breast-feeding interrupts the unrelenting estrogen effect on breast tissue. It may also be due to the improved circulation within the breasts. Accumulation of carcinogens may be decreased by breast-feeding—good for the breast, though of course passing them on to the baby, who may or may not absorb them from his or her gut.

One notable study of women in an aquatic Asian society, where they typically paddled canoes from one side and had a tradition of breast-feeding only from the opposite breast, found that these women developed much more breast cancer in the breast not used for breast-feeding.

A 1994 study by Newcomb and associates reported in the *New England Journal of Medicine* suggested that if all women who have children breast-fed for more than a total of twenty-four months, the number of premenopausal breast cancers would be reduced by 25 percent.[91]

Choose Early Pregnancy; Avoid Abortion

Though this is not the current Western trend, having babies at a younger age is also protective. Never being pregnant increases your risk, but if you have your first child after age 35, you have an even higher risk. Pregnancies that are interrupted by induced, but not spontaneous, abortion may place you at a 50 percent higher risk of developing breast cancer.[92] However, studies about this relationship are inconsistent, and may be related to reporting bias in control subjects, who are reluctant to admit having had an abortion.[93]

Avoid Birth Control Pills

You may increase your risk for breast cancer if you take oral contraceptives. A recent huge European review of fifty-four epidemiological studies conducted in twenty-five countries of 53,297 women with breast cancer found a 24 percent increase in risk with current usage of birth control pills, slowly dropping back to baseline ten years after stopping.[94] If you have a family history of breast cancer, the danger is even greater. A 2000 study in the *Journal of the American Medical Association* found that women who had a mother or sister with breast cancer and who had ever taken the pill had a 3.3 times higher risk than women who have never taken them.[95] However, those cancers that do occur in women who have ever taken the pill tend to be found in a less advanced stage than in women who have never taken the pill. However, you are safer to choose a diaphragm or a condom.

Avoid Estrogen Replacement Therapy

There is solid evidence that postmenopausal use of hormone replacement therapy (HRT) increases your risk for breast cancer. Analysis of data from the Nurses' Health Study found an increase of 32 percent for current users compared to women who had never used HRT. Risk increased by 46 percent for current users who had taken HRT for five years or longer.[96] The combination of estrogen plus a progestin (combined hormone treatment) has been found to be even riskier than using estrogen alone. The Nurses' Study found that for each year of use, the risk of breast cancer increased by 9.0 percent for combined use and by 3.3 percent for estrogen alone.[97] The older you are and the longer you have used HRT, the higher your risk. Risks rapidly decrease to baseline after discontinuance. Put in more understandable terms: If you are a woman 60 years of age, not taking HRT, your risk of developing breast cancer in the next five years is 1.8 percent; if you have taken HRT for five years and are currently taking them, your risk is 3 percent.[98] Follow the guidelines for alternatives to these drugs, given below.

Consider Not Wearing a Bra and Avoiding Underarm Deodorants and Antiperspirants

The scientific rationale for these recommendations is only preliminary, but early findings make the possibility of an association worth considering.

Cross-cultural, historical, and recent survey evaluation supports a connection between bra use and increased breast cancer rates. Singer and Grismaijer's book *Dressed to Kill* documents their retrospective investigation that looked at thousands of women with a history of breast cancer and compared their bra-wearing habits with a group of women with no history of breast cancer.[99] They found that women who wore a bra more than twelve hours a day, but not to bed, had a 1 in 7 chance for developing breast cancer. Wearing a bra less than twelve hours a day reduced the risk to 1 in 152 and those who rarely or never wore a bra had only a 1 in 168 risk!

Those who wore a bra more that twelve hours per day were found to be twenty-one times more likely to develop breast cancer. Ninety-nine percent of all breast cancer patients were found to wear their bras more than twelve hours daily, compared with only 8 percent of the women who did not develop breast cancer. Eighteen percent of those developing cancer wore their bras to bed, compared with only 3 percent who didn't. Women who had cancer were twice as likely to have red marks on their skin or other problems caused by tight bras, compared to women who did not develop cancer.

The bra's effect on breast tissue may be related to restriction of lymphatic flow, necessary to keep tissue healthy. Although Singer and Grismaijer's study and conclusions have not been accepted by the medical establishment because they were not supported by a recognized research institution, are not medical doctors, and did not control for other risk factors, including breast size, which has been found to be associated with cancer risk and for which bra wearing may be a marker,[100] the book is well worth reading.

Wearing a bra does *not* prevent sagging; sagging is a natural consequence of the shift from glandular tissue to fat that accompanies aging, best prevented by diet and exercise. By restricting movement, the natural circulation of blood and lymph throughout the breast is compromised when a bra is worn. The benefits of exercise in breast cancer prevention indicate another connection to lymph flow and breast cancer, though further investigation is needed.

" 'In Russia bras cost an absolute fortune. And in India and Pakistan the bra is a serious status symbol,' said a spokesman for the Salvation Army, explaining the "bra bank" that the international aid group is setting up," *Newsweek* reported.[101] Perhaps this and other well-meaning organizations need to be informed about the potential harm of exporting our fashions to countries currently enjoying lowered risk for breast cancer.

Further investigation of this link is clearly needed. Meanwhile, you may want to try life without a chest cummerbund and see how much better you feel. Except for some women with very large breasts—and even for them—most women eventually find it more relaxing. Preventive medicine may require a cultural change in this area, to the benefit of both your health and your sense of well-being.

One woman put it this way: "The moment I discovered that a bra was simply a social convention, mine was gone forever. If men had to wear something similar—such as a jock strap all day long—perhaps they would never have invented them!" As a woman, you may wish to continue the bra tradition, but if comfort is the issue, you may find that you do adjust to the ease and freedom of going without, and begin to prefer it.

If you do wear a bra, you may do best to choose one of 100 percent cotton, and choose, wherever possible, cotton for your other garments as well. Synthetic materials act like magnets to trap the radioactive radon in our environment, increasing your radiation exposure; a link between radon and breast cancer is now being researched.

Association of underarm deodorants and/or antiperspirants has also been suggested, but further research is needed.

Use Massage

By increasing local lymph and blood circulation for proper cell maintenance, in a manner similar to exercise, regular gentle massage of the breast may help prevent breast cancer. Further investigation to document this possibility is needed.

Expose Yourself to the Sun—Moderately

Moderate sun bathing may be protective. Women who live in sunnier portions of the United States have lower breast cancer rates, as well as lower rates of cancer of the colon. Vitamin D may have some protective action for the immune system; in laboratory studies, it suppresses the growth of breast cancer cells.[102] Just make certain to take your sun exposure moderately, and don't burn.

Avoid Radiation

This is an ironic recommendation, but fifteen years after their treatments, women who had radiation to cure Hodgkin's disease have now been found to be developing breast cancer at an increased rate.[103] For a further discussion of the relationship of breast cancer to previous radiation, see Dr. S. Austin's book, *Breast Cancer*, as listed in the Resources section at the back of this book.

Avoid Electric Blankets

Women who keep their electric blankets on all night have been found to have a slightly increased risk for breast cancer. Waterbeds, due to their electrical heating units, may pose the same risk. The mechanism may be a suppression of the normal nightly rise in melatonin secreted by the pineal gland. Melatonin is suppressed by electomagnetic fields in rat experiments. It has been found to diminish rat breast tumor cell growth.[104]

If You Are Premenopausal, Schedule Your Surgery Late in Your Menstrual Cycle

Current studies are conflicting, and the National Cancer Institute says that at this time it is premature to schedule operations according to your menstrual cycle, but several reviews have found a significantly better disease-free survival for premenopausal women operated late in their cycle.[105] A report from Guy's Hospital in London found that the survival rate was 84 percent in women with breast cancer who had their operations toward the end of their cycles, compared to 54 percent in those who were operated in an earlier phase.[106] The unopposed estrogen of the early part of the cycle may promote tumor cell dissemination.

If you are still having periods, and you do need surgery for breast cancer, play it safe and be certain to schedule it in the later part of your menstrual cycle; counting day 1 as the first day of bleeding, day 14 is average for ovulation, so choose between days 20 and 30, to be certain to place it at a point in the cycle where progesterone is at a high level.

Surgical Approaches to Breast Cancer

Cheryl, a 46-year-old divorced therapist and mother of two teenage daughters, was very knowledgeable about healthy lifestyles, and sensitive to her own body. Soaping herself in the shower, she noticed a small, slightly tender lump in the upper area of her right breast. She reported it to her primary care doctor, who recommended a surgical consult. The needle biopsy did not show cancer, though close follow-up was recommended. One year later, the lump was slightly larger, and an open surgical biopsy found it to be a small cancer.

After two weeks of careful consideration, including getting opinions from several specialists, she chose breast conservation therapy (described in the following section). The treatment required removing more tissue from around her biopsy site, an armpit lymph node biopsy, and follow-up radiation to the breast.

Determined to make the experience as positive as possible, Cheryl requested an operating room with a view, that classical music be played during her operation, and that her surgeon and anesthesiologist whisper encouraging statements to her when she was under and emerging from general anesthesia. Cheryl went home the same evening, and sailed through her recovery period. Her wound healed very quickly, and she had no limitation of arm movement. Radiation treatments did not cause any problems, other than uncomfortable but temporary "sun burning." She declined chemotherapy, and has been cancer-free for the last five years.

Treatment Options

Making a good plan for treatment of your breast cancer involves a lot of work to research and understand the various options with their pluses and minuses as they pertain to your specific tumor and stage. Following is a brief overview of the basic approaches. This general discussion will be followed by detailed analysis of each specific surgical technique, often the first step in a combined treatment program with radiotherapy and chemotherapy.

Without Any Treatment

After diagnosis, without any treatment, you have only a 20 percent chance of surviving five years and a 0 to 3 percent chance of living ten years. A breast cancer can either grow slowly or rapidly, depending on a complex relationship between the tumor and your resistance to it. The usual pattern of local progression is that your tumor would enlarge and eventually erode the skin over it, producing a malignant ulcer very difficult to treat. Spread of the cancer to distant sites would eventually interfere with your lung, liver, bone, and/or brain function.

Tumor Removal Without Further Treatment

Simply removing your tumor without follow-up mastectomy or radiation treatment is not generally recommended. Mastectomy reduces the local recurrence rate to less than 3 percent. After local tumor removal without radiation treatment, local recurrence develops in 40 percent of all cases; with radiation, the rate is only 10 percent.[107] Some controversy exists about whether radiation adds anything to your ultimate life expectancy. This is because, if your disease reappears in your breast, you could then have a mastectomy, which would virtually eliminate the possibility of cancer recurring yet again locally. Most studies have found your chance for survival does not change with radiation, because this is determined by the presence or absence of distant spread.[108] However, a recent report does suggest you may have a small increased risk of dying if you have a recurrence in the breast.[109]

Ongoing studies are now looking for tumor features that could predict the safety of omitting X-ray treatment after local excision. If you have DCIS, it may be acceptable to forgo the radiation if you have a small tumor with a favorable cell type and negative margins on your surgical specimen, as described below. It may also be possible if you have a small invasive tumor and are postmenopausal.[110]

It seems to generally make sense that if you choose to avoid a mastectomy, you should add X-ray treatment, since this gives you the best chance to ultimately preserve your breast. Ask your doctor about your specific tumor and the latest information about your risks if you are determined to avoid radiation treatment.

Standard Treatment Options for Noninvasive Cancer

Two currently proven options are available for treatment of noninvasive cancer (DCIS). If you are one of the 15 to 30 percent of women with breast cancer found in this form, you can choose between local tumor removal followed by radiation treatment, commonly called breast conservation therapy (BCT), or total mastectomy, as described below. In general, you should choose one of these treatments, since if you had local removal of DCIS without further treatment, you have a 20 percent chance of tumor recurrence in five years (up to 63 percent at fourteen years), and if it recurs, 50 percent of the time it returns as an *invasive* tumor, with a less favorable prognosis.[111] If you have local removal plus radiation treatment, the invasive recurrence rate at ten years is reduced to 5 to 7 percent and risk of dying is only 1 to 3 percent, while if you have a mastectomy, this risk is 1 to 2 percent.[112] Mastectomy is usually recommended if you have a large tumor with high nuclear grade and involved margins after lumpectomy.

Treatment of DCIS is controversial because the natural history is not well understood, long-term results with different types of treatment are few, and in reality, many different kinds of tumors with different aggressiveness are grouped under the heading "DCIS." Although there are no prospective randomized trials, some studies have tried to determine whether removing the tissue at the site, along with follow-up radiation treatment, is necessary for *everyone* with this type of breast cancer. Recent evidence indicates that if a small, localized DCIS is of the "non-comedo" type, has a low nuclear grade, and is completely removed surgically, X-ray treatments are probably unnecessary. A 1999 study by Silverstein reported in the *New England Journal of Medicine* indicated that if the margins are clear of tumor cells by at least 1 millimeter (preferably at least 10 millimeters), radiotherapy is of no benefit.[113] If the margins are involved or close, a second (or third) surgical reexcision may still allow you to avoid radiation treatment or mastectomy if good margins can ultimately be attained. Since spread to armpit lymph glands is very rare (2 to 7 percent) in DCIS, you need not have a biopsy of those lymph nodes. Discuss latest results with your doctors.

Standard Treatment Options for Early Invasive Breast Cancer

If you have an early invasive tumor, you can also choose between BCT and mastectomy, usually accompanied by armpit lymph node biopsy. Although removing armpit lymph nodes may not affect overall survival, it is an excellent method to prevent later tumor appearance in the armpit (less than 1.5 percent), as well as to provide the best information about your prognosis and possible value of further treatment with chemotherapy or hormonal treatment.

The need for armpit node evaluation and treatment is currently a very hotly debated topic and the recommendations are changing. Recent studies indicate if you have a small tumor that can't be felt—less than 1 centimeter in diameter—with the favorable cell type and nuclear grade characteristics described earlier, you have a very low likelihood of spread (less than 5 percent) and you may appropriately choose to avoid the added discomfort of the armpit operation.[114, 115] Other studies are now looking for other tumor features that would predict the likelihood of armpit or distant spread for larger tumors. If your nodes are not enlarged on physical exam, and your subsequent treatment with chemotherapy or hormonal therapy (based on results of other tumor tests) would not be changed regardless of armpit node findings, or if you are an older woman or have serious medical problems and therefore would not be recommended to undergo chemotherapy, you may not need the armpit operation. A 2000 study from National Cancer Institute of Italy of 401 breast cancer patients treated without axillary dissection or radiation found that in tumors less than 2 centimeters there was only a 5.3 percent chance of later needing an axillary operation for recurrence whereas if the tumor was more than 2 centimeters the chances were 18.4 percent.[116]

"Sentinel" Lymph Node Biopsy and Early Invasive Breast Cancer

This new technique has been developed to identify and biopsy only the "sentinel" lymph nodes, or the first nodes draining the tumor and therefore most likely to contain tumor spread if present. If results are negative, it allows you to avoid most of the objectionable side effects of the standard armpit biopsy procedure. If positive, you should have the full standard lymph node removal operation, since a 50 percent chance exists you have more positive nodes—which should be removed to prevent local recurrence and allow more accurate staging.

Although techniques vary somewhat, you may first receive an injection of radioactive tracer into the region of the tumor, previous biopsy area, or area underneath your nipple. This is followed by a scan in the X-ray department that identifies the "hot spots" where the tracer is first picked up. The spots are marked on your skin. You then go to the operating room where your surgeon may also inject a tracer blue dye. Once picked up by lymphatics, the tracer is carried to the nearest lymph nodes, called the "sentinel nodes" draining the breast. After making a small incision, your surgeon can identify the correct nodes by using a handheld "Geiger counter" probe and/or visualizing the nodes that have turned blue. The specimen is then given to the pathologist for immediate examination. If it contains tumor cells, a standard armpit node operation usually follows; if none are found, the incision is closed. This technique can be used both with breast conservation therapy and mastectomy.

So far, sentinel node biopsy is not considered standard treatment, because long-term results of more than five years are not yet available, but as favorable research studies are being reported, more and more surgeons are learning to use it and offering it to their patients. In the near future it is likely to replace the standard lymph node biopsy for most women with smaller tumors who show no evidence of lymph node spread on physical exam.

There are several advantages to this procedure. The incision is smaller, and you experience less pain. It can be done under local anesthesia. Only one to three or four nodes are removed. Damage to skin nerves that would cause your arm, shoulder, and chest wall discomfort is unlikely. Few nodes are removed, so that your chance of arm swelling is minimal. The nodes provided to the pathologist can be more intensively scrutinized with special stains, so that a more accurate diagnosis of true positivity or negativity can be achieved.

Potential disadvantages are that it is a technically demanding procedure, with a surgeon learning curve. In a small percentage of cases, the tumor spreads to a higher node without landing first in the sentinel node, and thus an error in staging can occur ("false-negative" result). This would potentially lead to undertreatment if you had positive nodes that were not found. You would then miss the chance to receive the benefit of adjuvant chemotherapy or radiation treatment.

Current studies indicate about 95 percent of sentinel nodes can be successfully located. Success may be increased if the original biopsy was of the needle variety rather than an open surgical biopsy, since the lymphatics are less disrupted.[117] However, 5 percent of women who do have tumor somewhere in their lymph nodes but not found in the sentinel nodes will be classified as false negative and may miss the benefit of adjuvant treatment.[118] On the other hand, 10 percent of the women who would be classified as negative on the standard node removal pathologic evaluation will be found to be positive on the more intensive investigation possible on the sentinel nodes and receive the benefit of adjuvant treatment that they otherwise would have missed.[119] Also, 8 percent of women have sentinel nodes outside the axilla, and in

3 percent of women with positive nodes, they are positive only in this location.[120] These may be found with the sentinel node technique but missed by the standard operation. This technique seems to be most applicable if you have an early cancer less than 2 centimeters with a low likelihood to have already spread.

Ask your surgeon if he or she has had experience with sentinel node biopsy. Authorities recommend that each surgeon should first perform at least ten to twenty such biopsies immediately followed by the standard operation to determine his or her accuracy. Even though your surgeon may be in an early part of the learning curve, a more experienced surgeon may be recruited to help with or "proctor" your biopsy.

In the near future, noninvasive techniques such as the PET scan may be refined to accurately determine your node status without the need for any type of biopsy. Current evidence indicates this may be useful if you are postmenopausal with a larger tumor, but not yet sufficiently reliable if you have a small tumor.[121]

If your tumor is more than 1 centimeter in size, or has spread to your lymph nodes, added follow-up chemotherapy and/or hormonal therapy will usually be recommended, regardless of whether you choose breast conservation therapy or mastectomy. If you are premenopausal, radiation therapy may be added to mastectomy if you have a large tumor or positive nodes.

Standard Treatment of Advanced Breast Cancer

If you have an advanced cancer that has already spread beyond the breast and armpit, you may need combined treatment with one or more of the following: chemotherapy, hormonal therapy, radiotherapy, and surgery.

Breast Conservation Therapy with Follow-Up Radiation

Breast conservation therapy (BCT) usually includes lumpectomy, or removal of the primary cancer, an armpit lymph node biopsy, and radiotherapy to the remaining portion of the affected breast. (See Figure 6.4.) Confusion of terms still exists: "local excision," "lumpectomy," "partial mastectomy," "segmental mastectomy," and "tumorectomy" all mean pretty much the same thing. "Conservation" means that the breast is preserved and does not imply the tumor is treated conservatively, or less aggressively, than with mastectomy.

BCT usually requires at least two surgical procedures. The first removes the tumor and may be done when you have an open excisional biopsy, or if your initial biopsy was of the needle biopsy type, at the same time you have the armpit lymph node biopsy (see below). The area of the tumor may need to be "reexcised" during another procedure if the final microscopic exam shows tumor cells may have been left behind.

When the tumor is close to the nipple, you can request it be removed through an incision at the edge of your areola, the dark part around your nipple, so the scar will be less apparent, However, the incision should be as close to the tumor as possible, so as to minimize the difficulty in removing it and the possibility of seeding tumor cells in the neighboring normal tissue.

The second procedure is the armpit lymph node biopsy. The operation is done using general anesthesia or local anesthesia with seda-

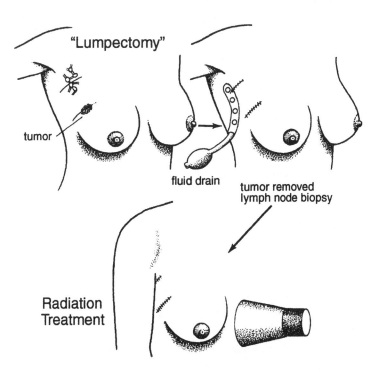

Fig. 6.4 Procedures involved in breast conservation therapy

tion and usually takes 45 to 90 minutes. If the earlier removal and analysis of your tumor indicated reexcision was necessary at the tumor site, this can be accomplished at the same time. To reach the lymph nodes, your surgeon makes a two- to three-inch incision just below the hair-bearing area in your armpit, which should not leave a conspicuous scar. The nodes that drain lymph fluid from the breast are removed, along with surrounding fatty tissue, and checked for cancer spread. Those nodes draining the arm are disturbed as little as possible. A soft plastic drain is usually placed underneath the skin and brought out through a separate one-quarter-inch incision. It is connected to a soft plastic fluid collection bulb that is easy for you to manage. The primary incision is then closed with sutures or skin tapes. This procedure can be done on an outpatient basis, though many women prefer to stay overnight. Your drain is removed after a few days. Postoperative recovery and complications are similar to those after mastectomy with lymph node removal (see page 220). The sentinel node biopsy procedure is likely to replace this procedure for women with smaller tumors.

After your incisions have healed, radiation therapy is given to the breast to kill any microscopic cancer cells left behind. An extra "boost" of radiation treatment may be given to the area of the tumor after the whole breast has been treated. Cancer cells are more sensitive to radiation than normal cells, because they are reproducing faster and are more likely to be in the radiation-sensitive stage of cell division. Usually five to six weeks of radiation, five days per week, is needed. If you have chosen to avoid the armpit node removal operation, the X-ray field may include the armpit, to destroy any tumor cells that may have spread there. To reduce the risk of tumor reappearance in the armpit and to minimize the risk of severe arm swelling, the armpit should be treated with surgery or X-ray, but not by both.

Newer techniques and equipment avoid most of the complaints of older forms of radiation treatment, such as a hard, smaller, tanned breast; breast swelling; change in skin sensation; damage to the heart and lungs; rib fractures; nerve irritation; and arm swelling. Arm swelling is much more common if you have X-ray treatment to the armpit area as well as the breast, especially if you have had a "complete" rather than a "limited" armpit lymph node removal. The long-term cancer-causing effects of the doses of X-rays used are still unclear, but so far this appears to be a safe form of therapy. Recently, X-ray treatment has been associated with a small increase in deaths from causes other than breast cancer, but this effect is balanced by a small reduction in the deaths from breast cancer.[122]

Since radiation therapy is an additional expense, breast conservation with follow-up radiation is more costly than total mastectomy alone, which is discussed in the next section. If plastic surgical reconstruction of the breast is added to mastectomy, however, the final costs are similar. A good-to-excellent appearance of the breast can be obtained in 90 percent of all patients who have breast conservation therapy with follow-up radiation.[123] If you are not satisfied with your result because of breast distortion or displacement of the nipple, you can consider plastic surgery correction.

Total Mastectomy

Total mastectomy is an operation that removes your breast but not the underlying muscles. This procedure greatly reduces the outdated "radical" mastectomy's side effects, which included loss of shape of the chest and shoulder, chronic stiffness and weakness of the shoulder, and arm swelling.

A *total mastectomy without armpit lymph node biopsy (a simple mastectomy)* is usually done for noninvasive DCIS or small cancers with very "favorable" characteristics. You may be able to have a simple mastectomy on an outpatient basis, although most women stay in the hospital for a day or two. After you are under general anesthesia, your surgeon removes the breast, including the nipple, using a six- to ten-inch incision, running laterally from a point near your breastbone to under your arm. (See Figure 6.5.) This incision is usually not visible when you wear a low-cut blouse. The underlying muscles are not disturbed. The surgery takes one to two hours to perform, and if you choose, your breast can be reconstructed during the same surgery, as described in the following section.

One or two soft plastic drains are placed under the skin and emerge through tiny incisions in your side. They are connected to plastic fluid collection bulbs. The primary incision is then closed with sutures or surgical tape. The drains are removed after a few days. It's unlikely you will have discomfort, requiring pain pills, for more than a week. Possible

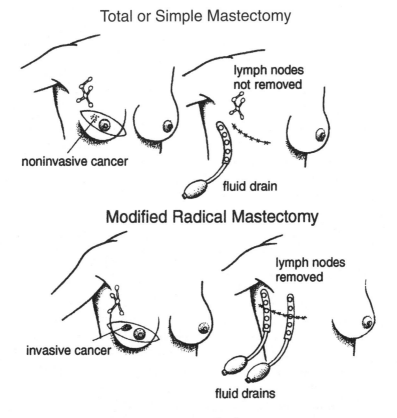

Total or Simple Mastectomy

lymph nodes not removed

noninvasive cancer

fluid drain

Modified Radical Mastectomy

lymph nodes removed

invasive cancer

fluid drains

Fig. 6.5   Procedures involved in mastectomy

complications of a simple mastectomy include blood or fluid collection under the skin and incision infection. If there is too much tension or a limited blood supply to the skin flaps, you may develop a rim of dead skin (epidermolysis) that turns black and eventually scabs and heals underneath. Occasionally, the incision will have to be revised. This problem is much more common if you smoke. You may have some numbness over the area, but your arm and armpit should not be affected. You should be able to resume your usual activities after two or three weeks.

The *skin-sparing mastectomy* technique, usually with immediate reconstruction using your own tissue, removes the nipple but very little breast skin. The tumor and rest of your breast is then hollowed out through the nipple opening. The remaining "skin envelope" is then filled with muscle and fat tissue transferred from elsewhere as described under breast reconstruction. The nipple is reconstructed later by borrowing skin from your upper thigh or elsewhere. For women with DCIS and smaller invasive tumors, this procedure is being increasingly used, with superior cosmetic results and equivalent cure rates.[124]

Most women with invasive cancers choosing *total mastectomy* also have an *armpit node biopsy* (a modified radical mastectomy). The operation takes one and one-half to three hours, under general anesthesia. Although some centers are doing this operation successfully on an outpatient surgery basis, most women stay in the hospital for one or two days afterward. Using an incision similar to that described above, your surgeon removes your whole breast, and reaches up to the armpit area to remove the armpit lymph glands draining lymph fluid from your breast. If you are having the sentinel node biopsy

procedure described above and it is negative for tumor spread, the full armpit operation may be omitted. A "limited" ("level 2") removal takes out only the ten to twenty lower nodes closest to the breast, and is preferred—unless some nodes are positive, in which case a "complete" ("level 3") removal of the highest nodes may be added. Underlying muscles are not removed. Two soft plastic drains are usually placed and brought out through the skin at tiny incisions below the primary incision. The skin is closed with stitches or surgical tape.

After being discharged from the hospital, you need to make several follow-up office visits to your doctor to monitor your healing and recovery, as well as go over the pathology report from the tissue removed. This will also be the time to discuss any further therapy.

Your drains are left in place for five to ten days, depending on the amount of drainage, then easily removed in the doctor's office. You can attend to them yourself at home, simply emptying the collapsible plastic collection bulb when it fills and then squeezing the air out of it to maintain suction. The incision area should be kept dry and covered for forty-eight hours, or longer if you wish. You may be asked to take sponge baths rather than showers until after the drains are removed.

You may need pain pills for a week or two after a mastectomy with lymph node biopsy. To avoid a stiff or "frozen" shoulder, moving your arm after surgery is important, though it should not be vigorous in the first week. A gradual exercise program of squeezing a rubber ball, bending and moving your elbow in a circle, "walking" your fingers up a wall, and combing your hair is recommended. It may take two or three months before your arm and shoulder regain a comfortable full range of motion. After four to eight weeks, once your healing is complete, you can wear a bra with a prosthesis inside.

Complications include problems with healing similar to those earlier described in the section on mastectomy without armpit node removal. In addition, difficulties may develop with the armpit part of the operation.

You may notice minimal or, rarely, severe arm swelling from interruption of the lymph This is ared with ay treat-l particu-statistics that per-A 1999 in New ts had a nference g the op-ally this gnificant t devel-kly and rtant to ury and fection, manent

percent ation in tion, in mpit, and/or in the inner part of the upper arm, because of removal or injury to sensory nerves during surgery. These unpleasant sensations usually decreased in a few weeks, but 18 percent of these patients had no improvement. Very rarely, important arm and shoulder nerves are damaged, which affects muscle function. Permanent limitation of range of motion of the arm or shoulder is also very unusual.

Fluid may continue to collect under the skin after the drains are removed (seroma). The NYU study found this to occur in 59.5 percent of their patients. If this happens, your doctor may need to remove the fluid using a needle one or more times. This is not painful, since the area will still be numb from the surgery or can be numbed with local anesthetic.

Over 80 percent of the women who have the standard armpit node removal operation experience at least one postoperative complication, and associated psychological distress is common.[126] The major attraction of the sentinel node biopsy procedure described above is that women without node spread can avoid these problems.

I recommend that you arrange a visit from a member of "Reach to Recovery," sponsored by the American Cancer Society, or "Why Me?," national organizations comprised of postmastectomy patients. These women are volunteers who have lived through the breast cancer experience and can provide support and advice about exercise, buying prosthetics, and adjusting to having had cancer. Also, find a support group through these organizations, your doctor, or the American Cancer Society. Further suggestions on how to find these groups in your geographic area are located in the Resources section at the back of this book.

Postmastectomy Reconstruction

The anatomy and function of the breast cannot be restored. However, the surgical state of the art has reached new heights in recreating a shape and consistency similar to your original breast. Age is no barrier. Good results can usually be obtained using one of the various methods to be described. Reconstruction should be considered a standard treatment option for most patients choosing mastectomy. All states now mandate that it be covered by health insurance, including Medicaid and Medicare. Many women, however, don't feel that reconstruction is necessary for their quality of life, and choose not to have this additional procedure.

Reconstruction may be performed at the time of your mastectomy or at a later date—even years later, if you wish. Immediate reconstruction is beneficial for psychological reasons, and it avoids the necessity of a second operation and hospitalization. Although it prolongs your operative time, and probably your hospital stay, it may ease your adjustment to surgery, and can make total mastectomy as emotionally acceptable as the breast conservation treatment previously described.

Recent studies suggest the cosmetic result is ultimately more pleasing if your reconstruction is done at the time of the original operation because there is more unscarred skin with which to work. Immediate reconstruction has a high rate of patient satisfaction. Reconstruction should be delayed if you have a high risk of complications at your incision site (as is the case with heavy smokers); if it would delay chemotherapy; or when postoperative radiation treatments have been recommended. The American College of Surgeons reported that in 1990, 7.2 percent of the women who chose mastectomy also chose reconstruction, and two-thirds had it done immediately.

No evidence exists to indicate having either immediate or delayed reconstruction affects your chances for survival. Indeed, your attitude about wanting reconstruction may change: of all women who at the time of surgery say they want to have later reconstruction, only one-third are still interested in the procedure six to twelve months later. The majority report being content to wear a prosthesis and avoid more surgery.

The goals of breast reconstruction are to match the size, contour, and nipple/areola of the other breast as closely as possible. They should appear the same under clothing. Scars are noticeable, although recently, new techniques such as the "skin-sparing" mastectomy that removes very little skin are minimizing the incisions.[127]

Three basic types of reconstruction are available. The simplest places a saline-filled silicone implant beneath your pectoral muscle, just as described in the section on breast augmentation. However, this method is rarely used, because most of the time there is not enough skin available to cover it and match your opposite breast.

If implants are chosen, a procedure called *tissue expansion* is usually used: a specialized implant is inserted under the skin and chest wall muscle during your original operation, or at a later date. Over several weeks, during postoperative office visits, it is gradually inflated with saline to stretch your tissues. You may experience mild discomfort during this period. When the desired breast size has been achieved by this process, the expander is surgically replaced with the "permanent" implant. This procedure can be done on an outpatient basis, under general anesthesia.

Your nipple and areola reconstruction is usually done later, when healing is complete. It can be performed by simply reshaping the local tissue with stitches and later tattooing it to make the new nipple and areola the same color as your natural one. Alternatively, skin can be taken from another site, such as your upper thigh, then transplanted to the reconstructed breast. These minor procedures can be accomplished under local anesthesia in your plastic surgeon's office.

Possible complications of prostheses include a fibrous scar that makes the tissue contract around the implant, infection, and implant leakage as described in the section on breast augmentation. Overall, the risk of a complication requiring surgical correction is 34 percent in five years.[128] No evidence suggests that having an implant increases your chance for a local cancer recurrence or causes a delay in finding it if one does occur.[129]

The third type of breast reconstruction operation brings a "flap" of your own skin, fat, and muscle into the breast area, to create a contoured mound similar to your opposite breast. Most plastic surgeons feel the aesthetic results with flaps are more natural and pleasing than with implants. The tissue can be "swung" up to the breast area on a "pedicle" containing an artery and vein, or transferred as a "free flap" with the artery and vein completely divided at the original site, then reconnected into an artery and vein located near the reconstruction. Three types of flap are commonly used. The most frequently employed procedure is called a *TRAM flap;* skin, fat, and muscle from your lower abdominal wall are brought up to the breast area, to create the new mound. This often has the added benefit of a "tummy tuck." A TRAM flap is a very involved, lengthy operation that may take three to four hours to complete. A scar will be noticeable in your lower abdominal skin. The *latissimus dorsi flap* uses some skin, fat, and muscle from your back. It is a simpler operation, used to create a small breast or cover an implant. You will likely have a noticeable scar on your back. The *gluteus maximus free flap* brings tissue from the lower part of one of your buttocks and is used in thin women where abdominal tissue is not plentiful. You may have some minor asymmetry in the buttocks. After flap reconstruction,

further minor "touch-up" procedures or liposuction can be used to fine-tune the result.

All of the flap procedures can have complications, such as tissue loss from poor blood supply. Serious problems are uncommon, though when they do occur, further surgery is usually necessary. You are at greater risk if you have high blood pressure, diabetes, are overweight, have previous scars in the area of the flap, or if you are a smoker unable to stop. Smokers undergoing breast surgery have a 30 to 50 percent higher incidence of wound complications than nonsmokers.[130]

Recovery after reconstruction depends on the procedure used: two to three weeks if you have an implant, and four to eight weeks after a flap.

When performed with skill, these choices all have acceptable results. They also have significant pros and cons. If you are interested in having your breast reconstructed, you need to have a frank discussion with your surgeon and plastic surgeon so you can become an informed decision-maker. Your expectations should be realistic. Be certain to inquire about the latest updates in procedures and implant materials.

Considerations to Help You Choose Your Treatment Program

Changes in lifestyle and diet; the use of visualization, meditation, and stress management; and a support group may improve your chances for cure and survival time. *These should be used in addition to, not as a replacement for, standard treatment.*

Determining the most appropriate treatment plan for you can be a very difficult and confusing process. You should consider all of the information you have learned about your tumor. You may well have a mixture of some favorable and some unfavorable prognostic factors. Many variations in breast cancer are seen; you will most likely have several treatment options and may not find any "best" answer. Your doctors will recommend those options that have equally good results in terms of cure. Others, although with a higher likelihood of failure, may seem better for you. Your perception of what is most important to your physical and mental health, and your quality of life, may be different from that of your doctors.

Most authorities agree that a team approach—utilizing the special skills of the surgeon, plastic surgeon, radiation oncologist, medical oncologist, cancer nurse-specialist, social worker, and psychologist—will lead to the best results. In some "breast cancer centers," these specialists are available for a group discussion of your options, with you and your family. This is the optimum approach. Also, it may be desirable for other members of your family, especially children, to receive counseling, to help them through this period.

Local Treatment of the Tumor

For more than 90 percent of all breast cancer patients, the cancer is discovered at an early stage, when the choice of treatment between mastectomy and BCT is unlikely to affect survival, but may affect quality of life. Although psychological studies of large numbers of patients have shown very little difference in overall emotional distress, you, as an individual, may have a more positive body image and feel more desirable after BCT. This is a very personal decision. In 1990 the National Institutes of Health assembled a panel of experts to update breast cancer treatment recommendations. The panel agreed that "breast conservation treatment is an ap-

propriate method of primary therapy for the majority of women with stage I and II breast cancer, and is preferable because it provides survival equivalent to total mastectomy and also preserves the breast."[131]

Both breast conservation therapy with radiation and total mastectomy have advantages and drawbacks. Mastectomy removes your whole breast, though reconstruction can be chosen. With breast conservation, a major operation is still usually necessary to remove your tumor and assess your armpit lymph nodes. Radiation then requires an extra five or six weeks of treatment, and adds additional expense. Radiation changes your breast somewhat, though modern techniques lead to better cosmetic results. This route is an especially good option if you have a small tumor. However, the long-term effects of large doses of radiation are still unclear; high doses of radiation at younger ages have been associated with an increased risk of some kinds of cancer later in life.

Consider the following information, then discuss it with your doctors and those close to you, before making your final decision.

BCT and mastectomy are basically equal in relation to five factors. These five factors are:

1. Cure and survival.
2. Complications.
3. Functional status.
4. Quality of life and sexuality issues.
5. Degree of psychological stress and adjustment.

There are three factors that favor having BCT over a mastectomy. These three factors are:

1. Your self-image may be better. You may not be happy wearing an external pros-

thesis, and you may feel anxious and depressed that mastectomy without reconstruction would be a permanent detraction from your appearance and quality of life. However, long-term follow-up studies of large numbers of women have found no significant advantage to BCT in regard to general psychological adjustment, anxiety, sexual function, and the quality of their relationships.[132] Your happiness and satisfaction with life before cancer treatment are a better predictor of your postcancer adjustment than whether or not you opt for breast conservation treatment.[133]

2. BCT requires less surgery and a shorter hospitalization time.

3. BCT may be more desirable than total mastectomy if you have large breasts, where removal of one will result in significant asymmetry, imbalance, and discomfort. (However, with mastectomy, you could have plastic surgery to reconstruct the affected side and reduce the opposite side to match.)

There are six factors that favor having a mastectomy over BCT. These six factors are:

1. Mastectomy is less expensive (without reconstruction).

2. Less time is required to complete treatment.

3. Mastectomy may be more desirable than BCT if you have very large, pendulous breasts which make uniform radiation dosages difficult.

4. A good cosmetic result is less likely with BCT if:
   • you have a relatively large tumor in a small breast.
   • you have a tumor greater than 4 centimeters.
   • your bra cup size is greater than B, as you may have greater fibrosis and retraction from radiation therapy.
   • you have a breast augmentation implant, since radiation may cause excessive scar formation around it.

   In these situations, mastectomy with reconstruction may give better results.

5. Mastectomy has a lower local recurrence rate than BCT; 3 percent with mastectomy versus 10 percent with BCT. Local recurrence rates are even higher after BCT if:
   • you have a tumor greater than 5 centimeters in size.
   • your mammogram shows diffuse microcalcifications involving more than one-quarter of the breast.
   • your tumor has an extensive intraductal component (EIC), where more than 25 percent of the invasive tumor is composed of noninvasive tumor within breast ducts and ductal carcinoma in situ (DCIS) is present in the surrounding normal tissue. The local failure rate increases up to 35 percent if your tumor shows EIC.
   • you are younger than age 35, when your risk for a local recurrence rate is 14 percent.

   Mastectomy can be done after a BCT local recurrence without proven difference in overall chance for cure.[134] Survival rates are the same.

6. If you are likely to worry constantly about cancer recurring in your breast, mastectomy is preferable.

There are six reasons BCT should not be chosen. These reasons are if you:

1. Have multiple cancers in different areas of the same breast.
2. Have involved margins after local excision (reexcision may be possible).
3. Have had prior radiation to the chest.
4. Have a skin disease such as lupus erythematosis or scleroderma, which causes severe reactions to radiation treatment.
5. Are in the first six months of pregnancy.
6. Are unlikely to follow through with treatment recommendations due to fear of radiation treatment, finances, difficulty in making return visits to see your doctor, or other psychosocial factors.

Adjuvant Treatment of Breast Cancer

Although mastectomy and BCT produce similar long-term survival rates, both may need to be combined with chemotherapy and/or the drug tamoxifen for best results, especially if your lymph nodes are found to be "positive" for cancer. Neither breast conservation therapy that includes radiation, nor mastectomy, provides treatment for tumor cells that might have spread beyond your breast and armpit.

The objective of *adjuvant chemotherapy* and *adjuvant hormonal therapy* following surgery is to treat tiny, undetectable deposits of malignant cells already spread to distant areas. This approach is intended to increase your chances for cure and survival *even though no direct evidence suggests you have any cancer left in your body*. Recommendations about whether and which type of adjuvant treatment you should have are determined by several factors: the stage of your cancer at the time it was found, which is a clue as to whether it has spread through your blood system; information from the pathologic examination of the breast (and probably lymph) tissue removed; and the known risks and benefits of the various drug combinations and hormones used. Most likely you will have a mixture of good and poor prognostic factors, and this makes decisions more difficult.

Tumor size and lymph node status are the primary factors on which a recommendation for adjuvant therapy is based. Your age, menopausal status, general health, and estrogen receptor status are secondary considerations. Other prognostic factors such as S-phase, DNA index, oncogene erb-2 expression, flow cytometry, and others may be incorporated into chemotherapy recommendations.

If cancer cells are found in your armpit nodes, or if your tumor is larger than 1 centimeter, adjuvant chemotherapy has been shown to decrease your chance for recurrence by 28 percent. The advantage is higher if you are below the age of 50, or have a poorer prognosis.[135] Looking at it another way, if without adjuvant chemotherapy your chances for recurrence are 30 percent, with treatment your risk will be cut by one-third to about 20 percent.

Different combinations of three to five anticancer drugs are used, and treatment generally takes four to twelve months, with a variety of treatment schedules depending upon the drugs used. Side effects are varied, ranging from mild to quite severe. They include premature menopause, nausea and vomiting, decreased white blood cell and platelet counts that leave you vulnerable to infections and bleeding, fatigue, hair loss, and, rarely, the growth of secondary cancers. With the addition of the alternative medicine approaches described earlier in this chapter, you may be able to lessen these side effects.

Adjuvant hormonal therapy following

surgery usually uses the drug tamoxifen (Nolvadex) to change your body's hormonal balance, to slow growth of any remaining cancer and/or cause it to recede. Similar to chemotherapy, it decreases your odds for recurrence by about 25 percent.[136] It has proven to be most beneficial in postmenopausal women with "estrogen receptor positive" tumors, as previously discussed. Taking tamoxifen for five years is recommended. Possible side effects include hot flashes (up to 25 percent), menstrual irregularities in premenopausal women, nausea, weight gain, vaginal dryness or increased secretions, blood clots, and depression. Less than 10 percent of the women taking tamoxifen discontinue the drug due to unpleasant side effects. Tamoxifen has been found to slightly *increase* the risk for uterine cancer, so it should not be used without good reason. A gynecological exam should be done before starting this drug, and on a yearly basis thereafter.

Tamoxifen has been shown to reduce the risk of another cancer in the opposite breast by 40 percent. As an added benefit, you develop better bone density and a more favorable blood lipid profile that may protect you against coronary artery disease. The Scottish Cancer Trial found a 50 percent decrease in heart attacks in women taking tamoxifen compared with those who did not.[137] Tamoxifen is now the leading-selling anticancer drug in the world.

Tamoxifen's potential role in preventing a first breast cancer in women at high risk has recently been documented. In 1992, the National Surgical Adjuvant Breast and Bowel Project began a study of 13,388 women without breast cancer, but at high risk in terms of age or other factors. They were randomized to receive either tamoxifen or a placebo for five years. Tamoxifen reduced the incidence of breast cancer by 50 percent. However, an increase in risk of uterine cancer and blood clots was found.[138] More study is needed to determine how greatly the benefits will outweigh the side effects. The U.S. Food and Drug Administration has recently approved the use of tamoxifen for women at high risk for breast cancer. Raloxifene (Evista), a drug developed to prevent osteoporosis, is now being investigated as an alternative to tamoxifen. It may have similar breast cancer prevention effects as tamoxifen but doesn't increase the risk of uterine cancer. However, it also increases risk for blood clots.

Unless you would like to be part of a prevention study, you should not choose adjuvant chemotherapy and hormonal therapy if it has been determined you have a low risk that your cancer had spread through the bloodstream, because the risks can be life-threatening. You are at low risk if you have a tumor less than 1 centimeter, with favorable tumor characteristics, and without evidence for spread to lymph nodes or elsewhere. In 1990 an NIH Consensus Development Panel recommended against routine adjuvant chemotherapy in these cases.[139]

If your tumor was near or grew into the underlying muscle, or had broken through the wall of any of your lymph nodes, radiation treatments called *adjuvant radiotherapy* may be recommended, even after mastectomy, to decrease your chances for a local recurrence of cancer on your chest wall or in your armpit. Recently, some evidence indicates that radiotherapy is useful if you are premenopausal and have positive lymph nodes or a large tumor.[140] Three to five weeks of treatment five days per week is the usual schedule.

If your tumor is very large or has other unfavorable characteristics when first discovered, you may be recommended to receive *induction* or *neoadjuvant* chemotherapy *before* planned surgical treatment. At this point, the tumor cells may already have spread, and it is important to treat them with chemotherapy as quickly as possible. Also, because of the size of the tumor, surgery may not be feasible. After the chemotherapy, the tumor may shrink to the point where mastectomy or even BCT might then be considered. Research is now investigating whether *most* women with breast cancer, even those with small tumors, would benefit from chemotherapy before any other treatment.

Since adjuvant therapy is a rapidly changing field, make certain you have the latest information from first, second, and third opinions, as discussed in Chapter 2. In addition, seek information from a major cancer research and treatment center, as indicated in the Resources section of this book.

Locally Advanced and Inflammatory Breast Cancer

Locally advanced breast cancer develops fixation to the skin or underlying chest wall, ulcerates, or has fixed, enlarged armpit lymph nodes. One type, called *inflammatory* breast cancer, occurs in 1 to 6 percent of all women with breast cancer. It looks very much like an infection, and the two are commonly confused. Typically, the breast is swollen, warm, pink or purplish, tender, and the skin develops tiny dimples like an orange. Unlike with an infection, no fever develops. These types of tumor have a poor prognosis, and are therefore initially treated with chemotherapy. Surgery can be done if the tumor shrinks sufficiently, and is often followed by radiation treatment for best results.

Recurrent or Metastatic Breast Cancer

If you are one of the 5 to 10 percent of patients who has a "local recurrence," a return of a cancerous lump at or near the site of your first cancer, and if further tests do not show it has spread beyond your breast, chest wall, or armpit lymph glands, you still may be cured by further surgery, radiation, chemotherapy, and/or hormonal therapy. If your first treatment was BCT, the standard recommendation would be for you to have a "salvage" mastectomy, after which your chance for living five years is 60 to 80 percent. In some cases, another local excision can be considered, rather than mastectomy. If you initially had a mastectomy, the chance for a local recurrence is reduced to 3 percent, but five-year survival after further treatment is only about 20 to 40 percent. The presence of simultaneous distant spread is the main determinant of survival.

If your tumor is found to have metastasized—that is, spread beyond both your breast and armpit nodes—either at the time of its initial discovery or after your tumor was first treated, it is considered to be beyond the bounds of cure by further surgery or radiation. Chemotherapy and/or hormonal therapy is then recommended, in the hope of delaying or reducing your symptoms and prolonging your life. Although many patients live much longer, at present, average survival time is two years,[141] and ultimate cure is unlikely using only these methods.

The controversial treatment of *intensive chemotherapy* followed by *bone marrow* or *stem cell transplant* is now being carefully evaluated as a means of prolonging life and possibly curing some women. The candidates are otherwise-healthy patients who have evidence of their cancer having spread to distant parts of the body. Also, studies are now under way that give this therapy to patients with a very high risk for, but without current evidence of distant spread (finding ten or more positive armpit lymph nodes is the usual indicator). This treatment takes about a month of hospitalization, and you first must endure aggressive chemotherapy to reach any cancer cells in your body. Your bone marrow, which is responsible for producing the white cells essential to your immune system, is destroyed by the high doses of drugs. Other sensitive body tissues are also affected. During treatment, you are, therefore, at high risk for serious infection and other complications.

New bone marrow, usually taken from your own body prior to the chemotherapy, is then reimplanted in your body to provide you with healthy marrow after chemotherapy. Another similar approach restores your marrow with stem cells harvested and saved from your own blood prior to chemotherapy. (Stem cells are a basic type of blood cell that create red and white blood cells, and also the platelets, which are essential for clotting.)

Results of these very expensive and controversial studies have been disappointing so far. For the average patient, no evidence shows that it is better than standard chemotherapy treatment in terms of quality of life and improved survival.[142] A 2000 study from the University of Pennsylvania found that in women who had a good response to standard chemotherapy and who then received high-dose chemotherapy after stem-cell transplant had no improvement in survival compared with the women who continued conventional treatment.[143]

The subject of chemotherapy is in a constant state of evolution. If you do develop, or are at very high risk for, distant spread, you need to discuss the latest treatment updates with a specialist in this field, and then obtain second and third opinions, as presented in Chapter 2.

Breast Cancer Follow-Up

Seventy-five percent of breast cancers that recur become known within two years and 95 percent by five years. If you have BCT, the timing of local recurrence may be much later. If no evidence of return of your disease has appeared after five years, a high likelihood exists you have been cured. However, relapse *can* occur even after ten years, making lifetime follow-up necessary. Also, once you have had one breast cancer, you have a 1 percent per year (25 to 30 percent lifetime) chance of developing a second new tumor in your other breast. The risk increases to 1.5 percent per year if you are over age 55.[144]

You need a personal follow-up schedule. In addition to careful breast self-examination (recurrent cancers are detected by the patient 70 percent of the time), schedule an examination by a physician every three months for the first year, every three to six months for the second year, every six months for the third through fifth years, and yearly thereafter. You also need a yearly mammogram. Other studies such as chest X-ray, scans, blood tumor markers, and liver enzyme blood tests are controversial in the absence of symptoms, and may just be a waste of time and resources since no benefit exists in treating recurrent cancer before symptoms appear. Any new pain or lump should be investigated.

BREAST CANCER SUMMARY

Prevention

Diet and Supplements

- Follow a low-fat, high-fiber diet.
- Avoid eggs, grilled and fried foods, sugar, and refined foods.
- Eat protective foods—soybeans, fruits and cruciferous and other fresh vegetables, and antioxidants.
- Avoid pesticides and industrial pollution—eat organically.
- Avoid alcohol and caffeine.
- Take vitamins and supplements—vitamins A, B_6, C, E, and selenium, and magnesium.
- Add mixed carotenoids, 25,000 IU daily.

Lifestyle

- Follow mammogram screening guidelines.
- Do breast self-examination monthly.
- Get regular exercise, 1 hour 3–5 times weekly.
- Quit smoking.
- Maintain optimum weight; monitor your shape.
- Breast-feed; choose early pregnancy; avoid abortion, birth control pills, and estrogen replacement therapy.
- Choose not to wear a bra; choose only cotton clothes next to your skin.
- Avoid underarm deodorants and antiperspirants.
- Expose yourself to the sun—moderately.
- Practice daily yoga stretches and breathing exercises.
- Use massage.
- Avoid radiation electric blankets.

Alternative Medicine Approaches

- If you are premenopausal, schedule your surgery late in your menstrual cycle.
- Use herbs and immune modulators—Hoxey formula, essiac, shark cartilage, chaparral, astragalus, echinacea, and garlic.
- Practice stress management, meditation, and visualization.
- Seek support from family, friends, and a support group
- Develop a "fighting spirit."
- Use acupuncture and practice qi gong.

Conventional Medicine Approaches

- Chemotherapy.
- Hormone therapy.
- Radiation therapy.

Surgical Approaches

- Local excision only.
- Breast conservation therapy: local excision and radiation treatment.
- Simple mastectomy.
- Modified radical mastectomy.
- Breast reconstruction.
- Standard armpit lymph node biopsy.
- Sentinel node biopsy.

CHAPTER 7

LUNG

Carole Hart, a 45-year-old dedicated writer and producer, a winner, along with her husband, of seven Emmy awards, had a 30-pack/year history of smoking. While in the midst of an intense new television production, she suddenly experienced repeated dizziness. Tests revealed the cause of her symptoms to be cancer in her brain, which had spread there from her lung. She began X-ray treatment of the tumors in her head, along with chemotherapy for the cancer in her lung.

She also began a course of alternative medicine techniques including hypnosis and acupuncture. She quit smoking, changed her diet using the low-fat, high-fiber approach given in Chapter 2, took the vitamins and other supplements recommended there, and began daily yoga stretches and meditation, along with deep breathing therapy. She experienced few side effects from her conventional treatments, and was soon again creating movies and television shows, being careful to continue her new, healthy lifestyle habits. Seven years later she was considered cured, with no remaining sign of any cancer.

Oh the sensation of it, the ritual. You can take a break, put your feet up, lean way back, and inhale slowly and deeply. Smoking has such potent short-term rewards that one in four Americans still smokes, despite the now widespread knowledge of its risk. Alternative medicine treatment methods, such as yoga breathing exercises, offer new hope: they can help you quit cigarettes successfully, or assist in your recovery from lung surgery should you need it.

"Lung" means "light" in many languages, and the word for "breath" and "spirit" is also often the same. The health of your lungs is especially important after surgery of any type, because it places special stress upon them. In this chapter, we discuss how to help keep them healthy, along with the treatment of surgical lung disorders, using conventional and alternative medicine approaches.

Cigarette smoking causes or aggravates most lung diseases. It is responsible for 80 to 90 percent of all lung cancers. Smoking's chronic irritation also leads to excessive secretions, and difficulty removing them, which can cause infections such as pneumonia, bronchitis, and bronchiectasis. Scarring from these processes causes the stiffness and destruction of normal lung tissue, which is called emphysema.

If you have smoked for twenty to thirty years, you will have destroyed one whole lung's worth of tissue. All surgery, especially of the lung, will be more dangerous for you. If you smoke, quitting is the most important step you can take to help you avoid or recover from lung surgery or any other operation. To help you stop, refer to the special section in Chapter 2 on quitting smoking through alternative medicine techniques.

The lungs, because of their moist environment, are prone to a variety of infections. Very effective antibacterial and antituberculosis drugs have made the need for surgery in infectious lung diseases quite rare. The most common operation currently performed on the lungs is done to remove lung cancer. Early detection of this cancer and its surgical removal give you the best hope for cure, though dietary measures and vitamins now offer some preventive and therapeutic promise.

How Your Lungs Work

Your chest cage can be thought of as a cylinder, surrounded on its outer edges by the ribs, cartilage, and breastbone (sternum). (See Figure 7.1.) The intercostal muscles connect your adjacent ribs to one another. The diaphragm, which is actually a muscle, makes up the lower boundary, separating the contents of the chest from those of the abdomen.

The diaphragm and intercostal muscles are the most important respiratory muscles. As your intercostal muscles contract, they flare your ribs up and out, increasing your chest's diameter, while the diaphragm pulls downward. These two movements act like a bellows, decreasing the pressure inside your chest cage so it becomes less than that of the atmosphere around you. Because air moves from areas of high pressure toward lower pressure, the air then flows through your mouth and nose into your trachea (windpipe) and lungs.

Your chest wall muscles and diaphragm relax at the end of each intake of air. Because the lungs are elastic, they then deflate, and air moves out of them in the process called exhaling. If you have emphysema, your lung's elasticity is mostly lost, so your muscles must use valuable energy to work to empty your lungs. The *pleura*, the smooth thin layer lining the inside of your chest cavity, secretes a small amount of lubricating fluid which allows the lungs to move freely within your chest.

Your lungs resemble an inverted tree, whose main trunk is the trachea and whose branches are the *bronchi*, often referred to as "bronchial tubes." The leaves are the millions of *alveoli sacs* where oxygen and carbon dioxide are exchanged. Lining your airways are cells that produce mucus to protect the tissue against the drying effects of air. Other specialized cells have attached *cilia*—tiny hairs that move back and forth to "beat" secretions and small inhaled particles toward your mouth, where they can then be coughed out or swallowed. This function, which is an important part of the lungs' self-cleaning process, is par-

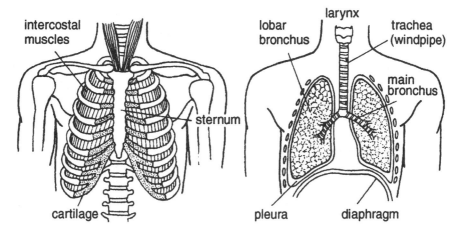

Fig. 7.1 The chest cage and lungs

alyzed by cigarette smoke, predisposing you to lung infection, especially in the postoperative period.

Each lung is divided into *lobes,* with three on the right and two on the left; each lobe has subdivisions called *segments.* Since they have no sensory nerves, your lungs cannot transmit pain. Early lung cancer is therefore especially difficult to detect, unless the sensitive pleura lining your chest cavity is irritated by the disease, in which case discomfort can be intense and localized.

The air around us contains 21 percent oxygen. Within the lungs, this oxygen diffuses through the walls of the alveolar sacs into the bloodstream, which circulates it to the body's cells. This is a critically important process; oxygen is necessary for maintenance of cell life and function. Meanwhile, the body's cells release carbon dioxide, a waste product of cell function. It is taken up by the blood in your veins, transported to the lungs, released across the alveolar wall into your airways, and finally exhaled. When all parts of this complex process are working normally, a wonderful balance exists.

Coughing, caused by irritation of the tissue

lining your airways, is an important mechanism for clearing out secretions and inhaled particles (called sputum). A cough may be "productive," with large amounts of sputum, as in patients with chronic bronchitis, or it may be dry and "nonproductive," as in smokers' cough. Coughing up blood is a sign of lung or airway disease. It can occur with irritative and infectious diseases, but is most worrisome because it may also be a signal of lung cancer.

How Lung Disease Is Diagnosed

Lung disease is diagnosed by history, physical exam, X-rays, and, if necessary, more complicated tests, as described below.

History

If you are having lung problems, a review of your smoking history, work environment, TB exposure, and the places you have lived and traveled should be explored with your physician. The amount an individual has smoked is expressed in *pack/years,* which is found by multiplying the number of packs smoked per day by the number of years smoked. If you have smoked two packs per day for forty years, you have an eighty pack/ year history. The risk for tobacco-induced diseases increases sharply with increasing pack/years.

Some areas of the world are associated with benign lung changes that can be seen on a chest X-ray; an example is the Southwestern United States, where nodules in the lung may be caused by "desert fever" (the medical name for which is coccidiomycosis). Generally, this condition does not require treatment.

Your home and workplace environment may have contributed to your lung problems. Inhalation of secondary smoke from others' cigarettes, coal dust, sawdust, and asbestos particles are but a few of the many hazards. Any smoke-filled or polluted environment can cause or accelerate lung disease.

Your doctor should ask questions about shortness of breath and your activity level; coughing patterns including type, color, and amount of sputum produced; and chest pain. You should provide information about past lung problems such as viral or bacterial pneumonia, TB, bronchitis, emphysema, and asthma.

Physical Exam

The sounds of breathing heard through your doctor's stethoscope can help in diagnosing your disease. Various disorders have characteristic sounds. "Thumping" on your chest produces typical sounds if the lung is emphysematous, collapsed, or solidified, or your chest cavity contains fluid.

Sputum Tests

Specimens of your sputum can be analyzed for microorganisms and malignant cells. An accurate result requires a deep cough, which may be stimulated by first passing a suction tube through your nose into your trachea (windpipe). This is somewhat uncomfortable. In some kinds of lung cancer, accurate diagnosis by sputum analysis is as high as 80 percent.

Chest X-Ray

The chest X-ray is the most revealing simple test in the diagnosis of lung disease. It helps to confirm your doctor's impressions after a physical exam, and also reveals subtle changes impossible to find by examination. Chest X-rays are particularly important if you are at high risk for cancer; that is, if you are more than 45 years old with a greater than twenty pack/year smoking history and/or a history of industrial exposures. If you are in this category, a reasonable screening program includes a yearly chest X-ray. Comparing present X-rays with those from previous years can pick up early changes not obvious on a single film.

CAT Scan

The CAT (CT) scan reveals the most detail about the lungs and chest cavity; nodules and tumors as small as 3 millimeters can be seen. A biopsy is necessary to arrive at an exact diagnosis when cancer is suspected.

Lung Function Tests

Because of the stress that general anesthesia and major surgery place on the lungs, if you are a smoker or have a history of lung problems, you may be required to undergo lung function tests before your operation. A simple way to test for lung function problems is to climb three flights of stairs. If you can do this without stopping because of shortness of breath, your breathing capacity is probably satisfactory for you to tolerate the general anesthesia required for many types of surgery. In addition, if you can blow out a match at a distance of six inches from your mouth without pursing your lips, you probably do not have an obstructive lung disease that would significantly interfere with your surgical outcome.

Lung function tests *(spirometry)* may be necessary if you fail these screening tests or have obviously significant impairment of your lungs. You breathe into a machine that measures the volume of air moved, and the rate at which you are able to move it. This quantifies the extent and effects of your lung disease. The test results help determine your risk for major surgery, particularly if lung tissue must be removed.

Blood Gases

If you are critically ill, the blood gases test is one of the most important of all medical measurements. Blood drawn from an artery is analyzed for its concentration of oxygen, carbon dioxide, bicarbonate, and its relative acidity/alkalinity. Results show how well your lungs, kidneys, and other vital systems are functioning. It may also be recommended if you are facing lung surgery, to determine your "baseline" respiratory status. The sample is usually drawn from an artery at your wrist; this puncture may be more uncomfortable than when blood is taken from a vein, but complications are rare.

Flexible Fiberoptic Bronchoscopy

Flexible fiberoptic bronchoscopy is useful for determining the cause and site of any bleeding in the lungs, evaluating suspicious X-ray findings, and finding the location of lung cancer if you have had a positive sputum test but no tumor has been seen on your X-rays. This test is performed under light sedation, with you lying on your back or side. Topical anesthesia is applied to your mouth and airway to stop your gag and cough reflexes. A flexible lighted tube containing a camera and tiny instrument channel is passed through your mouth and windpipe, and then down the airways (bronchial tubes) of both your lungs. The views of the inside of your lungs as seen by the camera can be projected onto a television monitor. Specimens of secretions can be collected and analyzed for organisms and malignant cells, and biopsies may be obtained from areas that look suspicious. Bronchoscopy is usually somewhat uncomfortable, and takes fifteen to forty-five minutes to complete. Rare complications include significant bleeding (1 percent) and death (0.01 percent).[1]

During this test, a *transbronchial biopsy* of lung tissue may be performed by placing the scope in the airway nearest lung tissue that appears to be diseased. A small needle is painlessly pushed through the bronchus wall and into the suspicious area, where cells are then collected for analysis. The most common complication, collapsed lung (0.5 percent), requires placement of a temporary chest tube.[2] See the description of the various types of chest tubes on page 238.

Transthoracic Biopsy

This is an outpatient procedure that may be recommended if a suspicious area is found in your lung close to the chest wall. Your doctor injects a local anesthetic and then, while watching on a CAT scan or fluoroscopic TV monitor, guides a needle through your skin and on into the questionable tissue, where a specimen is taken. This technique is particularly useful in diagnosing your cancer cell type if you are a poor risk for surgery, if you have an inoperable tumor, or if you are thought to have a type of cancer best treated by radiotherapy or chemotherapy. It allows you to avoid open surgical biopsy. Complications of this procedure include collapsed lung, seen in 10 to 15 percent of biopsy patients, when air leaks from the lung into the chest cavity at the site of the needle puncture, collapsing the lung. If this happens, you have a 10 to 20 percent chance of needing a chest tube, to suck out the air and reexpand the lung, until the leak seals in a day or two.[3]

Mediastinoscopy

Mediastinoscopy is performed in patients with proven or probable cancer to determine their chances of being cured by surgery. This test can be done on an outpatient basis. After you are given local anesthesia plus a sedative, or general anesthesia, a rigid scope is introduced through a small incision at the base of the front of your neck and is pushed into your upper mediastinum (the space between the lungs), where a search is made for cancer spread to that area. Positive findings would make it unlikely you would be cured by surgery, so you can avoid a useless operation. Mediastinoscopy takes from fifteen to forty-five minutes. Rare complications (2.3 percent) include excessive bleeding and collapsed lung, which may require an operation or placement of a chest tube to control.[4]

Thoracoscopy

The ultimate method of diagnosis, thoracoscopy, can be done in an outpatient setting. After you are given general anesthesia, a small scope is introduced through a three-quarter-inch incision between your ribs, and the chest cavity is examined directly. Usually two secondary smaller incisions are made to pass instruments. Tissue can be removed for immediate microscopic examination. A biopsy of lung tissue obtained through thoracoscopy may be necessary to diagnose a suspicious nodule or if you are thought to have rare or difficult-to-culture infectious organisms that cannot be diagnosed in any other way. Complications include significant bleeding (1.9 percent) and collapsed lung (3.4 percent), which may require a chest tube or operation to treat.[5] Postoperative pain can be treated with pain pills, if necessary.

Exploratory Thoracotomy

This "open" surgical procedure gathers the same information as thoracoscopy, but is done through a much larger incision and requires a few days in the hospital. It is necessary when a definite diagnosis, or the possibility of a surgical chance for cure of a known cancer, cannot be determined in any other way. If the findings indicate that further surgery is advisable, it can be carried out at the same time, through the same incision.

Collapsed Lung

A collapsed lung (*pneumothorax*) develops when air leaks from your lung into your chest cavity, causing your lung to collapse. Spontaneous rupture of a small "bleb" (bubble) at the top of your lung is the most common cause of this problem. Blebs can be present at birth, or arise in association with a lung disease that blocks your airways, such as emphysema caused by smoking.

Pneumothorax occurs four times more often in men, usually those in the 20 to 40 age range. Smoking, coughing spells, and a slender, tall build are predisposing factors. The most common symptom is pain, followed by shortness of breath. Rarely, severe shortness of breath is a signal of a "tension pneumothorax," in which air that has leaked out of the lung and into the chest cavity is trapped, producing increasing pressure, which pushes the heart toward the opposite side, interfering with its function. This is a life-threatening situation requiring emergency treatment.

Alternative Medicine Approaches to Collapsed Lung

Megan, a 25-year-old nurse, was feeling a great deal of pressure and strain because of her father's prolonged terminal illness. She had been working odd hours, and also traveling long distances to see him. Sudden, sharp chest pain and shortness of breath in the middle of the night caused her to rush to the emergency room. A small pneumothorax was discovered, and she was treated on an outpatient basis. An alternative medicine doctor suggested she begin daily practice of yoga to reduce her stress, as well as attend group support sessions to release her emotions about her father's impending death. She suffered no further problems.

Surgical treatment is necessary for a collapsed lung. However, alternative medicine offers the following strategies for prevention.

Practice Stress Management and Yoga Breathing Exercises

Since some episodes of spontaneous pneumothorax appear to be induced by stress, stress reduction may be a means of preventing its occurrence; techniques of stress manage-ment are discussed in Chapter 2. If you live far from medical care, I recommend preventive surgery, as described below, after a first episode. Needless to say, if you smoke, you should quit. Follow the guidelines on how to quit smoking given in Chapter 2.

The yoga breathing exercises are especially suited for strengthening the lungs in a gentle manner. Follow the guidelines given in Chapter 2, practicing three or four times a day for ten to fifteen minutes.

Practice Visualization

Visualization may assist in your treatment. Follow the guidelines given for deep relaxation and visualization given in Chapter 2. For example, imagine your lungs as a large bunch of balloons crowded inside a small room. They are being pushed to one side by air leaking from one of them. See the leaking balloon being mended with a strong patch, then all the excess air leaving the room by a special one-way revolving door. Now image the balloons dancing gently in the room, and at the same time feel your lungs easily filling and releasing their air.

Surgical Approach to Collapsed Lung

John, a college student, while cramming for a final examination, suddenly felt pain in the right side of his chest, and became short of breath. He thought he was having a heart attack, and called 911. The medics did an EKG (electrocardiogram), which was normal, but they could not hear good breath sounds from his right chest. John was taken to the nearest emergency room, where a chest X-ray showed a completely collapsed right lung. A tube was inserted into his chest cavity and the air sucked out, quickly reexpanding his lung and relieving his symptoms. His roommate brought his books, and he was able to continue his studies while connected to a chest tube and suction device. The treatment was successful, and John was able to be discharged in three days, in time to take his exam.

Surgical therapies for spontaneous pneumothorax depend on the amount of air leakage and lung collapse, the severity of your symptoms, and whether you have had a previous episode. A small, stable leak with minimal discomfort can be simply observed, because the leaked air will usually be gradually and naturally reabsorbed. If mild discomfort is present without shortness of breath, the air may be sucked out by inserting a small catheter (tube), which is then immediately removed. If your symptoms are moderate, a small tube with a flap valve (Heimlich valve) may be placed while you remain an outpatient. This tube prevents buildup of air in the chest. Coughing and deep breathing forces air out of the tube, while the valve prevents air from coming back inward when you inhale. The tube may be removed in a day or two, after the leak has sealed.

Eighty-five percent of patients with collapsed lung require a larger chest tube because of significant discomfort, shortness of breath, or the presence of a large pneumothorax. Hospitalization is then necessary. After local anesthesia, your doctor makes a three-quarter-inch skin incision, then inserts a three-eighth-inch tube between your ribs and on into your chest cavity. It is attached to an underwater seal, flap valve, or suction apparatus that prevents air from going back into the chest through the tube. A chest tube is quite uncomfortable, and pain medication will probably be necessary. After the air leak has been sealed for twenty-four hours, which usually occurs within a few days, the tube is removed.

You will probably be advised to have a curative treatment if you have an air leak that is prolonged; if you have a pneumothorax on both sides; if large lung bubbles, or "blebs," are seen on your X-rays; or if you live some distance from medical attention or do a lot of traveling. If you wish to avoid surgery, irritative agents can be introduced through the chest tube in an attempt to make your lung adhere to the inside lining of your chest cavity, but the success rate of this is less than that for surgical techniques (78 to 91 percent by chest tube compared to 95 to 100 percent for surgical interventions).[6]

If your pneumothorax is treated successfully without surgery, there is a 15 to 20 percent chance it will recur. If it does, you should be treated to prevent another episode. If you are not treated, you are likely to have even more episodes, which could be very dangerous.

The operation to treat or prevent recurrent pneumothorax is performed under general anesthesia. In the past, surgeons have used an "open" six- to eight-inch incision placed between the ribs on the front or side of your chest. Currently, this operation is usually done with a thoracoscope, a small lighted tube with a TV camera that is inserted through a three-quarter-inch incision between your ribs. Various small instruments can be introduced through the scope. The goal of the surgery is to produce adhesions (thickened scar tissue) which "glue" together the lung and lining of the chest cavity. This will prevent lung collapse, should another air leak develop. Abrading your lung surface with coarse gauze and introducing irritants such as talc accomplish this end. If blebs are found, they can be removed. If a leak is still present, it can be sewn closed.

A chest tube is required for a few days after surgery, and you usually can be discharged within a week. Complication and mortality rates for this surgery are low. If the thoracoscope can be used, you can go home in two or three days and your postoperative recovery is much more rapid. Ask if your surgeon has had experience with this newer technique.

Lung Cancer

Television personality Morton Downey Jr. thought he was above it all. Even though statistics relate that if you smoke, your chances of developing lung cancer are one in ten, he loudly and publicly ridiculed those who suggested that he and others quit. However, after he developed pneumonia, and an X-ray revealed he had an early lung cancer, he changed his life completely. He quit smoking immediately, and even began to make commercials to encourage others to stop.

The American Cancer Society estimates that there will be 169,400 new lung cancers diagnosed in 2002 and 154,900 people will die as a result.[7] Excluding the usually curable skin cancer, it is second to colon cancer as the most common form of cancer, and is the most common cause of cancer death in the United States for both men and women, accounting for 28 percent of all cancer deaths.

Lung cancer is one of the most difficult of all cancers to treat. Because of the extent of their disease, 50 percent of all patients have no chance for surgical cure at the time they are diagnosed. At present, less than 13 percent of all lung cancer patients are able to be cured.[8] However, alternative medicine offers new hope, and in early reports, survival is ex-

tended in those who use these adjuncts in addition to conventional therapy.[9]

Cigarette smoking has long been known to be the number one cause of lung cancer; it is now held accountable for 80 to 90 percent of all cases. Nine out of ten men and seven out of ten women who die from lung cancer were smokers. Cigarette smoke contains many carcinogenic chemicals that cause chronic irritation of airway lining cells. Cells become damaged, reproduce abnormally, then progress to outright cancer. If you are an average smoker, your risk is increased nine to ten times, and if a heavy smoker, ten to twenty-five times.[10]

Lung cancer rates have been increasing steadily for the past thirty years. The rate of increase is highest in women, who are rapidly approaching men in what once was overwhelmingly a man's disease. Recently, the incidence has decreased in men, but continues to climb in women. Women's increased smoking rate is responsible, and since 1987 lung cancer surpassed breast cancer as the most common cause of cancer deaths in women. Women's lungs are more susceptible to lung damage and carry a much higher risk than for men with the same pack/year smoking history. Nonsmokers exposed to secondhand smoke at work or in the home are at increased risk. Lung cancer rates are higher in African-American men, men living in cities, and people with a history of TB.

Some industrial, occupational, and environmental air pollutants also cause lung cancer. Iron, chromium, and nickel workers have a higher incidence as do those exposed to coal tars, chloromethyl ether, arsenic, and uranium. Radiation, radon, and asbestos exposure increases the risk.

Lung cancer is "silent" in its early stages, though it may be curable if discovered then.

However, by the time symptoms appear and suspicion is aroused, the average cancer has been present for more than two years, making the chance for cure so difficult.

Your first symptom of lung cancer may be an irritating cough or a streak of blood in the sputum. The tumor may block a small bronchial tube, causing pneumonia in the lung tissue beyond the blockage. Chest pain and shortness of breath indicate a more advanced tumor that has invaded neighboring sensitive tissues or has affected a large amount of the lung. Occasionally, the first symptom is caused by the cancer's spread to the brain, bone, or liver.

Early Detection of Lung Cancer

If the diagnosis could be made within the first few months after a lung tumor has formed, a much happier outcome could be obtained. Unfortunately, studies screening people without symptoms with periodic chest X-rays and analyses of sputum for tumor cells have not shown any benefit in reducing mortality. Since these tests are unreliable and expensive, the American Cancer Society and the National Cancer Institute do not recommend them unless symptoms develop. CAT scan screening is being investigated but is not yet recommended because of cost. A recent study in *Lancet* used low-dose CT scan to screen 1,000 apparently healthy current and former smokers over age 60. Seventy-four percent of the twenty-seven cancers found by this method were not seen on routine X-rays.[11] Hope exists, and research goes on, to discover a blood test marker for lung cancer that would be applicable to the general population for this common cancer. If you are or have been a smoker, ask your doctor about screening options.

Establishing a Diagnosis of Lung Cancer

When lung cancer is suspected, you need a full workup to establish your diagnosis. If cancer is found, further testing is required to determine its cell type and whether or not it has spread. Most of this information can be found without your needing major surgery. The workup will enable your physician to determine whether you still have a chance to be cured through surgery or, if not, what your best available treatment options would be.

The first steps in your diagnostic workup are chest X-rays and sputum analysis. X-rays may provide a probable diagnosis, but a tissue sample is usually required to confirm it. Eighty percent of the time, bronchoscopy can visualize your tumor and provide a diagnosis through a biopsy. If these tests do not provide adequate tissue for analysis, and if your tumor is accessible, you can have transthoracic needle biopsy.

Mediastinoscopy determines if you can be helped by surgery. If this test finds that the tumor has invaded or spread to glands outside the bounds of a surgical cure, an operation can be avoided (this is the situation in 50 percent of cases).

Occasionally, it is impossible to arrive at a definite diagnosis or know the extent of your disease through these methods. "Exploratory" surgery must then be performed. Often, this can be done using the thoracoscope.

Cell Type and Staging of Lung Cancer

There are four major cell types of lung cancer. *Squamous cell* or *epidermoid* lung cancer starts in bronchial lining cells and is the type most closely associated with smoking. *Adenocarcinoma* arises from glandular cells of the bronchi and has a somewhat worse prognosis. They are about equally common, totaling roughly 70 percent of these cancers. *Undifferentiated small cell* or *oat cell* (20 percent) and *undifferentiated large cell* (10 percent) are the other major types. Since small-cell cancer has usually spread by the time of diagnosis, surgery is rarely useful.

Lung cancer of all types is "staged" according to the size of the primary tumor, its location, the degree of invasion of adjacent tissues, the presence or absence of spread to lymph nodes and their location, and the presence or absence of metastasis (spread to distant tissues).

Staging information helps in determining which forms of treatment are recommended, along with your prognosis. Some areas of controversy exist and technology and knowledge are rapidly advancing; if you are found to have lung cancer, you need to consult with specialists in surgery, radiotherapy, and chemotherapy. Ask to have your case and treatment options discussed at your hospital's "tumor board conference."

Table 7.1 gives you a *general* idea about your chances for cure and probable life expectancy. These figures are derived from the experience of thousands of patients who have undergone various forms of treatment. Cir-

cumstances specific to your case may make these figures different for you.

Alternative Medicine Approaches to Lung Cancer

Ninety percent of the people who smoke cigarettes do *not* develop cancer: what is *different* about the 10 percent who do? By contributing to a less-competent immune system, diet and stress may play important roles in the development and progression of this difficult cancer, and dietary changes and stress management hold promise for its prevention and treatment. The stress of his talk show being canceled may have contributed to the development of Morton Downey's lung cancer. Following are several alternative medicine approaches to preventing or treating lung cancer.

Quit Smoking

Of course, this is the first best thing you can do, and the alternative approaches to quitting smoking given in Chapter 2 may help you accomplish it. One of the most striking illustrations about smoking, passed on to me by a spa owner, is that after the spa's "Smoke-

TABLE 7.1.
Prognosis of Lung Cancer[12]

	Percent of Patients Surviving 5 Years	Percent of Patients in This Stage
All Patients	14.5%	
Not Staged	8.5%	14%
By Stage		
Localized to lung	48.0%	15%
Lymph node spread	21.4%	24%
Distant spread	2.5%	48%

Enders Weekend," the Jacuzzi has to be drained and cleaned, because of the yellow residue sweated out by the participants! Nicotine yellows your fingers, and even your sweat. When I finally quit smoking, one of the unhealthy habits I had picked up in medical school, I circled the date in red on the calendar, and used toothpicks and chewing gum to help. In addition, I began practicing the yoga techniques discussed in Chapter 2. These help the body and mind relax, and enabled me to quit for good.

Eat Foods Rich in Vitamin A and Take Vitamin A Supplements

The possibility that antioxidants in the diet could have an influence upon who develops lung cancer was first appreciated after a report in 1981 from the Rush-Presbyterian-St. Luke's Medical Center in Chicago. Researchers there found that in almost 2,000 Western Electric employees, 25 of the 33 lung cancer victims had diets relatively low in carotenoids, the form of vitamin A found in dark green and yellow vegetables.[13] A number of other studies have also supported this connection.

Certainly, then, eating foods high in vitamin A may provide protection. Other antioxidants including vitamins C and E may also help protect the lungs against the harmful effects of tobacco smoke. Whether or not simply taking supplements can have the same effect is less clear. Research carried out at the National Cancer Institute found that high doses of vitamin A increased the activity of white blood cells.[14] White cells are felt by many researchers to remove cancerous cells. Vitamin A deficiency may cause immunosuppression. Vitamin A supplementation may be immunoenhancing, even in those who are not deficient. Vitamin A seems to be especially promising in the treatment of all types of tumors of the cells that cover the body's surface and line its cavities, of which lung cancer is one.[15] Research in the use of vitamin A, its derivatives, and beta-carotene, has led many authorities to recommend that lung cancer patients take vitamin A in conjunction with whatever treatment program is followed. Although beta-carotene supplements were recently indicated not to help in prevention, when mixed with other carotenoids, they may give protection. With your doctor's approval and monitoring, you may begin with 10,000 IU of vitamin A and 25,000 IU of mixed carotenoids daily, along with a diet rich in vitamin A foods. Follow the diet and vitamin guidelines given in Chapter 2.

Eat Foods Rich in Vitamin E

A report on 29,000 male smokers in Finland found that those with high blood levels of alpha-tocopheral, the most active form of vitamin E, reduced their risk of lung cancer by 19 to 23 percent.[16] The proven effects came from foods rich in vitamin E such as soybeans, nuts, sunflower seeds, wheat germ, and whole grains, rather than from vitamin supplements.

Avoid Saturated Fat

Nonsmoking women who eat a diet high in saturated fats (tropical oils, meat, dairy products, and hydrogenated vegetable oils) have up to five times increased risk of developing lung cancer as those nonsmoking women who eat a leaner diet. A low-fat diet may also be protective for everyone else.[17]

Practice Stress Management

Stress may play a role in the onset and progression of any cancer.[18] Follow the stress reduction techniques in Chapter 2.

Practice Visualization

Try exercises such as this one: Imagine your lungs as a bunch of grapes in which some grapes have become waxy and hard. Pick out these grapes, place them in your garbage disposal, and grind them up. Now, while seeing all the remaining grapes as healthy, at the same time, feel your lungs as completely well and free of any disease. Send your white cells like white knights throughout your body to check and make certain no waxy grape seeds are left anywhere else, and then leave these white cells stationed throughout your system to prevent any future return.

Conventional Medicine Approaches to Lung Cancer

Lung cancer generally responds poorly to radiotherapy (X-ray treatments) and chemotherapy. These treatments can be considered in terms of "curative" primary treatment; "adjuvant" treatment administered in combination with surgery in hope of increasing the cure rate; or "palliative" treatment of incurable disease that is aimed at slowing tumor growth and/or relieving distressing symptoms.

Surgery is the treatment of choice, whenever possible, in localized cancers and some that have already spread to lymph glands. Sometimes surgery is not an option because of the tumor's location, distant spread, or if you are not a surgical candidate because of severe underlying lung disease. If the tumor appears to be confined to the chest, radiotherapy is occasionally curative, with a five-year survival rate of 15 percent.[19]

After surgery, radiation treatment may increase your chance of cure if your cancer is found to have spread beyond the tissue removed. It may also be beneficial as "adjuvant" therapy; that is, given after surgery when all of the cancer seems to have been removed but the probability of a local recurrence is high. Since *small-cell* tumors tend to spread to the brain, preventive brain radiotherapy is usually recommended with this type of lung cancer. At this point, no proven benefit exists for adjuvant chemotherapy; however, ongoing studies may find valuable drug combinations in the future.

Both radiotherapy and chemotherapy are useful in "palliating," that is, relieving lung cancer symptoms. Radiotherapy, delivered to the site of the tumor, has an 80 percent chance of temporarily shrinking your tumor, opening up blocked air passages, relieving pain, and/or being otherwise beneficial. It may prolong your survival by several months. Cancer that has spread to the bones, causing pain and/or threatening to cause fractures, can also be controlled with radiation treatments. Chemotherapy produces some beneficial response in 70 to 90 percent of small-cell cancers and in 30 to 40 percent of the other cell types.

Both radiotherapy and chemotherapy have significant side effects that must be balanced against the hoped-for response.

Surgical Approaches to Lung Cancer

Frank, a 65-year-old stockbroker with a 90 pack/year history of smoking, had a screening chest X-ray that showed a small (three-eighth-inch) nodule in the lower lobe of his left lung.

The spot was not present on his chest X-ray two years before. Exploratory surgery proved that it was a cancer, without any evidence of having spread. The lobe containing the tumor was removed. Frank recovered easily and wisely used his hospitalization as a time to stop smoking.

As physicians, we find it very frustrating not to be able to help a patient. So often, we see smokers whose disease is found too late to be cured by surgery. Also, smokers in general have a much harder time recovering from routine operations on other parts of their bodies. If you smoke, and you could see what we see—lungs stiffened, fibrotic, and blackened with the soot of smoke—perhaps it would help spur you to quit.

A "coin" lesion is a small lung nodule that can be seen on a chest X-ray. It should be treated as a malignancy until proven otherwise. If you are in a low-risk group and the nodule appears benign on the X-ray, a period of observation is indicated. If repeat follow-up X-rays show no change over a two-year period, the nodule is very unlikely to be a cancer. If your chest X-ray shows a new coin lesion with indeterminate characteristics, or if you are a smoker, you should have a full diagnostic workup.

If your coin lesion is a cancer, you have the most favorable prognosis for operability and ultimate cure. If you undergo curative surgery, you have a 50 percent chance of being alive at five years, three times better than the usual lung cancer prognosis. Coin lesions can usually be treated by a lobectomy.

Unfortunately, most lung cancers are not coin lesions. They are larger, have invaded neighboring tissues, and/or have spread to distant areas through the lymph system or bloodstream. Modern diagnostic staging techniques have limited the number of patients undergoing useless lung cancer surgery for incurable tumors. Nowadays, only about 50 percent of all patients with lung cancer have an operation. Sixty-five percent of these patients are able to have an operation with attempt to cure, where all of the known tumor is removed. Fifteen percent have small amounts of tumor that is not, or cannot be, completely removed; this type of operation is termed palliative rather than curative. After surgery begins, 20 percent are found to have inoperable tumors that cannot be safely removed, so the procedure is terminated.

If surgery to attempt a cure is possible, *with all known tumor removed,* you have an excellent chance of being cured. If the tumor has not spread to lymph nodes in the removed tissue specimen, your cure rate is about 70 percent; if nodes were involved, about 50 percent.[20] Most recurrences of lung cancer become evident within one to three years after a curative operation. If you have no evidence of recurrent disease for five years after surgery, you are probably cured.

If you decide to have surgery, preoperative testing includes lung function tests, analysis of blood gases, and exercise tolerance tests. These predict how well you will withstand the proposed operation, and how much tissue can be removed without posing a threat to your life, or leaving you with so little functioning lung tissue that your activities would be severely restricted.

For the surgery, you are brought to the operating room and given general anesthesia. After the breathing tube is inserted, you are rolled on your side. Major lung surgery is usually performed through a ten- to twelve-inch incision between the ribs, running from beneath the shoulder blade to your side. A rib-spreading instrument provides a wide opening. A rib may have to be removed to give better access, but this does not cause any postoperative problems. Lung cancer surgery includes removing part or all of one lung, along with the adjacent lymph glands. *Pneumonectomy* removes the whole lung, and may be necessary if the tumor is in the central part of the lung or close to the main bronchus. (See Figure 7.2.) *Lobectomy* removes one of the two (left) or three (right) lobes of one lung and is now the most common operation for lung cancer. Recently, thoracoscopic techniques have been used to perform lobectomies for favorable cancers.

If your other lung is fairly normal, you should be able to exercise moderately even after one of your lungs is completely removed. However, if like most lung cancer patients, you have been a heavy smoker, your remaining lung tissue may not be able to handle the load after removal of one whole lung or lobe.

A *segmental resection* removes one section of a lung lobe, and may be used if you have limited lung function. A *wedge resection* simply takes out the tumor, along with a small margin of adjacent tissue. This latter procedure may be performed if you have very poor lung function that would make even segmental resection dangerous. Thoracoscopic techniques are now being used for segmental and wedge resection of small peripheral lung tumors, and in cases where only a small amount of lung tissue can be removed safely.

The local cancer recurrence rate does increase significantly when smaller amounts of tissue are removed. However, for smaller tumors, the survival rates may be similar to those for a larger operation. In general, lobectomy is the procedure of choice if your lobe's bronchus is tumor-free where it joins the rest of the airway tree and you can tolerate that amount of tissue being removed, as deter-

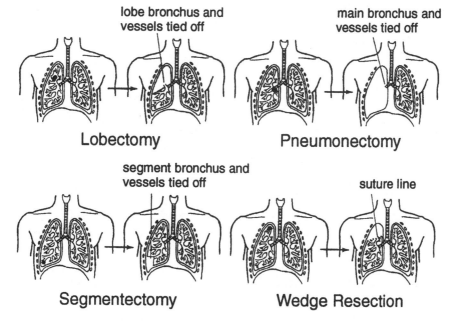

Fig. 7.2 Types of lung cancer surgery

mined by preoperative lung function tests. Lobectomy has a significantly improved cure rate for tumors larger than 3 centimeters when compared with operations that remove less tissue.[21] In any operation for lung cancer, adjacent tissue, such as the chest wall lining, the sac covering the heart, and the diaphragm, must be removed if the tumor has invaded it. In addition, a biopsy of the lymph glands near the main bronchus and trachea is usually performed.

Postoperatively, you awaken in the recovery room, and a short time later are moved to the ICU (intensive care unit). The breathing tube, left in place until you need no further breathing assistance, can usually be removed after the effects of anesthesia have worn off. If you are debilitated or have poor function in your remaining lung tissue, the tube may be necessary for several days, or even longer. Lines and tubes monitor your EKG, lung and cardiac function, blood pressure, and urinary output. Once you are off the ventilator (the machine that regulates your breathing) and are in stable condition, you can be moved out of the ICU.

Unless you have had a pneumonectomy, where chest tubes are not used, one or more tubes will have been inserted through your chest wall, between the ribs, and into the chest cavity. These tubes are connected to suction bottles to ensure against lung collapse from an air leak or fluid accumulation. Leakage is monitored by watching for small bubbles bubbling up through a "water seal" in the bottle.

Although the chest pain after your surgery will decrease your desire to do so, you *must* cough and breathe deeply. These actions mobilize your airway secretions, which otherwise tend to become thick tenacious "plugs" that block airways, leading to lung tissue collapse and infection. In addition to deep breathing, several other techniques may be used to help remove the secretions: suctioning the upper airway using a catheter passed through your nose or endotracheal tube; repositioning you in bed periodically; and "percussion," which is the tapping of the chest wall by a specially trained nurse or respiratory therapist. If these are not effective, your doctor may need to use a small flexible bronchoscope to suck out the plugs. You may be given an "incentive spirometer," a plastic tube containing a Ping-Pong ball that you try to push up the tube by forceful blowing or inhaling. It encourages deep breathing and also generates airway pressure to keep your lung tissue expanded. Frequent chest X-rays are needed to assess your lung's response to surgery and postoperative events.

Postoperative pain can be significant. It can be managed by an epidural block, IV patient-controlled pain medication (PCA), or intramuscular or oral pain medication (see page 126).

Most likely, you can begin eating and be out of bed on the first postoperative day. You can walk around either connected to the chest tube suction device or with the tubes detached from it and clamped for short periods. Smoking should be *strictly* forbidden, because it irritates your lung tissue, causing increased secretions and decreased ability to move them out of your airways. Chest tubes are simply removed at your bedside, in one to several days, after air leakage and fluid drainage have stopped. Walking and moving around become much less awkward. You should be able to be discharged five to ten days after surgery.

You should see your doctor in office visits until your incision is well healed and your lung function optimized. If you did not already stop smoking before surgery, use the hospital stay as a starting point.

Pneumonectomy has a mortality rate of 5 to 8 percent, while lobectomy carries a 2 to 5 percent risk. These numbers depend on the extent of your disease, the amount of function of your other lung, your general condition, and the expertise of your surgeon and available postoperative care. Most deaths that occur during and after surgery are due to lung or heart disease. The most frequent complication is a postoperative air leak, which may develop through defects in closure of small airways or lung tissue. Small leaks are quite common; most of them stop in a few days, but 5 percent of patients develop a persistent leak. An accumulation of fluid can develop after your chest tube is removed. If small, not enlarging or producing symptoms, it can be simply observed. Most disappear in days or weeks. Larger accumulations of air or fluid require replacement of the chest tube. Troublesome but temporary cardiac arrhythmias (irregular heartbeats) develop in 10 to 20 percent of cases.

Cancer Spread to Lungs from Other Sources

The lungs are one of the most frequent areas to which other types of cancers spread, since they contain a network of tiny blood vessels that can trap tumor cells circulating in the blood. Many patients who have undergone curative treatment for their primary tumors elsewhere in the body are subsequently found to have a suspicious lung mass. This may be either diagnosed at the time of the original treatment or at a later date.

The question then arises whether removing this lung deposit would be beneficial, especially if you have no other evidence of a tumor. If a careful diagnostic workup shows no other sign of cancer, evidence suggests an aggressive surgical approach is warranted. Cures in the range of 30 to 40 percent can be obtained in these cases. The most favorable results are in patients whose lungs have tumor cell deposits from colon, breast, kidney, testicle, or the sarcoma type of cancers.

LUNG CANCER SUMMARY

Prevention

Diet and Supplements

- Follow a low-fat, high-fiber diet, rich in vitamins A and E.
- Avoid saturated fat.
- Vitamin A, 10,000 IU daily.
- Vitamin C, 1,000–2,000 mg, 2–3 times daily.
- Vitamin E, D-alpha, 400 IU daily.
- Mixed carotenoids, 25,000 IU daily.

Lifestyle

- Don't smoke.
- Practice daily yoga.
- Practice stress management.

Alternative Medicine Approaches

- Follow the preventive guidelines, above.
- Acupuncture, hypnosis.
- Visualization.

Conventional Medicine Approaches

- Chemotherapy.
- Radiotherapy.

Surgical Approaches

- Open surgery, thoracoscopic surgery.
- Wedge resection.
- Segmental resection.
- Lobectomy.
- Pneumonectomy.

CHAPTER 8

HEART

Joe, a 48-year old lawyer, had just gone through an extremely difficult divorce and custody battle. He began to notice some tightness in his chest while he was jogging. At first, he blamed it on indigestion. Finally, when it kept reappearing, he sought a medical diagnosis. A stress test showed an abnormality, and a follow-up angiogram (artery X-ray) revealed one diseased artery, which was 70 percent blocked. His cardiologist suggested a bypass operation, or an angioplasty.

However, the doctor warned that once the angioplasty had been performed, Joe's artery would be permanently scarred, making long-term disease more likely. In addition, he had found that 20 to 40 percent of angioplasty stent procedures block up by six to twelve months and that, while Joe's chest pain symptoms would likely be relieved, his risk for myocardial infarction and death would not be reduced. Undergoing bypass surgery likewise would be only a temporary solution, since up to 50 percent of these procedures close up by five to ten years.

Joe decided instead to first attempt a trial of the Ornish Program for heart disease reversal, which involved changing his lifestyle: He altered his diet, increased the regularity of his exercise, commenced daily yoga, and joined a support group. His pain disappeared within a week, and retesting one year later showed complete reversal of his arterial blockage.

The heart, the symbol and essence of life itself, serves us faithfully, with little fanfare, until its health is in jeopardy. However, in recent years, knowledge about the association of lifestyle and this problem has provided reliable information for both preventing and reversing heart disease. In this chapter, we will inform you about how to bypass the bypass whenever you can, make a choice about which surgical procedures are best if you must have operative treatment, and begin a program to prevent future problems.

You, like most people, may have felt heart disease just wouldn't happen to you. That's what popular *Who Wants to Be a Millionaire?* host Regis Philbin thought. He regularly noshed on lots of meat, hamburgers, cheeseburgers, and French fries. "I guess I was asking for it," he said. "Although, you know, you always think it could never happen to you. I thought I was in shape—but I found out I really wasn't." At age 58, Regis needed emergency angioplasty to unblock an occluded heart artery, which became evident when it gave him severe chest pain during filming aboard a Carnival cruise ship. "I was scared," he said. "That was the closest I've ever been to anything major. And as I was wheeled into this room with all those doctors and equipment, I was intimidated. Anything could go wrong. All of a sudden, I felt very much alone, hoping everything would be all right and worrying about my wife and family."[1]

Heart disease, the number one health problem and cause of death in modern Western society, is responsible for more deaths than all other diseases combined. While bypass surgery inserts channels around the obstacles, angioplasty opens the heart vessels from within, by nonsurgical balloon techniques, a sort of "Roto-Rooter" technique. These are the most common major procedures performed on adult American men and, increasingly, on women as well.

The most likely surgery of any kind that may be recommended to you during your lifetime is the coronary bypass operation. However, the good news is that now you have a good chance of preventing and reversing coronary disease by other means than surgery. The Ornish Program for heart disease treatment has now become so well accepted among cardiologists it is no longer considered alternative medicine, but is a fruitful example of the rapidly evolving field of integrative medicine.

After rising rapidly during the first part of this century, the incidence of heart disease has declined nearly every year since 1950—probably owing to decreased consumption of animal fats, less smoking, and better control of high blood pressure. However, heart disease is still at epidemic proportions, with nearly one out of ten people in our population currently suffering from it.[2]

One in five American men has a heart attack before the age of 65, and half of them are dead within a year. Men ages 35 to 55 have five times the death rate from heart disease that women do, because females are largely protected by estrogen before menopause. Women also have lower levels of meat consumption, and have, in the past, had less job stress, stress-related hypertension, and cigarette use. Soon after menopause, though, their rate of heart disease rapidly increases. Overall, as women's lifestyles have changed, their rates have begun approaching, or even surpassing, that of men.

The buildup of restricting "atherosclerotic" fatty plaque in the arteries of the heart, and its subsequent rupturing and/or clotting, is still thought to be the major immediate causes of coronary heart disease, although the mechanism for this process is being debated. Spasm of coronary arteries, even without plaque buildup, during times of stress, is an additional important contribution to flow reduction and subsequent heart attack.

Plaque buildup is mainly correlated with excess fats in your diet; when fats were restricted during wartime, the rate of heart disease plummeted, and coronary heart disease is very rare in vegetarians.

What about the diet doctors such as Dr. Robert Atkins who promote high-fat, low-carbohydrate regimens for weight loss? Their assertions are not backed by accepted science. Although some patients may achieve short-term weight loss and lower cholesterol levels due to calorie restriction, the long-term effects of these regimens have not been studied, and the weight of research itself strongly now supports the conclusion that high fat intake in the long run is associated with increased plaque buildup in the arteries of the heart.

"Invasive" treatment of coronary artery disease is a multibillion-dollar-a-year industry, and many surgeons, cardiologists, hospitals, and technological support personnel have financial incentives to recommend it. The self-interest aspect may be difficult to separate from valid medical reasons for performing bypass and angioplasty.

Patients' symptoms *are* initially relieved by these procedures in 90 percent of cases. However, no evidence exists that these expensive and potentially complicated procedures actually *prolong* life expectancy. One study, by Tu and colleagues, published in the *New England Journal of Medicine* in 1997, compared the treatments of elderly patients with heart attacks admitted to hospitals in the United States and Canada. Despite U. S. patients receiving 5.2 times as many coronary angiograms, 7.7 times as many angioplasties, and 7.8 times as many bypass procedures as the Canadian patients, the one-year survival rates were virtually the same.[3]

Four large prospective randomized studies comparing "conservative," limited use of angiography and revascularization (angioplasty or coronary artery bypass) with "aggressive," routine use of angiography and revascularization for acute coronary syndromes, studying more than 6,400 patients, have shown that the aggressive approach does not reduce the incidence of nonfatal reinfarction or death, and in fact may be more dangerous.[4] In addition to their expense and risk, *some studies show that as many as 30 to 50 percent of all patients have a return of symptoms within five years after a bypass operation. After an angioplasty, 40 to 60 percent of all patients have recurrent symptoms within four to six months.*[5]

As our society ages, and as decisions regarding treatment of heart disease correspondingly increase, we must grapple with cost-containment and quality-of-life issues. Is bypass or angioplasty always necessary when it is recommended to you? Can alternative medicine regimens allow you to avoid these relatively dramatic and risky procedures? Studies have now shown that 80 to 90 percent of the patients who faithfully follow diet, exercise, and lifestyle modification treatment plans, as instituted by Dr. Dean Ornish, obtain pain relief and improved heart function.[6]

Immediately after comedian and talk show host David Letterman's five-way heart bypass operation, his surgeon told him, "I had a really good feeling while I was doing it." Letterman later told his audience that those are exactly the kind of words you want to hear after that type of life-threatening emergency surgery. Certainly, bypass surgery can sometimes be lifesaving, and an appropriate choice for you. However, in the procedure, a small buzz saw is used to cut through your breastbone. Your ribs are spread open, then your heart stopped for up to one-half hour, while shoelace-size veins taken from your legs are sewed around blockages. When you can, you may first wish to consider a trial of changing your lifestyle instead.

And even if you do choose to have surgery or angioplasty, you will *still* need to develop

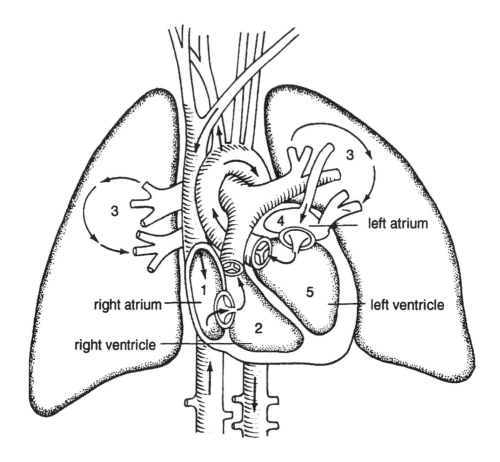

right atrium

right ventricle

left atrium

left ventricle

1. Blood from body returns to right atrium.

2. Right ventricle pumps blood to lungs.

3. Blood reaches lung: carbon dioxide is released; oxygen is taken up.

4. Blood from lungs returns to left atrium.

5. Blood is pumped to body by left ventricle.

6. Blood reaches body tissues: oxygen is released; carbon dioxide is taken up.

Fig. 8.1 The anatomy and functioning of the heart

eating habits and ways to handle your stress that will maximize your chances for long-term health and help prevent reappearance of your disease—especially since the bypass grafts and angioplasty-treated arteries tend to clog up much faster than your original arteries. Taking certain supplements after angioplasty may help you avoid reclosure.

How Your Heart Works

The heart is a muscle about the size of your fist, with four hollow chambers: the *right atrium* and *right ventricle* and the *left atrium* and *left ventricle*. (See Figure 8.1.) When it contracts, blood is squeezed out, while the four *heart valves* keep flow moving in a forward direction. When the heart relaxes, more blood can flow into its chambers.

Your blood is pumped from the right side of the heart to the lungs, to acquire oxygen and release carbon dioxide. It then returns to the heart's left side, to be pumped out to the body's tissues, where the oxygen and other nutrients are distributed, and carbon dioxide and waste products picked up.

The heart pumps continuously, and therefore requires more blood flow itself than any other muscle or organ in your body. It has its own system of blood vessels, the *coronary arteries*, that supply oxygen and nutrients to its thick muscular walls, and to the electrical tissue responsible for coordinating contraction. (See Figure 8.2.) The *left main coronary artery*

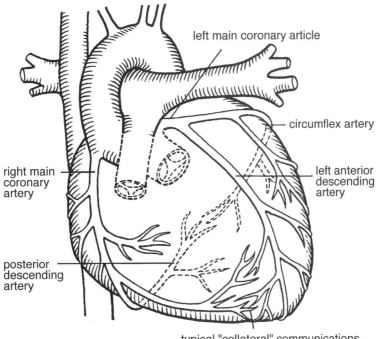

left main coronary article

circumflex artery

right main coronary artery

left anterior descending artery

posterior descending artery

typical "collateral" communications

Fig. 8.2 The coronary arteries

supplies the left front part of the heart. It quickly divides into the *left anterior descending artery*, the major supplier of the left side of the heart, and the *circumflex artery*, which provides blood to the lateral and sometimes inferior outer wall of the left ventricle and front part of the *septum*, the muscular wall between the right and left ventricles. The *right main coronary artery* and its branch, the *posterior descending artery*, feeds the back of the heart, as well as the lower part of the septum and right ventricle.

The major arteries are connected by branches called *collaterals*. If one artery is blocked, the degree of development of these collaterals (i.e., how much they can take over the blocked artery's function) determines whether you experience symptoms.

Your heart beat rate and force of contraction are affected by exercise, brain activity, hormones, stress, and medication. Physical activity causes your body's muscles to demand more nutrients; the healthy heart responds with a quicker rate and stronger contractions. Meditation and sleep reduce your body's demand on the heart to a minimum, while the common "dietary drugs"— caffeine and cigarettes—speed the heart, creating more work for it.

In this chapter, we focus on coronary artery disease, since it is, by far, the most common cause of heart disease. Because the heart and the vascular system (your veins and arteries) together make up the circulatory system, you may also want to read Chapters 10 and 11 for a more complete understanding of the entire system and the problems that afflict the arteries both in the heart and elsewhere in the body. Primary difficulties with the heart's rhythm, valves, and the muscle itself, which require surgery, are much more intricate, and therefore outside the limitations of this book.

Coronary Artery Disease and Atherosclerosis

Atherosclerosis comes from the words *athere*, meaning "mush" or "porridge," and *skleros*, which means "hard." Atherosclerosis is a generalized, usually progressive disease in which a sludgelike material builds up within the walls of your arteries, where it blocks normal blood flow. Atherosclerotic deposits begin as soft yellow streaks, which become harder, more fibrous, and calcified over time. In the United States, children raised on the usual American diet have been found to have streaking in their arteries at as early as one or two years of age. Most of us have begun this process by early adulthood. The end result can be partial or complete blockage of one or more of the coronary arteries. (See Figure 8.3.)

Atherosclerosis, by blocking blood flow in arteries, is the underlying cause for more death and illness in this country than any other disease. If it is found to cause symptoms in one area, such as with circulation to your legs, it is probably present in your other organ systems as well. Most patients with vascular problems die of their underlying heart disease regardless of which part of the body developed the first symptoms.

Japan and other countries consuming a low-fat diet have only one-fifth the U.S. rate of atherosclerosis. Genetic differences cannot account for this, since those who move to the United States soon acquire our rates of disease, although stress may also influence this shift.

The combined elements of diet, smoking history, family history, blood pressure, and ability to handle stress all play important contributory roles in the atherosclerotic process. As noted, evidence now supports the conclu-

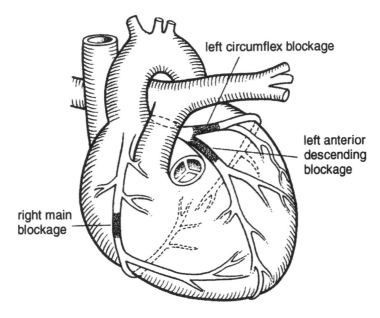

Fig. 8.3 Types of blockages in coronary artery disease

sion that atherosclerosis is both clearly preventable and reversible by dietary and lifestyle modifications or by medication.

Atherosclerosis and Cholesterol

Half of persons who have heart attacks in this country have "normal" cholesterol levels. But that is simply because the baseline cholesterol is too high. The average level is 200, and a steep incline in heart disease follows anything higher than 150. In the Framingham study of who develops this problem, no one was recorded as having a heart attack who maintained a cholesterol level under 150.[7]

Cholesterol is a waxy material composed of fat and fatty acids. It would be both impossible and undesirable to remove all cholesterol from your body, since 1,000 milligrams are synthesized in the liver each day. Cholesterol is necessary for vital cell processes, but the liver produces enough on its own; excess

taken in your diet contributes to atherosclerotic disease. Your total blood cholesterol level depends upon genetics, the amount of cholesterol and fats in your diet, the quantity produced by your liver as a result of other dietary factors, and your acute and chronic levels of stress. Cholesterol is also increased by obesity and lack of regular exercise.

High levels of cholesterol and saturated fats in the typical American diet are associated with our high rate of atherosclerotic disease. Only foods from animal origin—meats, poultry, dairy products, seafood, and eggs—contain cholesterol; vegetables, fruits, grains, and beans have none. However, fats from any source, including palm oils and most margarines, collectively contribute to your total cholesterol level, and to your subsequent risk for atherosclerosis.

It's so hard to know what to eat these days. When you read the papers, you are bombarded by the "latest" research, much of it contradictory. One study shows one thing, another demonstrates the opposite. What can you rely on about heart disease and cholesterol?

Your "lipid profile" shows the levels of the types of cholesterol that make up your total cholesterol. Cholesterol is a solid substance which must be attached to other compounds, called lipids, in order to become liquefied enough to move through your bloodstream. The bulk of cholesterol is carried as *low-density lipoprotein (LDL) cholesterol*. LDL is "bad" because it is the type of cholesterol that builds up in the walls of your arteries.

Triglycerides are a form of fatty acids. A high level of triglycerides also correlates with risk of accelerated atherosclerosis. This kind of fat is related to simple sugar intake, alcohol, lack of exercise, and diabetes.

High-density lipoprotein (HDL) cholesterol, is another compound that carries cholesterol, but it serves as a "good" substance. It acts as a "scavenger" to take cholesterol from overloaded cells to your liver for elimination through the bile and to eventually leave your body in the stool. A high HDL level (greater then 45 mg%) therefore increases your resistance to atherosclerosis. HDL levels can sometimes be increased by regular exercise.

If you are over the age of 20, you should know your total cholesterol level and lipid profile, and have them taken each year. A total cholesterol level of less than 200, LDL of less than 130, and triglycerides of less than 200 are frequently cited as desirable to maintain. However, these recommendations are based on the averages of our culture and are too high to be healthy.

You should work to keep your levels well below these averages to lower your risk of developing atherosclerosis. If your total choles-

terol level is above 150, it puts you at increased risk. However, your total cholesterol level is not as important as the *ratio* between total cholesterol and HDL cholesterol. Most of us are born with a total cholesterol level around 60 to 75, with a matching HDL level, so that our HDL to total cholesterol ratio begins at about 1:1. Consumption of cholesterol-containing foods changes this ratio as we grow, elevating the total cholesterol and decreasing the HDL. Research has shown that a ratio lower than 1:2.5 (meaning less than 2.5 times as much total cholesterol as HDL) provides excellent protection. Achieving this ratio usually requires an HDL level of more than 75.

Your arteries are not simply passive pipes that get clogged. The lining cells allow fats carried by the blood to actually enter the arterial wall. When the blood cholesterol goes above a safe level, the lining cells become overwhelmed, and allow excess fat to be *stored* within the artery wall. To the surgeon's eye, this region appears as a slightly raised yellow area, called a fatty streak.

As such a streak enlarges, the cells break down and cholesterol deposits accumulate outside the cell wall, producing a solid core called a *plaque,* which can protrude into the channel of your blood vessel. Calcium is deposited in the area of the injury, where it hardens and produces a narrowing and restriction to blood flow.

As atherosclerotic disease progresses, the artery's muscle layer is destroyed, fibrous tissue develops, the vessel loses its elasticity, and your artery becomes rigid. This in turn contributes to high blood pressure. The cholesterol plaque surface may break down, producing a raw "ulcer," which promotes blood clotting and a subsequent vicious cycle. Eventually, when the channel is so small that blood flow is significantly reduced and cells are deprived of sufficient oxygen and nutrients, your symptoms may begin.

You can develop *thrombosis* (a blood clot) when platelets and blood clot on a plaque suddenly block blood flow completely. Sluggish flow beyond the blockage then increases the likelihood of further clotting. Threat to your life or limb may result, depending on the site of the block and whether adjoining arteries can compensate for it.

New theories explaining the onset and development of plaque have been put forward: that lack of the vitamin folic acid in the diet raises homocysteine levels, as discussed below, and/or that infection or other injury also contribute to the atherosclerotic process.

Bits and pieces of cholesterol, platelets, and/or blood clot can break off the surface of a plaque and travel in the bloodstream. These chunks are called *emboli*. If they are larger than the smallest blood vessels (the *capillaries),* they can eventually travel to an area where they may produce a sudden blockage. This is the most common cause of strokes.

Atherosclerosis and Inflammation

Newer theories propose a relationship between inflammation and the formation of plaque in your arteries. C-reactive protein (CRP) is a protein in your blood that participates in and is a marker for inflammation. It has been found to be elevated in some patients with heart attacks, and may help predict your risk. The antiinflammatory effects of aspirin, and at least some of the lipid-lowering drugs, such as atorvastatin (Lipitor), may help explain their success in preventing coronary heart disease. Bacterial infection, nicotine ef-

fects, and high blood pressure may also contribute to inflammation in your arteries. Antibiotics may also serve to provide protection; further research is needed.

Angina

You have a little tingling down your left arm. You feel slightly short of breath when you climb the stairs. You get a little indigestion while exercising. Could this mean you have heart disease?

Angina means "heart pain," discomfort produced when the heart muscle does not receive sufficient oxygen or nutrients to keep up with its needs. If your coronary arteries are narrowed or blocked by atherosclerotic deposits or a clot, or go into temporary spasm, the resulting pain may cause you to stop what you are doing. This lessens the demand on your heart, and your angina then usually disappears. The most common events that bring on angina are vigorous physical activity, body coldness, emotional stress or excitement, sexual activity with its physical and emotional demands, and overeating, when your digestive tract requires more cardiac output, especially when this is followed by exercise.

Angina's typical tightness, crushing, or squeezing pain may be centered beneath your breastbone or in your left chest, and it may radiate into your jaw, left shoulder, or arm. It may be accompanied by sweating, nausea, and pale or gray discoloration of the skin. The amount of activity required to produce symptoms is determined by how severely your coronary artery is narrowed; angina does not commonly occur until there is at least a 75 percent narrowing in an artery. If the blockage reaches 90 percent, angina may be experienced even without any precipitating event.

Seventy-five percent of the individuals who develop angina remain *stable,* with pain that is predictable and easily relieved. If you are one of these, although you are still at risk for a heart attack and sudden death, you have time for a trial of the alternative medicine treatments.

The other 25 percent of those who experience angina have increasingly frequent and intense *unstable* angina. If the blockage in these cases is not quickly reversed, a heart attack is likely to occur. Early angioplasty or surgery is then necessary.

How Coronary Artery Disease Is Diagnosed

Diagnosis of coronary artery disease can be very quick, easy, and inexpensive based on your history, physical exam, and EKG. However, often other more expensive tests may be necessary to characterize and quantify the problem, especially if an invasive form of treatment is being considered.

History and Physical Exam

Your doctor's initial investigation should include a careful medical history and physical examination. Your doctor should look for any recognized risk factors for coronary artery disease including smoking history, high blood pressure, diabetes, high cholesterol levels, sedentary lifestyle, and family history of heart disease. A thorough discussion of symptoms includes questions about the type and location of your chest pain, any accompanying shortness of breath, leg swelling, or fainting spells, what brings on your symptoms, and what you have been able to do to relieve them. Most other medical problems confused with heart disease can thus be eliminated.

Your doctor takes your blood pressure and pulse, listens to your heart and lungs with a stethoscope for characteristic sounds caused by heart disease, and gives you a general medical checkup.

Blood Tests

In addition to measurements of your total cholesterol, LDL cholesterol, HDL cholesterol, and total cholesterol/HDL ratio, the newer tests of homocysteine blood level and C-reactive protein can help assess your heart disease risk.

Chest X-Ray

This shows heart size, position, and shape to help diagnose hypertension (high blood pressure), heart failure, and heart valve disease.

Electrocardiogram

The *electrocardiogram,* which is easy, quick, painless, inexpensive, and produces no complications, has been—and will most likely continue to be—the mainstay of heart diagnosis. For this test, you lie on an examining table with your shirt off. Electrodes that sense electrical impulses are attached by tape or suction cups to several sites on your chest. An EKG machine picks up these impulses, produced as your heart contracts and relaxes, then traces them as lines on a rolling strip of graph paper. Representative samples are cut out and assembled for a permanent record. The test is completed in a few minutes. Your heart's rhythm, and the effects of medications, body chemistry imbalance, hypertension, acute heart attack, and scarred areas from old heart attacks can all be seen.

A *Holter monitor* is a small portable cassette tape recorder that records your EKG over a twenty-four-hour period as you go about your normal activities. It may catch intermittent abnormal tracings.

EKG Exercise Stress Test

Since half of all angina patients have a normal resting EKG, but only show abnormal EKG patterns during periods of increased cardiac demand, the *EKG exercise stress test (stress cardiogram)*, has been developed to determine how your heart responds to increased physical exertion. If you have intermittent symptoms, or are at increased risk—especially if you plan any activities that would accelerate the work of your heart, such as an exercise program—you should have a stress test.

For this procedure, you are hooked up to an EKG machine and asked to walk on a moving, inclined treadmill or ride a stationary exercise bike, usually for ten to fifteen minutes. Speed and steepness are increased, to heighten the physical exertion required to keep up with the moving surface. The goal is to see how your heart responds to the demands of physical activity, by getting it to beat at a rapid rate, which has been predetermined by your age or other factors. If EKG abnormalities or chest pain develop, the test is stopped.

Even if you have no symptoms, a stress test may help your cardiologist find early heart disease, and enable recommendations to be made for a safe rehabilitation exercise program. A very small danger exists that the demands of this test could *precipitate* a heart attack (in 1 out of every 10,000 cases), so it must be carefully monitored, and you should stop if you feel any fatigue or pain at all.

Thallium Exercise Stress Test

In the *radioactive thallium stress test,* radioactive particles are injected into your bloodstream through a vein. A scanner then takes multiple X-ray pictures of your heart, showing its circulation as blood and isotope spread through its tissues. Your heart may receive an appropriate amount of blood during rest, but blocked vessels may not be able to supply its needs during exercise. To test for that possibility, this scanning is done immediately after you have exerted yourself by walking on a treadmill or peddling a bicycle, while you are hooked up to an EKG machine, and then four hours later at rest. A "cold" spot seen on the exercise scan but not on the resting study indicates an area of heart muscle not getting adequate blood flow, and therefore at risk, though still alive. Cold spots on both scans indicate a dead area of scar tissue from an old heart attack.

Echocardiogram

The painless *echocardiogram (sonogram)* reflects sound waves from your heart's surface and chamber walls, providing a picture of the size of the heart chambers, heart muscle thickness, and valve structure. Abnormal contractions and clots within the heart chambers may be seen, as well as valve dysfunction. This test is quick, painless, relatively inexpensive, and does not require X-ray exposure.

Echocardiogram Exercise Stress Test

This test uses the same technology as the echocardiogram, to look at your heart's wall motion at resting baseline and just after you have exercised. A normal response shows increased contractility in all of the walls.

Worsening regional wall contractility indicates inadequate blood supply to that area. This test, which will often provide the same information as the thallium stress test and add additional data about valve function, does not require radiation, and is much cheaper.

Stress Testing with Drugs

If you are unable to exercise for an EKG, thallium, or echocardiogram stress test, you may be given an intravenous drug that mimics the effects of exercise on your heart. *Persantine* is a medication that increases blood flow to heart muscle supplied by normal arteries. Any area to which an obstructed artery is attached would not receive increased flow, and this would be reflected in the thallium test reading. *Dobutamine*, another drug, causes the heart to beat faster and with more forceful contractions. EKG changes may reveal any inability of your heart to keep up with its circulation needs under these conditions. First you undergo a baseline study, the drugs are then administered as a substitute for exercise, and the test repeated.

Gated Radioisotope Ejection Fraction Test

In this test radioactive particles are injected intravenously and a scanner picks up the emissions over your heart. The amount of blood your heart ejects with each beat is measured by computer. This gives an assessment of how well your heart squeezes, reflecting coronary artery circulation, damage from previous heart attack, muscle disease, or valve problems.

PET Scan

In this type of scan, radioactive dye is injected into your arm vein, then special color-coded three-dimensional pictures of blood flow to all parts of your heart are taken. These indicate the ability of your coronary arteries to supply blood to each of the areas of your heart. This is the most precise *functional* test of the competence of the heart's arteries, and has the advantage of being "noninvasive," meaning no devices are placed in the heart, making it a less risky test. Since the equipment to perform a PET scan is expensive, it is currently available at a limited number of centers nationwide.

Electron Beam CT Scan of Coronary Arteries

This new noninvasive screening test may be useful if you have no cardiac symptoms or known heart disease. It measures calcium in the walls of your coronary arteries. In less than a minute it gives you a "calcium score" that can predict your risk for a heart attack in the next five years. You can use this information to provide a stimulus to institute needed lifestyle changes as discussed in this chapter.

Coronary Angiography

This exam, also known as *cardiac catheterization,* is an X-ray procedure that outlines your coronary blood vessels as blood flows and your heart pumps. A motion picture is captured on tape for later analysis. Unusual patterns, areas of blockage, and the extent of collateral arteries developed can be clearly demonstrated. Because this test is expensive and has potential complications, it should only be done if heart bypass surgery or angioplasty is being considered.

For an angiogram, you must lie on an X-ray table, hooked up to a heart monitor. After mild intravenous sedation, your radiologist or cardiologist prepares your groin (or occasionally your arm) with an antiseptic and gives you local anesthesia in that area. A needle is placed into an artery and a small catheter (plastic tube) inserted through the needle. Using X-ray guidance, the catheter tip is manipulated into the desired location in your heart. A small amount of dye is then injected and a series of X-rays taken. The dye injection may cause a mild heat sensation in your arm, leg, or chest. Sedatives and painkillers can be given to blunt the unpleasantness, but you must remain awake.

Cardiac catheterization takes from thirty minutes to two or more hours, and may be mildly to very uncomfortable. It can be performed as an outpatient if no treatment, such as angioplasty or surgery, is found to be necessary.

This catheterization carries a small risk of complication (1 in 200 to 300 tests). Irregular heartbeats may be caused by irritation from the catheter; severe dye reaction develops occasionally; heart attack may occur; or the catheter may perforate the heart wall. Risk is higher if you have severe coronary artery disease.

The radiologist or cardiologist must puncture a high-pressure artery in your groin, in order to pass the catheter. This may cause a bruise, sometimes extending all the way to your knee, that may take a week or two to go away. Infection sometimes develops at the catheter puncture site. Rarely, a "false aneurysm" or leak from the puncture site develops. This can usually be treated without surgery. Even more rarely, an artery blockage occurs at the puncture site or elsewhere that must be fixed surgically.

How do you decide whether to risk the possibility of such a complication, or even losing your life, in the process of taking a test to diagnose disease? If you have chest pain that has suddenly accelerated from a baseline level, or is present even at rest, immediate bypass or coronary angioplasty may be needed to prevent a heart attack and sudden death. If you have just had a heart attack and emergency surgery or angioplasty is contemplated to reduce its size or prevent extension, or if you have persistent pain after a heart attack, an angiogram is warranted. The most common reason for bypass or angioplasty is disabling angina not controlled by nonsurgical treatment.

If you are not considering immediate surgery or angioplasty, you may choose to have the less-invasive tests, and use a trial of alternative approaches first. If the lifestyle change program or medication fails, an angiogram can then be done to determine whether surgery or angioplasty would be appropriate.

Alternative Medicine Approaches to Coronary Artery Disease

Wilson, *a doctor specializing in internal medicine and the authors' cousin, was a 33-year-old when he had his first heart attack. He underwent a three-vessel coronary artery bypass procedure. After his surgery, despite a strong family history of early deaths from heart disease, he continued to smoke two packs of cigarettes per day. He did not lose his excess weight, and maintained a strenuous work schedule. Wilson didn't know how to relax. He also suffered through two painful divorces. Ten years later, his bypass grafts clotted, and he died on the operating table during a second emergency heart bypass operation, leaving behind a third wife and three young children.*

Coronary artery bypass surgery carries enormous physical and psychological consequences. When faced with this operation, you, too, might take a second look at soy.

No doubt many persons benefit from their bypass procedures. However, several studies have shown that bypass surgery does not always get people back to work. Some continue to think of themselves as sick, and do not return to being fully functional individuals.[8] Even though the bypass has relieved their pain, a feeling of depression and illness remains. Whether or not you choose a bypass or angioplasty, your best chances for restoring your experience of wellness are by making changes in your lifestyle.

The lifestyle approach to coronary artery disease has been pioneered by Dr. Dean Ornish, myself, and others, who in the "Lifestyle Heart Trial" studies showed that using this approach can reverse this disease. As Director of Stress Management Training at the Preventive Medicine Research Institute, while working with Dr. Ornish from the outset of this research, I personally witnessed its remarkably quick benefits.

One of my patients, for example, used to watch television programs he didn't like rather than get up to change the channel, since he didn't have a remote control device, and he would experience angina just from crossing the room. After only two weeks on the Ornish regime, he was walking two miles with no chest pain!

Although blockage in the coronary arteries may be caused by atherosclerotic plaque (fatty buildup), an acute clot, or spasm of the muscle in the coronary artery wall, these problems are themselves precipitated by dietary and other lifestyle factors.

Fat and cholesterol in the diet, and perhaps refined sugar, are now thought to be mainly responsible for the plaque that clogs coronary arteries. In addition, acute spasms in an artery can be caused by psychological stress (transmitted via the brain and hormonal messengers), by nicotine from cigarette smoking, and by the excess fats in the blood. Angioplasty and surgical treatment are based on treating

the disease as it exists at that point, and does nothing to prevent the postsurgical progression of your atherosclerosis. Therefore, *surgery is doomed to eventual failure unless the underlying causes are removed.*

Dr. Ornish's Lifestyle studies have been able to show that it is possible not only to treat angina patients effectively without drugs or surgery, but also to shrink the plaque in the arteries enough to assure sufficient blood flow to improve the heart's functioning. Also, changes in cholesterol levels may induce more favorable coronary vessel relaxation, allowing improved flow within weeks to months before plaque decreases in size.[9]

The plaque does not need to be reversed completely; even a small decrease in blockage is usually sufficient to provide enough increased blood flow to improve function sufficiently to make you symptom-free. In a landmark study reported in the *Journal of the American Medical Association* in 1998, comparing the Lifestyle program with routine coronary care prescribed by cardiologists, Dr. Ornish reported the average decrease in diameter blockage was 3.1 percent after five years in the Lifestyle experimental group, compared with an average *increase* in diameter blockage of 11.8 percent in the group following standard coronary treatment recommendations. The frequency of angina attacks was decreased by 91 percent at one year and 72 percent after five years in the Lifestyle group, results comparable with those of bypass surgery and angioplasty. In contrast, the group of patients receiving routine coronary management had a 186 percent increase in angina at one year and a 35 percent increase after five years, even after many of these patients had had coronary bypass operations.[10]

In Dr. Ornish's studies, measurements of blood pressure, ability to walk on a treadmill, and the amount of blood ejected with each heartbeat were all improved. Blood pressure and heart medications could be eliminated or reduced, and in most cases, cholesterol levels fell below 150 mg%.[11]

A five-year follow-up study published in 1995 by Ornish and collaborators in the *Journal of the American Medical Association* compared PET scan heart muscle circulation abnormalities before and after treatment in patients randomized to the Ornish program versus the "usual care" prescribed by cardiologists. They showed a decrease in size and severity of abnormalities on PET scans in the Ornish treatment group and an increase in abnormalities in the "usual care" group.[12] Only 1 percent of the patients in the study group had worse results after five years, compared with 45 percent of those in the usual care group.

In other words, these studies have shown that *it is possible to take a sick heart and halt or reverse the progression of disease in 99 percent of all patients and make it healthy again without drugs or surgery.*

Have you been recommended to have a bypass or angioplasty? Are you wondering if you would be eligible for the Ornish Lifestyle program with your particular disease pattern? Do you wonder if you would have the self-disciple to follow the program's strict requirements? Is there a practitioner in your area trained in the Lifestyle program and able to achieve similar results to Dr. Ornish himself? Yes, it's very likely that you are eligible, that you would be able to adhere to the program, and that there is a Lifestyle program near you. Dr Ornish's nonprofit Preventive Medicine Research Institute has trained a large number of practitioners and institutions around the country. Study results from the Multicenter Lifestyle Demonstration Project indicate that the enrolled patients were motivated to maintain the lifestyle changes required by the program and, working with other trained providers, were able to achieve results similar to those of Dr. Ornish described above. Seventy-seven percent of patients who were eligible for coronary bypass or angioplasty were able to avoid them for at least three years by following the Lifestyle program.[13] Mutual of Omaha found this saved $29,529 per patient. Results also showed that patients who began the program after surgery or angioplasty were able to reduce their need for another procedure.

Also, the program works for patients of all ages while the risks of angioplasty and bypass increase with age. In May 2000, the U.S. government's Health Care Financing Administration implemented a demonstration study in eleven medical centers across the country to determine if the Lifestyle program is a safe and cost-effective alternative to invasive treatments. Eighteen hundred selected Medicare patients with angina and increased risk for heart attack and considered candidates for angioplasty or bypass in the near future will be enrolled. If you have symptoms and are over age 65, ask your doctor if you are eligible.

If your situation is acute, with progressively worse pain, then angioplasty or surgery may be justified. But a supervised trial of diet, lifestyle change, and stress reduction therapy makes best sense for most persons with stable symptoms.

If you do choose angioplasty or an operation, or medications, such as nitroglycerin or calcium channel blockers, which dilate the coronary arteries or reduce the heart's workload, you do nothing to affect your underlying atherosclerosis. *Lifestyle change is needed for all heart patients.* Following are the elements involved.

Quit Smoking

When you start any lifestyle treatment program, such as the Ornish program, you must first stop smoking. A vast amount of data supports the view that smoking accelerates atherosclerosis and coronary artery disease. Smoking lowers "good" HDL cholesterol, reduces oxygen supply, and causes abnormal and irregular heartbeats, high blood pressure that increases oxygen need by the heart, damage to blood vessel lining cells, and platelet stickiness and clumping that is more likely to plug blood vessels. Smokers have more angina, are two to three times more likely to have heart attacks, and 70 percent more likely to have a fatal complication when they do.

If you are a smoker, you should also consider its effects on your family, friends, and coworkers. If you are a nonsmoker, you may have some educational work to do, since second-hand smoke is also bad. In 1992, the American Heart Association reviewed the literature and concluded that "the risk of death due to heart disease is increased by 30 percent among those exposed to environmental tobacco smoke at home and could be much higher in those exposed at the workplace, where higher levels of environmental tobacco smoke may be present."[14] In the largest study of nonsmokers married to smokers, the risk of death from heart disease in the nonsmoking spouse was found to be increased by 20 percent over that of a person with a spouse who was also a nonsmoker.[15]

Because it is very difficult to quit, most persons need help from family, friends, and/or professionals. If you are trying to stop, yet are surrounded by people who smoke, it is even more difficult. See the section on how to quit smoking in Chapter 2. In the beginning, two

sessions a day of the yoga stretches, deep relaxation, breathing exercises, meditation, and visualization are recommended. Hypnosis and acupuncture have also been found to be successful. If you have difficulty quitting on your own, seek out a support group that can keep inspiring you to do what is healthy. You may benefit by taking a vacation, or attending a yoga retreat.

Don't be discouraged if you are not immediately successful, since persistence pays off. Studies have shown that even if you fail, the more times you try, the more likely you are to ultimately reach your goal. Surprisingly, the increased cardiac risk from smoking decreases rapidly after you stop. It is significantly diminished by one year, and close to baseline at three years.[16] Conquering this addiction is worth any difficulties: it is the most important thing you can do for yourself.

Decrease Your Fat and Cholesterol Intake

Many people have heard of—and patterned their eating habits after—the "prudent" American Heart Association diet. *But that is not enough:* It gets you, as Dr. William Castelli of the famous Framingham Study puts it, merely from "galloping-galloping" coronary artery disease to "galloping" coronary artery disease. Simply removing visible fat from your plate will not enable you to drop your cholesterol level below the danger range. Red meats have fat among the fibers, and even chicken and fish have enough fat and cholesterol to raise your body's levels to the danger zone—felt by Drs. Castelli, Ornish, and others to be anything above 150 mg% total cholesterol. No one in the Framingham Study, which has followed 20,000 people over thirty years, has ever experienced a heart attack while having a cholesterol level below 150 mg%.[17] That means if you decrease your cholesterol to below 150 mg% and maintain it there, you effectively make your risk as low as possible.

Some studies have shown that the body can excrete only about 500 milligrams of cholesterol per week.[18] The typical American diet consists of 800 to 1,000 milligrams of cholesterol per *day*. Two hundred and fifty milligrams are present in one egg. Major dietary modification is required to reverse the damage of high cholesterol intake. Some of the early studies of cholesterol made the mistake of not reducing intake low enough to show the benefits of such change. In Dr. Ornish's program, ingestion of cholesterol is restricted to the negligible amounts found in nonfat dairy products. No other cholesterol sources— meats, chicken, and fish—are included in the diet.

Substitute Monounsaturated for Saturated Fats

Saturated fats constitute more than 10 percent of calorie intake in the typical American diet. This type of fat is highest in total cholesterol and LDL. Progression of coronary artery disease is strongly influenced by intake of saturated fats.[19] You can minimize saturated fats by using vegetable oils obtained from canola oil or olive oil. These are relatively high in monounsaturated fats and low in saturated fats. A study of subjects taking a Mediterranean diet that replaces animal with vegetable fats, and is high in olive oil, fruit, and vegetables found a 79 percent decrease in heart attack and cardiac deaths compared to control subjects taking a standard low-fat diet.[20] However, even though this diet is a

step in the right direction, its preventive power is not as great as the Asian diet, which is lowest in added fats, or the full vegetarian, oil-free Ornish approach.

Cholesterol levels can also be decreased by substituting polyunsaturated corn and soybean oils for saturated oils, but this does not lower levels as much as the oil-free diet. The solidified form of vegetable oils found in shortenings and commercial baked goods contain omega-6 fatty acids, which actually raise total cholesterol and LDL. Just how much oil you can safely add to your diet to fully prevent heart disease has yet to be determined.

Fish oils are rich in polyunsaturated omega-3 fatty acids, which increase HDL levels. Fish consumption has been correlated with decreased risk of coronary artery disease in many epidemiological studies. A study published in the *New England Journal of Medicine* found that men who ate an average of 35 grams of fish a day (8 ounces per week), over a thirty-year period, had a 38 percent decreased risk of dying from a heart attack (67 percent less of not dying suddenly from one) compared to a nonvegetarian population who ate none.[21] A recent *Journal of the American Medical Association* editorial concluded that "the existing evidence suggests that consumption of fish once a week will help prevent coronary heart disease and therefore should be a component of a healthy diet. It also appears justified to advise patients with cardiac disease to consume 2 fish servings per week. These levels of fish consumption not only may help reduce coronary heart disease mortality, but may also favorably influence all-cause mortality."[22]

It is the ratio of omega-3 to omega-6 fatty acids that helps determine whether plaque will form. Certainly, avoiding foods with relatively more omega-6 oils, such as meats, and increasing omega-3 intake from fish will move you in the right direction.

However, you are at an even lower risk if you avoid cholesterol-containing foods altogether. Flaxseed oil, canola oil, walnuts, and the green vegetable purslane, although not as concentrated, are more optimum sources of omega-3 fatty acids, because they contain no associated cholesterol.

Increase Your Fiber Intake

Several prospective studies have shown that dietary fiber decreases your blood levels of total cholesterol by 5 to 10 percent, and LDL by 6 to 12 percent (with minimal effect on "good" HDL). Fiber acts by binding fats you do eat in your digestive tract so they are excreted with the stool rather than absorbed.

Epidemiological and prospective studies have found a significantly reduced risk for heart attack and death from coronary heart disease in men and women in higher fiber intake groups, particularly from cereal sources.[23]

You can reach the daily recommended level of fiber by taking 3 tablespoons of bran, or three servings of whole grain or whole-grain products. You need not buy expensive fiber supplements, and should be skeptical of advertisements; oat bran gives no more protection than any other form of bran. Other rich sources of fiber include fruits (especially apples, pears, and citrus fruits), legumes (peas, beans), and vegetables. One study showed that adding eggplant to your diet may also lower your cholesterol level.[24]

Choose a Vegetarian Diet

Aside from its lack of cholesterol and concentrated undesirable saturated fats, a vegetarian diet also protects you from coronary artery disease by the effects of its plant proteins. Soy protein has been studied extensively. J.W. Anderson and coworkers, in the *New England Journal of Medicine,* reported an analysis of many studies considering the effects of soy protein on blood lipid levels. They found that an average intake of 47 grams per day of soy protein (three or four servings) decreased total cholesterol by 9.3 percent, LDL by 12.9 percent, and triglycerides by 10.5 percent, while increasing "good" HDL cholesterol by 2.4 percent. Those persons with the highest initial baseline levels had the largest reductions—up to 24 percent.

Animal protein has other undesirable effects. Dr. Frank Sachs and his colleagues at the Harvard research labs took individuals already eating a vegetarian diet and added meat protein, disguised in biscuits, so that the participants would not know they were eating it.[25] Not only did blood pressure and cholesterol levels rise, but *anxiety* levels also became elevated—even though the study was designed to take into account any suspicion the participants might have had about what they were eating. (It was a double-blind, crossover research design.) This indicates that components in meat may lead to increased restlessness and anxiety, another very significant observation with implications for the health of our species and planet.

Reduce Your Salt Intake

High dietary sodium (salt) is associated with high blood pressure and stroke. If you are overweight, you are at particular risk for heart disease if you have a salt habit. A nineteen-year prospective follow-up study published in 1999 in the *Journal of the American Medical Association* found a 61 percent increased risk for cardiovascular disease death in the over-weight group with higher salt intake.[26]

Avoid Refined Sugars

Some research has shown a correlation between the incidence of heart disease and ingestion of sugar and other refined foods.[27] Both sucrose and fructose have been documented to increase cholesterol production, as well as triglyceride levels. Diabetics have increased rates of heart disease.

Increase Your Antioxidant Intake

A diet rich in foods containing the antioxidant vitamins C and E and beta-carotene, such as fruits, tomatoes, and vegetables, helps provide protection to your arteries by preventing lipoprotein oxidation and accumulation of plaque.

Green and black teas contain significant levels of antioxidants, and black tea has been found to be associated with a lower risk for heart disease, probably by increasing elasticity of blood vessels via these antioxidant effects. Choose decaf teas, and add skim or soy milk, to neutralize tannic acid levels.

Take Supplements

Vitamin E has been found to reduce the risk of heart attack in men.[28] The daily recommended dose is 400 IU of the D-alpha type.

Vitamins B_6 and folic acid decrease the blood level of homocysteine, an amino acid routinely produced by the body, which damages the cells of blood vessel walls, causes atherosclerotic plaque buildup, and predisposes to thrombosis. Dr. Eric Rimm of Harvard, in a study of 80,082 women in the Nurses' Health Study over a fourteen-year period,

found that the risk of coronary heart disease was decreased by 45 percent in those women with the highest intake of folate and vitamin B_6, compared with those having the lowest intake.

They found that large segments of this population have insufficient dietary intake of folates and B_6 to prevent cardiovascular disease, and that women who regularly used multiple vitamin supplements, as the major source of these vitamins, did best. They concluded that intake *above* the currently recommended dietary allowances may be important. Ingestion of 400 mcg of folic acid and 3 mg of vitamin B_6 per day are required to minimize cardiac disease.[29]

Similarly, a 1998 editorial in the *New England Journal of Medicine* recommended a 400 mcg dose of synthetic folic acid per day by vitamin supplements and/or food fortification, in addition to that consumed in a healthy diet.[30] Take a balanced vitamin B-complex capsule containing 400 mg of folic acid and 50 mg of vitamin B_6 per day.

Oral contraceptive pills antagonize the effects of B_6, folic acid, and other nutrients that affect homocysteine metabolism. This mechanism may be responsible for the increased blood clots and vascular damage associated with the pill, so if you are taking them, be sure to follow these supplement recommendations.[31]

Garlic supplements in the form of allicin-standardized garlic powder tablets have been shown in seventeen of twenty placebo-controlled studies to have significant cholesterol-lowering effects (about 10 percent).[32] Unfortunately, deodorized garlic does not give as much protection. Daily supplementation is suggested at two tablets three times daily—taken just *before* your meals; if you take them at the end of a meal, they sit on top of your food, and you are more likely to be aware of their odiferous nature.

Vitamin C deficiency has been implicated in cardiovascular disease[33]; the daily recommended dose is at least 1,000 mg. The amino acids carnitine and methionine are also considered protective by some investigators; the dosage should be 500 mg three times daily.[34] The mineral chromium was demonstrated to reduce buildup of plaque, and to lower cholesterol; intake should be 200 mcg twice daily.[35] Some researchers feel that the antioxidant vitamins, particularly selenium,[36] also help prevent atherosclerosis; follow the guidelines for these and other supplements detailed in Chapter 2.

Instead of Alcohol, Choose Relaxation Techniques and Red Grape Juice

I know that some studies have supported alcohol use, but I believe that relaxation training is a much better route to prevent heart disease. Further research, comparing persons who drink moderately with those who regularly practice yoga stretches and meditation would clarify this, but currently the widespread health dangers and significant side effects from excess alcohol intake in our society do not warrant recommending it as a way to cope with heart disease. Alcohol-related problems are the number one cause of hospital admissions in this country.

Dr. Rimm and colleagues, in a 1996 review of twenty-five studies of the relationship of alcohol consumption and coronary heart disease, confirmed that moderate alcohol intake substantially reduces the risk of coronary artery disease and heart attack.[37] The benefit varies among the studies, but is about approximately 45 percent reduced risk overall. How and why alcohol accounts for this is not en-

tirely clear, but it has been shown to increase HDL levels and temporarily decrease blood coagulability. Social support and relaxation may be additive to the effects of the alcohol per se. If you regularly practice yoga and other stress-management techniques, and join a support group, you may be able to avoid the side effects of this route to heart disease risk reduction.

The currently recommended optimum amount of alcohol to take seems to be about one or two drinks a day for men and one a day for women. One drink translates to 1 ounce of hard liquor, 4 ounces of wine, or one 12-ounce bottle of beer. Some evidence suggests that red wine is better than white wine, which is better than beer, which in turn is better than hard liquor, although Dr. Rimm's study concluded that all alcoholic drinks are linked with lower risk. Of course, alcohol in excess has some adverse effects on the heart and other organ systems, as well as social and psychological implications and cannot be recommended routinely. *However, women who drink even one glass of wine per day have an elevated risk for breast cancer.* Some researchers believe that red grapes may provide a substitute for alcohol's HDL and clotting effects, avoiding the downside of this controversial risk reduction practice. Further investigation of this nonintoxicating grape connection is needed.

Exercise Three to Five Times per Week for One Hour

Age is a risk factor that cannot be reduced. Especially as you reach the 40- to 50-year age range, you should be conscious of exercise patterns. Many studies have shown that moderate regular exercise reduces your risk of heart disease and stroke, and you live longer.

Exercise has a favorable effect on many of the known risk factors for coronary artery disease—high blood pressure, diabetes, obesity, and cholesterol. It increases "good" HDL cholesterol. In men and postmenopausal women with HDL and LDL levels that place them at high risk for coronary artery disease, Marcia Stefanick and coworkers from Stanford found that exercise was necessary in addition to a low-fat diet to significantly reduce "bad" LDL cholesterol.[38]

However, sudden vigorous activity, particularly in cold weather, can severely strain your heart. Many persons—about 50,000 each year—drop dead from acute heart attacks or heart rhythm disturbances induced by shoveling snow or similar exertion. Exercise programs should start modestly and increase at a safe rate, based on your progress and capability. Persons with known heart disease should be closely monitored. If you are over age 50, you should have a stress test prior to starting an exercise program, to detect any unsuspected disease.

Your aerobic exercise program may consist of one hour of vigorous walking, swimming, riding a bike, or similar activities. Strength and flexibility training such as lifting weights and yoga or tai chi are also important. However, you needn't necessarily work up a sweat to benefit. A report from the Nurses' Health Study found that a 35 to 40 percent risk reduction was possible with three hours of brisk walking each week; as much benefit as one and one-half hours of more vigorous jogging, aerobic dance, and so forth.[39]

Monitor your heart rate, and aim to exercise for twenty minutes after it reaches a rate of 200 minus your age. For example, if you are 55 years old, exercise at a rate of 145 (200 - 55) beats per minute. Initially, do this three times per week, and gradually increase to five times per week. The Ornish program prescribes mild to moderate aerobic exercise for three hours each week. Walking is the recommended form of exercise.

Maintain Your Optimum Weight

Obesity places extra stress on your heart, contributes to the worsening of coronary atherosclerosis, and shortens your life expectancy. If you have gained more than 20 pounds during your adult years, you are at a higher risk for heart disease. Mortality from heart attacks is particularly increased when excess body fat is distributed to give you an "apple" rather than a "pear" shape. If most of your increased weight is in your belly, you are an apple; if in your thighs and hips, you are a pear. The difference in fat distribution may be hormonal, or reflect the liver's ability to process excess fats in the diet.

Regular exercise and dietary modification are both necessary for weight control. Follow the approaches in Chapter 2 to help you achieve and maintain appropriate weight.

Treat Hypertension and Diabetes

Damage to arteries caused by high blood pressure accelerates atherosclerotic heart disease. Use the Ornish program, and follow the guidelines given in Chapter 2. If your blood pressure does not respond, take medication to keep it in the normal range—140/90 or less.

Diabetics are more prone to accelerated atherosclerosis and complications of coronary artery disease. If you have diabetes, dietary change and weight loss alone may help you eliminate this problem. Following the Ornish approach is the optimum treatment for diabetics.

Practice Stress Management and Yoga Daily

Stress has been implicated as a *critical* contributor to the accumulation of fatty buildup and the occurrence of spasm in the coronary arteries. Any outpouring of adrenaline places increased burden on the heart by accelerating its rate and increasing blood pressure. Half of all heart attack victims have had a major stressful event within the previous forty-eight hours.[40]

More heart attacks occur on Monday than any other day of the week. Forty percent of all heart attacks occur during travel, which is often a stressful time. Shorter men have more heart attacks than taller men, perhaps because shorter men may experience higher stress levels in a culture that associates height with power, particularly in the business world. Retirement is one of the most major of life changes, and may put some persons at increased risk for illness.

The story of Paul "Bear" Bryant, the winningest college football coach in history, is significant. Within thirty-seven days of his retirement, he was dead from a heart attack. He had said morosely to his friends just a day before his death "No more Saturdays," and he complained that he had nothing more to which he could look forward. Edger Bergen, the ventriloquist known for his performance with puppet "Charlie McCarthy," died from a heart attack just two weeks after officially putting Charley in a box and retiring from show business. Retirement, especially, means that you should be careful to follow the stress management program in Chapter 2.

Tony Cannigliaro, a well-known ballplayer for the Boston Red Sox, was in excellent health, running eight miles a day, when he learned that the restaurant he owned, located in California, had been damaged by mud slides. While rushing to the Boston airport, he suffered a severe heart attack. Subsequent tests showed that his arteries were perfectly clear but had undergone spasm in response to the stress, causing his heart attack.

As noted, stress may lead to heart attack even if cholesterol plaque in the arteries does not limit blood flow. When angina is caused by spasm, coronary artery bypass grafting is of little value. Control of spasm can be achieved by stress reduction training, yoga, and biofeedback, along with the aforementioned dietary changes.

The number of times per day you feel angry or frustrated has been found to be one of the most predictive indicators of your risk for a heart attack.[41] The authors' father is a good example of the relationship of stress, especially anger, to heart disease. He had a heart attack while watching a basketball game. It was the playoff game between Kentucky and North Carolina; he was living in Kentucky, and they were losing. When asked whether he got angry during games, he was unaware of it. However, our mother pointed out he was always yelling at the coach and the players on the other team. Now, fortunately, he is a devoted follower of the Ornish alternative treatment plan.

Excitement due to *happy* events, such as sexual activity, sports events, movies, or even vacations can also increase demands on the heart, and we should be wary of "too much" of even a good thing. A recent three-million-dollar Virginia lottery winner dropped dead from a heart attack within twenty-four hours of his win. A careful look must be taken at all the stress-producing factors in your life and, if possible, adjustment and retraining should be a priority.

The journal *Science* reported another dimension of this phenomenon. Monkeys fed a high-cholesterol diet developed partial coronary artery blockages. When the animals were stressed, the blocked areas grew two and a half times as large. Nonstressed vegetarian monkeys initially did not have as much blockage, but when they were stressed, their plaques also enlarged two and a half times. However, these vegetarian animals still did not develop plaque large enough to give them significant heart problems.[42] The lesson from this study is that even if you can't learn to control your stress level, a vegetarian diet may protect you from disease.

Stress can also raise your cholesterol levels. Studies have shown that when April 15 rolls around, the blood cholesterol level of tax accountants rises, even though they are eating the same diet.[43] Indianapolis 500 race car drivers likewise have higher cholesterol levels after their races than before, sometimes as much as 50 mg% above that of two hours previously.[44]

Relief of stress may protect you from plaque formation. In a remarkable chance finding, a Chicago study discovered that one group of rabbits fed a plaque-producing diet did not develop as much plaque as the other groups receiving the same diet did. It turned out one of the laboratory technicians was taking those animals out of their cages at night, talking to and petting them.[45] It also works the other way around: Owning a pet may protect you by reducing *your* stress. Those who own pets are more likely to survive their heart attacks, and persons who obtain a pet after a first heart attack are less apt to have a second one.[46]

As part of the Ornish Heart Disease Reversal Program, daily stress reduction classes are taught, using yoga stretches, deep relaxation, breathing exercises, visualization and imagery, and meditation. Patients are advised to use these techniques for an hour each day. Yoga practitioners have long known that the mind influences the body. It was not until the 1960s, however, when Elmer and Alyce Green from the Menninger Clinic took Western technology to India, to study yoga masters there, that the importance of this became an accepted part of Western medicine. Biofeedback was born, merging technological recording devices with the relaxation and mental control of the yoga tradition. For optimum stress management, an hour per day of these techniques is recommended, as described in Chapter 2.

Regular aerobic exercise is also one of the best ways to reduce chronic anxiety or depression, so both active exercise and yoga are recommended.

Socialize More Often; Join a Support Group

A high hostility level has been found to predispose young adults to coronary artery calcification.[47] Hostility, social isolation, and depression have been found to be major risk factors for developing heart disease. They also affect prognosis once heart disease is present. This may partly explain why frequent social activities, such as attending church regularly, increase your chances for surviving a heart attack by 60 percent.[48] Even belonging to a bowling league that meets once a week lowers your risk. Frequent use of the first-person words "I," "me," and "mine" during an interview correlated with increased isolation and was found by Dr. Lawrence Scherwitz to be an effective indicator of a person too socially isolated for his or her own good health.[49] Joining a support group or getting help from a psychologist or psychiatrist may be lifesaving.

Practice Visualization

Visualization may be useful to help open your coronary arteries. For your daily practice, pick a quiet time and place. Do each of the elements given in Chapter 2. Choose any image that assists you to clean your arteries. As one example, imagine your heart as a huge cavern full of pirates' treasure, and your coronary artery as a narrowed passageway to the diamonds and gold. Months earlier, you had found an ancient map underneath a funny-looking rock while jogging through a tropical rain forest. You now find yourself only a hundred feet away from your prize. The passage becomes too small for you to squeeze through (the pirates of the eighteenth century must have been four feet tall). You have a pick and shovel, and you slowly enlarge the passage, and then progress forward to pick up the treasure.

Try Other Approaches

Chelation, a process in which the chemical ethylene-diamine-tetraacetic-acid (EDTA) is given through an intravenous drip, has been proposed to help clear atherosclerotic plaque from arteries. No double-blind scientific evaluation has confirmed this, but some studies do show benefit,[50] and many individuals report improvement of their symptoms. Research in this area is planned, but as of now, no long-term research had yet determined whether life expectancy is improved, or whether ongoing

chelation can cause serious side effects, such as possible damage to the kidneys, as is suspected. Since, as previously discussed, dietary change and lifestyle modification is usually enough to achieve reversal of heart disease, this expensive and not fully tested treatment may be best reserved for those unable or unwilling to change their diets. If you are in this category, you should seek out the latest information on chelation, listed in the Resources section at the back of this book. Make certain your treatment is supervised by your doctor.

Conventional Medicine Approaches to Coronary Artery Disease

Conventional management of coronary artery disease includes lifestyle changes such as weight control, exercise, cessation of smoking, good nutrition, and careful management of general medical problems, particularly hypertension and diabetes. Specific drugs that directly affect the heart, cholesterol level, and blood coagulability can be added if necessary. The ultimate conventional approach to managing severe coronary artery disease is coronary angioplasty and stenting.

Drug Treatments

Drugs have been extensively studied and used to prevent and treat heart disease. Although an in-depth discussion is outside the scope of this book, since most heart patients take one or more of these drugs, the basic concepts will be outlined. In general, the goal is to decrease the imbalance between the heart muscle's demand for oxygen and the ability of its arteries to meet this need. Following are the drugs most commonly used by heart patients.

Nitrate Drugs

These drugs, including nitroglycerin (Nitrostat), isorbode (Isordil), and various paste and patch forms, relieve angina by a blood pressure–lowering effect that decreases the heart's workload. They also increase the flow of blood through diseased coronary arteries, thereby supplying more oxygen to the muscle tissue. They block spasm, and produce maximum dilation of the coronary vessels, by paralyzing the tiny muscle cells in the vessel wall. Nitroglycerin is the best-known drug in this class. When placed under the tongue during an angina attack, it acts very rapidly—relieving pain within a minute or so. Unfortunately, the effect lasts for only twenty to thirty minutes, though this should be long enough to stop the precipitating activity that brought on the angina. Nitroglycerin can also be used in a skin paste or patch form (Nitro-Dur, Nitro-Bid Ointment), which allows it to be slowly absorbed, providing protection over six to eight hours. Side effects from nitroglycerin, such as headaches and dizziness, may be bothersome.

Beta-Blockers

Beta-blocking drugs, such as propranolol (Inderal), metoprolol (Lopressor, Topral), and atenolol (Tenormin), diminish the heart's response to adrenaline and other circulating stimulators. This decreases the heart rate, force of contraction, and blood pressure, and thereby the heart muscle's workload and demand for oxygen. The diseased vessels do not need to supply as much blood flow.

Beta-blockers have been documented to decrease the incidence of repeat heart attacks. However, a price is attached to using these drugs for angina pain reduction. They leave your heart unable to increase output, which may cause weakness, easy tiring, and shortness of breath. Suddenly stopping of one of these drugs gives you increased risk of heart attack and sudden death. Other distressing side effects are nausea and impotence. Some beta-blockers have fewer of these side effects, so you should ask your doctor about them.

Calcium Channel Blockers

Calcium channel blocking agents, such as diltiazem (Diltia, Cardizem, Dilacor), verapamil (Calan, Covera, Isoptin), and nifedipine (Adalat, Procardia) do not produce the beta-blockers' side effects, and have been found to be especially useful in angina caused by coronary artery spasm.

Calcium dissolved in body fluids plays a role in muscle cell contraction. The calcium channel blockers inhibit its movement across muscle cell membranes, preventing muscle spasm in the coronary vessel walls. They also decrease the heart muscle's force of contraction and, thereby, its need for oxygen. These drugs may also slow the progression of atherosclerosis.

However, some calcium channel blockers have recently been implicated in an increased risk of heart attacks following their use for treatment of hypertension. Their exact role in the future depends on further research to determine which patients may be at this increased risk.

Other drugs also may be used to control blood pressure, heart failure, and heart rhythm disturbances, all of which are important because they decrease demands on the heart and increase its efficiency. If you have an enlarged heart or heart failure, derivatives of a drug called digitalis, and diuretics such as

Diuril and Lasix (medications that decrease fluid pressure in your tissues by increasing urine output), may be used to control these problems. This will lower your heart's oxygen needs, preventing angina.

Cholesterol-Lowering Drugs

As noted above, cholesterol is an important factor in forming plaque that narrows the arteries in the heart and the rest of the body. Several types of cholesterol-lowering drugs decrease the rate of progression of atherosclerosis, halt it altogether, and even reverse it in some patients. They also stabilize rupture-prone plaques, and decrease the likelihood of blood clot formation. Even small amounts of plaque reversal, as seen on angiogram, can lead to a marked decrease in angina and risk for heart attack and death. Many studies have shown the benefits of these drugs, and found their effects proportional to the reduction in total cholesterol and particularly LDL.

Niacin (vitamin B$_3$) is an inexpensive drug that decreases total cholesterol level and increases HDL. Its mechanism of action is poorly understood. You may experience the side effects of facial flushing, fatigue, and skin discoloration. The rapid-release type of niacin, rather than the sustained-release form, should be chosen, because the latter has been associated with liver toxicity.

Cholestyramine (Questran) and colestipol (Colestid) bind with bile acids in the intestine, removing these acids with the stool. This increases the body's breakdown of cholesterol, decreasing blood cholesterol levels. These drugs can cause constipation and gastrointestinal disturbance.

The "statin" drugs, more expensive medications that decrease cholesterol levels, such as gemfibrozil (Lopid), simvastatin (Zocor),

pravastatin (Pravachol), and atorvastatin (Lipitor) have been shown to be beneficial. In three five-year studies involving 15,000 persons, cholesterol-lowering drugs decreased heart attack deaths by 31 to 42 percent, and the need for coronary angioplasty or bypass surgery by 37 percent. Strokes and deaths from any cause were also reduced. One study included persons with symptoms of heart disease and elevated cholesterol,[51] one looked at patients with previous heart attacks but traditionally average cholesterol levels,[52] and the other at persons with high cholesterol but no history of coronary artery disease.[53] All these research projects showed significant benefit.

The recent Air Force/Texas Coronary Atherosclerosis Prevention Study showed that benefit from a Step I low-fat diet (30 percent calories from fat) and a "statin" cholesterol-lowering drug is even extended to healthy middle-aged and older men and women with average total cholesterol, average (bad) LDL but below-average (good) HDL levels. It found a 37 percent decreased risk of first heart attack, unstable angina, and death from coronary heart disease; a 33 percent reduction in the need for coronary revascularization; and a reduction in overall stroke mortality. This study indicated that approximately 6 million Americans not currently treated would benefit from cholesterol-lowering drugs.[54] Another 2000 study reported in the *New England Journal of Medicine* found that statin treatment of men with coronary disease with low (good) LDL levels resulted in a 24 percent reduction in the combined outcome of death from coronary disease, nonfatal heart attack, and stroke. These results were thought to be related to increased HDL and lower triglyceride levels.[55]

The National Institutes of Health's National Cholesterol Education Project guideline for beginning drug therapy if you don't already have heart disease is an LDL greater than 190 if you have less than two risk factors for cardiovascular disease and 160 if you have two or more risk factors. It is 130 if you already have heart disease.[56] However, these drugs are expensive ($900 to $1,800 per patient per year) and may produce side effects such as liver and kidney damage. Since increased cholesterol levels are usually responsive to lifestyle manipulation, we suggest you begin these drugs only if you are at high risk and fail a trial of the dietary changes, weight loss, and other alternative medicine approaches.

Hyperthyroidism, liver disease, or diabetes may elevate cholesterol. When these conditions are treated, cholesterol levels can be brought under control. If you have familial hypercholesterolemia, a genetic tendency to produce too much cholesterol, cholesterol-lowering medication may be needed.

Drugs Affecting Blood Clotting

Low-dose aspirin, by decreasing platelet "stickiness," is beneficial in protecting against clot formation and the complications of ulcerated plaques. It provides protection in the brain and heart circulation, and its regular use is also advised by many doctors for leg circulation problems.

Taking an aspirin every day, or every other day, was found to decrease first heart attacks in men over age 50 by 44 percent in the Physicians' Health Study.[57] It also has been shown to decrease second heart attacks, strokes, and cardiovascular deaths in both men and women by 25 percent.[58] The U.S. Preventive Services Task Force recommends that men over 40 take aspirin whenever the risk for coronary artery disease outweighs the risk of aspirin complications. The Nurses' Health Study suggests that this recommendation is as beneficial for women as for men.

If you are at increased risk for coronary artery disease or stroke and you cannot take aspirin because you are sensitive to it or taking other drugs that would be incompatible with it, the more expensive drugs dipyrimidol (Persantine), ticlopidine (Ticlid), or clopidogrel (Plavex), which have an effect on platelets, can be substituted.

Estrogen Replacement

Estrogen replacement after menopause increases HDL, the "good" cholesterol, by up to 15 percent, decreases LDL, the "bad" cholesterol, by 15 percent, and decreases the amount of LDL incorporated into coronary arteries. It also improves the dynamics of coronary blood vessel elasticity, allowing increased flow. A study by M. K. Hong and associates found an 87 percent reduction in the prevalence of coronary artery disease as seen on an angiogram in postmenopausal women taking estrogen replacement.[59] A review of thirty-two epidemiological studies demonstrated that estrogen replacement decreases the risk for heart disease in postmenopausal women by 44 percent.[60] However, there may be no benefit for women with established coronary disease. A 2000 report from the Nurses' Health Study demonstrated no beneficial effect, at least in the short term in women who already had coronary disease.[61] In fact, in the first year of HRT treatment, the Heart and Estrogen/Progesterone Replacement Study of 2,763 women with established coronary disease found an increased risk of coronary events, though a benefit was found in the fourth and fifth years.[62]

The general trend to place postmenopausal women on estrogen to prevent cardiovascular disease, menopausal symptoms, and osteoporosis is unfortunately accompanied by an increased risk for breast and endometrial cancer, as well as blood clots and gallbladder disease. Fortunately, both heart disease and osteoporosis can be prevented by following the dietary recommendations given in this chapter and Chapter 2, and the side effects of menopause can be controlled by less dangerous means, such as vitamins, herbs, and exercise. See Chapter 19 for further discussion of the HRT debate. See also Dr. Michael Murray's book *Menopause: How You Can Benefit from Diet, Vitamins, Minerals, Herbs, Exercise, and Other Natural Methods (Getting Well Naturally).*[63]

Angioplasty and Stent Treatment

Angioplasty is a procedure that opens blocked blood vessels by use of a balloon-tipped catheter—inserted through an artery in the arm or groin—that is manipulated into the area of the blockage. When the balloon is expanded, the narrowed area is squeezed or cracked open to enlarge the channel. (See Figure 8.4.) Since angioplasty for blocked coronary vessels was first introduced in 1977, it has assumed a prominent place in the management of this disease. It is estimated that in 1999 more than 1.3 million coronary revascularization procedures were performed worldwide, almost twice as many as the estimated 700,000 surgical coronary bypasses.[64]

Stents are tiny wire mesh tubes that are collapsed onto the balloon catheter, then carried to the narrowed area. The balloon acts to expand the wire mesh to a rigid position, that props the artery open. (For a futher discussion of this, see "Radiologic Catheter Techniques to Treat Artery Disease" on page 295.) A 2000 *JAMA* review of published studies found that stents have been shown to reduce the need for repeated coronary procedures by 35 to 75 percent, reduce restenosis in coronary arteries by 20 to 55 percent, reduce the need for later coronary bypass, and are now used in 80 percent of all angioplasty procedures in the United States.[65] It is estimated that more than 500,000 patients received stents in 1999.[66] Unfortunately, no trial has yet shown that stents reduce risk of myocardial infarction or risk of death.[67] In fact, several studies have shown increased risk for these complications when compared with balloon angioplasty alone.[68] It is hoped that emerging stent technology along with use of newer drugs will extend the short-term benefits of stents into long-term decrease in mortality.

Thrombolysis is a procedure that may prevent or diminish heart muscle death if you are having a heart attack, and may be lifesaving if begun early in its course. Medication (tissue plasminogen activator—TPA) can be dripped through a coronary artery catheter to dissolve a fresh blood clot. To get these drugs working as soon as possible, they can be given intravenously in emergency rooms and even by 911 crews on site, with radio/telephone supervision from an ER doctor. For most patients, this approach is likely to be much more available and timely than angioplasty by an experienced team. After thrombolysis, angioplasty and stenting can be used to treat any underlying remaining blockage. However, if an experienced team is rapidly available shortly after the onset of an acute heart attack, emergency angioplasty and stenting have been shown to have long-term results that are superior to thrombolysis alone.[69]

Not all patients qualify for angioplasty because the disease may be too diffuse (especially if all three major vessels are involved), it may not be possible to reach the constricted

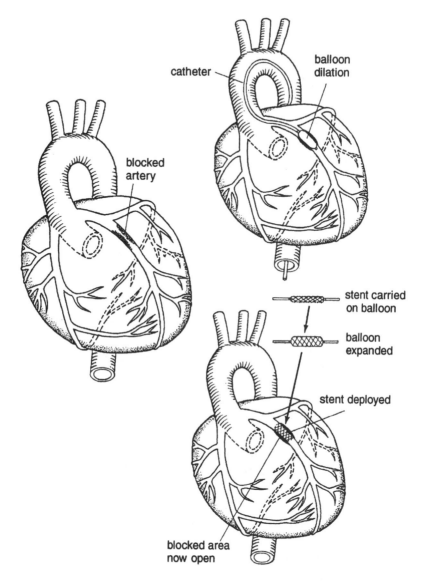

Fig. 8.4 Procedures involved in coronary artery balloon angioplasty and stent treatment

area with the catheter, or it may be too stiff or angulated to dilate; however, when angioplasty is successful, as it is in more than 90 percent of all cases initially, it can eliminate your symptoms and help you avoid the bypass operation. At the time of the procedure, you have a 3 percent risk that artery damage, rupture, or a clot can make you worse, and a 1 to 2 percent chance you will then need an emergency bypass. The acute mortality is 1 percent.

Unfortunately, one-third to one-half of patients' arteries reblock within six months, necessitating a repeat angioplasty or surgical bypass. Reblockage and the need for emergency bypass caused by complications of angioplasty have been dramatically reduced when stents are used.[70] Be sure to ask about the latest results. Once you have had angioplasty, with or without a stent, your artery is less likely to respond fully to the Ornish reversal program.

Two studies published in *Circulation* in 1997 document that you should choose an experienced angiographer or cardiologist, and have your procedure in a hospital that performs a large volume of these interventions. Steven Ellis and his associates found that complications including induced heart attack, death, and need for emergency bypass, were 9.3 percent in the group performed by the operators who did the lowest volume compared to only 2.9 percent in patients in the highest volume operator group.[71] James Jollis and his group studied 97,478 angioplasties done by 6,115 physicians in 984 hospitals. They found that low-volume physicians had higher rates for their patients needing to go on to bypass surgery, and low-volume hospitals were associated with higher rates of bypass surgery and death. They also found that more than 50 percent of physicians and 25 percent of hospi-

tals failed to meet the minimum-volume guidelines first published by the American College of Cardiology/American Heart Association (50 angioplasties per physician and 200 per hospital) and that these patients had the worst outcomes.[72] The best results are when the physician performs 225 to 270 cases annually.[73]

Surgical Approaches to Coronary Artery Disease

The CABG or "cabbage" is the standard surgical procedure for treating coronary artery disease not responsive to medical or alternative management. Recently, variations have become available that attempt to reduce some of the discomfort and drawbacks of the classic procedure.

Coronary Artery Bypass Grafting

An open heart operating room may present the most fascinating and mesmerizing theater in the world today. Usually harmonious, but at times chaotic, the action is ever-changing. A surgical team of six to eight members is clustered around different centers of activity. In the center of the room, under the glare of overhead lights, your chest is spread wide open by rigid retractors. All eyes focus on the purple, motionless heart. The surgeon's skill is demonstrated by fluid and graceful movements which rapidly place stitches between your heart's diseased artery and the bypass graft, which will bring increased blood flow to tissue previously starved for oxygen. Assistant surgeons facilitate by retracting, sucking up blood, cauterizing bleeding, and tying and cutting stitches. The scrub nurse guards trays full of special instruments, wordlessly passing the correct one to the surgeon's outstretched hand. A second team may be simultaneously "harvesting" a portion of your leg vein, for the vein bypass graft or grafts.

Meanwhile, away from the center of action, other team members perform duties critical to your life. The specially skilled cardiac anesthesiologist is responsible to keep you in a deep sleep, with all your muscles relaxed and motionless. Just as essential is the monitoring of critical lung, kidney, and brain function, adjusted when necessary by the use of respirator settings, fluid rates, and medications. The heart/lung pump machine technician shifts flow rates and pressures to ensure that your body's organs receive oxygen and nutrients when your heart is not performing its duties.

A few hours after you are put to sleep and your heart arrested comes the most dramatic point in the whole performance. The grafts have been placed. Will the heart successfully resume its rhythmic pumping when it is warmed and kick-started? A collective sigh of relief signals successful return of efficient contractions. The team's blood pressure and heart rates return to normal, and the levity begins as the incisions are closed. Last night's baseball game is detailed, hospital politics argued, and the latest joke retold.

More than 700,000 coronary artery bypass grafting (CABG or "cabbage") operations were performed worldwide in 1999.[74] This operation is now used in the 20 to 40 percent of angina patients whose symptoms cannot be controlled by drug therapy, and who still have enough pain to interfere with daily life. If your angina does *not* respond to either medication or alternative therapies, and angioplasty is not possible, you have an indication for surgery.

This operation is successful in initially eliminating or reducing angina in more than 90 percent of all patients.[75] Randomized studies have shown that coronary bypass is more effective than medical treatment in relieving angina, improving exercise and work capability, and improving overall quality of life.[76] If you have had a heart attack at an early age, or have continued angina after a heart attack, you may also benefit from surgery. It may also be advised soon after a heart attack to prevent further damage. Compared to angioplasty, and stents, coronary bypass is followed by less angina, less recurrent coronary artery blockage and need for further procedures, and fewer late heart attacks. Also, it is preferred for diabetics on drug or insulin therapy with more than one diseased coronary artery who need an initial procedure.[77] However, it is more expensive, $44,200 (1992) versus $21,700 (1993) for angioplasty,[78] requires more hospital time, and has more operative deaths, complications, strokes, and early heart attacks. Overall, the five-year mortality of 11 percent is about the same.[79] Evolving technology is steadily improving the results of both techniques.

Will your *life expectancy* be extended with coronary artery bypass grafting? Large studies have indicated that if you have angina with mild exertion or at rest, you will survive longer with coronary artery revascularization, rather than conventional medical therapy.[80] An analysis of all the randomized studies comparing bypass surgery with conventional medical therapy indicated that almost all patients benefit from revascularization.[81] The appropriate answer probably depends on the location and extent of your disease, as determined by coronary angiography. In general, the more coronary vessels that are found to be diseased, the more beneficial bypass surgery is compared to medical treatment alone. If you have disease in your left main coronary artery or in all three arteries, you may clearly expect to live longer after CABG. If you have only one or two diseased arteries, you probably would not extend your longevity by surgery unless these vessels are more than 75 percent blocked or you have impaired left ventricular function. If you have only one artery diseased, and it is not the left main coronary, you should not undergo bypass surgery unless you have lifestyle-limiting angina. If your angina is relieved by medical treatment and lifestyle changes, you may achieve comparable or even increased longevity, by not having surgery.[82]

If you choose bypass surgery, you are brought to the operating room on a stretcher. Six or eight doctors, nurses, and technicians, are all very busy setting up machines and instruments for the operation. After you are under general anesthesia, a breathing tube and various wires and catheters are placed to measure blood pressure, body temperature, cardiac and lung function, and urine output. An incision is made in your sternum (breastbone) from the base of your neck to your upper abdomen. Other incisions may be made in your leg(s) to "harvest" (remove) veins for the bypass grafts.

Instruments called retractors are used to spread the sternum, so your heart is easily accessible. Since the structures are so delicate, and the surgical technique must be precise, this operation usually is not performed on a beating heart. The heart is bathed in a potassium chemical solution and cooled with ice water to stop it. Blood is taken from a catheter placed in the large vein entering your heart (vena cava) and shunted through a *cardiopulmonary bypass machine*, also called a heart/lung machine, which takes over the functions of your heart and lungs while the operation is in progress. Here carbon dioxide is exchanged for oxygen, then blood is pumped back to your body through a tube placed in your groin.

Coronary artery bypass grafting can use either a piece of vein taken from your leg (most common), or an artery from within your chest (internal mammary artery), arm (radial artery), or abdomen, for the conduit to reroute blood flow around a blocked artery. Artificial plastic grafts cannot be used. Your diseased artery is opened beyond where it is blocked, in a relatively normal area, so that the graft can be attached, with many fine stitches. Several blocked areas can be bypassed during the same operation, using one or more grafts. Figure 8.5 illustrates some of the possible hook-up configurations. Once surgery is complete, the heart is rewarmed, stimulated with drugs, and may be shocked to get it going again. After usual rhythm and pumping action returns, you are taken off the bypass machine. The breastbone incision is closed with wires, and the skin with stitches or staples. The surgery takes from two to five hours, depending on the complexity of the procedure.

You awaken in the recovery room or special cardiac surgery intensive care unit, and are closely monitored until all of your body functions are stable. Your family can visit once you are settled in. Four to twelve hours later, after you are wide awake, and strong enough to no longer need support from the lung ventilator, the breathing tube is removed, and you can talk. You can probably be out of bed and start eating on the first day after the surgery. When intravenous medication drips are no longer necessary, and your organs are functioning well, you are transferred out of intensive care to a "step-down" unit where intermediate monitoring is available, and then to a regular hospital room.

Pain associated with your chest and leg incisions is usually controlled by IV medications

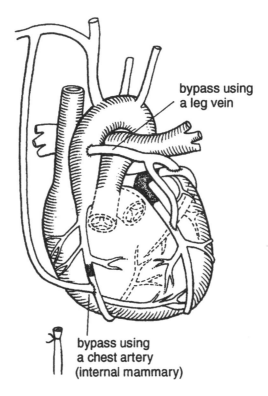

bypass using
a leg vein

bypass using
a chest artery
(internal mammary)

Fig. 8.5 Types of coronary artery bypass graft hookups

for the first few days, and then you are switched to pills. Some leg swelling may persist for weeks, due to the incisions required to harvest your leg veins used for the bypass grafts. Neighboring blood vessels easily compensate for the missing vein (or chest artery if you had this type of graft), without long-term side effects. You can probably be discharged in five to seven days.

Your cardiac surgeon and cardiologist should see you in follow-up office visits to ensure good healing and heart function. You should be instructed on how to begin a graduated exercise program, and can probably return to work in six to eight weeks.

Complications include all those common to a major operation, as well as several spe-

cific ones: the inability of the heart to resume normal activity after it is rewarmed, stroke, bleeding from the graft stitches, and infection in the chest or leg incision. Risk for complications depends on the degree of your heart disease, your overall health, and the skill of the operating team. The mortality rate is generally 1 to 4 percent, but may be higher for older, poor-risk patients and for less-active surgical teams. Complications and mortality for second CABG operations are twice as high because of technical difficulty caused by scar tissue and sicker patients.

As with angioplasty, you should choose an experienced heart surgeon and a high-volume hospital. E. L. Hannan and colleagues studied the relationship between the number of procedures performed by heart surgeons and hospitals and the mortality rate for all bypass surgeries in New York State in 1989. They found that both surgeon and hospital volumes were significantly related to mortality rate. Surgeons who performed 180 or more procedures and hospitals with 700 or more had a mortality rate of 2.67 percent compared with a rate of 4.29 percent for those with lesser volumes.[83] *You should become familiar with the success and reputation of the team chosen for your surgery; they should perform at least 150 to 200 bypass operations a year.*

After surgery, your bypass grafts can themselves become blocked, due to complications or progressive atherosclerosis. Veins block up faster than arteries used for bypass because veins have a thinner, less well protected wall. Five to twenty percent of all vein grafts block in the first year. Thereafter the rate is 2 to 4 percent per year, reaching 22 to 30 percent at five years and 50 percent at 10 years.[84] Stent placement in a narrowed bypass graft may be beneficial, and reduce your need for repeated procedures.[85] Artery grafts do much better. Their blockage rate is only 5 percent at one year, 6 percent at eight years, and less than 15 percent at ten years.[86] After fifteen years, one in seven patients who have vein grafts require reoperation. This is twice the rate for patients having at least one internal mammary artery graft.[87]

Overall, after a first CABG operation using vein grafts, 90 percent of all patients survive for five years, 80 percent for ten years, and 58 percent for fifteen years. After internal mammary graft CABG procedures, the survival is better, 89 percent at ten years.[88] These results are generally better than for medical treatment, although the results tend to become similar after ten years. All of the statistics looking at long-term follow-up of medical treatment, angioplasty, and bypass surgery are based on technology that may now be outdated, so you can expect better results in the future.

Beating Heart Bypass

An approach to avoid the complications of the bypass pump is currently a hot topic. Some surgeons are doing bypass operations on coronary arteries with the heart still beating. "Beating heart bypass" presumably avoids known pump-related complications of postoperative neurologic dysfunction, emboli of blood clots and debris, and the diffuse inflammatory response produced when blood contacts the artificial surfaces of the bypass pump circuitry. Inflammatory mediators may affect the heart, lungs, kidneys, brain, and gastrointestinal tract organs. Not all patients are candidates for this procedure, it may be difficult to do a full revascularization, and most cardiac surgeons haven't had experience with it. More studies need to be evaluated but it looks promising.[89]

Transmyocardial Revascularization

Transmyocardial revascularization (TMR) is a new, and at this point experimental, technique that may prove beneficial if you have failed medical treatment and cannot have angioplasty or bypass surgery because of the diffuse nature of your coronary artery blockages. Often such patients have already had one of these techniques, but still have symptoms or are in danger.

The chest is opened through a small incision between the ribs. Unlike for bypass surgery, it is unnecessary to stop the heart or connect the patient to a heart/lung machine.

The surgeon then uses a computerized laser device to burn fifteen to forty 1-millimeter holes through the one-half-inch wall of the left ventricle. This allows oxygen-rich blood from the left heart chamber to directly enter into the tiny spongy areas between the muscle fibers, rather than having to circulate through diseased coronary arteries to get there. The blood clots, and forms a plug, where it meets the air on the heart's outer surface, thereby preventing a leak. Recovery is much quicker than after the CABG procedure.

Initial results are promising. In a study of 200 patients at eight medical centers, 80 percent had relief of angina, 52 percent were able to decrease their medications, and hospitalizations were decreased by 70 percent. The mortality rate within thirty days after TMR is 8 percent, but the results after one year are much better than after medical treatment alone.[90] Long-term results are unknown. You can ask the department of cardiac surgery at a major medical center to find where this procedure is available in your region.

Minimally Invasive or Limited-Access Heart Surgery

Two procedures are being developed and evaluated to determine if coronary bypass can be done safely and effectively using small incisions, minimal overall trauma, and a quick recovery time, as an alternative to traditional bypass techniques.

Port-access coronary artery bypass (PAC-CAR or PORTCAB) requires that your heart be stopped and you be placed on a heart/lung machine just as in the standard CABG procedure. Several small holes are made in your chest wall, so that ports can be placed to pass a camera and instruments through to reach the heart, similar to laparoscopic surgery in the abdomen. While watching on a TV monitor, your surgeons connect bypass grafts to the coronary arteries beyond blocked areas, just as in the standard CABG procedure. The obvious advantage is less trauma and a quicker recovery. The disadvantage is less access to reach all areas of the heart.

Minimally invasive coronary artery bypass (MIDCAB) avoids the use of the heart/lung machine. Surgery is performed while the heart is still beating. Usually, only one or two arteries are bypassed. The operation uses ports similar to PORTCAB, but also a small incision directly over the artery to be bypassed. Your surgeon directly views the artery while the graft is sewn in place, rather than by watching on a TV camera. The big advantage is avoidance of the possible complications of stopping the heart and using the heart/lung machine, as well as quicker recovery. The disadvantage is the technical difficulty of working with tiny arteries and suture material while the heart is moving.

Both of these options are in their early developmental stages at many medical centers. So far, results haven't been as good as standard procedures,[91] with decreased graft success and increased stroke, heart infarction, reoperation, and death rate. These procedures cannot be recommended outside an experimental study until more experience is gained and the data analyzed. At this point, they are also both still much more invasive than coronary angioplasty.

CORONARY ARTERY DISEASE SUMMARY

Prevention

Diet and Supplements

- Follow a low-fat, high-fiber vegetarian diet—less than 5 g cholesterol and less than 10 percent of calories from fat (less than 14 g fat daily).
- Substitute monounsaturated for saturated fats.
- Avoid refined sugars.
- Reduce your salt intake.
- Vitamin C, 1,000–2,000 mg, 2–3 times daily.
- Vitamin E, D-alpha, 400 IU, 2 times daily.
- Vitamin B-complex capsule containing 400 mcg of folic acid and 50 mg of vitamin B_6 daily.
- Garlic powder tablets, 2 tablets, 3 times daily.
- Carnitine and methionine, 500 mg, 3 times daily.
- Flaxseed oil, 1 tablespoon daily.
- Coenzyme Q10, 150 mg daily.
- Red wine or grape juice, 1–2 glasses daily.
- Green and black decaf teas, add skim or soy milk.

Lifestyle

- Don't smoke.
- Practice daily yoga.
- Exercise 1 hour, 3–5 times a week.
- Maintain optimum weight.
- Practice stress management.
- Socialize more often.

Alternative Medicine Approaches

- Follow the preventive guidelines, above.
- Weekly support group, socialize more often, attend church services, learn to have a longer fuse on anger.
- Practice visualization.
- Try chelation (controversial).

Conventional Medicine Approaches

- Treat hypertension and diabetes.
- Alcohol, 1–2 drinks daily.

Medications

- Nitrate drugs—nitroglycerin, nitropaste, Nitrostat, Isordil, Nitro-Bid.
- Beta-blockers—propranolol, metoprolol, atenolol, Inderal, Lopressor, Tobral, Tenormin.
- Calcium channel blockers—diltiazem, nifedipine, verapamil, Adalet, Calan, Procardia, Cardiziem.
- Cholesterol-lowering drugs—niacin, cholestyramine, Questran, colestipol, Colestid, gemfibrozil, Lopid, pravastatin, Pravacid, simvastatin, Zocor, atorvastatin, Lipitor, clofibrate, Atromid.
- Drugs affecting blood clotting—aspirin, dipyrimidol, Persantine, ticlopidine, Ticlid, clopidogrel (Plavix).
- Estrogen replacement—Premarin, Estrace, Estraderm.

Procedures

- Balloon angioplasty, stenting.
- Thrombolysis.

Surgical Approaches

- Coronary artery bypass—heart bypass machine, "beating heart" bypass.
- Limited Access Heart Surgery—PAC-CAR, MIDCAB.
- Transmyocardial revascularization.

ARTERIES

My Leg

My leg is gone now but I shouldn't cry
It was either that or possibly die
And efforts were made for almost a year
Surgery after surgery to keep arteries clear
Hoping for the best but prepared for the worst
On May 21 the bypass burst
Tied off to stem the flow, then evaluated,
Amputation was ordered and operated
A new life of learning I now undergo
Adapting to a pace painstakingly slow
While I learn to maneuver with crutches and such
Urged on by dear ones who care so very much
I struggle with my stump as I carry on
Fighting the "phantom pains" in a foot that's gone
Waiting for the day when I'm finally fit
With an artificial leg and can get around on it
My heart cries for the Surgeon who did his best
To keep two usable legs on this Mr. W
It's like an artist's mural, where he gave his all
Then had to return and tear down the wall
My big consolation out of this ordeal
It may sound silly but it's for real
My leg is educating Interns at "U-Dub"
While my formal learning was a high school "grad"
My left leg got a chance that I never had
It went to college, if only as a tool
For research at Washington's Medicine School
                                    Wendell H. West

Wendell West is an active 61 years old, but still addicted to cigarettes despite years of suffering at their expense. He had gone through terrifying discomfort and lifestyle limitations generated by a series of failed leg artery operations. His sense of humor is a major support, and he expressed it in the above poem.

Vascular disease and its threat of amputation and stroke are frightening to contemplate. Alternative medicine brings new help, offering approaches which focus on prevention. You may be able to completely avoid an artery operation, or use these methods to convalesce more quickly from one. You also may not have to undergo stroke prevention surgery, or recover more fully from the devastation of a stroke should it develop.

As we will present in detail, your options in surgery have also expanded, giving you new possibilities for full return of function. Operating on the arteries and veins, other than the heart, called "peripheral vascular surgery," was until the 1950s limited to the tying off of traumatized, bleeding vessels, and amputations. Since then, techniques have been developed to replace diseased segments of arteries using your own veins, or graft material made of plastic. Hundreds of thousands of such vascular operations are now performed each year. Virtually any of your major blood vessels can be repaired, replaced, or bypassed, and your blood flow restored.

Very often, such surgery on your blood vessels is a triumph. You can resume satisfying activities, with your self-confidence and self-esteem regained. However, these procedures treat only your symptoms, not your underlying disease. One operation can lead to another if you do not also address the causative lifestyle factors.

Practically every person facing vascular surgery has a long history of smoking. The typical high-fat American diet is also a major contributor. If you stop smoking, you are two to four times more likely to have successful results. If you change your diet and follow other lifestyle recommendations, you may immediately begin to *reverse* your symptoms.

Diabetes is often a major contributing factor to artery problems, as high blood pressure is to strokes. Alternative medicine contributes a new range of techniques for tackling these problems.

In this chapter, we will focus on disorders of the arteries to the legs and brain; vein problems are considered in the next chapter. If you have been told you have vascular disease but are not facing an emergency, we both agree you can safely embark upon a trial of the alternative medicine approaches, since you have a good chance your symptoms will get better without your having to undergo surgery.

How Your Arteries Work

The richly colorful blood, bright red and full of promise, moves with the steady push of the heart out into your limbs, allowing you to stretch them and walk, run and twirl, and even, occasionally, jump for joy. Each of these movements directly depends upon the health of your blood vessels.

Blood serves as your body's transport medium, and the blood vessels are its highway. The heart, by pushing the blood through your vessels to all parts of your body, allows your organs to keep in touch with one another. Blood distributes oxygen, nutrients, hormones, and other substances to your body's cells. The cells exchange their waste products for this input, and use these materials to give them energy and direction for their specific functions.

If blood flow is cut off, the cells served by the obstructed vessel begin to slow down, and their toxic waste products build up. Eventually, after running through temporary alternative energy sources, these cells cease to function altogether, and they die. Some such cells, like the brain neurons and heart muscle cells, have very high energy needs, so that interruption of their blood flow produces effects almost immediately. Other cells, such as those comprising skin, bone, and skeletal muscle, can survive several hours of interrupted flow.[1]

The *aorta*, the large artery emerging from the heart, gives off major branches to your body's organs. (See Figure 9.1.) The first are the *coronary* arteries, serving the heart muscle itself, then those to the brain and the arms; next it turns downward through the chest, and enters the abdomen. From there it sends offshoots to the abdominal organs, and finally divides, to supply the legs.

Throughout most of your arterial system, small arteries serve as interconnections be-

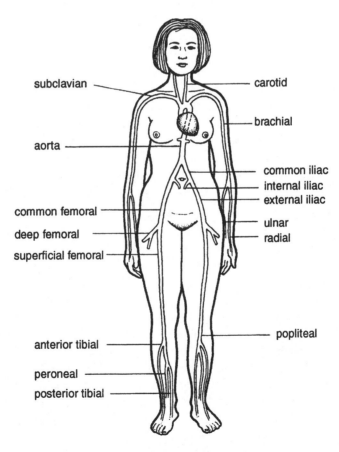

subclavian

carotid

brachial

aorta

common iliac

internal iliac

external iliac

common femoral

ulnar

deep femoral

radial

superficial femoral

popliteal

anterior tibial

peroneal

posterior tibial

Fig. 9.1 The main arteries of the body

tween the various larger arteries and their branches, so that some protection is provided should one artery become blocked or damaged. When an obstruction appears slowly, these smaller collateral vessels enlarge to carry more blood, which thus bypasses the blocked artery, routing the blood back into the main channel. If your natural collaterals are not sufficient, bypass surgery creates a similar effect.

Artery Disease

The arms and hands are well protected against arterial blockage by rich collateral vessels, making problems in these areas very unusual.

The classic symptom of arterial peripheral vascular disease is pain in the legs associated with exercise, the result of your muscles not getting enough oxygen and nutrients to meet their increased needs. The medical term for this is *claudication*, which means limping, and describes the pain that develops when you are walking. *Claudication distance* refers to the typical distance you can walk before symptoms are felt. Usually the ache disappears after you rest for a few minutes, and you can then continue on, repeating the walking and resting cycle. Only 5 percent of all patients with claudication eventually face amputation.

If you experience discomfort even while resting, the situation is more ominous, and your limb may be in danger. This serious problem is worse at night, when blood pressure tends to decrease, and less blood reaches the diseased area. Called "rest pain," it is usually felt in the toes and front of the feet, and may force you to get out of bed—to walk around, or hang your leg over the edge of the bed—in order to restore the flow of blood

into your lower leg and foot. Skin ulcers and minor leg wounds that do not heal also indicate poor circulation, and possible need for surgery to bring more blood to the affected areas. Fifty percent of patients with this type of problem eventually face amputation.

If blood supply to your nerves is decreased, you may experience other symptoms, such as numbness and tingling. Impotence can be caused by associated decreased circulation in your pelvic vessels, while compromised circulation to your intestines creates abdominal pain, most often after meals, when your digestive system creates higher demands for blood. Strokes and heart attacks develop if the blood supply to your brain or heart is interrupted.

A dangerous reduction in the blood supply to a particular area of the body may not always produce symptoms until the damage is already severe. One common example is the kidneys, where decreased circulation can cause insidious loss of kidney function as well as high blood pressure.

If you have arterial disease, you are most likely to have a slow, progressive increase in symptoms. You therefore have time to obtain an exact diagnosis and consider your alternatives. However, the onset of problems from blocked arteries can also be rapid, and even threaten your life and limb, such as when a thrombosis (blood clot) or embolus (migrating piece of clot or cholesterol) suddenly obstructs one of your arteries. In these cases, you may need immediate surgery.

The most common cause of arterial vascular problems is *atherosclerosis*—a usually progressive disease in which a sludgelike material builds up within the walls of the arteries throughout your body. (See Chapter 8 for a full discussion of the atherosclerotic process.) The combined elements of diet, smoking, diabetes, family history, blood pressure, and ability to handle stress all play important contributory roles. As discussed in Chapter 8, evidence now suggests that atherosclerosis is both preventable and reversible by dietary and lifestyle changes, or by drug treatment.

How Artery Disease Is Diagnosed

The diagnosis of arterial vascular disease begins by your doctor taking a careful history of your symptoms, lifestyle, and associated diseases, followed by a thorough physical examination.

History

Your doctor should ask you questions about the type and exact location of your symptoms, such as pain, cramps, tingling or numbness, cold sensations, and impotency, as well as when they started, how they have progressed, what brings them on, and what (if anything) you have been able to do to relieve them. Also very important, is how any limitations impinge on your work requirements and lifestyle, preventing you from doing what you need or like to do.

You should discuss the main risk factors of smoking, diabetes, hypertension, and high cholesterol levels. Attention to these may allow you to avoid surgery. Report any past history of heart disease or strokes, and any medications you are taking.

Physical Exam

Your skin should be examined for a number of factors: the presence of discolorations and ulcers; warmth; the time it takes for pinkness to return after squeezing the blood out; and the time required for blood to return to your superficial veins after they are first emptied by elevation, then placed in a dependent position. A stethoscope can find "bruits," the harsh sounds produced by blood flowing through a narrowed area. Key checkpoints are the arterial pulses felt in the neck, arms, groin, behind the knees, and feet. Differences in one arm or leg, when compared with its opposite, may be significant. Your abdomen is examined for evidence of an aneurysm.

Doppler Exam

In the initial vascular evaluation, your doctor may use a *Doppler flow probe* to listen to your blood pressure and flow patterns. This relatively inexpensive handheld device can take pressure measurements even when pulses cannot be felt. The Doppler works by bouncing sound waves off a column of moving blood cells. While you lie on the exam table, a blood pressure cuff is placed around each ankle and pressures taken while the doctor listens for blood flow at two points on each foot. These measurements are then compared with your arm blood pressures. The exam requires no needles or incisions, is painless, and quick. Doppler pressures can be taken at rest and after exercise; the results provide an indication of the severity of disease, its location, and the need for surgery. The Doppler probe can be attached to a recording device to print out a tracing of your blood flow pattern for further analysis.

After finishing the initial evaluation, your doctor may suggest other tests to further pinpoint your problem, depending on what is suspected and what sort of surgery might be necessary.

Ultrasound

In the *ultrasound (sonogram)* exam, you lie on a table while the examiner passes a probe over your body searching for blood vessels. The probe sends out high-frequency sound waves, which are then recorded as they bounce off the blood vessels. Some waves reflect back from the front wall of the vessel, while others pass through the channel to bounce off the back wall. The sonographic computer constructs an image based on the difference in the time it takes for the waves to hit the two sides. Completely noninvasive, quick, and painless, sonography is particularly good at diagnosing a dangerous aneurysm (a ballooned-out artery). However, it does not provide information about blood pressure or flow.

Duplex Doppler Exam

This test, the most sophisticated and revealing of the noninvasive options, combines the sonography and the Doppler probe to provide *both* a moving picture of blood flow in the artery and a picture of its wall. You lie on a table while the technician runs a probe over the area in question and a computer constructs images from the signals it picks up. This will provide information about the location of a blockage, how significant it is in reducing blood flow, and the condition of your other vessels above and below any blockage.

If you are facing a decision about whether to undergo an angiogram (an invasive diagnostic procedure) or reconstructive surgery, you will probably have this test first. The duplex Doppler is also useful for "surveillance" studies, which may be performed periodically after surgery to look for the development of problems within a grafted artery. If any are found, they can then be corrected before they cause complete graft failure.

CAT Scan

This exam is helpful in diagnosing an aneurysm, and is the most accurate indicator of its size. However, because it is expensive and involves X-ray exposure, you should avoid a CAT scan whenever possible, and request sonography instead.

Angiogram

This test produces an X-ray picture of your blood vessels and is the standard against which all other tests are measured. You most likely will be recommended to have an angiogram prior to vascular surgery because it gives your surgeon the most precise information—or a "road map," detailing the surface characteristics and sites of diseased vessels. However, since angiography is "invasive," meaning catheters (small tubes) are introduced into your arteries, and therefore carries a small risk of complications, it should *not* be performed unless you are seriously considering surgery. You should not have this test if you do not have significant symptoms that warrant surgery, if you are not a surgical candidate because of medical problems, or if you do not want an operation.

Angiography is usually an outpatient procedure. During the test, you must lie still, on your back, on a hard X-ray table. You are given mild intravenous sedation. After skin preparation with an antiseptic, a local anesthetic is injected into the tissues under your groin skin crease (or rarely, it may be injected in your arm, if your groin vessels are blocked). A specially trained "invasive radiologist" places a needle in the artery, and then a long, thin flexible catheter is inserted through the needle and manipulated to an area above your diseased vessel, while the radiologist watches its progress on a TV monitor. Dye is injected through the catheter, and a series of X-rays are taken as the dye travels through your vessels.

Discomfort may be caused by the needle puncture and catheter manipulation, and the dye injection can cause sudden artery irritation, which is felt as hot, burning pain. Luckily, it usually lasts only for a few seconds, until the dye is cleared. Such pain may be minor when small dye volumes are used in small vessels, but it can be significant in the larger aorta and limb arteries. However, intravenous medications can be given to make you drowsy and take the edge off the pain. Depending on what information is necessary, this test takes from thirty minutes to an hour.

In some cases, your radiologist may be able to *treat* a partial or even complete blockage with special catheters immediately after an angiogram, while you are still sedated and on the exam table. This allows you to avoid surgery. After the procedure is completed, the catheter is withdrawn.

Although the complication rate of angiography is very low, its dangers are real and should be understood. Major problems occur in 1 to 2 percent of exams. They include bleeding from the artery puncture, a blood clot which can block the artery at the puncture site, or migration of this clot to cause blockage downstream. Emergency surgery may be needed to repair these problems and—very, very rarely—loss of life or limb can follow.

MRA Scan

The expensive *magnetic resonance angiogram scan* for blood vessels may be useful in rare situations if your vessels cannot be seen well on any other test, or if you cannot be given the dye necessary for standard angiography because of dye allergy or problems with your kidneys. This test uses a strong magnet to affect your tissues, producing an X-ray-like picture, but it is not as precise as a standard dye angiogram.

Alternative Medicine Approaches to Artery Disease

Claude, a 57-year-old architect, began to notice his calf muscles aching when he played his weekly tennis game at the club. He had a 40 pack/year history of cigarette smoking, along with discoloration and hair loss of his lower legs, both signs of circulatory insufficiency. A Doppler exam showed narrowing in the arteries to both legs. He tried chelation, an unproved alternative approach popular with some of his friends, where a chemical agent EDTA is given intravenously. It is thought to attach to and remove the calcium in the blockages, thereby shrinking the plaque, and thus improving circulation. He felt somewhat better, but his symptoms did not completely disappear.

Claude decided to change his lifestyle. He quit smoking, and began to follow the full Dean Ornish reversal program, outlined in Chapter 8. He reported to me: "I have never felt better in my life! Even when I don't have any disease left, I will continue my yoga classes, exercise, and diet changes, just to feel the way I now do when I get up in the morning, and all day long." A follow-up Doppler exam showed remarkable reversal of his arterial narrowing.

Everyone is at risk for atherosclerosis. Lifestyle changes or medications can reduce your risk. Family history or complications from other diseases, such as diabetes, can also predispose your cells and blood vessels to wear out prematurely. But a "healthy" lifestyle, as described in Chapters 2 and 8, can slow progression or even reverse your vascular problems.

Atherosclerosis is usually a widespread disease; if you have symptoms in your legs, you probably also have coronary artery disease, a more important determinant of your life expectancy. Vascular surgery is always palliative, since it only relieves symptoms, sometimes just temporarily, and does not cure your underlying overall atherosclerosis. In effect, it is simply a temporary local plumbing job—to restore circulation, prevent expansion and rupture of the pipes, and avoid damage from blockage caused by detached and migrating bits of sludge. After one pipe is fixed, another may still cause problems.

In general, vascular surgery should be reserved for complications of atherosclerosis that threaten your life or limb, or produce symptoms severely affecting your lifestyle. In any case, you will still need to follow the dietary and other changes to assure the best success of your surgery and to prevent progression of your disease.

I have witnessed the success of the Ornish Heart Disease Reversal Program in quickly reversing symptoms of claudication. Shrinking of atherosclerotic plaques in humans has been documented to occur when lifestyle changes are made. The most important approach to treating your disease is to adopt that program for prevention and treatment of atherosclerosis. See Chapters 2 and 8 for more information. Following are other excellent measures to take.

Quit Smoking

As noted, most vascular disease is caused or made worse by smoking. Even a small amount of nicotine, even one cigarette, induces blood vessels to contract, making their channels smaller, creating *a measurable de-crease in blood flow to your tissues. Your cells suffocate.* as oxygen in the blood is replaced by carbon monoxide. Your platelets become more prone to cause blood clotting. In addition, toxic compounds in smoke directly injure your vessel lining, promoting initiation and acceleration of atherosclerosis.

If you are a smoker, the first, most important step is to quit. *Nothing you could do is more important!* Should you have surgery, its success—and avoidance of a future operation—is much more likely if you quit. Your life expectancy is likewise improved. The relaxation and stress management techniques discussed in Chapter 2 may give you some help in quitting; especially see the section there on how to use alternative medicine techniques to help you stop smoking.

Smoking also increases blood cholesterol levels and lowers HDL (the "good" cholesterol), compounding the damage. Without cessation of smoking, all other lifestyle changes and medical treatment are of little help. *If you smoke, you should make quitting the number one priority in your life.*

Lower Your Fat and Cholesterol Intake

Drs. Dean Ornish and Neal Blankenhorn have been able to show that many patients with peripheral arterial disease were able to stabilize their atherosclerotic deposits using a low-fat diet.[2] The Monitored Atherosclerosis Regression Study has shown that progression of peripheral artery disease (specifically, carotid arteries in the neck) can be reduced, and even reversed, with a low-fat, low-cholesterol diet and lifestyle modification.[3]

After changing their diets, many patients have found marked relief of their leg symptoms within even as short a time as a week or two. Small dietary changes do not provide this effect, so you will need to follow the full Ornish program, under the supervision of a doctor trained in this approach.

Before or after you develop this disease, keeping a yearly record of your total cholesterol, total cholesterol/HDL ratio, and triglycerides, can help determine your need for further change in your habits.

Add Vitamin E

Vitamin E has been found by one study to be an effective agent in the treatment of leg pain accompanying exercise.[4] The recommended dosage is 400 IU daily of the D-alpha form. Use of this vitamin should be coupled with the dietary changes, discussed in Chapters 2 and 8, that aim at halting progression and reverse arterial blockages.

Control High Blood Pressure

High blood pressure also hastens progression of atherosclerosis. The increased pressure produces mechanical injury to the vessel's lining cells, causing a thickening of the lining. *High blood pressure requires careful control,* with attention to diet and medication. If you make a serious effort to make changes in your diet and stress management, you have an 85 to 90 percent chance of blood pressure control without medication.

Exercise Regularly

Exercise decreases total cholesterol, possibly by increasing the levels of "scavenger" HDL, the fraction of "good" cholesterol that acts like a garbage collector in the bloodstream. Exercise also stimulates the formation of extra collateral vessels around blocked areas.

Maintain Your Optimum Weight

Weight reduction decreases the demands on muscles suffering from a limited blood supply. Therefore, if you are overweight, a weight-loss diet, combined with exercise, may help you walk farther. Follow the program given in Dr. Dean Ornish's *Eat More, Weigh Less* book; it has an 80 to 90 percent success rate.

A number of studies have shown that overweight people who are "apple" shaped, that is, carry their weight in the abdominal area, are at higher risk for cardiovascular disease than those who are "pear" shaped, that is, carry their weight in their hips and thighs. If you have an "apple" shape, weight loss may be especially key to your health and longevity in relationship to circulatory disease.

Practice Stress Management

Stress has been shown to elevate cholesterol, independent of diet. For further information on the stress-disease connection, please refer to Chapters 2 and 8.

Yoga postures, relaxation, and breathing exercises are particularly beneficial to atherosclerotic patients, for several reasons. The gentle stretches help improve blood and lymph flow to your limbs without causing excessive demand for blood. Deep breathing and meditation actually diminish the needs of your cells for blood. Relaxation itself acts to lower cholesterol.[5] Directions for these practices are found in Chapter 2.

Investigate Chelation

Although this method of treatment is expensive, and its safety and efficacy have not been scientifically proven, many people have believed it helpful to them. Review the latest research.

Practice Visualization

You can do exercises such as the following: picture your arteries as a system of plumbing that has, over time, become clogged with rust. Imagine yourself wielding a strong Roto-Rooter, removing any blockage from the system. Image this, and feel it happening within your body. Then see yourself also as adding no further rust from your diet or stress.

Conventional Medicine Approaches to Artery Disease

Conventional nonsurgical management of symptoms from blocked arteries includes stopping smoking, exercising, taking good care of your feet, practicing careful management of medical problems such as diabetes, and taking drugs that affect the arteries and blood coaguability. It also includes direct treatment by angioplasty and stenting.

Foot Care

Careful protection of your feet, especially in cold or damp weather, is especially important if you have poor circulation. Areas with borderline blood supply do not heal well, so you must pay special attention to seemingly minor wounds, corns, and ulcers, to prevent invading infection and gangrene.

Marion, a 65-year-old diabetic who lives by herself, developed a fever, and started to feel her blood sugar getting out of control. Her doctor found a pebble in her foot that had caused a severe infection. It had probably been there for a week! After surgery to remove several toes, two weeks in the hospital, and almost losing her whole foot, she now has special shoes, and makes certain to examine her feet each morning and night.

Diabetics frequently have problems with their feet, since this disease affects nerves, causing decreased sensation in the foot and toes. The foot's protective pain mechanism against trauma is then lost, and scratches, bruises, and minor skin irritations are not prevented from further trauma by the sensation of discomfort. Since tight shoes and overlay from neighboring toes and toenails are not felt, extremely difficult-to-treat pressure sores may form that may require months of careful attention to heal. Neglect may lead to bone infection, gangrene, and ultimately, amputation.

If you are diabetic, you are also significantly more subject to atherosclerosis, and your body's ability to heal wounds and fight off infection is diminished. In addition, if you run increased blood sugar levels, it provides a more favorable environment for bacteria and fungus growth. Such bacterial infections are responsible for one-half of all major leg amputations in diabetics; obstructive athersclerotic arterial disease accounts for the rest.

If you have diabetes, you must therefore be extremely protective of your feet. Make twice-a-day foot examinations and care a part of your daily routine. If you have difficulty seeing your feet or trimming your nails safely, get someone else to help you. Since excessive moisture is damaging, don't soak your feet for more than a few minutes. Use mild soap and warm water and dry carefully, especially between your toes.

Because your sensation may be decreased to heat and cold, avoid thermal injury by not using a heating pad or hot water bottle on your feet. Don't put your feet in hot water—test it with your finger first. Avoid going outside in cold or rainy weather. If you must, wear warm, insulated, waterproof shoes.

Always wear shoes and socks, even at home. Well-cushioned slippers should be chosen. If you tend to form calluses, get special shoes or inserts to avoid pressure on those areas. Double-layer hiking socks, especially designed to prevent blisters, are an extremely good investment. They are available at sporting goods stores. Shake hard particles out of your shoes and avoid high heels or pointed toes. Be especially careful with new shoes, which tend to produce blisters. If you have dry, flaky skin, use a bland moisturizing lotion. Don't use skin powder, since it may cause excessive drying.

See your doctor if you notice any blister, discolored area, crack, cut, ulcer, swelling, or drainage.

Drug Treatments

Medication may be helpful in decreasing your symptoms, as well as slowing the progression of your disease. The conventional drug treatment with medications affecting blood clotting and accomplishing cholesterol lowering, to prevent progression of atherosclerosis, is discussed in Chapter 8.

Aspirin, by its effect on platelets, helps prevent blood clotting in narrow and damaged arteries. If you have circulation problems, you should take an aspirin a day unless there is a medical reason not to.

Pentoxyphylline (Trental) is a medication that acts by making red cells softer, thereby presumably allowing them to "squeeze" through narrowed areas more easily. It may have other effects also. Two to three months of taking this medication may be needed to determine whether it will help you, since it affects only new red blood cells as your body

manufactures them. If you have pain on walking, you have at best a 50-50 chance it will help you make it a bit farther.

Cilostazol (Pletal) is a new drug and only the second after Trental to be approved by the FDA for claudication. It dilates blood vessels, decreases platelet clumping, and improves cholesterol ratios. A large randomized trial showed patients taking Pletal had a 47 percent improvement in walking distance compared to 12.9 percent for the placebo group. After sixteen weeks, they were able to walk about 100 yards farther than before starting the medicine,[6] at a cost of about $80 per month. It seems to be more effective than Trental.

Radiologic Catheter Techniques

The development of high-tech catheters that can be passed through a large needle into the area of disease has made treatment of constricted arteries possible without "open" surgery. Usually performed by a specially trained "invasive" radiologist or angiographer, the procedures are similar to the one previously described for angiography, in Chapter 8. In the most common and least expensive technique, called *angioplasty*, a balloon-tipped catheter is passed through a groin artery into the narrowed area. (See Figure 9.2.) The balloon is inflated to reach a preselected diameter, after which it will not enlarge any farther. The balloon inflation compresses atherosclerotic plaque, and the artery stays dilated once the balloon is removed. The dilation process is painless.

The best angioplasty results have been obtained in short blockages in the pelvic iliac arteries; 95 percent are still open at one year and 80 percent after two. These results are almost as good as those obtained through

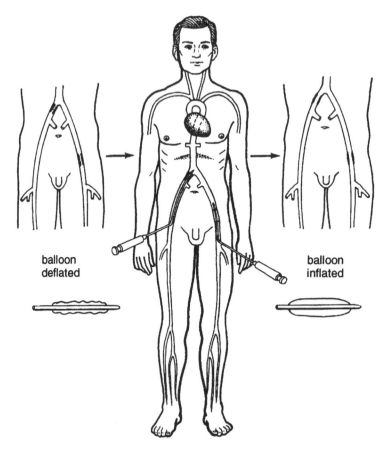

balloon
deflated

balloon
inflated

Fig. 9.2 Procedures involved in balloon angioplasty

surgery, but the complication rate is much lower. Results of dilation in the smaller arteries of the leg are not as good as those from surgery, 28 to 60 percent success at intermediate follow-up,[7] but angioplasty may nonetheless be tried, especially if you cannot have an operation. Even if the vessel does not stay open for very long, it may provide enough increased flow to allow an ulcer to heal. In any case, no bridges are burned by trying dilation: the procedure may be repeated, or reconstructive surgery can be performed later. Catheter techniques have also been used with kidney and coronary artery disease. Risk of causing a stroke limits its use in brain circulation disorders.

Stent placement has now been added to balloon angioplasty. A stent is an expandable metal tube that is carried to the area of narrowing by the angiography balloon catheter. (See Figure 9.3.) The balloon is then used to expand the stent against the inside of the narrowed area. The stiff metal keeps the artery from contracting again once the balloon is removed. Results have been favorable for treating disease in large vessels, but less so in smaller ones.

Another approach to opening narrowed,

or even completely blocked, blood vessels without surgery is the use of the *atherectomy catheter* or "Roto-Rooter." This catheter acts like a drill to grind down or remove the plaque with a diamond or laser tip. The technique is quite expensive, and more dangerous than simple balloon angioplasty. Sometimes it is used in combination with balloon angioplasty to open up fully blocked channels: the Roto-Rooter removes enough plaque to allow the balloon to be passed.

Although it is appealing in concept, atherectomy suffers from the same major problem as do all of the other catheter techniques. They produce physical damage to the inside of the artery, which then goes on to heal with a thickening process *(intimal hyperplasia)* that tends to produce recurrent narrowing. Much research is now under way as to how to control healing, so it will not cause repeat blockage. If this obstacle is overcome, much of vascular surgery may be replaced by catheter techniques.

Thrombolysis is a catheter technique used to dissolve blood clots that are blocking circulation, often in a previously functioning graft. A blood clot–dissolving drug is injected through a special catheter into the area of the clot. Surprisingly, this approach may work days and even weeks after the block occurs. If it is successful, the underlying problem may then be corrected by catheter technique or surgery, preventing a repeat blockage. This procedure is especially useful when clots have formed in the smaller vessels of the leg and foot or hand, and may "open up" vessels on which surgery would have been impossible.

Alice was a 65-year-old woman who underwent a successful groin-to-below-knee bypass using one of her own veins as the bypass graft. Two years later, she suddenly developed a return of her symptoms, which were worse than before her surgery. She waited two days before telling her surgeon, fearing another operation would be necessary. When she could stand the pain no longer, she came to the hospital; an angiogram showed a clotted graft, as well as clots in several blocked arteries in her lower calf and foot. She was in danger of losing her leg. Happily, the clots were completely liquefied once an angiographic catheter was inserted and a clot-dissolving drug dripped through it. The underlying problem was then found, and corrected by a balloon catheter technique, avoiding a second surgery.

While a radiographer is performing a catheter procedure, surgical backup must be

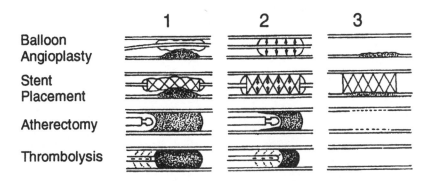

Fig. 9.3 Catheter techniques for opening narrowed or blocked arteries

available; a surgeon should be familiar with your case before catheter use is attempted. You have a 2 to 5 percent chance of developing a complication such as embolus, thrombosis, or rupture of the artery, that would require an emergency operation to repair the damage.

Surgical Approaches to Artery Disease

Gladys, an 82-year-old great-grandmother, was barely able to walk across the room before her legs gave out from restricted blood flow. She thought she was too old and useless, and that expensive surgery would be a waste. Finally cajoled by her grandchildren, she consented to an operation to repair her leg arteries, and now happily walks her dog through her neighborhood.

You and your surgeon should carefully weigh the decision whether or not to have surgery on your leg arteries. Generally, an operation is not recommended if your symptoms are minor, since an unsuccessful procedure could result in *worse* problems. This advice is especially true for smokers and diabetics, who face a high probability that their vascular disease will gradually become worse. They should therefore not "use up" their veins, suitable as future bypass grafts, unless their symptoms are severe, or a leg is in danger.

Sometimes I wonder if I should even operate on patients with this disease who won't stop smoking, as the results are so much worse. Some surgeons won't operate on current smokers. I try to talk all of my patients into quitting, and it is really frustrating when they don't.

Most persons with mild leg pain associated with walking do very well without surgery,

and can successfully learn to live with their disease. *Few patients with mild symptoms eventually require surgery.* Eighty percent of people who develop pain with exercise either show no further increase in symptoms, or they actually get better. The other 20 percent do not immediately progress to the point of severe symptoms or tissue loss, which would require an operation. Only 5 to 7 percent, usually heavy smokers and/or diabetics, ultimately must have a reconstructive procedure to avoid amputation.

If you do choose surgical reconstruction, it should be because you need it to relieve *present* symptoms—not to prevent your problems from getting worse in the *future*. Atherosclerosis is progressive, and surgery cannot stop its course. Surgical treatment for mild symptoms is ill advised, because it may fail, due to progression of your disease above or below the treated site, and an initial procedure may limit your options for reconstruction at a later date, when your symptoms may be more severe.

Symptoms that interfere with job requirements or walking more than a few steps usually indicate the need for an angioplastic or surgical procedure to improve blood flow; those that limit your "joys of life" constitute a gray area. You may be unhappy about not being able to walk two miles a day without stopping—and this may be a very important part of your life. Another person may be content to live with navigating no more than one-half block at any time. If no threat to your limb is present, you yourself should decide when and whether your symptoms and accompanying restrictions on activity warrant surgery and its risks. If you have severe, lifestyle-limiting symptoms, or if your circulation is so poor you are facing loss of your limb (evidenced by pain at rest, skin ulcers, or gangrene), you need a vascular reconstructive procedure.

John, a 70-year-old part-time real estate sales-man, whose wife had died a few years ago, developed an artery blockage that prevented him from walking more than 100 yards. His main joy in life was golf. Even though he could not stop smoking, he made a convincing case that he should have surgery so that he could walk around the golf course with his cronies two or three times a week.

Richard, an octogenarian, prided himself on looking and acting twenty years younger. He had received a penile implant a few years ago, when pelvic circulation problems caused impotence; but it wasn't until a leg artery became blocked and he could no longer keep pace with his square-dancing partner that he opted for vascular surgery. A bypass put him back on the dance floor.

You shouldn't deem yourself too old, too sick, or too useless to qualify for an operation. Such negative judgments slow you down and, undoubtedly, make it more difficult for you to deal positively with your recovery.

Thomas, a previously vigorous 88-year-old, became home-bound after developing two very painful toe ulcers. He felt he was too old, and that having diabetes and previous heart attacks made him unsuitable for surgery. After he had suffered for several months, his family practically dragged him to the surgeon's office. It was determined a bypass would be reasonably safe, and could be accomplished without difficulty, and he was soon back to walking around his neighborhood.

If you are considering surgery, diagnostic evaluation by the techniques described earlier should first be used to determine whether surgical reconstruction is possible. Angiography is the most accurate way to locate the blocked area, and provide a "road map" for the planned reconstruction.

The most common sites of arterial blockage are in the aorta and iliac arteries in the abdomen, the superficial femoral artery in the groin and thigh, the popliteal artery behind the knee, and tibial arteries in the calf. A very important requirement for successful surgery is that you have reasonably good arteries below the major blockage, necessary to accept the increased blood flow from the procedure. If more than one level of blockage is discovered (i.e., in both the abdomen and thigh arteries), the one closer to the heart is usually repaired first. The results of the increased flow are then assessed before proceeding further. If your symptoms disappear, nothing further need be done; if not, more surgery is required. The specific operative techniques are described in the following sections.

Endarterectomy

Endarterectomy is a surgical technique that removes plaque obstruction from an artery. An opening is made in the artery, the plaque separated and removed from the artery's muscle layer with fine forceps and scissors, then the opening closed. If the resulting channel appears to be narrow, the opening may be closed using a widening "patch" made of vein or plastic material. Endarterectomy is most suitable for short narrowings in larger arteries. It avoids the need for a plastic bypass graft, which carries with it a small risk of graft infection. Endarterectomy is most commonly used in the carotid artery in the neck, to prevent stroke.

Unfortunately, if you have leg circulation problems, you are not likely to be a good candidate for this operation, since your disease is probably widespread. Endarterectomy over a long length of diseased artery is more likely to fail than a bypass.

Bypass

Bypass is the most common technique used to treat an obstructed area anywhere in the body. A bypass graft is a new "pipe" placed from above to below the blocked area, thereby carrying blood around the blockage. The vessel above the graft provides the "inflow" blood and the vessel below the graft the "outflow" or "runoff" pipe to carry the increased flow.

Surgery is most successful when the inflow and outflow vessels are relatively normal. Unfortunately, since atherosclerosis is usually widespread, the surgeon must often deal with problematic outflow in small vessels, which are not optimal for surgical bypass attachment. Most grafts that ultimately fail do so because of progressive disease in the outflow vessels, or within the graft itself. This slows the flow through the graft to the point where the blood clots spontaneously.

A bypass graft may be fashioned from one of your veins, or from plastic material. In the large arteries above the groin, plastic grafts are preferred because they are immediately available, inexpensive, and easy to work with, and they hold up well in this position. However, if a bypass is performed below the groin, especially if the graft must cross the knee joint, grafts created from veins are preferred, since they perform better. This is because leg arteries are smaller and blood-flow

rates naturally slower than those in the pelvis. Blood flowing slowly is more likely to clot, especially if flowing over a rough surface. Slow-flowing blood is less likely to clot in a vein graft with naturally smooth vessel-lining cells that inhibit clotting. Small plastic grafts are more likely to fail, as the plastic surface is more thrombogenic and blood is more likely to clot in them at lower blood-flow rates. Also, compared to vein tissue, plastic tends to stimulate more of an overgrowth of scar tissue at the point where the graft is sewn to the natural artery. This causes a narrowing that is more likely to result in a critical flow restriction in a small diameter plastic leg graft than in a larger graft used in the pelvis.

The saphenous vein, the longest vein in the body, extending from ankle to groin, is most often used for a bypass graft. Veins from the arms can be chosen if the saphenous veins have already been employed, or are too small or diseased. If necessary, several vein pieces can be sewn together to make one bypass graft. Your body will do quite well without having these veins in their original places, since you have multiple alternate veins for blood to return to the heart. Recently available are specially processed veins taken from cadavers that can be used if you have no suitable veins available.

Specific Abdominal Artery Bypass Operations

Blockage of the aorta or iliac vessels in the abdomen may produce leg pain felt in your calf, thigh, and buttocks. Men may suffer impotence if the aorta and/or both internal iliac arteries are blocked. If possible, a nonsurgical radiologic balloon catheter technique may be employed in these arteries with success rates of 80 to 90 percent at five years if stents are used. If surgery is necessary, a bypass or endarterectomy can be performed, with excellent results; 95 percent of all grafts are open at one year and 90 percent at five years. Bypass is a fairly major operation, and carries a mortality rate of 1 to 5 percent. If you have significant medical problems, you may not be a good candidate for this surgery. Your surgeon may feel your heart cannot withstand the strain created by clamping and unclamping of your aorta. If you have poorly functioning lungs or kidneys, you also have a higher risk.

Alternative routes are available for bypassing blockages of the aorta and iliac vessels if you are one of those at risk because of heart, lung, or kidney problems. However, the long-term results are not as good, because such grafts are longer, providing more resistance to flow. They are also more subject to trauma and infection. Bypass grafts from the armpit artery to the groin artery (axillary/ femoral) and from one groin to the other (femoral/ femoral) can be performed under local anesthesia if necessary, with very little strain on the heart and other organs. These grafts are termed "extra-anatomic" because they do not follow the anatomic route of the bypassed artery. Routed through a tunnel beneath the skin, these grafts are vulnerable to external compression, which can clot off the graft, especially if you have low blood pressure.

For a bypass operation, you are admitted to the hospital on the morning of your surgery. After you are anesthetized, a tube is placed into your windpipe, another in your bladder, and possibly, another through your nose into your stomach. A blood pressure monitoring line may be placed in an artery near your wrist, and an intravenous catheter passed near or into your heart to monitor its function. If you are having the typical ab-

dominal artery procedure, a long incision is made from your breastbone to near your pubic bone. The aorta and iliac vessels are then exposed through the abdominal cavity. Alternatively, an incision may be made from the tip of the lowest rib on one side to near the middle of your abdomen—the so-called "saber slash." In this incision, the abdomen is not actually entered; the lining of the abdominal cavity, the intestines and organs are pushed forward to expose the vessels.

The exposed arteries are evaluated for the best places to sew in the graft or, perhaps, to remove constricting plaque(s) by endarterectomy. A blood anticoagulant is given to prevent blood from clotting during the time its flow is interrupted. The aorta and iliac vessels are clamped, and openings made in them. A plastic graft is sewn from the aorta to the iliac vessels, bypassing the blockage. (See Figure 9.4.)

If your iliac vessels are found to be too narrowed for satisfactory outflow, the graft is sewn to your femoral vessels in the groin through separate incision(s). Once the hookups are completed, the clamps are removed and improved blood flow is restored downstream. Your incisions are then closed.

Operating time can vary from two to four or more hours. Most operations can be completed without a blood transfusion. You will probably wake up in the recovery room, and have a short stay in the ICU. It may take three to five days before all of your tubes and IVs are removed and you can eat solid food. Pain can be controlled for the first few days by an "epidural" catheter in your back, or by intravenous or intramuscular injections. After a few days, oral pain pills should be enough. You can probably be out of bed the day following surgery, and home in four to seven days.

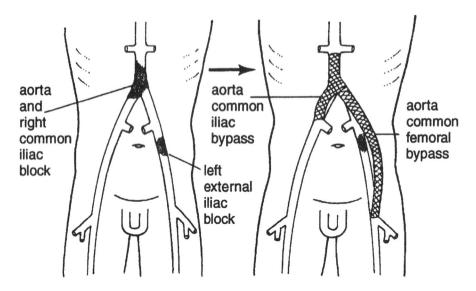

Fig. 9.4 Placement of bypass grafts extending from aorta to iliac artery and from aorta to femoral artery

After discharge, your surgeon should see you, to ensure that blood flow through your graft and into your legs is optimum, and that your incisions are healing well. Your legs will usually feel better immediately, and you should be feeling very comfortable after a couple of weeks.

Specific Leg Artery Bypass Operations

The main artery in the groin divides into two main branches. The superficial (meaning closer to the surface) femoral artery carries blood to your lower leg, while the deep femoral artery supplies the muscles of your thigh. Blockages in leg vessels typically cause cramping pain in the calf when walking.

Disease in the superficial femoral artery may not produce symptoms even when totally blocked, because the deep femoral artery carries one-half the blood flow to the leg and has many connections with the popliteal artery at the knee. These "collateral" vessels may en-

large to carry more blood, thus forming a "natural" bypass for the diseased artery. However, if the deep femoral and/or the popliteal or calf arteries also have significant blockages, or if the block in the superficial femoral artery develops rapidly, your body may not have sufficient time to develop communications among the other arteries to compensate. In this case, you may have symptoms.

If you choose to have surgery for femoral/ popliteal disease, a bypass from your groin to the popliteal artery above or below the knee, using a saphenous vein graft taken from your leg is the usual recommended procedure. (See Figure 9.5.) The best results are obtained when a good vein graft is available and your popliteal and calf vessels are still open.

Disease in the smaller arteries *below* the knee is more difficult to treat surgically than that in the larger arteries, and is the most common cause of amputation. If one of the three calf vessels is open below a blocked area, or if an open ankle vessel is providing

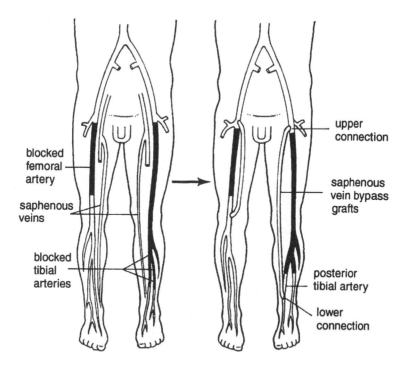

Fig. 9.5   Placement of bypass grafts extending from the femoral artery to the popliteal artery and from the femoral artery to the tibial artery

blood to the foot and toes, you have a good chance for a successful "distal" (toward the farther end of the leg) bypass. But I recommend this only in attempt to save a threatened leg or foot, or if you are able to walk only very short distances. If you choose this surgery simply to relieve pain that occurs when you exercise, and the graft fails, you may be worse off, and might even face amputation because of the inability of your surgical wounds to heal.

For leg bypass operations, you are admitted to the hospital on the day of surgery. You may have a "vein mapping," in which a duplex Doppler locates the best veins to be used for the bypass graft, then marks your skin so your surgeon can easily find them. You may choose to be asleep, or request a spinal anes-

thetic with sedation. A bladder catheter is used, but more extensive monitoring devices are usually unnecessary unless you are a high-risk patient.

Incisions are made in your groin, and above or below your knee, to access the vessels for the bypass attachment. For calf artery blockages, the lower incision is placed farther down the leg. Other separate incisions may be necessary to "harvest" the vein for the graft. Some surgeons make one long incision from groin to knee. After an anticoagulant is given to prevent your blood from clotting, your arteries are opened. The graft is attached by stitches to one artery, passed through a tunnel under your skin, and sewn in place to the other artery. After the graft is tested and determined to be successful, all incisions are closed. The operation may take an hour and a half to four or more hours, depending on the condition of your arteries and the quality of the vein used for the bypass.

You will most likely be returned to your regular room after spending an hour in the recovery room. Pain can be controlled with an epidural catheter, or intravenous or intramuscular injections. After a day or two, pain pills should be adequate. You should be up and walking the following day, and home in two to five days. If you can take aspirin, you should take one tablet per day to help prevent clotting, since this has been shown to reduce failure by approximately one-third.[8] If you can't take aspirin, a newer antiplatelet drug, Ticlid or Plavex, may be indicated.[9] If a plastic or long vein graft was used, or you are otherwise considered at high risk for bypass failure, you may be placed on long-term anticoagulants to decrease the chances of blood clotting within your graft.

Your surgeon should follow you very closely in office visits, to ensure your graft is working well and your incisions heal satisfactorily. Ankle blood pressure measurements are checked with each visit. Your leg should feel better immediately, though the incisions will be sore; it is common for them to ooze thin, pinkish fluid for a couple of weeks. Your leg will have a tendency to swell from a combination of the effects of the newly increased blood flow and the surgical incisions. This problem can last for a month or two, and needs to be controlled by elevating your leg as necessary.

Ninety percent of vein grafts placed above the knee remain open after one year, and 70 percent after three years. If leg or arm veins are not available for use as grafting material, plastic grafts may be used *above* the knee,

though results are 10 to 20 percent poorer than when vein grafts are used. Results of calf or foot bypass with a vein graft are not quite as good as the more commonly performed above-knee bypass; the success rate is 80 percent after one year and 50 percent after three years. Using a plastic graft for these bypass grafts produces poor results and is not recommended. The probability of success decreases with increasing disease in your "runoff" vessels; if you continue to smoke, the figures are much lower. If your graft fails, you have a 50 to 60 percent chance that further surgical reconstruction will be successful[10]; if not, you have a 25 to 30 percent chance you will require an amputation. Deaths from this surgery are rare.

Laparoscopic and Endovascular Bypass Surgery

Laparoscopic techniques to place bypass grafts around obstructed arteries are being pioneered in a few institutions around the world. Diseased aorta, iliac, and even arteries in the legs have been bypassed using small incisions and special instruments. The hope is for less risk and blood loss, fewer problems with leg swelling and other complications, and a quicker recovery. It will be several years before these techniques, if found to be superior, will be generally available.

Endovascular techniques can be used to pass "internal stent-grafts" from within the artery itself to areas of narrowing and blockage. Please see the discussion under aneurysm on page 307. However, the results with angioplasty and stenting are already quite good and less expensive. It may be that endografts will be proven superior when long or diffuse disease needs to be treated.

FAILURE OF VASCULAR RECONSTRUCTION

If you continue to smoke, you have two to five times the risk of early and late graft failure. These figures hold true for plastic and vein grafts and for grafts involving the aorta, iliac, femoral, popliteal, and tibial regions.[11] If you are unable to stop smoking, you are three times more likely to need an amputation at five years.[12]

Early failure of your graft can occur within hours, days, or weeks. If this happens, it is usually due to severe obstructive disease or to technical difficulties during the procedure. Your bypass will not stay open if inadequate inflow or severe obstruction develops in outflow vessels, or if the graft itself is of poor quality. If an early failure does happen, another operation—an attempt to find and correct the cause of failure—is usually indicated, with a success rate varying from 50 to 90 percent.

Failure of a bypass after months or years is usually caused by buildup of fibrous tissue at the connection sites and/or ongoing progressive atherosclerotic disease, which restricts blood inflow or outflow to the graft. Progressive narrowing of the graft itself may also be due to atherosclerosis. Eventually, blood flow in the graft may be slowed to the point of clotting. A return of your symptoms, or a decrease in how far you can walk before pain appears, indicates a problem with your graft, and a need for evaluation.

You can help prevent graft failure by returning to see your surgeon for careful follow-up exams, which should include blood pressures taken at the ankle, along with intermittent routine "surveillance" studies with the noninvasive duplex Doppler probe. This routine can identify a deteriorating, yet salvageable, graft even before symptoms develop. Early identification of problems is key, and repair of your graft with balloon angioplasty or relatively minor corrective surgery is much more successful if it can be undertaken before the graft fails completely.

Walter, *a 79-year-old diabetic, on a routine one-year follow-up duplex Doppler exam, was found to have a narrow spot in his groin-to-foot vein bypass graft. The blood pressure in the foot was only slightly reduced, and he could not sense any changes in his walking ability. The graft was able to be repaired under local anesthesia in outpatient surgery, and he was still doing well two years later.*

Amputation

Major leg amputation, above or below the knee, may be necessary if you have uncontrollable pain, infection, gangrene, or a severe traumatic injury. If you are facing amputation, you should first see a vascular surgeon, to assess any possibility for reconstruction. If you are in relatively good health, surgery to save your leg should be attempted, even if the chance for success is not great. Similarly, if it seems unlikely you will be able to walk again using a leg prosthesis, corrective surgery should be tried. On the other hand, if your mobility is already restricted due to a stroke or severe arthritis, or if you have a very short life expectancy, it makes little sense to undergo a bypass that might not work.

Obviously, the prospect of amputation is

very upsetting to you and your family. At least initially, you must depend upon the help of others. Physical, emotional, and financial concerns must be attended to, with support from family, medical personnel, and social workers. Most younger patients, especially those requiring amputation because of a traumatic injury, are able to resume relatively normal lives with the help of an artificial limb, after a period of rehabilitation.

Unfortunately, amputation is most often necessary in the elderly, in generally poor physical condition with widespread atherosclerotic vascular disease, who then must face severe disability for their remaining lifespan. Fortunately, rehabilitation and support services can ease the effects of amputation, so whatever months or years you have left can be made useful and enjoyable. Every effort must be made to maximize quality of life.

Minor amputations, of toes and parts of the foot, leave little disability. Amputations following an injury usually heal well, and those required for gangrene or nonhealing ulcers also usually heal if you have a relatively good blood supply at your ankle level.

When it is obvious that major amputation is necessary, it should be at below-the-knee level if you have a good chance for wound healing, since this site gives the best rehabilitation. This amputation allows you to walk with a prosthesis, balance when sitting up, and transfer from bed to wheelchair more easily, especially if you are elderly. Most below-the-knee amputations done because of injury or a tumor heal well; 10 to 30 percent of those performed because of vascular disease do not, and require further amputation above the knee. If you do not have vascular disease, surgical mortality—death within one month of the operation—is very low; if you have vas-cular disease, mortality is 10 percent, usually from underlying heart disease.

Above-the-knee amputations are necessary when skin ulcers or infection are present in the area where a below-knee amputation would be done, or when it seems unlikely you have enough blood supply to heal at that location. Because of more severe vascular disease, the surgical mortality rate is higher than for below-knee amputations: 10 to 30 percent.

If you were able to walk before amputation, you should be considered for an artificial limb. Before your prosthesis is fit, you need to exercise daily, to develop muscle strength and ensure your muscles do not permanently contract. However, if you are elderly or infirm, especially if you have an above-knee amputation—where walking with a prosthesis requires twice as much energy expenditure and better balance than a below-knee prosthesis—trying to use an artificial limb may be a waste of time and effort. You may prefer to walk with crutches or use a wheelchair.

ARTERY DISEASE SUMMARY

Prevention

Diet and Supplements

- Eat a low-fat, high-fiber diet.
- Vitamin E, D-alpha, 400 IU daily.
- Vitamin C, 1,000–2,000mg 2–3 times daily.

Lifestyle

- Control high blood pressure.
- Control high cholesterol.

- Control diabetes.
- Don't smoke.
- Exercise 1 hour, 3–5 times weekly.
- Maintain optimum weight.
- Take good care of your feet.
- Utilize stress management.

Alternative Medicine Approaches

- Follow the preventive guidelines, above.
- Join a weekly support group.
- Practice visualization.
- Chelation (controversial).
- Coenzyme Q10, 150 mg daily.
- Pycnogenol, 500 mg daily.

Conventional Medicine Approaches

- Foot care.
- Medication—aspirin, pentoxyphylline, Trental, cilostazol, Pletal.
- Radiologic catheter techniques—balloon angioplasty, stenting, thrombolysis.

Surgical Approaches

- Endarterectomy.
- Bypass—vein graft, plastic graft.

Aneurysms

When an area within an artery loses its resistance to pressure and expands like a balloon, an *aneurysm* forms. Both the muscle and elastic layers of the arterial wall weaken. Cigarette smoking, which causes damage to the arterial wall, is a common cause of this problem. Genetics may play a role; therefore, if a member of your family is diagnosed with an aneurysm, you are more likely to develop one, and should be screened regularly for it after age 60. High blood pressure, which increases forces within a weakened area, may

contribute to aneurysm formation. Such elevated pressure can also create an increased rate of expansion once an aneurysm has formed.

Aneurysms are subject to four complications. *Rupture* occurs when the arterial wall gives way and blood leaks into adjoining tissue. *Thrombosis* happens if a blood clot within the dilated area completely blocks the channel. *Embolus* is produced whenever a blood clot or debris breaks off and migrates downstream, eventually blocking a smaller artery. Lastly, the expanding aneurysm can compress or erode adjacent tissues, such as nerve, vein, bone, or internal organ.

Abdominal Aortic Aneurysm

The abdominal aorta is by far the most common location for aneurysm formation, though aneurysms may develop in the groin, leg, or any other artery. In fact, the presence of one aneurysm demands the search for more. Twenty percent of patients with abdominal aortic aneurysms also have others.

Two percent of Americans develop an abdominal aortic aneurysm. Each year, fifteen thousand Americans die from its rupture—it is the tenth most common cause of death in men over age 50. A genetic predisposition has been found. About 20 to 25 percent of patients have a close relative with an aneurysm. It is a disease of aging and rare before the age of 55. Men are affected four times more often than women, probably because of their higher rates of smoking, hypertension, and accelerated atherosclerosis.

Only about 50 percent of aneurysms produce symptoms prior to rupturing. A sensation of vague discomfort, or a pulsation or "heartbeat" in the upper abdomen, can be a signal. As the aneurysm grows larger, it may put pressure on or erode the vertebrae, causing back pain.

If you have a small aneurysm—or a large belly—your diagnosis may be difficult, though 80 percent of aneurysms *can* be felt. Your doctor should examine for an aneurysm as a routine part of your yearly physical examination, especially if you are a smoker, have high blood pressure, or have a relative who had an aneurysm. Aneurysms are sometimes coincidentally detected when abdominal X-rays are obtained for other reasons. By far the quickest and easiest way to determine the presence and size of an aneurysm is by sonography. A CAT scan provides the most accurate information about size; but since it is much more expensive than the sonogram and increases your exposure to X-ray, it is rarely recommended.

If surgery is planned, you may receive preoperative angiography, to assess the upper extent of the aneurysm, look for others, and determine whether abnormal kidney arteries are present. If you have poorly controlled high blood pressure, the radiologist should look for a narrowed kidney artery that might be the cause, and could be corrected at the time the aneurysm is repaired. Angiography is especially useful if you have symptoms of obstructed arteries beyond the aneurysm, since it helps determine where to connect the graft downstream.

Alternative Medicine Approaches to Abdominal Aortic Aneurysm

The most important contribution of alternatives is in the prevention or reversal of any underlying causative atherosclerotic disease or high blood pressure. Both of these increase the likelihood of formation, then enlargement and rupture, of an aneurysm. Follow the guidelines given in the previous chapter, for preventing and reversing heart disease.

If you have an aneurysm of less than 5 centimeters that is not producing symptoms, it can reasonably be observed with sonograms every four to six months to document its stability. If your lifestyle change program is working and the size remains constant, you may be able to avoid an operation. However, you will need to continue to be monitored.

Following are the most significant alternative medicine contributions for preventing abdominal aortic aneurysms or keeping them from expanding once they have formed.

Quit Smoking

Cigarette smoking acts to accelerate atherosclerosis by increasing carbon dioxide in the blood and lowering oxygen levels and by interfering with local repair mechanisms by constricting capillary flow. You can use alternative approaches to help you quit for good; see Chapter 2, especially the section "Quitting Smoking."

Maintain Optimum Blood Pressure

High blood pressure, especially over time, takes its toll on the abdominal aorta. You can act to achieve and maintain appropriate blood pressure with the help of alternative approaches. Your nutritional choices, weight, reactions to stress, and amount of exercise can all impact your blood pressure. Follow the guidelines in these areas given in Chapter 2.

Change Your Diet

Following a low-fat, high-fiber vegetarian diet can help prevent both high blood pressure and atherosclerosis. Adding garlic, onions, celery, tomatoes, broccoli, carrots, and the spices anise, fennel, oregano, black and red pepper, and saffron may also be helpful; further research is needed.

Take Supplements

Certain supplements may help you maintain suitable blood pressure. Calcium citrate, 500 mg, and magnesium citrate, 250 mg, may be taken two times daily. Garlic lowers both blood pressure and cholesterol; take two capsules of odor-free garlic twice daily.

Practice Stress Management and Yoga Daily

As considered more fully in Chapter 2, yoga and other stress management techniques can assist you in changing your body's physiology and can directly help lower blood pressure that is too high. Develop a daily practice.

Surgical Approaches to Abdominal Aortic Aneurysm

Marvin thought the thumping he felt below his ribs was just caused by his heart beating. When he developed a backache, he thought he had a slipped disk, and went to see his doctor. He was stunned to learn that the pulsation and discomfort were caused by an enlarging aneurysm pressing on his spine. He was told the weakened area was ready to blow out, like a bald tire, and he was recommended for surgery without delay. Worried about losing time from his grocery business, Marvin was still pondering this advice a few days later when he developed severe abdominal pain and passed out. Luckily, his wife Ann was present and called 911. Within forty-five minutes, he was in the operating room, where his ruptured aneurysm was successfully repaired. Had the leak occurred while he was driving his car or reeling in a salmon, Ann might have been left to tend the store by herself.

Aortic Aneurysm Repair

About 15 percent of aneurysm patients require emergency surgery. A ruptured or symptom-producing aneurysm must be operated on as soon as possible. If such symptoms develop, like sudden severe back pain, dizziness, or fainting, you should go to a hospital immediately and be in the operating room within minutes after arriving. Depending on whether you are in shock from sudden loss of blood, and if you have other medical problems, your risk of mortality from emergency surgery varies from 30 to 90 percent, with most deaths caused by uncontrollable bleeding.

Since aneurysms tend to develop in elderly people who also have other medical problems, particularly cardiovascular disease, and since the corrective procedure places major stress on all organ systems, most surgeons are cautious about operating on aneurysms. Many studies have examined the natural history of aneurysm formation, with the goal of determining when the risk of rupture outweighs the risk of surgery. It appears that the risk of rupture if you have an aneurysm less than 4 centimeters in diameter is only about 2 percent.[13]

Once an aneurysm reaches 5 centimeters in size (the aorta is normally less than 2.5 centimeters—one inch—in diameter) most surgeons recommend operative repair. The five-year risk for rupture increases to 25 percent for an aneurysm 5 to 5.9 centimeters in diameter, 35 percent if 6 to 7 centimeters, and greater than 75 percent if more than 7 centimeters.[14] Studies have shown that at greater than 5 centimeters the risk of rupture and death is substantially higher than that of the operation itself. Smaller 4- to 5-centimeter aneurysms may also rupture, so many surgeons advise earlier surgery if you are in good health. The risk for a smaller aneurysm rupturing is higher if you have emphysema or diabetes.[15] If repeated sonograms show that a smaller aneurysm is expanding at a rate of more than one-half centimeter per year, it should be repaired.

The operation for this disorder and the postoperative recovery are very similar to those for blockage of the aorta or iliac vessels, described on page 300. The graft is sewn into the aorta above and below the aneurysm, or as a "Y" graft into the iliac or groin arteries, depending on the state of the vessels beyond the ballooned-out area. (See Figure 9.6.)

The mortality rate for surgical repair of a aneurysm before it ruptures is very low: less than 5 percent. Most deaths are actually caused by complications of an underlying cardiac disease. Significant complications occur in 10 to 15 percent of patients, requiring a re-operation in 2 percent. The best results are obtained by surgeons who do this type of surgery frequently, and who have access to modern intensive care units. Later problems related to the graft include graft infection, separation of stitches at the hook-up site (false aneurysm), and graft blockage. Impotence follows surgery in about 10 percent of male patients, due to interruption of some pelvic nerves or decrease in blood supply to the pelvic organs. After successful surgery, you

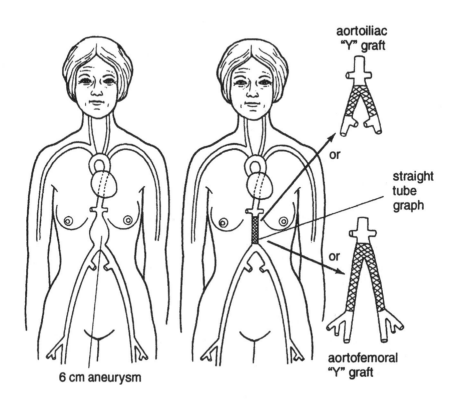

aortoiliac
"Y" graft

or

straight
tube
graph

or

aortofemoral
"Y" graft

6 cm aneurysm

Fig. 9.6 Placement of graft in aortic aneurysm repair

have the same life expectancy as similar individuals who have never needed aneurysm surgery.

Endovascular Stent Grafts

Currently minimally invasive "endovascular" techniques, where grafts are passed by catheters through small groin incisions then manipulated inside the arteries to the area of disease and tacked in place by stents, is an exploding, controversial area of technology that holds much promise for the future. Clinical trials at academic medical centers are now working out the technical challenges and complications, and defining this new approach's role.

If you have an aneurysm, to be a candidate for this procedure your aneurysm must have specific characteristics in terms of shape, configuration, and you must have usable groin and pelvic arteries in order to pass and fasten the graft safely. So far, it seems that with the latest grafts, somewhere from 50 to 80 percent of all aneurysm patients would qualify for an attempt using this technique.[16] A 1998 study reporting initial experience from the Massachusetts General Hospital found this procedure was completed successfully in 77 percent of the patients in whom they attempted it.[17] More recent results from several centers find that it can be completed successfully in more than 95 percent of eligible patients.

Hoped-for benefits include decreased risk, pain, sexual dysfunction, expense, and a quicker recovery when compared with the standard large incision "open" operation described above. Patients with severe medical problems with large aneurysms who were previously thought to be unfit for the standard open repair may qualify for this approach. A large multicenter trial reporting on 250 patients found the procedure mortality rate and expense about the same as the standard open repair but significant reduction in complications, a shorter hospital stay, and an earlier return to function in these patients.[18] The average patient is out of bed and eating within twenty-four hours, home in two or three days, and back to normal activities in two weeks.

Long-term results, although promising, are as yet the big unknown. Patients receiving these grafts must be followed with CAT scans every six months indefinitely to look for leaks, recurrent aneurysm formation, and graft displacement. About 15 to 20 percent of patients will need a secondary endovascular procedure to correct these problems and about 2 to 4 percent will need to be eventually converted to a standard open graft.[19] In follow-ups of 1,046 patients in a national multicenter trial, there have been seven late graft ruptures, a rate projected to be 2.6 percent at two years.[20] It's quite interesting to hear vascular surgeons respond when asked what kind of procedure they would select if they had an aneurysm that needed repair. About half respond they would choose the standard operation and half the endovascular approach.

This new technology will likely play a very prominent role in the management of vascular disease in the future. Ask your surgeon about the latest results, and if it is an option available in your area for your particular problem. Again, to get the good results as described, a team combining the skills of the vascular surgeon and interventional radiologist with extensive experience with these techniques is necessary.

Stroke

A stroke, called in medical terms a *cerebral vascular accident,* or *CVA,* is a shocking event. You feel helpless, whether you are a witness or a victim. What is encouraging is that by means of alternative methods you can take action to prevent this difficulty, or use effective alternative techniques to help you recover.

Stroke is the third leading cause of death in the United States, accounting for 10 percent of all deaths. An estimated 731,000 persons have a stroke each year with 4 million living survivors.[21] Many are severely debilitated, and the psychosocial expense is immense. The incidence of stroke is growing, caused by an increasing prevalence and less adequate control of key cardiovascular risk factors.[22] The National Stroke Association Stroke Prevention Advisory Board identified six important risk factors: high blood pressure, previous heart attack, heart rhythm disturbance, elevated blood cholesterol, diabetes, and narrowing of the carotid arteries. Lifestyle factors identified are smoking, use of alcohol, diet, and physical activity.

In about 80 percent of patients, atherosclerotic plaque is responsible. Most atherosclerotic strokes result from disease located in the surgically accessible carotid arteries in the neck. Strokes can be prevented if this blockage is diagnosed and treated before it reaches critical levels.

Surgery that aims to prevent stroke has had an astonishing increase within the last two decades. If you or someone in your family is faced with a recommendation for surgery to prevent stroke, it is especially important you obtain as much information as possible. In the following sections, we present ways in which you can possibly avoid this dangerous surgery, and determine when the risks of the operation are worth it.

One-half of all strokes appear without prior symptoms. As will be discussed, large numbers of individuals who have various degrees of carotid artery narrowing, without symptoms, are now being followed to see if patterns of stroke-proneness can be identified.

Blood Circulation of the Brain

The brain derives its blood supply from four vessels. (See Figure 9.7.) The two *internal carotid arteries* serve as the major source of blood supply to the two hemispheres. The two *vertebral arteries* supply the brain stem. The carotids normally carry 90 percent of the blood flow to the brain; the vertebrals 10 percent. All four arteries join to form a circle on the undersurface of the brain—the *circle of Willis*—that gives off major branches to each area.

This arrangement is very useful: If blood supply is restricted by disease in one or more of the four vessels, the others will usually increase their flow volume, maintaining supply to the branches of the circle. Unfortunately, the circle is incomplete in 80 percent of all people, owing to congenital lack of development of part of the circle, and those with an incomplete circle do not fully have this safety net.

Atherosclerotic blockage to the brain develops in two ways. Blood flow may be reduced by partial constriction or complete blockage of one or more of the four major arteries. Alternatively, a diseased area may form an atherosclerotic ulcerated plaque, and then bits of blood clot, platelet, or cholesterol debris migrate until they get stuck in vessels with a slightly smaller diameter. This latter type of blockage, affecting small brain arteries, is thought to happen far more commonly than reduced blood flow caused by obstruction in a major vessel.

Three smaller branches, the *anterior, middle,* and *posterior cerebral arteries,* take off

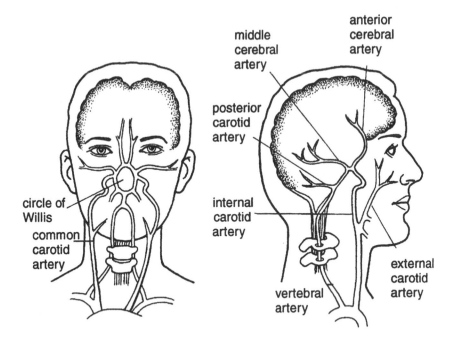

Fig. 9.7 The main arteries of the brain

from each side of the circle of Willis to supply specific brain areas. Very little communicating circulation exists between these vessels. Migrating debris can lodge and block flow, so that with a major blockage, the neighboring vessel is rarely able to restore enough circulation to prevent cell death. Each blocked artery produces specific and unique stroke or symptom patterns.

How Brain Artery Disease Is Diagnosed

Brain artery disease is diagnosed by a careful history, physical exam, and other more sophisticated tests.

History

Your doctor will need to take a very detailed history to help determine the cause of your symptoms. Many different organ and systemic problems can mimic brain artery disease. Typically confused with this disease are heart rhythm disorders, degenerative neurologic disease, drug toxicities, body chemistry imbalance, and a myriad of other problems. Questions pinpoint the location, onset, frequency, duration, and severity of symptoms, as described below. General medical problems such as diabetes, hypertension, heart disease, and known vascular disease should be discussed, as well as your smoking, alcohol, and, exercise habits. Be sure to list all the medications you are taking.

Symptoms of brain artery disease are very diverse, depending on which area of the brain is affected. If the blockage affects the carotid artery's ability to distribute blood, the classic picture includes weakness, paralysis, and loss of sensation. You may experience visual disturbances, such as changes in your field of vision, double vision, and blindness. Interference with thought processes, including an inability to speak, or to comprehend or express oneself (a condition called "aphasia") may develop. This "carotid distribution" of symptoms accounts for 80 to 90 percent of all symptom patterns.

Ten to twenty percent of symptoms are in the "vertebral distribution," affecting the back part of the brain. Problems arising from diseased arteries in this area are less clear, and frequently are confused with symptoms caused by heart disease, emotional disturbance, or neurological diseases. Dizziness, fainting, buzzing in the ears, lack of coordination, drowsiness, lethargy, slurring of speech, swallowing difficulty, or paralysis of one side of the face and the opposite side of the body may be present. Double vision or loss of parts of the visual field can occur. "Drop attacks," sudden loss of strength in the legs, may also follow.

Symptoms can be temporary or permanent. Temporary problems, termed *transient ischemic attacks (TIAs),* indicate lack of blood supply, caused by temporary decreases in circulation following the migration of small bits of debris that block a small brain vessel. The debris dissolves, or neighboring circulation overcomes the temporary block, and your symptoms disappear. A TIA, by definition, lasts less than twenty-four hours. *Reversible ischemic neurologic deficits, (RINDSs)* are similar though less-common events that may last from twenty-four hours to several days, but are completely reversible. The term "stroke" indicates brain cell death and symptoms that are not reversible, though they may be relieved through rehabilitation.

Physical Exam

Your physical examination includes a general check of your heart, neurologic, and vascular systems as well as a specific search for problems in your neck arteries by your doctor feeling and listening with a stethoscope. Your doctor may find a "bruit," a harsh sound caused by turbulent flow through a constricted or diseased area in the carotid artery. However, the mere presence of a bruit does not necessarily indicate this area is the source of your symptoms. This point is especially important, because it is the origin of much confusion about who should be operated upon, as we shall discuss shortly.

Tests to Exclude Nonvascular Causes

Since neurologic symptoms and strokes are caused by many different vascular and nonvascular problems, an accurate diagnosis must be made before a course of treatment can be chosen. To differentiate between these causes of neurological symptoms, you may be recommended to have a complete heart workup, including an EKG and a twenty-four-hour Holter monitor recording, to look for rhythm disturbance. A Holter monitor is a small pack worn on a belt, with wires connecting it to electrodes on your chest. The unit is portable, so that you can go about your day—and sleep through the night—while wearing it. Neurologic diseases can be screened for by EEG or brain wave test, CAT scan, or MRI scan. Blood tests may be requested to look for chemistry imbalance.

Once cardiac and other nonvascular causes have been eliminated and it becomes clear that you do have vascular disease, its nature and location must be determined, as well as whether it is best treated by surgery or medical management.

Duplex Doppler Exam

The easiest and most commonly used noninvasive study is the *duplex Doppler exam.* In this painless test, a sound probe is pressed against the skin over each carotid (vertebral) artery, and a computer then constructs a picture from sound waves bounced off the moving column of blood within it. This test can estimate blood flow reduction and turbulence caused by partial blockage, but is not as valuable in determining whether you have plaques and ulcers likely to shed pieces that would create an obstruction.

Brain Angiography

Four-vessel brain angiography gives a clear picture of blood flow and vessel wall characteristics. If you are being considered for surgery, you may be studied in this way, to provide a detailed map of the carotids and ensure no other brain abnormalities are present that might account for your symptoms. Recently, however, with improvements in duplex Doppler technology, most vascular surgeons are *not* requesting preoperative angiography for most of their patients, thereby avoiding its cost and potential complications. Discuss your specific case with your surgeon.

Brain angiography is usually performed by threading a catheter through a needle placed in a groin artery, since it is easiest to show all four brain vessels by this route. The arm can also be used. The procedure is similar to that for evaluating artery disease (see page 288). Newer techniques utilize computers to form sharper images while using less dye, which reduces the discomfort and risk of the procedure. The major complication rate is 1 percent, and the death rate 0.5 percent. The possible complications include stroke, temporary neurologic symptoms, and local problems from the catheter puncture site, such as bleeding, infection, and vessel thrombosis; the latter requires emergency surgery for repair.

Angiography should not be performed unless you are considering a surgical solution.

Brain MRA

Magnetic resonance angiography is being developed as a noninvasive way to show blood vessels more precisely, and may eventually replace angiography, therefore avoiding need for dye and catheters. So far, it is less useful than the Doppler exam.

Alternative Medicine Approaches to Prevent Stroke

As a young child, I watched as my mother and grandmother cared for my grandfather, who had suffered a debilitating stroke owing to high blood pressure. It was painful for everyone. He had been a prominent surgeon, chief of surgery at his town's hospital. But now he couldn't talk. I missed having a grandfather to play with, to share my growing love for the practice of medicine; I never got to hear him tell the unique stories of his life. We as a nation can act to prevent such losses, by changing our lifestyle habits.

Fifty percent of all patients who develop a major stroke do so without warning signals. Paying attention to preventing stroke, by addressing the risk factors associated with it, is the very best first effort we can make.

In addition, once you have an asymptomatic carotid bruit, you may also be able to avoid very risky carotid surgery by changing your lifestyle. If you have had intermittent neurologic symptoms or a minor stroke, you must seek evaluation and conventional medical or surgical treatment, but alternative medicine offers much hope in helping you recover.

Most TIAs are a result of atherosclerosis, occurring as a widespread disease in your body. Your chance of dying from atherosclerosis-induced heart disease is far greater than that of dying of a stroke. Still, stroke is the third leading cause of death; it causes 10 percent of all deaths, and drastically affects the quality of life of stroke survivors. Following a dietary and stress reduction approach acts to prevent both heart disease and stroke. Following are the most promising methods for alternative prevention of stroke, to be used along with the methods discussed in Chapters 2 and 8.

Control Your Blood Pressure

High blood pressure is the most common and controllable risk factor for stroke, and maintaining optimum blood pressure substantially reduces your chances of having a stroke.[23] Blood pressure readings are composed of two numbers: The first, termed the systolic measurement, is the highest level of pressure in your arteries at the peak of your heart's beat. This level should ideally remain below 140. The second number, the diastolic, reflects the pressure in your arteries when your heart is at rest and should stay below 90. If your pressure runs above either of these numbers and you reduce it by as little as 5 points, you diminish your risk by 42 percent.[24]

Changing to a low-fat, high-fiber diet can help you lower your blood pressure and keep it down, often more successfully than with medication. Begin a daily stress management program and maintain optimum weight, often all that is needed to get your blood pressure down. You can easily follow your blood pressure at home with an inexpensive electronic or manual monitoring device.

Change Your Diet

Evidence from animal and human studies indicates that atherosclerotic plaque is reversible and specifically in the carotid arteries.[25] Chang-

ing to a low-fat, high-fiber diet, with lots of fruits and vegetables, may not only halt progression of the disease, but also actually reverse it. Information from the Nurses' Health Study published in 2000 in *JAMA* found that women with the highest whole grain input had a 31 percent decrease in risk for stroke when compared to those with the lowest intake.[26]

A diet deficient in fruits and vegetables can increase your risk of stroke. A 1999 study reported in *JAMA* from the Nurses' Health Study (5.8 servings per day) and the Health Professionals Follow-Up Study (5.1 servings per day) found a 31 percent decrease in stroke in the groups with the highest intake of fruits and vegetables—especially cruciferous and green leafy vegetables and citrus fruits and juice compared to those in the lowest intake groups. An increment of one serving per day was found to decrease risk by 6 percent.[27]

Eat lots of fruits and vegetables—at least five servings per day—and foods containing fiber—at least six servings per day. Follow the dietary instructions given in Chapter 2.

Control Your Cholesterol

This is an important risk factor for stroke. By narrowing arteries and causing plaque debris that can break off and migrate to block brain arteries, cholesterol acts to precipitate strokes. Know your cholesterol level and work to keep it at a healthy level, as described in Chapter 8.

Control Your Diabetes

Diabetes is linked to increased risk of stroke by epidemiologic and laboratory evidence. It accelerates the process of atherosclerosis, promotes plaque formation, and has harmful effects on LDL and HDL cholesterol levels. Although it has not yet been proven that the rigorous control of blood sugar levels decreases your risk for stroke, further evidence may prove that it does. The National Stroke Association recommends tight control, as it is known to decrease risk for nerve, kidney, and eye damage. Work with your doctors to ensure optimum control.[28]

Take Supplements

Increased intake of beta-carotene, vitamin E, and other antioxidants may help prevent strokes in several ways. If neurologic symptoms are the result of artery blockage, rather than hemorrhage, taking supplements to prevent clotting may be helpful in preventing stroke, or helping treat it once it has occurred, although you should be monitored by your doctor. Vitamin E has been shown to be more effective than aspirin in preventing clot formation.[29] States with higher levels of selenium are associated with decreased risk for stroke; the Atlantic states, lowest in selenium, comprise the "Stroke Belt."[30] Lowered clotting was found with supplementation of 200 mcg per day.[31] In animal experiments, the addition of omega-3 fatty acids, found in flaxseed oil, decreased brain damage from stroke.[32] Recommended supplementation is one tablespoon of flaxseed oil daily.

Increased blood levels of homocysteine, associated with deficiencies of folate, vitamin B_6, and vitamin B_{12}, damage carotid artery lining cells, causing narrowing, and may be associated with stroke.[33] Take a balanced vitamin B-complex capsule containing 400 mcg of folic acid, 50 mg of vitamin B_6, and 50 mcg of vitamin B_{12} per day.

The herb ginkgo biloba has shown ability to prevent strokes.[34] It appears to act via improvement of blood flow and decreased viscosity. Usual dose is 40 mg, three times daily.

Drink Tea

A fifteen-year study of 552 British men reported a 70 percent reduction in stroke in the group that drank 4.7 cups of black tea daily, compared with men who only drank 2.6 cups. Tea contains flavonoid antioxidant compounds, and seems to be protective for coronary artery disease as well.[35] Just make certain to add milk or soy milk, to neutralize the cancer-causing tannins found in black tea.

Maintain Your Optimum Weight

Excess weight itself is a risk factor for stroke. The mechanism may be connected to the documented relationship between higher weight and higher blood pressure, or to independent factors such as changes in baseline hormone levels—for example, of cortisol—associated directly with elevated weight.

Just losing weight may be all you need to get your blood pressure and hormones back into the normal range and keep them there. Even as little as five to ten pounds may make a difference.

A very successful weight-loss program that has been scientifically documented is the one described in Chapter 2 of this book and detailed in Dr. Dean Ornish's book *Eat More, Weigh Less*. Persons who choose to follow such a program—which consists of a vegetarian, low-fat, high-fiber diet accompanied by exercise, daily yoga, and group support—have shown an 80 to 90 percent success rate in losing the necessary offending pounds and then maintaining appropriate levels, according to research presented in the book. Refer to the dietary, exercise, yoga, and group support guidelines given in Chapter 2 of this book to help you achieve and maintain your goal.

Exercise

Regular exercise has been shown to reduce the risk of stroke, as well as that for premature death and other cardiovascular diseases. This benefit is present even for light to moderate exercise such as walking, although some evidence suggests that increasing the level and duration may add additional benefit.[36] A 2000 Nurses' Health Study reported in the *Journal of the American Medical Association* found a 34 percent decreased risk for stroke with thirty minutes of vigorous exercise every day. The benefits were the same for brisk walking as for more vigorous jogging or aerobics. However, walking at a casual pace was not as beneficial.[37]

Avoid Excessive Alcohol Intake

Evidence indicates that light to moderate drinking may have some beneficial effects. It may act by increasing HDL cholesterol levels and decreasing platelet aggregation and fibrinogen levels. A 1999 Physicians' Health Study reported in the *New England Journal of Medicine* found a 21 percent decreased risk for as little a one drink of beer or wine per week. Increased intake, up to one drink per day, did not provide further benefit.[38] Other studies have found risk reduction ranging from 20 to 60 percent, both in men and women. If you drink, limit your intake to one or two drinks per day. Binge drinking and heavy drinking of three or more drinks per day are associated with increased risk for hemorrhagic stroke.[39] However, according to a Consensus Statement from the National Stroke Association, if you are a nondrinker, you should not be encouraged to start.[40]

Quit Smoking

An analysis of thirty-two studies found smokers to be at 50 percent higher risk than nonsmokers, and the more you smoke, the higher your risk.[41] The Framingham[42] and Nurses' Health Study[43] both showed the risk of stroke from arterial blockage to decrease to that of nonsmokers two to five years after quitting. Inhaling other people's smoke also increases your risk for acute stroke[44]—another reason to pursue a smoke-free environment at home, at work, and in public places. Follow the guidelines given in Chapter 2 to help you stop.

Avoid Oral Contraceptives

A meta-analysis of sixteen studies looking at the relationship between birth control pills and stroke published between 1960 and 1999 was reported in *JAMA* in 2000. Current use was found to be associated with 2.75 times the risk for stroke. The risk was significant, 1.93 times, even with the smaller estrogen dose preparations used today.[45] Even though the absolute risk is small, 1 stroke per 24,000 users per year, this is another reason to use other methods for birth control.

Control Your Temper

A seven-year Finnish study found that the incidence of stroke was twice as high in men who experienced outbursts of anger, when compared with those who controlled their tempers.[46] Follow the stress reduction techniques described in Chapter 2.

Use Acupuncture

This is one of the most promising alternative medicine approaches for stroke recovery. Relief from paralysis has been documented in

Chinese studies.[47] Its action for prevention deserves further study.

Practice Yoga and Tai Chi

These approaches can help your brain find alternative connections, and keep your muscles flexible. They provide stress management, and are part of the Ornish Heart Disease Reversal Program, which can apply to stroke prevention and reversal as well. See Chapter 8.

Practice Visualization

This technique may also be of particular benefit in stroke recovery, helping your brain to establish new pathways. Use any image that applies to your particular deficit, following the guidelines given in Chapter 2. Repeat your practice every few hours.

Conventional Medicine Approaches to Prevent Stroke

Conventional medical treatment to prevent stroke includes stopping smoking; controlling high blood pressure, heart disease, and diabetes, as discussed in the section on the alternative medicine approaches to prevent stroke; and taking medications.

Drug Treatments

Drugs found to have an established benefit in reducing risk of stroke are those that decrease the tendency of blood to clot and that lower cholesterol.

Blood Thinners

Medical treatment with the anticoagulant warfarin (Coumadin), which inhibits blood clotting, has been shown to reduce the risk of stroke by 68 percent in patients with atrial fibrillation, and is recommended for long-term use by the National Stroke Association if you fibrillate and are more than 75 years old or have the specific risk factors described above.[48] It is also indicated if you have had a heart attack, and have developed fibrillation, left ventricular function disturbance, or a blood clot in your left ventricle within several months after your heart attack.[49]

Aspirin is now the main form of medical treatment for brain artery disease, since it is safer than standard anticoagulant drugs. However, it, too, has a major complication rate of 1 percent per year. It exerts its anticoagulant-like, or "blood thinning," effect by causing the platelets in your blood to become less sticky, and therefore less likely to pile up on an ulcerated plaque and serve as a source of emboli. Studies have shown that aspirin decreases the TIA rate, and decreases the risk of nonfatal stroke and death from vascular disease in persons at high risk by about 25 percent.[50]

Too much aspirin inhibits vessel wall prostacyclin, a protective agent that prevents clotting. It can also irritate the stomach, and has been associated with ulcers. The optimum dosage of aspirin has not yet been fully determined, but is currently felt to be one baby aspirin (81 mg) per day.

Clopidogrel (Plavix) decreases platelet clumping and has been found to be 8.7 percent more effective than aspirin in decreasing stroke, heart attack, and death from vascular disease in persons at high risk.[51] This drug's safety is similar to that of aspirin.

Cholesterol-Lowering Drugs

The coenzyme A reductase inhibitors or cholesterol-lowering "statin" drugs decrease the risk of stroke after a heart attack and are recommended by the National Stroke Association.[52] A 2000 study in the *New England Journal of Medicine* found a 23 percent reduction in risk in patients who had previously had a heart attack or unstable angina.[53] See the discussion in Chapter 8.

Control Diabetes

The complications of diabetes increase your risk of stroke. Especially if your blood sugar is not well controlled, your rate of atherosclerosis can accelerate, leaving your arteries less pliable. This can induce high blood pressure or predispose you to clot formation.

Simply losing excess weight can help bring type II diabetes under better control. Follow the guidelines for diet, exercise, yoga, and group support given in Chapter 2.

Angioplasty Balloons and Stents

The use of carotid artery balloon angioplasty and stenting, similar to its application in the heart and leg circulations, discussed in Chapter 8 and above, is an emerging controversial technology to prevent stroke without a surgical operation. This approach has always worried surgeons because of the danger of balloon manipulation causing plaque debris to embolize or travel to brain arteries, thereby causing stroke or death. At this point, the technology hasn't advanced to a stage where it can be recommended, because results so far have been much worse than surgery.[54] However, with new technology on the horizon, this may prove to become a safe technique.

Surgical Approach to Prevent Stroke

Richard *was sitting in his chair watching television when part of the screen appeared to go dark. He started to push himself out of the*

chair, but found his left arm was very weak, and he went nowhere. He tried to call his wife, but could not find the words. After fifteen minutes, the TV screen gradually filled in, strength returned to his arm, and he was able to tell his wife what he had experienced. Richard's doctor did some tests, then referred him to a vascular surgeon, who ordered a duplex Doppler exam, which showed a narrowing in the carotid artery in the right side of his neck. He underwent uneventful surgery to eliminate the problem.

A *transcient ischemic attack,* such as the one Richard experienced, is a temporary event. If you have experienced one, you run a major risk of stroke, unless you undergo treatment. If you have had one TIA, your chances are about fifty-fifty of developing a stroke *before* having another TIA. A very large study, from fifty medical centers, studied 595 patients who had experienced a TIA, loss of vision in one eye, or a nondisabling stroke in the presence of a 70 to 99 percent carotid artery blockage. The researchers concluded that carotid artery surgery was highly beneficial in these patients. They found a 17 percent decreased incidence of stroke in the first eighteen months in the group randomized to undergo carotid artery surgery, compared to the nonsurgical group. Surgery produced a reduction in the stroke rate to 7 percent, versus 24 percent in the group treated medically.[55] Also, surgery reduced the risk for impairments in vision, fluency of speech, language comprehension, swallowing, arm and leg function, and ability to shop and visit outside the home.[56]

When TIA symptoms are clear-cut and correlate with findings of a 70 percent or greater artery blockage on duplex Doppler or angiography exams, little question exists about your need for an operation. Recent evidence suggests benefit from an operation even when the blockage is in the 50 to 69 percent range.[57] Although surgery does not produce a significant increase in life expectancy, because of the underlying risk of death from atherosclerotic heart disease, the *quality* of remaining life is much better.

However, the mortality rate for patients who already have significant cardiac disease and then undergo carotid artery surgery is as high as 8 percent. If you fall into this category, you would probably do better with nonsurgical management.

The most common surgical approach to prevent stroke is *carotid endarterectomy*. This surgical procedure removes carotid atherosclerotic plaque and debris, which is usually well localized to the easily accessible area in your neck where the common carotid artery divides.

You are admitted to the hospital on the morning of surgery. Carotid endarterectomy can be performed under local or general anesthesia. If general anesthesia is used, a breathing tube is placed after you are asleep. Some surgeons prefer you remain awake, so your brain function can be assessed by them asking you questions during the time your artery is clamped.

Your surgeon makes an incision along the muscle running from the collarbone to just behind the ear. (See Figure 9.8.) This exposes the common, internal and external carotid arteries. The dangerous part of the operation occurs when your artery is clamped and unclamped. Two potential hazards follow. First, while the artery is closed off, your brain may not receive enough blood from its other blood vessels. To avoid this problem, many surgeons routinely use a "shunt" bypass tube that allows blood flow to continue while the artery is cleaned out. Other surgeons avoid this technique, unless evidence has been found that

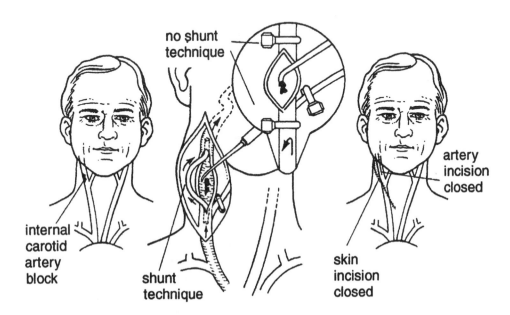

Fig. 9.8   Procedures involved in carotid endarterectomy

blood flow is critically decreased, because they feel that the manipulation of the shunt tube is more likely to cause the other major danger during the surgery: allowing bits of debris to migrate into your brain, where they can cause stroke.

After clamping, the vessel is opened and the diseased plaque carefully removed with forceps and fine scissors, leaving the artery with a smooth lining. The artery is then closed with stitches. The skin incision can subsequently be brought together with staples, skin clips, stitches, or skin tapes. Some surgeons routinely place a small plastic drain in the incision to prevent the possibility of a blood clot (hematoma) that could threaten breathing. It comes out a day or less after the operation.

Carotid endarterectomy requires forty-five to ninety minutes to perform. Postoperatively, you must be closely monitored—especially your blood pressure—for several hours, because severe complications can occur during this time. You may spend some time in intensive care, and can probably go home in one to three days. You may have some swelling, bruising, and stiffness in the neck for a week or two. You should see your surgeon at office visits, to ensure that no complications develop, and that your incision heals satisfactorily.

A recommendation for surgery to prevent stroke should not be taken lightly. Nationwide, the combined major complication and death rate from carotid endarterectomy is reported to be about 8 percent. Even the best reports indicate a 1 percent mortality and 1 percent risk of permanent stroke. Unreported outcomes are undoubtedly much higher, since poor results do not tend to be publicized. Your risk of dying or having major complica-

tions or a stroke from the surgery varies with your general medical status, the extent of disease in your brain's circulation, and the experience and skill of your surgeon and medical center. Heart attacks occur in 0.5 to 4 percent of endarterectomy patients, and are the leading cause of death.

Other possible complications include bleeding into your neck incision, and damage to nerves in your neck, which could cause hoarseness, permanent skin numbness, drooping of the side of your mouth, sagging of your shoulder, and deviation of your tongue to one side.

Surgery and "Asymptomatic" Bruits

At times, modern screening technology reveals more information than medicine knows how to handle. Many persons who have never had symptoms are found to have neck "bruits" (turbulent sounds found by placing a stethoscope over an area of partial blockage), or other noninvasive test results suggesting the presence of brain artery disease. Bruits are simply a general indicator of widespread vascular disease. A few persons with bruits do go on to develop TIAs and strokes, but most do not. The question of what you should do if you are one of these patients is most controversial.

In the early 1980s, vascular and neurosurgeons were operating on just about everyone they could find with a neck bruit, whether they had symptoms or not, with the idea this would protect against strokes. However, widely publicized studies soon showed an unacceptably high rate of strokes or death from the operation itself, and it became clear that the chance of developing a stroke was higher *with* surgery than without it. Carotid endarterectomy then developed a very bad reputation, and use of this procedure almost came to a halt.

Since that period, much has been learned about the natural history of an asymptomatic bruit. In the 1990s clinical trials showed that when patients are properly selected, a clear benefit is accrued from this operation, and a dramatic rise in the rates of this procedure has followed dissemination of this information.

If you have a bruit, your carotid artery should be watched very carefully, via periodic noninvasive Doppler exams. If your narrowing reaches 60 percent, you should consider an operation, since the risk of stroke *then* becomes substantial. Solid evidence now suggests that preventive surgery reduces the relative risk for stroke in men by 66 percent and women by 17 percent over five years, compared to medical treatment alone, in patients with a greater than 60 percent blockage of a carotid artery.[58] The American Heart Association recommends surgery if you have greater than 60 percent blockage *provided* you are carefully selected, the surgery is done by a surgeon and medical center who have a documented surgical complication and death rate of less than 3 percent, and postoperative management of modifiable risk factors is present.[59]

A national study of Medicare patients has shown that hospitals where carotid endarterectomy is performed more frequently have better results, and that Medicare patients' operative mortality is substantially higher than that reported in the clinical trials.[60] The National Institutes of Health also recommends that this operation should be done only by surgeons who have demonstrated mortality and major complication rates of less than 3 percent. Much discussion in vascular surgery circles and the medical literature has focused on the desirability of individual surgeons and hospitals to document their results and make this information available to prospective patients. Ask your surgeon if he or she has this information.

Carotid Surgery After Stroke

Twenty percent of all patients die as a result of their first stroke, usually within the first few days. After about six weeks, a stroke is considered to have stabilized—in other words, the tissue swelling will have resolved, no further changes from that stroke follow, and any effects will likely be permanent. The "completed" stroke may leave mild or profound deficits, with many degrees in between, depending on how much and what specific part of the brain is affected.

Except in cases of profound stroke, brain tissue remaining within the vascular field of the diseased artery is in jeopardy for another stroke. Your chance of developing another stroke is 10 percent at one year, and almost 50 percent at five years. This is the biggest risk to your life, since the mortality of a second stroke is much higher than with the first; about 50 percent of all stroke patients eventually die from another one. If you have had a stroke, after a period of stabilization, you need to consider diagnosis and treatment to prevent future strokes.

Duplex Doppler, angiography, and CAT scan help pinpoint the cause of the stroke, and determine whether surgery is indicated, and when it is safest. Surgery can then be carried out, as discussed above.

STROKE SUMMARY

Prevention

Diet and Supplements

- Follow a low-fat, high-fiber diet.
- Balanced vitamin B-complex capsule containing 400 mcg of folic acid, 50 mg of vitamin B_6, and 50 mcg of vitamin B_{12} per day.
- Vitamin E, D-alpha, 400 IU daily.
- Vitamin C, 1,000 mg 2 times daily.
- Bioflavonoids, 1,000 mg daily.
- Selenium, 200 mcg daily.
- Flaxseed oil, 1 tablespoon daily.
- Garlic, 8 mg allicin daily.
- Ginko biloba, 40 mg 3 times daily.
- Switch from coffee to herb tea, or decaf black or green tea.

Lifestyle

- Don't smoke.
- Control high blood pressure.
- Control high cholesterol.
- Control diabetes.
- Exercise regularly: 1 hour, 3–5 times weekly.
- Maintain optimum weight.
- Avoid excess alcohol intake.
- Avoid oral contraceptives.
- Control your temper.

Alternative Medicine Approaches

- Follow the preventive guidelines, above.
- Try acupuncture.
- Practice daily yoga, tai chi, qi gong.
- Use visualization.

Conventional Medicine Approaches

- Blood thinners—aspirin, warfarin (Coumadin), ticlopidene, Ticlid, clopidogrel, Plavix.
- Cholesterol-lowering drugs—niacin, cholestyramine, colestipol, gemfibrozil, Lopid, pravastatin, simvastatin.
- Carotid stent.

Surgical Approach

- Carotid endarterectomy.

C H A P T E R 10

VEINS

Increased abdominal pressure caused by straining to pass small firm stools has been singled out as a major cause of varicose veins.

Denis Burkitt, M.D.

Janet, a 30-year-old executive vice president of a bank, was disturbed by varicose veins at her ankle that were large enough to show from beneath her nylon stockings. They also began to ache a bit after a long day. She thought about surgery, but she first decided to explore alternative medicine. After a review of her nutritional intake, found low in fiber and too high in fats, she began eating significantly increased amounts of raw foods. She also began a supplement program, and implemented the other suggestions given below. Within a month, the veins diminished enough to cause her no further cosmetic difficulties or pain.

If you are embarrassed to wear shorts or a swimming suit because of the condition of the veins in your legs, or your veins cause you discomfort, you may be considering vein surgery. Disorders of the leg veins are *very* common in the Western world, and uncommon in the East. They may range from seemingly trivial spiderlike skin blotches or dilated superficial veins with only cosmetic significance to huge, distorted, and painful varicose veins, ulcers, or even vein blood clots that can migrate and block your lung's blood circulation.

In addition to providing dietary and other lifestyle suggestions for preventing the formation of these abnormal veins, in this chapter we will review alternative medicine research which suggests that a number of agents and activities may actually give you a chance for reversal of these disorders. A broader understanding of the relationship of diet and lifestyle to the health of your veins has provided a fresh way of thinking about these annoying and sometimes serious problems.

We both recommend an initial trial of alternative approaches, before you choose surgery. For severe venous disease you should wear surgical support stockings for the rest of your life anyway, with or without surgery. Most symptoms can usually be relieved through the sole use of such stockings and other simple, nonsurgical measures. In some circumstances, however, you may find that surgery may still be worthwhile, and several options are available.

How Your Veins Work

Your *arterial system* carries oxygen and nutrient-rich blood to your tiny, one-cell-layer-thick vessels, the *capillaries*. The capillaries then connect your arteries to your *venous system*, which returns blood to your heart and lungs. Smaller veins join with larger branches until they reach the *vena cava*, the largest of all veins, an inch in diameter, which empties directly into your heart.

Your veins consist of "*superficial*" and "*deep*" systems. (See Figure 10.1.) What we see when we look at our arms and legs are the superficial veins. This superficial system is at low pressure. In contrast, the deep system, surrounded by muscles, carries blood at high pressure. *Communicating veins,* which connect the superficial with the deep system, have valves to protect the superficial veins from the high pressure of the deep veins.

Two mechanisms provide the force for venous blood flow. First, some of the pumping

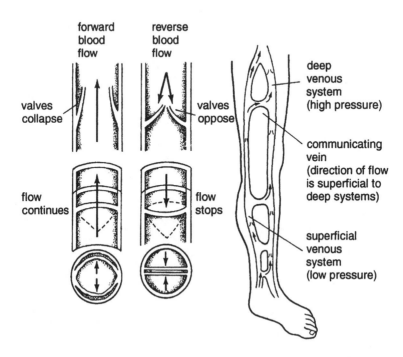

Fig. 10.1 The anatomy and functioning of the veins in the leg

pressure of the heart is transmitted to the veins through the capillary bed. Second, through a combination of muscle action and the *venous valves,* your every movement squeezes the veins, pushing blood back toward your heart. The one-way valves within the veins prevent your blood from flowing backward.

If you stand motionless for a prolonged period, the force of gravity tends to cause fluid and blood to leak out of your capillaries and small veins; if you have no mechanism to compensate for this, the fluid and blood then pools in your lower legs, injuring the surrounding tissues and eventually causing skin ulcers. However, when you are active, the muscle pump and valve system act together to rapidly reduce the pressure of gravity, restoring upward flow, protecting your veins and tissue.

When these vein valves are absent, defective, or destroyed, the efficiency of this important system is decreased, and varicose veins form. Even in individuals with normal valves, inactivity eliminates your muscle pump, leading to leakage of fluids and subsequent leg swelling. Exercise and yoga stretches stimulate local muscle action, and thus can play an important role in prevention and treatment of vein disorders.

Varicose Veins

Varicose veins are enlarged, elongated, and tortuous superficial veins that appear almost exclusively in the legs. (See Figure 10.2.) As noted above, they result from abnormally high pressure in the veins caused by lack of or

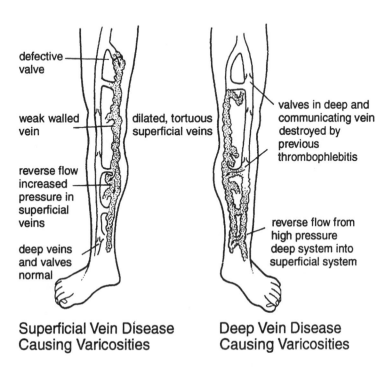

Superficial Vein Disease Causing Varicosities

Deep Vein Disease Causing Varicosities

Fig. 10.2 Types of varicose veins

damage to the vein valves. The severest varicose veins are formed when disease has destroyed the valves in your deep venous system. The pressure in your deep veins is increased, and the valves in the communicating veins weaken, transmitting high pressure into the superficial system. Such elevated pressure dilates these veins, and eventually renders their valves incompetent.

Risk for vein disease increases with age, so that while only 1 percent of the people in the United States less than 20 years of age have varicosities, 50 percent of those older than 50 years have them.

Your occupation and lifestyle influence your chances of developing varicose veins. Jobs requiring prolonged standing such as waitressing, or store clerking—or even being a surgeon—increase the risk. Anything that elevates your abdominal pressure may be harmful. For example, rickshaw drivers, compared to other males in their society, despite a high-fiber diet, have high rate of formation of varicosities, because their continuous heavy lifting causes chronically increased venous pressure.[1]

Risk for varicose veins is much higher in women, probably reflecting hormonal influences on the vein wall. Pregnancy often aggravates varicosities, when elevated hormone levels may weaken these walls. Late in pregnancy, increased blood volume and the enlarged uterus's compression of pelvic veins act together to increase venous pressure.

Heredity may raise your risk for varicosities. The inherited defect may be a vein wall weakness, or the valves may be absent, few in number, or defectively constructed, resulting in a similar increase in venous pressure and vein dilation. Still, even if you inherit the tendency to develop varicose veins, you may be able to prevent them by following a high-fiber diet, along with the other simple measures presented below.

Varicose veins can cause a variety of problems, though often, you may have no symptoms at all, even with apparently extensive disease. On the other hand, what appears to be minimal disease can cause some people a great deal of discomfort. You may experience aching, tiredness, heaviness, mild swelling, muscle cramps, itching, and burning. Such symptoms are usually worse toward the end of the day, especially after prolonged standing or sitting, and are minimized in the mornings. Women often have increased problems around menstruation. Most of this discomfort can be promptly relieved by elevation of your legs.

Simple superficial varicose veins rarely cause leg swelling or skin problems. The "stasis" changes of dark discoloration, scaling, itching, and skin oozing, ulceration, and infection, are associated with the long-standing effects of increased venous pressure transmitted from the deep venous system. "Stasis ulcers" usually develop on the inner surface of the lower leg, just above the ankle. They are notoriously difficult to heal, and tend to recur.

How Varicose Veins Are Diagnosed

Varicose veins can usually be diagnosed just by history and simple physical exam. The duplex Doppler exam may be requested to look at your deeper veins and valve function. Rarely, a venogram is necessary.

History

Your doctor should ask about your symptoms, their severity, what makes them worse, and what you have done to relieve them. A past history of leg trauma or deep venous blood clots may give clues that you have damaged deep vein valves. Family history of varicose veins is common. You need to discuss your smoking history, medical problems associated with blood-clotting tendency, work requirements, and lifestyle choices.

Physical Exam

Your doctor should examine and feel your veins. One leg larger than the other may indicate long-standing deep venous valve damage. A variety of simple tests using rubber tourniquets and the Doppler device can help locate defective valves and communicating veins, which may be allowing reverse flow from the deep to superficial systems.

Duplex Doppler Exam

The *duplex Doppler exam,* as described on page 290, is the best noninvasive test for a sophisticated look at the venous system. It can show blockages, reverse flow through damaged valves, and blood clots.

Venogram

In unusual cases, a more invasive test, the *venogram,* may be necessary to help your surgeon locate abnormal veins. Dye that can be seen on X-ray is injected into a vein in your foot and pictured as it goes up the leg and into the pelvis. Abnormal valves, vein patterns, blockages, and blood clots can be seen. Venography is somewhat uncomfortable, since the dye is irritating to the veins; it can cause a thrombophlebitis, a painful inflammation of the veins. However, such a result is rarely significant now with less irritative contrast dye.

Alternative Medicine Approaches to Varicose Veins

In most cases, even very unsightly veins can become greatly diminished with changes in lifestyle. You may also find these modifications helpful for your overall health, and worth a trial, before you choose a surgical procedure. Following are the most promising approaches.

Change Your Diet

As noted above, varicose veins are *not* ubiquitous in human cultures. Although about one-fifth of the world's adult population has varicosities, including 50 percent of older Americans and Europeans, these vein problems are very rare in cultures that eat a high-fiber diet.

If you are consuming three meals per day and do not have two or three easy-to-pass bowel movements interspersed throughout the day—the result of a diet with adequate fiber—your colon can become congested and full of stool, so that it presses on the large pelvic and abdominal veins, causing increased pressure within them, and transmitting that high pressure to the veins in your legs. Any accompanying straining at stool also elevates your venous pressure. Pushing forcefully at stool has been strongly associated with both varicose veins and diverticular disease of the colon—the small outpouchings of the colon lining that can become inflamed or bleed, discussed in Chapter 15.[2]

Even during pregnancy, women who eat a high-fiber diet do not develop varicose veins as frequently as women on a low-fiber diet[3]—making this an especially important time to switch to increased fiber. In general, varicosities during pregnancy recede after delivery, and can temporarily be treated with support stockings, along with the lifestyle measures listed below.

Since more than 50 percent of persons with varicose veins have no symptoms, especially if you are one of these, a trial of natural approaches may always be your best first step, to see if you can ameliorate any cosmetic problems without resorting to surgery. A number of studies have documented that, after a switch to higher fiber in the diet, both appearance and symptoms associated with varicose veins improve. Follow the dietary guidelines given in Chapter 2, including fresh whole fruits and vegetables and whole grains. Especially to be avoided are refined white flour and sugar, which contain no fiber at all, and can particularly act like wallpaper paste to congest your colon. You can choose soy cheese, which does have fiber, instead of that made of dairy, which has none. If you are still not having easy bowel movements, adding several tablespoonfuls of fresh-ground flaxseeds to your daily food intake should give you easy passage, along with vital essential fatty acids, as presented in Chapter 2.

Take Supplements

Low levels of several vitamins have been associated with the development of varicose veins, particularly *vitamins A, C, E and the bioflavonoids*. Vitamin C and E supplements may help strengthen vein walls, decreasing their tendency to stretch and incapacitate valves when faced with increased pressure. Take 5,000 IU of vitamin A daily, 1,000 mg vitamin C complex with bioflavonoids, two to three times daily, and 400 IU vitamin E, one to three times daily. See Chapter 2 for further discussion of supplements.

Blood flow and venous appearance were found to be improved with the antioxidant Pycnogenol.[4] The usual dosage is 150 to 300 mg daily.

The herbs centella asiatica extract (containing 70 percent triterpenic acid) 30 mg,

three times a day, ruscus aculeatus (butcher's broom) extract 100 mg, three times daily, and escin (horse chestnut seed extract) 10 mg, three times a day, have been found very useful in preventing and treating varicose veins by strengthening the vein wall, increasing its tone, and reducing venous leak.[5]

An analysis of all available double-blind, randomized controlled trials of oral horse chestnut seed extract as symptomatic treatment for patients with chronic venous insufficiency was reported by Drs. Max Pittler and Edward Ernst in *Archives of Dermatology*. They found this treatment superior to placebo, and as effective as standard medications in reducing leg swelling and symptoms of leg pain, itching, and feelings of fatigue and tenseness.[6]

The enzyme bromelain, found in pineapple and papaya, exhibits fibrinolytic effects, at a dosage of 500 mg daily, and can be especially helpful if you have already developed thrombophlebitis.[7] The herbs *bilberry, garlic, ginger, hawthorn, onions, cayenne,* and *parsley, at dosages of 500 mg daily,* may provide cofactors that help improve your circulation and help you avoid blood clot formation.[8]

Maintain Your Optimum Weight

Excess weight is itself a risk factor for varicose vein formation.[9] See Chapter 2 for optimum dietary and alternative medicine approaches to help you achieve your best weight, and reduce the stress associated with maintaining that accomplishment.

Exercise Regularly and Practice Yoga

Whenever you can, to prevent vein problems, you need to avoid sitting or standing for long periods without movement, and implement a regular exercise program into your lifestyle. Movement and exercise enlist your muscle pump, keeping your superficial venous pressure to a minimum. Try to do active exercise three to five times per week.

Yoga practices are especially useful in the treatment of varicose veins, since they systematically squeeze all the major muscle groups, moving your circulation most effectively; they are presented more fully in Chapter 2. The shoulder stand is the most important of the postures, and you should gradually increase holding the full or modified pose ten to fifteen minutes twice daily.

Elevate Your Legs

Putting your legs up is important. Elevation counters gravity, assists venous return, and decreases pressure, promoting the clearance of fluid that causes leg swelling. At night you can elevate your legs by putting four- to six-inch blocks under the foot of your bed. If you can, put your feet up during the day, particularly if you have a severer case. The principle is to elevate your lower legs above the level of your heart, so that your blood and lymph fluid can "run downhill" to your heart instead of backward to your feet.

Don't Cross Your Legs

Kicking the habit of crossing your legs at the ankles and especially the knees is the first thing you should do if you have varicose veins. Crossing interferes with the upward flow of blood, increasing the pressure inside the veins. Increased pressure causes them to dilate, elongate, and twist. If you do this as part of your yoga practice, make certain to have a soft cushion beneath your buttocks, ease into it gradually, and stay no longer in the posture than you are completely comfortable.

Use Magnets

The ache of varicose veins may be diminished by the application of magnets. You can simply apply a small disk magnet, available at health food stores, or use magnetic insoles in your shoes. Further research is needed.

Practice Visualization

Visualization may be helpful. As an example, you may choose to imagine your veins as if they were a watering system on a large lawn. Excessive pressure from the large hoses is causing the smaller ones to twist and enlarge. Turn down the tap, and see all of the flow as easy, gentle, and relaxing. In your mind's eye, picture your veins as normal and perfectly competent, and at the same time, feel this happening within your body.

Take Other Measures

Position during bowel movements may also contribute to varicosities; a discussion of alternatives is located in the section on hemorrhoids later in this book. Persons with varicosities should avoid tight-fitting clothing, which puts pressure on the abdomen and thus interferes with venous return.

Stress may play a role in this disease, since holding tension in your muscles acts to interfere with good venous circulation. Practice the stress management program given in Chapter 2.

The development of both hemorrhoids and varicose veins may also reflect congestion in the liver and the gallbladder. A liver-gallbladder flush, as described in Chapter 13, may therefore assist in your healing, and help prevent recurrence.

Conventional Medicine Approaches to Varicose Veins

In addition to leg elevation, the conventional medicine approaches to varicose veins are support stockings and injection sclerotherapy.

Support Stockings

Wearing a good elastic support stocking provides carefully controlled pressure against diseased superficial veins and, in effect, performs the same function muscles do for the deep system. The enlarged, tortuous veins are collapsed, eliminating stagnant pools of blood, and blood is prevented from running down to your feet through incompetent valves. Flow in the deep veins is promoted, and the net effect is to decrease venous pressure, preventing capillary leak. Your skin, which may have become thin and delicate, is supported and protected against injury.

If you have minimal disease, you may get away with cheap, over-the-counter "support hose." However, if you have significant varicosities and symptoms, you need high-quality elastic surgical support stockings. Stockings with different amounts of counterpressure, depending on the extent of disease present, are available only with a doctor's prescription. Unfortunately, these stockings cost from $20 to $50 for the toe-to-calf type, even more for the models that include the thigh, or a "body stocking." However, they are well constructed, and with proper care can be expected to last from six to twelve months.

Problems can develop with the stockings. A poor fit can create a tourniquet effect, making matters worse. The stockings may be difficult to pull on and remove, particularly if you are elderly or have arthritis. Even a well-fitting stocking can be uncomfortable and hot, especially in warm weather.

In addition, a trade-off exists between the beneficial effects of these stockings and their obvious cosmetic challenge. However, most people don't require more than a toe-to-calf stocking, even if varicosities are present above this level, since the highest venous pressures occur in the lower leg; it is extremely rare to develop skin problems or swelling above the knee. Shorter stockings, after a period of adjustment, are usually acceptable if they are well fitted. Expensive thigh level and body stockings are often abandoned as too much trouble.

If severe stasis changes or skin ulceration occurs, an Unna boot can be used to heal the acute problem. The Unna boot is a wrap, similar to an Ace bandage, impregnated with a paste containing zinc oxide, calamine, and other ingredients to promote healing. It is in turn covered with an Ace bandage, which provides compression. It should be changed every five to ten days. After healing occurs, a prescription surgical support stocking should be worn thereafter, to prevent recurrence.

Joe, an 80-year-old retired Navy cook, had for years noticed a brown discoloration, and enlarged veins, above the inside of his right ankle. One day, he scratched an itching area and, over a five month period, watched the scratch slowly develop into a two-inch ulcer, despite the usage of various over-the-counter topical preparations. He eventually showed it to his doctor, who sent him for a surgical consultation. The surgeon recommended tying off the veins that were contributing increased venous pressure to the ulcer bed, followed by a skin graft to cover the ulcer. Alternatively, the option of trying to heal the ulcer through the use of a series of Unna boots was ex-

plained. Joe was fearful of surgery, and its expense, and chose the Unna boot route. After eight months of weekly boot changes, the ulcer eventually healed. He then became extremely careful to wear his surgical support stocking whenever he was on his feet, to prevent recurrent problems.

Sclerotherapy

Sclerotherapy is an office procedure, requiring fifteen to thirty minutes for each treatment session. While you stand, several small needles are placed into the distended veins. You then lie on an examining table, and your doctor injects an irritating sclerosing solution into each varicosity, causing vein wall inflammation. The vein is next collapsed by an external elastic compression (Ace) bandage, which must be worn for several weeks. The vein walls permanently seal together. You can walk immediately after the procedure. Usually, you experience only minimal discomfort.

You should follow up with your doctor in a week or so, to see the effect of the injections and determine if more are necessary. The whole process can be time consuming, since usually not all veins can be treated at once. Often many office visits, injections, and wrappings over several weeks or months are required. The main advantage of this procedure is that, if successful, you can avoid an operation and scars.

Possible complications include blood clots from vein irritation, and allergic reactions. If the sclerosing solution leaks out of the vein, the adjacent tissue may shrink, leaving a depression. Your skin may become discolored, and a skin ulcer that can be difficult to heal can develop. Such complications can leave you with a worse cosmetic result than that with which you began. The varicosity recurrence rate is also higher than with surgery.

Although sclerotherapy is widely used in Europe, not many American surgeons have been trained to use this technique on typical, larger varicosities. Sclerotherapy, as well as a laser, is more frequently used to treat small, superficial, cosmetically objectionable "spider veins," and for limited recurrent varicosities after surgery. Many dermatologists and plastic surgeons offer these procedures.

Surgical Approaches to Varicose Veins

Maria, a 36-year-old mother of five, developed varicose veins that became larger and more painful with each succeeding pregnancy. Her symptoms were partially relieved with a body-stocking type support hose, but she decided she would have surgery as soon as possible after her final child was born. She is happy with the results, and wears nonprescription support stockings to prevent a return of her problem.

In most cases, symptoms associated with varicose veins can be eliminated by support stockings. Surgery is thus rarely necessary. However, surgery may be recommended if you have significant symptoms not controlled with support stockings, very large varicosities, bleeding from veins which have eroded through the skin, nonhealing ulcers despite appropriate conservative management, or recurrent blood clots in your superficial veins (phlebitis). Your choices include ligation and excision, or ligation and stripping.

Prior to the surgery, most surgeons request a duplex Doppler exam of your veins. This is to determine if you have incompetent valves in your greater and lesser saphenous veins and to locate any incompetent communicating veins between your superficial and deep venous systems, which would need to be treated for best results.

On the day of surgery, you are admitted to the hospital in the morning. Your veins are carefully marked with an indelible marker so your surgeon can easily find them when your leg is elevated and the veins collapse. Your operation can be performed under general or spinal anesthesia, or local anesthesia if the varicosities are confined to a small area.

In *ligation and excision,* sections of diseased superficial veins are removed through multiple one-quarter-inch incisions up and down your legs. (See Figure 10.3.) A small one-inch incision is made in the groin and the diseased greater saphenous vein tied off, to prevent reverse blood flow back down the leg. If the lesser saphenous vein is diseased, it is tied off behind the knee. If your major veins are normal, the surgery is limited to removing the grossly visible clusters of varicosities through one-quarter-inch incisions. Normal veins, which may be needed later for bypass grafting, can be left undisturbed. This method has a higher rate of recurrent varicosities than when stripping is added.

Classic *ligation and stripping* is the same as ligation and excision except that after the vein is tied off in the groin, a flexible stripping instrument is passed within it down to your knee or ankle. A one-half-inch incision is

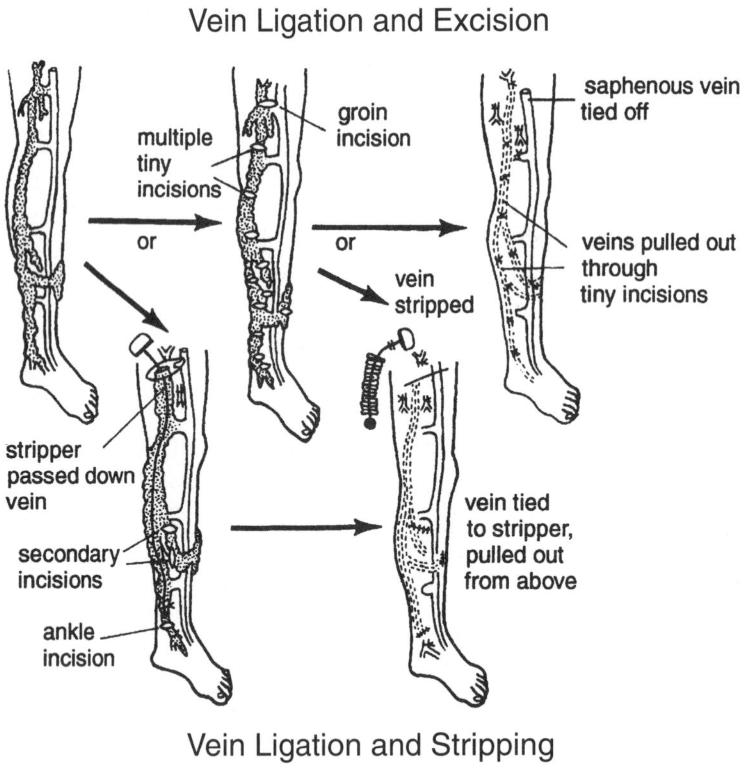

Vein Ligation and Excision

multiple tiny incisions

or

groin incision

or

vein stripped

saphenous vein tied off

veins pulled out through tiny incisions

stripper passed down vein

secondary incisions

ankle incision

vein tied to stripper, pulled out from above

Vein Ligation and Stripping

Fig. 10.3 Procedures involved in vein ligation and excision, and vein ligation and stripping

made and the vein tied to it. The stripper and vein are then pulled out through the groin incision, separating it from its bed and branches. Side branch varicosities are removed through multiple small incisions as above. This method has a higher incidence of uncomfortable postoperative nerve sensations than simple ligation and excision, especially with stripping below the knee.

Normally, the superficial venous system carries only 15 percent of the return blood flow from the leg, and after surgery, this flow is easily handled by the deep venous system.

After the operation is completed, the incisions are closed with stitches, staples, or skin tapes. Your leg is wrapped in an elastic bandage from toe to high thigh, to keep the disrupted veins collapsed and prevent blood from accumulating under your skin. You will be encouraged to walk as soon as possible, to prevent deep vein clots from developing. Only a few patients stay overnight.

After surgery, you should avoid sitting with your feet down, elevate the foot of your bed, and wear the elastic wrap. Your surgeon should see you in a week or so, to evaluate the effects of the operation and to ensure that your incisions are healing satisfactorily. The elastic bandage can be shortened to the calf level, and will need to be worn for several more weeks. To avoid recurrent varicosities, you should wear a support stocking, although you may be able to use one of the cheaper, nonprescription varieties if your disease is mild. Work can be resumed as soon as you are comfortable. Persistent varicosities that didn't disappear with the original surgery can be removed as a minor outpatient procedure using local anesthesia, or treated by sclerotherapy.

Some postoperative swelling and bruising is usual, most of which should disappear in a few weeks. Complications include *hematoma,* a blood clot under the skin, and problems with incision healing. Injury to skin sensory nerves can cause numbness and disturbing burning, shooting pain, though this is rarely a persistent problem.

The success rate of varicose vein surgery is 80 to 90 percent, with recurrence ranging from 10 to 30 percent, depending on the completeness of removal of the superficial venous system. If the varicosities are caused by deep venous system disease, the permanent success rate is much lower, and you should wear surgical support stockings for the rest of your life.

VARICOSE VEIN SUMMARY

Prevention

Diet and Supplements

- Follow a low-fat, high-fiber diet.
- Multivitamin, particularly including vitamins A, C, E and the bioflavonoids.
- Vitamin C, 1,000–2,000 mg.
- Psyllium powder, 1–2 tablespoons daily.

Lifestyle

- Utilize daily yoga postures, especially inverted poses.
- Utilize stress management.
- Maintain optimum weight.
- Exercise regularly: 1 hour, 3–5 times weekly.
- Elevate your legs; don't cross your legs.
- Utilize a squatting position on the toilet.
- Avoid tight-fitting clothing.

Alternative Medicine Approaches

- Follow preventive guidelines, given.
- Vitamin A, 5,000 IU daily.
- Vitamin C complex with bioflavonoids, 1,000mg 2–3 times daily.
- Vitamin E, 400 IU 1–3 times daily.
- Pycnogenol, 150–300 mg daily.
- Primary Herbs: *Centella asiatica*, 30 mg 3 times daily; *escin*, 10 mg, 3 times daily; butcher's broom *(Ruscus aculeatus)*, 100 mg 3 times daily; bromelain, 300 mg daily.
- Secondary Herbs: as teas, or added to diet: gotu kola, bilberry, garlic, ginger, hawthorn, onions, cayenne, parsley.
- Bromelain—in pineapple and papaya.
- Horse chestnut seed extract.
- Homeopathics: arnica, aconitum, carbo veg, hamamelis, pulstilla.
- Magnets.
- Liver flush.
- Visualization.

Conventional Medicine Approaches

- Support stockings.
- Sclerotherapy.

Surgical Approaches

- Ligation and stripping.
- Ligation and excision.

CHAPTER 11

ESOPHAGUS

*Now good digestion wait on appetite
And health on both.*

William Shakespeare

Hattie was typical of someone suffering from heartburn. At age 65, she had experienced a burning sensation in her stomach region for years, had spent a fortune on antacids, was sleeping propped almost upright, and still could find no ongoing relief from her stomach distress. She contemplated surgical correction of her esophageal reflux, but decided at the last minute to at least try one more time to solve her problem without a scalpel.

She began the alternative medicine program given below: a low-fat, high-fiber diet, combined with substituting herbal chamomile tea for her daily caffeinated coffee and tea. For the first few days she had a bit more gas and frequent bowel movements, but after two weeks she was a new person. No more pain, better sleep, and more energy were her rewards. She felt so much better she then began volunteering at her local hospital, to teach others about the rewards of alternative medicine approaches.

At least once in your life, you, too, have probably suffered from classic "heartburn," a significant burning feeling in your chest, which often follows a large or spicy meal. "Heartburn" is a misnomer; what is burning is not your heart, but your esophagus. Occasionally, an "affair of the heart" can cause digestive distress, but the only actual connection between heartburn and the heart is that both are located in your chest.

The esophagus is usually a silent organ, and we take the ability to swallow for granted. When esophageal difficulties do develop, the fundamental process of nourishing your body can be jeopardized, creating severe psychological stress. Fortunately, except for cancer of the esophagus, most esophageal problems can be treated quite successfully by the new contributions of alternative medicine, which address the roots of the problem. Simply attacking heartburn with antacids or acid-inhibiting drugs, although it may help at times to eliminate your symptoms, avoids attention to the important underlying factors, discussed below.

If you do choose them, newer surgical techniques are much less invasive, and utilize the laparoscope to provide faster recovery, smaller scars, and less pain.

How Your Esophagus Works

In the past twenty or thirty years, much has been learned about the esophagus's mechanical function—its specific muscular contractions that enable you to swallow, its response to stimuli, and the critical relationship of its pressure to that of the stomach. Influences of the nervous system and hormones on the esophagus are not yet as well understood.

Many tests and devices have been developed to help sort out esophageal disease from other problems that may give you similar symptoms. These have helped pave the way for safer and more effective use of the alternative medicine approaches, medications, and surgery discussed in this chapter.

Your esophagus is a muscular tube that extends from the middle of your neck, at the back of your throat, down through your chest, behind your lungs and heart. (See Figure 11.1.) It descends through your diaphragm (the muscular wall that separates the lung cavity from the abdomen), and on into the upper part of your abdomen, where it joins your stomach. It is fourteen to seventeen inches long, and about three-quarters to one and one-half inches in diameter—although it can expand to two inches wide when food or liquid is passing through. Like the rest of your gastrointestinal tract, the esophagus has a soft pink lining and outer muscle layers, some arranged in a circular pattern, and some running lengthwise. Its muscular activity is not under your conscious control, although muscle contractions occur in response to swallowing, which is, of course, a voluntary activity.

Two pinch-valves, called *sphincters*, are located at each end of the esophagus. These are normally closed. The *upper esophageal sphincter* prevents food, liquid, and swallowed secretions from "refluxing"—returning up into your mouth or throat, where you could breathe them into your lungs. When you swallow, this pinch-valve must relax in a coordinated way to allow the contents of your mouth to pass through. Likewise, your *lower esophageal sphincter* prevents your stomach's acid from returning upward, where it would irritate or injure the esophagus's sensitive lining. It must relax as well, at the right time, to allow any swallowed material to pass at the proper moment.

Both of these valves must also relax to allow for belching or vomiting, important protective mechanisms for releasing distress whenever your stomach becomes irritated or distended. Most of the problems of the esophagus are a result of dysfunction of these valves, or a lack of coordination of the wavelike contractions that are created when you swallow.

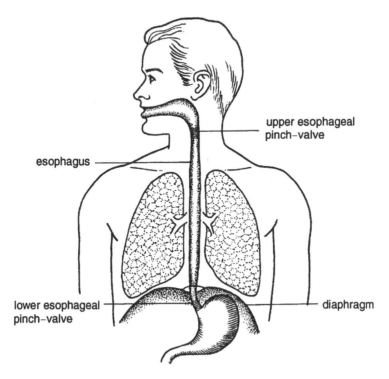

Fig. 11.1 The anatomy and location of the esophagus

How Esophageal Disease Is Diagnosed

Expensive and uncomfortable tests are usually not needed if your symptoms are typical of simple heartburn (see page 337). However, since esophageal difficulties can occasionally be caused by serious disease, you should not simply reach for antacids, or try other remedies on your own. This is especially true if you have difficulty swallowing or a sensation of food sticking in your throat.

Esophageal disease is diagnosed by history, physical exam, X-rays, esophagoscopy, and if necessary, more sophisticated tests of its muscular coordination and pinch valve function.

History and Physical Exam

Your doctor should perform a detailed investigation of your symptoms in relation to your eating habits, activities, and discomfort patterns. Location, intensity, and duration of pain are important, as well as when it typically occurs. Be sure to report difficulty or pain on swallowing, sensation of food or liquids sticking in your throat or chest, and return of sour, acid, or solid material to your mouth that may indicate problems with your esophagus. Frequent attacks of bronchitis, hoarseness, or pneumonia may be caused by this refluxed material being breathed into your airways while you are sleeping. During the physical exam, your doctor feels your neck and abdomen for masses, looks in your mouth, and listens to your chest with a stethoscope.

If your symptoms are worrisome, or persist after a trial of the conventional and alternative medicine programs described later in this chapter, you will need further tests.

Esophagogram

An *esophagogram* is a test where you swallow a barium solution (clay that shows up on X-ray) as your radiologist watches on a TV monitor. X-ray films are taken and a videotape can be made to record your esophageal contractions. The radiologist will be looking for narrowing of the esophagus, abnormalities in contraction or pinch-valve relaxation, reflux of stomach contents back into your esophagus, and signs of cancer. For this test you stand against, or lie on, the X-ray table, and roll into various positions as you swallow the barium. This test takes only a few minutes, and is comfortable and safe.

Esophagoscopy

For an *esophagoscopy*, you lie on your side while the doctor maneuvers a flexible three-eight-inch scope through your mouth, into your esophagus, and on into your stomach. This allows a close look at the lining of your esophagus. The doctor can determine whether reflux from your stomach into your esophagus is present, and can pass small instruments through the scope to take biopsies for microscopic study. Esophagoscopy is somewhat uncomfortable, though not usually painful. A local anesthetic is used to numb the back of your throat and knock out your "gag" reflex. Mild intravenous sedation is commonly given. It takes five to fifteen minutes, and is

available on an outpatient basis in most hospitals and many doctors' offices. This test does carry some risk: The danger of a major complication is about 0.2 percent and includes significant bleeding and perforation (puncture) of the esophagus, more likely if a biopsy is performed.[1]

Esophageal Manometry

This test is performed by having you swallow a small plastic tube that measures pressures at different places in your esophagus. It assesses the function of your lower esophageal pinch-valve and looks for abnormalities in the contraction waves. It is safe, only slightly uncomfortable, and does not require hospitalization. Because of the sophisticated equipment and the medical expertise required, it may not be available in all hospitals. This test is necessary if you are considering esophageal surgery to correct swallowing difficulties or severe reflux, as described in the next section.

Esophageal pH Testing

If there is some doubt about the cause of your symptoms, you may be asked to have a twenty-four-hour test that records the relative acidity/alkalinity of your lower esophagus. A tiny tube with a pH sensor is passed through your nose and on into the esophagus then positioned just above your stomach. The tube is connected to a small recorder that you can wear on your belt. If you have symptoms of heartburn when your esophagus tests acid, there is good evidence that stomach contents returning to your esophagus are causing the symptoms.

Hiatal Hernia and Esophageal Reflux

"Sliding" hiatal hernias are quite common, affecting 50 percent of the American population over the age of 40. This type of hernia (outpouching) occurs when the junction of your stomach and esophagus balloons up (slides) through the opening where your esophagus passes through your diaphragm, forming an outpouching. Individuals with a weakness in the tissue normally holding this junction below the diaphragm are predisposed to hiatal hernia. The problem may be present at birth, or develop with advancing age or chronically increased pressure in the abdomen. You may be predisposed to its development if you are overweight, pregnant, strain when urinating or having a bowel movement, practice frequent vigorous exercise, or wear tight clothing.

Gastroesophageal reflux (GERD) is the term used to describe the return of your stomach contents back into your esophagus when the pressure within the stomach exceeds that of the lower esophageal pinch-valve. Esophageal reflux and a hiatal hernia often go together, and until recently the hernia was thought to be the main cause of reflux. However, studies have shown that the real cause of reflux is an "incompetent" lower esophageal pinch-valve, not a hiatal hernia per se—although a hernia may be an additive factor. Older surgical procedures focused on repairing the hiatal hernia and not the pinch-valve. The results were poor, and surgery for reflux problems thus had a bad reputation. Several surgical procedures now focus on restoring the competence of the lower esophageal pinch-valve, with excellent results.

Reflux happens occasionally in most people, and is usually associated with increases in intra-abdominal pressure transmitted to your stomach through vigorous movements such as exercise, heavy lifting, bending, coughing, or stooping that cause the contents of your stomach to flow back into the esophagus. However, a few waves of esophageal contraction rapidly move the acidic material back into your stomach, and you feel no pain. Saliva, which contains bicarbonate, helps to neutralize this misplaced acid.

If you have more severe reflux, you experience "heartburn" in your chest, as the stomach acid splashes up. The acid irritates the tender wall of your esophagus, which lacks the protective mechanisms found in your stomach. The typical burning and wavelike pain underneath your breastbone are often worse at night after a large meal, and may also be precipitated by lying down or being active in a way that tends to increase the pressure in your abdomen.

The pain from symptomatic reflux can sometimes be quite severe, even simulating a heart attack. Frequent, prolonged exposure of your esophagus to stomach acid inflames and thins its lining. Your esophagus then becomes even more sensitive to the reflux material, so that your symptoms are more rapidly and frequently produced. This condition is commonly referred to as *esophagitis*, which means an inflammation of the esophagus.

People with chronic reflux usually have three problems: decreased resting pressure in the lower esophageal pinch-valve, a shorter length of this high pressure pinch-valve zone, and inadequate increase in pinch-valve pressure when pressure in the stomach increases from eating or straining. Their pinch-valve is said to be "incompetent."

Studies show decreased esophageal pinch-valve stimulation by nerves and/or hormones in people with chronic reflux. They secrete less *gastrin*, a hormone produced by the stomach that increases lower esophageal pinch-valve pressure in response to meals. Also, they do not effectively clear refluxed material through swallowing and esophageal contractions, so that it remains in contact with the sensitive esophageal lining for prolonged periods.

If you have chronic reflux, you can develop significant complications. The acid may erode your esophageal lining, producing bleeding from the raw surface. An ulcer may form and, rarely, perforate through the esophageal wall. As the chronically inflamed and irritated esophageal lining contracts with fibrous scar tissue, a "stricture" or narrowing can develop. The first evidence of this is usually a sensation of food sticking in the throat—most often meat, because of its high density. As the narrowing increases, you begin to have difficulty swallowing soft foods, then liquids. Another danger is that you may breathe refluxed stomach material into your trachea and lungs, producing hoarseness, bronchitis, and pneumonia. This is more prone to occur at night, when you swallow less frequently.

Heartburn can be a serious symptom. A recent study from Sweden found a correlation between the increasing severity, frequency, and duration of reflux symptoms and increasing risk of esophageal cancer. Those patients with the severest symptoms had a risk 43.5 times that of persons without symptoms.[2] Because of continual irritation, the normal surface lining cells of the esophagus may transform into another type of cell (a condition called *Barrett's esophagus)*, found in 10 percent of patients with chronic symptoms, which has a 0.5 to 1 percent per year risk of the adenocarcinoma type of esophagus cancer.[3] This type of cancer has increased at a rate higher than any other type of cancer in the United States.

If you have symptoms of severe heartburn or swallowing problems that can lead to or be caused by a malignancy, you need to be investigated by esophagoscopy and biopsied before embarking on treatment for your reflux symptoms.

Alternative Medicine Approaches to Hiatal Hernia and Gastroesophageal Reflux

This disorder almost always responds to an alternative medicine program. "Lifestyle modification is the first step in treating reflux esophagitis," Dr. Donald Castell, chief of gastroenterology at the Bowman Gray School of Medicine, has stated. Many authorities agree that you should try to avoid surgery for heartburn whenever possible. Although about 20 percent of the adults in the United States have heartburn on a weekly basis, less than 5 percent of persons with typical reflux esophagitis should ever need an operation.

Importantly, the mere presence of a hiatal hernia does not mean you must treat it, either medically or surgically. Less than 10 percent of all individuals with a sliding hiatal hernia have any significant symptoms of reflux. On the other hand, 5 to 20 percent of those who suffer from heartburn don't have a hiatal hernia at all, but rather just an incompetent lower esophageal pinch-valve.

Alternative medicine treatment of reflux is intended to produce three changes: increase the pressure within the lower esophageal pinch-valve; decrease the pressure in the stomach and abdomen; and change the nature of the reflux material so it is not as irritating to the esophageal lining. The following are three of the most promising new alternative approaches to accomplish this.

Eat a High-Fiber Diet

The most important element in alternative medicine approaches for heartburn is the addition of fiber. Lack of adequate fiber in your diet is the most likely cause of both your esophageal reflux and hiatal hernia formation.

"The hypothesis that fiber-depleted diets are a factor in the causation of hiatal hernia is consistent with all that is known of the disease," summarized Dr. Denis Burkitt, British researcher on fiber. Dr. Burkitt argues that a high-fiber diet can both prevent and treat reflux and hernias. Fiber helps by both eliminating straining as you pass your stool, and diminishing the amount of acid in your stomach.

Because abdominal pressure is increased whenever you push down against a stool either too dry or too viscous, your stomach may be forced up through your diaphragm, or acid backed up into your esophagus. Abdominal pressure during straining can become three times as high as the pressure in your chest; such an increase is higher than that caused by weight lifting.

One study of West Africans eating high-fiber diets revealed only 4 hiatal hernias in 1,000 persons screened—more than 100 times less than the rate found in the United States.[4] Relief of symptoms may be obtained by the simple addition of bran or ground flaxseeds to your diet. Replace your white flour bagels, croissants, doughnuts, and English muffins with ones made from whole wheat flour, or other whole grains, and substitute whole ripe fruit for sugary desserts.

Human stomachs have a low level of acid, when compared to the carnivores, whose stomachs contain ten times as much. Eating meat causes our stomachs to pour forth acid to try to digest it, more than what the stomach evolved to carry; the chimps, gorillas, and apes, our closest genetic relatives, rarely eat meat. The chronically high excess acid levels associated with a meat diet diminish gastrin production, decreasing esophageal pinch-valve pressure, and thereby increasing the likelihood of this caustic acid reflecting into the lower esophagus. Switching to a vegetable-based diet may quickly solve your problem.

Fatty foods also delay stomach emptying, thus increasing the potential for reflux. Diets relatively high in protein from sources such as lentils and other legumes are best, because they increase your pinch-valve pressure.

If you suffer from heartburn, you may also be sensitive to other common dietary elements known to decrease lower esophageal pinch-valve pressure. Alcohol, even in moderate amounts, is a culprit. Coffee, including the decaffeinated variety, also lowers this pressure, and so is a very frequent cause of heartburn; it also increases stomach acid, making it a double offender. If you are a coffee person, giving up coffee, or at least cutting down on your intake, as difficult as it may be to do, may be all that is needed to help relieve your symptoms. Chocolate, orange juice, tomato juice, garlic, onions, cabbage, mint, and salty, spicy, fried, or fatty foods also act to lower your pinch-valve pressure.

A diet high in simple carbohydrates such as sugar and white flour can worsen your reflux symptoms, by stimulating acid production without adding neutralizing fiber. If you are suffering from reflux, try eliminating these items and you may watch your pain disappear without the scalpel.

Because dietary change can often yield quick, satisfying results, with no risks or unpleasant side effects, it seems worth a trial. You can find directions for a basic, tasty high-fiber, low-fat diet in Chapter 2.

Change Your Habits and Medications

Cigarettes and other tobacco products lower esophageal pinch-valve pressure and stimulate stomach acid. If you smoke, quitting can be especially important to relieving your heartburn.

Many medications decrease lower esophageal pinch-valve tone: Estrogen, progesterone, and steroids can all act this way. Birth control pills or postmenopausal hormonal therapy should be avoided if you have pinch-valve problems. Drugs such as antihistamines, narcotics, antiasthma medications, and calcium-channel-blocker heart medications can also predispose you to reflux.

Make Posture and Exercise Changes

Increased pressure in the stomach and abdomen tends to overcome weak lower esophageal pinch-valve pressure, so that certain positions can make your reflux worse. Lying down adds the force of gravity, and large meals, simply because of their mass, increase pressure within the stomach. The combination of a large evening meal with lying down afterward can give you such severe reflux symptoms at night that they wake you from sleep.

Several measures should be used to counteract these factors: Eat only small amounts at a time; eliminate large meals; and eat nothing for three to four hours before lying down. Raise the head of your bed on six-inch blocks, to enlist gravity to counteract stomach pressure. Avoid tight clothing such as girdles, belts, or jeans that increase intra-abdominal pressure. Take care to limit bending, stooping, coughing, and heavy lifting, especially after meals. If you can control it, try not to belch, since it may bring more acid into contact with your esophagus. These simple actions may dramatically relieve your symptoms.

The way we in the Western world sit on the toilet also increases intra-abdominal pressure, more than the squatting posture used in some other cultures. Hiatal hernia, with its contribution to reflux, is very rare in the traditional cultures where the knees are drawn toward the chest during bowel movements. You may want to try loosely squatting by bringing your legs up toward the toilet seat or using a small stool to support your legs, and thus reduce your abdominal pressure.

Reflux, from both pressure on the stomach and hormonal changes, may become more apparent during the latter part of the menstrual cycle, and especially during the last three months of pregnancy. Some studies have shown that up to 25 percent of all pregnant women have daily symptoms caused by reflux. So, if you are pregnant, alternative medicine measures are especially important for prevention and treatment.

Change Your Diet

When your stomach contents are less acidic, reflux symptoms and the damage to your esophagus caused by reflux are reduced. Smoking, alcohol, caffeine, and fatty foods stimulate acid production, and should be eliminated. Irritating foods like orange and tomato juice and highly spiced dishes should be reduced. A high-fiber diet moves food more quickly through the digestive tract, so it does not sit as long in the stomach, where it would increase acid production and the possibility of backward flow. Addition of bran to your diet, therefore, has a natural antacid capacity.

Use Other Natural Remedies

Other natural remedies to aid digestive flow and prevent reflux are fresh papaya or papaya tablets, yogurt, aloe vera juice, and the herbs chamomile, licorice root, ginger, fennel, anise, slippery elm, marshmallow root, coriander, plantain, and sage. Because it reduces lower esophageal pressure, mint tea is *not* recommended. The herbalist Jethro Kloss described fennel as "one of the thoroughly tried remedies for gas and acid stomach." In India, anise is often given at the close of a meal to assist digestion. These herbs can be added to your meals, chewed afterward, or taken as teas. Start with one capsule or cup of tea after each meal. Ginger and chamomile teas drunk with or after each meal are especially helpful.

Maintain Your Optimum Weight

An excess of abdominal pressure, associated with increased weight, may help push the stomach out of its normal positioning with respect to the diaphragm. Follow the dietary guidelines in Chapter 2, to reach and maintain your optimum weight.

Practice Stress Management and Visualization

Heartburn occurs more commonly when you are tense, nervous, or under stress. The relaxation program described in Chapter 2 offers important protection for your digestive tract. One study showed visualization produced a 70 percent decrease in stomach acidity.[5] In another study, patients with increased stomach acid who looked at blotting paper and imagined "absorbent dryness" were able to decrease their stomach acid in just ten days.[6]

Use Hypnosis and Acupuncture

Hypnosis may be helpful in the relief of this problem, although research results are pending. Similarly, acupuncture may provide amelioration of symptoms, but although case reports have indicated success, further research is needed in this disorder.

Use Chiropractic and Osteopathy

These modalities may help relieve symptoms by relaxing abdominal pressure enough to allow the stomach to drop back into its proper position.[7]

Use Homeopathy

The homeopathic remedy nux vomica, made from the seed of an East Indian tree, may relieve symptoms of reflux esophagitis; other commonly used remedies are ferrum phos, calacarea carbonica, and hepar sulph. You may need the assistance of an experienced homeopathic practitioner.

Conventional Medicine Approaches to Hiatal Hernia and Gastroesophageal Reflux

Conventional medicine treatment includes many of the lifestyle changes discussed in the alternative section, as well as the following types of medications.

Antacids

Liquid or tablet antacids such as Maalox (magnesium and aluminum based), Mylanta (calcium and magnesium based), Tums (calcium based), Amphogel (aluminum based), and Rolaids (calcium and magnesium based) are popular over-the-counter remedies. These brands are available in various combinations of ingredients, so be sure you read the labels. They may be especially effective in neutralizing stomach acid and relieving heartburn when one to two teaspoons or tablets are taken one to three hours after meals and before bed. However, antacids containing aluminum compounds may contribute to aluminum poisoning, suspected to be a contributing factor in senile dementia.[8] Despite the popular recommendation that taking antacids can help you prevent osteoporosis, no evidence proves this, and in fact, chronic excess use of calcium carbonate antacids may cause kidney stones.[9] In addition, these antacids have a strong rebound effect: As their effect in lowering acid content wears off, the stomach secretes even more acid. Those antacids containing sodium are not recommended for patients with high blood pressure. Diarrhea or constipation are common side effects of any effective antacid; too dramatic a decrease in acidity may also set the stage for infection, since normal levels of stomach acid prevent invading bacteria or viruses from growing in the digestive tract. Because of their many side effects, use over-the-counter antacids only for quick relief on an occasional basis.

Gaviscon, a combination-ingredient antacid, produces a neutralizing layer that floats on top of your stomach contents. When reflux develops, this neutral solution is pushed upward first, providing protection to your esophagus.

Acid Blockers

The over-the-counter drugs cimetadine (Tagamet), ranitidene (Zantac), and famotidine (Pepcid) and the prescription drugs omeprazole (Prilosec) and pantoprazole (Protonix) block acid production by 70 to 95 percent, and can be chosen if you are not responsive to other nonsurgical methods. These drugs are especially effective if taken at bedtime because they block acid production completely for four to twelve hours. However, the long-term side effects of blocking stomach acid production are unknown; therefore, they are probably best used only for short periods. If you do need long-term treatment with powerful acid blockers, your doctor should check you for *H. pylori* infection, and treat it if necessary, since the combination of lack of stomach acid and *H. pylori* infection can increase your risk for stomach cancer.[10] (For a further discussion, see page 374.)

The prescription drug metaclopramide (Reglan) increases lower esophageal pinch-valve pressure, as well as encouraging stomach emptying, thereby decreasing stomach pressure. Since it has frequent side effects such as drowsiness, fatigue, and anxiety, its use should be restricted to the 10 percent of patients who do not respond to the previously described lifestyle changes or acid-blocking agents.

Surgical Approaches to Hiatal Hernia and Gastroesophageal Reflux

Careful nonsurgical management and alternative medicine approaches are effective in treating 95 percent of all individuals with symptomatic reflux esophagitis. If you have uncomplicated esophagitis, you should consider surgical treatment only after three to six months of faithful and supervised conventional medical and alternative medicine therapy.

If you have an esophageal narrowing, or stricture, it may be possible to nonsurgically dilate it with a balloon catheter tube passed through an endoscope during esophagoscopy (see page 351). This is an outpatient procedure. Dilation should be followed by good alternative medicine and conventional medical management, to prevent recurrence.

If treatment fails despite your best attempts at lifestyle and medical management and you are still miserable, you can look to a surgeon for relief. Also, you may wish to choose surgical treatment if your symptoms are controlled but you are facing a lifetime of expensive medicines such as omeprazol (Prilosec), with their unknown long-term side effects. If you have a narrowing (stricture) or bleeding, or if a biopsy shows that constant irritation has produced the Barrett's precancerous transformation of the cells lining your esophagus, you need surgery. Delaying surgery in these cases makes the operation more difficult and dangerous, especially if it must be performed on an emergency basis.

The *Nissen fundoplication* procedure is the surgical operation most often used to prevent reflux. It is designed to achieve a pressure in your lower esophageal pinch-valve higher than that in your stomach, thereby preventing the contents of your stomach from moving back up into the esophagus. This operation is now most commonly performed with a laparoscope. In fact, the number of operations for reflux has substantially increased because of its success, along with patient and referring physician enthusiasm for the use of a laparoscopic to replace the traditional "open" procedure.

General anesthetic is needed for the Nissen operation. The surgeon uses three or four one-quarter to one-half-inch incisions to pass the special camera and instruments into the upper abdomen, then manipulates and sews the tissue while viewing the surgical area on a TV monitor.

First, the "outpouched" junction of your stomach and esophagus is pulled back into the abdomen. Because pressure within the abdomen is higher than that in the chest, your esophagus pinch-valve pressure is increased, discouraging reflux. Second, the esophageal opening in your diaphragm, which may have been weakened or stretched by a hiatal hernia, is closed more tightly, to help prevent the junction from sliding up into the chest (which is otherwise likely to happen because of the lower pressure in the chest). Third, and *most important,* part of the upper stomach is wrapped and stitched around your lower esophagus to create a valve mechanism, so that increased pressure within your stomach will squeeze it off, preventing reflux. Altogether, this technique compensates for the previously incompetent lower esophageal pinch-valve.

If your Nissen operation is done by the "open" method, your surgeon makes a five- to eight-inch up-and-down or crosswise incision in your upper abdomen, although a chest incision is sometimes used under certain conditions.

The Nissen procedure may take from one to two hours. You awaken in the recovery room with a tube running from your nose down into your stomach, to keep the pressure in your stomach low for a day or two. Postoperative discomfort can be controlled with intravenous painkillers until you are able to drink fluids and take pain medication, usually initially in elixir form. Your symptoms of heartburn should disappear immediately. Some swelling in the area of the "wrap" at the lower end of your esophagus may limit your swallowing for a few days or weeks, so you must resume your regular diet cautiously. You can usually be discharged from the hospital in one to three days after the laparoscopic procedure, or four to six days after the open approach. You may have some incisional discomfort, and should avoid driving or vigorous exercise until you are completely comfortable. You should be able to return to work in a week or two.

If the "wrap" is made too tight, you may have an unpleasant "gas-bloat syndrome," with excess gas and inability to belch or vomit, although this is seen in less than 5 percent of all cases.

The laparoscopic procedure decreases your hospital stay and produces much smaller scars, less pain, and a quicker overall postoperative recovery. The mortality rate is less than 1 percent.

After the older open Nissen operation, 5 to 10 percent of all patients experienced a recurrence of their symptoms, and the percentage increased to as high as 25 percent over time. Long-term results from the laparoscopic approach are not yet known, but early results are better than the open procedure. Quality of life assessment is an excellent global way to evaluate the effect of an operation and compare it to other forms of treatment. An Emory University study of 181 laparoscopic patients who completed preop and postop questionnaires determined that they obtained relief of their symptoms and scored significantly higher on all health categories tested after surgery. They did not develop postoperative side effects that had a significant impact on their perceived quality of life. Additionally, they found that surgery may be more effective than medical therapy at improving quality of life for patients with gastroesophageal reflux disease, including those who reported that their symptoms were well controlled with medication preoperatively.[11]

GASTROESOPHAGEAL REFLUX SUMMARY

Prevention

Diet and Supplements

- Eat a low-fat, high-fiber, vegetarian diet.
- Eat bran, 3 tablespoons daily.
- Avoid caffeine, alcohol, mint, chocolate, tomato and orange juice, garlic, onions, cabbage, salty, spicy, or fried foods, sugar, white flour.
- Add yogurt to your diet.

Lifestyle

- Don't smoke.
- Maintain optimum weight.
- Avoid estrogen, progesterone, steroids, antihistamines, narcotics, antiasthma medications, calcium channel bockers.
- Avoid lying down after meals and eating late at night; elevate head of bed.
- Try the squatting position on the toilet.
- Practice daily yoga.
- Practice stress reduction.

Alternative Medicine Approaches

- Follow the preventive guidelines, above.
- Drink herb teas—chamomile, licorice root, ginger, fennel, anise, slippery elm, marshmallow root, coriander, plantain and sage, 1 cup, 3 times daily.
- Fresh papaya or papaya tablets, yogurt, aloe vera juice.
- Digestive enzymes, 1–2 tablets, 3 times daily.
- Hypnosis and acupuncture.

- Chiropractic, osteopathy, homeopathy.
- Visualization.

Conventional Medicine Approaches

Medications

- Antacids—Mylanta, Maalox, Tums, Amphogel, Rolaids, Gaviscon.
- Acid blockers—cimetadine (Tagamet), ranitidine (Zantac), famotidine (Pepcid), omeprazole (Prilosec).
- Stomach-emptying drugs—metaclopramide (Reglan).

Surgical Approach

- Nissen fundoplication—laparoscopic, open.

Esophageal Cancer

Esophageal cancer is the eighth most common cancer worldwide. An estimated 13,100 new cases of esophageal cancer will be diagnosed in the United States in 2002 with 12,600 deaths.[12] This is a very difficult malignancy to treat, with overall cure rates of only about 10 percent. (See Table 11.1.) Several reasons account for this. Since symptoms do not appear until about 75 percent of the esophageal channel is blocked, diagnosis is usually delayed to the point where most tumors have already spread beyond the possibility of a cure. Lymphatic drainage of the esophagus spreads cancer rapidly along its wall, and from there it goes on to lymph nodes in the abdomen, chest, and neck. Because the esophagus is in close proximity to delicate vital structures such as the heart and lungs, esophageal cancers also tend to invade in a way that makes surgical removal impossible. These factors have led some surgeons to conclude that the goal of surgery should usually be to relieve symptoms rather than to attempt a cure.

Persons at high risk for esophageal cancer include those with esophageal scar tissue causing narrowing, injury from caustic substances such as lye, transformation of lining cells due to reflux irritation (Barrett's esophagus), esophagus muscle contraction disorders, and especially, heavy drinkers and smokers.

Hope for decreasing death rates lies in the preventive measures described earlier in this chapter, and in early diagnosis. Barrett's esophagus can be treated with laser or thermal devices and will probably become the

TABLE 11.1.
Prognosis of Esophageal Cancer[14]

	Percent of Patients Surviving 5 Years	Percent of Patients in This Stage
All Patients	13.7%	
Not Staged	12.6%	24%
By Stage		
Localized to esophagus	27.0%	25%
Lymph node spread	13.3%	27%
Distant spread	2.2%	25%

standard of care to eliminate the risk from this disease.[13] Cure rates of 40 percent or more can be attained if tumors are found while they are still small and confined to the esophageal lining. However, no symptoms are present at this stage. Since the incidence of esophageal tumors in the United States is only 1 per 100,000 persons per year, it is impractical and not cost-effective to screen the entire population. Some medical centers have begun to use screening techniques on high-risk groups. If you fall into one of these groups, ask your physician about screening by esophagoscopy.

The earliest symptom of esophageal cancer is difficulty swallowing—first of solids, then of liquids. Pain, bleeding, and weight loss indicate advanced disease. If you have swallowing difficulties, you need X-ray studies and an esophagoscopy that includes a biopsy.

Alternative Medicine Approaches to Esophageal Cancer

Since certain ingested carcinogens are thought to be the most important causes of esophageal cancer, you can take action to help prevent this disease and possibly to assist in your recovery, and prevent recurrence.

Following are the most important alternative medicine approaches.

Quit Smoking

A strong correlation exists between esophageal cancer and cigarette use. For example, rates of this cancer are much lower in Seventh-Day Adventists, who do not smoke as a rule. You can utilize alternative techniques to help you quit for good. Follow the guidelines given in Chapter 2, especially those under the heading, "Quitting Smoking."

Avoid Alcohol

Especially when combined with smoking, alcohol use increases the risk for this cancer. The alcohol itself may dissolve carcinogens, such as cigarette smoke, increasing their cancer-causing effects on the sensitive esophageal lining. The rates of esophageal cancer are greater in France, with its relatively high alcohol consumption, and lower in Seventh-Day Adventists, who do not generally use alcohol.

Change Your Diet

Esophageal cancer is more common in individuals with nutritional deficiencies; this may be an addictive factor in alcoholics.

Geographic factors seem to play an important role in rates of this cancer, and dietary choices may explain this. Japan has four to five times the U.S. rate, some provinces in China have ten times the incidence, and some villages in Iran twenty times as much. The exact cancer-causing nutritional factors in these regional differences are not completely clear, but consumption of black tea, which it is taken without added milk, may contribute to the higher rates of this cancer. A study of regular tea drinkers in China found that those who drink green tea had a 60 percent decreased incidence of esophageal cancer. Green tea contains polyphenols, felt to protect against cancer in general by blocking enzymes that produce cancer-causing substances.[15]

Teas other than those made from herbs have large quantities of tannic acid, a known carcinogen. Adding milk to tea counteracts this acid's effects and seems to fit cultural variations in the cancer pattern. The English, who generally add milk to their black tea, have a low risk for this form of cancer.

General recommendations for the prevention of cancer—including adopting a diet low in fat, high in fruits and vegetables, and minus refined sugars—are further discussed in Chapter 2.

Conventional Medicine Approaches to Esophageal Cancer

X-ray treatment is most often the best approach for tumors in the upper one-third of the esophagus, where surgery is quite difficult. An operation is preferred for tumors in the lower two-thirds. Increasing emphasis is now on "combined" treatment plans using surgery, radiation, and chemotherapy where recent studies have demonstrated promising results with localized disease. However, not all patients are able to complete such therapy, due to the onset of toxic, occasionally life-threatening, side effects. Five-year survivals of 14 to 26 percent have been reported.[16] You should discuss the latest information with specialists in this area.

If your tumor has spread beyond the chance for surgical cure, radiotherapy can be used to relieve symptoms of pain and swallowing difficulty caused by tumor blockage. This treatment is successful in 80 to 90 percent of all cases. Also, passing a plastic tube through your tumor into your stomach or removing part of the tumor using cautery or laser through an esophagoscope may relieve the blockage. This can be an outpatient procedure, using local anesthesia and intravenous sedation. It may not allow pain-free swallowing, but 80 percent of the patients who receive these tubes can leave the hospital and receive further care at home.

Surgical Approach to Esophageal Cancer

Treatment of esophageal cancer aims for cure whenever possible. If that is not realistic, then it tries for relief of symptoms and freedom from swallowing difficulty. The first successful removal of an esophageal tumor was performed in the 1930s. Since then, vast improvements in surgical technique have enabled more patients to survive the surgery, although little improvement in cure rates has been seen. Surgery does provide the only hope for cure, and is more effective than radiation treatment in relieving symptoms.

Before you can be considered for surgery, a CAT scan and a sonogram using a probe passed into the esophagus on the end of a tube need to be performed to determine whether your tumor has spread to your distant lymph glands, organs, or adjacent vital tissues. Such spread means the cancer is incurable, and that the best form of treatment is one which will relieve symptoms with fewest side effects. Thirty to forty percent of all patients are in this category when they are initially diagnosed. If a good chance for cure by an operation seems possible, true of 60 to 70 percent of all patients when first seen, you should have surgery. In cases that are uncertain, where your tumor is large or appears to be encroaching on neighboring tissues, radiation before surgery may shrink the tumor, making removal possible.

Surgery undertaken with the goal of curing the cancer includes removing most of your esophagus, as well as adjacent lymph glands and other tissue. You must have general anesthetic for this operation. Your surgeon makes an up-and-down or crosswise incision in your upper abdomen and another in your chest or neck, depending on what part of your esophagus is involved. After part of your esophagus is removed, your stomach is brought up to connect with the remaining portion of your esophagus. (See Figure 11.2.) Rarely, a seg-

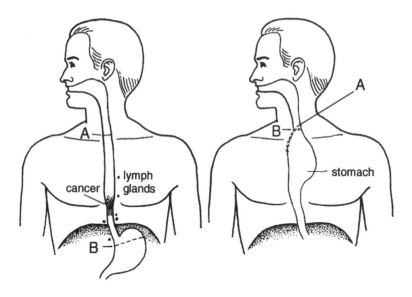

Fig. 11.2 Procedures involved in esophageal cancer surgery

ment of the small bowel or colon may be used to bridge the gap between your esophagus and stomach. This operation may take three to five hours to complete.

You wake up in the recovery room with a tube through your nose into your stomach, to keep pressure from building up there; another in your chest cavity to keep your lungs expanded; and a bladder catheter to monitor your fluid balance. Postoperative discomfort is best handled with an epidural catheter or intravenous painkillers. The chest tube and bladder catheter can be removed after two or three days; the nasal tube is usually left in for five to seven days, until an X-ray shows satisfactory healing between the remaining esophagus and stomach. Then you can begin a progressive diet. You will most likely be discharged after eight to fourteen days. Full recovery will take several weeks more.

Complications include those associated with any major surgery, as well as breakdown of the sutures joining the esophagus and stomach, and infection developing in the chest or abdomen. If a complication occurs, another operation may be necessary. The overall mortality rate for this surgery is about 2 to 6 percent.

ESOPHAGEAL CANCER SUMMARY

Prevention

Diet and Supplements

- Follow a low-fat, high-fiber, vegetarian diet.
- Avoid sugar, alcohol, and black tea without milk.

Lifestyle

- Don't smoke.
- Avoid alcohol.
- Practice stress management.

Alternative Medicine Approaches

- Follow the preventive guidelines, above.
- Follow alternative adjuncts, given in Chapter 2.
- Practice visualization.

Conventional Medicine Approaches

- Radiotherapy.
- Chemotherapy.

Surgical Approach

- Esophagectomy.

CHAPTER 12

STOMACH

There is nothing in the world more shameless than this cursed belly! It forces a man to remember it, in spite of dire distress and sorrow of heart.

Homer

Diagnostic precision goes hand in hand with endoscopy, but the literature suggests that it's as important to look at the patient as it is to look at the ulcer. . . . To know why and who could be just as important as knowing where and how big.

Louis Goldman, M.D.[1]

Your stomach hurts. You wonder if it could be an ulcer. You can't function with the discomfort, so you consider taking one of the widely advertised antacids, or even contemplate surgery. You have plenty of company.

The most commonly used over-the-counter type of medicines in the United States are antacid preparations, taken not only to treat heartburn, as described in the previous chapter, but also in an attempt to assuage any sort of "dyspepsia" (indigestion)—in an effort to calm our national stomachache.

The "gnawing within" of ulcer disease can make you desperate for relief. A Houston man was given a five-year prison sentence for "stealing" an ulcer operation. He was uninsured, so he assumed the identity of a friend, checked into the hospital under that name, had his ulcer surgically treated, and only was caught afterward, by the hospital chaplain!

Between 20 and 40 percent of the population in the Western world suffers regularly from upper abdominal symptoms of chronic or recurrent pain, bloating, fullness, nausea, regurgitation, heartburn, belching, and/or loss of appetite, although up to 60 percent of these persons have no specific organic cause found on diagnostic evaluation.[2] Half of all Americans use antacids occasionally to combat such symptoms, three-fourths of those who take them are habitual users, and *1 in 10 Americans takes antacids every day*.

The most frequently doctor-recommended type of drug in the United States is that of the acid-blocking medications such as *cimetidine (Tagamet)*, which also can now be obtained over-the-counter. Stomach pain is thus a true national problem, with over $1.3 billion spent on prescription drugs for it each year.[3]

However, an actual ulcer is the underlying cause of dyspepsia only in a minority of persons with stomach discomfort. Excess stomach acid is implicated in most ulcers, and treatments are directed at neutralizing or decreasing acid output.

The use of acid-blocking drugs has dramatically changed conventional recommendations for ulcer treatment. Also, a specific bacterium, *Helicobacter pylori*, found to be associated with most ulcers, has led to antibiotic treatment for this disease. With these treatments, surgery is rarely necessary.

Alternative medicine offers a comprehensive new approach to your stomach. These modalities can be utilized separately, or as complements alongside other regimens, to address the important underlying factors contributing to the bacterial infection in the first place, as well as to the excess acid production and other factors associated with ulcer formation.

Should you consider having an operation to relieve your distress? We both agree that the pros and cons of ulcer surgery should be carefully considered before you decide whether or not to seek a surgical solution. The laparoscope does provide a more attractive surgical option for those few who do not find relief through alternative and/or conventional medical management. However, application of the alternative medicine suggestions given below is often all that is needed for elimination of your stomach distress.

How Your Stomach Works

The stomach has always fascinated surgeons, and much research has centered on how stomach secretions are regulated, stimulated, and inhibited. Controlled by complex interactions of nerves and hormonal stimuli, it is subject to diseases and complications requiring precise techniques and surgical judgment.

Your stomach, resembling a large J-shaped sausage, and the *duodenum*, the upper portion of the small intestine that connects to your stomach, are located in the upper part of your abdomen. The stomach is the thickest and most muscular part of the digestive tract. It can contain from a few tablespoons to a quart or more of food and liquid. Partial breakdown of these materials takes place by mechanical churning, along with the action of stomach-produced acid and enzymes.

Two pinch-valves, or sphincters, control inflow and outflow. When the *esophageal sphincter*, at the junction of the esophagus and the stomach, relaxes, food and liquids pass into the stomach; when it is closed, your stomach contents are kept from passing back up into your sensitive esophagus. (See Figure 12.1.) The *pyloric sphincter*, at the junction of the stomach and duodenum, helps regulate outflow, preventing rapid emptying of large food particles into the intestinal tract.

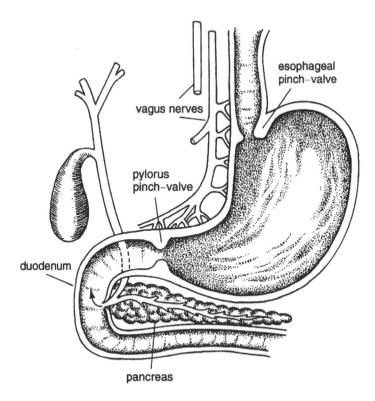

Fig. 12.1   The stomach and duodenum

The most important nerve supply to the stomach travels through the *vagus nerves,* which influence its secretion and movement. The stomach's blood supply is very rich, as might be expected in such an active organ, and this explains the copious bleeding that follows once an ulcer erodes into underlying blood vessels.

Your stomach contains one million acid-producing cells, along with other cells that generate *pepsin,* the stomach's major digestive enzyme, and *gastrin,* the stomach's main hormone. *Mucin cells* secrete a thick, strong mucus which protects your stomach lining cells from irritants, as well as from its own acid and digestive enzymes.

The concentration of acid inside the stomach chamber is a million times that of the interior of its lining cells. Maintaining this incredible difference in acidity without damage to delicate cells takes a large amount of energy and cell work. Some chemicals like alcohol, aspirin, ibuprofen, cortisone, and bile salts tend to break down your cells' ability to resist autodigestion.

Your stomach secretes up to three quarts of acidic and digestive fluids each day! A constant low flow rate continues between meals. Food stimulates a huge increase in output, allowing concentrated stomach acid and powerful enzymes to split apart and digest most food ingredients.

It's truly a wonder that your stomach does not digest itself! The stomach's major defenses against this occurring are the mucous covering of its inner surface, the unusually tight junction between its lining cells, and the ability of these cells to prevent acid from getting through their walls into the more fragile interiors.

Other factors that play a lesser role in your defense against autodigestion are the acid-neutralizing capacity of body secretions such as the bicarbonate present in saliva, bile, and pancreatic juice, along with buffers—most notably, fiber and proteins—present in food broken down by the digestive process.

Taking time to chew your food may seem like a simple motherly suggestion, but it *is* quite important, since it mixes in buffering saliva.

How Stomach Disease Is Diagnosed

The most common stomach diseases that might be causing your symptoms are gastritis (an inflammation of its lining), ulcer, and cancer. Chronic indigestion, belching, vomiting, sharp or aching upper abdominal pain, and bleeding into the gastrointestinal tract can result. However, disorders in the esophagus, gallbladder, pancreas, and other systems can cause a similar picture and must be considered. Your history and a physical exam may be all that is necessary to differentiate a stomach disease from other possible causes, but you are likely to need X-rays and endoscopy as well.

History

Your doctor should ask a series of questions about any symptoms you might have. Report what seems to bring on your problems, and what you may have done to relieve them. Smoking and alcohol intake and pre-

scription and over-the-counter medications may play a role.

Stomach pain can take many forms, varying from a vague feeling of indigestion or discomfort to a distinct burning, wavelike pain in the central part of your upper abdomen that may move through to your back. Discomfort can be worse *between* meals and at night, and may be relieved by eating or by antacids, which temporarily buffer the acid. It can also be worse with meals. Belching, vomiting, hiccups, and stomach distention may be signs of underlying stomach disease, affecting the stomach's motility and outflow. Loss of appetite, weight loss, or anemia may be your first sign. Bleeding from the stomach may produce a tar-hued stool, or vomiting of bright red blood or "coffee grounds"—colored material. Cancer may not produce any early symptoms.

Physical Exam

Your examination should begin with a general medical exam, particularly including a check for abdominal tenderness, any mass or enlarged lymph glands, and blood in your stool.

If your symptoms are minor and occasional, you can safely avoid more extensive tests, and go directly to trying alternative and conventional medical therapies, under your doctor's supervision. However, if you have significant pain, or your symptoms persist despite these remedies—especially if you are older than 50—more testing may be necessary. Although it is a great temptation to use new "wonder drugs," such as the powerful acid suppresser omeprazole (Prilosec), it is unwise to take them without knowing exactly what you are treating. Such a practice may result in inappropriate treatment and/or complications.

Or it may delay your getting an accurate diagnosis until advanced disease, even cancer, becomes obvious.

Upper GI Series

The *upper GI (gastrointestinal) series* is the best first test. After you swallow a thick liquid barium (clay) mixture which shows up on X-ray, you lie on an X-ray table and roll from side to side. Your radiologist watches on a fluoroscope machine (which creates X-ray motion pictures) and takes X-rays of the outlines of the inside of your esophagus, stomach, and duodenum. The size, shape, movement pattern, rate of emptying, and surface changes caused by ulcers, polyps, and tumors can be seen. Unfortunately, the GI series may miss 25 to 35 percent of duodenal ulcers, because they are hidden by the normal irregularities in this area. The upper GI series is not painful, can be accomplished in five to fifteen minutes, and has no significant complications.

Endoscopy

The most informative test for investigating upper gastrointestinal problems is *endoscopy*. After receiving a throat spray to eliminate your gag reflex, you lie on your side while a long, flexible, lighted scope is inserted through your mouth, then guided into your esophagus, stomach, and duodenum. A thorough, direct examination can be made, and suspicious areas biopsied with tiny instruments passed through a channel in the scope. A small bit of tissue can also be taken, to look for evidence of the bacterium *Helicobacter pylori;* this is the most accurate way to make such a diagnosis.

Endoscopy can be accomplished in twenty to thirty minutes. Your doctor's manipulation of the scope is uncomfortable, although it should not be painful. You can be sedated, but must be kept awake enough to cooperate in swallowing and changing positions on the examining table. Complications are rare: Perforation of the gastrointestinal tract happens in 1 in 1,000 endoscopies, and an emergency operation is usually required. Your overall risk of mortality is only 1 in 10,000.[4]

Peptic Ulcer Disease

An ulcer is essentially an open sore in the inner lining of your stomach or duodenum, varying in size from a fraction of an inch to more than two inches in diameter. It can be shallow, but also may create a hole through the full thickness of your digestive tract's wall. "Peptic" is the word associated with most stomach and duodenal ulcers. It means "to cook, or digest." Peptic ulcer is four times more common in the duodenum than in the stomach, probably because the lining of the duodenum is less adapted to protect itself against acid.

Peptic ulcer disease (PUD) has been recorded for at least 2,500 years. Since 1955, for a combination of reasons not clearly understood, a steady decline in this disorder has taken place; since 1970, it has decreased by 50 percent. Ulcers that do develop are less virulent and easier to treat, which may be the result of today's earlier and better treatment. This disappearing ulcer trend, however, is evident only in so-called developed countries, such as the United States and Western Europe.

Changing patterns of diet and cigarette smoking may have contributed to these decreasing ulcer rates. Stress is considered a major cause for ulcer disease,[5] and overall stress levels in the West have certainly not diminished. However, it may be that certain types of stress—especially that accompanying changing from a rural to an urban society—are particularly ulcer-provoking. Western culture may have passed through this stage. Developing nations such as those in Africa and South America are now experiencing a rapid rise in their rates of peptic ulcer disease.

No specific "personality type" or socioeconomic status has been firmly linked to peptic ulcer disease. A genetic component may be present, since close relatives of ulcer patients have three times the risk. Men are much more likely to develop ulcers and their complications, and still comprise 80 to 85 percent of the persons requiring surgery, but the women's rate is fast increasing. For unknown reasons, perhaps related to stress, ulcers tend to be worse in the spring and fall.

Certain medicines may be implicated in the development of an ulcer. Most notorious are the antiinflammatory drugs such as aspirin, ibuprofen, and cortisone, which break down the stomach's resistance to autodigestion. Alcohol has direct irritative and acid-increasing effects, and smoking and coffee drinking are known to stimulate excess acid production.

As mentioned, the bacterium *Helicobacter pylori* has been found to be associated with many ulcers, and is now felt to be the most important single precipitating factor, although infection with the organism may need to interact with other factors to cause an ulcer to form. Many ulcers do occur without the presence of *H. pylori*. You can be checked for it by a simple blood test.

As noted above, peptic ulcer disease is usually diagnosed by its typical symptoms and an upper GI (gastrointestinal) series X-ray. Occasionally, endoscopy may be needed, especially if an ulcer is suspected but not seen on an X-ray, or to ensure that the ulcer does not contain cancer. Unless surgery is contemplated, more complicated diagnostic tests are unnecessary.

Although far fewer patients need surgery since the advent of the various modern treatment methods, these medical therapies may provide only temporary control of the underlying ulcer-producing factors, and some patients eventually still need surgery for chronic ulcers or complications.

Alternative Medicine Approaches to Peptic Ulcer Disease

If your symptoms are not severe and you are monitored by your doctor, surgery for peptic ulcer disease is rarely necessary, and very effective conventional medicine regimens exist for the nonsurgical treatment of ulcer disease. Therefore, alternatives are mainly directed at prevention. You still have a 5 percent risk of requiring surgery for sudden excess bleeding, perforation, stomach outlet blockage, or unresponsiveness to medication. Because ulcers also have a tendency to recur, even if you choose to treat your disorder with drugs or an operation, you may also benefit from an alternative medicine program, to prevent return of your disease.

If you do choose or require partial removal of your stomach, you are at higher risk of cancer of the stomach in the remaining portion, most likely due to changes in the lining of the stomach that follow this procedure. This risk may also be diminished via application of the lifestyle changes given below.

At least one study suggests that the more you understand about your disease, the more likely you are to do well: Patients given pictures of ulcers, a discussion of pain control, and medication reported decreased disability and diminished interference in their daily lives from ulcer pain.[6]

Following are the most important alternative medicine contributions to prevention and treatment of ulcer disease.

Quit Smoking

If you smoke, stopping is the most important single step you can take to prevent and treat your ulcer disease. Within the last twenty years, the fact that ulcers have become much less common may partly be due to an accompanying decline in smoking rates. Ulcer risk used to be quite low in women, but as their smoking habits have increased, so has their ulcer rate. Nicotine increases stomach acid secretion, the predisposing factor for many peptic ulcers. In addition to causing ulcer formation, nicotine and carbon monoxide (which is produced by smoking) also interfere with ulcer healing. The *New England Journal of Medicine* has reported that getting patients to quit smoking may be the most important factor in preventing ulcer relapse—more significant than taking the widely prescribed acid-blocking drugs, which do not protect against relapse once they are stopped.[7] The risk of dying from an ulcer complication is also increased in smokers.

Avoid Alcohol

Alcohol is known to be associated with ulcers, probably by its direct and indirect effects on the stomach lining cells, as well as its negative influences on immune function.

Change Your Diet

It seems particularly ironic that the most prescribed medicine in this country, at great expense, must be given simply because of our American habit of eating meat and dairy products, along with not enough fiber, as dis-

cussed in the previous chapter, and again below. You may wish to reassess your dietary choices, and tackle this disorder at its roots, rather than simply take medication.

Increase Fiber

Lack of fiber in your diet may be a major contributing factor to your ulcer disease. X-ray studies show that the volume of your stomach contents is greater after you eat whole-grain bread than after you eat white bread, with better mixing of the stomach contents. This improved mixing and volume allow your stomach's acid to be neutralized before it pours into your duodenum, whose lining has much less resistance to acid. Similarly, stomach acidity has been found to be higher with a meal of refined cornmeal than whole cornmeal, and white rice has less buffering capacity than whole-grain chappatis (an unleavened bread). A low-fiber diet also causes food to move *faster* from your stomach into your duodenum, carrying more acid with it, so that ulcer-causing conditions are generated even if you secrete normal amounts of acid. One study divided ulcer patients into two groups: Those fed a low-fiber diet had a relapse rate of 80 percent within one year, while the high-fiber group had only a 45 percent relapse rate.[8]

Once your ulcer has begun to heal, two to three weeks after diagnosis, you can begin to add fiber to your diet, as described in Chapter 2. Start with a teaspoon of bran added to each meal. Foods best for your initial healing period are described in Chapter 2.

Decrease Fat and Meat

Fat in your diet, especially from red meat, may contribute to your ulcer disease. It may also help explain the recent lower incidence of ulcers, as Americans have begun consuming less red meat.

Meat particularly stimulates acid secretion. Carnivores have ten times as much resting stomach acid as humans, and meat in the human stomach may simply produce too much acid for its design. *Vegetables cause an acid response that is only 60 percent that of meat.*

Forty percent of duodenal ulcer disease can be explained simply by excess acid; the other 60 percent seems to be due to a defect that allows stomach acid to pour into the duodenum, out of synchronization with the output of neutralizing alkaline bile and pancreatic secretions. A diet high in meat and fat and low in fiber may combine to do just this.

You can help treat and prevent ulcer disease by switching to the low-fat, high-fiber diet described in Chapter 2, and this change may be all that is needed to heal your disease and prevent its return.

Drink Raw, Fresh Cabbage Juice

Cabbage juice is a remedy traditionally used in Europe, and many people attest to its benefits. Up to a quart a day, taken in divided doses, is said to speed healing by increasing the growth of protective mucin-producing cells. Cabbage juice may be mixed with carrot juice to make it more palatable, and give you an extra source of vitamin A.

Restrict Acid-Stimulating Foods

Cream and milk products, originally the mainstays of ulcer treatment, have been shown to provide little buffering protein and, in fact, may stimulate more acid than they neutralize. Cream, which contains fat, causes an increase in acid production by delaying stomach emptying. Ulcer patients treated with

a milk-based diet have been shown to have a higher death rate than other patients. Alcohol directly increases stomach acids, and beer is second only to milk as a cause of increased stomach acid produced by the liquids you drink. Coffee, even the decaffeinated variety, increases stomach acids, and so may be a major offender. The incidence of stomach ulcers is sixty times greater in South India than in North India, and the difference in coffee consumption may be partly responsible.

At least initially, you should avoid spicy foods. A diet that eliminates refined foods, especially sugar, greasy foods, salt, citrus, sodas, and any other food that gives you symptoms, is especially important during your first month of healing. Also, you need to avoid raw foods during this time.

Frequent small meals, another traditional recommendation, actually *repeatedly stimulate acid production.* Three small-to-moderate-sized meals is the best plan.

Restrict Some Medications

Certain medications may predispose you to an ulcer. Aspirin is the most common, and regular users of aspirin have four times the ulcer rate of nonusers. Many over-the-counter medications are "hidden" sources of aspirin, so you should check the labels of all your medicines. Cortisone, prednisone, ibuprofen, and many other prescription drugs can also cause an ulcer, which will heal after the medications are discontinued. Check with your doctor about the necessity of using these drugs.

Practice Stress Management

Looking at the physiology of your stomach and its acid secretions may be searching in the wrong place for the origin of your ulcer: This disease may truly begin in your head. Chronic anxiety may overstimulate your vagus nerves so that, in turn, your stomach simply produces too much acid. Rather than relying on antacids or other drugs, you may do best by treating your underlying emotional stress.

Dr. William Beaumont was the first to discover the mind-body connection of the stomach. In 1930, at the University of Massachusetts, he studied the stomach secretions of a man who had recovered from a gunshot wound to the stomach, but who still had an opening from his stomach out through his skin. Dr. Beaumont noted that whenever the patient became angry or upset, acid poured forth from his stomach.

The relationship between mind and stomach has now been one of the most studied of all psychosomatic interactions. Ulcers have been found to be more frequent in people who have a strong urge to receive gratification through their hard work, who are usually very sincere and dutiful. Such people readily become frustrated if they do not receive the appreciation they feel is due them from their colleagues or superiors. If these feelings are internalized and not expressed, a chronic stress syndrome, which includes overactivity of the parasympathetic nervous system—including the vagus nerves—is induced. The frustration-ulcer link has been demonstrated in humans, in large studies.[9]

Ulcers are found more commonly in men, though in recent years the ratio has changed from ten-to-one (male to female) to four-to-one. Interestingly, the ratio was the opposite in Victorian times, when ulcers in women outnumbered those in men by ten-to-one. Emotional stress may be a factor in these differences. Ulcers tend to be more common in the spring and fall—times when stress may be more acute. High-strung persons with long-standing anxiety or emotional tension may be especially likely to smoke, as well as eat poorly, contributing to the other risk factors for ulcer development. Often the loss of a loved one can precipitate an ulcer, especially in children or teenagers. Persons with happy marriages have been shown to be at decreased risk for ulcer formation.

Even the Bible records an understanding of the relationship of our minds to our stomachs: Proverbs 15:17 says, "Better is a dinner of herbs where love is than a fatted ox and hatred with it" (although the problem may also be due to the fatted ox). During World War II, the residents of central London were bombed severely and regularly, but air-raid shelters and warnings were provided. The citizens' sense of support and relative safety may have accounted for a 50 percent decrease in ulcer disease. However, in peripheral London, which was much less bombed but also less well organized, a 300 percent *increase* in ulcers was noted.

If you have already developed an ulcer, it is less likely to heal if you remain distressed.[10] Since the nature of these emotional connections has been determined, a number of relaxation and visualization measures have been used to assist in the healing of peptic ulcers. Your frustration, fear, tension, and worry need to be addressed, and regular stress management exercises practiced.

Biofeedback has been successful in treating ulcer disease. Patients taught biofeedback have been able to reduce the amount of acid in their stomach.[11] In another study, 70 percent of patients with gastritis (inflammation of the stomach lining caused by increased acid or decreased resistance to acid) were improved after visualization training. In just ten days, one patient lowered his acid secretion to normal using a visualization technique where he looked at blotting paper and "imagined its absorbent dryness."[12] Hypnosis may achieve similar results. In yoga studies, practitioners were shown to be able to reduce stomach acid.[13]

Ulcers can be induced in mice and rats by causing them stress. Any type of relaxation activity that allows you to completely release yourself from tension and to refresh yourself would likely be helpful. Simply remembering to take a deep breath every so often can be a quick, portable relaxation measure, giving your emotions a rest. You can find details on how to practice stress management in Chapter 2.

Get a Good Night's Rest

Lack of sleep has been associated with increased risk for ulcer, probably by impairing wound healing through effects on the immune function and elevation of cortisol levels.[14] See Chapter 2 for help with getting a good night's sleep.

Take Supplements

Deficiencies of a number of vitamins and minerals have been associated with ulcer disease. One study found a direct correlation of vitamin A in the diet and ulcer disease: a higher intake produced lower disease rates.[15] Addition of vitamin A to the diet of animals who were stressed was also found to provide a protective effect and, when added to antacid therapy, doubled the healing rates.[16] Vitamin A has been shown especially useful in preventing the stress ulcers suffered by burn victims.[17]An effective intake should be 20,000 IU daily, but have your doctor monitor your liver function if you take a higher dose.

Vitamin B_6 may help prevent breakdown of the stomach lining cells. When mice are physically restrained so they cannot move at all, they become so stressed that they develop ulcers. In one study, some of the mice were given an injection of vitamin B_6 before being immobilized. Only 10 percent of these mice developed ulcers, compared with 50 percent of the control group who had received none.[18] Take 50 mg daily.

Bioflavonoids inhibit histamine release, may help protect against bleeding, and have been used as adjuncts in the treatment of ulcers, at doses from 500 to 1,500 mg, one to three times daily. Healing was found to be faster in a bioflavonoid-treated group when compared to a control group, and recurrences were less common.[19] Patients with peptic ulcer have also been found to have decreased levels of vitamin C, and rats treated with vitamin C develop fewer ulcers.[20] Take 1,000 mg, three times a day. Vitamin E administration has been found to prevent ulcers in animals, and may also be helpful in humans.[21] Take 400 IU daily.

Zinc helped patients in one study experience three times as much healing, as well as reduced pain.[22] Take 50 mg, three times daily. To prevent nausea, zinc should be taken with food.

Start with one of these supplements, and add others as needed. See Chapter 2 for further information on the use of vitamins and other supplements.

Use Herbal Remedies

In addition to chamomile tea, I recommend DGL-licorice, 2 droppersful three times daily. Systematic studies of such herbal therapies for ulcer disease are scant, although some reports of success with the herbs echinacea, fenugreek, goldenseal, licorice root, and slippery elm have appeared.[23] You can take these as teas, or 500 mg capsules, one to three times daily. Aloe vera gel may help soothe and heal ulcers. Take one to three capsules or table-spoons of liquid three hours after meals. Acidophilus yogurt may be beneficial, as long as it is low in fat. Cardamon, coriander, and flaxseeds soaked overnight can be added to your diet. The herb meadowsweet (spirea ul-maria) is very popular as a treatment in Europe, and can be taken as 500 mg capsules or tea, three to four times a day. The herb chamomile can be taken as tea every few hours, and it not only often soothes your stomach, but also may help to relax you if you are a tense, ulcer-prone person having a hard day.[24] It has antidepressant effects in the brain.

Use Homeopathy

Homeopathic remedies may be useful in ulcer disease, though no published studies are currently available; the usual remedies are nux vomica and arsenicum album. Homeo-pathic treatments should be individualized, and are best administered by an experienced homeopath.

Conventional Medicine Approaches to Peptic Ulcer Disease

If the alternative medicine approaches are not entirely successful, you can add the fol-lowing well-proven conventional medicine treatments.

Antacid Treatment

Antacids, which neutralize the acid already produced by your stomach, have been the past mainstay of the conventional medical treatment of ulcer disease. Some products contain calcium, in itself shown to stimulate acid secretion. Some Alka-Seltzer products, marketed to relieve acid indigestion, should be used with caution, since they contain as-pirin, which can in fact induce ulcer forma-tion.

Modern antacid preparations are a combi-nation of magnesium and aluminum hydrox-ide, which are effective acid buffers. Side effects—diarrhea from the magnesium and constipation from the aluminum—tend to counteract each other, so that your bowel function remains relatively normal. You can change the relative proportion of each by try-ing different formulas. Don't take these con-tinuously, however, since they can deplete the body of phosphate, thereby causing bone soft-ening. The aluminum may also be detrimental to your body, although not much of it is ab-sorbed: some studies have implicated it in cases of Alzheimer's disease.[25]

Antacids taken between meals are effective for only ten to twenty minutes. If ingested with meals or afterward, they tend to remain in your stomach for a longer time, and are ef-fective for two to four hours. Recommended dosage is one to two tablespoons, one to three hours after meals. Several studies have indi-cated that antacids have about the same pain relief as a placebo ("fake" medicine with no therapeutic effect, except through your mind), and may not speed healing by much, so their general use by doctors has decreased, and acid-blocking drugs are now preferred.

Bismuth, an ingredient in many over-the-counter stomach medications, helps eliminate *H. pylori,* known to be often associated with ulcer disease.

Modern Drug Treatment

The H-2 acid-reducing drugs cimetadine (Tagamet), ranitidene (Zantac), famotidene

(Pepcid), and nazatadine (Axid) and the proton pump inhibitors and omeprazol (Prilosec) and lansoprazole (Prevacid) are now the most frequently prescribed drugs in the United States, and have revolutionized conventional ulcer treatment. These drugs block the action of the acid-producing cells of your stomach, and thereby counteract acid stimulation by the vagus nerves, gastrin hormone, and stress. Cimetadine and ranitidene reduce acid output by about 70 percent, famotidene by 90 percent, and omeprazol by 90 to 100 percent.

These drugs decrease your symptoms almost immediately, and promote healing of your ulcer: 50 percent of ulcers are gone within three weeks and 70 percent within six weeks. You may experience one or more side effects, such as dizziness, headache, diarrhea, constipation, impotence, breast enlargement in males, or mental changes—all of which are reversible when the drug is stopped. At this point, these drugs are fairly costly: $35 to $65 per month of treatment.

Twenty-five million people in the United States have now taken cimetadine (Tagamet). The main limitation is that acid-blocking drugs do not address your underlying ulcer-causing factors, and have a high incidence of ulcer recurrence when you stop taking them. To counteract this, some doctors are recommending ongoing "maintenance" treatment at reduced dosage, at bedtime only. However, symptomatic treatment is more appropriate than routine prophylactic treatment because only half of patients will have more than one recurrence within the first year after ulcer onset, and the best solution may be to use these drugs only if symptoms recur. Maintenance use of these drugs should be reserved for those who relapse in the first three months after healing, have return of symptoms three or more times per year, or who have had a bleeding complication. If you do need maintenance treatment, your doctor should check you for *H. pylori* infection, and treat if necessary, since the combination of lack of stomach acid and *H. pylori* infection can increase your risk for stomach cancer.[26] In order to maximize the possibility of a permanent cure, you should include the alternative medicine recommendations described on page 360.

Protective Barrier

Sucralfate (Carofate) is a drug with an entirely different mechanism of action. A bland compound of aluminum sulfate sucrose, it is taken orally and adheres to and protectively coats the raw ulcer surface, forming a barrier against acid, pepsin, and bile salt for six to twelve hours. The success rate of sucralfate is similar to that of cimetadine and ranitidene. In addition, treatment is much cheaper and side effects are minimal, although experience with the drug is more limited.

Helicobacter Pylori Infection Treatment

The bacterial organism *Helicobacter pylori* is commonly found in our stomachs. Approximately 10 percent of Americans under the age of 30 and 60 percent over the age of 60 are infected with it. However, the bacteria has been found in 90 percent of patients with duodenal ulcers, 80 percent of those with stomach ulcers, and in almost 100 percent of patients with chronic gastritis or stomach inflammation.

Evidence that *H. pylori* is not just an innocent bystander comes from studies showing that eradication of the organism with antibiotics, when added to acid-blocking treatment, is remarkably more successful in the rapid healing of duodenal ulcers than acid-blocking treatment alone. Notoriously difficult-to-heal gastric ulcers also respond faster, with a dramatic reduction in recurrence rates. A 60 to 90 percent duodenal ulcer recurrence rate within twelve to eighteen months after initial acid-blocking therapy alone is reduced to 2 to 12 percent when antibiotics are added. A 1997 study showed that if patients taking aspirin and NSAIDs (Motrin, etc.) were excluded, the recurrence rate after successful eradication of *H. pylori* in duodenal and gastric ulcer patients was essentially zero at ten years.[27]

If you have an ulcer, you should be examined for *H. pylori* infection.

Surgical Approaches to Peptic Ulcer Disease

Juan, *a 58-year-old recent immigrant from Latin America, developed severe upper abdominal pain the day before coming to the emergency room. X-rays showed air in his abdomen, and in the operating room he was found to have a hole in his duodenum, the first part of the small intestine, just past his stomach outlet, caused by a perforated peptic ulcer. The hole was surgically closed with stitches and a "patch" of neighboring tissue. He recovered well, and afterward carefully followed the alternative medicine recommendations, given on page 360, to avoid the danger of a recurrent ulcer.*

Alternative and/or conventional medical treatments can heal most peptic ulcers. However, despite recent advances and the trends toward decreasing rates and severity of ulcers, you may still require surgery. Rarely, you may need an operation if medical treatment is unable to control your disease (in which case it is termed "intractable"), or more likely, if you suddenly develop a life-threatening complication, such as bleeding, obstruction, or perforation.

The decision to undergo nonemergency surgery for a persistent but uncomplicated ulcer may be quite difficult; you need to seek experienced medical judgment. Ask your doctor the following questions: How severe is my ulcer? What are the chances I will develop a complication? Has maximum alternative and conventional medical management been given adequate trial?

Generally, you should not persist too long with unsuccessful alternative or conventional medical management, since if a complication were to develop, it would necessitate more difficult and dangerous surgery. If you have symptoms that cause interruption of your daily activities, if you are frequently forced to lose time from work and family, or if you consume large amounts of antacids and antiulcer medications, you have an intractable ulcer that may do best with surgical treatment. Some ulcers are simply less likely to respond to medical management, and are more prone to complications. Your ulcer is more likely to require surgical repair if it has penetrated into your pancreas, is located at the outlet of your stomach, has previously caused a complication, or is greater than one inch in size. Ulcers in children, teenagers, persons over the age of 65, alcoholics, the mentally retarded, and the emotionally disturbed also more commonly need surgical treatment.

Bleeding is the most common ulcer complication requiring surgery, and the leading cause of death in ulcer patients. If your ulcer eats into your intestinal wall's tiny blood vessels, a slow ooze of blood, evidenced by black, tarlike stools, can develop. (See Figure 12.2.) If one of your larger arteries is penetrated, bleeding can be massive, making your stools maroon or red, and causing you to vomit bright red blood.

Most bleeding episodes can now be controlled without surgery. Medical management with antacids and acid-blocking medicines, such as omeprazol, are used initially. However, if significant bleeding continues, further steps must be taken. Typically, this involves endoscopy: A flexible endoscope is introduced through your mouth into your esophagus, stomach, and duodenum. Using tiny instruments passed through the scope, the bleeding site then can be cauterized (sealed with an electric current) or injected with a blood vessel–constricting chemical, with an 80 to 85 percent success rate. If necessary, you can be given replacement blood. Intensive medical management may then heal your ulcer. Bleeding reoccurs in 15 to 20 percent of the patients initially controlled this way, and another attempt at endoscopic control is warranted, with an 84 percent long-term success rate.[28] However, if your bleeding is not controlled by these means, you must be taken quickly to the operating room, where the bleeding can be stopped with surgical sutures.

If your bleeding is controlled without surgery, you must consider the likelihood of an eventual recurrence. About 33 to 50 percent of those who have bled once bleed again within five years. If you have had two episodes of bleeding requiring hospitalization and transfusion, you should consider surgery.

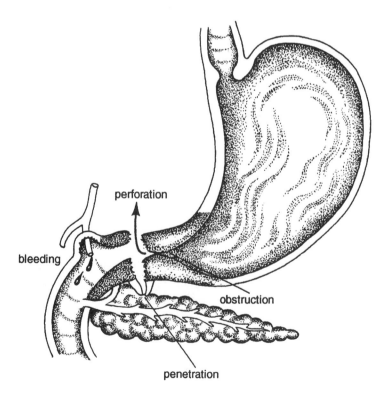

Fig. 12.2 Ulcer complications requiring surgery

Acute perforation usually requires immediate surgery. This occurs when an ulcer erodes through the full thickness of your duodenal wall, allowing stomach acid and other contents to spill into the abdominal cavity. The acid "burns" the tissues, causing sudden, severe pain. Without surgery, shock, infection, and abscess may result. However, about 50 percent of perforated ulcers are quickly "sealed off" by neighboring tissues so that if you are not too sick, a trial of stomach decompression with a tube passed through your nose into your stomach, acid blockers, and antibiotics, is warranted.[29]

Obstruction occurs when swelling from an acute ulcer or scarring from a chronic ulcer blocks your stomach outlet, preventing normal passage of the stomach's contents into the duodenum. Your stomach can dilate, occasionally to an enormous degree, and you may experience persistent vomiting. You must then be hospitalized, and your initial treatment will include a stomach suction tube passed through your nose, intravenous fluids, nutritional replacement, and ulcer medication. In a few days, after the acute component subsides, you will need surgery if scarring at the ulcer site has caused a persistent blockage.

Many great names in surgery are associated with research on stomach acid production and the subsequent development of acid-reducing surgical procedures. In the early days, removal of two-thirds to three-quarters of the stomach and its acid-producing cells was routine. In the 1940s and 1950s, the vagus nerves were recognized to be important in stimulating stomach acid production. As a result, *bilateral trunkal vagotomy*—which involves cutting the main trunks of both vagus nerves—became the mainstay of ulcer surgery. Three operations constitute the great majority of acid-reducing procedures performed in the

world today: *vagotomy and pyloroplasty, vagotomy and antrectomy,* and *highly selective (parietal cell) vagotomy.*

Vagotomy and pyloroplasty is the most common ulcer operation performed in the United States. The vagus nerves' acid-stimulating function is eliminated by cutting the main trunks of the two nerves, which reduces your total acid output by 50 to 70 percent. Since nerve supply to your pyloric pinch-valve is also interrupted and resulting spasm could cause outlet obstruction, a division of its circular muscle, called *pyloroplasty,* is also performed. The chief advantages of this operation are its ease, speed, and safety. The disadvantages are an increased risk of unpleasant symptoms that can develop after surgery, such as "dumping" (the rapid emptying of the stomach, causing sweating and nausea), diarrhea, and recurrent ulcers. These are discussed in further detail on page 371.

Vagotomy and antrectomy involves surgical removal of the lowest third of your stomach, the antrum, where cells that secrete the acid-stimulating hormone gastrin are found, as well as the cutting of both vagus nerve trunks. (See Figure 12.3.) Your acid output is decreased by 85 percent. The chief advantage of this procedure is that it has the lowest rate of recurrent ulcer formation. Its disadvantages are that it is relatively difficult to perform, you have increased risk if you are in poor health or undergoing surgery in an emergency, and increased chance of postoperative "dumping" and diarrhea.

Highly selective (parietal cell) vagotomy, the most widely performed ulcer procedure in England and Western Europe, has now become popular in the United States. Only those vagus nerve branches that go to the acid-producing portion of your stomach are cut, and the rest of your stomach retains its

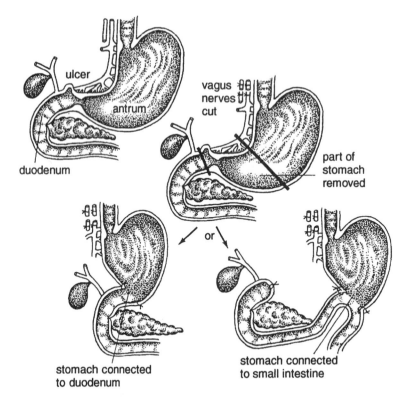

Fig. 12.3 Procedures involved in vagotomy and antrectomy

nerves, so that the pyloric pinch-valve can function normally and relatively normal stomach emptying is preserved. Acid secretion is reduced by 30 to 50 percent. Your stomach is not opened, which avoids the possibility of stitches breaking down after surgery. The procedure can be difficult and time-consuming. Compared to the other operations, its advantages are that it is the safest (less than 1 percent mortality) and has the lowest rate of the side effects of "dumping syndrome" and diarrhea (1 to 2 percent). However, ulcers recur at a relatively high rate, 5 to 20 percent. Recently, some surgeons have performed this operation through the laparoscope, which decreases the size of scars and discomfort, and speeds recovery.

Each of these techniques has its advantages and disadvantages, so you and your surgeon need to decide what the most important considerations are for you. At times, of course, the wisest decision can be made only after your surgeon has begun the operation and can thoroughly assess the anatomical factors involved. A presurgical discussion of the options will enable the surgeon to have your wishes clearly in mind. If you have an *H. pylori* infection and yet need surgery for a complication such as perforation, a less radical procedure can usually be selected with treatment of the infection after surgery to prevent recurrence.[30]

Vagotomy and pyloroplasty is relatively safe and quick, and because it is easily combined with tying off of a bleeding vessel, it is the method to choose if you are elderly, a poor surgical risk, or actively bleeding. It does carry a 5 to 10 percent recurrent ulcer rate. If you have a severe ulcer or elevated stomach acid output, you have a higher chance of developing a recurrent ulcer, and therefore should choose vagotomy and antrectomy, the "maximum" operation to reduce your acid output, with the lowest rate of ulcer recurrence (1 to 2 percent).

Most surgeons believe that the highly selective vagotomy is the safest operation, and therefore, it has gained wide popularity. It can now be performed through the laparoscope, lessening your postoperative discomfort and recovery time. However, this procedure has not been used extensively in emergency operations, and most surgeons do not have much experience with this technique, especially using the laparoscope. The recurrent ulcer rate after a highly selective vagotomy may be as high as 20 percent, but you can always choose another surgical technique later if medical treatment is unsuccessful.

The mortality rate of peptic ulcer surgery depends less on the specific procedure than whether a complication requires emergency surgery (which results in a 5 to 10 percent mortality rate) or not (1 to 2 percent mortality).

Early complications within the first few hours or days of surgery include bleeding, breakdown of the stomach stitches, intra-abdominal infection or abscess, intestinal obstruction, and incision infection. In these situations, a repeat operation may be necessary.

"Dumping syndrome" occurs when too-rapid emptying of your stomach contents into your small intestine causes dizziness, flushing, sweating, nausea, and headache. Dumping is experienced occasionally by up to 75 percent of patients whose surgery has eliminated the pyloric pinch-valve function, although only 20 percent have it with annoying frequency. Five percent require significant dietary restrictions. In 1 percent, the symptoms are so severe that corrective surgery must be undertaken.

Diarrhea episodes are experienced to some degree by about 50 percent of patients who have had a trunkal vagotomy. The reasons for this are not well understood. Usually the diarrhea is intermittent, tends to lessen with time, and is not a great problem. In 5 percent, it may require treatment. Drugs such as Imodium, which slow your intestinal movements, are useful if you have such an attack.

Alkaline reflux gastritis and *esophagitis* are caused by bile and pancreatic juice returning into the stomach or esophagus as a result of loss of pyloric pinch-valve function. This produces pain after eating, nausea, and vomiting. Up to 25 percent of patients experience such episodes occasionally, but less than 1 percent need corrective surgery.

A recurrent ulcer is more easily treated than severe dumping, diarrhea, or alkaline reflux after complete trunkal vagotomy. Therefore, highly selective vagotomy should be your first choice if you need surgery for an uncomplicated ulcer.

For all three procedures, you are given general anesthesia. The surgeon makes an up-and-down incision from your navel to your breastbone, or an upper abdominal crosswise incision below your ribs. The procedure may take one to three hours.

You awaken in the recovery room, and may need to spend a day or two in an intensive care unit until it is certain you have no immediate complications. You are given intravenous fluids, have a bladder catheter to monitor your urine output and fluid needs, and possibly a breathing tube for twenty-four hours or more, until you are proven strong enough to breathe satisfactorily without aid.

You most likely need a tube down your nose into your stomach, connected to a suction bottle to suck out air and secretions. This tube decreases the danger of your stomach distending, which would stress the healing line of stitches, and also prevents vomiting. The tube is usually necessary for two or three days. When it is removed, you can begin to take small amounts of liquid or soft food, and advance to a regular diet, usually by the fourth to sixth day after surgery.

You can probably leave the hospital in five to seven days. Your convalescence should include lots of rest and nonvigorous exercise. Diet must be individually tailored, depending upon how your system adapts to your new digestive tract arrangement. You can expect to eventually regain your old eating patterns with only minor restrictions. After a few weeks, you should begin to regain the weight lost during your illness and hospitalization. Forceful exercise should be avoided for about three months. Several return visits to your surgeon are advisable during this period.

If you have a highly selective vagotomy through a laparoscope, your recovery progress will be rapid and you will probably be able to eat in a day or two and then be discharged from the hospital. Postoperative physical restrictions are minimal, and you may soon return to work.

Nonpeptic Stomach Ulcer Disease

John was a 55-year-old Native American who took aspirin for several weeks for upper back pain, which he believed was caused by arthritis. He passed maroon-colored stools for three days before he became dizzy and saw his doctor. He was anemic, with his blood count only one-third normal. Endoscopy found an ooz-ing stomach ulcer, 2½ inches in diameter, which had penetrated into his pancreas, thereby causing the back pain. After removal of one-third of his stomach, including the ulcer, he recovered completely.

Not all ulcers in the stomach are peptic ulcers caused by excess acid production. In fact, many patients do not secrete much acid at all. Unlike peptic ulcers, the frequency of this type of ulcer is *not* decreasing. Stomach ulcers are now believed to be due to the stomach lining's protective mechanisms somehow becoming defective. This type of ulcer is especially common in smokers, alcoholics, and persons taking antiinflammatory medicines. Alcohol, aspirin, steroids, and other antiinflammatory drugs, as well as the return of your duodenal contents back into your stomach, may produce injury to your stomach lining cells, or may inhibit their natural protective mechanisms. This makes them more vulnerable to the effects of acid and enzymes, promoting ulcer formation. *Helicobacter pylori* infection may also play a role.

Symptoms of stomach ulcers and methods of diagnosis are similar to those for peptic ulcers. If you have a stomach ulcer, you need to have it biopsied with an endoscope, since 5 to 10 percent of such ulcers appear within a stomach cancer.

Alternative Medicine Approaches to Nonpeptic Stomach Ulcer Disease

The alternative medicine approaches to nonpeptic stomach ulcer disease are similar to those given for peptic ulcer disease. However, they may be less successful because recurrences are more common, unless your disease is caused by a specific medication that can be discontinued. Please see the alternative medicine approaches for peptic ulcer disease.

Following are the most important alternative medicine approaches to nonpeptic stomach ulcer disease.

Change Your Diet

Fat in your diet, by slowing the passage of food through your digestive tract, may allow for reflux (backing up) of bile into your stomach. Switch to a low-fat, high-fiber diet, as given in Chapter 2.

Take Supplements

Decreased levels of vitamin B_6 have been found in patients with these nonpeptic stomach ulcers.[31] Vitamin B_6 may help prevent the breakdown of your stomach lining cells. You can begin by taking 50 milligrams daily.

In a study of stomach ulcer patients who had no evidence of zinc deficiency, the group given 90 milligrams of zinc three times daily exhibited three times the healing rate as the other group, as well as more complete healing.[32]

Conventional Medicine Approaches to Nonpeptic Stomach Ulcer Disease

The conventional medical management of nonpeptic stomach ulcer disease is similar to that for peptic ulcer disease; recurrences are more common, unless your disease is caused by a medication that can be discontinued. Please refer to the section on the conventional treatment of peptic ulcer disease.

Surgical Approach to Nonpeptic Stomach Ulcer Disease

Surgery is usually performed for a complication of bleeding, perforation, or obstruction, as well as if it is suspected you may have an underlying malignancy, even if your ulcer biopsies are negative. Usually one-third of your stomach nearest its outlet (the antrum) is removed, along with the ulcer. Your vagus nerves are not cut unless your ulcer is associated with high acid output or is very near the outlet. If you are in poor medical condition, simply removing the ulcer, combined with a trunkal vagotomy, may be the safest procedure.

Recently, stomach ulcer operations, including highly selective vagotomy, have been performed with the use of the laparoscope. So far, the indications for choosing this technique, and its results, are unclear.

STOMACH ULCER DISEASE SUMMARY

Prevention

Diet and Supplements

- Follow a whole foods, low-fat, high-fiber, vegetarian diet.
- Bran, 3 tablespoons daily.
- Avoid trigger foods: fatty meats, refined sugar, spicy foods, salt, citrus, sodas.
- Vitamin A, 20,000 IU daily.
- Vitamin B_6, 50 mg daily.
- Vitamin C, 1,000 mg, 3 times daily.
- Vitamin E, D-alpha, 400 IU daily.

Lifestyle

- Don't smoke.
- Don't drink alcohol.
- Avoid trigger medications: aspirin, nonsteroidal antiinflammatory drugs, cortison, ibuprofen.

- Practice stress management.
- Get a good night's rest.

Alternative Medicine Approaches

- Follow the preventive guidelines given.
- Bioflavonoids, 500–1,500 mg 1–3 times daily.
- Zinc 50 mg, 3 times daily.
- Licorice, deglycyrrhizinated, 380 mg tablets, chewed 3–4 times daily, 20 minutes before meals.
- Cabbage juice—raw, fresh, 1 quart daily.
- Avoid cream and milk products, coffee, and raw foods.
- Add cardamon, coriander, and flaxseeds to your diet.
- Herb teas, such as chamomile, echinacea, fenugreek, goldenseal, licorice root, slippery elm, meadowsweet, as tolerated.
- Aloe vera gel, 1 capsule or tablespoon, 3 hours after meals.
- Non-fat acidophilus yogurt.
- Homeopathy, such as nux vomica, arsenicum album.
- Biofeedback.

Conventional Medicine Approaches

- Antacids—magnesium hydroxide, aluminum hydroxide, Mylanta, Maalox, bismuth.
- Acid-reducing drugs—cimetadine (Tagamet) ranitidene (Zantac), famotidene (Pepcid), and omeprazol (Prilosec).
- Protective barrier—sucralfate (Carofate).
- *Helicobacter pylori* infection treatment.

Surgical Approaches

- Vagotomy and pyloroplasty.
- Vagotomy and antrectomy.
- Highly selective (parietal cell) vagotomy.

Stomach Cancer

Stomach cancer is the world's number two cancer killer. In the United States and Western Europe it was very common in the first half of the twentieth century, but for unknown reasons is decreasing. However, in 2002 it still will account for 21,600 cases and 12,400 deaths in the United States.[33] Genetics, environment, and diet may be predisposing factors. Miners and other workers who inhale carcinogenic dust and fumes are at higher risk. The incidence of stomach cancer is seven times higher in Japan, where consumption of smoked and pickled foods, soy sauce, and the tannic acid in black tea, unbuffered by milk, increases that culture's contact with known carcinogens. Barbecued foods contain nitrate compounds, known to promote stomach cancer. *Helicobacter pylori* infection may also play a role. If you have pernicious anemia, a condition in which no stomach acid is produced, or if you have had previous stomach trauma from ingesting caustic acid or alkali, or previous stomach surgery, you are at higher risk.

Stomach cancer has an overall cure rate of only 21 percent. (See Table 12.1.) Early diagnosis offers you the best chance for cure, although your early symptoms may be quite subtle. Eventually, you may experience pain, weight loss, bleeding, obstruction, and/or perforation. Tumors that ulcerate are usually diagnosed earlier and are more frequently cured. Diagnostic studies include endoscopy with biopsy, along with a CAT scan to look for evidence of spread.

Alternative Medicine Approaches to Stomach Cancer

You can take action to help prevent or possibly assist in the treatment of stomach cancer

TABLE 12.1.
Prognosis of Stomach Cancer[34]

	Percent of Patients Surviving 5 Years	Percent of Patients in This Stage
All Patients	21.8%	
Not Staged	13.4%	15%
By Stage		
Localized to stomach	59.0%	21%
Lymph node spread	21.7%	31%
Distant spread	2.3%	33%

and the prevention of its recurrence by utilizing alternative medicine techniques. Follow the guidelines given for preventing and treating esophageal cancer in Chapter 11.

Following are the most promising alternative medicine approaches to esophageal cancer.

Quit Smoking

Cigarette smoking may encourage the formation of stomach cancer by increasing carbon dioxide and decreasing oxygen in the blood, by impairing local blood flow repair mechanisms because nicotine constricts small blood vessels, and through the carginogenic action of smoke itself. You can help yourself quit smoking for good by using the alternative medicine tools discussed in Chapter 2, especially in the section, "Quitting Smoking."

Avoid Alcohol

The rates of stomach cancer are higher in those who regularly consume alcohol. You can use alternative medicine's various techniques of stress reduction and relaxation as a substitute for alcohol consumption; see Chapter 2 for details.

Change Your Diet

Dietary carcinogens in salty, pickled, smoked, or barbecued foods, are thought to contribute to the development of stomach cancer. Fresh fruits and vegetables, garlic, and green tea may act preventively.

Three grams of garlic per day (about one clove, either raw or cooked) seem to protect against stomach cancer. At the 1999 annual meeting of the American Association for Cancer Research in Philadelphia, Aaron Fleischauer reported on a meta-analysis of eight epidemiological studies looking at garlic intake and stomach cancer. A 50 percent reduction in stomach cancer was found among populations that ate garlic-rich diets, compared to those that ate little garlic.[34]

Conventional Medicine Approaches to Stomach Cancer

When surgery is not possible, or not likely to be curative, you can consider chemotherapy and radiation. These treatments may give you a chance of increasing your lifespan by several months. With newer combinations of drugs and more advanced radiotherapy technology, better results may be obtained in the future. As with other forms of cancer, you should seek the latest information from medical, radiological, and surgical cancer specialists.

Surgical Approaches to Stomach Cancer

Unless you have evidence of widespread disease, the treatment of your stomach cancer should be surgical, if it appears safe to remove it. Even if you cannot be cured by surgery, an operation offers you the best chance for relief of the symptoms of bleeding and obstruction.

Your case must be considered in a frank discussion with your family and your doctor before an operation is chosen. If you decide to have surgery, you have a 50 to 70 percent chance that all or most of your tumor can be removed. If all visible tumor can be removed and it has not spread to your glands or invaded the full thickness of your stomach wall, you have a 60 percent chance you will be cured. If your lymph nodes are involved, or if you have invasion of the full thickness of the wall, your chance for cure drops to 20 percent. The average life expectancy after a noncurative operation to relieve symptoms is ten to twelve months. When surgery is not possible, this is decreased to two to three months.

The most common operation for stomach cancer, *subtotal gastrectomy,* can be performed in 80 percent of all cases, and removes 60 to 80 percent of the stomach. In 20 percent of all patients it is necessary to perform a *total gastrectomy,* that takes out all of the stomach. Surprisingly, most patients can adapt satisfactorily no matter how much stomach must be removed.

You will be admitted to the hospital the morning of your surgery. General anesthetic is necessary. The surgeon makes an up-and-down incision from your navel to your breastbone, or a crosswise incision below your ribs.

After exploring for evidence of tumor spread and determining how much stomach must be removed, your surgeon frees up the stomach from neighboring tissue, dividing its blood and lymph vessels and nerves. The duodenum, or first part of the small intestine, is divided just past the stomach's pyloric pinch-valve, and the stomach near its upper end, or across the esophagus if the whole stomach must be removed. Lymph nodes associated with the stomach and sometimes the spleen are also removed. Continuity of the intestinal tract is re-established by the small intestine being sewn to the remaining part of your stomach, as in a vagotomy and antrectomy. If the stomach is totally removed, the small intestine is sewn to the end of your esophagus. These procedures generally take one to four hours to complete. Possible complications associated with stomach cancer surgery are the same as for stomach ulcer surgery. The overall operation mortality rate is 5 percent.

The experience with laparoscopic-assisted gastric surgery for early gastric cancer is promising,[35] but very few patients in the United States would qualify because most have advanced disease, and few U.S. surgeons would feel comfortable with this technique at this point in time.

Recovery from stomach cancer surgery is similar to that described for recovery from peptic ulcer surgery. However, since a larger portion of the stomach has been removed, initially you will have to be more careful to eat smaller amounts of food more frequently. Eventually you should be able to regain your old eating patterns, with some restrictions. Even if all of your stomach must be removed, you should be able to eat a fairly regular diet. The first part of your intestine will dilate somewhat to assume some of the stomach's storage capacity. You will need to eat smaller volumes and may find that you need to avoid certain foods as determined by trial and error. If all of your stomach has been removed, you will need regular vitamin B_{12} injections.

STOMACH CANCER SUMMARY

Prevention

Diet and Supplements

- Follow a high-fiber, low-fat diet.
- Eat plenty of fresh fruits and vegetables.
- Eat fresh or cooked garlic, one clove daily.
- Avoid black tea taken without milk.
- Avoid salty, pickled, smoked, or barbecued foods.
- Avoid alcohol.

Lifestyle

- Don't smoke.

Alternative Medicine Approaches

- Follow the preventive guidelines above and for esophageal cancer in Chapter 11.
- Hypnosis, acupuncture, aromatherapy, and the other immune adjuncts presented in Chapter 2.
- Visualization.

Conventional Medicine Approaches

- Radiotherapy.
- Chemotherapy.

Surgical Approaches

- Subtotal gastrectomy.
- Total gastrectomy.

GALLBLADDER

"But wait a bit," the Walrus said:
"Before we have our chat;
For some of us are out of breath,
And all of us are fat!"

Lewis Carroll

The indelible image of President Lyndon Johnson, while he was in the White House, lifting up his shirt to show reporters the long scar from his gallbladder operation, is a testament to how often this painful problem afflicts Americans. Half a million of us have our gallbladders surgically removed every year.

It is ironically appropriate that gallbladder surgery is sometimes even termed the "bread and butter" operation of general surgeons, because it provides bread and butter for their tables—and it may be our American love of butter and other high cholesterol foods that causes this prevalent problem in the first place.

"Fair, fat, female, and forty" is the stereotype for persons most likely to develop gallbladder disease, and excess fats and lack of fiber in the diet are the likeliest underlying causes. Evidence suggests that changes in diet can be effective in not only preventing, but perhaps treating gallstones, along with other alternative medicine therapies.

If you must have surgery, laparoscopic removal of the gallbladder, which requires only tiny incisions, causes little discomfort, and is followed by a quick recovery, has revolutionized the standard surgery for this disease in just a few short years.

Gallbladder disease is the most common reason for major abdominal surgery in the United States today. Operative removal of the gallbladder is very safe in most patients; the surgical death rate is less than two per thousand overall, and even lower if you are in relatively good health.[1] Still, this means that up to 850 people may die each

379

year as a result of their gallbladder operations—as artist Andy Warhol did. You *can* act to keep your gallbladder from forming stones, and utilize alternatives to treat this disease. In this chapter, we will discuss the different approaches to preventing and treating gallstones, so you can choose what is most right for you.

How Your Gallbladder Works

Your gallbladder, a pear-shaped outpouching of your liver's bile duct system, stores bile produced by your liver cells. (See Figure 13.1.) The golden bile is collected by ducts within the liver, and then a portion of it is stockpiled in concentrated form, an ounce or two at a time, within the gallbladder.

When fat enters the small intestine from your stomach, it stimulates release of the hormone cholecystokinin, and your gallbladder contracts. The concentrated bile is then squeezed out and passed by way of the common bile duct into your small intestine, where it helps with digestion and absorption of fat. Most bile is reabsorbed in the last part of your small intestine, and returned to your liver to be reused. Some bile also serves to help excrete body waste products, such as pigments from old decomposed red blood cells, as they are discharged along with the bile in your stool.

Gallstones

Since most people with gallstones do not have symptoms, 20 million Americans, or eventually 15 to 20 percent of us, simply walk around not knowing we are carrying such stones in our gallbladders. Rare before age 20, they increase in frequency with advancing age, affecting one in three persons after age 70.

Gallstones are three to four times more common in women, and twice as frequently found in users of birth control pills, both probably a result of the female sex hormones' contribution to increased cholesterol concen-

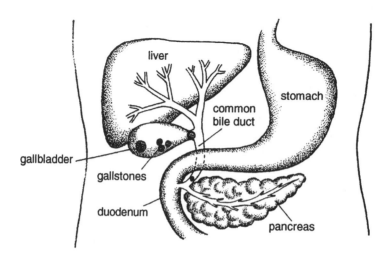

Fig. 13.1   The location of the gallbladder

tration in bile. Individuals who are over-weight secrete increased cholesterol into their bile, and so also have a higher incidence. Medical conditions such as sickle cell anemia, bowel absorption disorders, and previous stomach surgery also predispose an individual to stone formation.

Several specific factors can promote gall-stone formation; secretion of abnormal bile is the most common and important of these. Eighty percent of gallstones are of the "cho-lesterol" type. In normal bile, cholesterol is present in a soluble, liquid form. For choles-terol to remain dissolved, a delicate balance must be maintained between the three main bile constituents: cholesterol, bile salts, and lecithin. Abnormal bile contains too much cholesterol relative to the other ingredients. Such "supersaturated" bile is present in "stone-formers" throughout adulthood, and precedes the formation of stones by many years. Supersaturated bile has a tendency to form crystals. Persons who form stones have higher concentrations of mucoproteins and other proteins in bile that can accelerate ini-tial crystal formation. Calcium, bile pigments, bacteria, and cellular debris then cluster around these crystals, and harden to form stones.

Much research has been conducted in an effort to determine exactly why certain per-sons form this abnormal bile. Some ethnic groups have an extremely high rate of stone formation. In Pima Indians, 70 percent of the women develop stones, usually at an early age, while the incidence in African-Americans is low. In some families, many members make stones. On the other hand, cross-cultural stud-ies suggest that a cholesterol-free, nonmeat and low-fat dairy diet, with high-fiber, by low-ering the relative cholesterol content of the bile, provides significant protection against stone formation regardless of genetic influ-ence.

Twenty percent of gallstones are "pig-ment" stones, created from the breakdown products of red blood cells. These are more common in persons with sickle cell anemia, other red cell abnormalities, and other dis-eases that destroy red cells.

Sluggish bile flow can also lead to the ex-cessively concentrated bile that promotes stone formation. In addition, poor contractil-ity of the gallbladder allows accumulation of debris and crystals, allowing them to grow rather than being flushed out into the intes-tine. During pregnancy and after certain types of stomach surgery, the gallbladder does not contract properly, making stone formation more likely.

The presence of *bacteria* in the bile adds to debris formation. Poor emptying of the gall-bladder enhances bacterial overgrowth, in-creasing opportunities for stone precipitation and the risk of serious infection.

How Gallbladder Disease Is Diagnosed

Gallstones are quite common and not nec-essarily the source of your symptoms. You will need a careful history, physical exam, blood tests, ultrasound test, and, rarely, other tests such as the CCK-HIDA scan and upper GI series to determine if your symptoms are caused by gallbladder disease.

History

Your doctor should ask a series of ques-tions about your symptoms, including how long you have had them, the frequency, sever-ity, and duration of attacks, what may have brought them on, and what you may have done to relieve them. Be sure to report any nausea, vomiting, fever, yellow jaundice, or changes in color of urine and stool. Information about your family history of stones, medical problems such as liver or ulcer disease, and medications may be important.

Two forms of gallbladder attacks can develop; you may have one or both. *Biliary colic* is usually less severe and of shorter duration than *acute cholecystitis*. The former occurs when your stone-containing gallbladder contracts and a stone is forced up against your gallbladder outlet, obstructing bile flow. Contraction against this obstruction increases pressure within the gallbladder and produces feelings of indigestion, nausea, and/or pain. Such symptoms usually come on rapidly, increase quickly to peak intensity in an hour or so, and are continuous. You feel pain most often in your upper middle abdomen, below your ribs or toward your right side. A typical attack of biliary colic usually begins a few hours after your evening meal (or any large meal), but can occur at any time. The attack ends after a few hours, or sometimes as little as thirty minutes. The gallbladder eventually relaxes, pressure decreases, and the stone moves away from its blocking position, ending the attack. Between attacks, you have few symptoms.

Fatty or greasy foods cause your gallbladder to contract, and so may precipitate these biliary colic attacks. However, since many people with normal gallbladders cannot tolerate fatty or greasy foods, indigestion after such meals does not necessarily mean you have gallbladder disease.

An acute cholecystitis attack is more intense and prolonged. Your gallbladder may be persistently obstructed by a stone, or it may have become inflamed by irritation from stones, increased pressure, or bacterial infection. You may experience nausea, vomiting, and continuous pain, mostly present in the upper abdomen, though it may radiate to your back or right shoulder. Chills or fever may develop. Typically, these attacks last many hours or days, causing you to visit your doctor or hospital emergency room, and may require an emergency operation.

In 5 to 10 percent of gallbladder attacks, the gallbladder becomes inflamed or otherwise diseased *without* the presence of stones. This diagnosis is difficult to make with certainty. Biliary dyskinesia, or abnormal gallbladder contractility, can cause symptoms similar to biliary colic without stones or pathologic abnormalities.

Physical Exam

Your doctor should feel your abdomen. If you are having an acute attack, pressing on your upper abdomen may produce excruciating pain; in some cases a swollen, tender gallbladder can be felt through the abdominal wall. Between attacks, you may experience some mild tenderness, or no discomfort at all.

Blood Tests

Blood tests reflecting liver function usually come back normal with simple gallstone disease. However, they are often requested, as they may suggest an unexpected complication such as a gallstone blocking the bile duct. If you are having an acute attack, blood tests are necessary to look for infection and pancreatitis from a stone blocking the pancreatic duct as well.

Ultrasound

The most common test used to diagnose gallstones is the ultrasound (sonogram). Ultrasound finds stones by identifying the "shadows" they cast when they block high-frequency sound waves. This test requires no X-ray exposure, and is a very rapid means of making a diagnosis, especially important if you are having an acute attack. The sonogram can also find abnormalities of the pancreas, liver, bile ducts, or kidneys that might mimic gallbladder disease.

CCK-HIDA Scan

This study is useful for diagnosing biliary dyskinesia when other studies appear normal. You are injected intravenously with hepatic iminodiacetic acid (HIDA), a radioactive isotope which is concentrated in your gallbladder. You are then given an injection of cholecysykinin (CCK), a hormone that causes gallbladder contraction. The percentage of isotope emptied is measured, and whether or not your symptoms are reproduced is noted. If this test is positive, you likely have biliary dyskinesia, and resolving your gallbladder should relieve your symptoms.

Upper GI Series

Many surgeons also request a preoperative upper gastrointestinal (GI) X-ray series if they suspect that symptoms seemingly due to gallbladder disease may actually be caused by an ulcer, esophageal reflux, or other stomach problems.

What Happens If Your Gallbladder Stones Go Untreated?

Seventy-five percent or more of gallstones are "silent," often found during examination for other problems. Each year, 2 percent of patients with known silent stones do develop symptoms.[2] Surgery, however, is generally not recommended unless this occurs. On the other hand, once your gallbladder has formed stones and caused symptoms, you are likely to experience increasingly frequent and severe attacks.

Complications of gallbladder disease can be quite severe, even fatal, without treatment,

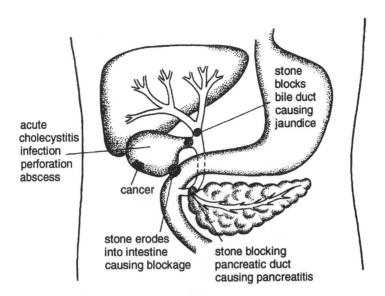

Fig. 13.2 Complications caused by gallstones

although they usually don't develop without the warning of preexisting symptoms. An obstructed gallbladder can become infected, may develop gangrene or a perforation (a hole that allows the contents of the gallbladder to leak out into your abdomen), or may form an abscess. (See Figure 13.2.) A stone can pass from your gallbladder into your bile duct system and obstruct flow of bile, causing jaundice, liver disease, or severe infection. If a stone in your bile duct blocks the outflow of pancreas secretions, it can cause an inflammation, called pancreatitis, which can be lethal. In rare instances, a large stone can pass all the way into your intestine and cause bowel obstruction. Gallstones present for more than twenty years are thought to be a possible cause of gallbladder cancer, which is found in 1 percent of the gallbladders that are removed.

Alternative Medicine Approaches to Gallbladder Disease

_____

Julie was an enterprising ultrasound technician with documented small gallstones. Rather than have her gallbladder removed, she decided to attempt a trial of the liver-gallbladder flush. She was able to use her skill at ultrasound to document the movement of her stones up and out of her gallbladder. She became stone-free, and then began following a low-fat, high-fiber diet, along with the other lifestyle changes given below, to prevent further gallstone formation.

_____

A gallbladder attack is very uncomfortable. Usually, it shows itself about twenty minutes after you eat a fatty meal, when you start to feel awful. You may wonder if you need surgery; or if you have been found to have stones incidentally on an X-ray or ultrasound, whether you should have them removed.

Dr. William Gracie of the University of Michigan studied patients with "silent" (non-pain-producing) gallstones. He found that most people with silent gallstones do *not* develop problems, and can go through life without complications from these incidental stones.[3] He recommended that unless your gallstones give you pain, they need not be removed, and he actually advised against it.

You may simply choose to live comfortably with your gallstones—since millions of Americans have them, and most never develop any problems. You also may want to try alternative medicine treatment to eliminate them. A trial of alternative medicine approaches may help turn symptomatic stones into silent ones—and save you from both an operation and other diseases as well. In all cases, however, you must be monitored by your doctor. Following are changes you can institute.

Change Your Diet

Happily, gallstones are *preventable* in most people. They are almost nonexistent in vegetarian populations.[4] Cholesterol is the chief component in 80 percent of the gallstones in the United States, and dietary cholesterol comes only from animal sources. A low-fat vegetarian diet reduces the amount of cholesterol collecting within your bile. Cross-cultural studies document a low risk for gallstones among populations eating this diet. The other 20 percent of the gallstones, which come from increased breakdown products of blood cells, are preventable only by treatment of the underlying blood disorder.

In addition to avoiding fats, an increase in

fiber, with three large bowel movements a day, is optimum for preventing gallstone formation. British researcher Dr. Denis Burkitt did extensive studies in different cultures showing that a high-fiber diet helps eliminate cholesterol by binding it, along with saturated fats, in your digestive tract. They are not then reabsorbed and stored in your gallbladder. By thus changing the composition of your bile, precipitation of stones is discouraged. Also, fiber decreases the formation of desoxycholic acid and also binds with it in the digestive tract, so that it can be eliminated with the feces. This increases the solubility of cholesterol in the gallbladder, discouraging and reversing stone formation.[5] Simple addition of bran to the diet has been shown to create a less fat-saturated bile. Take three tablespoons a day.

Diets too high in legumes with water-soluble fiber increase gallbladder cholesterol saturation and are associated with an increased risk of gallstone formation. You should be moderate in your intake of beans, peas, and other vegetables with seeds in pods if you have gallstones or are at high risk.[6]

Fatty, greasy, and fried foods, which trigger especially forceful gallbladder contractions, are the classic precipitators of biliary colic and particularly should be avoided. These foods may transform silent gallstones into symptomatic ones. Avoid all animal products, and do not add oil to your foods. Follow the guidelines for a low-fat, high-fiber diet given in Chapter 2.

Eliminate Food Allergies

Avoiding foods to which you are allergic has been found in some studies to relieve symptoms of gallbladder disease. These foods may cause an allergic reaction within the walls of your bile ducts, partially obstructing bile flow from the gallbladder, and thus act to precipitate attacks.[7] One initial study found 100 percent relief of symptoms when patients eliminated foods to which they were allergic. First, the subjects were placed on a diet of beef, rye, soy, rice, cherries, peaches, apricots, beets, and spinach. After one week, foods were added. The most common ones which gave symptoms were eggs, pork, and onions. Other allergenic items were fowl, milk, coffee, citrus, corn, beans, and nuts. Reintroducing eggs caused attacks in 93 percent. Such allergies may be diagnosed by skin or blood tests, or you can follow an elimination diet, reintroducing foods one by one and noting if your symptoms return.

In general, eat a high-fiber diet, including whole grains, whole wheat breads, salads, beans, unless you have an allergy to them, and bean sprouts. Avoid green peppers, cabbage, tomato sauces, and cucumbers, along with any other foods you know to bring on symptoms. This change of diet alone may free you from pain, and thus help you avoid the need for surgery.

Take Supplements

Studies of Native Americans, who genetically have an exceptionally high rate of gallstone formation, have shown that adding *lecithin* to the diet decreases stone formation. Increased bile lecithin increases cholesterol solubility, discouraging cholesterol solidification in the gallbladder, preventing stone precipitation.[8] The recommended dose is 1,200 milligrams of lecithin, three times daily. Another study showed that gallstones dissolved in humans using *choline* (one of the B vitamins) and lecithin. The amount of choline was 500 mg three times daily.[9]

Vitamin C may protect against gallstone formation.[10] Dosage is 500 mg three times daily. Addition of garlic and onion to the diet may lower cholesterol and thus reduce gallstone risk.[11] You may take two garlic oil capsules daily, 500 mg each, to make certain of this effect. Magnesium, 200 to 500 mg three times daily, by relaxing the musculature of your gallbladder, may help relieve your pain during a gallbladder attack, and keep your stones from causing you further pain.

Avoid Birth Control Pills

Taking birth control pills doubles your risk of developing gallstones. If you cannot use a more natural method such as a diaphragm or condom, make certain you follow the low-fat, high-fiber diet given in Chapter 2.

Maintain Your Optimum Weight

Gallstones are rare in persons who maintain their optimum weight.[12] Being overweight may affect fat metabolism, causing an alteration in bile composition, predisposing to stone formation. However, you should lose your extra weight gradually, no more than one to two pounds per week, as rapid weight loss leads to a rapid increase in the size of stones and increased risk for symptoms. You can use the recommendations from Chapter 2 to assist you in getting to your correct weight.

Exercise

Although the mechanism is unknown, exercise reduces the risk for symptomatic gallstones. A 1999 study reported in the *New England Journal of Medicine* analyzing data from the Harvard Nurses' Study found a 31 percent decreased need for cholecystectomy in the group of women with the highest rate of recreational physical activity as compared with those in the lowest group. Follow the recommendations in Chapter 2.

Practice Stress Management

Stress may also contribute to stone formation. Cholesterol has been shown to increase at times of stress—independent of diet—and stress-reduction exercises such as yoga are documented to lower cholesterol levels. A good program that helps you relieve tension is important. See Chapter 2 for details.

Use the Liver-Gallbladder Flush

The liver-gallbladder flush is a traditional naturopathic treatment to naturally empty the gallbladder of stones. It causes the gallbladder to contract, pushing the stones out into the small intestine, where they can be eliminated with the stool. It can be used to eliminate silent stones, but must be modified, as noted below, for an acute attack. *This procedure should be performed only under a doctor's direct supervision.*

For silent stones, begin the flush by taking two droppers of dilute liquid phosphoric acid, available in health food stores, three times daily, for one week, ahead of time. This has the effect of improving muscle relaxation in the gallbladder. On the day of your flush, start at lunchtime, by eating only a large green salad, with nonfat dressing.

The next step is to take an enema, with two tablespoons of Epsom salts mixed into the enema water. Once absorbed, the Epsom salts, which contain magnesium, relaxes the musculature of the gallbladder. The enema also acts to relieve pressure in the digestive tract. Blood needed for the processing of your food can be diverted from your intestines to protect and repair your gallbladder. In addition to the enema, you can take one to two tablespoons of Epsom salts, or 200 to 500 mg of magnesium citrate, by mouth, to assist this process.

Eat one-half of a grapefruit for supper. After that, drink only citrus juice, to avoid further stimulation of your gallbladder, and allow your body to focus its blood supply on solving the problem. Just before bed, take one-half cup of pure, unrefined olive oil, followed by a glass of grapefruit or orange juice, and immediately lie on your right side with your right knee up.

Small stones have been documented to safely pass by this method, but since stones could, in theory, subsequently lodge in your bile duct, making it necessary to remove them by the use of a flexible scope passed through the stomach into the bile duct or by surgery, make *certain* your doctor supervises you. No scientific studies are yet available for this method of treatment.

During an acute attack, eliminate the phosphoric acid preparation. Rub castor oil on your abdomen, over the point of pain. Take the Epsom salts or magnesium by mouth, follow it right away with the olive oil, and lie on your right side. If your pain does not quickly subside, see your doctor immediately.

Practice Visualization

Imagine your gallbladder like a small bag containing some dark green waxy marbles. See the bag relaxing, and the marbles moving easily out into your intestines, and then out of your body. Next see the bag filled only with easily flowing beautiful light green liquid. Hold this image in your mind, while feeling it happen within your body.

Conventional Medicine Approaches to Gallbladder Disease

There are two conventional medicine approaches to gallstones that are not generally recommended unless you are at a very high risk for or are too debilitated to undergo surgery. The advent of the laparoscopic surgery technique has made their usage exceedingly rare.

Drug Treatments

Drug treatment has not reached the point where gallbladder disease can be reliably cured or its dangerous complications avoided. Medications such as ursodiol (Actigal) do dissolve stones in 30 percent of patients with noncalcified, cholesterol stones less than 2 centimeters in diameter, but require many months to work, and the stones tend to reform in more than 50 percent of all patients once the drug is stopped. This treatment is generally not recommended unless you are at high risk for surgery.

Shock Wave Lithotripsy

This method for eliminating gallstones is similar to that commonly used to treat kidney stones (see page 704). You lie in a water bath. The stones are localized on a sonogram, and then high-energy focused shock waves cause them to break apart. You then pass the fragments out through your intestines. Passage can be painful and cause complications. Even if this technique is successful, new stones are likely to form, since the underlying stone-forming process is not treated. It can be attempted if you are too debilitated to undergo surgery. The advent of the laparoscopic surgery technique has made lithotripsy usage extremely rare.

Surgical Approaches to Gallbladder Disease

Theresa, a 32-year-old emotionally disturbed woman with a terrible fear of doctors and hospitals, began experiencing almost daily attacks of biliary colic. It took her social worker and surgeon a great deal of time and effort to convince her to consent for removal of her gallbladder. She underwent an uneventful laparoscopic operation, and returned to her group home four hours after waking up from anesthesia. She did not even need to take postoperative pain medication.

Maureen, a 24-year-old Native American woman, was two months pregnant when she developed severe abdominal pain and vomiting. An ultrasound showed her gallbladder was full of stones, and her pancreas was also enlarged. This "gallstone" pancreatitis was nearly fatal, requiring two weeks in Intensive Care and causing her to miscarry. Once she had recovered sufficiently, she had her gallbladder removed.

If you have an attack of acute cholecystitis that is not getting better with a short trial of medical management, you need emergency surgery. In general, if you have recovered from an attack of acute cholecystitis or pancreatitis caused by a gallstone, you should have your gallbladder removed as soon as possible after the diagnosis is made, unless you have had a recent serious illness. For the most part, you should also have surgery if you have recurring attacks of *biliary colic*, because delay only subjects you to attacks that are increasingly more frequent and dangerous. The chances of developing a complication or re-

quiring emergency surgery increases as time passes.

Alternative medicine approaches should *not* be used to delay your seeking surgical advice. Many times, patients see a surgeon days after the onset of an acute cholecystitis attack, by which time they have abscessed, gangrenous, or perforated gallbladders. In these cases, surgery is more difficult, a laparoscopic approach may not be possible, and you are more likely to have complications. Diabetic and elderly patients may be especially likely to have a rapidly deteriorating course. Seek medical consultation *before* you embark on any course of treatment.

If you have typical attacks of biliary colic but have a normal ultrasound, ask to be checked for biliary dyskinesia. If your CCK-HIDA scan indicates abnormal gallbladder function, there is 94 percent chance of improvement or even resolution of your symptoms with cholecystectomy.[13]

If you have experienced only *mild* biliary colic attacks, and are otherwise healthy, you may choose a trial of alternative medical therapy, and then wait and see what happens. To pursue this option safely, you must fully understand the risk of the trial and how to identify its failure, and you must be under medical supervision.

Gallbladder surgery has undergone a tremendous revolution in the past several years: More than 80 percent of cholecystectomies (gallbladder removal operations) are now performed with a laparoscope. If you have not had a complication from the gallstones, the chances are 95 percent that a laparoscopic procedure can be successfully completed.

After you have been given general anesthesia, a three-quarter-inch incision is made just above or below your navel, and carbon dioxide pumped into your abdomen. This gas inflates your abdomen like a balloon, lifting your abdominal wall away from your organs and creating a "working" space for your surgeons. A port—a hollow tube through which instruments can be passed—is then placed through this incision, and a tiny TV camera threaded through it. (See Figure 13.3.) A second three-quarter-inch incision is made in the upper midabdomen, two one-quarter-inch incisions in the right side of the abdomen, and ports for surgical instruments inserted in each. While the camera relays images of the action onto a TV screen, allowing your surgeon to "see" what he or she is doing, the gallbladder is manipulated and detached from its bed on the liver, and its duct attachment to the liver bile duct cut and tied off. The gallbladder is then pulled out through one of the incisions. After the ports are removed, the incisions are closed with dissolvable inside stitches, and the skin with skin tapes.

Make certain you choose a surgeon with lots of experience with laparoscopic surgery, since excessive injuries have been reported with novice or occasional users of this technique.

Until laparoscopy became common, "open" cholecystectomy had been the classic operation for gallstones. For this procedure, an incision four to six inches long is made crosswise under your ribs on your right side, or up and down in the center of your upper abdomen. The surgeon can then see the gallbladder and remove it. The incision is closed with sutures, staples, or skin tapes. In 2 to 5 percent of all cases, a laparoscopic cholecystectomy must to be converted to the open procedure, because of difficulty in seeing the gallbladder through the TV camera, abnormal or unclear anatomy in the surgical area, inability to complete the operation safely because of scar tissue or bleeding, or discovery of large stones in the bile duct.

Both the laparoscopic and open procedures remove your whole gallbladder. If only

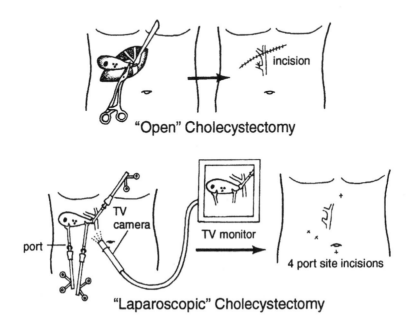

Fig. 13.3   Procedures involved in open and laparoscopic gallbladder surgery

its stones were taken out, you would soon form more, and your symptoms would return. During the operation, your surgeon may also perform an X-ray to look for stones that may have migrated out of the gallbladder into the liver bile duct system, and which could later cause a bile duct blockage or pancreatitis. If they are small, they can be flushed out during the operation or will usually pass spontaneously. If larger stones are discovered, they may be removable by laparoscopic techniques in 50 to 90 percent of all cases or the procedure may have to be converted to the open type and the stones removed by opening the bile duct. Alternatively, the stones may be removed at a later date by the nonsurgical endoscopic retrograde cholangiopancreatography (ERCP) procedure. A scope is passed through the mouth, then on through the stomach into the duodenum, where the distal end of the bile duct is visualized. The stones are then pulled out from below using special instruments introduced through a channel in the scope. This technique is successful in 90 to 95 percent of cases.

After your gallbladder is removed, a soft three-eighths-inch plastic drain is sometimes placed, extending from the area of your surgery through your skin. This prevents accumulation of bile and blood by sucking the fluids into a soft plastic bulb at the exterior end of the drain. The drain is usually removed within a day or two. If your bile duct must be opened to remove stones, a rubber tube called a "T-tube" is placed in the duct to relieve pressure by diverting bile. The T-tube is brought through your skin and connected to a bile-collecting bag, then removed in your surgeon's office about three weeks after surgery. Neither of these tubes is necessary for most simple gallbladder operations.

Bleeding, bile leak, damage to your bile duct system, and infection are possible complications of cholecystectomy. Complications of elective gallbladder surgery are rare: 3 to 5 percent overall. However, they increase with age, and are five times as high for emergency surgery. The overall complication and mortality rate of laparoscopic surgery is a little less than the open procedure, but risk of major bile duct damage is higher (about 1 in 200 to 500 cases).

You can do several things to avoid postoperative complications from this surgery. Breathing deeply and coughing to bring up secretions—even though this is uncomfortable—act to keep your lungs fully expanded and help prevent pneumonia. Getting out of bed and walking promotes circulation and prevents blood clots in your legs, as well as aiding in quicker restoration of your bowel function.

If you have an open procedure to remove your gallbladder, you may have discomfort requiring pain medication for several days. You can usually begin eating on the day following surgery, rapidly progress to a regular diet, and be discharged from the hospital in one to three days. In laparoscopic operations, patients are usually discharged a few hours following surgery, although you may choose to stay overnight. No increase in complications has been seen with early discharge. You will probably be more comfortable in your own home, and costs are less.[14] Postoperative pain is much less with the laparoscopic method, though pain pills may be necessary for a few days. Recovery time is typically a few days to a week, compared to two to four weeks following the open procedure.

After discharge, you should see your surgeon for one or more office visits, to make certain your incisions have healed well, and you have no complications.

What Happens After Your Gallbladder Is Removed?

If you were having symptoms attributed to gallbladder disease, you have an 85 percent chance for relief after it is removed. The more "classic" your symptoms of biliary colic or acute cholecystitis, the more likely a successful result. If your symptoms were vague, such as indigestion, nausea, gaseousness, or poorly localized discomfort, the outcome is less certain. You may have been suffering from another common problem often confused with gallbladder symptoms, such as esophageal reflux, irritable bowel, or gastritis.

Since your gallbladder served a function, you may well ask how your life will be affected after it is removed? The previously concentrated bile delivered to your intestine when your gallbladder contracted in response to food is replaced by a more continuous, less concentrated flow directly from your liver. Most people notice no difference in digestion, and do not develop any other symptoms. About 5 to 10 percent do notice a slight change in bowel frequency and consistency, and say their stools are greasier. No specific postoperative dietary restrictions are needed, other than following the suggestions in the alternative medicine section to prevent related illnesses.

GALLBLADDER DISEASE SUMMARY

Prevention

Diet and Supplements

- Follow a low-fat, high-fiber diet.

- Eat garlic and onion regularly in your diet.
- Lecithin, 1,200 mg, 3 times daily.
- Vitamin C, 500 mg 3 times daily.

Lifestyle

- Maintain optimum weight.
- Exercise regularly: 1 hour, 3–5 times weekly.
- Avoid birth control pills and hormone replacement therapy.
- Utilize daily yoga.
- Utilize stress management.

Alternative Medicine Approaches

- Follow the preventive guidelines, above.
- Check for food allergies, especially to eggs, pork, or onions.
- Choline, 500 mg, 3 times daily.
- Garlic oil, 500-mg capsules, 2 times daily.
- Magnesium, 250–500 mg, 3 times daily.
- Liver-gallbladder flush.
- Acupuncture, hypnosis, homeopathy, magnets.
- Visualization.

Conventional Medicine Approaches

- Drug treatment: ursodiol (Actigal).
- Shock wave lithotripsy.

Surgical Approach

- Cholecystectomy—laparoscopic, open.

CHAPTER 14

PANCREAS

Surgeons call the pancreas the "tiger of the abdomen," because operations on it are difficult and complication rates high. We know less about the pancreas than about other parts of the digestive tract. It is a sensitive, unpredictable organ that has stymied scientists who have attempted to conduct research on it.

You can take definite lifestyle and alternative medicine steps to help prevent your pancreas from developing a surgical disease, and to assist it back to health once it has become impaired.

How Your Pancreas Works

Your pancreas is a leaf-shaped organ that lies behind the stomach at the back of the abdomen, against the spinal column. (See Figure 14.1.) It has two major nutritional functions. Its *exocrine* cells secrete digestive enzymes, water, and bicarbonate, which neutralize stomach acid and help break down dietary fat and protein into tiny molecules, more readily absorbable through the digestive tract lining. Every day, the pancreas secretes more than two pints of this juice into your digestive tract.

A ductal system runs through your pancreas, collecting the enzymatic secretions from the exocrine cells. Tiny ductules empty into larger ducts, that finally pass into the main pancreatic duct, which empties into the upper part of your small intestine. The pancreas is divided into *head*, *neck*, *body*, and *tail* regions.

A normal pancreas has the capacity to produce a greater quantity of bicarbonate and enzymes than is necessary for digestion. Because of this ability, you may not develop symptoms until 85 to 90 percent of it has been destroyed. When disease has

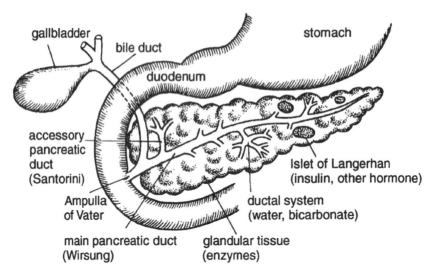

Fig. 14.1   The anatomy and location of the pancreas

progressed to the point that enzyme production is insufficient to break down the fat you eat, your stool becomes greasy, loose, and buoyant, and has an offensive odor.

The endocrine cells of your pancreas secrete insulin. This hormone allows your cells to take in sugar, which supplies the energy for their vital cell activities. Insulin is the most important blood sugar regulator. It is released when your blood sugar rises, causing a subsequent decrease in these levels; conversely, it is decreased when your blood sugar falls, thereby bringing the levels back up. Diabetes is usually caused by the malfunction of insulin production and regulation.

Diabetic symptoms, such as excessive thirst, frequent urination, and fatigue, develop whenever insulin output is deficient. Rare hormone-producing tumors may produce excessive insulin levels, causing a wide range of symptoms due to low blood sugar.

Pancreatic pain, caused by inflammation or a tumor, is felt in the upper abdomen, and may radiate to the back. It may be worse when lying down and better when leaning forward, and vary from mild discomfort to incapacitating pain. Symptoms such as nausea, vomiting, abdominal bloating, fever, and weight loss may occur with pancreatic disease, but they can also be symptomatic of disorders of other abdominal organs. Jaundice—yellowing of the skin—is a common sign of pancreatic cancer, and is produced when tumor obstructs bile flow at the point where the bile duct travels through the head of the pancreas.

Most signs and symptoms of pancreatic disease are nonspecific; that is, they can also be caused by many other problems. Therefore, your doctor should complete a careful analysis of your medical history, a physical examination, and do diagnostic tests before arriving at a diagnosis.

How Pancreatic Disease Is Diagnosed

There are many steps in diagnosing pancreatic disease, some as simple as a history and physical exam, and some involving tests that are quite complicated.

History

Your doctor should ask a series of questions about any symptoms you may have, as just described. Unexplained weight loss, back pain, and jaundice are frequently associated with pancreas disease. Important information includes your history of alcohol intake, medications, known gallstone disease, and any of the rarer medical causes of pancreas disease.

Physical Exam

Your doctor should examine your abdomen for an upper abdominal mass or tenderness as you lay flat on the exam table. However, since the pancreas is difficult to feel, as it lies deep behind your stomach, tucked underneath your ribs, the doctor is not likely to feel it unless it is significantly enlarged.

Blood Tests

The levels of the pancreatic enzymes amylase and lipase in your blood may be elevated in many types of pancreatic disease. Your response to treatment can be monitored as these levels change.

Sonogram and CAT Scan

These are the two most important noninvasive ways of visualizing your pancreas. A sonogram analyzes sound waves as they penetrate and reflect off the gland. A radiologist or sonogram technician passes the sound wave probe over the skin on your abdomen. Abnormalities produced by swelling, pockets of fluid, and tumors can be detected in this way. X-ray exposure and intravenous injections are not required. This is an inexpensive,

painless test that takes about fifteen minutes. However, ultrasound may have a hard time picturing the pancreas as much of it is obscured by overlying bowel gas.

The CAT scan is a computerized X-ray test which may be enhanced by an intravenous injection to outline your blood vessels, and by your swallowing a barium contrast liquid to image the intestinal tract. Pancreatic abnormalities as small as one-half to one inch in diameter can be seen. The CAT scan gives a much clearer picture of your pancreas and adjacent organs than a sonogram does. However, it does involve exposure to X-rays and is much more expensive.

Endoscopic Retrograde Cholangiopancreatography

Endoscopic Retrograde Cholangiopancreatography (ERCP) is a key test for diagnosing pancreatic and gallstone disease. It may also be therapeutic; procedures can be performed as part of an ERCP that may relieve your symptoms and enable you to avoid surgery. An ERCP is usually necessary if you are scheduled to undergo pancreatic surgery.

The procedure is performed by a gastroenterologist in a radiology or endoscopy suite. You are lightly sedated, though you must be able to cooperate by rolling from side to side as you lie on the examining table. Local anesthesia is used to numb your throat and eliminate your gag reflex. A flexible fiberoptic viewing scope is inserted through your mouth and then maneuvered through your upper digestive tract, to the area of the pancreatic duct, while your doctor watches on a TV monitor. A tiny plastic tube is passed into the duct, and dye is injected through it to make it show up on X-ray. Films are then taken to show the size and shape of your pancreatic and liver bile duct systems; these may reveal blockages, dilations, and/or cysts.

If stones are found, they can usually be removed by passing tiny balloons and wire baskets through the scope and manipulating the stones into the intestine, so they will pass on out of the body with the stool. If the bile duct is found to be narrowed where it opens into the intestine, it can be enlarged by cutting some of the muscle or scar tissue constricting it. This procedure is called a *sphincterotomy* or *papillotomy*. If a tumor is found during an ERCP, it can be biopsied and a stent (a small tube) inserted through it and left in place to prevent the tumor from obstructing the bile duct. These procedures may enable you to avoid surgery. Stones formed in the gallbladder that have moved into the bile duct are often removed by this method, before or after the laparoscopic surgical removal of the gallbladder.

ERCP is somewhat uncomfortable, and takes twenty to ninety minutes to complete. You should feel back to your baseline a few hours afterward, and may either go home or stay overnight, depending on what was found and if any cutting procedure was done. A 1 to 2 percent chance of bleeding or perforation of the bile duct follows when a sphincterotomy is done as part of the test. If a cut was made in your duct, you should avoid aspirin or blood-thinning medication for one week. Inducing acute pancreatitis is also a possibility.

Magnetic resonance cholangiopancreatography, a new noninvasive way to image the pancreas and the pancreatic and bile ducts, has some advantages and some disadvantages when compared with ERCP. In this procedure, you are placed in a large magnet and images are obtained for computer processing. No injections are necessary and you should experience no pain. It currently has limited availability, and no other therapeutic or diag-

nostic procedures such as a biopsy can be performed, as with ERCP. In the future, it may replace need for ERCP in many cases.

Percutaneous Transhepatic Cholangiography

Percutaneous Transhepatic Cholangiography (PTC) may be useful if you are jaundiced because of a complete blockage of the bile duct system. Most often PTC is performed to help determine whether the blockage is caused by stones within the duct or by a tumor. You lie on an X-ray examining table, and receive light intravenous sedation and local skin anesthesia. A thin needle is inserted through your skin, into the liver, and on into a bile duct. Dye is then injected, which enables the bile duct system to be outlined on X-ray films.

If you are found to have a blockage, pressure can be relieved by passing a small drainage catheter through the needle and into the bile duct. The catheter is left there, and a small soft plastic bag connected to the external end of it, to collect bile. In this way, jaundice can be relieved without surgery, and the severe itching that accompanies it alleviated. PTC is mildly uncomfortable, and takes thirty to sixty minutes to perform. Possible complications are bleeding, bile leak into the abdominal cavity, and infection.

Pancreas Needle Biopsy

This procedure procures a piece of your pancreas for examination under a microscope, without need for surgery. The test is done with local anesthesia and mild sedation as you lie on an X-ray table. A thin needle is passed through your abdominal wall and on into your pancreas, using a sonogram probe or a CAT scan as a guide. Pancreas cells, or a solid piece of tissue, are then removed. Surprisingly, it produces little discomfort, and complications are rare.

Endoscopic Ultrasound

A close look at the pancreas can be obtained by passing a scope into the stomach and duodenum. An ultrasound catheter is then passed through the scope to create images of the pancreas and surrounding structures. Guided biopsies of abnormalities can be accomplished. This is a very good way to determine the extent of a pancreas tumor and whether it is able to be removed safely by surgery.

Acute Pancreatitis

Acute pancreatitis occurs when pancreatic enzymes are released and activated within the gland itself, leading to inflammation. The swelling that accompanies this condition can be mild and limited, or devastatingly destructive. Extensive areas of the pancreas may dissolve, and life-threatening bleeding can occur. Fluid cysts and infected abscesses may form in the injured areas. While this process is centered in the pancreas, its effects may be widespread, because of fluid loss, circulating enzymes, and substances accompanying tissue breakdown that are toxic to the heart, lungs, and kidneys.

Acute pancreatitis has many different causes, though in the United States, it is usually precipitated by gallbladder stones or alcohol consumption. A gallstone may pass out of the gallbladder and migrate to a point where it blocks the pancreatic duct. Pancreatic enzymes then become activated within the pancreas, and acute pancreatitis results. The way in which alcohol creates this condition is not

fully understood. Experimental evidence from humans is lacking, though it is believed alcohol may reach the pancreas through the bloodstream and thus irritate it. In up to 25 percent of all cases, no antecedent factor can be found, though injury to the abdomen, a viral infection, or drugs other than alcohol may all contribute to its development.

Your symptoms from acute pancreatitis may vary from a dull ache to disabling pain in the upper abdomen. The pain may also be felt in your back. Since bowel function is slowed by the irritation, nausea, vomiting, and abdominal bloating are quite common. You may develop temporary diabetes.

Alternative Medicine Approaches to Acute Pancreatitis

Jules, a 52-year-old actor and heavy cigarette smoker, had gained weight over the past twenty years. He decided to embark on a quick-weight-loss scheme that included only a small amount of fruit, vegetables, occasional fish, and no grains. He continued to drink and smoke heavily. Jules was losing weight nicely, but one night he suddenly awoke with severe abdominal pain and nausea. A visit to the emergency room at his local hospital revealed an attack of acute pancreatitis as the cause. Most likely, it had been brought on by his "crash" diet, combined with his alcohol and cigarette use. He was able to avoid surgery, and used the time in the hospital to quit smoking and drinking, and began a program of taking digestive enzymes and the mineral chromium, along with regular, balanced meals. He not only recovered fully from his pancreatitis, but was then able to maintain his proper weight, stay off cigarettes and alcohol, and enjoy a much healthier sense of well-

being. His acting was also much more satisfying than before his illness.

———————

Ninety-five percent of all cases of acute pancreatitis heal without surgical treatment, because swelling of the gland does not result in significant tissue destruction or bleeding. After the inflammation subsides, your gland returns to normal.

During an attack of acute pancreatitis, you must be hospitalized, since you must not eat, to avoid further stimulation of the pancreas until all your symptoms have cleared up, and fluids must therefore be given intravenously. Usually, you stay a week or so in the hospital.

During this time, and to prevent acute pancreatitis from developing or returning, you need to attend to the elements of a healthy lifestyle. Following are the most important for acute pancreatitis.

Avoid Alcohol

Pancreatitis can often be traced to alcohol use. See Chapter 2 for alternative medicine approaches to achieving and maintaining stress management to help you successfully quit, through such measures as a good diet, acupuncture, massage, and yoga. Support through a group such as AA is essential.

Change Your Diet

Since stones from your gallbladder can precipitate this problem, follow the guidelines given in the previous chapter, on the prevention of gallbladder disease, along with the high-fiber, low-fat dietary recommendations given in Chapter 2, to help you avoid forming any gallstones, or eliminating any that already exist.

Take Digestive Enzymes and Other Supplements

To assist you while your pancreas is not working properly, digestive enzymes and the mineral chromium help you digest your food and keep your blood sugar levels steady. Take two to six multienzyme tablets, such as Ultrazyme as discussed in Chapter 2, per meal and 200 mcg of chromium one or two times a day. Follow as well the other supplement guidelines given in Chapter 2, to support your immune system.

Practice Stress Management, Visualization, and Imagery

Follow the principles given in Chapter 2 for stress reduction, visualization, and imagery. You may wish to use a specific imagery practice, such as the following: Imagine your pancreas as a beautiful beach, with some areas of stranded garbage washed ashore. Get some large bags, collect all of the debris, and take it to the local recycling center, located in your liver. Now, in your mind's eye, see your pancreas as well and healthy, at the same time as you feel this happening within your body.

Surgical Approaches to Acute Pancreatitis

Surgery is rarely considered *during* an episode of acute pancreatitis. It is only recommended if you develop extensive destruction of the gland or a pancreas infection, or if your condition is getting worse despite intensive medical treatment. If surgery becomes necessary, the most important goal of your surgeon is to remove dead tissue and establish drainage, so the toxic products can be removed from the abdomen. Much more commonly, if the acute pancreatitis was caused by gallstones, surgery is strongly recommended *after* the acute episode subsides. The gallbladder and its stones should be removed, usually through the laparoscope, as soon as possible to prevent further attacks, ideally during the same hospitalization, as described in the preceding chapter.

If you have complications from acute pancreatitis, you may require surgery after the acute episode subsides. Inflammation may cause blockage of your pancreas ducts, and continued secretion behind the blockage may lead to *pseudocyst* formation. These cysts occur in 5 to 20 percent of patients with acute pancreatitis. Smaller cysts often disappear spontaneously, but they can grow, producing pain, bowel obstruction, and life-threatening complications by hemorrhaging or rupturing into the abdominal cavity. A *pancreatic abscess* can form in destroyed pancreatic tissue or in a pseudocyst that has become infected, as happens in about 5 percent of all cases. This complication accounts for two-thirds of all deaths from acute pancreatitis.

A pseudocyst may be successfully treated by sonographic- or CAT scan–guided drainage catheters, passed through the abdominal wall, using local anesthesia. However, these catheters often become plugged, and the pseudocyst then recurs.

If one of these complications requires surgery, it must be performed under general anesthesia. Most likely, you will already be in the hospital being treated for the acute pancreatitis. A breathing tube is placed in your trachea (windpipe). Intravenous lines in your neck and arms permit the administration of fluids and medications and monitor heart function, and a small catheter (tube) in an artery at your wrist is placed to monitor your blood pressure and blood gasses. A small drainage tube is placed through your nose into your stomach and another into your bladder. Your surgeon then makes a crosswise incision under your ribs, or one up and down the midline, from your breastbone to your navel.

Your surgeon examines your pancreas to determine which type of operation is best. One of three surgical options can be chosen for treating an uninfected pseudocyst, depending on its size, location, and thickness of the cyst wall. Rarely, the whole cyst may be removed. It can also be drained *internally* by making an opening in it, along with a similar aperture in the stomach or intestine, then sewing them together so that the cyst contents drain directly into the gastrointestinal tract. Or if the cyst wall is too thin to hold these stitches, it can be drained *externally*, using soft rubber drain tubes to carry the fluid outside the body.

If your surgeon is operating to remove extensive amounts of dead pancreas or finds an abscess, as much dead and infected tissue as is safely possible is removed, then multiple drain tubes are placed through the abdominal wall to draw away any further infected material and secretions. The abdominal wall is then closed with stitches. If an infection was found, the skin incision must be left open to prevent an incision infection. It will heal in a week or two, and necessitates dressing changes.

You wake in the recovery room and will likely spend a few days in an intensive care unit. The breathing tube may be left in place for a day or two. Stomach and bladder tubes are also necessary for a few days. Soft plastic drains placed through the abdominal wall are usually removed after several days, but may be necessary for much longer, depending on the amount of drainage and whether it contains infection or pancreatic secretions. If your incision has been left open, you will need two or three dressing changes a day.

Once your gastrointestinal function returns, you can resume eating. Until then, your nutritional needs are met by intravenous solutions, or an intestinal feeding tube. Hospital stays for pancreatic surgery usually last ten to fourteen days, and perhaps much longer if a pancreatic infection is present. After discharge, you need to see your surgeon for several postoperative visits, until all tubes are removed, and you and your surgeon are satisfied with the results. Full recovery takes two to three months.

Chronic Pancreatitis

In the United States, most cases of chronic pancreatitis are caused by alcoholism. Unlike acute pancreatitis, which is often precipitated by an alcoholic binge, chronic pancreatitis does not develop until after at least five to ten years of daily drinking. Alcohol causes blockages within the pancreatic ducts, chronic inflammation, and formation of excessive amounts of fibrous tissue that interfere with the gland's functioning.

Upper abdominal pain is the most common symptom of chronic pancreatitis. The pain is usually made worse by eating, because of resulting pancreatic stimulation. When you can't eat, weight loss and nutritional deficiency follow. Addiction to pain medications is very common. Destruction of the gland and fibrosis cause deficient digestive enzyme output, leading to malabsorption of fat and proteins. Symptoms include indigestion and soft, greasy, smelly stools. Deficient insulin output causes diabetes.

Alternative Medicine Approaches to Chronic Pancreatitis

Mark, *a 57-year-old creative writer and English professor, enjoyed lecturing to his eager young college students, and was frequently nominated for teaching awards, though secretly he longed for time to focus on his own writing. He comforted himself through his difficulties by consuming at least one or two bottles of wine every night. After some years, he noticed bloating in his abdomen, accompanied by occasional pain. Tests revealed a chronically inflamed pancreas, and his doctor advised him he would need an operation if he didn't quit drinking alcohol.*

At first, he found stopping impossible, but finally, he joined Alcoholics Anonymous. He discovered it a much more satisfying and friendly community than he had thought possible. He then quit his teaching job, to live on his pension and travel. Mark reveled in adequate time to write and sell his books, as well as to write for and about the many inspiring people he met in recovery.

You can act to help prevent and treat chronic pancreatitis and avoid its recurrence by the application of alternate medicine measures. Following are the most important alternative steps you can take.

Follow the Advice Given for Acute Pancreatitis

Alternative medicine therapy should address the underlying disease whenever possible; if you have been drinking alcohol, stopping is the most important first step. A high-fiber, complex-carbohydrate diet low in fat and free of refined sugars, is also important. In addition, the supplement program outlined in Chapter 2, especially the multi-digestive enzymes discussed there, such as Ultrazyme, two to six tablets at each meal, may help relieve your symptoms.

Vitamin E has been shown to be of benefit, reducing the pain associated with chronic pancreatitis.[1] Start with 400 IU, three times daily.

Meditation, yoga, acupuncture, and the other alternative medicine therapies noted for their ability to relieve pain, as discussed in Chapter 2, may also be helpful.

Practice Visualization

Imagine your pancreas as a mound of clay on a potter's wheel. It has become filled with burrows and pebbles. You are a sculptor, and can easily smooth out and remove any areas of congestion. Once you have restored the clay to perfection, you make it into a beautiful bowl, and enjoy a delicious meal of your favorite foods—in just the right amounts. Hold this image in your mind, and at the same time feel it happening within your body.

Surgical Approaches to Chronic Pancreatitis

Jordan, a 55-year-old army sergeant, had a long history of drinking, which destroyed his first marriage and alienated his family. He developed constant abdominal pain, which led to further drinking, as well as narcotics addiction. Eating made his symptoms worse, so he avoided food, and his weight dropped from 170 to 120 pounds. His life was saved when he met Doris; Jordan said she gave him "a reason for living." She brought him to a doctor. Studies of his pancreas showed an obstructed, dilated pancreatic duct. Surgery drained the duct, relieving the pressure. His pain disappeared, and he was able to eat and regain his lost weight. He conquered his addictions, and stopped smoking as well. After a bypass procedure to relieve a blockage in his right leg caused by years of tobacco abuse, he can now accompany Doris on long hikes in the Cascade Mountains.

Medical treatment of chronic pancreatitis is not as effective as that of acute pancreatitis, because of the permanent changes in the gland caused by the chronic fibrosis. In persons whose disease is caused by alcohol abuse, continuing to drink will make matters worse. However, stopping drinking improves symptoms in just 30 percent of patients. Surgical treatment is recommended only if you have severe pain. Surgery can provide relief, but it will not restore pancreatic function once permanently destructive changes have developed.

Two types of surgical procedures can be used. The one your surgeon recommends depends on the anatomical changes in your duct. If a dilated (swollen) main duct can be effectively drained, pressure can be relieved. On the other hand, if the ductal system is not dilated, then most or all of the diseased gland must be removed in order to provide pain relief. Ultrasound tests, a CAT scan, and ERCP may be performed before surgery, to determine the site and nature of ductal dilation, whether there are pseudocysts, as well as give your surgeon a "road map" for dealing with this difficult organ.

Surgery for chronic pancreatitis is done using general anesthesia. Preoperative preparation and the incision are the same as for acute pancreatitis.

A drainage procedure is the preferred surgical approach whenever possible, since no pancreatic tissue is removed with this method. The most common method of drainage is accomplished by making an incision in the enlarged pancreatic duct, as well as in a piece of small intestine, then sewing the openings together so that pancreatic secretions can freely drain into your intestine, reducing pressure within the pancreas. If your main pancreatic duct is not enlarged, or if disabling pain persists after a drainage procedure, part or all of your pancreas must be removed. Soft plastic drain tubes are placed through the abdominal wall and connected to collection bulbs. Finally, the abdominal wall is then closed with stitches.

Recovery is similar to that for surgery of acute pancreatitis except that it should be much quicker and smoother, since pancreatic infection is rarely encountered in chronic pancreatitis. Hospital stays for this pancreatic surgery usually last five to ten days.

The drainage operation is fairly safe, and pain is relieved or significantly decreased in 70 to 80 percent of all patients. The mortality and complication rate when part or all of your pancreas must be removed is higher than that for a drainage procedure: the initial surgery itself is more hazardous, and the problems related to the loss of pancreatic function more difficult to control. Relief of pain is successful in 70 to 90 percent of all cases.

Patients who continue to drink alcohol often have trouble with medications, and many die as a result of diabetic complications. Attempting to save a part of the pancreas may help avoid these problems, but also may be less effective in relieving pain. The mortality rate from the drainage operation is 3 percent, versus 5 to 10 percent when part or all of the pancreas is removed.[2]

Pancreatic Cancer

Pancreatic duct cancer is the fifth most common cause of cancer death in the United States. In 2002 an estimated 30,300 new cases and 29,700 deaths will be recorded.[3] Overall, the incidence and mortality rates have slightly decreased over the last two decades, although there has been a small increase among African-American women. The lifetime risk is slightly higher in women, primarily because of a longer life expectancy. This cancer is uncommon before the age of 45, though quite frequent after age 65.

Diet has also been implicated as an important factor in pancreatic cancer. Evidence from epidemiological studies implicates animal fat as a primary contributor.[4] In Japan, a marked increase in dietary fat intake has taken place since 1950. During this period, a fourfold increase in pancreatic cancer has been documented. Eggs and full-fat milk also show associations. Excess protein, as found in meat-based diets, has also been implicated.[5] In addition, intake of sugar has shown a correlation.[6] White bread consumption increases risk, while higher intake of raw fruits and vegetables lowers it.[7] Some researchers speculate that the vitamin C in fruits may be responsible for their protective effects.[8] Mormons and Seventh-Day Adventists, who avoid cigarettes, meat, coffee, and alcohol, have very low rates of pancreatic cancer.

This cancer has been found to be six times more common in persons whose blood levels are low in lycopene, an antioxidant chemical found in foods that gives the red color to fresh red fruits and vegetables.[9] Diets low in the antioxidant vitamin A group also put persons at higher risk. Although this connection remains controversial, coffee drinking, both regular and decaffeinated, has been implicated as a contributing cause; some studies have shown an even higher incidence in decaf users.[10]

Pancreatic cancer is more than twice as common in tobacco smokers, indicating that a pancreatic carcinogen is probably present in smoke. Persons frequently exposed to petroleum products and fumes are at higher risk.

This cancer has also been associated with alcohol intake—beer with both sexes and wine with women—especially more than six beers per day.[11] Cirrhosis of the liver is a known risk. Chronic pancreatitis increases the risk. Environmental exposure to radiation, chemicals, or petroleum products has also been documented.[12] Previous surgery on your stomach,[13] or if you already have diabetes, also increases your risk.

Unfortunately, most pancreatic cancers do not produce symptoms until the tumor has advanced to the point where a surgical cure is impossible. Occasionally, early tumors located in the head of the gland compress the bile duct, causing obvious jaundice at a potentially surgically curable stage. Tumors in the body or tail of the pancreas are almost always incurable because no early symptoms are present. Almost all cancers that cause pain are beyond cure, since they have already invaded neighboring vital organs. (See Table 14.1.)

The pain of pancreatic cancer is usually felt in the upper abdomen, and may radiate to the back. Jaundice is the first symptom in 10 to 30 percent of cases, and develops at some time during the disease in 90 percent, because the tumor eventually compresses the bile duct. By the time of their diagnosis, 70 to 90 percent of all patients have experienced weight loss.

No good screening procedures are available for pancreatic cancer. A diagnosis of pancreatic cancer is considered if you have upper abdominal pain, weight loss, or a mass that can be felt in the upper abdomen. Sonogram and CAT scan are the most accurate first tests. ERCP or PTC may be necessary to pinpoint the cause and location of a bile duct obstruction. Endoscopic ultrasound with biopsy may provide diagnostic tissue and help determine whether a cancer can be safely removed.

TABLE 14.1.
Prognosis of Pancreatic Cancer[14]

	Percent of Patients Surviving 5 Years	Percent of Patients in This Stage
All Patients	4.3% (20.0% 1-year)	
Not Staged	3.2%	19%
By Stage		
Localized to pancreas	16.2%	8%
Lymph node spread	7.3%	23%
Distant spread	1.5%	51%

If you are thought likely to have pancreatic cancer, and surgery is not being considered because it would not be curative or you are in poor health, a needle biopsy can obtain a bit of tissue for microscopic exam. However, a cancer-negative report from such tissue analysis can be misleading, since the needle may have missed the tumor tissue. A diagnosis can usually be made without surgery. However, in many cases when pancreatic cancer is very likely, you may have exploratory surgery and removal of the pancreatic mass without a firmly established diagnosis before the operation.

Alternative Medicine Approaches to Pancreatic Cancer

Miles, a stockbroker on Wall Street, was living a stress-filled life, and had a thirty-four-year history of chain smoking. He began to notice distention in his abdomen, and, thinking it simply indigestion, started popping Tums. However, his problems did not go away, and an exploratory operation showed inoperable pancreatic cancer. He changed his job, commenced a macrobiotic vegetarian diet, stopped smoking, drank carrot juice, took supplements, and began daily meditation, breathing exercises, and yoga postures. Despite the dire expectations associated with his diagnosis, he was alive and well five years later, with no sign of continuing cancer.[15]

Alternative medicine approaches may be helpful in both the prevention and treatment of pancreatic cancer and the avoidance of its recurrence. Changes in lifestyle may affect the growth rate of a tumor once it has developed; further research is needed.

Following are the most promising alternative measures for the prevention and treatment of pancreatic cancer.

Quit Smoking

One-third to one-half of all pancreatic cancers are caused by smoking,[16] and could be prevented if we as a nation simply stopped smoking. After you have quit, your risk for developing this cancer gradually goes back to normal. If you smoke, try the alternative medicine approaches given in Chapter 2 to help you quit for good.

Avoid Red Meats, Eggs, and Other High-Fat Foods

As noted above, strong evidence suggests that the carcinogenic elements of meats contribute to this disease, as well as their high fat content. Ingestion of eggs and dairy products (other than nonfat) also have shown a correlation with this disease. Follow the high-fiber, low-fat diet given in Chapter 2. A low-fat vegetarian diet, as described in Chapter 2, is felt by some researchers to prolong life.[17]

Eat Plenty of Fresh Red Fruits and Vegetables

As noted, the high content of the antioxidant lycopene may make these foods especially protective against this cancer.[18] Add five servings of tomato-based sauces per week.

Avoid Coffee and Other Caffeine-Containing Beverages

The suggested association of coffee to pancreatic cancer risk has not been established, but indicates our habits may be worth changing. You can use the herb tea substitutes suggested in Chapter 2.

Take Supplements

The general supplement program also outlined in Chapter 2 may be helpful.

Vitamin A has demonstrated an antitumor potential in preliminary studies. Dr. Hans Nieper of Hannover, Germany, has reported anecdotal success in treating this disease using a combination of vitamins, carrot juice, vegetarian diet, and various immune stimulators.[19] For further discussion of alternative medicine therapy for prevention and treatment of cancer, see *Choices in Healing*, by Dr. Michael Lerner, and *Beating Cancer with Nutrition* by Patrick Quillin, and *Dr. Gaynor's Cancer Prevention Program*, as listed in the Resources section at the back of this book.

Utilize Other Alternative Adjuncts, and Seek Updates

Acupuncture, deep relaxation, breathing exercises, yoga postures, and the other adjuncts given in Chapter 2 may be utilized to relax your body and decrease your need for pain medication.

Dr. Bernard Bihari, a researcher in New York City, has found some initial success in treating pancreatic cancer using 3 mg per day of Naltrexone in a special time-release formula. However, further research is needed.

The Gonzales program is also being evaluated for its case-reported benefits. The Gonzales program is a combination of dietary change and supplements pioneered by Dr. Nicholas Gonzales. For more information on the program, contact Dr. Gonzales in New York City at 212-213-3337.

Practice Visualization

Imagine your pancreas as a beautiful garden. In it, some large but fragile weeds have been growing. You are very fit and strong, and having a great time weeding out these interlopers. Now your garden looks beautiful, the weeds are sitting in the compost pile, and with your feet propped up, you are enjoying some nice iced herb tea, while surveying your radiantly healthy pancreas-garden. Picture this, as you feel it happening within your body.

Conventional Medicine Approaches to Pancreatic Cancer

Most patients with pancreatic cancer are not candidates for curative surgery. The following treatments may be useful if surgery is not a good option.

Internal Stent Bypass

Recently, a strong trend has developed to use a nonsurgical *internal stent* to treat bile duct obstruction. This is a rigid tube passed through the cancer that keeps the bile channel open as the tumor grows. (See Figure 14.2.) A gastroenterologist can place the tube with the help of a flexible scope passed through your mouth, similar to ERCP, described above. At times, a radiologist may pass the stent during the PTC procedure. Although potential complications can follow from the insertion of a stent, this is probably preferable to a bypass operation to relieve your symptoms, especially if your life expectancy is short, since the procedure mortality and complication rate as well as hospitalization time are much less than those for the operative route.

Chemotherapy and Radiotherapy

Chemotherapy and radiation treatments alone cannot cure cancer of the pancreas, but they may be helpful in relieving symptoms

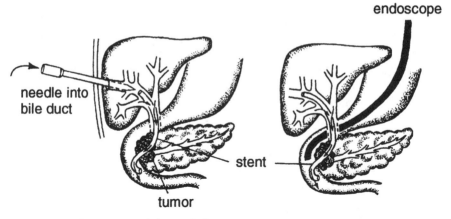

Fig. 14.2   Procedures involved in internal stent bypass for pancreatic cancer

and prolonging survival by a few months. These options may be recommended as the only treatment if you have advanced disease or after surgery if it is obvious you have not been cured.

Recently, the addition of chemotherapy and radiotherapy to potentially curative surgery has been shown to be of significant value in increasing life expectancy and cure rates. If this is the case for you, you should strongly consider this approach.

Surgical Approaches to Pancreatic Cancer

Of all patients with pancreatic cancer, only 10 to 20 percent are candidates for having it removed surgically. However, if you qualify, you have only a 30 to 45 percent chance that a "curative" operation can be attempted once your abdomen is opened and explored. If pre-operative tests do not indicate the tumor has spread widely, and that it can be removed safely, you should choose surgery, since it provides your only chance for cure. However, even if an operation is possible, you have only

about a 10 percent chance to live five years; a 20 percent chance if no spread is found because microscopic nests of tumor cells may be left behind; but only a 5 percent chance if pancreatic lymph nodes are involved. However, if your tumor is smaller than 2 centimeters without nodes involved, your chance for survival increases to 35 percent.[20]

These dismal statistics have sparked controversy about whether surgical cure should even be attempted, since you may be more likely to die from a complication of the surgery than to be cured of your disease by the operation. It is generally agreed you should not undergo surgery if your tumor has spread to the liver or lymph nodes beyond the pancreas; it has invaded neighboring vital organs; or you are not in good health. The arguments in favor of a curative attempt, if you have a localized tumor, are surgery gives the only chance for cure, and even if a cure is not achieved, you will survive longer, with fewer symptoms. Another argument is that the more favorable tumors located in the bile ducts and duodenum in neighboring areas are often impossible to distinguish from those in the head of the pancreas.

You might be deprived of a chance for cure if your surgeon has a bias against curative surgery. I favor an attempt at curing pancreatic cancer through an operation whenever possible.

Surgery to remove a pancreatic cancer is the most difficult and complicated procedure of all abdominal surgery. Several studies have shown that results are much better with surgeons and hospitals with a lot of experience with this disease. In 1996, the U.S. National Commission on Cancer found a surgical mortality rate of 19 percent in hospitals with less than ten cases per year, compared with 3 percent where more than ten were performed. Likewise, a study of all procedures done to remove pancreas cancer in the state of Maryland from 1990 to 1995 showed a nineteen times increased risk of dying at a low-volume hospital as compared to a high-volume hospital.[21]

It is very important for you and your family to sit down with your surgeon and frankly discuss this difficult disease and his or her experience with it. Each treatment has its merits and drawbacks. If you choose surgery, you should have a voice in how aggressive you want your surgeon to be, since he or she may not be able to really see the extent of the disease or gauge the danger of surgery until after the operation has begun. Gambling for a cure may also carry a higher chance of complications. It is important that your surgeon has an understanding of your wishes prior to surgery.

After you are under general anesthesia, a breathing tube is placed in your windpipe to control your breathing. Intravenous lines in your neck and arms permit the administration of medications and monitor heart function, and an arterial line in your wrist measures your blood pressure and blood gasses. Drainage tubes are placed in your stomach and bladder.

You may first undergo a laparoscopic exam through small incisions to determine if there is evidence for cancer spread to your liver, lining surfaces of the inside of your abdomen, or distant lymph nodes that would make it unwise to proceed with the operation. Laparoscopy has been found to reveal unsuspected metastases in 31 percent of patients examined prior to planned pancreatectomy.[22]

Your surgeon then makes a crosswise incision under your ribs, or one up and down the midline, from your breastbone to your navel. Next, several exploratory tests are done to determine if you indeed have a chance for cure, and whether the operation can be performed safely. These procedures check for tumor spread and invasion into neighboring vital organs. The two main types of curative operations remove either part or all of the pancreas.

Total Pancreatectomy and the Whipple Procedure

The pancreas may be totally removed or, more commonly, part of the body and the tail may be saved (a *Whipple procedure*). (See Figure 14.3.) The disadvantage of removing all of the pancreas is that after surgery you will have diabetes and must rely on insulin injections and digestive enzyme tablets. The Whipple procedure maintains enough pancreatic function to avoid these problems. No higher cure rate has been obtained when all of the gland is removed, but the rate of surgical complications may be slightly lower. As Figure 14.3 indicates, several suture lines are necessary to reconnect the biliary tract, stomach, intestine, and whatever portion of the pancreas is left. The operation requires four to eight hours to complete.

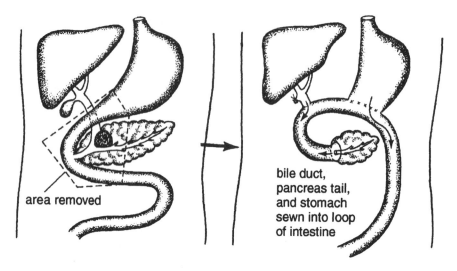

area removed

bile duct,
pancreas tail,
and stomach
sewn into loop
of intestine

Fig. 14.3 Whipple procedure for pancreatic cancer

You wake in the recovery room and likely spend a few days in an intensive care unit. The breathing tube may be left in place for a day or two. Stomach and bladder tubes are also necessary for a few days. Soft plastic abdominal drainage tubes are usually removed after several days. Tiny plastic tubes may have been placed through the abdominal wall into the bile and pancreas ducts. These drain bile and pancreatic juice, promoting healing by preventing pressure buildup in the ducts and stabilizing the line of stitches connecting the ducts to the small intestine. The tubes are attached to soft plastic collection bulbs and usually stay in place for several weeks, but you can easily take care of them at home.

You can resume eating after four to seven days, once your gastrointestinal function returns and healing seems satisfactory. Until then, your nutritional needs are met by intravenous solutions, or an intestinal feeding tube. Hospital stays for pancreatic surgery usually last ten to fourteen days. You need to make several postoperative visits to your sur-

geon's office, until all tubes are removed and you and your surgeon are satisfied with the results. Full recovery takes six to eight weeks.

The mortality rate from the Whipple procedure is 2 to 5 percent in the best studies at high-volume hospitals. Complications arise in 25 to 35 percent of all cases, such as leakage from the pancreatic or bile duct suture lines, problems with stomach emptying, and incision infection. Most complications are not life-threatening.

You have a 65 to 80 percent chance your tumor will be known to be incurable when first found. In this case, if you are otherwise healthy, you may choose to have palliative surgery. If the tumor can be safely removed, you may live longer and more comfortably, but you risk that operative complications might make you worse.

Bile Duct and Stomach Bypass

Alternatively, a pancreas with a tumor can be left in place, and a bypass procedure performed to relieve bile duct obstruction and the severe itching and pain that accompany the resulting liver distention. In this operation, the bile duct above the blocked area is sewn to the intestine. If it appears the tumor might soon block the stomach outlet, a stomach-to-small-intestine bypass can be done at the same time. Recovery from a bypass procedure is much quicker and simpler than after a Whipple operation, but the operative mortality and complication rates are similar.

PANCREATIC CANCER SUMMARY

Prevention

Diet and Supplements

- Follow a low-fat, high-fiber diet.
- Eat lots of fresh fruits and vegetables.
- Avoid coffee.
- Vitamin A, 10,000 IU daily.
- Vitamin C, 1,000–2,000 mg, 2–3 times daily.
- Vitamin E, D-alpha, 400 IU daily.

Lifestyle

- Don't smoke.

Alternative Medicine Approaches

- Follow the preventive guidelines, above.
- Use hypnosis, acupuncture, aromatherapy, and the other immune system adjuncts given in Chapter 2.
- Practice visualization.

Conventional Medicine Approaches

- Bile duct stent.
- Chemotherapy.
- Radiotherapy.

Surgical Approaches

- Whipple procedure—partial pancreas removal.
- Total pancreas removal.
- Bile duct and stomach bypass.

COLON

> *. . . cancer of the bowel is very prevalent in meat-eating areas like North America and Western Europe, while it is extremely rare in vegetarian countries such as India. In the United States, for example, bowel cancer is the second most common form of cancer (second only to lung cancer), and the people of Scotland, who eat 20 percent more beef than the English, have one of the world's highest rates of cancer of the bowel.[1]*
>
> Vistara Parham

In our Western culture, heart and gallbladder operations are freely discussed, and may even be considered somewhat "status" surgeries. However, surgical procedures performed below the belly button have been another matter, rarely mentionable at all, until recent efforts have been made to bring the colon into national consciousness.

We in the United States enforce rather rigid toilet training, and from that time onward the smells and waste products of our colons are associated with aversion, secrecy, and embarrassment. Because of the dread of a rectal exam, many people avoid even this simple, lifesaving screening. President Reagan's surgery for a cancerous colon polyp, performed while he was in office, and the colon cancer of news anchor Katie Couric's husband and of baseball player Darryl Strawberry have made it more obvious how frequently disorders can develop in this portion of the body.

When working normally, your large intestine, rectum, and anus are actually wonderful organs. In some other societies, they are openly and freely discussed, and competitions to see who can pass the most gas are a source of widespread revelry, rather than our furtive and embarrassed jokes; in the nineteenth century, one enterprising

French entertainer even made a career out of playing this "instrument."

The colon can be prone to a variety of physically and psychologically caused disturbances, and surgery to treat these diseases is very common. However, you *can* take active steps to *prevent* these diseases, as we will discuss in this chapter.

Colon inflammations, infections, partial obstructions, bleeding, and pain often respond quite well to nonsurgical treatment. In many cases, a trial of alternative medicine therapies, such as changes in your diet, exercise, and stress management habits, may be all that is needed to help you avoid the scalpel.

How Your Colon Works

Your *colon*, also called the "large bowel" or "large intestine," is the fourth major organ in the digestive tract highway. Food (or more accurately, its undigested remains) enters your colon after passing through your esophagus, stomach, and small intestine, the "small bowel."

The colon is usually four to five feet long. With chronic constipation, it may markedly elongate, becoming twisted and tortuous; colitis causes it to become thickened and shortened. The junction of your small and large bowels lies in your right lower abdomen, where the muscular *ileocecal valve* prevents bacteria and the other contents of the large bowel from traveling backward into your small bowel. (See Figure 15.1.)

The *cecum*, two to four inches both in diameter and in length, is the first and widest part of the colon. The notorious *appendix* is attached to the lower end of the cecum. The *ascending colon* passes up to the *hepatic flexure*, a 90-degree turn to your left; the *trans-*

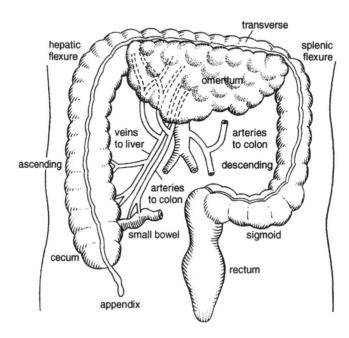

Fig. 15.1 The anatomy of the colon

verse colon follows, across to the *splenic flexure*, a 90-degree turn downward. The *descending colon* is next, leading into the *sigmoid colon*, an S-shaped floppy segment that joins your rectum. The sigmoid, the narrowest part of the colon (one to two inches wide), has the highest likelihood of becoming obstructed by twisting, inflammation, or tumor.

The wall of your colon consists of three layers: the lining, or *mucosa*, made of cells that absorb or secrete various substances; the *muscle layer*, which has an inside portion of fibers arranged in a circular fashion and an external portion with longitudinal fibers; and the *serosa*, your colon's smooth outer covering. A layer of fat called the *omentum* attaches to your transverse colon. Referred to by surgeons as the "watchdog of the belly," it hangs down into your lower abdomen, and helps to "wall off" or isolate any diseased area by adhering to it. The *mesentery*, a sheet of tissue which contains the colon's blood vessels, lymphatic channels, and nerves, attaches your bowel to the back of your abdominal cavity.

Your colon does not have nerves that normally provide sensations. Thus it will not give you symptoms unless it is swollen, stretched with gas, blocked, or inflamed, whereupon you may feel a dull ache or cramp in the central or lower part of your abdomen. If an inflamed area touches the sensitive inside lining of your abdominal cavity, you feel pain at that point.

Three basic functions—*absorption, excretion,* and *stool storage*—are the contribution of the colon. Most absorption of water and nutrients is accomplished in your cecum and ascending colon, so that by the time your stool reaches the transverse and descending portions, it is semisolid or solid.

Your small bowel squirts one and one-half to two quarts of liquid (unabsorbed food residue) into your colon each day! About 90 percent of this total is then absorbed back into your body as the liquid passes through, so that your daily stool usually measures only one-fifth to one-half of a pint. The *portal vein system* carries substances absorbed from your digestive tract to your liver, which continues the processing of carbohydrates and proteins so they can be utilized by the body. *Lymph channels* accompany these veins; as a result, tumors tend to spread to the liver by this route.

Your body excretes waste products through your stool. Stool contains various bile acids and blood breakdown products, unabsorbed dietary ingredients, and bacteria normally found in the large intestine. *More than 90 percent of your stool volume is bacteria.* The storage function of your colon allows you to go about daily activities with little concern for the timing of bowel movements.

We all pass an average of one-half to one pint of gas per day. Intestinal gas, medically called "flatus," is about 90 percent swallowed air, which we take in with eating, drinking, talking, and just swallowing—most of the time without realizing it. Some "gassy" foods, such as the infamous beans and cabbage, do increase flatus output, because your colonic bacteria act upon them to produce extra gases.

Your colon has its own muscular activity, different from that of the progressive, orderly pattern of your small bowel. The colon contracts in segments, with individual parts squeezing in an uncoordinated fashion. However, during defecation, most of your lower colon contracts all at the same time, to empty itself. If a part of your colon contracts against or pushes on an already-contracted segment, which is especially common when you are anxious, it produces an area of increased pressure that you may sense as a cramp. Eating itself induces your defecation reflex, and *a bowel movement soon after every meal, as seen in children and dogs, is now felt to be a sign of optimum colon health.*

Changes in your bowel habits—stool frequency, consistency, ease of elimination, unexplained constipation or diarrhea lasting more than a few days, and especially any blood or mucus in your stool—should prompt you to seek medical attention. Narrowing of your stool or a sense of incomplete emptying of your bowel can be signals of cancer.

Colon problems can cause generalized or localized pain, which may vary in type from severe and sharp to cramping or dull aching. Subtle symptoms include loss of appetite, nausea, nutritional disturbances, weight loss, lack of energy, tiredness, and dizziness. Many people avoid seeking medical attention until such symptoms interfere with their lifestyle. However, as with most diseases, early diagnosis before irreversible changes or disastrous complications evolve can be lifesaving.

Alternative Medicine Approaches to Keeping Your Colon Healthy

A new perspective was brought to bear on all colon disease by the research of Dr. Denis Burkitt, who discovered the importance of the now well-known high-fiber, high-bulk diet to help maintain the colon's health. Despite one recent study, which did not show a relationship between higher fiber intakes and prevention of colon disease, much scientific evidence continues to support this connection.

As considered in Chapter 2, Dr. Burkitt and others concluded that our bodies probably evolved for, and do best on, a vegetarian diet. Our nearest genetic relatives, the chimps, gorillas, and apes, mainly follow this diet, and flourish on it. Some anthropological evidence even suggests that the first humans were probably fruit and nut gatherers, not hunters, and meat-eating may have been a later, unhealthy addition. Certainly the eating of meat per se did not account for our greater intelligence than apes or you would see lions and tigers at Harvard and Yale.

Burkitt specifically studied various populations in Africa and England, comparing stool size, consistency, frequency, and content. He then analyzed the incidence of colon disease. The stools of African villagers were two to three times as large as those of the English, as well as softer and more frequent. As the villagers moved to cities and changed from their traditional diet, their stools changed toward the typically Western, harder and less frequent, variety. This alteration correlated directly with increased incidence of various colon diseases.[2]

Small, hard stools and infrequent movements have been shown to elevate intracolonic pressure, thought to be the most important factor in the production of diverticulosis—the ballooning out of small pouches from the wall of the colon that can cause pain, infection, and bleeding. Difficulty in the passage of small, hard stools also leads to the various anal and rectal problems, such as hemorrhoids, fissures, and infections. (See Chapter 17.)

In addition, with a low-fiber, meat-based diet, complicated interactions of dietary constituents, bile acids, and intestinal bacteria may produce cancer-causing substances. If your intestines have a long transit time (i.e., food moves through slowly) and you have bowel movements infrequently, these carcinogens become concentrated, and remain in contact with your intestinal lining for more extended periods of time. Recent research suggests specific benefits are derived from the fermentation residues of a high-fiber, low-fat diet.[3]

Anthropological debate aside, statistics and studies from many angles have now testified to the benefits and increased desirability of this diet in prevention of an extraordinary number of diseases, from heart attacks and arthritis to cancer. Although an occasional study has not supported this thesis, the overwhelming majority of research strongly has found in its favor. This evidence seems now especially significant for colon disorders. Adopting a high-fiber, low-fat vegetarian diet may help you prevent diverticuli, colitis, and cancer of the colon.

Your daily requirement of fiber is about 20 to 40 grams, equal to three tablespoons of bran, three servings of whole-grain bread, or its equivalent in other grains. It would take three *loaves* of white bread to give you this amount of fiber. And even if you could eat that much, it would still be unhealthy, because it would probably cause sufficient constipation to put you at risk for disease. White flour bagels, croissants, doughnuts, pasta, et cetera, should be replaced with their whole-grain equivalents.

You can roughly gauge whether your colon is being protected by the size and number of bowel movements you have each day. If you eat three meals, three bowel movements should be coming out each day, totaling about a pound to a pound and a half of stool. When you sit on the toilet, you should be able to just relax and whistle; if you have to grunt and strain, so does your colon, and this can be a signal of impending disease. If vegetables are the main courses at your meals, and all other foods are side dishes, you should easily produce one, two, or even better, three stools per day.

In the past, medical authorities have been tolerant of variations in bowel patterns, considering a range of from one movement per day to one per week as normal and acceptable, but the latter is now seen in a new light, as a cause for concern. If changing your diet, as elaborated in Chapter 2, and adding a few tablespoons of whole miller's bran to each meal, doesn't produce two to three movements each day, be sure to seek further medical advice.

Your toilet habits also play an important part in maintaining your colon's health. Ideally, you should be able to defecate soon after you feel the urge. For many people, the pattern is established like clockwork, with a sensation of need coming at the same time each day. Of course, bowel activity is easily interrupted by changes in diet or daily routine, most typically found when traveling. If you delay defecating, it can lead to constipation, increased pressure within your colon, and subsequent difficulty with stool passage—and thus the other, more serious problems caused by chronic constipation.

In summary, your diet is the most critical factor in your stool size, consistency, frequency and chemical content, and thus your colon's health. Take care of yourself by following the guidelines for optimum diet given in Chapter 2.

How Colon Disease Is Diagnosed

John, a 53-year-old physician who had been lax in following the cancer-screening guidelines he recommended for his own patients, had never even had a rectal examination.

After his younger sister was found to have colon cancer, and his wife pressured him to be checked, he underwent a screening sigmoidoscopy. A three-quarter-inch polyp with malignant changes was successfully removed through the scope, and no further treatment was necessary. He then began a regular screening program for early detection of any additional growths.

Diagnosis of colon disease involves a good history and physical exam, a check for blood and possibly abnormal organisms in your stool, and often X-rays, scans, and a scoping procedure. The following are the key exams.

History

Your doctor should know all about your usual bowel pattern and any changes. Symptoms described above, especially abdominal pain, bloating, cramping, and local tenderness are important. Mention any self-medications or treatment you may have tried, and how they may have affected your symptoms. Stool that is loose, watery, or contains blood, mucus, or pus needs to be investigated. Any family history of colorectal cancer needs to be revealed.

Physical Exam

Your colon physical exam begins with your doctor feeling your abdomen for areas of tenderness, masses, and liver enlargement. Next is the digital rectal exam, the first, easiest, and quickest screening exam for colorectal cancer. Approximately 15 percent of these tumors are located within reach of your doctor's examining finger. A stool specimen can be taken to test for blood. The exam can be performed on a special flexible table, or simply with you lying on your side.

Stool Occult Blood Test

This simple test looks for blood not grossly visible in your stool, an important clue, since the fragile surface of a tumor or polyp often sheds tiny amounts of blood. Occult blood testing is positive in 2 to 5 percent of all patients who are screened routinely. Of these patients, 30 to 40 percent have benign polyps and 2 to 10 percent prove to have a cancer. However, since a tumor may not bleed, or do so only intermittently, only 60 percent of colon cancers can be found by this method. Still, occult blood testing is the best simple screening test now available, and *once you are over the age of 50, you should have your stool tested for blood every year.* Routine yearly stool screening, followed by colonoscopy in positive tests, has been estimated to be able to reduce colorectal cancer mortality by 33 percent *if the recommendations are faithfully followed.*[4]

Easy and inexpensive, the occult blood test consists of a kit of cards with small squares of test paper on which to smear stool samples. You test two sections of your stools for three days. The cards are mailed back to your doctor, who treats them with a chemical stain that turns blue if blood is present. For the most accurate and reliable test, you must be on a meat-free, high-fiber diet for a day or two prior to and during the test period. This avoids falsely positive tests from the blood in meats, and the fibrous roughage irritates the surface of any possible tumors or polyps, to cause detectable bleeding. Any positive test indicates you need further diagnostic exams, including sigmoidoscopy and a barium enema or colonoscopy.

Sigmoidoscopy

One in five hundred patients over the age of 40 who has no symptoms but still chooses to undergo routine screening *sigmoidoscopy* is found to have colon cancer. In the area of the colon and rectum examined, such screening sigmoidoscopy may reduce deaths from colorectal cancer by two-thirds.[5]

This test is easily performed in most doctors' offices. A lighted tube is inserted into your rectum and lower sigmoid colon. A one-inch wide, rigid, ten-inch-long scope is commonly used, but a narrower, flexible twenty-five-inch scope has a better diagnostic capability and may cause less discomfort.

Sigmoidoscopic examination is uncomfortable, though not usually painful. It takes two to five minutes using the rigid scope, and ten to twenty minutes with the flexible scope. The exam may be conducted without any preparation on your part, or you may be asked to take a liquid diet, laxatives, or an enema. You lie on your left side, or kneel with hips flexed and head down. Alternatively, you may be positioned on your back with your feet up in stirrups. Your doctor inflates air through the scope to expand your rectum and colon, which helps in passing the instrument and in seeing your bowel lining. This air may cause some cramping, but intravenous sedation is rarely needed.

During sigmoidoscopy, your bowel lining can be biopsied, cultures taken for microorganisms, and small polyps removed; 50 percent of all cancers and 80 percent of all polyps can be found by this method.

Colonoscopy

News anchor Katie Couric chose to be filmed while having this screening test, to em-phasize its ability to check the entire length of the colon. It is now the mainstay for diagnosing colon disease occurring above the reach of the sigmoidoscope. After preparation with a liquid diet and bowel-cleansing solution, you lie on your left side on the examination table. You will probably be given mild intravenous sedation. A long, flexible scope, three-fourths-inch in diameter, is then inserted through your anus. You may be asked to turn from side to side to help in passing the scope, which can then be manipulated to view all the way to your cecum 95 percent of the time. Taking ten to sixty minutes to perform, colonoscopy is sometimes uncomfortable, though it should not actually be painful. Biopsies, tests for infection, and removal of polyps can all be accomplished during this procedure.

Complications of sigmoidoscopy and colonoscopy are more common if biopsy or polyp removal has been performed. Significant bleeding occurs in 7 to 25 cases per 1,000 exams, though it rarely requires surgery, since it usually stops spontaneously or can be controlled by other methods. If perforation happens, as it does in 2 to 4 cases per 1,000 diagnostic exams, and 3 to 10 per 1,000 polypectomies, it may necessitate emergency surgery. Overall, the mortality rate is 1 in 10,000 diagnostic exams.[6]

Barium Enema

In the *barium enema* test, you lie on an X-ray table while a rubber tube, with a balloon to prevent back flow, is placed in your rectum. A liquid barium (clay) mixture is passed through it and up to your cecum, outlining your colon. You are asked to roll from side to side, while your radiologist watches on a fluoroscope television monitor and takes several X-ray pictures. Polyps, tumors, twisted or constricted areas, diverticular outpouchings, and lining changes suggesting various types of inflammatory disease can be identified. A *barium enema with air contrast* introduces air into your colon after you have evacuated most of the barium. This latter exam gives the best definition of subtle lining changes, and finds small polyps and tumors. The examination takes ten to twenty minutes, and may be uncomfortable, though it should not hurt. The risk of colon perforation is 1 in 50,000 cases.

Scans

CAT scans and ultrasound (sonogram) scans may be helpful if you have an acute inflammatory diverticulitis, to see if it has caused an abscess that will need to be drained. These along with other more expensive and sophisticated tests such as MRI, PET, and nuclear isotope scans may be indicated if you have or have had cancer, to help with diagnosis and plan treatment.

Screening for Colorectal Cancer

Screening methods now available should prevent most deaths from colorectal cancer both by diagnosing early cancers when they are curable and by removing polyps that may transform to cancer as they enlarge over a period of years. Unfortunately, less than one person in three for whom screening is recommended in the United States is screened by *any* appropriate method.[7] Take advantage of the proven benefits.

The American Cancer Society recommends one of the following five screening options for individuals after age 50 with *no* known risk factors for colorectal cancer:

1. Annual test for occult blood in the stool and flexible sigmoidoscopy every five years
2. Flexible sigmoidoscopy every five years
3. Annual test for occult blood in the stool
4. Colonoscopy every ten years
5. Double-contrast barium enema every five years

A digital rectal exam should be done at the same time as sigmoidoscopy, colonoscopy, or double-contrast barium enema. Although colonoscopy is more expensive, uncomfortable, and less likely to be covered by insurance companies for screening, it picks up more disease than flexible sigmoidoscopy. Recent studies comparing screening flexible sigmoidoscopy with colonoscopy have found that sigmoidoscopy alone may fail to lead to diagnosing 62 percent of all tumors or significant polyps in the upper part of the colon above the reach of this scope.[8]

If you are at *increased* risk because of having a close family member with colon or rectal cancer—especially if it was diagnosed before the age of 55—you should have a colonoscopy (or sigmoidoscopy and air-contrast barium enema) between ages 35 and 40 and have it repeated every five years. You are also at higher risk if you have a history of polyps or inflammatory colon disease, or have had previous colon, breast, ovarian, or uterine cancer. If you fall into one of these categories, you must be screened more frequently, in consultation with your doctor.

Of course, if you have rectal bleeding or a change in your bowel habits, you should immediately see your doctor.

Diverticular Disease

Catherine, a 68-year-old, had a severe problem with diverticular disease, including a ten-day hospital stay for acute diverticulitis five years before. Since then, she had suffered from severe constipation, requiring daily laxatives and manual stool extraction every other day. After not having had a bowel movement for five days and becoming extremely bloated, she required an emergency operation, in which a narrowed part of her colon had to be removed. She then began producing three soft stools per day.

A *diverticulum* is a small pocket created when the internal layer of your colon pushes out through its muscular wall, at the potentially weak site where a small artery penetrates to carry blood to the lining. (See Figure 15.2.) Increased pressure within your colon over a long period of time is thought to produce this ballooning. Usually, many diverticula are formed, mostly in the sigmoid colon.

In the West, *diverticulosis*—the term for simply the presence of these pockets—is a common disease of aging. Unusual before the age of 40, when it is found in less than 2 percent of the population, thereafter, it steadily increases, so that after age 50, 20 to 30 percent of us have some diverticuli, and by age 80, the rate is more than 50 percent. If problems develop, they usually begin in the 50–60-year age range. It has been estimated that 0.5 to 2 percent of the 20 to 30 million Americans with diverticuli require hospital admission.[9]

Diverticulosis does not generally produce symptoms, though you may feel occasional cramping, abdominal pain and tenderness. *Diverticulitis*, developing in an estimated 20

percent of persons with diverticuli, is inflammation within a diverticulum, caused by trapped fecal material or by high pressure within the outpouching, creating swelling and interference with blood supply, causing significant symptoms. A "miniappendicitis" can result, with local inflammation obstructing neighboring diverticuli and starting a chain reaction.

If this process remains localized, your symptoms may be minimal. But if the infection creates an abscess, you become increasingly sick, with abdominal pain (usually worst in the lower left side of your abdomen), loss of appetite, fever, nausea, vomiting, diarrhea, or constipation. If your inflamed diverticulum is not "walled off" by adjacent tissue, it may perforate and spread infection into your abdominal cavity, a severe surgical emergency. It can also form a tunnel, or *fistula*, into another hollow organ such as your bladder, uterus, vagina, or small bowel; this requires surgical repair.

Scarring produced by repeated episodes of inflammation may lead to your bowel becoming narrowed, perhaps causing partial or complete bowel obstruction. If a small artery within the wall of your diverticulum is eroded, you can develop intestinal bleeding.

Diagnosis of diverticular disease is made by a barium enema, sigmoidoscopy, or colonoscopy examination. A CAT scan or sonogram may be necessary in acute diverticulitis, if an abscess is suspected.

Alternative Medicine Approaches to Diverticular Disease

Susan, a 65-year-old secretary, first became aware of a problem with her bowels when she began to notice an intermittent slight ache in

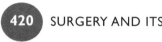

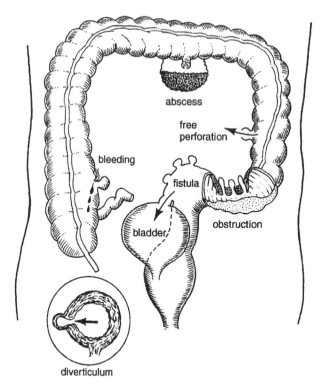

abscess

free
perforation

bleeding

fistula

bladder

obstruction

diverticulum

Fig. 15.2 A diverticulum and the complications it can cause

her left lower abdomen, accompanied by increased gas, constipation, and a bloated feeling. Her barium enema X-rays showed the presence of many diverticuli. She chose a trial of alternative medicine approaches, gradually adding more fiber to her diet. Since she disliked cereal, she simply added two small bran muffins to her breakfast routine, along with eliminating all white flour products and caffeine. Soon she was having two to three very easy bowel movements per day, and had no further episodes of abdominal discomfort.

Suppose you were to take a small lump of clay in your hand, and squeeze very hard. What would happen? The clay would start to

ooze through your fingers, where the pressure could be relieved. If your stool content is too thick, and the strain too great, you will begin to form diverticuli.

Before agreeing to elective surgery, you may wish to first adopt the following changes, to try to achieve symptom relief; and if you do choose surgery, you will still need to institute them anyway, to prevent further problems.

Change Your Diet

A high-fiber, low-fat, vegetarian diet can be used to treat diverticulosis with good results. As noted above, Dr. Denis Burkitt and others have demonstrated the role of diet in the formation of diverticuli. Diverticulosis, as well as most other colon diseases, is very rare in Africa; in England the rate is high, though lower in the vegetarians there who consume high-bulk diets.[10] Autopsies performed over the years in the United States have shown a huge increase in the incidence of diverticuli, from occurring in 5 percent of the population in 1910 to 56 percent in 1980. This correlates with our cultural change to more refined food, in the currently typical American diet. In Eastern countries such as Japan, Korea, and Iran with typical high-fiber, less refined diets, the diverticula prevalence is only 0.6 to 1.6 percent.[11]

Diverticuli form when your colon has to create high-pressure contractions as it struggles to pass hard, low-bulk stools. Laboratory experiments have shown that persons with diverticulosis have much higher intracolonic pressures, as well as abnormal spastic contractions. With a shift to a high-fiber diet, these wave patterns return toward normal.[12] Prior to understanding this relationship, the conventional Western doctor's dietary treatment recommendation for patients with diverticular disease was the exact *opposite*—a low-fiber diet, which in effect had been making matters worse. Studies of symptomatic diverticulosis patients who change to a high-bulk, bran-type diet have shown that 90 percent remain symptom-free for five years, and are also less likely to develop complications of their disease.[13] Take wheat or bran fiber with each meal, 10 to 20 grams per day, and also increase your liquid, fruit, and vegetable intake. Ten grams of fiber is present, for example, in a bowl of bran cereal. Choose one free of sugar. See Chapter 2 for details of an optimum diet.

Exercise Regularly

A study from Harvard Medical School investigated the relationship of physical activity and symptomatic diverticular disease in more than 47,000 men participating in the Health Professionals Follow-Up Study. A 43 percent decreased risk for symptomatic episodes was found in the most vigorous group compared to the least active group. *The participants who watched the most television and video had the highest risk.* The combination of inactivity and a low fiber intake increased risk by 156 percent.[14] Although the exact mechanism of this protective effect is unclear, exercise is known to decrease intestinal transit time, meaning that the food moves through your bowel more quickly, thus not allowing high pressure areas to develop.

Practice Visualization

First, practice stress reduction. Try exercises such as the following: Imagine your colon as a long pipe that has a number of small bubbles along its length. See the bubbles as collapsing, and the pipe becoming strong and straight. Hold this image in your mind, while at the same time feeling it within your colon.

Conventional Medicine Approaches to Diverticular Disease

If you have chronic diverticular disease, the usual recommendation is to add extra fiber to your diet, so that your stools easily pass without your needing to generate a lot of colonic pressure. However, if you have acute symptoms or a complication, you still may be able to avoid emergency surgery. The following approaches may get you through the crisis.

Antibiotics and Bowel Rest

Conventional treatment consisting of a liquid or low-fiber diet that gives your intestines a rest and is less likely to block an inflamed area, along with oral antibiotics, is successful in treating 70 to 100 percent of initial attacks of uncomplicated acute inflammatory diverticulitis. Most can be resolved without hospitalization; they subside in a few days. However, with more severe attacks you must be hospitalized and have intravenous fluids and antibiotics, as well as close observation for development of complications.

After the resolution of your acute symptoms, slowly institute the high-fiber diet discussed in Chapter 2, since it has been shown to decrease the chances for further attacks.[15]

In general, you have only a 25 percent chance of ever having a second attack, usually within two years of the first. If such a second attack is severe enough to require hospitalization, it indicates your disease has progressed to the point at which the likelihood of your having recurrent symptomatic attacks reaches 90 percent. Since medical treatment is so much less effective, surgery may then be justified.

Catheter Abscess Drainage

If you have an abscess, it may be possible to treat it with antibiotics if it is small and you are not very ill. Or, it may be possible to have it drained by the passage of an ultrasound- or CAT scan–guided drainage tube through your abdominal wall into the abscess cavity. This may help you avoid emergency surgery and a temporary colostomy. Elective colon resection can be performed later, after the emergency.

If bleeding develops in a diverticulum, 80 percent of the time it will stop spontaneously. You can be watched closely in the hospital, and have bowel rest, IVs, and blood replacement. If your blood pressure is unstable, or the bleeding is massive, continues, or reappears, you must have surgery.

Surgical Approaches to Diverticular Disease

Howard, a 65-year-old, was puzzled to notice bursts of air and a burning pain when he urinated. His doctor had him drink a glass of orange juice into which was mixed a tablespoon of powdered charcoal. Only a few hours later, he saw black particles in his urine. In the operating room, he was found to have a "fistula"—a connection between a diverticulum in his sigmoid colon and the top of his bladder. A piece of colon was removed, and the hole in his bladder closed. He recovered without further problems.

If you develop one of the complications of diverticulitis—such as an abscess, perforation, obstruction, fistula, or uncontrolled hemorrhage—you need surgery. Surgery is more controversial if your symptoms are less severe; a trial of alternative medicine approaches is warranted before you decide to have an operation. Preventive procedures in the absence of symptoms are *never* indicated.

You must consider surgery if you have recurrent attacks of acute inflammatory diverticulitis, since your chances for a complication increase with each succeeding occurrence. Complications appear with 25 percent of second attacks, and 60 percent of subsequent significant episodes. If you were to require an emergency operation, your complication rate would be markedly increased. A temporary colostomy would be usually necessary, along with a second operation to remove it, increased hospital time, and more time lost from work.

As a general guideline, you should choose elective surgery if you have:

- Recovered from an attack of complicated diverticulitis.
- Had two attacks of uncomplicated acute inflammatory diverticulitis.
- Symptoms from a single attack lasting more than a month.
- Test results impossible to differentiate from cancer.

If you are younger than 40, you should consider surgery sooner, because the disease is usually more severe and has a greater tendency toward recurrence and complications.

Two types of surgery are available to treat areas of the colon damaged by diverticulitis.

Partial Colectomy

If your surgery can be done on an elective basis, a one-stage partial colectomy, or removal of the diseased part of the colon with immediate reconnection, is the best operation. Your chances for permanent relief of symptoms are 95 percent. The mortality rate is 1 to 2 percent, increasing with age and overall poor health. The usual hospital stay is five to seven days, and you can be back to work in four to six weeks. Currently there is a trend to do this operation even in an emergency setting if your surgeon feels it is safe to do so. (For a discussion of partial colectomy, see page 430.).

Partial Colectomy with Temporary Colostomy

If emergency surgery must be performed without bowel preparation, most surgeons still recommend removal of the diseased segment of your colon, with the creation of a temporary colostomy. Later, another operation can remove the colostomy and reconnect the bowel. The mortality rate for emergency surgery is 5 to 35 percent, depending on the type of complication, timeliness of the surgery, and your overall health, and total hospitalization time is stretched to one to three weeks, with two to four months lost from work. (For a discussion of partial colectomy, see page 430. For a discussion of colostomy, see page 446.)

DIVERTICULAR DISEASE SUMMARY

Prevention

Diet and Supplements

- Follow a high-fiber, low-fat diet.
- Drink 8–10 large glasses of water daily.
- Bran, 3 tablespoons daily.
- Psyllium, 1–2 tablespoons daily.

Lifestyle

- Exercise regularly: 1 hour, 3–5 times weekly.

Alternative Medicine Approaches

- Follow the guidelines for prevention, above.
- Chamomile tea, every 2–3 hours.
- Slippery elm, 500 mg, 1–2 times daily.
- Flaxseed oil, 1–2 tablespoons daily.
- Practice visualization.

Conventional Medicine Approaches

- Antibiotics and bowel rest.
- Catheter abscess drainage.

Surgical Approaches

- Partial colectomy.
- Partial colectomy with temporary colostomy—for complication.

Bowel Obstruction

Mechanical bowel obstruction is a serious matter, necessitating emergency surgery if it cannot be relieved by conservative measures. Eighty-five percent of all large bowel obstructions are caused by cancer or narrowing from diverticular disease, the other 15 percent by twists, hernias, or other less-common diseases. If the obstruction is not relieved or decompressed, the danger of a "blowout"—pressure behind the blockage blowing a hole in your intestinal wall—is great, and carries with it a high mortality rate.

Your signs and symptoms of bowel obstruction can include progressive abdominal distention (swelling) that may appear over a few days, lack of passage of stool and gas, nausea, vomiting, and abdominal pain.

Hospital treatment is required. To prevent further distention and vomiting, a plastic tube is first placed through your nose into your stomach, to suck out air and secretions. Intravenous fluids are usually necessary, to replace the large amount of body fluids pooling within the swollen bowel. If a question exists about the extent of the obstruction and need for emergency surgery, X-rays, CAT scan, a sigmoidoscopy or colonoscopy, and/ or a barium enema may be needed.

If you have a *complete large bowel obstruction*, an emergency operation to relieve the blockage avoids perforation, as well as problems caused when body fluids accumulate inside the bowel and bacteria proliferate in them. A temporary colostomy is then usually needed. If the obstruction is partial or incomplete, surgery can be deferred until the bowel has been cleaned out and you are in the best possible shape. In this case, a temporary colostomy can generally be avoided.

Some obstructive processes can actually be treated by sigmoidoscopy, colonoscopy, or barium enema. In *volvulus*, the colon spirals on itself, similar to the way an inner tube or balloon can be twisted. If it can be untwisted by sigmoidoscopy or barium enema, emergency surgery can be avoided; such measures are effective in about 80 percent of all cases. Recurrence is a problem in 30 to 50 percent, with increasing likelihood of another volvulus after each recurrence. However, if you are elderly or a poor risk for surgery, it may be less dangerous to wait for the next attack (which may also respond to conservative treatment) rather than risk a surgical mortality of over 10 percent.

Inflammatory Colitis (Ulcerative Colitis and Crohn's Disease)

Marcy, a 16-year-old, developed severe pain in her right lower abdomen during an all-night party. When seen in the emergency room, she had symptoms typical of appendicitis, and so was sent to surgery, where it was found her small intestine and the first part of her colon were swollen and inflamed, typical of Crohn's disease. After her operation, she began medical treatment, which included medications and changes in her diet.

———————————

First, a definition of terms. *Acute colitis* is caused by infection from bacteria, viruses, or parasites. *Inflammatory colitis* is thought to be caused by a disorder of the immune system. These two disorders can be confused because acute colitis causes inflammation and inflammatory colitis can be acute. Although acute colitis is a common problem, it is very rarely treated with surgery and therefore won't be discussed here.

Chronic *inflammatory colitis (inflammatory bowel disease* or *IBD)*, has two varieties: *ulcerative colitis* and *Crohn's disease*. Both are enormously challenging diseases, in which you may suffer from such severe diarrhea and cramping that your entire life can be disrupted. Fortunately, they often respond to alternative medicine approaches. If you do require surgery for ulcerative colitis, newer techniques may allow you to retain your rectal function.

Colitis predominately affects young people, with an average age at diagnosis of 23 years. It is thought to be caused by a disorder of the immune system, in which an antibody mistakenly identifies the colon itself as "foreign" and attacks it. Why this happens is unknown, though stress and diet may be precipitating factors. Some racial and hereditary predisposition is also apparent, with the highest incidence occurring in those of Jewish descent. One-third of all patients have a close relative with the disease.

Crohn's disease can appear in your small intestine, colon, and/or rectum, with the inner lining, muscular layer, and outside covering of your bowel all affected. Ulcerative colitis involves only the inner lining of your colon and rectum, not your small intestine. Both disorders may cause enough inflammation to cause abdominal pain, distention, diarrhea, and bleeding. They also may be complicated by perforation, abscesses, obstruction, and/or fistula (creation of an abnormal passage to the skin or another organ).

Inflammatory colitis patients may develop nutritional problems, weight loss, growth disturbances, and complications outside the colon. These are thought to be due to the faulty immune system also attacking other parts of your body. Forty percent of all colitis sufferers develop hepatitis; arthritis and eye problems are also common. Less frequent problems include bile duct obstruction, kidney stones, phlebitis (inflammation of the veins), canker sores, and severe skin disease.

Crohn's disease affects your colon in a "skip" fashion, with normal areas interspersed between diseased ones. Twenty percent of Crohn's cases involve your colon alone; both the colon and small bowel are diseased in 30 percent; and 50 percent of patients have only the small bowel affected. Ulcerative colitis may involve your rectum alone ("ulcerative proctitis," 10 to 15 percent of the time), or your rectum and progressively more colon, until your whole colon is involved ("pancolitis," seen in 30 percent of all patients).

A diagnosis of IBD is made on the basis of your symptoms, along with your doctor finding typical patterns of colon and rectal swelling and inflammation through a barium enema, sigmoidoscopy, colonoscopy, and/or colon or rectal biopsy.

Ulcerative colitis follows three clinical patterns. In 10 percent, it first appears in a *fulminant* manner, with rapid onset, severe symptoms, and a high rate of complications that necessitate emergency surgery. The most common form, seen in 70 percent of all patients, is a *chronic intermittent* disturbance characterized by periods without symptoms alternating with acute attacks. A third form, seen in 20 percent, is *chronic and continuous*, giving you persistent symptoms of diarrhea and abdominal pain. Crohn's disease tends to be intermittent, with only occasional acute attacks.

If narrowing of your bowel develops from either disease, you will have symptoms of partial obstruction: persistent cramping, abdominal pain, distention, and diarrhea exacerbated by eating.

Crohn's disease and ulcerative colitis are similar diseases, often causing identical symptoms and similar findings on examinations. In fact, in 10 percent of IBD cases the specific disease cannot be differentiated. In practice, therefore, alternative and conventional medical approaches to treatment are the same. The surgical approaches, however, are quite different, unless an emergency procedure is necessary. Ulcerative colitis can be cured by an elective operation, but surgery should be avoided in Crohn's disease, where further disease flare-ups are likely.

Alternative Medicine Approaches to Inflammatory Colitis

Joan, a 55-year-old real estate agent, had a long history of frequent bowel movements, occasionally accompanied by blood. Having exhausted the conventional treatments with little relief, she decided to try an alternative medicine approach. She started on the diet given in Chapter 2, being especially careful to avoid refined sugars and dairy products. Within a few short weeks, she was completely free from symptoms for the first time in twenty years, and thereafter continued with normal bowel function.

A bland diet, free of milk products, may be useful in helping control the diarrhea episodes that accompany acute IBD. You may also find benefit from the following alternative medicine approaches to your chronic colitis.

Correct Nutritional Disturbances

Multiple factors contribute to the severe nutritional abnormalities in IBD patients. Weight loss occurs in 65 to 75 percent of all sufferers. You will need to pay close attention especially to your caloric and protein intake.

Avoid Refined Sugar

Studies have shown that persons who develop colitis have a higher intake of refined white sugar than do people in the research control groups.[16] Refined sugar consumption has been shown to depress your immune function.[17] Foods made with refined white sugar generally also lack fiber, and are low in zinc, important for the healing process.

Avoid Fast Foods

A Swedish study found that persons who ate fast foods two times or more per week had a 3.4 times higher rate of Crohn's disease, and 3.9 times higher risk for ulcerative colitis.[18]

Change Your Diet

A number of studies have indicated that refined foods, which lack fiber, may be more common in the pre-illness diets of colitis patients. Treatment with a high-fiber diet has been shown to be beneficial.[19] It may act by providing a better balance of colonic bacteria. See Chapter 2 for instructions on converting to a high-fiber diet.

Eliminate Allergenic Foods

Your bowel may be sensitive to certain foods. You can note any symptoms brought on by the various food items, and be tested for food allergies. A number of studies have shown that eliminating the offending substances—usually wheat, gluten, dairy (especially cheese), and meats—eliminates symptoms.[20]

Take Supplements

Patients with IBD have been found to be deficient in many vitamins. In general, you should take more than the daily recommended daily dosages. Mineral supplements are also indicated.

Folic acid, one of the B vitamins, may be particularly helpful. Recommended dosage is usually 500 to 800 mcg daily.[21]

Vitamin A deficiency may act to allow the bowel wall to become more permeable to bacteria, placing stress on the immune system, so that it becomes disordered and attacks the bowel lining itself.[22] Recommended levels of vitamin A are 10,000 IU daily, with your doctor's supervision.

Zinc deficiency has been found in colitis patients, and its usefulness in treating the disease is documented.[23] It has also been shown to be especially helpful in treating the eye symptoms associated with colitis. Recommended dosage is 50 mg, three times daily.[24]

Vitamin C deficiency may be associated with fistula formation in colitis.[25] Begin with 500 mg daily, and increase as needed, with supervision.

Flaxseed oil and fish oil contain substances found to have antiinflammatory effects. Experimental evidence suggests that they may be useful in the treatment of ulcerative colitis and Crohn's disease. Fish oil has been shown to decrease clinical severity of ulcerative colitis by 56 percent and allow a decrease in standard medications.[26] This study used fifteen Max-EPA capsules per day. In Crohn's disease, fish oil decreased recurrent acute inflammation attacks by 41 percent in one study, in which three enteric-coated capsules of the fish oil preparation Purepa were given three times per day.[27]

Use Herbal Remedies

Chamomile tea is quieting to the bowel; three to four cups may be consumed per day.[28] Other herbs with anecdotal support include goldenseal, licorice root, gentian root, papaya leaf, myrrh gum, Irish moss, fenugreek, and ginger root.[29] Doses begin with one capsule or cup of tea, three times daily.

Practice Stress Management

Stress has been shown to be related to the onset and reccurrence of symptoms. In one study, patients with colitis showed less ability to handle disorder in their lives, and bleeding episodes can be correlated with feelings of hopelessness.[30] Practicing regular relaxation may therefore be important, and you may find stress management and yoga relaxation techniques especially helpful. See Chapter 2 for details.

Quit Smoking

Although smoking doesn't seem to affect the colon in patients with Crohn's disease, it does increase small bowel inflammation and symptoms.[31] See Chapter 2 for help with quitting.

Practice Visualization

Try exercises such as the following: See your colon as a garden hose whose inside has become thickened and frayed to the point where bits of rubber have begun to come out with the water. Soothe and strengthen the inside of the tube with healing salve, and add rubber patches wherever needed. Then see the hose in its final form as perfectly strong and healthy. Image this sequence, while feeling it happen within your abdomen.

Use Acupuncture

Interestingly, acupuncture has been shown to create movement in the omentum (the mobile layer of fat and lymph tissue attached to the stomach and colon), so that it can perform its protective function more quickly and effectively. Such mobility may help to reduce inflammation and increase the effectiveness of the immune system.[32]

Conventional Medicine Approach to Inflammatory Colitis

Both ulcerative colitis and Crohn's disease are treated with similar regimens. The aminosalicylic acid drugs sulfasalazine (Azulfidine) and mesalamine (Pentasa, Asacol, Rowasa) have an antiinflammatory effect and are used in mild to moderate disease. They can be given in pills, or via enema or suppositories (Rowasa). They help prevent relapses, though are not very effective in severe acute attacks. The corticosteroids prednisone (Deltasone, Meticorten) and prednisilone (Prelone, Pedia-

pred) are more effective in severe acute attacks. They decrease inflammation and modulate immune response, but have significant side effects. Budesonide, a new, safer steroid preparation, represents an important advance. Because it has high topical activity and is poorly absorbed, it causes fewer side effects.[33] However, it is still undergoing clinical trials and not yet approved by the FDA for use in Crohn's disease.

If you have ulcerative proctitis (inflammation of the lining of the rectum) only, you may get along quite well by just placing steroid foam in your rectum whenever your symptoms develop. Side effects are present with any drug regimen, but they are most troublesome with chronically used steroids. Therefore, if steroids are frequently required, a drug that suppresses the immune response, such as azathioprine, methotrexate, or cyclosporin A may decrease relapses and allow you to stop or reduce your steroid dosage. The antibiotics metranidazole (Flagyl) and ciprofloxacin are useful in active Crohn's disease.

The search for the best treatment regimens for acute attacks and to prevent recurrence is a rapidly changing field. Exciting research being conducted into the mediators of inflammation and the immune system provides much hope that better drugs will soon be available to provide long-term control. A single infusion of infliximab (Remicade), a monoclonol antibody against tumor necrosis factor, decreases symptoms in about two-thirds of all Crohn's disease patients but does not induce a sustained remission. Growth hormone injections may also have a similar short-term benefit. If you have inflammatory colitis, you need to develop a trusting relationship with a gastroenterologist who has a special interest in IBD.

Surgical Approaches to Inflammatory Colitis

Bill, *a 28-year-old police officer with a fourteen-year history of ulcerative colitis, had problems tolerating medication and such frequent need to pass diarrhea-like stools that it was interfering with his job performance. He decided to have surgery. First, he had his whole colon removed, and the end of his small intestine brought out through his abdominal wall, where contents could be collected in a stoma bag. A few months later, he also had his rectum lining taken out, sparing the muscles which affect his ability to control stool passage. His small intestine was taken down from his abdominal wall and a pouch created from it, which was then sewn to his anus. He soon became well, with good voluntary bowel function, and is back in his car patrolling our streets.*

Some indications for colitis surgery are obvious, such as need to treat the life-threatening complications of bowel perforation, abscess, obstruction, massive hemorrhage, or when medical management fails to control a severe attack. Ten percent of all colitis patients do end up needing emergency surgery.

When your requirement for surgery is not so urgent, the decision is more difficult. The usually recommended surgical procedure for ulcerative colitis is dramatic: total removal of your colon and rectum. You should therefore first try alternative medicine and medical management. However, if you are still miserable, evidence suggests that your quality of life can be significantly improved to equal that of the general population, if you choose early surgical intervention.[34]

One-third to one-half of all patients with ulcerative colitis and 70 percent of those with Crohn's disease eventually do require surgery. The average interval between onset of disease and surgery for ulcerative colitis is nine years.

Surgery does *cure* ulcerative colitis. However, if you have Crohn's disease and the affected area of your colon is removed, you have a 40 percent chance it will reappear. Even if all of your colon is taken out, you have a 10 percent chance of recurrence in your small bowel.

If you have a chronic form of IBD, your decision about surgery should be made on the basis of a careful analysis of your medical history, quality of life, and prospects for future disease and complications. You should understand both your risks and your possible benefits. When surgery is undertaken in an "elective" situation, the mortality rate is less than 1.5 percent. But if you delay it and an emergency arises, surgical mortality can be as high as 40 percent.

If you have ulcerative colitis, your risk for developing cancer is a critical consideration. The earlier the onset, the longer your disease is present, and the more of your colon it involves, the higher your chances for cancer. After ten years, the cancer rate is only 3 percent. After thirty-five years of disease, 30 percent of the patients with all of their colon involved and 40 percent whose onset of disease was by age 15 develop cancer.[35] If you have ulcerative colitis and do develop colon cancer, your chance for a cure is lower than for a colon cancer patient who does not have ulcerative colitis.

Therefore, if you have had total colon involvement with ulcerative colitis for more than ten years, you should consider surgery. You have much better options now than years ago, thanks to improved surgical techniques, stomal appliances, and stomal therapists. Alternatively, you may choose very close monitoring, including yearly barium enemas or colonoscopies. A currently favored option is to biopsy several areas of the bowel through colonoscopy, recommending surgery if you are found to have *dysplasia* (premalignant changes in your colon lining).

One of three surgical procedures can be chosen, depending on the type of inflammatory colitis you have.

Partial Colectomy

This may be your solution if you have Crohn's disease and only a section of your colon is involved. The diseased section is removed and the neighboring healthy bowel joined together.

Total Proctocolectomy with Permanent Ileostomy

This procedure cures you of ulcerative colitis. However, as previously noted, if you have Crohn's disease, you are relieved of your colon symptoms, but face a 10 percent risk of recurrence in your small bowel.

This operation removes all of your colon, rectum, and anus. A permanent "ileostomy," or opening of the small bowel onto your skin, is created. An ileostomy is usually placed in your right lower abdominal wall. (For a discussion of proctocolectomy with ileostomy, see pages 444.)

Proctocolectomy with Ileoanal Pouch

This is the most frequently recommended operation if you choose surgery for ulcerative colitis (*not* Crohn's disease) and are generally healthy. All of your colon and most of your rectum are removed, leaving the portion of the rectum containing the muscular squeeze valve mechanism, the sphincter, which gives you the ability to control defecation. The diseased lining of the rectum is then stripped out and a "reservoir" made out of the end of the small bowel, bringing it through the rectal muscular sphincter mechanism and sewing it to the anus. (For a discussion of proctocolectomy, see page 446. For a discussion of the ileoanal pouch, see page 448.).

INFLAMMATORY COLITIS SUMMARY

Prevention

Diet and Supplements

- Follow a low-fat, high-fiber diet.
- Avoid refined sugar.
- Avoid fast foods.
- Eliminate allergenic foods, such as wheat and dairy.
- Folic acid, 500–800 mcg daily.
- Vitamin A, 10,000 IU daily.
- Zinc, 50 mg, 3 times daily.
- Black currant oil, 500–1,000 mg daily, or fish oil, 3–4 grams daily.

Lifestyle

- Don't smoke.
- Practice daily yoga postures.
- Practice stress management.

Alternative Medicine Approaches

- Follow the guidelines for prevention, above.

- Chamomile tea, 3–4 cups daily.
- (DGH), 300 mg 3 times daily.
- Goldenseal, licorice root, gentian root, papaya leaf, myrrh gum, Irish moss, fenugreek, and ginger root; doses begin with one capsule or cup of tea, three times daily.
- Vitamin C, 500 mg daily, increase as needed with supervision.
- Fish oil capsules (Purepa), 3 capsules, 3 times daily.
- Flaxseed oil, 1 tablespoon daily.
- Use acupuncture, hypnosis.
- Practice visualization.

Conventional Medicine Approaches

Medications

- Aminosalicylic acid drugs—azulfidine, mesalamine (Pentasa, Asacol, Rowasa).
- Coticosteroids—prednisone, prednisilone, budesonide.
- Immune surpressers—azathioprine, methotrexate, cyclosporin A, infliximab (Remicade).
- Antibiotics—metranidazole (Flagyl), ciprofloxacin.

Surgical Approaches

- Partial colectomy (for Crohn's disease).
- Total proctocololectomy with permanent ileostomy (for ulcerative colitis and Crohn's disease).
- Proctocolectomy with ileoanal pouch ileostomy (for ulcerative colitis and Crohn's disease).

Colon Polyps

Colon polyps, growths of the intestinal lining that protrude into the channel of your colon, are thought to be caused by dietary, chemical, bacterial, viral, and/or genetic factors. They are found in 10 percent of all Americans undergoing routine screening sigmoidoscopy. *At one time or other, by early to middle adult life, up to 30 percent of our population has intestinal polyps.* They tend to grow in the lower part of your colon and rectum, and 90 percent are within reach of the flexible sigmoidoscope.

Two types of polyps are distinguished: *hyperplastic polyps* are tiny, and do not enlarge or cause problems, while *adenoma polyps* may enlarge and may be premalignant. Adenoma polyps less than one-half inch in size have a 3 percent rate of cancer within them; those one-half to one inch have a 10 percent risk; and greater than one inch a 50 percent rate. Adenoma polyps can be flat or nodular, forming on a stalk with a narrow base. A *villous adenoma polyp*, usually flat, has a malignancy rate of 15 to 40 percent, which does not seem to vary with its size. Polyps are usually "silent"—that is, they do not produce symptoms—but can sometimes cause bleeding, obstruction, and diarrhea.

Alternative Medicine Approaches to Colon Polyps

If you do choose this course of treatment, you still must be monitored by your doctor, and follow the screening guidelines in the previous section. The following are additional guidelines to follow.

Change Your Diet

Dietary fat increases free oxygen radicals, which may cause abnormal activity in colorectal lining cells. Epidemiological studies have shown a correlation between blood cholesterol levels and colorectal adenoma polyps.[36] Dietary cholesterol comes from animal fats.

Polyps in your colon may also be caused by dietary elements interacting with hereditary factors. Heredity may predispose your colon to form polyps via a genetic mechanism, but whether they develop or become malignant may depend on the presence of factors in your diet that encourage polyp formation or transformation of their cells toward malignancy. Since some studies have correlated the same dietary elements—a high-fat, low-fiber diet—with polyp formation, as in colorectal cancer, and a polyp may take up to fifteen years to become malignant, more research is needed to show if polyps themselves can be reversed and malignancy prevented by shifting your nutrition. A prudent change in diet may help prevent both disorders.

Take Supplements

Laboratory, clinical, and epidemiological evidence indicates that calcium helps prevent colorectal polyps. A recent randomized double-blind clinical trial of calcium supplementation (1,200 mg calcium carbonate per day) in addition to normal dietary intake found a 17 percent reduction in the number of patients who developed polyps and a 24 percent reduction in average number of polyps in the supplement group.[37] Epidemiological studies have also shown a protective effect of vitamins A and E.[38]

Regression of existing polyps as well as prevention of new ones is possible by supplements of 2,000 to 3,000 mg of vitamin C daily and 400 IU of vitamin E three times daily.[39]

Avoid Alcohol and Tobacco

A Health Professions Follow-Up Study found that smoking within twenty years prior to colonoscopy increases your risk of a small polyp by 200 percent, and smoking more than twenty years in the past increases your risk for a large polyp by 138 percent.[40] Colorectal cancer risk is also increased. Therefore, even if you do not smoke now, if you have ever smoked, particularly when you were a teenager or young adult, you especially need to follow the screening recommendations given above. To help you quit smoking, see the guidelines in Chapter 2.

Alcohol use gives you three times the risk for a polyp, when compared to a nondrinker. Combined smoking and alcohol use have been found to make you twelve times more likely to develop colonic polyps.[41]

Conventional Medicine Approach to Colon Polyps

All adenoma polyps identified through sigmoidoscopy or colonoscopy should be removed through the scope, as discussed on page 417. Available evidence strongly suggests that eliminating these polyps prevents future cancers.[42] In addition, studies have shown that people who are regularly screened for polyps—with removal of any of the adenoma variety found—have a decreased incidence of death from colorectal cancer compared to those who do not have these procedures.[43] If you have had a polyp removed, you should be closely followed: The National Polyp Study reported a 58 to 87 percent reduced incidence of death by regular follow-up screening colonoscopy.[44]

Surgical Approaches to Colonic Polyps

If you have polyps larger than one-half inch that cannot be taken out safely through the scope, they must be biopsied and closely followed, or else surgically removed. Two approaches are available to surgically remove a polyp that may be benign.

Colotomy with Polyp Excision

In the colotomy procedure, your surgeon opens your bowel, removes the polyp with a small area of surrounding normal bowel wall, and simply closes the incision. During the operation, the excised specimen is examined by the pathologist to ensure the polyp is benign. If it is malignant, a standard colectomy for cancer is then performed, while you are still on the operating table.

Colectomy

This procedure should be chosen whenever it is likely your polyp is malignant, based on its appearance as seen through the scope, even if your initial biopsies were benign. A standard cancer colectomy with lymph node drainage area is performed. (For a discussion of partial colectomy, see page 430.)

COLON POLYPS SUMMARY

Prevention

Diet and Supplements

- Follow a high-fiber, low-fat diet.
- Keep your cholesterol below 170.
- Calcium 1,200 mg daily.
- Vitamin C, 2,000–3,000 mg daily.
- Vitamin A, 10,000 IU daily (with supervision).
- Vitamin E, D-alpha, 400 IU 2–3 times daily.
- Avoid alcohol.

Lifestyle

- Avoid tobacco.

Alternative Medicine Approaches

- Follow the preventive guidelines, above.
- Vitamin C, 2,000–3,000 mg daily.
- Vitamin E, 400 IU, 3 times daily.
- Practice visualization.

Conventional Medicine Approach

- Colonoscopic polypectomy.

Surgical Approaches

- Colotomy with polyp excision.
- Colectomy.

Colorectal Cancer

Margaret, a 44-year-old woman, had a father, two uncles, sister, and brother who developed colon cancer. Her own cancer, in the right colon, was found and removed at age 41. She then moved to Seattle, where, years later, screening colonoscopy found another cancer in her left colon. It was then removed, along with the rest of her colon. Her two daughters, ages 20 and 24, were then screened by colonoscopy.

One in seventeen Americans (6 percent) develops cancer of the colon or rectum, and 40 percent of those so diagnosed die from it. It is thus responsible for 10 percent of all cancer deaths, making it second only to lung cancer in its lethal effects. Incidence rates have declined in the 1990s, probably because of increased screening and colon polyp removal. An estimated 148,300 new cases will be diagnosed in 2002 and there will be 56,600 deaths.[45] *You can take action to lower your risk for this cancer, and prevent recurrence once disease develops.*

Diet and heredity are the two major factors known to play a role in the cause of this cancer. Our Western diet, high in animal fat and low in fiber, is the nutritional profile for population groups with a high incidence of colorectal cancer. Consumption of beef and other red meats is especially correlated. Inadequate intake of fruits and vegetables also plays a role. Smoking, particularly at an early age, increases your risk—and the more you smoke, the higher your jeopardy. Unlike with most other cancers, this risk stays with you even after you stop smoking.[46] However, even though increased risk remains after you stop, your risk decreases with each successive year.[47]

If you have a close family member with colon cancer, you have a 10 to 20 percent lifetime risk, which becomes even higher if your relative developed the cancer before age 55. Twenty percent of all patients with colon cancer have this familial incidence, accompanied by a tendency for cancer at an earlier age, and for multiple tumors. Because family members are exposed to similar dietary and other environmental factors as well as sharing genes, it is hard to determine the relative importance of each component in causing this cancer.

Other factors increasing your risk include a history of ulcerative colitis or Crohn's disease, colonic adenoma polyps, and breast, uterine, or ovarian cancer. Physical inactivity may contribute.

Your prognosis is directly related to the stage or extent of your disease when it is found. (See Table 15.1.) If your tumor is discovered through screening tests, before symptoms develop, the cure rate is twice as high than if you are treated after symptoms appear. *The key, then, is to be diagnosed and treated before you have symptoms.*

Review the American Cancer Society screening recommendations for early diagno-

TABLE 15.1.
Prognosis of Colorectal Cancer[50]

	Percent of Patients Surviving 5 Years	Percent of Patients in This Stage
All patients	61.1% (55.0% 10 yr.)	
Not staged	34.8%	6%
By stage		
Localized to colorectum	89.7%	37%
Lymph node spread	64.4%	38%
Distant spread	8.3%	20%

sis of diseases of the colon and rectum on page 418. Thirty percent of all North Americans over the age of 60 have polyps, and 5 percent of these polyps are malignant. It is very important to follow recommendations to find this very common cancer at an early stage. Most such cancers are felt to arise from previously benign polyps. If these can be diagnosed and removed through a sigmoidoscope or colonoscope, it may save you from ever developing a cancer or needing an operation. An 85 percent decrease in lower colon and rectal cancer incidence was found in a twenty-five-year study where 18,000 patients underwent annual sigmoidoscopy and removal of polyps, when present.[48] Another report from the National Polyp Study found a decreased death rate from colorectal cancer when screening with polyp removal was performed.[49]

Colorectal cancers are typically slow-growing, with tumor size doubling every two years. Thus, you may have had this cancer for several years before you feel any symptoms. If discovered during this asymptomatic phase, most tumors are still localized to the bowel, and can be cured by surgery.

Once symptoms do appear, about 50 to 70 percent of the time the cancer has spread to lymph nodes, and about 15 percent of the time to the liver or beyond. If all colorectal cancers are considered, at least 56 percent have spread by the time treatment is instituted, and the overall survival is 61 percent at five years and 51 percent at ten years.

Early symptoms of colorectal cancer may be quite subtle: dull aching pain (the most common symptom) is present in 50 percent. You may also experience abdominal distention (swelling), a change in bowel habits with episodes of constipation or diarrhea or both, a sense of incomplete emptying of the bowel, narrowing of the stool, loss of appetite, and/or unexplained weight loss. Blood in the stool can be detected in only about 60 percent of all cases. In 30 percent, visible bleeding is the first signal of colon cancer. If you see blood in your stools, even if thought to be due to hemorrhoids, you should have a flexible sigmoidoscopy. If this test doesn't pinpoint the source of bleeding, you should have a full colonoscopy evaluation, since a significant chance exists of the cause being a cancer or polyp.

About 10 to 15 percent of the time, your tumor can be felt on rectal exam. Sixty percent can be seen on flexible sigmoidoscopy; colonoscopy finds almost 100 percent.

Alternative Medicine Approaches to Colorectal Cancer

Diane, *a 43-year-old attorney, had a strong family history of colon cancer. She was still shocked when, during her yearly physical exam, her doctor discovered an early rectal cancer. Fortunately, it could all be surgically removed, and her bowel reconnected, which allowed her to avoid a colostomy. Then she changed her diet, to a low-fat, high-fiber vegetarian one, and instituted the supplements and stress reduction program described in Chapter 2. She continued to be regularly screened by follow-up blood tests and colonoscopies, and was doing well five years later, with no further sign of cancer. Diane made certain all her other family members also received regular screening, as well.*

Fortunately, alternative medicine approaches give much hope for both preventing colon and rectal cancer, and helping prevent its recurrence. If you already have a tumor, you need to first have it surgically removed. However, changing your diet and taking some other alternative measures may help you avoid its return. Following are the most important alternative medicine measures to help prevent and treat colorectal cancer.

Change Your Diet; Especially Avoid Beef

"The prospect of using diet to prevent cancer recurrence looks pretty favorable," stated Dr. Frank L Meyshens Jr., director of the cancer center at the University of California at Irvine.[51] For both prevention and treatment, follow the guidelines for a basic good low-fat, high-fiber diet, given in Chapter 2. The strong association between high-fat, low-fiber diet and cancer of the colon and rectum has been well established. The amount of *beef* you eat is particularly associated with colorectal cancer. Highest consumption of beef is found in northern Scotland, which has the highest colorectal cancer rate in the world; Australia has the second highest per capita intake of beef, with the second highest incidence; and the United States is third in the world for both beef intake and rates of this cancer.

As the Japanese population, traditionally with low risk, is now eating more steaks and burgers, their colorectal cancer rate is increasing. One study found that your risk of colon cancer is four times higher if you are male and eat beef daily, and 2.5 times higher if you are female and go for the hamburgers every day.[52] The Nurses' Health Study also found that the group of women with the highest animal fat intake had two and one-half times the risk of developing colon cancer compared to those with the lowest intake.[53]

Diet is an important regulator of cholesterol levels, bile acid production, and the types of bacteria that live in the colon. Evidence suggests that factors in the breakdown products of bile, acted on by normal colon bacteria, may play a role in the development of this cancer; these are proven carcinogens in laboratory animals. The concentration of such substances in the stool is highest in colorectal cancer patients and groups that eat the typical Western diet.

In our culture, white flour is everywhere: bagels, pizza, bread sticks, croissants, doughnuts, pancakes—the list goes on and on. However, taking in such carbohydrates without any fiber places your colon and rectum at risk. Research indicates that with our usual slow intestinal transit and small stools, relatively prolonged contact of relatively more concentrated carcinogens with the bowel lining cells occurs.[54] Dietary fiber increases stool volume, dilutes potential carcinogens, and speeds transit time, thereby exerting a protective effect.[55]

Although two recent studies[56,57] haven't found a relationship between dietary fiber and colorectal adenomas (the precursors of most large bowel cancers), these trials followed patients for only three or four years, a period that may be much too short to demonstrate an effect. Also, there are questions as to whether the study participants actually complied with their recommended diet and whether the dietary changes were sufficient to make a difference. The preponderance of prior studies has found a protective effect. In a study from Finland, a high-fiber diet decreased the concentration of stool carcinogens and lowered colorectal cancer risk, despite this population's high fat intake.[58] A University of Toronto combined analysis of thirteen studies looked at the effects of dietary fiber on colorectal cancer incidence. Individuals eating an average of 31 gms of fiber per day had half the incidence of colorectal cancer as those eating only 10 grams per day. The researchers concluded that in the U.S. population, an increase in dietary fiber intake of 13 grams per day (a 70 percent increase) could decrease the colorectal cancer incidence by 31 percent, or 50,000 cases annually.[59]

Therefore, we Americans, with our stools one-third the size and transit times twice as long as low-risk native Africans eating an unrefined, high-fiber vegetarian diet, put ourselves at unnecessary risk. In contrast to Africans, African-Americans, whose diet typically includes less than one-half the fiber of the already high-risk white American diet, have an even higher risk for colorectal cancer than do white Americans, before age 70.[60] Insist on whole grains for all your breads and pastries, and add supplemental fiber to your diet.

A high-fiber, low-animal-fat diet may also be protective in other ways. Serum cholesterol and its breakdown products in the bile are decreased. The bacterial types are changed, with an increase in the relative amounts of oxygen-requiring versus non-oxygen-requiring bacteria; the former are known to be associated with *decreased* cancer risk.

Adding nonfat plain yogurt to your daily diet may be helpful. It gives you the additional benefit of optimum colonic organisms, because it contains lactobacillus acidophilus bacteria to replace more harmful types. Yogurt also changes the stool's acid-base balance, reducing bacterial enzyme activity that creates carcinogens.[61]

Both total fat intake and total calorie intake are associated with a higher risk for colorectal cancer, so you will need to become aware of what foods you choose with reference to these factors. Since so many fat-free alternatives are now available at the super-

markets, avoiding fats has become much easier. You will also need to be aware of avoiding excess calorie intake, especially since refined sugar, which decreases immune protection, is so often added to fat-free items to increase their taste. Choose a fat-free, sugar-free bran muffin or cereal.

If you already have colon or rectal cancer, you should also switch to a high-fiber diet. In initial research, addition of 13.5 grams of fiber to the daily diet of colon cancer patients after removal of their tumors slowed growth of colon cells, felt to help prevent future cancers.[62] Further research is needed on the results of this diet when thus used as an adjunct to therapy.

Eat Fruits and Vegetables

A diet high in fruits and vegetables has consistently been shown to be associated with a lower risk for a number of cancers, colorectal included.[63] You may be able to reduce your risk of this cancer by simply making certain to eat five servings of each of these elements per day.

Naturally occuring carotenes, vitamins C and E, selenium, flavonoids, rutin, quercetin, myricetin, lutein, lycopene, limonene, and other citrus flavones, found in citrus fruits, along with the fiber found in these foods are some of the number of elements now felt to be responsible for this effect, by their differing effects upon the immune system, their antioxidant effects, or their ability to help the body ward off the bad effects of environmental influences.

Limit Sugar Intake

Sugar consumption has consistently been linked to the risk of colorectal cancer, specifically in a dose-response fashion.[64] The exact mechanism of this correlation is as yet unknown, although refined sugars, by raising the blood sugar even in normal individuals, may interfere with white cell activity, which is necessary to both prevent polyps formation and defend against irregular cell formation. Further research is needed.

You can substitute whole fresh fruit for refined sweets; see Chapter 2 for further dietary details and suggestions for how to accomplish this goal.

Add Garlic to Your Diet

Three grams of garlic per day (about one clove, either raw or cooked) seems to protect against colorectal cancer. At the 1999 annual meeting of the American Association for Cancer Research in Philadelphia, Aaron Fleischauer reported a meta-analysis of eight epidemiological studies looking at garlic intake and colorectal cancer. A 30 percent reduction in colon cancer was found among populations that ate garlic-rich diets, when compared to those with little garlic intake.

Take Supplements

Given the strong evidence for progression of colon polyps to cancer, take supplements shown to prevent polyps: calcium, 1,200 mg per day; vitamin A, 5,000 IU per day; and vitamin E, 400 IU per day. Colorectal cancer patients have been specifically found to have a lower intake of vitamin E.[65] Colon cancer risk has been shown to be decreased in men taking supplemental vitamin D and calcium.[66]

A correlation between colorectal cancer and a deficiency of the mineral selenium has been reported.[67] The highest colon cancer incidence is in the Northeastern United States, where the soil is deficient in this mineral. In the Western United States, where selenium is plentiful, rates are one-third lower. Experiments with animals and epidemiological studies have shown that selenium has a specific protective effect against the development of colon cancer.[68] The recommended dosage is 200 mcg daily.

Add 500 mg of magnesium and one dropperful of phosphorus liquid daily, to assure adequate intake of these nutrients.

Quit Smoking

Carcinogens inhaled in smoke or ingested in saliva reach the bowel lining cells by the bloodstream and directly through the intestine. The same risk holds true for cigarette, cigar, and pipe smokers. The earlier you started, the increased number of years, and the more you have smoked, the higher your risk. If you smoked more than thirty-five years ago, even if you subsequently stopped, you are twice as likely as a never-smoker to develop colon and rectal cancer. Women smokers are 40 percent more likely to die from colorectal cancer than those who have never smoked and men have a 30 percent higher risk. It has been estimated that smoking is responsible for 15 percent of all deaths from colorectal cancers in the United States.[69] The good news is that if you stop smoking now, your risk will decrease with each succeeding year.

Avoid Alcohol

Colon cancer patients have also been found to have a higher intake of alcohol.[70] Beer has been especially linked to rectal cancer.[71] See Chapter 2 for guidelines to quit for good.

Exercise Regularly

A recent study from the surgeon general analyzed twenty-nine studies looking at the relationship between colon cancer and physical activity. It concluded that "the research on occupational and leisure-time or total physical activity strongly suggests that physical activity has a protective effect against the risk of developing colon cancer."[72] Men who work at sedentary jobs have a 60 percent higher risk for this cancer compared with those whose jobs require a high level of activity.[73] If you, like most of us, have a sedentary job, you can reduce your risk by daily exercise. See Chapter 2 for help in establishing a regular exercise regime.

Practice Visualization

Try exercises such as the following: Imagine that any cancer cells within your body are weak and small, and striped. The white cells of your immune system are strong and vigilant. They carry special sensors that can locate any striped cells, which they—like Pac-Man—then chew up and swallow. Scan through your body to make certain no striped cells are left, and leave many white cells in place to prevent their return.

Conventional Medicine Approaches to Colorectal Cancer

Along with the preventive measures just discussed, the following medications can be added to further reduce your risk.

Aspirin Therapy

A study from Harvard Medical School found that taking two or more aspirin per week for twenty years reduces the risk of colon cancer by 44 percent in women.[74] Another showed a 32 percent reduction in colorectal cancer in men taking aspirin two or more times per week.[75] Aspirin may stop the growth of polyps, which can slowly enlarge and become malignant. Another prospective study of more than 600,000 men and women taking low-dose aspirin sixteen or more times per month demonstrated a 50 percent lower death rate from colon cancer.[76]

Hormone Replacement Therapy

HRT may reduce the risk of colon cancer. A meta-analysis of studies addressing the association of HRT with the risk of developing or dying from colorectal cancer found a 33 percent decreased risk of developing and 28 percent decreased risk of dying from colon cancer. There was no association with rectal cancer. Protection was limited to recent users, taking HRT at the time of the study or within the previous year.[77]

Radiotherapy in Combination with Surgery

In two instances, radiotherapy may be recommended along with surgery. First, if your tumor appears large and fixed to adjacent tissues, so that removal is anticipated to be difficult and dangerous, *preoperative* radiotherapy may shrink it, making it easier to remove. This is especially true for rectal cancer, and may help you avoid a colostomy. In some cases, radiation may also destroy tumor spread to lymph glands. If after initial evaluation, eventual radiation need is anticipated, it causes fewer complications when given preoperatively. There is a growing trend toward preoperative treatment even in smaller rectal tumors. A meta-analysis of studies looking at the effect of preoperative radiotherapy on rectal cancer reported in the *Journal of the American Medical Association* in 2000 found a 29 percent reduction in cancer-related mortality and a 51 percent decrease in local recurrence.[78] Many authorities now consider this "standard of care" that should be given to every patient with rectal cancer.

Second, in rectal cancer, if the pathology specimen taken during surgery shows tumor invading through the rectal wall or spreading to your lymph glands, *postoperative* radiation has been shown to decrease the possibility the tumor will recur in your pelvis. It may also increase your overall chances for surgical cure.

Chemotherapy in Combination with Surgery

Reports indicate that chemotherapy given after surgery may increase your chance for cure by up to 33 percent if your tumor has spread to your lymph nodes. This treatment may also be recommended, although the benefit is less clear, if your tumor has invaded the full thickness of your bowel wall, but not yet spread to lymph nodes.[79] A combination of both chemotherapy and radiation therapy may also improve your survival if you have a rectal tumor.

Surgical Approaches to Colorectal Cancer

Turner, a 54-year-old, 350-pound man, underwent removal of his rectum and anus, along with the creation of a permanent colostomy, for treatment of the largest colorectal cancer I had ever seen. Fortunately, although it was the size of a cantaloupe, the tumor had grown inward into the center of his rectum, rather than outward through the wall, and no spread appeared in his lymph nodes or elsewhere. Four years later, he remained cancer-free.

Surgery, the treatment of choice for colorectal cancer, offers you techniques that are the product of many decades of careful study. More people than ever before are surviving these operations, thanks to better operative and postoperative monitoring, control of co-existing medical problems, and understanding of your body's response to this specific surgical stress.

In up to 95 percent of all patients, colorectal tumors can be surgically removed, and 85 percent of the time you can be operated on "for cure," meaning that your surgeon removes all visible disease, along with your adjacent lymph node drainage system. Such an operation removes any cancer that may have spread locally, and also provides information to "stage" your disease, to help decide whether or not postoperative chemotherapy and/or radiotherapy is recommended.

However, surgery has gone about as far as it can go, curing this cancer in about 50 percent of all patients, with no further technical breakthroughs anticipated. The most important factor in determining your cure rate is not the surgery itself, but the extent to which your tumor has invaded and spread at the time of your operation.

As with many other operations, results of rectal cancer surgery are best with surgeons who have been specially trained, or do a higher volume of these operations.[80] The unfortunate problem of local tumor recurrence after a "curative" rectal cancer removal can be dramatically reduced from more than 25 percent to less than 5 percent by the use of a "total meso-rectal" excision technique, developed by colorectal surgeons.[81]

If your tumor has spread so that a cure cannot be anticipated, removal of the tumor is still advisable. This avoids eventual problems of obstruction, bleeding, and pain, and ensures the best possible quality of your remaining lifetime.

Following are the operative procedures used to remove colon cancer, depending on its exact location.

Partial Colectomy

This is the most common operation for colon cancer; the tumor and some normal colon on both sides of it are excised. The veins and lymph nodes draining this part of the bowel are also taken, to look for and remove cancer that might have spread there. Usually, one-fourth to one-third of your colon is taken out. In most cases, your operation can be performed without need for a colostomy. (For a discussion of partial colectomy, see page 430.)

Low Anterior Resection

If your tumor is in the upper two-thirds of your rectum, it can usually be removed along with the distant part of your colon, the two ends then sewn or stapled together, similar to partial colectomy. Some tumors in the lower third may also be removed this way. Preoperative X-ray treatment may increase your chances for a successful operation if your tumor is locally advanced. (For a discussion of low anterior resection, see page 444.)

Abdominal Perineal Resection with Colostomy

If your tumor is within one to two inches of the anal opening, your anus and rectum usually must be removed and a permanent colostomy created. If you do have such a low-lying rectal cancer, however, you may have three other options: local excision through your anus, radiotherapy, or a combination of the two. These procedures treat tumor in your bowel wall, but cannot access or treat cancer that may have spread to your lymph glands or elsewhere. (For a discussion of abdominal perineal resection with colostomy, see page 444.)

Local Excision

If you have a rectal cancer, and if you are elderly, have incurable disease, are not suitable for surgery, or might have trouble dealing with a colostomy, local treatment may be your best choice. Even without these constraints, it may also be reasonable to request local excision if your rectal tumor is small. Statistically, if the tumor does not invade through the full thickness of the rectal wall and its cells do not have poor prognostic characteristics, you have only a 12 to 22 percent probability of having it already spread to your lymph glands.[82] Local treatment, therefore, may be adequate. If your tumor is more than five inches from the anal opening, however, the possibility of surgical perforation into your abdominal cavity makes local excision dangerous. If your cancer is larger than two inches or involves more than one-half the rectal circumference, local excision is also not advised. Intrarectal ultrasound and magnetic resonance imaging (MRI) techniques are being developed, and may turn out to be the best way to determine whether you are a good candidate for local excision.

Pre- or postoperative radiation can be added to increase your chance for cure if your tumor is shown to have invaded into the bowel muscle. Radiation therapy uses an external beam or an X-ray source placed within your rectum next to your tumor.

In a 1990 analysis of sixteen studies of local excision published in the medical literature, the local recurrence of the tumor was 19 percent and the cancer-free five-year survival was 89 percent. If local excision was unsuccessful, later additional surgery then cured 56 percent of these cases.[83] In comparison, for similar cases of rectal cancer confined to the rectal wall, five-year survival for the more standard abdominoperineal resection is 85 to 98 percent.

Complications and side effects of local removal are only about 1 percent. This is much less than abdominoperineal resection, and a permanent colostomy is avoided. A local procedure may even be performed on an outpatient basis. (For a discussion of local excision, see page 448.)

Colorectal Cancer Follow-up

You should have careful follow-up after your surgery. As many as 50 percent of all patients with colorectal tumors treated for surgical cure develop a recurrence. Most such reappearances become evident within the first two to three years. After five years, the return of the tumor is unlikely, and you can be considered cured. However, your chance of developing another colorectal cancer in your lifetime is about 5 percent, so you should have another colonoscopy one year postoperatively, then every three to five years thereafter.

A blood test called the CarcinoEmbryonic Antigen (CEA) has been shown to be useful in some patients, as an early indicator of recurrent colorectal cancer. If your CEA level is normal postoperatively, and then begins to rise, it suggests your tumor has returned. Sixty percent of such rises are detected before symptoms develop. Although the exact method of postoperative testing in terms of blood tests, scans, and X-rays is controversial, you should probably at least have your CEA checked every three or four months for the first two years.

If such testing shows only "limited" recurrent tumor in your liver or lungs, or near the site of the original cancer, it may be worthwhile to have this tumor surgically removed, when it is possible to do so. A recent study of 1,247 patients with colon cancer found that 44 percent developed recurrence, and 41 percent of these patients had only limited disease, qualifying them for a second operation. At surgery, all known tumor deposits could be removed in 75 percent, if the recurrence had been detected before symptoms occurred, compared with only 30 percent if the tumor was detected only after symptoms developed. Whenever all known tumor could be removed, 35 percent of these patients were still alive after five years.[84]

If you have symptoms of recurrent colorectal cancer that has already spread beyond the chance for surgical cure, it may still be useful to have "palliative" surgery, chemotherapy, or radiotherapy to at least temporarily relieve your symptoms.

COLORECTAL CANCER SUMMARY

Prevention

Diet and Supplements

- Follow a low-fat, high-fiber diet.
- Eat fruit and vegetables.
- Avoid beef.
- Take garlic, one clove raw or cooked, daily.
- Limit sugar intake.

- Eat bran, 3 tablespoons daily.
- Psyllium, 1–3 tablespoons daily.
- Calcium, 1,200 mg daily.
- Vitamin A, 5,000 IU daily.
- Vitamin C, 1,000–2,000 mg, 2–3 times daily.
- Vitamin E, D-alpha, 400 IU daily.
- Vitamin D, 400 IU daily.
- Selenium, 200 mcg daily.
- Magnesium, 500 mg daily.
- Phosphorus liquid, one dropperful daily.

Lifestyle

- Follow screening guidelines for blood in stool, sigmoidoscopy, colonoscopy, barium enema.
- Don't smoke.
- Avoid alcohol.
- Exercise 1 hour, 3–5 times weekly.
- Utilize daily yoga postures, especially the inverted poses.

Alternative Medicine Approaches

- Follow the preventive guidelines, above.
- Practice visualization.
- Join a weekly support group.

Conventional Medicine Approaches

Prevention

- Aspirin therapy.
- Estrogen replacement therapy.

Treatment

- Radiotherapy.
- Chemotherapy.

Surgical Approaches

- Partial colectomy.
- Low anterior resection.
- Abdominoperineal resection and colostomy.
- Local excision.

Colon Operations

Prior to elective surgery, your colon must be cleaned out for the operation. A liquid diet for two to three days, along with enemas and a strong laxative such as magnesium citrate or sulfate, removes feces and diminishes the number of bacteria. A combination of antibiotics effective against most of the bowel bacteria is taken by mouth the day before your operation. This is necessary because, while these organisms are a normal part of the colon, they can cause serious infection if they invade the rest of the abdominal cavity or contaminate the incision. All of these preparatory measures act together to reduce your risk for postsurgical infection to less than 10 percent.

The Go-Lightly prep is another common bowel preparation method. On the day before your operation, you drink three to four quarts of a nonabsorbable solution, until your output into the toilet is clear. Complete cleansing is accomplished in two to four hours. This is a very efficient method, though many people cannot force themselves to drink the unpleasant mixture, and it can only be used if you are in fairly good health, without bowel obstruction.

You are admitted to the hospital the morning of surgery. A small epidural catheter may be placed in your back, to enable easy administration of postoperative pain medication.

General anesthesia is almost always used

in colon surgery. After you are anesthetized, a breathing tube is placed into your windpipe and a catheter into your bladder. You may also have a nasogastric tube through your nose into your stomach. Usually, your incision is made from midway in your upper abdomen to just above your pubic bone, depending on which part of your colon needs to be removed.

Following are the operations that are performed for the different colorectal diseases discussed in this chapter.

Partial Colectomy and Low Anterior Resection

Partial colectomy, or *colon resection,* is the most common colon operation. It is used for cancer, Crohn's disease, infections, obstructions, and bleeding or gangrene from insufficient blood supply. *Low anterior resection* is quite similar, except that part of the upper rectum is also removed; it is chosen for colon cancer or large benign polyps. If these procedures are performed on an emergency basis, or if technical difficulty is present, you may also need a temporary colostomy (see page 446).

After you are on the operating table and asleep under general anesthesia, an up-and-down, six- to ten inch incision is made from your mid-upper to lower abdomen. Your diseased colon or rectal segment is then removed. (See Figure 15.3.) If you have cancer, your bowel's veins and lymph node drainage tissue also must be removed. The cut ends of your normal bowel are connected by one or two layers of stitches or staples.

A nasogastric tube may be left in place for three to five days, to prevent stomach dilation, abdominal distention, and vomiting,

until your bowel activity returns. Most surgeons do not use routine nasogastric tubes, placing them only postoperatively when necessary. A tube in your bladder monitors urinary output, helping with fluid replacement and preventing bladder overdistention. If you are debilitated, you may be given liquid nutritional support through a special "hyperalimentation" intravenous line (see page 132). If your abdomen contained infection or was contaminated by stool during the operation, the strong "fascia" inner layer of your abdominal wall incision will be closed with stitches, but your skin may be left open, to reduce the risk of incision infection. The skin may then either be closed a few days later with skin tapes, or left to heal on its own.

You should be able to resume oral intake by the second to fifth postoperative day, and go home by the fifth to tenth day. Your bowel movements may be looser and more frequent for the first few weeks or months, depending on how much and which part of your bowel was removed. If the majority of your colon remains, your stool eventually regains its usual texture. If most of your colon had to be removed, your stool will usually stay soft, and your bowel movements become more frequent. In general, as time passes, your remaining colon will take over the water absorption and fecal storage functions of the portion removed, and your stool will return to normal.

Abdominal Perineal Resection with Colostomy and Proctocolectomy with Ileostomy

Abdominal perineal resection is performed for rectal cancers located very near the anal opening. After you are anesthetized, an up-and-down incision is made from just above

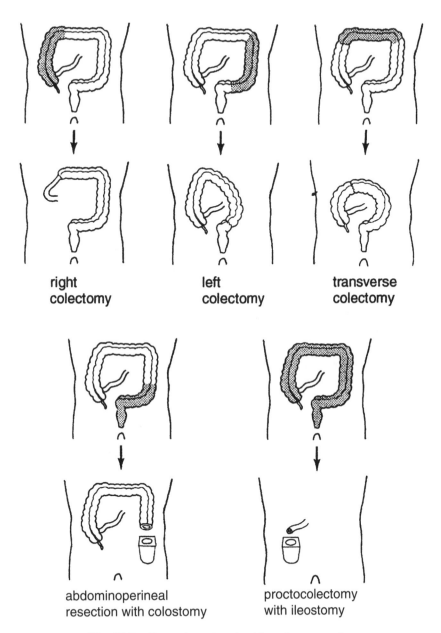

right
colectomy

left
colectomy

transverse
colectomy

abdominoperineal
resection with colostomy

proctocolectomy
with ileostomy

Fig. 15.3 Procedures involved in colon operations

your umbilicus to the pubic region, with a second elliptical incision around your anus. Your rectum and anus are removed, along with local blood vessels and lymph gland tissue. A permanent colostomy (see below) is made, usually using the left side of your colon. You awaken with a plastic bag (referred to as a "stoma" appliance), fastened over your bowel where it emerges from your abdominal wall. The anal incision is closed with stitches. One or two drains may be left for five to ten days, and a bladder catheter for four to seven days. You should be able to eat in three or four days, and be discharged home after six to ten days.

Total proctocolectomy removes all of your colon, rectum, and anus, and creates a permanent ileostomy, an opening of the small bowel onto the skin (see page 447). It is usually performed if you have inflammatory bowel disease, or *a polyposis syndrome,* in which you have numerous premalignant polyps. The incisions and pre- and postoperative course are similar to that of abdominal perineal resection, except that the ileostomy is usually placed in the right lower abdominal wall.

If performed electively, these are relatively safe operations. They have a mortality rate under 1.5 percent, a 10 percent chance of incision infection, and a 5 to 10 percent rate of incision healing problems.

Since nerves affecting your bladder and sexual function lie in the area of these operations, you may experience temporary or permanent dysfunction postoperatively. Problems with urination are quite common, although they usually clear up within a week or two. Rarely, male patients require a prostatectomy, (see page 576), to relieve bladder outlet obstruction. Problems with urinary continence

occur in 5 to 10 percent of all patients after cancer surgery.

Five percent of the men who undergo this type of surgery for benign rectal disease, and fifty percent of those with rectal cancer, experience retrograde ejaculation—discharge of ejaculate into the bladder rather than out the penis. Inability to achieve erection, seen in 5 to 20 percent of the cancer patients, is rare in those with benign disease. In women who have undergone these operations, bladder problems are extremely rare, inability to achieve orgasm is unusual, but painful intercourse may persist. The ultimate determining factor in sexual function may be more your libido (sex drive) than the physical effects of the surgery.

Colostomy

A *colostomy* is a temporary or permanent opening of your bowel onto your abdominal wall, through which stool is eliminated. A permanent colostomy is required whenever your anus and rectum are removed. Temporary colostomies may be performed if you have bowel obstruction, perforation, or trauma. Removal of a temporary colostomy and reconnection of your bowel ends is usually done one to four months after the temporary procedure.

After treating the underlying colorectal disease, your surgeon removes a circle of skin one inch in diameter, from your abdominal wall. The exact site is carefully chosen to be away from scars and skin creases, which could interfere with the sealing of the colostomy bag. Also, it is important that you can see the opening and reach it easily for postoperative management. Most often, the site chosen is in the lower left part of your abdomen, just above or below the belt line. Other positions can work just as well.

When you awake from surgery, you have a temporary plastic appliance covering the bowel opening or "stoma," to collect intestinal contents. Postoperatively, your exposed bowel is swollen, but it eventually shrinks to a permanent size of about one inch in diameter. The external surface has no sensation. The colostomy is usually elevated above your skin surface, to ensure a snug fit so the appliance will not leak onto your abdominal wall. A special belt may be used to hold this appliance in place. Its contents can be emptied by opening the closed-off end, or a snap-away bag used, which can be changed completely. While in the hospital, an "enterostomy" nurse instructs you in how to care for it.

New plastics, adhesives, and mechanics have made for more reliable, odorless, and smoothly functioning colostomy appliance systems. The cost of the materials is about $2 to $3 per day. Skin problems are fairly common at the site, but these usually heal. Obesity and chronically increased abdominal pressure, especially in those who do heavy lifting or have a chronic cough, increase the complication rate. In 5 percent of all colostomies, surgical revision is necessary because of poor blood supply, retraction under the skin surface, or scarring that narrows the opening.

After healing is complete, you can choose one of two methods to manage your colostomy, depending on your lifestyle and wishes. The simplest is to just allow it to empty freely into the colostomy appliance, worn at all times. Or you can irrigate at regular intervals, thereby establishing a regular bowel-emptying pattern. Then you do not need to wear the appliance, merely covering the stoma with a piece of gauze between irrigations. This second method requires forty-five to sixty minutes of bathroom time each day (or every other day in some patients), as well as some manual dexterity. Using an irrigating bag and nozzle, one to two pints of warm water is infused, stimulating colon contractions and emptying. Your stool then runs through a funnel into the toilet. Infusions may have to be done two or three times, with periods of waiting in between, before the colon is fully emptied. Most irrigators are quite successful and happy with this latter technique.

After a few months, most patients accept their colostomy, and develop a smoothly functioning routine to care for it. They recognize it is, in fact, lifesaving, or is providing relief from previously lifestyle-limiting symptoms. Ostomy clubs, composed of patients with colostomies or ileostomies, can help you with the necessary technical advice, as well as provide important psychological support. Participation is highly recommended. The American Cancer Society has a program for patients with permanent colostomies. See the Resources section of this book for information about this and other choices for assistance.

Ileostomy

After your entire colon and rectum have been removed for treatment of colitis, multiple polyps, or cancers, an *ileostomy* is created from the last part of your ileum or small bowel. The opening is usually placed in your right lower abdomen, above or below your belt line. The procedure is similar to a colostomy, except that an ileostomy must be devised to protrude an inch or so above the skin surface, to ensure a snug fit of the bag. The contents of the intestine at that point are liquid and highly irritative, and would otherwise cause skin problems at the opening. Output is generally continuous, so you must wear an appliance bag, which is periodically drained into the toilet through a stopcock. Ten to twenty percent of all ileostomy patients develop problems with bag fit, narrowing of the opening, or a hernia, which require surgical revision.

An alternative to the standard ileostomy is the *continent ileostomy*, (also called a *Koch pouch)*. Your surgeon uses a portion of intestine to create an internal storage pouch, along with a valve mechanism to prevent continuous drainage. You do not have to wear an appliance, but instead can drain the reservoir several times a day by placing a tube through the valve. A high complication risk, with 20 to 50 percent of these patients requiring surgical revision, means the procedure should be attempted only by surgeons with special training and experience. The ultimate success rate is about 75 percent, but this operation should be chosen only if you are young, a good surgical risk, and do not have Crohn's disease.

Ileoanal Pouch

If you have ulcerative colitis (*not* Crohn's disease) or a multiple colon polyp syndrome, you may choose to save your anal sphincters and avoid an ileostomy by having a "pouch" instead of a proctocolectomy. This procedure is usually performed in two or three stages. Preoperative preparation is similar to that described for colectomy. After you are anesthetized, an eight- to ten-inch up-and-down incision is made from your umbilicus to your pubic bone. The diseased colon and part of the rectum are removed, saving the rectal muscular sphincter mechanism so you can maintain your stool control. A temporary

ileostomy is then created. Usually you can begin to eat two to four days after your operation, and be discharged after five to ten days.

In the second stage, performed a few months later, your incision is reopened and your rectal lining stripped from its underlying muscles; then a storage "pouch" created from your small intestine and sewn to your anal lining. The ileostomy is removed during this stage, or at a later third operation. This procedure maintains your bowel movements in the "normal" manner and still avoids the threat of future colorectal cancer. Generally, you can begin to eat after a few days, and be discharged in five to ten days.

The ileoanal pouch procedure may be difficult, and has a complication rate of 15 percent, mostly from bleeding and infection in the operative area or recurrent episodes of inflammation within the pouch. Careful follow-up and several visits with your surgeon are necessary to ensure satisfactory healing and function. Since your stool will be more semi-solid than solid, you have to defecate several times a day. Dietary restrictions and medications may be necessary for a satisfactory bowel pattern. Continence may be a problem, resulting in a leaky, wet, chronically irritated anus. Decreased fertility has been noted in women.[85] However, quality of life is better than with an ileostomy stoma, and you have a 96 percent chance for a satisfactory outcome.[86]

Local Excision

Local excision, performed through the anus, is the usual treatment for benign polyps of the rectum, and is an alternative to abdominal perineal resection if you have a small cancer low in the rectum. Local excision may also be chosen if you are very ill or elderly, for relief of pain and bleeding when your cancer is beyond curing, or if you refuse to have a permanent colostomy and are willing to assume the risks of a lesser chance of cure.

You are admitted to the hospital on the day of surgery. You can have this operation under general or spinal anesthesia.

You are positioned on your back, with your legs up in stirrups, or on your stomach. A bladder catheter is usually placed after you are anesthetized. Your tumor is carefully removed, along with a full thickness of bowel wall and some surrounding normal tissues; then the defect closed with stitches. In some cases, instead of the tumor being removed with a scalpel, it is destroyed by electrocautery or a laser beam (a procedure called *fulgeration*) in one or more staged treatments. Most likely, you can be discharged the same day, or after a day or two, with little postoperative discomfort.

You need to be followed very closely by your surgeon, who should periodically reexamine the area where the tumor was removed for signs of recurrence.

Laparoscopic Colon Surgery

Colon operations using the laparoscope, or assisted with the laparoscope, are now being pioneered by some surgeons, though they are not yet widely accepted by most, owing to their difficulty, the "learning curve" to become good at them, and with cancer, lack of long-term results to assure that they are as effective as standard surgery. Results have been favorable in terms of smaller incisions, less pain, a shorter hospital stay, and a quicker return to normal activities, but not yet for reduced costs. Preoperative preparation and postoperative follow-up are the same as for standard operations.

Surgeons doing laparoscopically assisted colectomy for diverticular disease have reported results as good as for the standard open procedure.

In laparoscopic surgery for cancer, controversy exists as to whether these methods will provide the same cure rates as for the standard "open" surgery. The main concern is that an "adequate" cancer operation would be more difficult, and that tumor cells could be implanted at the laparoscopic port sites. Initial reports have been encouragingly on a par with the standard operations. However, since the answer won't be known for several years, the standard procedures are still the safest at the present time.

Complications of Bowel Surgery

The overall mortality rate of elective colon surgery is less than 3 percent, and about 6 percent after emergency operations.

Surgical complications of bowel surgery can become evident soon after the operation, may appear later during your hospital stay, or even after you go home. Bleeding within the abdomen or abdominal wall may (rarely) require a return to the operating room. Colostomy or ileostomy problems, related to blood supply or retraction under the skin surface, occasionally need surgical revision within the first few days. If breakdown of the suture line—where the cut ends of the bowel were sewn together—occurs, reoperation may be necessary. This is more likely with a low anterior resection (10 percent). Incision infection, the most common problem, is caused by contamination by bowel bacteria during the operation. Reopening the skin incision, draining the pus, rinsing the area, and changing the dressings are necessary. Intra-abdominal infection or abscesses must be drained through the placement of drainage tubes, placed either through the skin by X-ray or ultrasound guidance or by surgery. Rarely, complete breakdown of the abdominal incision closure occurs. A surgical reclosure is then usually needed.

Bowel obstruction, appearing early or late postoperatively, can be caused by temporary swelling at the bowel reconnection site, twists, or adhesive bands of scar tissue formed after surgery, or narrowing in a segment of bowel with inadequate blood supply. Occasionally, reoperation is necessary.

An incisional hernia develops in about 10 percent of all cases, and may have to be surgically repaired. This problem is discussed in Chapter 18.

CHAPTER 16

APPENDIX

If you're like most people, you probably assume that appendicitis strikes out of the blue, with no provocation. But you'd be assuming wrong.

Mark Bricklin, editor, *Prevention*

An appendicitis attack *can* seem to come out of the blue. If you do develop it, we both agree surgery is your best option for treatment. You should have an operation whenever the diagnosis of appendicitis is a significant possibility. However, newer diagnostic techniques have made its discovery much more precise, helping you avoid the scalpel whenever possible.

In this chapter, we will help you know what to expect and when you should be checked for this disease. By following the dietary recommendations of alternative medicine, you can act to prevent yourself from needing an appendix operation—the most common general surgery you may face. If you do need surgery, you can ask about the laparoscopic method, which can minimize your scar and make your recovery quicker and easier.

Your appendix is a "vestigial" organ. At one time in human evolution it may have been much larger and aided intestinal digestion and absorption. Now that it is smaller, it has no known function, though since it is filled with lymph tissue, it may play an as-yet-undiscovered role in local or distant immune activity.

Like the rest of the digestive tract, your appendix is dependent for its health upon your diet, and optimum choices may help you avoid surgery. Added fiber offers important specific prevention in this area. Even after surgery, you still should make this change in your diet, to prevent problems with other portions of your digestive tract, and the rest of your body as well.

Anatomy of Your Appendix

The appendix appears very innocent, a pink appendage located near the junction of your small and large intestines. (See Figure 16.1.) About the size of your smallest finger, two to five inches in length and one-quarter to one-half inch in diameter, it may be oriented in many different ways, from up behind your ascending colon to dropping down into your pelvis. It has the same sort of lining and muscle layers as your small bowel and colon (see page 413).

Appendicitis

Infection arising in the appendix, termed *appendicitis,* affects 7 percent (one in fifteen) of the U.S. population. It is the most common surgical disease of the abdomen in all age groups. Most of the complications of appendicitis develop if you delay in seeking medical

attention or otherwise do not receive prompt diagnosis and treatment, validating our recommendation for early surgery whenever abdominal complaints and tests are suggestive of appendicitis.

Appendicitis is usually triggered by an obstruction in the cavity of your appendix. Swollen lymph tissue in the appendical wall, stool, debris, ingested foreign material, parasites, or tumor can cause this blockage. As the appendix distends, bacteria overgrow and the resulting increased pressure causes loss of blood flow and eventually gangrene of its wall. In 25 percent of the cases, as time passes and the tissue breaks down completely, dangerous and potentially lethal *perforation* develops. A local *abscess* may form if the process is surrounded and walled off by neighboring tissue, but if not, infection can spread throughout your abdomen. Without any treatment, 5 to 10 percent of patients would die from infection, while almost 100 percent of the others would suffer severe complications.

Appendicitis happens most often in early adulthood, usually between the ages 20 and 30. However, it is also seen in young children

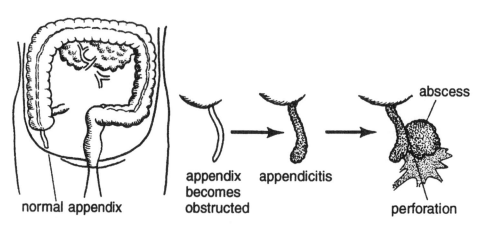

normal appendix · appendix becomes obstructed · appendicitis · abscess · perforation

Fig. 16.1 Normal and diseased appendix

and the elderly, in whom it is particularly dangerous because diagnosis is more difficult and may be delayed. Additionally, in a young child, the neighboring organs and tissues are not very adept at surrounding the appendix to keep the infection localized, making generalized infection more common, so that by the time surgery is performed, the appendix has already freely ruptured in more than 50 percent of cases. In women, particularly young girls, the resulting adhesions or scar tissue from such a perforation can interfere with fallopian tube function, causing infertility.

If you are elderly, your appendicitis may likewise be misdiagnosed and surgery delayed, since your pain may not be well localized or intense, you may have little or no fever or rise in white blood count, and constipation may be your only complaint. Perforation occurs in two-thirds of those with appendicitis over 65 years of age.

How Appendicitis Is Diagnosed

In most people, the symptoms of acute appendicitis usually advance fairly rapidly, and need for medical attention and surgery becomes obvious within twelve to twenty-four hours. Occasionally, the course is more prolonged, though rarely for more than forty-eight to seventy-two hours. It usually initiates a classic chain of symptoms. At first, you feel the pain produced by the distention of your obstructed appendix in the *central* portion of your abdomen. Continuing distention usually next causes loss of appetite, then nausea, and finally vomiting. As local inflammation progresses, and the local sensitive lining of the inside of your abdominal wall is irritated, your discomfort shifts, becoming localized in the *right lower* part of your abdomen.

If your colon or bladder is irritated by the nearby inflammation, diarrhea, pain on urination, or a frequent urge to urinate may follow. Low-grade fever may be present, usually not much higher than 100 degrees, unless you have an abscess or perforation. Movements such as walking, sitting, and tightening your abdominal muscles usually cause pain. Pressure on your right lower abdomen generally causes severe distress and muscle tightening, and sudden release of hand pressure over the irritated area also causes significant discomfort.

Unfortunately, this standard picture of appendicitis develops in only 60 to 70 percent of all cases. You may experience little pain or fever, or you may have severe symptoms with apparently minimal disease. Your surgeon's alertness to and experience with the varied presentation of appendicitis is the key to your getting an early diagnosis, very important to be obtained before perforation occurs.

Although extensive testing is usually unnecessary, time consuming, and may be misleading, the following information is useful in making a correct diagnosis.

History

Your physician will ask a series of questions designed to sort out appendicitis from the several other conditions that can produce a similar picture. You will be asked questions about what you last ate before your symptoms began, the timing and progression of symptoms, and if you've had fever or chills, nausea or vomiting, diarrhea or constipation.

It is important to report if you've ever had any symptoms like this before, your current menstrual period status (could you be pregnant or have just ovulated), and what you may have done to treat yourself. Your physician will need to know about any medical conditions you might have, medicines you normally take, and any prior abdominal operations.

Physical Exam

A nurse will take your *vital signs* (temperature, heart rate, and blood pressure). The doctor will listen to your lungs and heart, and for sounds produced by intestinal movements. You will be put through a series of movements that test for intra-abdominal irritation. Your doctor will press on your abdomen to see if there are signs of inflammation (involuntary tensing of your abdomen in response to pressure and a sharp pain with the sudden release of pressure). Rectal and pelvic exams are usually done, and a stool specimen is checked for blood.

Lab Tests

Blood tests for red and white blood cell counts are necessary. Your white count is usually elevated, but this is a test upon which your doctor cannot rely. A urine analysis is done to check for signs of infection or kidney stone. If you are a woman of child-bearing age, a check for pregnancy is ordinarily required.

X-Rays and Scans

Plain X-rays of the abdomen show abnormal findings in about 50 percent of cases, but in most patients, this test is not specific for appendicitis. With atypical symptoms, or in cases in which other problems such as diverticulitis or ruptured ovarian cyst are likely, a sonogram or CAT scan may help in the diagnosis.

There is a trend for emergency room physicians to order CAT scans on almost everyone with a suspicious history and physical exam for appendicitis, even before calling a surgeon. There is some evidence that making an early diagnosis in positive cases and sending the other patients home can save money for hospitals and avoid unnecessary surgery for patients.[1]

Alternative Medicine Approaches to Appendicitis

We were sitting in the park on a lovely Sunday afternoon, two high school friends enjoying intimate talk time. I watched as Susan, my companion, consumed an entire bag of pistachio nuts, along with a package of cheese and a hot dog, and nothing else. The next day, I heard that she was in the hospital, having just had her appendix urgently taken out.

You can take action, using alternative medicine choices, to help prevent appendicitis. Once you have developed this disorder, however, since the surgery is now quite simple via laparoscopy, you should opt for an operation, to prevent the dangerous complication of rupture. But you can request that your appendix not be removed "incidentally," or "routinely," when no disease is found within it, just because you are having an abdominal procedure for some other problem. The full use of the appendix may yet be discovered, and just in case, you can keep yours in good shape.

Following are the most promising steps you can take to help prevent appendicitis.

Change Your Diet

As noted earlier, appendix removal, the most common general operation in young people in Western cultures, may be almost totally preventable. Intake of dietary fiber has been closely linked to this disease. None of the foods my friend Susan had chosen for lunch contained enough fiber, the portion of plant material that passes easily through the digestive tract.

Consciously selecting a high-fiber, low-fat diet may help you keep your appendix healthy. The combination of fat and not enough fiber—nuts are one of the vegetarian foods relatively higher in fat and lower in fiber—most likely accounted for my friend's precipitant problem.

Foods lacking in fiber—most notably meats, cheeses, and white flour products—have been found to be more apt to block the appendix. A high-fiber, vegetarian diet acts to keep bulk flowing freely through the bowels, so that impaction in your appendix is less likely.

Dr. Denis Burkitt studied the vegetarian population of Kashmir and found that during the course of twenty years, only two cases had occurred.[2]

Avoid Constipation

The subtle constipation associated with appendicitis can be a warning signal. Aim for two to three easy-to-pass daily bowel movements; follow the dietary guidelines in Chapter 2 to achieve this.

If you have developed appendicitis and need surgery, you should still look at your diet and make certain you achieve a fiber intake of five to ten fresh fruits and vegetables daily, along with the equivalent of three tablespoons of bran, either as fat-free, sugar-free muffins, cereal, or whole grain bread.

If you have had to have your appendix removed, you should especially be certain to work up to an intake of 20 to 40 grams of fiber per day.

Take Supplements

If you still suffer from constipation despite a change in diet, you may find relief by adding powdered bran or psyllium seed to your food. Start with a teaspoon, increasing only gradually as needed, and make certain to take extra water along with the additional fiber.

Exercise Regularly

Regular exercise, by encouraging local and systemic blood and lymph flow, can help prevent constipation. Follow the guidelines given in Chapter 2.

Practice Stress Management and Yoga Daily

Stress may play a strong role in bowel function; the fight-or-flight response can cause diarrhea followed by constipation. The regular practice of yoga postures has been shown to relieve constipation from whatever the cause. Follow the guidelines given in Chapter 2.

Conventional Medicine Approaches to Appendicitis

Occasionally, patients first seek medical attention long after the onset of acute appendicitis. This may be because they had an atypical presentation with few early symptoms, they or their doctors think it is just the flu or another problem, they don't have insurance and are worried about hospital costs, or they are far from health resources.

Five to ten days later, by the time the diagnosis is correctly made, they usually have had a perforation with an abscess that is kept localized by being "walled off" or surrounded by neighboring organs and tissues. They usually have pain localized to the lower right area of the abdomen, and a mass is found on physical exam and scans. In this situation, it is more hazardous to operate because the inflammation tends to glue the tissues together, and damage may occur to the surrounding tissues when trying to extract the appendix. If this is your predicament and you are not seriously ill or have an intestinal obstruction, the following course of action is preferable to surgery.

Antibiotics

You will be admitted to the hospital for intravenous antibiotics and close observation. This approach is usually successful, and after a few days, you can be discharged to complete a course of oral antibiotics at home.

Abscess Drainage

If you have a large abscess, antibiotics alone may not be successful. It may be possible for a radiologist to pass a small drainage catheter through the skin to evacuate the abscess. If not, a surgical drainage operation will likely be necessary.

Interval Appendectomy

If you have had appendicitis treated medically, there is a high likelihood that the disorder will occur again. Therefore, your physicians will probably recommend that you have your appendix removed a few months later, after the inflammation resolves. This can ordinarily be done laparoscopically in day surgery.

Surgical Approaches to Appendicitis

Judy, a 25-year-old hairdresser, was awakened at 5 A.M. by pain in the middle of her ab-domen. At first, she simply assumed she was having menstrual cramps a bit early. She did think it unusual when she vomited, and then had no appetite for breakfast. As the hours passed, she felt progressively worse. When the pain shifted to her right lower abdomen and she could not walk comfortably, she went to an emergency room. Since she had experienced previous tubal infections, the ER doctor ordered a sonogram exam, which showed normal tubes, but also revealed a swollen appendix. I was called, and by 6 P.M., Judy had her appendix removed with the use of a laparoscope; she was back to work cutting hair just three days later.

You should understand that when you agree to surgery for suspected appendicitis, you have a chance something else, or even nothing abnormal, may be found. A different problem, which would have required surgery *anyway*, is seen in 15 percent of these cases. Until recently, when operating for acute appendicitis, a surgeon's "legitimate" rate for finding normal appendixes was 15 to 20 percent; though in young women and children, because of other problems that mimic appendicitis, up to 40 percent was acceptable.

However, at the present time, with the use of diagnostic ultrasound and limited CAT scans, the accuracy should be considerably higher. Using CAT scan, a recent study reported in the *New England Journal of Medicine* achieved greater than 95 percent accuracy and reduction in hospital costs.[3]

Still, a surgeon with a 100 percent "positive" rate would be suspected of waiting until the picture was too obvious, thereby delaying surgery, risking gangrene and perforation with potentially devastating complications. Therefore, it is considered much safer for your surgeon to remove some normal appendixes than to risk putting off removal of a diseased one.

Open appendectomy is usually performed under general anesthesia, through a two- to three-inch incision in the right lower part of your abdomen, just above your hip bone. (See Figure 16.2.) You may request the lower, easier-to-hide "bikini" incision, though this may make your operation technically more difficult. If your diagnosis is in doubt, and other problems likely, an up-and-down, midline "exploratory" incision may have to be used.

You may ask for a laparoscopic appendectomy, which uses three or four one-quarter- to three-quarter-inch incisions. Your scars are more pleasing. If difficulties or other problems are encountered, the laparoscopic procedure can always be converted to the "open" method. A recent analysis of seventeen randomized trials comparing the classic open and laparoscopic procedures found an advantage in less postop pain, fewer wound infections, and quicker recovery for the laparoscopic option, though it was more expensive. However, hospital stay and intra-abdominal infection rates were similar.[4]

Laparoscopic appendectomy is most applicable for diagnosis and treatment in patients with atypical histories and findings on physical exam, where problems other than appendicitis can be more easily seen than by the open technique. For example, women with pelvic infections, ruptured ovarian cysts, or tubal pregnancies, which frequently mimic

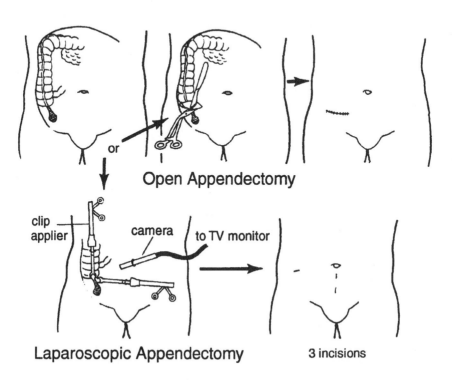

Fig. 16.2 Procedures involved in open and laparoscopic appendectomy

appendicitis, can be diagnosed and treated less invasively. In obese patients, it is easier to examine the whole inside of the abdomen with the laparoscope, and large open incisions can be avoided. Discuss with your surgeon the desirability of this technique for your particular situation.

During the surgery your appendix is removed at its junction with the colon and the "stump" is tied off. The muscles and skin are closed with stitches. A "subcuticular" closure, using dissolving stitches covered with skin tapes, gives the best cosmetic result. If you have developed perforation, as seen in 25 percent of all patients, your abdominal cavity is first irrigated with warm fluid to remove infected material, the muscle layers closed, and your skin left open to prevent infection. Your incision is treated with dressing changes, and can usually be closed with skin tapes three to four days later. If a well-defined abscess is present, you may need drains, brought out through a separate incision, then slowly removed over several days.

You awaken in the OR or the Recovery Room, and shortly can move to your room. An ICU stay is rarely necessary. If your appendicitis is uncomplicated, you should be able to immediately resume a regular diet, and be discharged the same day or after a short hospital stay. Pain is rarely severe, and can be managed by prescription or over-the-counter pain pills. You may return to school or nonvigorous work in a few days to a week or two, and resume normal activity after a few weeks. If you have had a laparoscopic appendectomy, you may be able to be discharged the same day, with minimal restrictions.

The postoperative complications of appendicitis include an overall mortality of less than 1 percent, infection from the appendix causing an abscess in the abdomen in 3 percent, and incision infection in 5 to 10 percent. The rates are highest if gangrene, perforation, or abscess is present at the initial operation.

APPENDIX SUMMARY

Prevention

Diet and Supplements

• Follow a low-fat, high-fiber diet.

Alternative Medicine Approaches

• Use enemas and hot packs.
• Use homeopathy and acupuncture.

Conventional Medicine Approaches

• Antibiotics.
• Abscess drainage through skin.

Surgical Approaches

• Open appendectomy.
• Laparoscopic appendectomy.

Anus and Rectum

In its collective wisdom, the U.S. government has spent over 50 billion dollars to study the backside of the moon, an area that has caused no one any suffering. But the same government has not spent one cent to study the backsides of its citizens to find out why they suffer from hemorrhoidal disease and what might be done to prevent painful piles.

Leon Banov, M.D.

Although not usually life-threatening, the very common disorders of the southerly end of your digestive tract can cause maddening itch or extreme pain, enough to interfere with your daily life.

Fifty percent of all Americans have enlarged hemorrhoidal tissue by age 40, and the incidence climbs higher with advancing age. As we shall see, our Western dietary and toilet habits are mostly to blame.

Napoleon's long-standing battle with hemorrhoids may even have kept him off his horse at Waterloo, delaying his entry into battle, perhaps costing him the war. Both President Carter and baseball player George Brett, while sitting in "seats" of power, experienced hemorrhoid difficulties that required urgent surgery.

As noted in Chapter 15, even though recent generations seem much less reticent to openly discuss sexual problems, secrecy and embarrassment often still surround our evacuations. New alternative medicine lifestyle change approaches for anal conditions can help you avoid a painful operation, and assist you in embarking upon a course of prevention of future problems.

How Your Anus Works

Your *rectum* is five or six inches long and is similar to your colon in structure though somewhat larger in diameter. (See Figure 17.1.) It acts as a holding area for your stool before its evacuation. Your *anus* is a muscular tube at the end of your rectum, one to two inches in length. Normally, a partial contraction, called "tone," is present in the part of your anus muscles over which you have no control, creating a pinch-valve, or *internal sphincter,* to prevent accidental passage of gas or rectal contents. Your anus and rectum together contain highly sophisticated nerve discriminators that can distinguish between solid, liquid, and gaseous contents. Without this ability, we hu-

mans would be spending much more of our lives in the bathroom, since we normally pass gas, on average, up to twenty or more times a day.

When stool or gas stretches your rectum, increasing the pressure to a certain level, the "defecation reflex" is stimulated. Your involuntary internal sphincter relaxes, and as your rectum contracts, contents pass. If you ignore these signals, by clenching the anus's surrounding voluntary muscles preventing stool passage, the reflex will subside, later to return less fully. If you don't listen to the "Call of Nature," your stool dries out, setting the stage for more difficult passage, and formation of the dreaded hemorrhoids and fissures.

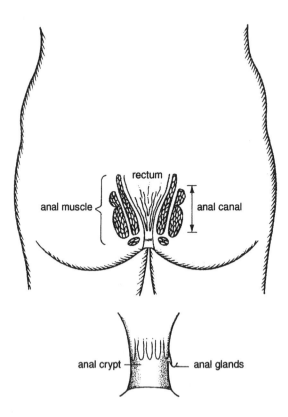

Fig. 17.1 The anatomy and location of the anus and rectum

Importantly, more tiny nerve endings are present per square inch in your anal region than in any other area of your body. Cushions of venous "hemorrhoidal" tissue are found inside the anus, and serve to aid in the maintaining of good continence; they become abnormal only when they enlarge and are displaced downward, as we shall see.

How Anal Disease Is Diagnosed

Anal disease is diagnosed by a careful history, physical exam, and a simple scoping test.

History

Your doctor's evaluation should begin with a very detailed history of your diet and bowel patterns, and include questions to elicit your specific symptoms, such as itching, pain, bleeding, discharge, change in stool size, a sense of incomplete evacuation, and unusual protrusions, swellings, or lumps with defecation. Ninety percent of the time, your doctor can make a diagnosis based on your history alone.

Hemorrhoids may coexist with other, more serious anal or rectal problems, such as tumors, polyps, and other diseases, so you need to have a full evaluation before you try any alternative medicine remedies on your own.

Anal Inspection and Digital Exam

Although it may seem awkward to you, you should not be embarrassed by an anorectal examination. Your doctor has likely seen it all in thousands of such exams.

No special preparation is necessary before your office visit. The exam can be carried out with you lying on your side on the exam table, or in the knee-chest position, where you kneel on your knees and elbows, or with your legs up in "stirrups." Most surgeons prefer to examine you in a "jackknife" position, lying on a special, flexible table. You kneel on a pad and lie forward on the table, which bends your hips and tilts your head down. You can request any position in which you would feel most comfortable.

The exam begins with the doctor taking a close look at your anal opening and the skin around it, as your "cheeks" are separated. Skin tags, cracks in the skin or fissures, external hemorrhoids, warts, infections, tumors, and other irritations may be seen. Sensation can be tested with a cotton swab. Next comes a *digital exam*, in which a gloved lubricated finger is inserted into your anal canal and lower rectum, to search for areas of tenderness, lumps, and any unusual thickening, and to test your muscle tone and ability to squeeze. Your stool should also be screened for traces of blood.

Anoscope

A lubricated *anoscope* is inserted, in order to give your doctor direct visualization of your anus. This exam takes less than a minute, should not be painful, and will be easier if you can consciously relax your muscles. Internal hemorrhoids, ulcers, infections, and other problems may be seen.

Sigmoidoscope

A straight *sigmoidoscopic exam* may sometimes be performed on your initial visit, to evaluate your rectum and lower colon, whereas a flexible sigmoidoscopy or colonoscopy (see page 417) is usually scheduled for a later date.

After completion of these simple examinations, your doctor can almost always explain your problem and suggest a course of treatment.

Hemorrhoids

Significantly, Preparation H, the over-the-counter hemorrhoid remedy, is the item most often shoplifted from drugstores. Does this signal its necessity in our culture, the embarrassment of actually having to purchase it, or both?

Hemorrhoids account for more medical visits than any other anorectal problem, and are responsible for 95 percent of all sudden bleeding associated with bowel movements. Persons with sedentary occupations, such as truck drivers, office workers, and even surgeons themselves, who must sit or stand in one place for long periods, have higher rates of hemorrhoids. Probably no woman in the United States who has given birth is completely free of them. Hemorrhoids are rare in children.

Two types of hemorrhoids can develop, each requiring different treatment. *External hemorrhoids* don't exist unless a blood clot develops in a vein at the anal opening, stretching and inflaming the exquisitely sensitive overlying skin. This type of hemorrhoid is covered with the flesh-colored lining of the lower one-third of the anal canal. If not surgically removed, its rubbery lump is gradually reabsorbed over a period of a few weeks, sometimes leaving a tag of skin behind. Your maximum discomfort is usually over after thirty-six to seventy-two hours.

Internal hemorrhoids, covered by the pink, moist lining of the upper two-thirds of the anal canal, consist of excessive swelling and downward displacement of the normal venous cushions inside your anal canal.

You may have some excess skin and folds around your anal opening. Much anal tissue labeled "hemorrhoid" is just such skin that has persisted after the swelling from previous problems has subsided. A better term is *skin tag*.

Years of repeated straining at stool, induced by a low-fiber diet, is now felt to be the major cause of hemorrhoids. At first, hemorrhoids were blamed simply on the human being's upright posture, but Dr. Denis Burkitt and others discovered ample evidence to refute this position, showing that native Africans and others who eat a high-fiber, low-fat diet are free of such afflictions. Even pregnant women in these cultures do not get hemorrhoids.[1]

Anatomically, internal hemorrhoids are *not* simply abnormally dilated veins of your rectum. This venous tissue, more like a sponge, is *normal*. In its original position, its spongy consistency gives your anus the ability to vary greatly in size with your stool diameter, which helps you maintain good continence. When it is displaced downward, the trouble begins.

Normally, your anal venous cushions are supported by strong connective tissue fibers, which attach your anal canal lining to the underlying anal muscles. With excessive pressure at defecation, the support tissue stretches, which allows the tissue to dilate and balloon into your anal canal. Straining at stool, coughing, heavy lifting, standing or sitting for long periods, and pregnancy all transmit high pressure to this tissue. With aging, your connective tissue fibers also weaken.

An internal hemorrhoid usually begins about the size of a grape. As it gets larger, the increased abdominal pressure from bearing down with bowel movements and the stool itself together act as a "ramrod" to push this tissue farther out of the canal. It may return spontaneously when the pressure is reduced, or you may have to push it back in with your fingers. You generally become aware of internal hemorrhoids by noting *painless* bright red bleeding when you pass stool. The bleeding often subsides in a few days, but may reappear whenever you stray from a good diet, become constipated, or have to strain to pass stool.

Alternative Medicine Approaches to Hemorrhoids

We both agree that symptomatic skin tags and internal and external hemorrhoids deserve a trial of alternative medicine therapies before you opt for any surgical treatment. Most hemorrhoids respond quite well to an alternative medicine program, and surgical procedures can be avoided. I (Sandy) have witnessed these measures to be most successful in my practice: I recommend you start with adding more fiber to your diet, avoiding caffeine, and applying calendula ointment, in addition to the other lifestyle changes given in this section.

Because surgical therapy for hemorrhoids can mean even more of a pain in the rear than that with which you began, lifestyle changes may be especially attractive in this light. The full surgical operation (hemorrhoidectomy) is a particularly painful choice. Your sensitive rectum hurts for weeks, and it has been reported to be one of the worst agonies you can endure, described as similar to the feeling you would have if you were "sliding down a banister that had turned into a razor," with your postoperative bowel movements feeling like "trying to pass a bucket of glass shards."

The following program of alternative medicine approaches serves for prevention of recurrence as well as treatment, *so even when you do choose a surgical approach*, you can help prevent a return of your disease.

Change Your Diet

Constipation is usually "at the bottom" of most hemorrhoids, even though you may not be aware you are actually constipated. Constipation is present whenever stools are too infrequent, too small, too dry, or too sticky.

Persons in countries which have good rectal health and low rates of hemorrhoids pass, on average, from a pound to a pound-and-a-half of soft stool daily, divided into two or three movements. Previously, it had been felt one bowel movement per day, or even every few days, was fine. Now fiber researchers feel this may be a sign of impending disease. Changing your diet is the most important step to relieve pressure in your rectum, to prevent and cure hemorrhoids without surgery.

When bran treatment was compared with placebo in fifty-one patients with hemorrhoids, within six weeks, the fiber group had improved frequency of bowel movements, the hemorrhoids had become smaller, and symptoms of pain and bleeding decreased.[2] Another study showed this treatment superior to surgical outcome.[3]

Your diet should be high in fiber-rich foods and low in the foods that do not contain fiber. Hemorrhoids may actually be one of those diseases where an "apple (or two) a day" in fact does "keep the doctor away." Meat, poultry, fish, eggs, and dairy products do not contain *any* fiber, and their high fat content causes them to pass too slowly through the digestive tract, making stools that are too dry and viscous.

Whole grains such as whole wheat breads and brown rice, along with fresh fruits and vegetables, are the best sources of dietary fiber. You can follow the dietary recommendations in Chapter 2, aiming to increase to a safer daily stool output, passed so easily you just sit on the toilet and whistle "Dixie" (or whatever tune you like), since no bearing down or strain is needed at all.

If needed, you can increase your fiber by eating a whole grain or bran cereal (choose one without added sugar), or by adding one to two tablespoons of whole bran or ground flaxseeds to your meals, increasing as needed to reach the desired stool output. Bran or psyllium have been found to be superior to nonbulk laxatives, as shown in one study where just three tablespoons of bran per day was mixed with food.[4]

Eight to ten glasses of water should be taken daily, especially when bran is added to your diet, since it absorbs water and thus helps keep the stool optimally moist, flaky, and less sticky. You may notice increased gas, bloating, and cramps when first adding bran to your diet; though such symptoms usually disappear as your digestive tract gets used to the healthy new bulk, it may sometimes be necessary to then back off and increase the amount slowly over days or weeks. Oat bran and oat bran cereal may cause less gas. Psyllium seeds or flaxseeds, soaked overnight in water, can be added to your cereal, beginning with a tablespoon and increasing as needed, to expand bulk.

Certain dietary substances are associated with increased risk for anal problems. Alcohol, citrus fruits, tomatoes, spicy foods, dairy products (especially cheeses), and spicy meats are very irritating to many people. Coffee, tea, chocolate, and caffeinated sodas, although having immediate laxative effects, act as *constipators* when their action wears off a few hours later; you may not even be aware of it, but instead of having two or three bowel movements per day, you have only one, placing your rectum at risk. Even decaf is a problem, since it still contains some 5 to 30 mg of caffeine, as well as irritating oils. Try to find an herb tea you like instead.

Laxatives, even herbal ones such as senna and cascara, often also paradoxically *cause* constipation when their effect wears off, and are not recommended—as noted above, bran and other bulk laxatives work better. Many medications such as pain relievers, antacids, blood pressure medications, tranquilizers, and antidepressants also may be implicated in constipation.

Vitamin K, necessary for blood coagulation, is manufactured by the friendly organisms normally living in our digestive tracts. Inadequate intake of green leafy vegetables, in combination with antibiotic or cortisone use, can cause a deficiency of this vitamin, increasing the tendency of your hemorrhoids to bleed. Make certain to eat a salad or other green vegetables daily. Taking acidophilus capsules or acidophilus yogurt, as noted below, can help fill your colon with friendly flora. Garlic has been shown to diminish the numbers of harmful bacteria.[5]

Blueberries, blackberries, and cherries contain high levels of proanthocyanidin and anthocyanidin, types of bioflavonoids that are part of the vitamin C complex, and can assist is optimum maintenance of your capillaries. Including liberal amounts of these in your diet may help prevent your hemorrhoids from bleeding.

Congestion in the liver, especially cirrhosis, causes backup pressure in abdominal veins, termed portal hypertension, and may contribute to enlargement of the veins of the rectum and anus. Fasting for a week or so (see pages 83–84) followed by the liver flush (see page 386) may help address this underlying problem.

Take Supplements

Supplements may assist in the body's wound-healing processes, helping prevent the skin and underlying tissue breakdown associated with hemorrhoids.

The C complex vitamins, especially the bioflavonoids such as rutin, and the pro- and anthocyanidins, are felt to decrease the fragility of capillaries.[6] One study showed diminished pain and itching of hemorrhoids within a few days of beginning ingestion of bioflavonoids.[7] Take 1,000 mg of vitamin C, three times daily, along with 1,000 mg of bioflavonoids. Vitamin E has also been reported to have an ameliorating effect, most likely from its ability to improve blood flow by decreasing coagulability without encouraging hemorrhage.[8] Begin with 400 IU daily.

The herbs marshmallow weed, collinsonia, and slippery elm, taken as tea or applied externally, have traditionally been used for relief. Begin with one of them, adding others only if needed. Take one capsule, three times daily.

To establish optimum bacterial content of your bowel, add garlic to your diet, as fresh or deodorized capsules, two capsules three times daily. Also add acidophilus, a friendly organism, to ensure optimum bowel flora. The acidophilus strains of yogurt can also be used, particularly if you have a history of antibiotic use. Take two capsules, three times daily, or eat one cup of acidophilus yogurt daily. One of the B vitamins, pantothenic acid, has been found to improve bowel function, lessen constipation, and improve wound healing.[9] Take 500 mg, three times daily. At times, deficiency of stomach hydrochloric acid may be present, contributing to constipation; your doctor can test for this. If you test low, take one or two digestive enzyme tablets, available at your local health food store, with each meal.

Use Homeopathy

The homeopathic remedies such as calendula cream 5 percent, nux vomica, sulfur, calcarea phosphorica, and ferrum phosphorica are often helpful; you can consult a homeopathic practitioner for the remedy most appropriate for you.

Maintain Your Optimum Weight

Obesity predisposes you to anal problems because chronic excess moisture forms around an anus deep-set between the buttocks. Itching, burning, and skin breakdown with subsequent bleeding can follow. A high-fiber, low-fat diet as discussed in Chapter 2 can best help you take the weight off and keep it off. Make certain to join a support group.

Exercise Regularly

Exercise is also a key to good anal and rectal health. As noted earlier, a higher incidence of hemorrhoids has been found in persons with more sedentary habits. Some authors suggest that "moving your buns" may be preventive and therapeutic—for this and other illnesses as well. Many different exercise programs are now available, so you might best join a group that suits your needs.

Practice Yoga Daily

Sitting for long periods increases pressure in the veins of your anus and rectum, and dries out the stool from the excess heat generated. By turning the body into the various yoga positions, this venous congestion is relieved.

A German study has shown that regular yoga practice effectively treats and prevents constipation, often at the root of hemorrhoid formation.[10]

The shoulder stand, abdominal lifts, forward bends, spinal twist, and yoga seal are the particularly recommended yoga postures. Time should be increased gradually to two to three minutes; the shoulder stand can be increased carefully and gradually, under supervision, up to ten to fifteen minutes, and practiced twice daily. See Chapter 2 for details.

Practice Stress Management and Visualization

Stress can cause us to ignore our bodily signals, and the body itself to slow its function.

Stress and worry act through hormones and the nervous system, increasing sympathetic tone and decreasing parasympathetic activity, to shut down the digestive tract. As many as 75 percent of patients with the alternating constipation and diarrhea of irritable bowel syndrome (also called "spastic colon") have been found to have abnormal personality tests.[11] Biofeedback, a form of stress management, has been successfully employed to relieve constipation.[12] Regular practice of the deep relaxation and breathing exercises, as well as other yoga techniques, may be able to help you move from tending to be "uptight" to a person whose movements are accomplished with grace and ease. Several studies have indicated benefit from visualization and self-hypnosis to help treat hemorrhoids.[13] See Chapter 2 for details of these practices.

First, practice deep relaxation, as given on

pages 43–46. You can then try this visualization: Imagine your hemorrhoid as a small balloon filled with air. Picture it releasing the air, and becoming completely flat. Hold this image in your mind, while feeling it happen within your body. Repeat several times daily.

Maintain Good Bowel Habits

Defecating when the urge arises is very important, though it may require all of us in the West to shift some deep cultural patterns. If we can begin to feel that we should honor bodily signals quickly, we can create a healthier climate for rectal function—one where it would be considered "good" manners to interrupt even a staff meeting, for example, to "take a call from Nature." Otherwise, the stool dries out and becomes more difficult to pass. As one old Himalayan saying suggests, "Under all conditions—go!"

Change Your Position During Defecation

What may be particularly important in hemorrhoid formation is the posture we in the West assume while on the toilet.

Sitting on a toilet seat, while it rests the legs, may in turn seat us in a position damaging to our rectums. It results in a marked increase in pressure on the rectum, which in combination with the small, hard, dry, and infrequent stools associated with the Western diet, cause the formation of hemorrhoids.

People in cultures that use the squatting position have a low rate of hemorrhoids. They also eat a high-fiber diet. Research to separate the relative importance of each variable has not yet been conducted.

While many of us who have traveled in Europe and Asia find the squatting toilets there a bother, they may save their users from ultimately more supreme discomfort. Special platform toilets are available, or you can draw up your knees or use a small stool to move more closely to a squatting position. In any case, you need to make certain to eat a high-fiber diet so that you will not have to strain, whatever position you take upon the toilet.

Make Hygiene Changes

Wiping with toilet tissue (especially perfumed) may be irritating to your sensitive bottom. Dabbing with moistened toilet tissue, cotton balls, or premoistened towelettes (e.g. Tucks, good for traveling), followed by patting the area dry, may give better cleanliness without irritation, skin breakdown, and bleeding. You may also try aloe-containing toilet tissue, which is my personal favorite. Aloe is a plant extract soothing to the skin, and this is by far the softest and gentlest toilet tissue currently available.

In many countries, such as France and India, washing the anal area with water after a bowel movement is routine. You, too, may find this very soothing; or try a shower or bath instead. Soap should be restricted, because it dissolves your skin's protective oil barrier, painfully exposing the sensitive nerve endings. Constant dampness must be controlled, since it aggravates all anal problems and may produce itching, erosion, and infection. Tight-fitting synthetic underwear or jeans prevent aeration, and may contribute to a moisture problem.

Use Local Treatments

A number of simple local measures can be used to relieve pain and assist in the healing of hemorrhoids. Internal hemorrhoids that have prolapsed outside your anus should be pushed back inside whenever possible. The "sitz bath" is simply a bath for the bottom, a way of thoroughly cleansing and soothing the anal region by sitting in a bathtub partially filled with warm water. The bath should be for twenty to thirty minutes, repeated two or three times daily, or more often as needed. Don't immerse your whole self; a local increase in heat from just putting your bottom in the water relieves spasm in the anal muscles, and the increased local circulation draws more white blood cells into the area for better healing and resistance to infection. Showers do not work as well.

A sitz bath followed by a cool application can provide extra pain relief. Ice packs are especially useful to relieve the pain of clotted external hemorrhoids, and are what allowed the baseball player George Brett to continue to play, before he had his surgically removed.

Moist big-size black tea bags can be applied locally to the anal area to provide a tightening effect from the tannic acid regular tea contains.

Witch hazel and aloe vera are traditional herbal remedies known to be effective and soothing when applied externally. One woman even reported benefit from application of packs of ground cranberries; perhaps their benefit was due to high concentrations of bioflavonoids, plus an astringent action. In Europe, remedies such as a slice of raw potato or garlic were traditionally placed in the rectum to shrink hemorrhoids, and in Eastern Europe and Russia a suppository was carved out of ice and inserted rectally. (Since the other alternative medicine measures given above are more convenient and soothing, these measures are *not* recommended.) I recommend you rub in castor oil, calendula ointment, or liquid vitamins A and E to provide for good lubrication.

Conventional Medicine Approaches to Hemorrhoids

The conventional approaches, the same as the alternative approaches, stress the maintenance of a soft, easy-to-pass stool that is not irritating. Dietary and lifestyle measures are essential. Also, the following can be added for painful flareups.

Stool Softeners and Bulking Agents

These over-the-counter preparations can be taken to help soften and bulk up your stool so that it is more regular and easy to pass. Both are available over-the-counter in drugstores and in health food stores.

Local Medications

These are often successful in shrinking swollen hemorrhoids. Preparation H, the over-the-counter favorite, contains an antiseptic, a live yeast cell derivative, and shark liver oil. Often, it seems to help you avoid surgery, though medical studies do not confirm its benefit.[14] Perhaps its popularity stems not from true effectiveness, but rather from the simple passage of time, which may ease the problem.

Medications containing cortisone, hydrocortisone, and its derivatives are helpful for temporary relief of itching but should be avoided for prolonged usage of more than a few days. They thin the skin, making it *more* susceptible to breakdown, fissures, infection, and exposure of underlying fragile nerve endings, leading to more itching and pain. Anesthetic ointments of the "caine" family, such as Nupercaine, may be helpful for acute discomfort. Many over-the-counter remedies produce sensitization, an allergic reaction that may make the underlying condition worse.

The most notorious offenders are topical antibiotics such as bacitracin and anesthetic ointments.

Sitz Baths

This easy, soothing self-treatment is a standard part of alternative, conventional, and surgical postoperative treatments. See the alternative section for directions.

Surgical Approaches to Hemorrhoids

Maria, a 60-year-old Cuban immigrant, was afflicted with hemorrhoids that popped out every time she had a bowel movement, sneezed, bent over, or climbed stairs. She had been embarrassed for years because of the need to reach around and push them back in many times during the day. She was cured with one painless rubber-banding session, and now wonders why she had to suffer for all this time.

Anal skin tags and internal and external hemorrhoids need to be distinguished, since their management is different.

Skin Tags

Tags rarely cause symptoms in themselves, although they may swell or be sore in reaction to another process such as an associated hemorrhoid or fissure. Surgery is not necessary, unless they cause a problem with hygiene, in which case they can simply be cut off in your doctor's office, using local anesthesia.

External Hemorrhoids

A clotted or "thrombosed" external hemorrhoid may cause enough pain to warrant you having it surgically removed. You feel the blood clot as a painful, rubbery, grapelike external lump. If a trial of alternative medicine measures does not produce relief, and your symptoms are severe, you can have your external hemorrhoid removed by a simple operative procedure. Rubberband and injection methods of treating internal hemorrhoids (see below) cannot be used on external hemorrhoids, because this tissue is very sensitive.

Treatment can usually be easily accomplished in your doctor's office or an emergency room. No preparation is necessary. You lie on your side, or facedown, on a flexed examining table. After local anesthesia, with or without light sedation, your doctor simply removes the clot and some surrounding tissue. The incision is left open, or closed loosely with a few stitches. Relief is immediate, although you may have some soreness in the incision for a few days. You can take sitz baths to help soothe the area. You will need to keep your stools soft and bulky, with stool softeners and bulk laxatives. Healing should take a week or two.

Internal Hemorrhoids

When lifestyle changes fail to relieve internal hemorrhoids and your bleeding, discomfort, or protrusion continues, several surgical approaches are available.

Rubberbanding

Rubberbanding is now the most common form of treatment for internal hemorrhoids, successful 80 to 90 percent of the time. You can have it performed during your initial office visit and exam, without any preparation. No anesthesia is required, since the bands are placed above the area in which you can feel pain.

You lie on your side or facedown on the flexed exam table. After the initial examination, your doctor uses an anoscope to visualize each enlarged hemorrhoid. A clamp is passed through a tiny stretched rubberband, grabs the hemorrhoid, and pulls it through the band, which is then released around its neck, depriving the encircled tissue of its blood supply. (See Figure 17.2.) One to three areas may be treated at one time. The strangulated hemorrhoid tissue dies and separates from the anal wall in three to seven days. The bands and tissue are then passed with the stool; a small amount of bleeding may be seen at that time. Discomfort should be mild, although you might experience some aching and need pain pills and stool softeners for a few days. I tell patients that "out of four patients who have banding, one has a lot of pain for a few days requiring pain medication and may lose a day or two of work; one has no pain; and the other two fall somewhere in between."

Complications of banding are very rare. Significant bleeding occurs in 1 percent of all cases. A few deaths have been reported, thought to be related to infection. Don't take aspirin or other blood thinners for two weeks and report any fever, inability to urinate, or passage of blood clots. After four to six weeks, you should see your doctor for a follow-up visit, to see if further banding is necessary.

You should request a trial of the banding procedure before considering surgical hemorrhoidectomy, since the expense, time needed for treatment and recovery, discomfort, and complications are much less.

Injection Therapy

This method is sometimes used for small hemorrhoids. An irritant chemical is injected

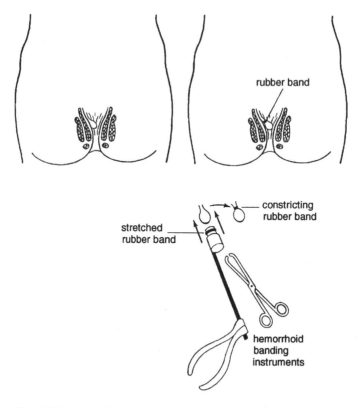

Fig. 17.2 Procedures involved in hemorrhoid rubberbanding

into the tissue surrounding the veins, causing scarring, which compresses and reattaches the tissue to the underlying muscle. The hemorrhoid shrinks, and its recurrence is prevented.

Surgical Excision

This is the classical "hemorrhoidectomy," which may be needed for extensive hemorrhoids, especially those crossing the anal opening and associated with large skin tags. It formerly entailed a three- to seven-day stay in the hospital, but is now usually performed on an outpatient basis.

You may choose local anesthesia, with or without light sedation, regional, or general anesthesia. Preparation may require a liquid diet for twelve hours prior to the operation, and an enema. You are on the operating table in the "jackknife" position, or with your legs up in the "stirrups" posture. From one to four "clusters" of enlarged hemorrhoid tissue are removed, your surgeon being careful to leave the anal muscle intact. The incisions are closed with stitches or left open to heal naturally by contraction and scarring. The operation generally takes from thirty to forty-five minutes, and you can probably be discharged after an hour or two of observation.

Postoperatively, you may experience a small amount of oozing, and pass some blood with your bowel movements. You can use a sanitary pad to protect your clothes. Your pain can be significant, for a few days to a week or more. Immediately after surgery, pain pills will probably be necessary, and an ice pack can be added to help control the pain and swelling. "Sitz baths"—sitting with your bottom submerged in a warm bathtub—are usually the best remedy, since they both soothe the area and relax any spasm in your anal muscles. You can repeat as often and for as long as you like. You may be more comfortable during your recovery sitting on a "donut," a round seat cushion available at most drugstores.

It is very important to make your bowel movements as easy as possible, to minimize your pain and fear of defecation, and avoid constipation and stool impaction. Use stool softeners and add extra bulk to your high-fiber diet. If necessary, drinking mineral oil, one tablespoon per day, can be used to lubricate your anal canal.

You should see your doctor in follow-up visits, until you have healed completely and are satisfied with the result. You can return to work whenever you are comfortable, though full healing and recovery may take from three to five weeks. Significant complications include excessive postoperative bleeding (1 percent), incision infection (1 percent), difficulty with continence (1 to 2 percent), and narrowing of your anal canal (4 to 5 percent).

Despite the hype of equipment manufacturers and the lure of new technology, *laser hemorrhoidectomy*, where a laser is used to remove the hemorrhoid tissue instead of a scalpel; *cryotherapy*, where a freezing probe destroys the tissue; and *heat coagulation therapy*, where the tissue is coagulated by an infrared probe, have no advantage and some disadvantages when compared with rubberbanding and standard surgical excision. These methods often cause increased pain and delayed healing, as well as a higher incidence of other complications.

---

*N*eal was a 35-year-old whose problems with hemorrhoids ran the gamut of treatment options and complications. He had large, circumferential, protruding, bleeding internal hemorrhoids along with very large skin tags. Well aware of the legendary discomfort of surgical hemorrhoidectomy, and worried about his ability to copay his hospital bill, he persisted with rubberbanding sessions for over a year, despite my advice to him that this method would not be successful. After one rubberbanding led to a quart of blood loss and an emergency room visit, Neal agreed to surgery. Unfortunately, ten days after his operation, he was again in the hospital with massive bleeding. Another trip to the operating room was required to tie off a bleeding vessel at the point where the previous stitch had dissolved. Soon, he was doing well, and began watching his diet.

HEMORRHOID SUMMARY

Prevention

Diet and Supplements

- Follow a low-fat, high-fiber diet.
- Drink 8–10 glasses of water daily.
- Avoid alcohol, citrus fruits, tomatoes, spicy foods, dairy products (especially cheeses), spicy meats, coffee, tea, chocolate, and caffeinated sodas.
- Bran, 3 tablespoons, or bran cereal daily.

- Psyllium, 1–2 tablespoons daily.
- Acidophilus capsules, 2 capsules, 3 times daily; or acidophilus yogurt, 1 cup daily.
- Garlic, as fresh or deodorized capsules, 2 capsules 3 times daily.
- Vitamin C, 1,000 mg, 3 times daily.
- Bioflavonoids, 1,000 mg daily.
- Vitamin E, 400 IU daily.

Lifestyle

- Maintain good bowel habits. Strive to have a bowel movement after each meal.
- Change your position during defecation.
- Maintain optimum weight.
- Regular exercise, 1 hour 3–5 times weekly.
- Practice daily yoga.
- Practice stress management.

Alternative Medicine Approaches

- Herbs—marshmallow weed, collinsonia, and slippery elm, taken as tea or applied externally, or one capsule, 3 times daily.
- Pantothenic acid, 500 mg, three times daily.
- Hygiene changes—aloe-containing toilet tissue; avoid soap, tight-fitting synthetic underwear or jeans.
- Moist black tea bags, applied externally.
- Witch hazel and aloe vera—applied externally.
- Castor oil, calendula ointment, or liquid vitamins A and E; rub them on, to provide good lubrication.
- Homeopathy—calendula cream 5 percent, nux vomica, sulfur, calcarea phosphorica, and ferrum phosphorica.
- Practice visualization.

Conventional Medicine Approaches

- Stool softeners and bulking agents— colace, Senicot, Surfact, Metamucil, Citrucel, Fiber Con.
- Local medications—Preparation H, cortisone, anesthetics, Nupercaine.
- Sitz baths.

Surgical Approaches

- Rubberbanding.
- Injection therapy.
- Surgical excision.

Anal Fissures

Mary, a 25-year-old secretary who had just lost her job, was also under a great deal of stress at home. After a bout of constipation and difficult passage of a large hard stool, she developed an acute anal fissure. The pain prevented her from sitting or moving around. She needed strong pain medication, spent most of her time in a warm bathtub, and the thought of having a bowel movement terrorized her. She did not feel she could wait for the effects of conservative management. A surgical anal sphincterotomy brought her immediate relief.

An anal fissure is a split in the lining of your anal canal, usually caused by the traumatic passage of a hard stool. It is such a common problem that most of us have experienced it. It is the most common cause of rectal bleeding in childhood, and painful rectal bleeding in the adult. Since delicate nerve endings and a bit of anal muscle are exposed, this condition may be accompanied by burning and stabbing pain with defecation, lasting fifteen minutes to an hour or more. The discomfort can be so severe it is impossible to sit or walk. A drop to a teaspoon of bright red blood may appear with each bowel movement as the split is reopened. Tissue swelling can produce a lump or skin tag that is often confused with a hemorrhoid.

The usual *acute* fissure that most of us get heals in a few days, aided by the alternative medicine management described below. However, if you develop a *chronic* fissure that will not heal, or you suffer repeated bouts of this problem, the underlying cause may be an overactive sphincter muscle mechanism causing high pressures and subsequently decreased blood supply, particularly posteriorly where there is a relative deficiency of blood vessels in most people. A normal-size stool passing through may be more likely to cause a rip. Stress may also play a role in fissure formation.

Alternative Medicine Approaches to Anal Fissures

Janet, a 25-year-old graduate student, was excited about going to Europe for the first time. But in order to finish all her work and get packed, she skipped meals and drank coffee instead. Just a few days before she was to board the plane, during a bowel movement, she experienced sharp pain, and discovered blood on the toilet tissue. A visit to the doctor revealed only an anal fissure, and she was placed on a regimen of plenty of bran cereal daily, more fluids, along with no further caffeine. She went off to have a great vacation, with no subsequent problems.

Avoiding surgery for your anal fissures is a very worthy effort, since this operation can be a significant "pain in the rear." In addition, it may make your problems worse, leave you incontinent for the rest of your life, and not prevent recurrences.

You can act to prevent and treat anal fissures by alternative means, which may also serve to help you avoid a return of your problems. The same alternative medicine approaches to hemorrhoids can be used for anal fissures. The following measures may offer further help.

Keep Your Stools Soft

If you are still having trouble with hard, small stools despite changing your diet, you may wish to try drinking one cup of dandelion tea three times daily to help keep your stools optimally soft.

Use Local Measures

Witch hazel is one traditional herbal remedy, now available in convenient herb-soaked pads, that may help to resolve the itching and bleeding of your fissures. This herb acts both as a venotonic, tightening your veins so they are less likely to bleed, and an antiinflammatory. Apply two to three times daily and after each bowel movement.

Castor oil is another local measure anecdotally reported to provide relief. Applications should be made after each bowel movement, at least two to three times daily until the problem has improved and then once daily as a preventive.

Practice Visualization

A specific visualization practice for anal fissures may also be helpful. For example, after you have performed the deep relaxation given in Chapter 2, imagine your anus like a sleeve with a tear in one side. See yourself carefully sewing up the rip, and your bowel movements passing gently and easily through the sleeve, past the new seam. Image this, and at the same time, feel it happening within your own body.

Conventional Medicine Approaches to Anal Fissures

If the lifestyle and alternative measures just discussed are unsuccessful in healing a fissure, the following conventional approaches may be successful in all but the most resistant fissure caused by an underlying sphincter dysfunction.

Stool Softeners and Bulking Agents

You should modify your diet to soften and bulk up your stool, so that it is more regular and easy to pass. This lessens the likelihood that passing a firm stool will traumatize the delicate anal canal and reopen a healing fissure. Both stool softeners and bulking agents are available over-the-counter from drugstores and from health food stores.

Sitz Baths

This simple treatment is likely to provide more relief than any other measure. For directions, see page 471.

Local Preparations

The "over-the-counter" local applications discussed for hemorrhoids can be tried. Creams or suppositories with cortisone should be avoided, since they tend to thin the tissue, predisposing you to further episodes.

Topical Nitroglycerin Ointment

This ointment, used at 0.2 percent strength, applied two or three times per day temporarily relaxes the anal sphincter and healing has been documented in two-thirds of all fissures treated this way. However, since it doesn't treat the underlying problem, recurrence is likely, but treatment can be successfully repeated.[15] Headaches are a side effect that may prevent its use in some patients.

Botulinum Toxin Injection

Recently there has been some success with botulinum toxin injection into the internal or external anal sphincter, which has the effect of temporarily paralyzing part of the muscle, thereby decreasing sphincter pressure at rest. Initial results are successful, without serious complications, but the long-term recurrence rate is uncertain.[16] A recent report from Italy described a 96 percent healing rate at two months with no recurrence at fifteen months follow-up.[17]

Surgical Approach to Anal Fissures

If your pain is so severe you can't carry out your normal activities, you may want a quicker solution than that provided by alternative treatments. Also, acute fissures that have not healed after three weeks of conservative treatment, recurrent severe acute fissures, and chronic fissures with scarred edges may require surgery to overcome the effects of the increased internal sphincter tone. By preventing muscle spasm, decreasing anal canal pressure, and increasing blood supply, lateral sphincterotomy relieves your discomfort and allows your fissure to heal.

Lateral sphincterotomy is the standard fissure operation in the United States. You can have it performed as an outpatient, under local, spinal, or general anesthesia.

You are positioned on the operating table on your side, facedown with hips flexed, or legs up in the "stirrups" position. After anesthesia, your surgeon makes a one-quarter-inch skin incision at the edge of the anus, then cuts about one-half inch of your internal anal sphincter muscle. (See Figure 17.3.) The fissure itself is not removed, but will go on to heal spontaneously in almost 100 percent of the cases. Associated enlarged skin tags can be removed at the same time. The operation takes about five minutes.

Discomfort after anal sphincterotomy is mild, and easily controllable with sitz baths and pain pills. Keep your stools bulky and soft. You should see your doctor after a week or two, to ensure that healing occurs and the anal muscle functions normally again. You have a 1 percent chance you will have problems with controlling gas, diarrhea, or stool after sphincterotomy.

ANAL FISSURE SUMMARY

Prevention

Diet and Supplements

- Follow the measures for hemorrhoids.
- Follow a high-fiber, low fat diet.
- Eat 5–7 servings of fruit daily.
- Eat a fresh salad daily, for a total of 5–7 servings of vegetables.
- Drink 8 large glasses of water.
- Avoid coffee, tea, sodas, chocolate.
- Drink dandelion tea, 1 cup, or 3–5 grams of dried root or 5–10 ml of tincture, 1–3 times daily, to keep stools soft.
- Bran, 3 tablespoons daily, or eat a high-fiber cereal daily.
- Psyllium, 1–2 tablespoons (start with 1 teaspoon in an 8-ounce glass of water, and increase as needed).

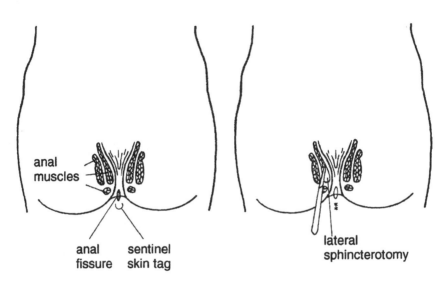

Fig. 17.3 Procedures involved in lateral sphincterotomy

- Acidophilus, 1–2 capsules, (29 billion organisms), 3 times daily.

Lifestyle

- Utilize the toilet in a squatting position.

Alternative Medicine Approaches

- Follow the preventive measures for hemorrhoids, and those above.
- Use witch hazel ointments or saturated wipes.
- Apply calendula ointment, HPUS 1X potency, 3 times daily.
- Use visualization.
- Practice stress management.

Conventional Medicine Approaches

- Stool softeners and bulking agents.
- Sitz baths.
- Local preparations—Preparation H, anesthetics.
- Topical nitroglycerin ointment.
- *Botulinum* toxin injection.

Surgical Approach

- Lateral sphincterotomy.

Anal Warts

Richard, *a 35-year-old gay man, developed anal itching and spotting of bright red blood with bowel movements. Examination showed multiple warts surrounding and within his anal canal. Initial treatment involved a trip to the operating room to remove all the visible warts with electrocautery.*

Despite initiation of safe-sex practices, he had evidence for recurrent warts on many of his monthly postoperative visits. Most of the recurrences could be treated in the office, though he did require one more operating room session. Eventually, he had no evidence of recurrence six months after his last treatment, and is considered cured.

Anal warts, called *Condylomata accuminata*, are caused by a human papilloma virus (HPV) infection. About 90 percent are transmitted by anal intercourse. In 10 percent of all cases, no obvious mode of transmission can be determined. These warts are usually elevated, with a cauliflowerlike surface or flat, and may be located in the skin around the anus and/or in the anal canal. There may be one or many. The moisture produced causes skin breakdown, with resultant symptoms of itching and burning. A small amount of bleeding may accompany bowel movements. Untreated, the warts may remain unchanged, grow in size and number, or disappear spontaneously. Long-standing warts very rarely become cancerous.

Alternative Medicine Approaches to Anal Warts

Both the surgical and conventional treatment of anal warts, although they may be initially successful, are often accompanied by intense pain and then followed by relapse. The alternatives discussed here have a direct effect upon the immune system and on the underlying root of the body's inability to rid itself of a pesky virus. In any case, these alternatives may be worth a try even if you choose an operation or drug therapy.

Use Homeopathy

The specific homeopathics traditionally used include caulophyllum, causticum, carcinosin, and thuja. You may need to consult with an experienced homeopath for individualized treatment.

Practice Visualization

For a specific visualization, first do the deep relaxation given in Chapter 2; then see your warts within your mind's eye like small heads of cauliflower. Imagine yourself applying a vanishing cream, and see them disappearing. Hold this vision, while at the same time feeling it happen within your body.

Conventional Medicine Approach to Anal Warts

There are several topical treatments that may be effective in controlling anal warts. They can be applied in solution, cream, gel, or film preparation in varying strength. Bi- and trichloroacetic acid work by direct tissue destruction. Podophyllotoxin (Condyline), podofilox (Condylox), and podophyllin (Podocon-25) have antiviral activity. Imiquimod (Aldara) works by modulating your immune system. Interferon (Alferon) has antiviral and immune-stimulating effects. It can be applied topically but may be more effective if it is injected into the warts. Cryotherapy with liquid nitrogen freezes the warts and may be the safest treatment during pregnancy. The anticancer drug 5-fluorouracil (Efudex) applied topically as a cream has also been reported to be effective but its safety in pregnancy is unknown. In general, these agents may or may not be effective for you. Some have proven beneficial in controlled trials with placebos and some have not. They need to be applied frequently to clear the warts and all have a significant recurrence rate. They all can produce local irritation, burning, itching, pain, and skin ulcers. Interferon can produce flulike symptoms. Topical agents are dangerous to use within the anal canal because of their effects on adjacent normal tissue. None of these treatments is as effective in wart clearance and prevention of recurrence as surgical procedures.[18] They also are not as painful and are less likely to cause scarring.

Surgical Approaches to Anal Warts

Surgical approaches include electrocoagulation, destruction by laser, and excision. These are office or ambulatory surgery procedures taking 10 to 20 minutes. No preparation is necessary. You can choose general, spinal, or local anesthesia, with or without sedation, according to the extent of the problem and your wishes. You are facedown on a flexed operating table or with feet up in stirrups. After anesthesia, your doctor removes the larger warts with a scalpel, electric knife, or laser. The smaller ones are destroyed with electric current or laser beam. The resulting small skin ulcers heal over in a week or two. Postoperative discomfort can be handled with sitz baths and pain pills, if necessary. You experience a discharge until skin healing is complete. There may be some permanent scarring.

You should see your doctor for careful follow-up examinations, for many months after the last wart has been seen. Recurrence of warts after one treatment is as high as 50 to 70 percent, which may be due to incomplete initial treatment, later activation of virus incubating in the anal tissue producing new warts, or reinfection from unprotected sexual contact. Any new warts can usually be treated in your doctor's office using local anesthesia.

Long-standing warts can undergo malignant change.

Anal Infections

A *perianal abscess* is an infection that begins in the tiny anal glands located just inside the anal opening. It may drain spontaneously into the anal canal or to the skin surrounding the anus. If it does not drain spontaneously, it can spread beneath the tough perianal skin deep into the tissues around the rectum causing a *perirectal abscess* that can be very serious and destructive. After an abscess is drained, either spontaneously or surgically, a 50 to 70 percent chance exists for a recurring abscess or the development of a chronic *perianal fistula*. A perianal fistula is an infected tunnel connecting the diseased anal glands with the perianal skin. Persistent pus discharge through a small nodule and local minor discomfort are its usual symptoms.

Alternative Medicine Approaches to Anal Infection

You can act to avoid an operation for persistent anal infections and save yourself from the additional pain attendant to such a procedure while at the same time helping prevent the possibility of recurrence of your disorder. Early anal infections generally respond to the alternative medicine approaches to hemorrhoids, given earlier in this chapter. In addition, you can try the following two methods, which many people find successful against anal infections.

Improve Your Overall Immunity

Changing your diet, using immune stimulators, and practicing stress reduction can all help boost your overall immunity so that your immune system can function optimally to fight infection. Follow the guidelines given in Chapter 2.

Practice Visualization

Visualization may also help. For a specific visualization, you may use this example: Imagine your anus is a meadow in the rain forest that has lately been receiving too much rain. Let the sun come out, and feel its healing warmth drying up any moist areas. Then see and feel your whole bottom area healthy, relaxed, and free of any distress.

Conventional Medicine Approaches to Anal Infections

Local treatment and antibiotics can be added to alternative measures to abort an early infection or to encourage it to drain spontaneously, but be sure not to delay seeing a physician, as you may develop a much more serious infection. The following conventional treatments may be successful.

Sitz Baths

Sitting in a warm tub results in more blood flow to the infected area, assisting your immune system in fighting the infection. It also may encourage the infection to "come to a head" and drain pus spontaneously, thereby avoiding the need for surgical incision. Sit in a warm tub for at least twenty minutes three or four times a day. You can actually sit there as long as you want, as it is also likely to decrease your discomfort.

Antibiotics

Although often responsible for delay in necessary surgical treatment, antibiotics may stop an early infection from extending. However, if there is much inflammation surrounding the focus of the infection, the antibiotic may be unable to reach the bacteria to counteract and destroy them.

Surgical Approaches to Anal Infections

Carol, a 28-year-old woman, worked in a crafts market. She had a four-month history of a draining nodule next to her anus, which proved to be the external opening of a perianal fistula. Lacking insurance, her first operation was done under local anesthesia on an office table. She was found to have an infected tunnel that traveled up along the outer side of her anal canal and appeared to pass through the muscle into the anal canal one inch above the anal opening. A complicated fistula was diagnosed, so I simply scraped the abnormal tissue from outside the muscle and left the muscle intact. I feared that cutting too much muscle (performing a fistulotomy) could cause problems with anal continence. The drainage persisted for weeks, despite most of the incision healing. She was returned to a hospital operating room and examined under general anesthesia, at which time she was found to actually have a simple extension burrowing under a small amount of muscle that could be safely cut. Now she is doing fine, with a healed incision, no drainage, and no problems with continence.

If a perianal abscess does not drain spontaneously early on, you need surgery. Time is lost trying to resolve the infection or "bring it to a head" with antibiotics and sitz baths. Tissue around the anus has few restricting barriers, so that infection may spread widely and deeply before "pointing" and breaking through the tougher skin; severe anal muscle damage or even life-threatening infection can be the outcome, especially if you are diabetic or debilitated.

Following are the techniques used to treat an anal infection, depending on the exact type and whether an abscess is present.

Incision and Drainage of an Anal/Rectal Abscess

Most anal infections can be drained on an outpatient basis, although if you have a larger abscess, you may have to stay in the hospital for a few days to ensure adequate drainage and healing. During your operation, you are on your side, facedown on a flexed operating table, or on your back with your legs up in "stirrups." Local, spinal, or general anesthesia can be chosen. The procedure usually takes five to ten minutes. Your doctor makes an incision over the area where the infection is closest to the skin surface. All pockets of infection must be eliminated. Sometimes, for larger abscesses involving the tissues adjacent to the rectum, a rubber drain or gauze "packing" is placed and slowly removed over a period of days. Usually, you feel much better immediately after the pus is evacuated and the pressure relieved. Postoperative discomfort is mild, and can be relieved with pain pills, if necessary. After surgery, you should take sitz or tub baths and massage around the incision to ensure that healing occurs "from the inside out," and not allow the skin to seal over the infected cavity. You should see your doctor for follow-up office visits until healing is complete, which may take from a few days to a week or two.

Anal Fistulotomy

Most anal fistula persist until surgery is undertaken. The *fistulotomy* operation can be done in outpatient surgery, under local, spinal, or general anesthesia. No preparation is necessary. During your procedure you will be facedown on a flexed operating table or on your back with legs up in "stirrups." The operation usually takes five to ten minutes. Your doctor "unroofs" the infected tunnel, while avoiding cutting a significant amount of anal muscle. The incision is left open. Treat the open incision with cleansings and dressing changes, as described for infected incision care on page 134. Complete healing may take several weeks, but discomfort is minimal. You will need to keep your stools soft and bulky. You should see your doctor in follow-up office visits to ensure that healing is complete and your muscle function is satisfactory.

Rarely, a complicated fistula may take a circuitous route, burrowing under a significant amount of anal muscle, and presenting the danger of postoperative incontinence if all of the overlying muscle is cut at one time. In this situation, a multiple-staged procedure is sometimes necessary, using a "Seton" suture or wire, which is progressively tightened over a period of weeks, thereby cutting through the muscle overlying the tunnel. Healing occurs behind the suture as it is advanced.

Curettage and Fibrin Glue Injection

Recently, injection of "fibrin glue," made from blood coagulation factors, into the fistula tunnel after scraping out its infected lining has been used to try to plug it up, after which healing by scarring can occur. This can eliminate the need to cut a significant amount of sphincter muscle that might cause problems with continence. Initial results indicate about a 70 percent success rate for simple and complicated fistula.[19]

ANAL INFECTION SUMMARY

Prevention

• See Hemorrhoid Summary.

Alternative Medicine Approaches

• See Hemorrhoid Summary.
• Visualization.

Conventional Medicine Approaches

• Sitz baths.
• Antibiotics.

Surgical Approaches

• Incision and drainage of an anal/rectal abscess.
• Anal fistulotomy.
• Anal fistula curettage and fibrin glue injection.

HERNIA

Tran, a 50-year-old Vietnamese refugee, was found to have hernias in both groins during a routine preemployment physical exam. Even though he was unaware of the hernias and had no symptoms, he had to have them taken care of to get the job, which involved lifting heavy boxes. He had them repaired by the laparoscopic technique using plastic mesh reinforcement. He had no problems after the operation and recovered quickly enough to be able to start work two weeks later without restrictions.

Hernias are a very common problem. On average, 2,000 groin hernia operations are performed in the United States each day. Described in some of the earliest historical writings, hernias have plagued the human race, it seems, since our upright posture was adopted. However, blame for hernias cannot be placed on stance alone: certain dietary, exercise, and smoking habits increase your risk.

When a structure pushes through a defect in its confining space, a small pocket, termed a hernia, is created. Most hernias appear through a weak spot in your abdominal wall musculature, which allows this outpouching, or sack, to form from the stretched inside lining of your abdominal cavity. Some of your intra-abdominal contents—bowel or fat—may pass into or along the side of this sack. A hernia may develop at any point where such a weakness is found.

In this chapter, we first present a discussion of underlying causative factors so you can use alternative medicine measures to prevent yourself from developing a hernia or, if you already have one, to help prevent the formation of another.

Until surgical repair was devised in the late nineteenth century, hernia sufferers wore elaborate "truss" (a word derived from "trouser") mechanisms that often *caused* more symptoms than they relieved and many people died as a result of hernia complications. If you already have a hernia, you can use this chapter to educate yourself. If, like many, you choose to avoid surgery, you assume a small risk for complications requiring emergency surgery. The several methods of hernia repair are based on the type of hernia you have, the condition of your tissue, and preferences of your surgeon.

Groin Hernia

Groin hernias develop in 5 percent of all males and 1 percent of all females. Three types can occur. The most common, *indirect inguinal hernia*, accounts for 60 to 80 percent of all hernias and is often present from birth, though it may show up only later in life. In males, a tongue of peritoneum, the thin layer lining your abdominal cavity, is pulled down with the testicle as it migrates from the abdomen into the scrotum around the time of birth. (See Figure 18.1.) Normally, this sack becomes a fibrous cord. However, if obliteration of it is incomplete, it can later enlarge, and your intra-abdominal contents slip in and out. An analogous development may be found in females, at the point where the round ligament leaves the abdomen to pass into the labia majora. Intestines, fat, or even one of the ovaries or fallopian tubes can then pass into this sack. Some indirect hernias may not

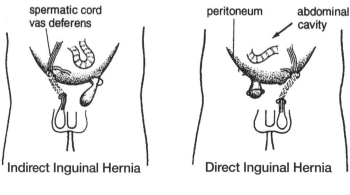

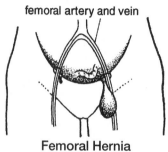

Fig. 18.1 Types of groin hernias

be present at birth, but form later in life as the tissues weaken.

Direct inguinal hernias are usually found in older people. They form when chronically increased intra-abdominal pressure and weakened tissues allow a bulge to develop just lateral to your pubic bone. Obesity, eating a low-fiber diet that forces you to strain during bowel movements, straining with urination because of an enlarged prostate gland, smoking or chronic cough, multiple pregnancies, or using incorrect lifting techniques contribute to formation of this type of hernia.

The third type of groin hernia, *femoral hernia,* is uncommon, occurring in only 3 percent of all hernia cases. Here a potentially weak area exists in your abdominal wall where your femoral artery and vein leave the abdomen to pass into your thigh. More common in women, these hernias are often related to the stress of childbearing, and are dangerous owing to their increased rate of bowel entrapment. Twenty percent of these hernias require emergency surgery.

Your hernia may not give you any symptoms, and you may be completely amazed to have it found on a routine physical exam. However, as time passes, a small hernia tends to increase in size, and you then begin to become aware of it.

The first symptoms are usually mild. When a loop of bowel or fat enters the sack, stretching the sensitive lining of the inside of your abdomen, you feel a dull ache, heaviness, dragging sensation, or twinge. A rapidly enlarging hernia may stretch or tear muscle, causing you more severe pain.

As your hernia enlarges, you may feel a soft lump between your pubic bone and scrotum or labia. In its early stages, this lump may appear only when you are straining, disappearing when you relax or lay down. Small hernias can be pushed back or "reduced" back into your abdomen without much difficulty. As the hernia gets bigger, reduction becomes more difficult and uncomfortable. A large hernia may extend down into your scrotum, reaching your testicle, attaining the size of a softball or even larger.

Your hernia can become trapped, or *incarcerated,* if it cannot be pushed back into your abdomen. If bowel is caught in the sack, *obstruction* may develop, and you would then experience nausea, vomiting, and bloating. If blood circulation to the trapped contents is blocked, *strangulation,* and even *gangrene,* would cause severe local tenderness, swelling, and redness.

How Groin Hernias Are Diagnosed

In most cases, the presence of a groin hernia is quite obvious. A bulge appears lateral to your pubic bone or the base of your scrotum or labia. Diagnosis, however, may be difficult if your lump comes and goes, and is not present when your doctor examines you. Also, early small hernias may give you symptoms, yet not have progressed far enough for you to find a noticeable bulge. Following are the methods used to diagnose this common problem.

History

Your doctor should ask about when you first developed symptoms, if any, or noticed a lump. If it was caused by some heavy lifting or other work-related activity, the circumstances must be clearly documented, since the cost to fix it may be covered by your state's "Labor and Industry" insurance laws. Precipitating factors such as smoking history, straining with bowel movements and urination, and exercise patterns should also be explored.

Whether the hernia reduces itself when you lie down or you have to struggle to push it back in is key to predicting its danger if not surgically repaired. Symptoms of abdominal distention and cramping are most worrisome.

Physical Exam

If not causing a visible lump, most groin hernias can be felt as a tap on your doctor's examining finger, pressed next to your pubic bone, while you are asked to perform the classic "turn your head and cough" and other straining maneuvers. A rectal exam and test of your stool for microscopic blood should be performed, to check for an enlarged prostate and colon cancer, both occasionally associated with hernia, especially in the elderly.

Scans

Ultrasound and CAT scans are sometimes ordered in obscure cases of chronic groin pain when a hernia is not obvious. However, they are more likely to be misleading than useful in diagnosing these hernias. Occasionally, an entirely different, unexpected diagnosis, such as an abdominal tumor, is found.

Alternative Medicine Approaches to Groin Hernias

*R*upert, *an 80-year-old businessman, still went to the office every day. He noticed a small painless lump in his right groin, which on examination by his doctor proved to be an inguinal hernia. Instead of surgery, he chose to wear a truss, and try homeopathy at the same time. His hernia has not gone away completely, but is smaller, he is symptom-free, and now simply has his doctor check it regu-larly to make certain no complications seem to be developing.*

Prevention is alternative medicine's key contribution to the problem of hernia. Since chronically increased intra-abdominal pressure is known to play an important role in its development, changing your lifestyle may prevent future hernias. Following are the available alternative medicine approaches to prevent groin hernias.

Change Your Diet

Eating a low-fiber diet that forces you to strain at stool causes the increased pressure associated with this problem. Eat a high-fiber diet, making certain to have 20 to 40 grams of fiber per day. Follow the dietary advice given in Chapter 2 to help prevent recurrence and, since you are at increased risk, formation of another hernia on the other side.

Maintain Your Optimum Weight

Avoiding obesity can help you prevent groin hernias. Extra weight puts extra strain on your tissues and thins the wall of your abdomen, making the formation of a groin hernia more likely. In addition, even if you have a groin hernia surgically repaired, you may find another one forming if you do not change this predisposing factor. Follow the dietary recommendations given in Chapter 2 to achieve and maintain your ideal weight.

Be Careful With Lifting

Hernias can develop gradually, the result of a combination of factors including the chronic use of poor form during lifting, or they can develop suddenly, the culmination of these influences combined with lifting a particularly heavy load. Taking the brunt of any lift in your legs by bending your knees and then centering your weight over your knees rather than simply leaning over and tensing your abdominal muscles can help prevent the strains that are associated with this disorder. See Chapter 22 for a further discussion of the proper form to use during lifting in the context of preventing back injury.

Quit Smoking

Both the effect of nicotine on small blood vessels, interfering with maintenance of your tissues, and the chronic cough that accompanies smoking can increase your risk for developing a hernia.

Exercise Regularly

You can build up the strength of your muscles and tissues, and do yoga postures to improve local circulation. One patient was able to cure a small hernia by pushing it back in while doing sit-ups to strengthen and enlarge the adjacent muscles so they would keep the rupture in place.

Practice Visualization

You can try visualization to keep your hernia under control. For example, imagine your hernia as a bicycle tube with a small area of weakness that has ballooned out. Your surrounding muscles are new Michelins called in to reinforce the area. Feel it tighten in your body as you hold this image in your mind.

Try Yoga, Acupuncture, Herbs, and Homeopathy

Once a hernia has formed, no scientific studies have been published to show actual reversal through alternative medicine approaches.

Mark Bricklin of *Prevention* magazine does relate that a traditionally used herb called "rupturewart" (*Herniare glabra*) was mentioned by Gerard, an eighteenth-century French herbalist, with "very many that have bursten restored to health by the use of the herbe."[1] The homeopathic remedies calcarea carbonica and nux vomica have been recommended.

Even though no proven reversal alternatives are presently available, unless your hernia is interfering with your lifestyle, is painful, or has developed a complication, you can choose to avoid surgery long enough to try for regression. Your hernia may never develop symptoms, and as long as it is monitored by your doctor to make certain it is not developing a complication, you can try acupuncture and homeopathy, along with a high-fiber diet and yoga postures, as given in Chapter 2, although no data as yet support their effectiveness.

Although deaths from simple hernia surgery are rare, they do exist. In addition to the risk of surgery, postoperative complications such as a hugely swollen scrotum, numbness, blood clots, infections, chronic pain, and permanent testicular atrophy (shrinkage) can be quite uncomfortable and alarming.

Hernias not causing any symptoms, often discovered in elderly men, are especially unlikely to cause complications. In most cases, they therefore do not need surgery. A 1977 report documented that men over age 65 with hernias have only a 0.3 percent per year (4 percent for their remaining lifetime) chance for a complication requiring emergency surgery. Overall, the chance of eventually dying from an emergency operation was 0.53 percent, comparable to a 0.3 percent risk of dying from elective surgery in this age group.[2]

Should you accept the risk of surgery to

prevent a future problem that might never happen? Many of my patients say they wish they had not delayed their hernia repair for so long, because it turned out they needn't have been concerned—the operation is so simple, relatively painless, and relief quick and complete. On the other hand, an albeit very rare example of what can go wrong when undertaking "minor" surgery for an asymptomatic problem is that of the president of a major Southern university who underwent an exploratory abdominal operation, initiated because of an undiagnosed shadow on an X-ray. No abnormalities were found, except for a small incidental groin hernia, one that had been giving him no symptoms, and had not caused the shadow. The surgeons decided that since they were in the abdomen already, they would correct the hernia. Unfortunately, a nerve to his leg was damaged while they were fixing it. When he awoke, he was unable to walk, and still spends part of his time in a wheelchair.[3]

By adopting alternative measures, you may be able to prevent your hernia from enlarging any further, and avoid surgery altogether. At the very least, you should make the above changes anyway, so you can prevent postsurgical recurrence or the formation of another hernia on your other side.

Conventional Medicine Approach to Groin Hernias

A "truss," designed to keep a hernia reduced, may be useful if you do not choose surgery, have a severe medical condition, or need temporary relief. Some patients have lived in harmony with their trusses for twenty or thirty years! However, trusses do not *cure* hernias, and may themselves cause more symptoms than they relieve. They are hard to

adjust, sweaty, can create skin problems, and may not even be successful in keeping your hernia reduced. A truss can also provide a temporary solution while you are exploring acupuncture, homeopathy, dietary change, and yoga, to alleviate your disorder.

Surgical Approaches to Groin Hernias

Mary, *a 75-year-old woman, developed a large painful swelling in her right groin. Hesitant about surgery, she waited two days to contact her doctor, who discovered a hernia. A piece of dead intestine was removed during surgery. Fortunately, she did well. During her hospital stay, she was found to have* another *hernia on the opposite side, which had not produced symptoms, and was advised to have it repaired, in a week or two. She declined, saying she had planned an important trip to see her sister, and would delay the operation until she returned. As it turned out, this hernia also developed intestine entrapment, and she had to have another emergency surgery while away on her trip.*

Most surgeons believe that groin hernias should be repaired, unless you have an acute illness or a serious chronic medical condition. Recommendation to have surgery is especially persuasive if you are young. Without treatment, hernias tend to become larger, and you are in more danger of entrapment, bowel obstruction, and strangulation. It is impossible to predict whether your particular hernia will cause such a complication, although femoral and indirect inguinal hernias carry greater risks.

Elective surgery for hernias causing symptoms is very safe in any age group, and your quality of life afterward is better. Emergency surgery carries a much higher recurrence, complication, and mortality rate. If you were to develop a bowel obstruction or strangulation, it would be very dangerous to delay your surgery for more than a few hours, which would be impossible if you lived far from a hospital or were several days into a backpack trip in the mountains, paddling a canoe down the Amazon, or traveling in outer space.

Groin hernia repairs are now performed on an outpatient basis, in marked contrast to years ago when a several-day hospital stay was the norm. Most insurance companies now will not pay for an overnight stay unless you have a complication. Some surgeons have even established complete surgical settings in their own offices and are performing hernia repairs at much less than half the cost associated with a hospital-based procedure. Studies have shown that with outpatient hernia surgery you have less need for medication, quicker recovery, and less time lost from work.

Most repairs are done using local anesthesia and IV sedation, though you can also choose general, spinal, or in a few places, acupuncture for your anesthetic. Many surgeons feel they can do a better repair under local anesthesia: your tissues retain their normal tone, making it easier to judge the degree of tension produced by the repair—too much tension is a major factor in hernia recurrence. You can be asked to strain and cough, so your surgeon can see how your repair is holding. Also, you can be up and walking sooner after a local.

You are wheeled, or walk, into the operating room, and climb up onto the operating table. You are then given the type of anesthesia you have chosen. Your surgeon makes a two- to three-inch incision above your groin skin crease. The hernia sack is removed or pushed back into your abdomen, then the weakened area in the abdominal wall is repaired.

The exact method of repair chosen to correct the weakness depends somewhat on the type of hernia you have and the condition of your tissue used in the mending. The two basic types of operation are those using your own tissue and those using mesh, a sheet of woven or knitted plastic material (see Figure 18.2), to patch over the weakened area.

Most surgeons I know now use mesh to repair most, if not all, hernias. We believe this type of repair gives the lowest recurrence rate (less than 0.5 percent compared with a rate of 5 to 10 percent without mesh), is less painful, and is quicker and easier than other repairs. The theoretical complications associated with placing "foreign" material into your body have not proven significant. Especially for huge or recurrent hernias, plastic mesh is now used routinely, with many variations in the way it is placed.

Your incision is closed with stitches, staples, or skin tapes. The operation takes from thirty to ninety minutes, depending on the type of hernia and repair performed. You can then climb off the operating table, or be wheeled into the recovery room for a short stay before going home.

"Laparoscopic" hernia repair is now also available in most areas. In this method, a piece of plastic mesh patches the defect, using a laparoscope to place it on the undersurface of the weakened area from inside your abdomen. The instruments and TV camera are placed through three one-quarter to three-quarter-inch incisions in the lower abdomen. Your surgeon manipulates the mesh while watching on a TV monitor. Most surgeons use general anesthesia. Proponents claim this

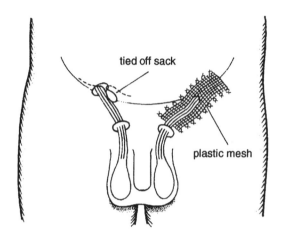

Fig. 18.2 Procedures involved in hernia mesh repair

technique causes less postoperative discomfort and allows a more rapid recovery. However, the procedure is more expensive, and at this point, it is uncertain whether it will prove to have comparable low recurrence rates, is cost-effective, or has any real advantage—other than smaller scars—over the standard, less-high-tech methods. It may be more applicable to fix recurrent hernias because it avoids the more difficult surgery when reentering the scarred area from the previous repair. I use this type of repair for recurrent hernias or when a repair is needed for hernias of both the right and left sides.

No matter which operation was performed, you may have significant discomfort in the area of your surgery for a few days. You can take oral pain medication, and use ice and an athletic supporter to decrease your swelling, relieve pain, and support your testicle.

Your operative site will be swollen to some degree, and your testicle may be mildly swollen and tender. Leakage of blood into your tissues, causing a black-and-blue bruise that may include your scrotum and penis, is harmless as long as you form no large space-taking blood clot; such a clot should be removed. If, after a few days, your incision becomes more swollen, tender, and reddened, an infection may be developing, and you should notify your surgeon.

The appearance of a "healing ridge" may alarm you, but this is simply a firm ridge of tissue beneath the line of your stitches, resulting from the normal healing process and most noticeable once your incision's initial swelling has subsided, a week or two after surgery. This healing ridge gradually softens and disappears. You may have a small area of decreased sensation below your incision caused by interruption of the fine network of skin nerves. Normal sensation usually returns over a period of months.

Surgeons disagree over how soon normal activities should be resumed after a hernia repair. Traditionally, you would have been excused from work for four to six weeks and advised to avoid strenuous activity for three months. Such recommendations would be extended if you had a recurrent hernia or did very physically demanding work. However, many surgeons now place no restrictions but advise avoiding any activity that causes pain. Your activities should be curtailed when you have discomfort, and can be increased after the soreness in your incision decreases. No evidence suggests that early vigorous exercise will ruin the repair, especially if mesh reinforcement has been used. You can return to work as soon as you feel that you can perform your duties comfortably.

Hernia repair is a very safe surgery. Mortality varies from 0.1 percent in elective cases to 10 to 12 percent in emergencies, with most deaths occurring in elderly persons who have developed strangulated intestine. Complications for elective surgery are seen in only 5 percent, though emergency surgery has a rate ten times as high. Complications are more common if you are over 60 years old. Your risk for a major heart or lung complication is greatly reduced if you choose local anesthesia.

A large incisional blood clot (hematoma) or infection occurs in 1 to 2 percent. Difficulty with urination, especially in older men with enlarged prostate glands, usually passes in a day or two, though a catheter may be required for a short time. Your testicle may be swollen and tender, especially if you had a large hernia extending into your scrotum. In less than 1 percent of all cases, the blood supply to your testicle is interfered with, causing testicle swelling, eventually followed by a permanent reduction in size (atrophy).

Damage to your local sensory nerves can cause temporary, sometimes permanent, lack of feeling in your scrotum, labia, or upper thigh. Rarely, a nerve reaction called a *neuroma* forms when a nerve is injured or trapped in scar tissue, and can produce persis-

tent pain. Significant chronic groin pain occurs in 1 percent of all patients. Very rarely, a surgical exploration to remove the trapped nerve can be considered.

Umbilical Hernia

An umbilical hernia occurs in 1 percent of all adults. An outpouching develops through a defect in your abdominal wall where your umbilical cord passed from your mother to you as a baby. Intestine or fat from within your abdomen or abdominal wall can pass into this sack. You may first develop this type of hernia during your own pregnancy. Other predisposing factors are obesity, chronically increased intra-abdominal pressure from a low-fiber diet, cough, constipation, urinary obstruction, or liver disease that creates fluid within your abdomen. Often small defects containing only fat do not cause symptoms whatsoever.

Diagnosis is usually obvious with the finding of a lump in or next to your umbilicus. However, if you are obese, this hernia may be difficult to find. Umbilical hernias can be more dangerous than other types of hernia because they often have small "necks." If the hernia is big enough to allow bowel into it, entrapment and strangulation of intestine can occur. Surgery is advisable at the time of your diagnosis if you have symptoms or bowel is involved. However, if the neck is quite wide and less likely to trap contents, and you are in poor health or wish to avoid surgery, you can wear a corset or girdle.

Alternative Medicine Approaches to Umbilical Hernias

Just as for groin hernias, prevention is the heart of what alternative medicine has to offer for umbilical hernias. If you already have an umbilical hernia, you generally need surgery to repair it. Once it is repaired, however, you can focus simply on preventive measures to avoid a recurrence.

Chronically increased intra-abdominal pressure is at the root of umbilical hernia formation, and you can take action to prevent further creation of such a hernia. The following alternative medicine approaches have proven successful for many people.

Change Your Diet

If you have enough fiber in your regular diet and can thus keep your bowels easy and regular, you can avoid the increased pressure associated with straining at stool that contributes to hernia development. Make certain to take in 20 to 40 grams of fiber per day; follow the general dietary guidelines given in Chapter 2 to act preventively or to avoid recurrence once you have formed a hernia.

Maintain Your Optimum Weight

When you weigh more than is appropriate for your frame, your tissues become stretched, thinned, and strained. Any small lift may be enough to tip the balance toward a hernia. You can prevent or reverse this predisposing problem by following the dietary guidelines given in Chapter 2. Consuming a low-fat, high-fiber diet will help you achieve and maintain a risk-free weight.

Be Careful with Lifting

The repeated stress of lifting can stretch and strain your abdomen and help set up an umbilical hernia. Proper lifting involves first bending your knees and then aligning yourself so that the bulk of your weight is centered over your knees rather than given to your abdominal muscles. See Chapter 22 for further discussion about the correct form to use when lifting.

Quit Smoking

Nicotine acts to constrict the small blood vessels, which interferes with the proper repair of your tissues and thus predisposes you to a hernia. In addition, coughing itself, often associated with smoking, can elevate your hernia risk. See Chapter 2 for alternative medicine solutions for quitting smoking for good.

Exercise Regularly

By improving general and local blood and lymph flow, exercise can help you maintain optimum tissue strength. This will prevent the tissue weakening that can set you up for an umbilical hernia. See Chapter 2 for exercise information and inspiration.

Practice Visualization

Visualization is a practice that can alter your body's blood and lymph flow to both help prevent and treat any altered physical state, even a hernia. After first relaxing yourself, imagine your abdomen as a smooth beach and your hernia as a sand drift. Imagine waves washing over the beach and smoothing out the drift. Picture this happening in your mind while at the same time feeling it being accomplished in your body.

Try Yoga, Acupuncture, Herbs, and Homeopathy

Yoga not only helps to relax your body, but stretches and strengthens the muscles and ligaments needed for lifting. You can also try acupuncture, the herb rupturewort (*Herniare glabra*), or the homeopathic *calcarea carbonica* or *nux vomica,* as recommended by a skilled homeopath. The reports of benefit remain anecdotal, making further research necessary.

Surgical Approaches to Umbilical Hernias

You can have your umbilical hernia surgery as an outpatient, choosing general, spinal, or local anesthesia. No preoperative preparation is necessary. Your surgeon makes a crosswise or up-and-down incision, usually just above or below or next to the belly button. Its length corresponds to the size of the hernia. After the sack is removed or pushed back into your abdomen, your abdominal wall defect is closed with stitches in one or two layers. Plastic mesh reinforcement may be required if you have a large or recurrent hernia, or if your tissue is weakened and the doctor fears stitches might cut through it. Your skin is closed with stitches, staples, or skin tapes. In some large hernias, your surgeon removes the belly button rather than making an attempt at reconstruction, avoiding a skin incision complication. The operation takes twenty minutes to an hour.

Postoperative discomfort can be handled with pain pills. Recovery and recommendations are the same as those after groin hernia surgery.

The mortality rate of elective umbilical hernia repair is less than 1 percent, but emergency surgery carries a mortality of 5 to 10 percent if dead bowel needs to be removed. Complications of incision infection or blood clot develop occasionally. Recurrences are unusual after repair, though risk is increased if you are obese, smoke, or have chronically increased intra-abdominal pressure.

GROIN HERNIA SUMMARY

Prevention

Diet and Supplements

- Follow a low-fat, high-fiber diet.
- Drink 8–10 glasses of water daily.
- Bran, 3 tablespoons daily.
- Psyllium, 1–3 tablespoons daily.

Lifestyle

- Don't smoke.
- Maintain optimum weight.
- Exercise 1 hour, 3–5 times weekly.
- Be careful in lifting.

Alternative Medicine Approaches

- Follow the guidelines for prevention, above.
- Practice visualization.

Conventional Medicine Approach

- External support—truss, corset.

Sugical Approaches

- Open repair with or without mesh reinforcement.
- Laparoscopic repair with mesh reinforcement.

Ventral and Incisional Hernias

Alice, *a trim 70-year-old woman, had a large midabdominal incisional hernia that was uncomfortable as well as an embarrassment to* *her, since she took much pride in her appearance. She had experienced some heart problems and had been advised by her internist not to have surgery. After several months of badgering her doctor, she was finally referred for a surgical opinion. The operation and its risks were explained, and she decided to have a repair with a large sheet of plastic mesh, and is now very happy with the results.*

A *ventral hernia* forms through a defect in your abdominal wall anywhere from your pubic bone to breastbone. If the hernia is between your umbilicus and breastbone, it is called an *epigastric hernia*. These hernias, like those in the groin or umbilicus, can be caused by chronically increased intra-abdominal pressure. You may have localized pain and discomfort or no symptoms whatsoever. Sharp pain and nausea may occur if a small piece of fat is caught in the defect as you lie down. If bowel is caught in the hernia, there may be intestinal obstruction and strangulation. Your diagnosis is made by the finding of a lump, more obvious when you strain. If you are overweight or have a small hernia, its discovery may be difficult.

Ventral hernias may be large or small. If the "neck" is narrow, you are in danger of bowel entrapment and strangulation, so you need this type of hernia repaired soon after it is found.

The very common *incisional hernia* can develop at any site where surgery has been performed, and a part or all of your incision may be involved. (See Figure 18.3.) You may have multiple defects, a "Swiss cheese" effect. Predisposing factors are previous wound infection, obesity, or when weakened tissue is subjected to sudden strain such as from cough or heavy lifting. Scar tissue may have formed

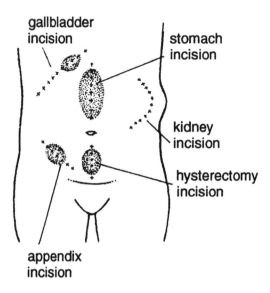

gallbladder
incision

stomach
incision

kidney
incision

hysterectomy
incision

appendix
incision

Fig. 18.3   Types of incisional hernias

between your abdominal wall and adjacent intestine, giving you twinges of pain. This sort of hernia tends to have a small neck, and is therefore prone to bowel entrapment and strangulation.

Surgical repair is usually advised for ventral and incisional hernias as they tend to enlarge, become uncomfortable, and can entrap bowel. They can also cause problems in breathing efficiently and the stretched, thin skin can break down. However, if the neck is wide, strangulation is less likely. If you have this type of hernia or a huge, recurrent, or multiple hernias, and are in very poor health, it may be wise to simply wear a girdle or corset to relieve your symptoms.

A *rectus diastasis* is a bulge in the area between your breastbone and umbilicus, caused by a separation in your rectus muscles that extend from your rib cage to pubic bone. It is sometimes caused by pregnancy. Although often confused with a hernia, this is not a true hernia, and carries no danger of bowel entrapment because no constricting neck is formed. You may still want an operation to bring your muscles back to normal position for reasons of comfort or cosmetic effect; however, the scar of your incision will be a trade-off.

Alternative Medicine Approaches to Ventral and Incisional Hernias

Once you have developed a ventral or incisional hernia, you may need an operation to fix it. However, you can act preventively to avoid a recurrence. Following are the most important steps you can take to prevent a ventral or incisional hernia.

Change Your Diet

A diet too low in fiber can act to increase abdominal pressure and straining at stool, both of which are associated with the formation of ventral and incisional hernias. Use the information given in Chapter 2 to assure that you take in from 20 to 40 grams of fiber per day and have easeful and plentiful bowel passage.

Maintain Your Optimum Weight

Once the fibers of the tissues of your abdomen have been stretched to the point where they cannot maintain their optimum repair, any small strain may contribute to the onset of a ventral or incisional hernia. See Chapter 2 for the dietary choices that can act to help you achieve and maintain your ideal weight, thereby cutting back on this risk factor.

Be Careful with Lifting

Making certain that when you lift an object you center the weight above your bent knees can act in a way to allow you to protect your abdominal muscles from ventral and incisional hernias. See Chapter 22 for more information on the proper form to use during lifting.

Quit Smoking

Nicotine affects the flow of blood through your tissues by clamping down on the small capillaries and increasing carbon dioxide content while decreasing oxygen amounts. Therefore, smoking is associated with weakened abdominal wall strength and an increased risk for formation of ventral and incisional hernias. See Chapter 2 for the best alternative medicine contributions to help you quit smoking and stay away from it.

Exercise Regularly

Optimum amounts of exercise act to give you protection against ventral and incisional hernias by helping your tissues become strong and pliant. In this optimum condition, should they be stretched or pushed, they will not allow a hernia to form. See Chapter 2 for further information on creating an exercise program for yourself.

Practice Visualization

Once a hernia has formed, you may be able to decrease its bulge by applying the power of a focused mind. For example, after first relaxing, picture a smooth pond with one bubble on its surface. Gently blow the bubble away and see the final polished surface. While you image this in your mind, feel it happening in your body. See Chapter 2 for more details.

Try Yoga, Acupuncture, Herbs, and Homeopathy

While no specific research supports the use of these modalities, case reports have indicated that some persons find benefit once a hernia has formed by the application of yoga postures, acupuncture, the herb "rupture-wort" (*Herniare glabra*), or the homeopathics *calcarea carbonica* or *nux vomica*, as recommended by an experienced homeopath. Further research may be warranted.

Conventional Medicine Approach to Ventral and Incisional Hernias

Your symptoms may be relieved by wearing a binder or corset that will give your abdominal wall support and prevent your abdominal contents from bulging out. The better, more durable types can be found at surgical supply stores listed in the Yellow Pages. They are usually adjustable by Velcro tabs. They may be worth a try if your physician believes your hernia is not likely to cause intestinal blockage or strangulation, and you wish to avoid surgery.

Surgical Approaches to Ventral and Incisional Hernias

Kevin, a 45-year-old Alaskan fisherman, underwent a stomach stapling procedure that was successful in reducing his weight from 350 to 225 pounds. Unhappily, he developed an incisional hernia which was repaired on four different occasions, twice with plastic mesh reinforcement. Eventually, the mesh eroded into a piece of small bowel and he developed an infected, open draining wound which put him out of work for six months before final healing occurred after two further operations.

Surgical repair of both ventral and incisional hernias is similar. The operation can be done without hospitalization if your hernia is small, though most larger hernias require a few days in the hospital. No preoperative preparation is necessary. You can be awake for a small hernia repair, using local anesthesia and intravenous sedation, but must be asleep if you have a larger one. Your surgeon will make an up-and-down or side-to-side incision directly over the bulge. The hernia contents are placed back into your abdomen and stretched and weakened tissue removed. If your tissue is strong, the defect is closed with stitches, but if it is wide or your tissue tenuous, plastic mesh may be used to bridge the abdominal wall defect or reinforce the repair.

Currently, a popular method for repairing large or difficult hernias places the mesh under the abdominal muscles on top of the peritoneum (lining of the abdominal cavity), thus the mesh is not in contact with bowel. It is anchored in place circumferentially by ten to fourteen stitches brought through the abdominal wall or internally by staples. Compared to other types of repair, the failure rate is very favorable (less than 5 percent), and patient satisfaction high, although initial discomfort is considerable, two to four or more days of hospitalization is required, and some patients experience long-term discomfort.[4]

Large hernia repairs are subject to fluid collections, especially if plastic mesh has been placed. One or two drains may be placed to prevent this. Thirty minutes to three hours are needed, depending upon size and complexity of your repair.

You may need injections to control immediate postoperative pain, but pain pills are usually satisfactory after a day or two. You can be out of bed the evening of your operation. Your abdomen may be tightened by the surgery and pain can further restrict your moving air, making you at risk for breathing problems and pneumonia. You should keep your lungs expanded by deep breathing and coughing to prevent these complications. If you smoke, it is best to stop a week or two days prior to your operation and not resume until you are fully recovered, or better yet, take this as an opportunity to quit.

Usually, you can begin eating on the first postoperative day. Drains, if any, are removed in two to four days and skin stitches or staples in five to ten days. Abdominal tenderness may last for a month or so. You are advised to avoid strenuous activity for four to eight weeks, though in some cases, permanent restrictions are necessary. Your surgeon will want to see you in follow-up exams until your incision has fully healed and you are satisfied with the result.

Complications of surgery include incision infection in 2 to 5 percent of all cases. If the newer plastic mesh is involved, draining the infection and local care, without removing the plastic, is usually successful. Very rarely, plastic mesh will erode through the bowel wall, leading to a leaking hole or fistula. This can present a serious problem, requiring further surgery to repair the bowel.

The hernia recurrence rate is 0.5 to 10 percent in repairs using mesh and up to 40 percent in those using your own tissue without mesh reinforcement.

Ventral and incisional hernias can now also be repaired using laparoscopic methods. You are under general anesthesia. Three or four one-quarter to three-quarter-inch incisions are made. A TV camera and surgical instruments can then be introduced. First, any adhering bowel is carefully dissected off the undersurface of the hernia defect and pulled back into the abdomen. Then a sheet of rolled-up mesh is passed through one of the ports then unrolled and sutured and tacked to the abdominal wall, covering and overlapping the defect from the inside. This procedure causes less postop discomfort than conventional repairs, a shorter hospital stay, recovery is quicker, and the scars may be more pleasing. However, though initial results are promising, the ultimate recurrence rate is as yet unknown. So far, the complication and recurrence rate is similar to the open repair.[5] Ask your surgeon if you would be a good candidate for this procedure.

Groin Hernias in Children

An indirect inguinal hernia occurs in 1 to 2 percent of all children, nine times more commonly in males. Frequently, it appears within the first year of life. When fluid or a piece of intestine or ovary is inside the sack, the hernia is evident as a swelling in the groin. The swelling may disappear whenever the sack contents slide back into the abdomen, but a thickening persists. The lump becomes larger whenever the child cries or strains.

Alternative Medicine Approaches to Groin Hernias in Children

Generally, since surgery to repair a groin hernia is very simple and safe, choosing operative repair for a child makes sense. However, alternative medicine has much to offer to help prevent genetically predisposing factors from being expressed as an actual hernia. Also, these steps may prove helpful whenever an operation is not possible.

Following are the most important alternative medicine approaches for groin hernias in children.

Choose an Optimum Diet

Adequate fiber in the diet may help prevent the formation of hernias. Enough fibrous foods should be included so that two to three easily passed bowel movements are accomplished each day. Since breast milk contains natural laxative agents, it is optimum to breast-feed for two to three years; such a practice also helps prevent childhood illnesses, due to the immunity factors in breast milk, and helps prevent obesity. Breast-feeding has multiple other benefits, including babies that are more content and have higher IQs. Breast milk should be the exclusive nutrition until age 6 months, when the teeth begin to develop. Then, high-fiber foods, such as fruits and vegetables, can be added. A vegetarian diet is best. Follow the guidelines for the best nutritional choices given in Chapter 2.

Maintain Optimum Weight

Excess weight may contribute to the tendency of this weakness to express itself as an actual hernia. The practice of breast-feeding, and then consuming a high-fiber diet, can help a child achieve and maintain ideal weight. Learning and applying good nutrition in childhood is also very helpful in the prevention of a whole host of adult diseases, including hernias in adulthood.

Teach Children to Lift Carefully

Teaching children to lift with their backs straight and knees bent may help to prevent the formation of a hernia. Lifting objects that are too heavy or bulky should also be avoided. For more information, see the discussion of prevention of adult hernias on page 493.

Surgical Approach to Groin Hernias in Children

A truss is not practical for children, so surgeons will usually advise early repair, even for very small babies, because these hernias tend to trap bowel and it is much easier and safer to do the operation on an elective basis. If the hernia becomes entrapped, an attempt can be made to reduce the hernia, usually successful on a sedated child. The operation should then be done in a day or two, as recurrent entrapment is a near certainty. The only reasons to delay surgery are if the baby is premature or has a cold, skin rash, or other acute illness.

The operation is an outpatient procedure under general anesthesia. A one-inch incision is made in the groin fat fold. The surgery is different than that in adults, in that only the sack is removed, and tissues do not usually need reinforcing. Usual operating time is fifteen to thirty minutes.

Postoperatively, the child has very little discomfort and no restriction on activity. Absorbable stitches placed beneath the skin are generally used to close the incision. In older children, vigorous activity may be uncomfortable for a week or two, but loss of time from school should be minimal. Some swelling and hardness in the incision may be present for a few weeks, along with temporary swelling of the testicle and scrotum.

Many surgeons recommend that the opposite groin be "explored" at the same time the known hernia is repaired, since the possibility of a second hernia developing later in life is 41 percent if the first hernia was on the left and 14 percent when on the right.[6] This likelihood is even higher in females. Chance of this decreases with increasing age; exploration of both sides usually isn't done after age six. The second exploration adds ten to twenty minutes to the operative time, and might save the cost and time involved in a second operation later in life. However, if the first hernia surgery is performed as an emergency, or the procedure was difficult, reconstruction of the other side should not be attempted, since the danger and consequences of bilateral spermatic cord or testicular damage outweighs its potential advantage.

The repair of a pediatric hernia is a very safe operation. Complications are rare. Injury to the spermatic cord or testicle occurs in 1 to 2 percent of all cases, much less for a surgeon experienced with pediatric hernias. If damage occurred on both sides, infertility could result. Incision infection occurs in less than 1 percent, and recurrent hernia is less than 1 percent.

Umbilical Hernias in Children

Umbilical hernias occur in 10 percent of all white and 40 percent of all black infants at birth. This type of hernia occurs through the abdominal wall opening where the umbilical cord passed from the mother to the baby. Usually, this defect closes by constriction of neighboring tissue shortly after the cord is severed. However, in some cases, the closure may take several months or years or not occur at all. For unknown reasons, slow closures are much more common in black children. About 80 percent of these defects do close by six years of age, though defects larger than three-quarters inch are less likely to do so.

If the defect is initially large or shows no signs of getting smaller at three to four years of age, most surgeons advise repair. In any case, this surgery should be done before the child reaches school age. Strapping or placing tape to hold the hernia in is *not* helpful in speeding closure, and may cause skin problems. It is unusual for pediatric umbilical hernias to entrap abdominal contents, but if this does develop, surgery is advised; such a complication tends to recur, and may lead to strangulation.

Alternative Medicine Approaches to Umbilical Hernias in Children

Since most of these hernias disappear on their own, the major contribution of the alternative approaches would seem to be to relax both the parents and the child and prevent the rush to an operation. Certainly, social pressure can be intense and may sway your decision. Meanwhile, following are alternatives to consider while waiting out nature's hand.

Maintain Optimum Weight

Excess weight can weaken the abdominal tissues, making it harder for an umbilical hernia to resolve on its own. Breast-feeding, up to age two to four years, is highly recommended to help prevent childhood obesity. See Chapter 2 for additional dietary guidelines to help your child achieve and maintain optimum weight.

Practice Stress Management and Yoga Daily

Both the child and the parents can find relief from the stress of an umbilical hernia while waiting for it to spontaneously resolve by the application of the stress management approaches discussed in Chapter 2. Deep relaxation and meditation can encourage a calm acceptance of body shape. Books and tapes on yoga practices for children are available from your local library or bookstore, or by calling 800-476-1347.

Surgical Approach to Umbilical Hernias in Children

Surgery for pediatric umbilical hernia is very easy and is accomplished in fifteen to thirty minutes. After the child is under general anesthesia, the surgeon makes a small, curved incision in the upper or lower edge of the umbilicus. The hernia contents are pushed back into the abdomen and the sack removed. The strong tissue surrounding the umbilical defect in the abdominal wall is then pulled together with stitches. The skin incision is usually closed with dissolvable stitches beneath the skin surface and skin tapes. The hernia recurs in less than 1 percent, since the tissue is quite sturdy. Complications are rare. The child may go home shortly after surgery with no limitations on activity. One return visit to see the surgeon is all that is usually necessary.

FEMALE REPRODUCTIVE SYSTEM

Why can't a woman be more like a man?

Alan Lerner

You don't need a hysterectomy. It can do you more harm than good. Those are strong words, but the fact is that more than 90 percent of hysterectomies [for benign diseases] are unnecessary.

Stanley West, M.D.

Currently, one out of every three American women ends up losing her uterus before age 60, and the numbers are steadily increasing, as the baby boomers age. Hysterectomy—removal of the uterus—is second only to cesarean section as the most common major operation performed upon women in the United States, and about 600,000 have this procedure each year.

If you are female, and if you have underlying fear of disease or suffer from significant pain or bleeding, you may worry about what is the right thing to do, especially if your doctor has recommended you have surgery. Importantly, rushing to have your uterine disorder treated surgically is not usually necessary; you can take time to assess all of your options. In this chapter, we present information to help you choose what is best for you. You may be able to obtain relief by trying alternative or conventional measures first, and thus avoid an operation.

Even in these relatively enlightened times, the female pelvis still often lives in the dark ages. Our Western traditions do not generally honor women's anatomy, as some civilizations have, and the uterus is often simply looked at as excess baggage, particularly after menopause. Multilayered cultural confusions, psychological inhibitions, and various outmoded beliefs about ovarian and uterine function contribute to this pattern. Emotional and physical satisfaction are counterbalanced by the strangeness, pain, or our simple sense of annoyance at the regular bleeding of even "normal" menstruation.

Alternative medicine's mind-body perspective seems especially important in the context of female pelvic disorders. Menstruation, labor and delivery, and menopause can all be seen as positive and natural events. If you are a woman and can learn to appreciate the female aspect of yourself, and feel comfortable with your periods or menopause, the stress-reducing aspects of this paradigm shift may itself help protect your health, or assist you in recovering from diseases in this area.

Unless you develop cancer, you do have a choice whether to have your uterus or ovaries removed. Many surgeons argue in favor of their removal, as we shall see, but rationale now also exists for keeping them both. In addition to the uterus influencing the production of estrogen by the ovaries, easing your transition through menopause, it also continues to produce hormones that contribute to brain tranquillity, and participates in orgasm as well as general bodily pleasure.

Many authorities suggest that up to 90 percent of the hysterectomies done for non-cancerous problems are unnecessary. Uterine removal is far more frequently performed in the United States than in any other country: the rate here is *twice* that of England. Although many women feel better after their hysterectomies, some experience significant side effects. Many common female ailments once solved by an operation can often now be successfully treated by alternative or conventional medicine, or an integration of both.

Not even all cancers require removal of the uterus; for example, if the cancer of the cervix is "carcinoma in situ," it can be removed locally, in an outpatient surgery center, without your having to lose your whole uterus. In 1990, BlueCross BlueShield began to ask its doctors and hospitals to voluntarily reduce the number of hysterectomies being performed, and many other insurance companies followed suit. The percentage of women undergoing hysterectomy has begun to decline in certain places, owing to some insurance companies actually refusing to pay for this operation unless it is for cancer.[1]

How can you know whether surgery is right for you? In the last few years, appreciation of the relationship of nutrition and stress to female pelvic illnesses offers much promise that changes in diet and lifestyle, along with other nonsurgical means, can very effectively help you avoid a number of pelvic diseases; or once they are present, even reverse them.

For example, simply changing your diet may influence your hormonal function, preventing a wide array of disorders. You can decrease your intake of foods high in fats, such as meat, poultry, and dairy products, which increase your body's production of estrogen. Excess estrogen is thought to help account for the current increases in uterine fibroids and endometriosis. These food choices also contain added estrogens from animal feed, contributing to female risk and potentially responsible for recent lowering of sperm counts in males.[2] You can instead increase your intake of foods high in *phytoestrogens*, found in many beans and vegetables. These estrogenlike substances assist in maintaining optimum estrogen activity while preventing excess estrogen buildup in the body. Many other cultures eat half of their foods from choices high in phytoestrogens, while in the United States, the standard diet contains less than 10 percent of foods containing these substances.

Encouraging news is also available on the operative front. If you do need or choose surgery, in the last ten years the number of minimally invasive gynecologic operations has skyrocketed, and now virtually every procedure can be performed using these techniques, giving you less pain, a smaller scar or scars, a shorter hospital stay, and a quicker recovery. Your sexuality can remain uninhibited and your general well-being restored.

Structure and Function of the Female Reproductive System

The female reproductive organs consist of two *ovaries*, two *fallopian tubes*, and the *uterus*, all which lie within the abdominal pelvic cavity, and the *vagina*, which connects to the external vulva. (See Figure 19.1.)

The flattened, walnut-sized ovaries sit behind and on each side of the uterus. These cream-colored glands hold hundreds of tiny immature *ovum* or *eggs,* which are present when you are born. The ovaries also produce the hormones *estrogen* and *progesterone.* Puberty marks the onset of the production of these hormones, which induces egg maturation, ovulation, fertility, and menstruation. These hormones also control development of the female characteristics of figure, breast development, and body hair.

Each month, usually from alternating ovaries, an egg matures, ruptures free from the tough covering of the ovary, and is picked up by the sticky, widened, open end of the fallopian tube lying right next to the ovary. The other end of the fallopian tube attaches to the upper part of the uterus. These pink tubes are about four inches long, and are lined with special cells whose hairlike processes wave the egg down the tube into the uterine cavity. The usual site for fertilization is within this tube.

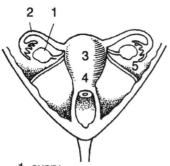

1. ovary
2. fallopian tube
3. uterus body
4. uterus cervix
5. suspensory ligament
6. uterus myometrium

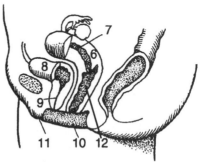

7. uterus endometrium
8. bladder
9. uretha
10. labia
11. clitoris
12. vagina

Fig. 19.1   The anatomy of the female reproductive system

The uterus, shaped like a small glistening pink pear, sits behind the bladder. Its lowest end is attached to the vagina and its upper part by ligaments to the pelvic side walls. It has two sections: the upper *body*, which holds the developing fetus if conception occurs, and the lower *cervix*, which opens into the vagina. Each month, estrogen and progesterone from the ovary act on the lining layer of the uterine cavity, termed the *endometrium*, gradually preparing a thicker nourishing site for implantation of a fertilized egg. Hormones also affect the mucus produced by the cervix, changing it from thick to thin, which allows sperm to pass through into the uterus.

If an egg is fertilized and does implant, hormones are then produced that provide stability to the uterine lining as the embryo matures. If not, the hormone levels fall and the lining sloughs off with menstruation. At menopause, when the ovaries stop maturing eggs, and the level of hormone production is decreased, menstruation ceases.

The thick outer layer of the uterus, called the *myometrium*, is muscular, and its contractions can be felt both during menstruation and childbirth. Uterine muscle fibers have the ability to grow and stretch enormously during pregnancy. At delivery, they contract on hormonal cue, squeezing the baby through the cervix. Also muscle, the cervix dilates from one-eighth inch to four or five inches in diameter, to accommodate passage of the head.

The *vagina* is the three- to five-inch tunnel that connects the uterus to the *vulva*, or external genitalia, which includes the *labia*, the skin folds around the vaginal opening, and the *clitoris*. It is the "birth canal" through which you saw your first glimpse of light—unless, of course, you arrived like Caesar, via "cesarean."

Healthy functioning of the female reproductive system is nothing short of miraculous, and disruption of its intricate system can cause intermittent or constant pain and discomfort, and irregular or abnormal bleeding.

How Disorders of the Female Reproductive System Are Diagnosed

Diagnosis of female disorders begins with a detailed history and simple physical exam. It may be necessary to follow your initial evaluation with some of the following more complicated tests.

History

Your doctor should ask about your menstrual history—when you had your first period (menarche), the usual number of days between the onset of blood flow, the number of days and the amount of bleeding with each period, and any associated symptoms. Irregular periods can have many causes. If you have been through menopause, your age at your last period and associated symptoms are included in your menstrual history.

Your sexual and reproductive history begins with questions about your sexual desire, frequency of intercourse and any associated problems or discomfort, age of initial intercourse, number of sexual partners, contraceptive method, and any sexually transmitted diseases you may have had. Next is a series of questions about pregnancies, if any. Your doctor needs to know in detail any difficulties you may have had in getting pregnant or in carrying through a pregnancy. If you are in your childbearing years, your desires about future pregnancy and birth control methods need to be discussed.

You should tell your doctor about any

vaginal bleeding not associated with menstruation, any foul discharge, pelvic pain, abdominal swelling, or discomfort on urination or during bowel movements. If you have a family member who has had ovarian cancer, be sure to let your doctor know, since about 10 percent of these disorders have a genetic basis.

Physical Exam

The basic gynecological physical examination includes careful assessment of your breasts, abdomen, vagina, uterus, fallopian tubes, and ovaries. For the "internal" or "pelvic" part of the exam, you will most likely be lying on your back with your legs up in "stirrups." You can leave your socks and/or shoes on, so that you are more comfortable. You might even try wearing cowboy boots, as some women have, just to keep a sense of humor and stay more relaxed on the examination table while your feet are in these awkward devices.

Your doctor first examines your vulva, vagina, and cervix with the aid of a plastic or metal vaginal speculum, placed in the vagina. This can be uncomfortable, though it should not be painful. A Pap smear is usually taken at this time, as well as a culture sample to look for abnormal bacteria, if indicated. Any abnormal ulcers or growths are assessed using simple biopsy techniques.

Next your doctor inserts two fingers into your vagina while simultaneously pushing down on your lower abdomen with the other hand, to feel your uterus and ovaries between the two hands. Enlarged fallopian tubes may also be felt. You may feel pressure, a dull ache, or a sharp twinge as the ovaries are compressed. If your abdominal muscles are relaxed, any abnormalities in size, contour, consistency, or sensitivity can usually be found

with this method. The exam is completed with a finger rectal exam, to evaluate the back wall of your uterus.

You can perform some of this examination yourself, using a vaginal speculum—which you can get from a surgical supply store without a prescription—and a mirror. A healthy cervix is shiny pink, with minimal discharge or oozing. Examination of the uterine body and the ovaries by self-exam methods is more difficult, though you may be able to feel them by squatting in a bathtub of warm water, and wiggling your fingers in your vagina at the same time as pushing with the other hand on your abdomen. In any case, no self-exam is a substitute for an exam by someone experienced in what is normal. A good time to try self-exam is right after your doctor has examined you and found everything just fine. This is valuable for learning what your cervix and the inside of your vagina look and feel like when they are normal, so that you can notice any changes.

Pap Smear

The Pap smear is absolutely pivotal to assessment of gynecological health, though debate continues about how often it should be done. During a routine pelvic examination, your doctor uses a cotton swab, a wooden blade, or a small wire brush to scrape a sampling of cells from the surface of the cervix, its opening into the uterine cavity, and the vagina. The material collected is placed on glass slides, then sprayed with a fixative. Analysis of the slides under a microscope is used to classify them into normal and increasingly abnormal ASCUS (atypical squamous cells of undetermined significance), LGSIL (low-grade squamous intraepithelial lesion), and HGSIL (high-grade squamous intraepithelial lesion). The Pap smear also can determine if an infection is present, as well as what your hormone status is, so that having one is a simple way to monitor your total cervical and vaginal health.

Should you have a Pap smear every year? Some cancers of the cervix are slow-growing, and can be seen on the Pap smear for several years before they become invasive, but some are not. We both recommend you have a Pap smear every year.

Sonogram or Ultrasound Tests

The transabdominal sonogram is a noninvasive test that produces a direct "sound picture" of your uterus, tubes, and ovaries. It can be used to confirm or follow a pregnancy. It can even tell the sex of the baby. You first must drink lots of water, to distend your bladder, making your pelvic organs more obvious. A handheld sound-wave probe is moved slowly over your abdomen. It sends out harmless high-frequency sound waves, which bounce off the structures; as they are reflected backward, they are picked up and displayed on a monitor. A small vaginal probe may also be used (EVUS—endovaginal ultrasound), to look from a different angle. Hysterosonography is a somewhat more complicated, invasive procedure where a tiny ultrasound probe is introduced into your uterine cavity for a closer view. These painless, relatively inexpensive tests take from fifteen to thirty minutes to perform.

Pelvic CAT and MRI Scans

The CAT scan takes a series of cross-sectional X-rays, to provide detailed pictures of the pelvic structures. Dye can be given intravenously, by mouth, and rectally, to make the tissues stand out more clearly. You lie on your back while the X-ray machine whirls in a circle around your body. The "spiral" CAT scanner is the latest innovation providing very high resolution, almost three-dimensional, images. The MRI, which utilizes a magnetic imaging process, is sometimes used to further assess pelvic structures.

Culposcopy

This is a precise way of diagnosing diseases of the vulva, vagina, and cervix. An instrument called a culposcope is used, allowing your doctor to look closely and microscopically at tissue suspected of being abnormal. Your vagina is usually first rinsed with a special mixture of dilute vinegar, causing abnormal, cancerous, or premalignant areas to appear as white patches. A biopsy can be directed right to that area, and if all malignant tissue can be removed, you can avoid further surgery.

Hysteroscopy

This test is done in your doctor's office, while your feet are up in stirrups. A very narrow lighted scope is passed into the vagina and directed through the opening of your cervix into the uterine cavity. Polyps, fibroids, other growths, abnormal anatomy, and scarring can be seen. This test can be done before a D&C (see page 506) to more precisely locate the cause of your problem.

Hysterosalpingogram

This is an X-ray test where dye is injected through the hysteroscope, thereby outlining the inside of the uterus and tubes. It is helpful in diagnosing abnormal anatomy and blocked tubes, common causes of infertility.

Culdoscopy

This is usually done in an operating room, under local anesthesia and sedation, while you are up in stirrups. A small scope is passed through a minute incision in the back of your vagina. Your pelvic structures are visualized to look for various abnormalities and small biopsies can be taken. This test has been pretty much replaced by laparoscopy.

Laparoscopy

This is now the best method to directly examine the outside surfaces of your uterus, ovaries, and tubes. It can be performed on an outpatient basis. You will likely need general anesthesia, though you can choose local, along with intravenous sedation.

You lie on your back on the operating table. After your skin is prepped with an antibacterial solution, your doctor makes a three-quarter-inch incision, right under your navel, so that afterward you have little visible scarring. A hollow operating "port" is passed through the incision into your abdominal cavity. Carbon dioxide is instilled through the port, to inflate your abdomen, creating viewing and working space. The laparoscope is then introduced through the port. Your doctor can view directly through the scope, or may attach a camera, and watch the image displayed on a television monitor. The operating table can be tilted head-down and side-to-side, so that your intestines can be slipped out of the way.

Special instruments can be passed through a channel in the laparoscope. Direct visualization of the female structures is quite simple, and biopsies can be taken if abnormalities are found. Fallopian tubal ligation to achieve sterilization is also made simple by this method: The tube is located and tied off, with

few complications. If you have had previous lower abdominal surgery, adhesions can limit the success of this procedure. A thorough laparoscopic exam generally takes thirty to sixty minutes.

The incision is closed with stitches or skin tapes. Once you are wide awake, you can leave the hospital with just a Band-Aid over the incision. You may have some soreness and bruising for a few days, but you should be able to resume your usual activities within a week.

Rarely, bleeding, infection, or bowel damage can follow use of the laparoscope.

Laparotomy

This procedure for gynecological diagnosis has mostly been replaced by the less traumatic and safer laparoscopy. Rarely, if your diagnosis can't be obtained from the laparoscopic exam, or if complications arise, then laparotomy is used: Your abdomen is opened up just as in major surgery, the pelvic structures observed, and when appropriate, treatment instituted.

Biopsy

Tissue must be taken for microscopic analysis whenever pelvic exam or any of the above other tests finds abnormally appearing areas of the vulva, vagina, cervix, or inside of the uterus. The following techniques are performed "from below," while biopsy of the ovary, tubes, and outer layer of the uterus are usually done directly during laparoscopy, or through a larger abdominal incision.

Punch Biopsy

Using local anesthesia, a small instrument cuts out, or punches out, a one-eighth- to one-quarter-inch piece of tissue. Bleeding is usually minimal, and the incision heals without need for stitches.

Directed Biopsy

This procedure uses the colposcope and staining techniques to focus the biopsy on specific tissue areas that have stained abnormally.

Loop Electrocautery Excision Procedure

Loop electrocautery excision procedure (LEEP) test employs a pencil-like attachment to a cautery machine, which has a small electrified wire loop. After your cervix is anesthetized with local anesthesia, the loop is used to remove tissue, while the cautery effect prevents bleeding. LEEP can be performed in your doctor's office. It is used as a treatment to remove abnormal tissue after culposcopy and biopsy has outlined the area of abnormal cells.

Cone Biopsy

This mostly outmoded technique removes a full circle of tissue from the cervical opening into the uterus. Usually this is only recommended after a persistently abnormal Pap smear, when the source cannot be identified by any of the above tests. Its use for *diagnosis* should be avoided, since it causes more bleeding and scarring, carries a higher risk of infection, and can cause problems with subsequent labor and delivery. It can be used as *treatment* for abnormal areas if they are too large for removal by other biopsy techniques, allowing you to avoid hysterectomy.

Endometrial Biopsy

This is an office procedure that does not require anesthesia. Your doctor passes a suc-tion straw through your cervix to sample the endometrial tissue of the inner lining of your uterus. It tests for causes of abnormal bleeding, and now is rapidly replacing D&C.

Dilation and Curettage

Dilation and curettage is more commonly called D&C. "Dilation" refers to stretching of the cervical opening to gain access to the uterine cavity, while "curettage" refers to scraping the uterine lining and contents. D&C has been used to control irregular menstrual bleeding, though other means are now preferred, and is a diagnostic tool to evaluate persons suspected of uterine cancer. It is also the procedure used in abortions or miscarriages.

Although most doctors and patients prefer general anesthesia, you may choose spinal, epidural, or local. Seaweed may be first implanted in your cervix, to soften it. Left in overnight, the seaweed allows dilation to be less painful, and general anesthesia can be avoided. This operation can be performed in day surgery, and you can be released in the afternoon.

You lie on your back with your feet up in stirrups. An operating speculum is placed in your vagina, then instruments of progressively increasing diameter ("sounds") are used to dilate the cervical opening. Small scraping instruments (curettes), or a suction apparatus, are employed to remove the lining of the uterus—the tissue normally shed during menstruation.

Postoperatively, you may have some bleeding and mild discomfort for a day or so. Complications include excessive bleeding (0.2 percent), infection (0.3 percent), and, rarely, perforation of the uterus (0.5 percent). Chance of a complication requiring hysterectomy for control is about 1 in 2,000 D&Cs. This operation does not increase your risk of painful periods or future miscarriage.

Dysfunctional Uterine Bleeding

Causes of bleeding specific to the uterus not associated with normal menstrual periods include those brought on by inflammation, infection, or irritation of the cervix, lining of the uterus, or fallopian tubes; endometriosis; problems of pregnancy including abnormal location of implantation of the fetus—medically termed *ectopic* pregnancy—normal intrauterine location of the pregnancy but with abnormal fetal or placental development, and spontaneous abortion; benign or malignant growths of the cervix, uterine body, fallopian tubes, or ovaries; systemic diseases or medications (aspirin, Motrin-type antiinflammatory drugs, Warfarin) causing abnormal red blood cells, platelets, or other clotting factors interfering with blood clotting; and hormonal abnormalities not related to the ovaries, such as thyroid disease. Excess menstrual bleeding can follow birth control pill use if the dose is too low for you, or, sometimes, after you quit taking them.

The most common cause of abnormal uterine bleeding is hormonal dysfunction, termed *dysfunctional uterine bleeding (DUB)*. The definition of DUB is excessive bleeding *without* a specific disease of the female organs, a systemic disease, or a drug-related blood-clotting disorder. DUB is caused by irregularities of the hypothalamic-pituitary-ovarian female hormone regulation and feedback mechanism that controls the menstrual cycle. Such irregular menstrual bleeding is quite common, and experienced by most women at some time. It may actually be a normal

physiological state at menarche, before the hormonal feedback mechanism is well developed, and again at menopause, when decreasing hormone production throws this mechanism out of balance. Since irregular uterine bleeding may also be a signal of serious disease, other causes must first be eliminated before you choose to treat it as simply DUB.

The Menstrual Cycle

Menstruation is *natural*. Our Western culture does not have a tradition of seeing this female function as beautiful, lovely, soothing. colorful, and artistic, as many societies have; the period is secret, shamed, or laughed at, as "on the rag." We now know that this sort of emotional stress certainly influences hormonal function.

The menstrual cycle is controlled by a complicated interaction between the brain's hypothalamus and pituitary gland, the ovary, and the lining of the uterus. Problems with menstruation and fertility can be due to abnormalities at any of these locations.

The hypothalamus is the link between the higher functions of your brain and your endocrine glands. It helps explain why stress can affect your periods: any emotional upset in your brain, changing your endorphin levels, can interfere with its key regulating function during puberty, adulthood, or menopause. On the other hand, stress management training and exercise, by increasing endorphin levels, can help assure proper hormonal function.

The hypothalamus regulates the pituitary gland, which secretes follicular stimulating hormone (FSH), which in turn causes the ovary to begin to mature a follicle (egg and its surrounding layers). Estrogen, produced by the developing follicle, is the main hormone acting in the first half of the menstrual cycle. It stimulates the lining of the uterus to increase in thickness from 1 millimeter to 5 millimeters, and develop more blood supply. Luteinizing hormone, from the pituitary, triggers ovulation and the formation of a corpus luteum from the follicle layers after the egg has been discharged.

Progesterone, secreted by the corpus luteum, dominates the second half of the cycle. It antagonizes the effects of estrogen, causing the uterine lining to stop growing and prepare itself for implantation of a fertilized egg. If fertilization does not take place, the corpus luteum degenerates, levels of estrogen and progesterone fall, and the lining sloughs off and is discharged with menstrual bleeding. Falling levels of estrogen and progesterone then cause the pituitary to once again secrete FSH, which in return influences the ovary to ready another egg, and thus initiate the next cycle.

A wide normal variation exists in the length of a menstrual cycle, number of days of bleeding, and the amount of blood lost during each period. The average cycle lasts twenty-eight to twenty-nine days. Normal deviations are defined to include cycles lasting from twenty-three to thirty-nine days, bleeding for two to seven days, and one to two tablespoons of blood loss.

Menorrhagia is the term used to describe excessive amounts of blood loss with each period. It is very difficult to accurately determine how much blood is shed, and it may seem like much more than it really is. However, if you pass blood clots or bleed for more than seven days, this suggests you have an abnormality that may lead to anemia. If excessive bleeding causes you to become anemic, you definitely need to be evaluated. DUB accounts for 80 percent of all cases of menor-

rhagia. *Metrorrhagia* is the term for frequent bleeding occurring at irregular intervals.

As noted, any excessive uterine bleeding or bleeding occurring outside the childbearing years needs to be thoroughly investigated by your doctor.

Evaluation of Dysfunctional Uterine Bleeding

DUB can occur *with* ovulation (15 to 30 percent) or *without* ovulation (70 to 85 percent). The first step in assessing DUB is determining whether you are ovulating regularly. Ovulatory cycles are more consistent, with a similar time interval between periods and number of days and amount of bleeding, than are those in which ovulation does not occur. They may be associated with premenstrual symptoms of mood swings, weight gain, and breast tenderness. Baseline body temperature charts indicate a one-half to one degree Fahrenheit increase in temperature around the time of ovulation. Women who bleed without ovulation usually do not have a regular cycle, cyclic symptoms, or change in basal temperature. They may experience irregular heavy bleeding or spotting.

If you are being checked for abnormal bleeding and it is not clear whether you are ovulating, you should have blood tests to determine your female hormone levels. If you are older than thirty-five, you should have an endometrial biopsy to obtain a tissue sample that will show if ovulatory hormonal effects are present.

If you are ovulating, assessment needs to ensure that the bleeding is not caused by an underlying organic problem, or is a side effect of medications such as aspirin or blood thinners. Blood tests can determine if hypothyroidism, liver disease, or anemia are present, or whether you have any problem with blood coagulation. Pregnancy (normal or ectopic), adenomyosis, fibroids, infection, or a tumor must be excluded. You should have a blood test for pregnancy, pelvic exam, Pap smear, and vaginal cultures. If the cause is not apparent on these simple tests, you may need a vaginal sonogram, hysterosalpingogram, hysteroscopy and biopsy, or D&C. *Any abnormal bleeding after menopause must be evaluated by endometrial biopsy or a D&C to eliminate the possibility of cancer.*

If abnormal bleeding occurs without ovulation (not associated with menarche or menopause), you may have an abnormality at any level of the hypothalamic-pituitary-ovarian feedback mechanism. Causes of imbalance include chromosome abnormalities, side effect of medications such as tranquilizers and antidepressants, chronic illness, obesity (fatty tissue converts other hormones into excess estrogen) or rapid weight change, very low calorie dieting, emotional stress (disrupts normal patterns in hypothalamus), and vigorous exercise. If you do not ovulate, you may show evidence of increased male hormone activity, such as excessive facial hair, acne, and decreased breast size.

In some patients who do not ovulate, polycystic ovary/ovarian dysfunction (Stein-Leventhal Syndrome) is responsible. This condition, which may be genetically inherited, is characterized by ovary enlargement, and is often associated with excessive hair growth on the face and body, obesity, and infertility. This syndrome seems to be due to irregularity in the hormonal feedback system between the ovaries and pituitary, and may be precipitated by stress.

If ovulation does not occur, and the cause is not clear after initial history and physical examination, you should be checked for hypothyroidism, liver and kidney disease, and diabetes. Blood levels of your pituitary and male and female hormones may need to be measured. Also, if ovulation has not been present for more than one year, you should have an endometrial biopsy, since you have an increased risk of endometrial cancer.

Alternative Medicine Approaches to Dysfunctional Uterine Bleeding

---

Noreen, a 46-year-old nurse, had endured heavy periods all of her life. As she began approaching the age of menopause, they became so frequent she considered just simply having her uterus removed as recommended by a gynecologist. However, she decided to seek a second opinion, and discovered that the uterus need not always be removed for relief of the problems she was having. If she were to select hysterectomy, she would be immediately free of her symptoms, but she could face a more abrupt menopause, with significantly severer symptoms such as hot flashes, since in one-third to one-half of all posthysterectomy patients, even if the ovaries are not removed, they cease to function.[3] If she were then placed on estrogen hormone replacement therapy (HRT), she would face an increased risk of breast cancer. She decided to try alternative medicine first, and obtained treatment from an acupuncturist. Within two months, her periods were regular again, and continued to be so until they ceased completely two years later.

If you are bleeding too much or too often from your period, it can be scary. However, you can take action to alleviate this situation, and thereby avoid the surgeon's knife.

What usually causes the hormonal fluctuations that lead to DUB, excessive menstrual bleeding from the uterus not related to a specific disease, making an operation seem necessary? Obesity, stress, inadequate or improper nutrition, lack of exercise, or too much exercise, are some of the risk factors that may create the conditions for this problem.

Alternative medicine may be effective to both prevent and treat DUB. If any suspicion of cancer exists, endometrial biopsy or D&C must be performed at least once, for diagnostic purposes. You will need close supervision from your doctor.

Most of my patients obtain relief quite quickly after initiating the following regimen. I recommend you adopt the complete combination of these lifestyle changes, particularly including avoiding caffeine and adding daily yoga practice.

Quit Smoking

Dysfunctional bleeding has been linked to smoking.[4] If you smoke, your first best step is to quit. Please see Chapter 2 for assistance in stopping for good.

Change Your Diet

Eating a healthful whole-foods diet low in fat and high in fiber may help restore your hormonal balance. Follow the guidelines given in Chapter 2. Eat citrus daily, especially the white pulp, which is high in bioflavonoids. Especially avoid caffeine, alcohol, sugar and other concentrated sweeteners, and dairy products.

Chronic yeast infections, related to refined sugar intake and antibiotic use, have been associated with the hormonal changes that may underlie dysfunctional bleeding.[5] Follow an anticandida program, strengthening your immune system by following the supplement guidelines in Chapter 2 and avoiding refined foods.

Eat Foods Rich in Phytoestrogens

Phytoestrogens are compounds found in plants that bind with estrogen receptor sites on cells. They provide a weak estrogenlike action, but without the imbalance often at the root of excess menstrual bleeding. Foods high in phytoestrogens include soybeans and soybean products such as miso and tofu, fennel, celery, and parsley. Carrots, thyme, licorice, and sarsaparilla can be added to the diet. Almonds and sunflower and pumpkin seeds, which contain phytoestrogens, may also be eaten, but should be taken in moderation, owing to their high-fat content.

Take Supplements

Take a good multivitamin to make certain you are receiving the full range of nutrients you need to assure proper hormone production.

Several studies have indicated that iron deficiency itself may cause excessive menstrual bleeding, and have found that supplementation with iron has corrected the problem.[6] Supplemental iron should be taken as ferrous sulfate, 325 mg three times a day. If your standard tests do not show you anemic or low in iron, ask for a serum ferritin blood test, which can uncover low iron stores not shown by other tests.

One study measuring serum vitamin A levels in seventy-one women with excessive menstrual bleeding found their levels to be slightly lower than those of controls. When they were given 25,000 IU of vitamin A twice a day for fifteen days, menstrual bleeding returned to normal in 57.5 percent, and was diminished in an additional 35 percent, making a total of 92.5 percent improvement. This effect was probably due to the influence of vitamin A on estrogen metabolism, achieving more appropriate levels.[7] Women on birth control pills have been found to have increased vitamin A levels, which may help account for these drugs' ameliorative effects on DUB. You may take a 5,000 IU dose of vitamin A for maintenance, but a higher dose for therapy must be under a doctor's supervision, since excess vitamin A can lead to liver damage.

Supplementation with vitamin C and bioflavonoids have been found to lower uterine bleeding rates.[8] Both are known to affect cell membrane functioning. The more absorbable bioflavonoids hesperidin, hesperidin methyl chalcone, and narigin, may be particularly useful. Dose varies individually, and usually ranges from 1,000 to 2,000 mg of each, three times daily.

Other researchers have suggested that free radicals (toxic by-products created when nutrition is suboptimal) may influence uterine bleeding, and they reported improvement in patients using 400 to 800 IU of vitamin E, an antioxidant, once daily.[9]

Occasionally, vitamin K deficiency may play a role in DUB, and therefore adding more chlorophyll-containing foods, rich in vitamin K, to your diet, such as dark green leafy vegetables, spinach, cabbage, and Brussels sprouts, has been reported to be helpful.[10] You may also take this in the form of liquid chlorophyll, one to three tablespoons daily, or vitamin K tablets, 300 to 500 mcg per day.

Zinc deficiency may also play a role; low serum zinc levels have been correlated with increased bleeding, and supplementation of 15 to 50 mg daily is recommended. Take extra calcium and magnesium, 500 to 1,000 mg of each. Likewise, a deficiency in essential fatty acids may interfere with appropriate hormone production; take flaxseed oil, one to two teaspoons daily, or borage oil capsules, 200 to 300 mg per day.

Use Herbal Preparations

The herb shepherd's purse (*Capsella bursapastoris*) has been studied in the treatment of excessive menstrual bleeding, and found to be useful.[11] Begin with one cup of the freshly made tea, one to three times daily; or one dropperful or capsule daily. The Chinese herb dong quai (*Angelica senensis*), sometimes called "the female ginseng," has been shown to help this disorder by influencing both estrogen and progesterone levels; recommended initial dosage is one to three capsules daily.[12] Similarly, the American Indian herb black cohosh (*Cimicifuga racemosa*) has been used, along with another herb, vitex (*chasteberry or viburnum*), one to three capsules or droppersful daily.[13] Papaya leaf has also been found to assist in controlling hemorrhage.[14] Begin with one capsule, three times daily. The herbs trillium and geranium can be taken in tincture combination with vitex, though research is inconclusive about their benefits; recommended dosage is one dropperful every fifteen to thirty minutes until bleeding stops, though not to exceed six doses. Cranesbill root (*Geranium maculatum*) is an herb traditionally used by Native Americans to treat excess bleeding.[15] The herb squaw vine was also utilized by Native Americans to treat this disorder, though no scientific study of its effectiveness has yet been conducted.

The most commonly used homeopathic preparations are sepia and lachesis, though this type of alternative treatment is best individualized by a homeopathic practitioner.

Optimize Thyroid Function

In 1982, Stoffer reported finding a link between thyroid deficiency and excessive menstrual bleeding.[16] The yoga program outlined in Chapter 2 has shown to correct low levels of thyroid deficiency without medication, but this approach must be monitored by your doctor.

Practice Yoga

The yoga postures act to change blood circulation to your internal organs, helping correct hormonal function and increase local nutrient supply for optimum repair work. Yoga postures assist in maintaining good circulation to the pelvis. Especially important are the forward bends and shoulder stand, deep relaxation, and alternate nostril breathing. See Chapter 2 for details of this program.

Maintain Your Optimum Weight

Excess weight can disturb hormonal regulation, and is associated with a higher risk of irregular menstrual bleeding. An active exercise program, yoga practice, and a high-bulk, high-fiber, low-fat diet, as outlined in Chapter 2, can be utilized to help you reestablish a good weight.

Exercise Regularly

Lack of regular exercise has been linked with excessive menstrual bleeding.[17] You will need to find the kind of aerobic program that appeals to you, and work out at least three times a week, for an hour. However, don't overdo it. Long hours of vigorous exercise can have an opposite effect, upsetting your hormonal balance: ovulation and menstrual difficulties are often experienced by marathon runners and professional athletes.

Practice Stress Management

Stress is notorious for interfering with the regular menstrual cycle.[18] A good stress management program allows your body time to rebalance itself after periods of strain. The various stress management techniques described in Chapter 2 may be helpful.

Try Other Measures

A short fast, with the added supplements suggested above, may help your body readjust its hormonal balance; directions for fasting are given in Chapter 2. Chiropractic or osteopathic care and massage may also be helpful adjuncts to treat your stress, and relieve physical tension in the pelvis that may contribute to the problem.

Placing your pelvis in a cold water bathtub, with your feet out, takes the blood from the surface of the body and sends it deep into the ovaries and uterus, to assist in their repair. Try this for one-half hour, two to three times per day. You can put on a sweater and read a good book; this alternative approach actually feels better than you might think, and is quite refreshing.

Practice Visualization

First do deep relaxation, given in Chapter 2. Then choose an image for visualization; for example, imagine your glands as instruments in a beautifully coordinated symphony orchestra. Picture the glands in your brain, the hypothalamus and pituitary, as the conductors, and your ovaries and uterus as responding perfectly to their direction. Image this, while feeling it happen within your body. If you are bleeding excessively, imagine yourself using a sponge to thoroughly dry the inner lining of your uterus, then picture the lining as calm and dry, so that no further bleeding occurs.

Avoid Hormone Replacement

Some doctors suggest that you take birth control pills or hormone replacement therapy (HRT) to prevent DUB, as well as to alleviate any other symptoms of menopause. However, since HRT is associated with increased risk for breast cancer and other risky side effects, you can avoid these problems by choosing alternative methods for treating any menopausal discomfort you may encounter.

One theory is that a symptomatic menopause may be a hallmark for adrenal or thyroid insufficiency. The adrenals can produce estrogen and progesterone, in adequate amounts to keep you free of symptoms during your menopause, if they have not been excessively affected by stress. Stress reduction, plus nutritional support, can allow these organs to achieve their optimal function, helping you through a healthy menopausal transition and maintaining your health once you are beyond it. Here are the current alternative medicine measures to replace HRT for treatment of menopausal symptoms:

- **Hot flashes.** Avoid caffeine; use the herb black cohosh, 500 mg two to three times daily; and take evening primrose oil, 500 mg two to three times daily. You may also try acupuncture, magnets placed over the adrenal acupuncture point on your foot, or color therapy. The homeopathics most often recommended are sepia and lachesis. Make certain to rest more, and add laughter, massage, yoga, and other stress relievers to your daily schedule.
- **Insomnia.** Avoid caffeine; take extra magnesium, 250 to 500 mg daily; and use the herbs passionflower, 500 mg; valerian, 500 mg; St. John's wort, 500 mg. Other herbs include chamomile, hops, scullcap, and lemon balm. Aromatherapy with lavender may also be helpful.
- **Depression.** Avoid caffeine, and use St. John's wort, 500 mg daily.
- **Heart disease.** Follow the Ornish Program, discussed in Chapter 8.
- **Osteoporosis.** This disease is uncommon in vegetarians. Follow the dietary and exercise guidelines given in Chapter 2.
- **Vaginal dryness.** One quarter cup of *soy* powder a day has been shown to reverse this problem. In addition, you may place a vitamin E capsule, 1,000 IU, in your vagina at night; it will dissolve, leaving the tissues optimally lubricated.

Conventional Medicine Approach to Dysfunctional Uterine Bleeding

Female hormone medications are effective in cases of resistant excess bleeding. Generally, estrogen-progesterone combinations or progesterone alone are used. Some of the medications can be given by injection, every one to three months. You can try birth control pills, which regulate your cycle and decrease menstrual bleeding by up to 60 percent. After three to six months on BCPs, you can stop to see if you begin ovulating. This program may be especially attractive if you desire contraception.

Medications such as ibuprofen (Motrin, Advil) and naproxin (Aleve, Naprosyn) have an antiprostaglandin effect, which increases blood clotting and constriction of uterine blood vessels, decreasing flow. Menstrual bleeding is diminished by 20 to 50 percent, but since they can produce the side effects of liver and kidney toxicity, these medicines should be used for only three to six months, at low dosages.

Danazol (Danocrine) is an expensive estrogen-blocking medication that may be tried in difficult cases, but it has male hormone side effects, such as weight gain, increased hairiness, and acne, making it of limited usefulness.

Surgical Approaches to Dysfunctional Uterine Bleeding

In general, surgical procedures are only necessary to help in diagnosing the cause of your DUB. The alternative and conventional approaches just discussed are much better means to treat it. Following are several techniques that may be recommended if other means fail.

Dilation and Curettage

The D&C used to be the mainstay of treatment of DUB, but it now is rarely indicated. It may be useful during an emergency, if you have a large amount of bleeding not responsive to other measures. This procedure empties the uterus of clots and endometrium, thereby helping to stop the hemorrhage. D&C may be recommended for women older than 35 years, who have very heavy bleeding, as a diagnostic test to rule out other uterine causes for bleeding. Occasionally, D&C may be worth trying as treatment, but it is curative only in a minority; in the rest, the problem simply develops again.

Endometrial Ablation

This newer procedure uses a laser or electrocautery to destroy the endometrium, inducing scarring and minimal regeneration of the lining. Its technique is similar to a D&C and is successful in eliminating or reducing bleeding in 70 to 90 percent of all cases.[19] Generally, it is used if you are not a good surgical risk for hysterectomy, and only if you are very certain you will not want to become pregnant in the future, since it eliminates this possibility.

Hysterectomy

This operation should be considered only if you have no response to other approaches, and if you are certain you do not want children. Twenty percent of all hysterectomies are done to treat DUB. (For a discussion of the hysterectomy operations, see page 537.)

DYSFUNCTIONAL UTERINE BLEEDING SUMMARY

Prevention

Diet and Supplements

- Follow a whole-foods, low-fat, high-fiber diet.
- Eat foods high in phytoestrogens, such as soy, celery, parsley, carrots, and sunflower and pumpkin seeds.
- Eat plenty of dark green, leafy vegetables.
- Multivitamins.
- Vitamin A, 5,000 IU daily.
- Vitamin C, 1,000–2,000 mg, 2–3 times daily.
- Bioflavonoids—hesperidin, hesperidin methyl chalcone, and narigin, 1,000–2,000 mg of each, 3 times daily.
- Vitamin E, D-alpha, 400 IU, 1–3 times daily.

- Zinc, 15–50 mg daily.
- Calcium, 500–1,000 mg daily.
- Magnesium, 500–1,000 mg daily.

Lifestyle

- Don't smoke.
- Practice daily yoga, especially the inverted postures.
- Maintain optimum weight.
- Exercise regularly: 1 hour, 3–5 times weekly.
- Practice stress management.

Alternative Medicine Approaches

- Follow the preventive guidelines, above.
- Sit with just the pelvis in a cool bath, 20–30 minutes, 2–3 times daily.
- Treat iron deficiency—ferrous sulfate, 325 mg, 3 times daily.
- Vitamin A in high doses under supervision.
- Vitamin K, 300–500 mcg daily.
- Herbs: shepherd's purse (*Capsella bursapastoris*), one dropperful or capsule daily or one cup of the freshly made tea, 1–3 times daily.
- Flaxseed oil, 1–2 teaspoons daily, or borage oil capsules, 200–300 mg per day.
- Dong quai, 500 mg, 1–3 times daily.
- Black cohosh (*Cimicifuga racemosa*), 500 mg, 1–3 times daily.
- Vitex (chasteberry), 500 mg, 1–3 times daily.
- Papaya leaf—1 capsule, 3 times daily.
- Chiropractic and/or osteopathic treatments.
- Short fast.
- Place pelvis in a cold water bathtub, 30 minutes, 2–3 times daily.
- Practice visualization.
- Avoid hormone replacement.

Conventional Medicine Approaches

- Female hormones—progesterone, estrogen-progesterone, birth control pills.
- Antiprostaglandins—ibuprofen (Motrin, Advil), naproxin (Naprosyn).
- Estrogen blocker—danazol (Danocrine).

Surgical Approaches

- D&C.
- Endometrial ablation.
- Hysterectomy.

Endometriosis

Endometriosis is one of the most common problems referred to a gynecologist, present to some degree in 5 to 10 percent of the female population during childbearing years, most commonly between ages 20 and 30. Endometriosis develops when the uterine lining tissue cells grow outside the uterus, where they respond to phases in the menstrual cycle, and so periodically bleed and cause other symptoms.

Although not cancer, these deposits, medically termed *endometriomas*, can act in similar ways, by invading local tissue and spreading over abdominal organs or even distantly, through blood vessels. Five percent of all women have symptoms of endometriosis. Pain in the pelvis, rectum, back, and as far as the upper abdomen or chest can let you know it is present. Other symptoms can include discomfort with menstruation or intercourse, irregular vaginal bleeding, or problems with conception. Endometriosis is reported to be present in as low as 20 percent to as high as 90 percent of the women who undergo evaluation for pelvic pain or infertility.[20]

The exact cause of endometriosis is not known, but it is associated with unrelenting stimulation by estrogen, and so is more common in women who have never been pregnant or who opt for pregnancy later in life. It may also be related to excess fat in the diet, which raises estrogen levels, and the added estrogen present in animal foods. Reflux menstruation, where endometrial lining cells back up through the tubes to reach and implant in the abdominal cavity, may play a role. A congenital predisposition for certain cells in the abdomen to differentiate into endometrial-like cells under the influence of estrogen may be present. This may explain how even men with prostate cancer can develop endometriosis if they are treated with high doses of estrogen, a fact favoring the excess estrogen theory as the underlying cause.

The diagnosis of endometriosis is relatively easy. Your symptoms tend to be cyclical, corresponding with phases of increased estrogen stimulation. However, symptoms may also be constant. Sometimes, tumorlike growths can be felt in the vagina, around the ovaries, uterus, or on the bowel during pelvic and abdominal exam. Enlarged, cystic masses can be seen on ultrasound exam. However, ovarian tumors can look similar, so that an exact diagnosis may require a laparoscopic exam and biopsy. The color of the nodular or scarlike implants vary widely, and may be clear, red, white, or blue-black to chocolate brown. Treatment can usually be carried out at the same time as laparoscopic diagnosis.

Ovarian cancer is more common in women who develop endometriosis, so that if you are found to have it, you will need frequent examinations and surveillance of your ovaries.

Alternative Medicine Approaches to Endometriosis

You may need no treatment at all if your symptoms are mild. Especially if you are near menopause, you may simply choose to "wait it out," since discomfort usually disappears then. However, because endometriosis tends to be a progressive disease, you should in any case observe the following guidelines. Most of them are aimed at decreasing estrogen stimulation of the endometrial implants.

Change Your Diet

A low-fat, high-fiber, whole-foods diet works by decreasing your body's production of excess estrogen. Follow the guidelines given in Chapter 2. Particularly avoid caffeine, sugar, added fats, salt, any animal foods, and dairy products.

Chronic yeast infections, located in the bowel as well as the vagina and often related to antibiotic use, can act to alter hormonal balance; avoid sugar and other concentrated sweets, and follow the supplement guidelines given in Chapter 2.

Eat Foods Rich in Phytoestrogens

Phytoestrogens are plant substances that bind to the estrogen receptor sites on cells, thereby lowering the effects of excess estrogen. Soybeans are especially high in these compounds; take at least one-half cup of a soy product daily.

Take Supplements

By changing estrogen feedback, supplements have been shown to diminish endometriosis. The most important include vitamin A, 10,000 IU, three times daily; vitamin C, 3,000 mg, three times daily; and vitamin E, 400 IU, three times daily. Also recommended are calcium and magnesium 1,000: 500 mg daily; borage oil, 500 to 1,000 mg, three times daily; and flaxseed oil, one to two teaspoons daily.

Use Herbal Preparations

By adding phytoestrogens, herbal preparations act to bring estrogen levels into balance. The Chinese herb dong quai, licorice root, and alfalfa, initially three to six capsules daily, are especially recommended. Beet leaf, burdock, and dandelion may also be added, one to three capsules daily to begin.

Maintain Your Optimum Weight

Excess weight is associated with excess estrogen production. Follow the dietary and stress management guidelines given in Chapter 2, and join a support group.

Use Other Measures

Sitting in a cold bathtub for twenty to thirty minutes two to three times daily acts to send your peripheral blood into your deeper pelvic area, increasing local concentration of white cells, so that your body is more able to muster its resources to self-correct this problem. Hot compresses followed by cold may be helpful for acute symptoms. Rubbing castor oil on your abdomen, then applying a hot water bottle for an hour each night, for a month or two, may also help to increase lymph flow, allowing the body to more optimally self-correct.

Acupuncture has been reported to help this condition, as well as homeopathy and massage. Individualize your treatment by seeking the help of a trained practitioner.

Practice Visualization

First follow the instructions for deep relaxation and visualization, given in Chapter 2. You might, for example, picture your endometrial implants as clumps of crabgrass growing in a beautiful lawn. Send your white cells to chew them up. Image this in your mind, and feel it happening in your body.

Conventional Medicine Approaches to Endometriosis

There has been a lot of research and experience using various drugs to treat endometriosis. If the alternative methods described above are not successful, you can consider the following.

Pregnancy

If you desire to and can become pregnant, this changes your natural hormone milieu, an action often mimicked by medications. Endometriosis tissue usually regresses and often does not return afterwards.

Pseudopregnancy

Creation of a "pseudopregnancy" by continuous use of estrogen-progesterone birth control pills for six to twelve months may be effective for mild-to-moderate endometriosis. This method relieves symptoms in 75 to 89 percent of all such cases.[21]

Progesterone alone is usually successful in relieving mild-to-moderate symptoms, but may give you the side effects of breast tenderness, nausea, fluid retention, or depression. This hormone can be taken in an inexpensive pill form or by injection. Pain is relieved in up to 90 percent of these cases.[22] Progesterone is usually recommended as the first medical treatment for endometriosis.

Drug Treatments

Danazol (Danocrine) is a medication that blocks the effects of the pituitary ovarian-stimulating hormones, thereby decreasing estrogen and progesterone production, and their promotional effect on endometrial implants. After six months of treatment, pain is relieved in 90 percent when disease is mild to moderate.[23] However, this expensive treatment gives bothersome side effects in up to 80 percent of all treated patients, such as excessive facial and bodily hair growth, weight gain, acne, and menopausal symptoms. Danazol also decreases HDL, the blood level of good cholesterol, increasing your risk of heart disease, and so should not be used for more than six months.

The newer medications leuprolide (Lupron), goserelin (Zolodex), and nafarelin (Synarel) block the release of pituitary ovarian-stimulating hormones, creating a "medical oophorectomy," which is reversible when the medication is stopped. Estrogen stimulation of the endometrial implants is thus blocked. These medications are given by injections under the skin or applied to the nasal passage lining, where absorption is rapid. They are effective in reducing pelvic pain in 90 percent of all cases, but also have a wide variety of unpleasant side effects similar to Danazol.[24] Because they can cause reversible osteoporosis, their use should be limited to six months.

Gestrinone is a new oral medication that can cause shrinkage of endometrial implants, and has shown effectiveness in relieving pain. Although there is limited experience with this medication in the United States, it has been widely used in Europe.

All these drug treatments provide only temporary relief, and your symptoms will likely return once the medication is stopped.

If infertility caused by extensive endometriosis is your main concern, advanced fertility techniques such as "superovulation" and in-vitro fertilization may be more effective than drug treatment.

Surgical Approaches to Endometriosis

Since this disease is on the increase, operations to remove or destroy endometriosis deposits are becoming more common. The usual first treatment of endometriosis is by conventional means, as just described. However, surgery may be useful if your endometriomas or endometriosis-associated scar tissue gives you recurring pain, obstructs your intestine, compresses your bladder, or interferes with your fertility. The following surgical approaches are the procedures most commonly used.

Conservative Local Excision

Conservative surgery is one of the most attractive and common treatments for endometriosis. Symptoms can be relieved, fertility enhanced, and all the female organs preserved. Small lesions can be treated by laparoscopic techniques. They are removed if they form a nodule or cyst, and destroyed by electrocautery or laser if they are flat. In some cases, with extensive disease and scarring, a larger, open abdominal incision may be necessary. After conservative surgery, your chance for relief of symptoms is 61 to 100 percent.[25] The rate of recurrent visible disease is up to 28 percent at eighteen months.[26]

Surgery may also restore your fertility if you had been unable to conceive because of *severe* endometriosis. It is successful in 50 percent of all women with such disease, and this improvement is much better than that of other forms of treatment.[27] It may even be beneficial if you have minimal to mild disease not actually blocking your fallopian tubes, but which may be contributing to your infertility. A 1997 report from Laval University in Quebec studied 341 infertile women with minimal to mild endometriosis found on diagnostic laparoscopy. Half of the women were randomized to a group that had destruction of their endometriotic implants with electrocautery or laser. This treatment added only thirteen minutes to the diagnostic part of the operation. The other group had diagnostic laparoscopy only. The investigators found that 30.7 percent of the women in the laparoscopic treatment group had become pregnant after thirty-six weeks compared to 17.7 percent of the women undergoing laparoscopy alone (a 73 percent relative increase). Overall, their conclusion was that the increase in thirty-six-week probability of pregnancy attributable to the laparoscopic treatment was 13 percent, and that one infertile woman in eight with minimal to mild endometriosis should benefit.[28]

Hysterectomy and Oophorectomy

Twenty percent of all hysterectomies are performed to treat endometriosis and adenomyosis (see page 520). This form of treatment removes the uterus, tubes and both ovaries, as well as treating endometrioma deposits. It is usually recommended when conservative surgery or alternative treatments are not effective or cause unacceptable side effects, or if significant symptoms persist after childbearing is completed. It is the most effective treatment for eliminating pain, successful in 90 percent of all cases.[29]

Leaving one ovary in place to prevent the side effects of decreased estrogen results in much higher recurrence rates and need for further treatment. Estrogen replacement medication, after removing the uterus and both ovaries, decreases the recurrence rate to less than 5 percent, although it has its own set of problems, discussed on pages 192 and 210.

The hysterectomy and oophorectomy operation can be done through an abdominal incision or through the vagina with laparoscopic assistance, depending on the size of the uterus and extent of disease. For a discussion of the hysterectomy operations, see page 537.)

ENDOMETRIOSIS SUMMARY

Prevention

Diet and Supplements

- Follow a low-fat, high-fiber, whole-foods diet.
- Avoid caffeine, sugar, added fats, salt, any animal foods, and dairy products.
- Replace meat and dairy with soy.
- Eat foods rich in phytoestrogens.

Lifestyle

- Maintain optimum weight.

Alternative Medicine Approaches

- Follow the guidelines for prevention, above.
- Vitamin A, 10,000 IU, 3 times daily.
- Vitamin C, 3,000, 3 times daily.

- Vitamin E, D-alpha, 400 IU, 3 times daily.
- Calcium, 1,000 mg daily.
- Magnesium, 500 mg daily.
- Flaxseed oil, 1 tablespoon daily.
- Borage oil, 500–1,000 mg daily.
- Dong quai, 500 mg, 3 times daily.
- Licorice root (DGL), 300 mg, 3 times daily.
- Alfalfa, 500 mg, 1–2 times daily.
- Beet leaf, 500 mg, 1–2 times daily.
- Burdock (*Arctium lappa*), 500 mg, 2–3 times daily.
- Dandelion, 500 mg, 2–3 times daily.
- Sit in a cool bathtub, 20–30 minutes, 2–3 times daily.
- Practice visualization.

Conventional Medicine Approaches

- Pregnancy.
- Hormones—estrogen-progesterone birth control pills, progesterone.
- Pituitary ovarian-stimulating hormone blockers—Danazol, Lupron, Zoladex, Synarel.
- Gestrinone.

Surgical Approaches

- Conservative local excision.
- Hysterectomy and oophorectomy.

Adenomyosis of the Uterus

Adenomyosis develops when the lining layer of the uterus, termed the *endometrium,* grows down into the deeper, muscular layers of the uterus, creating an enlarged, spongy, tender uterus. Excess bleeding during and between menstrual periods commonly follows.

No consensus exists on the effectiveness of medical treatment. Birth control pills often control adenomyosis if symptoms are mild, and can be continued until menopause when symptoms naturally decrease. They shouldn't be used in smokers, who would be placed at high risk for development of blood clot complications. Hysterectomy is usually recommended for moderate to severe discomfort.

You may try the general alternative medicine approaches given above and in Chapter 2, but no research has yet been conducted on their effects with this disorder.

Uterine Fibroids

Uterine fibroids are benign muscle tumors of the uterine wall. They are very common, affecting 20 to 25 percent of all women by age 40, and 50 percent overall. They are much more common in black women. While the cause isn't clear, they seem to be dependent on estrogen, since they are rare before menarche and often regress after menopause. They may also be related to excess fat in the diet.[30]

Fibroids vary in size and location. They can develop in the inner layer of muscle, bulging into the uterine cavity, or from the outer muscle layer, enlarging into the pelvis. (See Figure 19.2.) A fibroid may even form a stalk and move about in the uterine cavity or pelvis. Size may vary from that of a pea to a golf ball or they may become even larger than a softball. Usually more than one is present.

While most fibroids do not cause prob-

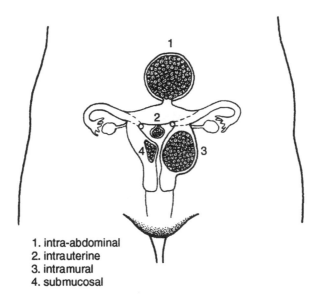

1. intra-abdominal
2. intrauterine
3. intramural
4. submucosal

Fig. 19.2 Types of uterine fibroids

lems, they can give you symptoms, such as excessive bleeding during or between menstrual periods, abdominal aching and fullness, pelvic and back discomfort, and pain during intercourse. They can interfere with fertility by blocking your cervix, uterine cavity, or fallopian tubes and can complicate a pregnancy; they carry two to three times the risk for spontaneous abortion. During labor and delivery, they may make a C-section necessary. If large enough, they can compress adjacent organs such as the rectum and bladder, causing bloating and problems passing stool and/or frequent or difficult urination. If a rapidly enlarging fibroid outgrows its blood supply, it can suddenly degenerate, causing severe pain. Very rarely, a fibroid may transform into a sarcoma, a type of cancer of muscular tissue. Although not causally related, women who develop fibroids are at four

times the risk for endometrial cancer, since ß both problems.

Fibroids can usually be diagnosed on pelvic and abdominal examination. They are easily seen on sonogram and CAT scan. Smaller fibroids bulging into the uterine cavity may require hysteroscopy to be identified. Laparoscopy may be necessary to ensure that no other disease is also present.

Alternative Medicine Approaches to Uterine Fibroids

If your fibroids are not causing you problems, they should be left in place, since they usually spontaneously resolve after menopause. Even if they enlarge, in most cases, as long as they do not create symptoms, they can be left alone. If you do have symptoms, however, following are the most promising alternative medicine measures you can take to diminish them. These approaches may also prevent uterine fibroids as well as reverse them.

Change Your Diet

A strong association between fibroid formation and excess fats in the diet may explain the pervasiveness of this disorder in the West.[31] Switch to a vegetarian diet, and eliminate dairy, alcohol, and sugar and other concentrated sweets. See Chapter 2 for dietary details.

Take Supplements

Some doctors have reported that vitamin E has been effective in reducing excessive bleeding.[32] Dosage should be 400 to 1,000 IU daily.

Other researchers have found that vitamin C may ameliorate the symptoms of fibroids.[33] You may take 2,000 to 3,000 mg, three times daily, of vitamin C complex, which should include bioflavonoids.

Add Herbal Remedies

The herbs trillium or viburnum, 15 to 25 drops three to four times daily, and shepherd's purse, three to four cups brewed as tea, fresh daily, or 15 to 20 drops of the tincture, have been found to be of help, especially for fibroid-associated excess bleeding.[34] Blue cohosh (*Caulophylum thalictroides*), two capsules two times daily, has been recommended.

Maintain Your Optimum Weight

Excess weight is associated with the increased estrogen levels that promote fibroids. Follow the guidelines given in Chapter 2 for the best diet, and practice stress management daily to avoid unhealthy food choices or quantities.

Exercise Regularly

Regularly exercising helps the endocrine orchestra to maintain its balance, and helps you to feel good, so that you can make healthy food and lifestyle choices. Follow the guidelines given in Chapter 2.

Practice Stress Management

A daily program of stress management helps the body to maintain optimum hormonal balance and repair. Follow the guidelines given in Chapter 2.

Psychological issues of anger or grief may contribute to circulatory congestion in the pelvis. You can explore these issues with a therapist or alternative practitioner, and during your daily meditation and visualization practice.

Practice Visualization

Visualization is one of the tools being explored for eliminating benign and cancerous growths, via mental stimulation of your own immune system and repair modalities. It needs to be practiced three to four times daily, as described in Chapter 2. First do the deep relaxation technique described on pages 43–46. Then picture in your mind, for example, that your uterus is a lovely pear that mistakenly has some small grapes attached. Imagine yourself gently removing all of these, and see the pear in perfect shape. Hold this image in your mind, and at the same time feel it happening within your body.

Maintain Balanced Thyroid Function

Formation of fibroids may be associated with underactive thyroid function. A lower basal body temperature may indicate diminished thyroid function even when blood levels are normal. You can use a yoga program, as given in Chapter 2, to help the thyroid return to optimum function.

Use Other Approaches

If you suffer from excessive bleeding due to fibroids, follow the recommendations on page 521. Adding acupuncture, chiropractic, homeopathy, and/or hypnosis to your treatment regimen may provide additional pathways to healing.

Discontinue Birth Control Pills or Estrogen Replacement Medication

Birth control pills and estrogen replacement treatment can stimulate fibroid growth by supplying estrogen. If this may be a factor for you, you can either stop them completely, using another form of birth control, or try lower doses or different preparations. See page 210–12 for alternatives to estrogen replacement treatment.

Conventional Medicine Approaches to Uterine Fibroids

There is really no long-term satisfactory drug treatment for fibroids. Recently, nonsurgical radiologic techniques have proven to be a viable alternative to surgery if your symptoms are not relieved by alternative measures. You can consider the following.

Drug Treatments

Medications such as Lupron, Zolodex, and Synarel suppress estrogen production by your ovary. They can shrink fibroids by 40 to 65 percent, but after treatment is stopped, the fibroids regrow to 88 percent of their former size within three months.[35] This approach may be useful in preserving fertility and defer-

ring hysterectomy until you no longer want to get pregnant. Such medical treatment may allow you to reach menopause, when natural shrinkage makes surgery unnecessary. However, these expensive medications should be used only for short periods of time, because of their side effects, which include hot flashes, mood swings, bone loss, decreased vaginal secretions, increased total cholesterol, and decreased HDL levels.

Fibroid Embolization

This new treatment is a minimally invasive technique to interrupt the blood supply to the fibroids, thereby causing shrinkage. It has the potential to substantially decrease the number of hysterectomies now being performed for fibroid problems. For older women, it can decrease symptoms until the natural fibroid shrinkage of menopause. The angiographic technique and possible complications are similar to that described on page 291. It takes sixty to seventy-five minutes to perform while you are lying on your back on an X-ray table. A specially trained "interventional radiologist" passes a small catheter through a needle into an artery in your groin, and then steers it into the arteries supplying blood to your uterus. Small solid particles are then injected through the catheter and plug the small branch vessels supplying the fibroid. The uterus has a well-developed blood supply, so that the flow from other vessels prevents the whole uterus from dying. This procedure can be done under local anesthesia with sedation, and you may go home later in the day or after an overnight hospital stay.

For most women, significant pain and cramping is associated with fibroid embolization, which may last for several days. This can usually be managed with pain and antiinflammatory medication. One-third of the patients develop fever and flulike symptoms for a few days, and 15 percent require a short hospital readmission for nausea and vomiting. Recovery is usually complete in a week or so, much quicker than the six to eight weeks after hysterectomy. A very small risk exists for uterine infection, which could require a hysterectomy.

The fibroids shrink about 50 percent. Success in improving symptoms of excessive bleeding and pelvic pain is about 85 to 90 percent within two months. Long-term success is not yet known, but appears very promising. Studies from Europe, where the procedure was developed in the early 1990s, and UCLA, where 400 procedures have been done since 1996, have not found regrowth of fibroids. Embolization doesn't appear to interfere with fertility, and births have occurred after it, but if you are planning future pregnancies, myomectomy, described in the next section, is the treatment of first choice. The potential for embolization treatment of infertility caused by fibroids is not yet known. A few women have experienced premature menopause, presumably because the blood supply to the ovaries was also blocked. If this procedure is unsuccessful, the other options for treatment presented here are still available.[36]

You can ask your gynecologist if fibroid embolization is available in your community, and if you would be a good candidate.

Surgical Approaches to Uterine Fibroids

Fibroids are the most common indication for hysterectomy, accounting for 30 percent of all cases. If you have excessive menstrual bleeding with resulting anemia, severe pelvic discomfort, problems caused by compression of adjacent organs, or infertility, you may need surgery.

The choice of a surgical treatment option should take into consideration your desire to retain fertility, how close you are to menopause, your medical condition, and the number, size, location, and rate of growth of your fibroids.

Following are the surgical approaches used to treat fibroids.

Myomectomy

Unless they are very large, simple removal of the fibroids, termed *myomectomy*, with preservation of your uterus, is now usually possible, though it is usually recommended only if you wish to maintain your fertility. Otherwise, hysterectomy is considered a better option, since less blood is lost and you risk fewer complications.

Myomectomy decreases your chance of having a miscarriage from 40 to 20 percent, and when it is performed because the fibroids are causing infertility, you have a 40 percent chance for a later pregnancy.[37]

Jane was a psychotherapist who did not wish to start her family until after her career was well established. In her early thirties, she was unable to become pregnant, and then discovered that the cause was several uterine fibroids. They were removed by myomectomy, through an abdomen incision. She now has three healthy daughters.

Myomectomy can be an outpatient procedure, or a day or two hospitalization may be necessary. You are given general or regional anesthesia. Two approaches may be used, depending on the size, number, and location of the fibroids. If they bulge into the uterine cavity, an approach through the vagina using a hysteroscope is possible. Your doctor can then cut them out through a small incision in the uterine lining, or destroy them with laser or electric cautery. This technique is effective in decreasing excessive bleeding in 70 to 90 percent of all cases.[38]

If your fibroids are large or arise from the outer uterine muscle layers, it may be necessary to approach the uterus through your abdomen. A laparoscopic technique can usually be used, but an open technique may be needed if you have large fibroids or pelvic scaring. One or more incisions is made in the uterus, and the fibroids "shelled out." The uterine incisions are closed with stitches.

Postoperatively, you may have some mild pelvic aching or cramping and a slight bloody discharge for a few days. Complications include excessive blood loss and uterine infection. Since more fibroids can develop after myomectomy, you have a 15 to 30 percent chance of requiring further surgery, usually hysterectomy.[39]

Hysterectomy

If you don't desire to maintain your fertility, hysterectomy is usually your best option to treat fibroids causing significant symptoms. Also, if your fibroid is enlarging rapidly or enlarges after menopause, suggesting the possibility of a uterine sarcoma, hysterectomy should be considered. It eliminates the possibility of future uterine malignancy, especially important if you plan to take postmenopause hormone replacement therapy.

Hysterectomy can be performed through the vagina if your uterus is small or through small abdominal incisions, with the aid of a laparoscope. An open abdominal approach may be best if your fibroids are large, or if you have other pelvic problems that need treatment or make laparoscopic surgery hazardous. These approaches require general anesthesia, a hospital stay of one day with laparoscope, or three to four days otherwise, and have a mortality rate of less than 1 per 1,000 cases. (For a discussion of the hysterectomy operations, see page 537.)

UTERINE FIBROID SUMMARY

Prevention

Diet and Supplements

- Follow a low-fat, high-fiber diet.
- Replace meat and dairy with soy.
- Vitamin E, 400–1,000 IU daily.

Lifestyle

- Exercise regularly: 1 hour, 3–5 times weekly.
- Practice stress management.
- Maintain balanced thyroid function.
- Maintain optimum weight.

Alternative Medicine Approaches

- Follow alternative approaches to excess menstrual bleeding.
- Vitamin A, 10,000 IU daily.
- Vitamin C, 1,000–2,000 mg, 3 times daily.
- Bioflavonoids, 1,000 mg daily.
- Herbal remedies—for excess bleeding: trillium and viburnum, tincture, 15–25

drops, 3–4 times daily; shepherd's purse tea, 3–4 cups daily; blue cohosh (*Caulophyllum thalictroides*), 10–20 drops daily.

- Practice visualization.
- Discontinue birth control pills or estrogen replacement medication.
- Do a liver flush.

Conventional Medicine Approaches

- Drug therapy—medications that suppress estrogen such as Lupron, Zoladex, and Synarel.
- Fibroid embolization.

Surgical Approaches

- Myomectomy.
- Hysterectomy.

OTHER BENIGN DISORDERS OF THE UTERUS

Prolapse of the Uterus

This problem occurs when the ligaments holding the uterus in place, as well as the muscles of the pelvic floor, weaken and stretch, allowing the uterus to move downward into and even out through the vagina. This laxity may also cause distortion of neighboring anatomy, with the bladder and rectum also displaced, giving you problems with urination and passage of stool. Prolapse often follows multiple pregnancies, and is the indication for about 15 percent of all hysterectomies.

If your prolapse is not causing you symptoms, no treatment is necessary. If your problems are mild, exercises to strengthen the muscles of the pelvic floor may be all that is necessary. Practice pelvic floor contraction exercises, every hour, and use the yoga program given in Chapter 2, working up to holding the shoulder stand ten to fifteen minutes twice daily. A plastic cylinder, called a *pessary*, can be placed in the vagina to hold the uterus in place. Various surgical uterus "suspension" procedures are available, which may provide relief, helping you avoid a hysterectomy. Some of these procedures can be performed using laparoscopic techniques.

Pelvic Inflammatory Disease (PID)

Acute or chronic infection in the fallopian tubes, uterus, and/or ovaries can cause fever, severe pain, pelvic scar tissue, and infertility. Antibiotics and drainage of any pus collections, through the vagina or by use of the laparoscope, are usually all the treatment needed. If the infection is localized, removal of only one tube and ovary may preserve your fertility. If the infection becomes chronic, with associated destruction of both tubes and ovaries, removing them, along with hysterectomy, may be recommended. If your disease has already caused infertility or future pregnancy is not desired, this may be the best treatment.

Endometrial Hyperplasia

This increased thickness of the cell layer lining the uterus is the reason for about 6 percent of all hysterectomies. If the cells become "atypical," they can progress to malignancy. If maintenance of fertility is desired, this condition can be treated with progesterone medication, after D&C has established that no cancer is present. If careful monitoring shows persistent hyperplasia, hysterectomy is indicated. Hysterectomy should be considered if endometrial hyperplasia is found after menopause.

Chronic Pelvic Pain

This very difficult problem accounts for about 10 percent of all hysterectomies. However, surgery should be the very last resort to treat chronic pelvic pain. It should be considered only after an extensive diagnostic evaluation has failed to find a cause that can be treated by other methods, and a trial of alternative treatment is unsuccessful. Gynecological problems, as well as muscular, skeletal, gastrointestinal, and urinary disease must be excluded.

Psychosomatic factors may play a role, so that a psychiatric evaluation may be useful before deciding on hysterectomy. If no other treatable cause is found, a six-month trial of antiinflammatory medication, birth control pills, and perhaps estrogen blockers should be tried. If all else fails, hysterectomy, with or without removal of tubes and ovaries, is successful in relieving or reducing pain in about 78 percent of carefully selected cases.[40]

Cervical Cancer

Cancer of the cervix is a common malignancy in women in the United States. There will be some 13,000 new cases and 4,100 deaths in 2002.[41] Incidence rates have decreased steadily over the past several decades.

Typically, the cells on the surface of the cervix undergo a slow progression from normal to "dysplastic," atypical but not malignant cells, and finally to frankly malignant ones. This process may affect the flat *squamous* cells that line the outer surface of the cervix (90 percent) or the mucus-producing *adenomatous* cells that line the opening into the body of the uterus (10 percent). After the cells become malignant, they may remain in a noninvasive, or *cancer-in-situ*, stage, also called *cervical intraepithelial neoplasia (CIN)*, confined to the surface of the cervix for an extended period of time, as long as ten to twelve years. However, 10 percent of the time the transformation to invasive cancer occurs in less than a year.

Eventually, an invasive and less curable phase develops, when the cancer cells invade deeply into the cervix and adjacent tissues. Malignant cells then come in contact with lymphatic and blood vessels and may invade into them. Clumps of tumor cells can break off and migrate through these vessels to distant parts of the body.

Since the cervix is constantly shedding cells into the vagina, abnormal premalignant cells can usually be found on a routine Pap smear. As many as 600,000 premalignant cases are diagnosed each year. If treatment is given at this point, the cure rate is 100 percent. The incidence of cancer-in-situ peaks during the ages of 20 to 30 years, while invasive cancer increases rapidly after age 25. Because of the Pap smear, cancer-in-situ is diagnosed more frequently than invasive cancer.

Most cases of cancer of the cervix are felt to be triggered by some agent in semen, or a sexually transmitted carcinogen. This conclusion is supported by several bits of epidemiological evidence. Cancer of the cervix is almost unheard of in nuns. It has long been known that women who have multiple sexual partners are at higher risk. The younger you are at beginning sex activity, especially if before age sixteen, the higher your risk. You are also at higher risk if you have had more than five children, used birth control pills for longer than five years, or have had a sexually transmitted disease. Women with the kidney disease glomerulonephritis have five times the risk, even if they are not taking immunosuppressive drugs, so that if you have this disease, you need to be more frequently screened.

Mothers and sisters of cervical cancer patients are at higher risk, so that if you have such a relative with this disease, you need more frequent monitoring. African-American women have nearly twice the risk as white women.

Mild cervical dysplasia is increasing, and deaths from cancer of the cervix have dramatically increased in women under 35. Use of the birth control pill may be partly responsible, along with the change toward earlier sexual contact and multiple partners.

The human papilloma virus (or HPV, type 16), which causes genital warts, is implicated as the most common agent to trigger the progression to cancer of the cervix. However, since 15 million women in the United States have HPV infection, and only 1 percent develop this disease, some other cofactor that affects immune function is probably involved. Poor nutrition, low socioeconomic status, and cigarette smoking are documented to increase your risk.

Cervical dysplasia and early cancer of the cervix produce no symptoms. Later in the disease, irregular spotting or a change in vaginal discharge may appear. Cervical cancer is highly curable if found early, when still localized, but much less so after distant spread develops. (See Table 19.1.) Screening programs that include regular pelvic exams and Pap smears have been shown to decrease mortality rates. The American Cancer Society recommends that all women who are sexually active or have reached the age of 18 have a yearly Pap smear and pelvic examination. After three consecutive normal smears the frequency may be decreased at the discretion of the physician.

Unfortunately, one-third of the women in the United States don't get regular Pap smears or follow screening guidelines. One-half of all woman diagnosed with cervical cancer have never had a Pap test. If you have an abnormal Pap smear, it should be repeated. If it remains persistently abnormal, you should have culposcopy, with biopsy of any abnormalities seen. If none can be found, further measures should be taken, as described under surgical treatment of cancer of the cervix.

If you are found to have cancer of the

TABLE 19.1.
Prognosis of Cervical Cancer[42]

	Percent of Patients Surviving 5 Years	Percent of Patients in This Stage
All Patients	69.9%	
Not Staged	52.4%	7%
By Stage		
Localized	91.9%	54%
Lymph node spread	49.1%	32%
Distant spread	14.6%	8%

cervix, the recommended treatment options depend on your stage, age, general health, and desire to retain fertility. Although seeming complicated, staging is a handy way of describing how far your tumor has spread. Your stage is determined by local biopsy, along with other tests, including X-rays, scans, and an examination and biopsy of intra-abdominal tissues by laparoscopy or open technique.

Within each stage, the treatment recommendations may be affected by the size of the tumor, as well as where it has spread. For later-stage disease, the possible options are many, and include different combinations of surgery, radiation, and chemotherapy. You need to have your specific case reviewed by a surgeon, radiotherapist, and chemotherapist who specialize in the treatment of gynecological cancer.

Alternative Medicine Approaches to Cervical Cancer

Jennifer, an active, energetic 45-year-old family physician, was so busy with her medical practice she neglected to have her own annual Pap test for several years. Finally, on examination, she was found to have moderate cervical dysplasia. Under her doctor's continued observation, she elected to try alternative approaches that included vitamins, an herbal vaginal pack, and a change in her lifestyle, which meant taking more time to exercise, eat properly, and practice stress management techniques. A repeat Pap test six weeks later showed marked improvement, and all of her subsequent tests proved normal over the following five years.

Finding that your Pap smear has come

back abnormal can be quite frightening. You need not panic—*half of all mild dysplasia reverts to normal on its own within one year without any treatment.* You may be able to reverse early and even mild-to-severe dysplasia by adopting an alternative medicine approach. However, you should undertake these approaches only under direct guidance from an experienced doctor, and make certain to be frequently monitored.

Since cancer of the cervix usually goes through a slow-growing, premalignant stage that can be detected by Pap smear, it may be reversed in the early stages using the following program, and even cancer-in-situ can be reversed.[43]

At present, the most important step conventional medicine recommends is that you make certain to obtain a yearly Pap smear. Early problems can be diagnosed and treated in your doctor's office, and you can prevent dysplasia from developing into cancer and avoid a hysterectomy. However, the Pap smear only detects abnormality, it's not a prevention or a treatment. You *can* take measures, such as the following, to prevent disease from developing in the first place, or reverse it once present.

Change Your Sexual Practices

Protecting yourself from contracting sexually transmitted disease (STD) is critical in preventing cervical cancer. Barrier methods of birth control such as condoms and diaphragms can help prevent virus contact, and spermicides have an antiviral effect. In addition, limiting sexual partners lowers your risk.

Don't Take Oral Contraceptives

Use of the birth control pills has been associated with a higher risk for cervical dysplasia.[44] Instead, use a diaphragm, and/or condoms for birth control.

Quit Smoking

An association has been found between smoking and risk of cervical dysplasia and cancer.[45] Smoking increases your chances of developing this disease by two to three times. Quitting smoking is the most important first step in an alternative medicine program. See Chapter 2 for further help in quitting.

Change Your Diet

Patients with dysplasia have been found to have lower than normal blood levels of vitamins A, B$_6$, C, folic acid, selenium, and beta-carotene, probably reflecting improper nutrition.

A low-fat, high-beta-carotene diet is believed to decrease your risk for cervical cancer.[46] It offers a better nutritional supply of naturally protective vitamins and minerals and may influence immune function, favorably affecting your resistance to the viruses that may cause this cancer, and increasing your ability to destroy cancerous cells. Such a diet, recommended to maximize immune function, is discussed more fully in Chapter 2.

Especially recommended are foods high in antioxidants, vitamin A, and beta-carotene, such as spinach, carrots, beet greens, sweet potatoes, cabbage, kale, broccoli, asparagus, wheat germ, lima beans, and other dark green, leafy vegetables.

Take Supplements

Taking supplemental vitamin A, beta-carotene, vitamin C, and folic acid may decrease your risk, and aid in the reversal process. Vitamin A is associated with the maintenance of healthy epithelium (outer layer of the skin), and has been studied in association with this epithelial-derived tumor. One study reports that retinoids, vitamin A derivatives, may be effective in preventing cervical dysplasia.[47] Reversal of early lesions has also been reported.[48] The usual recommended dose is 10,000 IU of vitamin A, once or twice daily, as supervised by your doctor.

One report suggests that vitamin C may help prevent cervical dysplasia.[49] The usual dosage recommended for this effect is 2,000 to 3,000 mg three times daily.

Folic acid, a B vitamin, may be deficient in cervical dysplasia patients, and has been found to reverse dysplasia in oral contraceptive users.[50] Dosage is usually 5 mg once daily, as supervised by your doctor.

Selenium is a mineral felt to have some anticancer, antioxidant effects. Recommended dosage is 200 mcg daily.

You may also benefit from inserting a vitamin A capsule into your vagina, up next to the cervix, twice daily. This local application of vitamin A may act to help the epithelium repair itself.

Use Herbal Preparations

Chaparral (*Larrea divaricata*) is an herb traditionally used by the American Indians for its antioxidant and immune system stimulation properties. It should not be utilized by anyone suffering from liver or kidney disease, so its use and dosage must be monitored by your alternative medicine doctor.

Use a Vaginal Pack

This is an herbal preparation, consisting mainly of the herb sanguinaria, which should be prescribed and administered by an alternative medicine doctor familiar with its use. It helps in the sloughing off of abnormal cells, and restoring health to the cervix. Research conducted by Dr. Tori Hudson at the Northwest School of Naturopathy in Portland, Oregon, showed that its application in combination with a general nutritional support program and dietary change, as outlined above, achieved reversal to normal of thirty-eight of forty-three abnormal Pap smear patients, ten of whom had carcinoma in situ.[51]

Practice Stress Management

Stress may play an important role in cervical cancer, since this cancer is felt to be largely triggered by a virus, and susceptibility to viral infections has been shown to be influenced by stress. You may have been exposed to the HPV virus, but whether your body is infected by it or can get rid of infected cells may depend upon your experience of stress in your life and what you choose to do to cope with it.

As discussed more fully in Chapter 2, stress means change, and since life is filled with change, life will always be innately stressful. Whether or not you develop a tumor depends upon a complex interplay of emotional, nervous system, and hormonal factors, which continually affect the ability of your immune system's white cells to both fight infection and remove abnormal cells once they are engendered.

Specific connections between our reponses to stress in general or to particular stresses and the onset of tumors is difficult to research, and may, in fact, never be fully documented. Initial reports of improved T cell counts, and numbers and activity of white cells in general, in response to stress management training, yoga and meditation, need to be followed up with further research. You may even be able to profoundly influence your body's own ability to remove a tumor once it has formed. Until the scientific explorations of these effects are more complete, you may still be able to take advantage of potential mind-body relationship benefits by following the guidelines given in Chapter 2, instituting stress management techniques into your daily lifestyle.

Practice Visualization

Follow the guidelines for deep relaxation and visualization given in Chapter 2. For example, imagine your cervix as a beautiful rose bud. On its surface is a small drop of dew. Imagine the sun coming out, and the dew disappearing. Now see the rose bud as clear and free of any problems, soft and radiantly lovely. Picture this in your mind's eye and, at the same time, feel it happening within your body.

Conventional Medicine Approaches to Cervical Cancer

Depending on the stage of your cervical cancer, you don't necessarily have to have a hysterectomy. Following are some options to consider.

Radiation Treatment

In early-stage cervical cancer, results of radiation therapy are equivalent to surgery. For very early tumors, the radiation can be given directly to the cervix in the form of "seeds" of radioactive isotopes placed into the cervix through the vagina, or by a standard "external beam" machine. However, the ovaries may be destroyed by this treatment, so that if you are a younger patient and want to save them, surgery may be the best option. Also, radiation may cause vaginal dryness and scarring.

Radiation is equally successful in midstage cervical cancer. Recent evidence suggests that radiotherapy in combination with chemotherapy is the preferred treatment for the later stages.[52] Both external beam and radiation seeds may be used.

Radiation to the pelvis may be recommended after radical hysterectomy if tumor has been left behind or has involved lymph nodes. Radiation to the whole abdominal area may be recommended if the tumor recurs after the original treatment.

Chemotherapy

Chemotherapy should be used in combination with radiotherapy for later-stage disease and when recurrence develops. It can also be used to relieve symptoms if cure is not possible.

Surgical Approaches to Cervical Cancer

Surgical treatment is preferred for early, preinvasive cancer-in-situ. Simple removal with a scalpel, electrocautery, laser vaporization, cryosurgery, or LEEP can be done in an office setting under local anesthesia. However, some controversy exists about the adequacy of these destructive techniques in terms of diagnosing and treating unsuspected *invasive* cancer. A conization procedure (see page 506) removes a deeper cone-shaped core of cervical tissue. The surgical specimen is more adequate to find undiagnosed invasive cancer, which would require a different treatment. However, this procedure may interfere with future pregnancy and has significant side ef-

fects, such as bleeding and pain. Local, spinal, or general anesthesia can be given. Simple hysterectomy may be the best choice if fertility is no longer desired.

Surgical options for superficially invasive (less than 3 mm deep) tumors include conization and simple hysterectomy. For deeper invasion (3 to 5 mm), radical hysterectomy, which involves removing more of the vagina, and examining pelvic lymph nodes for spread, is recommended. For midstage cervical cancer, radical hysterectomy is the surgical procedure of choice. The chance for cure is 85 to 95 percent in these small cancers.

For midstage cervical cancer, your options are radical hysterectomy and lymph node removal, radical hysterectomy plus radiation, and radiation with or without chemotherapy, depending on size of tumor and presence and location of lymph node spread. For late stages, radiotherapy with chemotherapy is recommended as the primary treatment. Surgery may be used for staging, by searching for spread within the abdomen.

The most radical surgery, called *exenteration*, is chosen in combination with hysterectomy when invasion of neighboring organs has taken place or recurrence of tumor has developed only in the pelvis after the original treatment. This operation may involve removing your fallopian tubes and ovaries, bladder, rectum, and/or vagina. Your stool and urine are then passed through openings created on the abdominal wall. Plastic surgical recreation of a vagina can be performed at a later time. The mortality rate of exenteration is about 5 percent. The chance for living at least five years is 50 percent. (For a discussion of all the hysterectomy operations, see page 537.)

CERVICAL CANCER SUMMARY

Prevention

Diet and Supplements

- Follow a low-fat, high-fiber, whole-foods diet, high in vegetables and fruits.
- Eat foods high in antioxidants, vitamin A, and beta-carotene, such as spinach, carrots, beet greens, sweet potatoes, cabbage, kale, broccoli, asparagus, wheat germ, lima beans, and other dark green, leafy vegetables.
- Vitamin A, 10,000 IU, 1–2 times daily, as supervised by your doctor.
- Vitamin C, 2,000–3,000 mg, 3 times daily.
- Folic acid, 5 mg daily, as supervised by your doctor.
- Selenium, 200 mcg daily.

Lifestyle

- Follow Pap smear screening guidelines.
- Change your sexual practices—use barrier methods of birth control such as condoms and diaphragms, limiting sexual partners.
- Don't take oral contraceptives.
- Don't smoke.
- Reduce stress.

Alternative Medicine Approaches

- Vitamin A capsule, intravaginally next to the cervix, twice daily.
- Herb chaparral (*Larrea divaricata*), monitored by your doctor.
- Sanguinaria vaginal pack, monitored by your doctor.
- Practice visualization.

Conventional Medicine Approaches

- Radiation treatment.
- Chemotherapy.

Surgical Approaches

- Local excision—scalpel, electrocautery, laser vaporization, cryosurgery, and LEEP.
- Conization.
- Simple hysterectomy.
- Radical hysterectomy.
- Exenteration.

Uterine Cancer

Cancer of the uterus is the most common form of female pelvic malignancy, comprising 6 percent of all cancers in women. It is more difficult to detect than cancer of the cervix, and takes two forms. The rare type, called *sarcoma,* arises in the muscle layer. The much more common form starts in the inner cell lining, the *endometrium.*

Cancer of the endometrium is the fourth most common malignancy in women in the United States: 39,300 new cases and 6,600 deaths will occur in 2002.[53] The incidence is nearly twice as high for African-American women as for white women. Estrogen exposure is the major risk factor for this malignancy. Early menarche and late menopause, failure to ovulate, never having children or having them at a late age, and use of postmenopausal estrogens increase risk. Adding progesterone preparations decreases the risk caused by using only estrogen for post-menopausal hormone replacement treatment. Also, a history of uterine atypical adenomatous hyperplasia (see page 526), diabetes, gallbladder disease, hypertension, obesity, and a high-fat diet increase risk. An increased incidence of this cancer is found in women who have had or are at high risk for breast cancer, or are taking the drug tamoxifen. Pregnancy and use of oral contraceptive pills decrease the risk.

Signs of cancer of the uterus are the same as those of cancer of the cervix, including bleeding or discharge unrelated to the menstrual period, and pain with urination, bowel movements, intercourse, or in the pelvic area.

Diagnosis of uterine cancer is usually made after typical symptoms or findings on a routine pelvic exam lead to further investigations. Pap smear is not reliable in detecting early endometrial cancer. A hysteroscopy with biopsy, endometrial suction biopsy, or D&C removes tissue for microscopic analysis. If cancer is found, further tests such as a sonogram or pelvic CAT scan are necessary to determine its extent.

Your treatment options and prognosis depend on the tumor's cell characteristics, stage, whether its cells respond to female hormones, and your overall health. (See Table 19.2.) If found in early stages, these cancers are highly curable by surgery.

Alternative Medicine Approaches to Uterine Cancer

Once cancer is present, the uterus must be removed. However, alternative medicine approaches such as the following may act to prevent this disease, as well as assist in its treatment.

Change Your Diet

The good news about cancer of the uterus is that this cancer has been found to be associated with a high-fat, low-fiber diet, and if you change your nutritional choices, you may substantially reduce your chances for developing it. If you already have cancer, a low-fat diet may lessen the possibility of recurrence.[54] Directions for this diet are given in Chapter 2.

Take Supplements

Supplements may act to improve your immune function. Suggested additions are vita-

TABLE 19.2.
Prognosis of Uterine Cancer[55]

	Percent of Patients Surviving 5 Years	Percent of Patients in This Stage
All Patients	84.0%	
Not Staged	49.1%	5%
By Stage		
Localized to uterus	96.1%	73%
Lymph node spread	62.7%	14%
Distant spread	25.8%	8%

min A, 10,000 IU daily; vitamin C, 2,000 to 3,000 mg three times daily, and selenium, 200 mcg daily.

Practice Stress Management

Stress may be a contributing factor to the development of uterine cancer. A combination of hormonal, nervous system, and emotional reactions may affect your immune system's ability to remove abnormal cells once they have formed. Further research is needed.

Local circulation of white cells to the uterine area to do maintenance functions may also be affected by stress, which shifts circulatory patterns to ready us for the fight-or-flight response.

Consciously invoking a relaxation response on a daily basis may offset the effects of the inevitable stressors of living; initial research has supported this. You can take advantage of the mind-body connection to your immune function by beginning a stress-management program as outlined in Chapter 2, and including yoga, relaxation, meditation, and other alternative medicine staples.

Practice Visualization

First do the deep relaxation, as given in Chapter 2. For example, imagine the white cells of your immune system as a host of angels, carrying light wands that are able to transform any abnormal cells back to normal. Have them search every area of your body, complete their work, and then set them to guard against future problems. Picture this in your mind's eye, and see it happening within your body.

Conventional Medicine Approaches to Uterine Cancer

The same as cervical cancer, uterine cancer in certain stages can be treated nonsurgically. Following are some techniques.

Radiation Treatment

X-ray treatment, utilized by itself for some early and late-stage cancers, is more often combined with surgical treatment for mid-stage disease to increase your chances for a good result. Such therapy may be given by external beam, or via radioactive pellets placed directly into the area of the tumor.

Chemotherapy and Hormonal Therapy

Cancer-killing drugs, female hormones (Megace, Provera), and hormone blockers (tamoxifen) can be given by pill or intravenously. However, they are usually given to patients with more extensive spread when surgery and radiation are not possible or likely to provide cure. You will need to discuss the latest information with your gynecologist.

Surgical Approaches to Uterine Cancer

Very early stage cancers can be treated by a D&C, followed by hormone therapy, or by hysterectomy.

Hysterectomy is the most common form of treatment for cancer of the uterus. *Total abdominal hysterectomy* removes both fallopian tubes, ovaries, and some pelvic lymph nodes, and usually cures localized cancers. If the lymph nodes and abdominal washings (irrigation fluid used to pick up free-floating tumor cells) are negative, no further treatment is necessary. A *radical hysterectomy,* which also removes part of the vagina, is done for later stages. In rare cases, a *pelvic exenteration* is recommended for tumors invading adjacent organs, or recurrent tumors. (For a discussion of the hysterectomy operations, see page 537.)

UTERINE CANCER SUMMARY

Prevention

Diet and Supplements

- Follow a low-fat, high-fiber diet.
- Replace meat and dairy with soy and other beans.
- Vitamin A, 10,000 IU daily.
- Vitamin C, 2,000–3,000 mg daily.
- Selenium, 200 mcg daily.
- Avoid black tea.

Lifestyle

- Practice stress management.

Alternative Medicine Approaches

- Follow the preventive guidelines, above.
- Add garlic, onion, and tumeric to your diet.
- Practice visualization.

Conventional Medicine Approaches

- Radiation treatment.
- Chemotherapy.
- Hormonal therapy.

Surgical Approaches

- D&C.
- Total abdominal hysterectomy.
- Radical hysterectomy.
- Pelvic exenteration.

Hysterectomy

You have many choices when it comes to having a hysterectomy. Do you really need it? Can you avoid an operation altogether? Can you safely keep part of your uterus? Will your sex life be improved, stay the same, or perhaps be made worse?

The answers to these questions will be considered in detail in the following pages. Final answers in some areas may currently be impossible, since different studies have produced contradictory results. We will consider all of the angles of these controversies to help you sort out the solution that is best for you.

Avoiding Hysterectomy

The uterus was historically seen as "its own animal," and corresponds to the flower and seed pod of the body. It actively participates in orgasm, with soothing and delightful rhythmic contractions. *Physiologically, a combined clitoral and uterine orgasm is impossible after a hysterectomy.* The cervix also produces prostaglandins, which provide for brain relaxation.

The uterus carries on a continuous feedback conversation with the brain and ovaries, helping your transition through menopause with much fewer symptoms. Women who have had a hysterectomy undergo menopause four years earlier than women who undergo spontaneous menopause, even if their ovaries were not removed.[56] Your uterus even acts to help your ovaries maintain some estrogen secretion after menopause. Anatomically, it aids in holding your other pelvic organs, such as the bowel and bladder, in place.

Although most women do just fine after a hysterectomy, depression, sexual dysfunction, weight gain, pelvic relaxation of the bowel and bladder, excessive hot flashes, night sweats, and insomnia may occur in some women. A 2000 *Lancet* report based on eleven studies found that women who had hysterectomy were 40 percent more likely to have problems with urinary incontinence than those who hadn't.[57] Some women find it harder to connect sexually with their partners, and the incidence of divorce is higher.[58]

Unless you have cancer, other, less disfiguring ways are now available to treat the various female disorders that have in the past led to the recommendation of hysterectomy. You *never* need to have your ovaries removed just because you are having your uterus taken out, unless they contain cancer. Follow the alternative medicine treatment guidelines related to your specific disease, and seek help from an alternative medicine specialist when necessary. Many books advising against hysterectomy can now be found in the women's section of larger bookstores.

Of course, women are not defined by the presence or absence of a uterus. If you have already had a hysterectomy, you can use the stress management, yoga, and visualization techniques given in Chapter 2 to help you regain a satisfactory orgasm based on clitoris function. Deep meditation exhibits the same brain waves as orgasm, so that if you find difficulty achieving sexual connection in your life, you may find this pathway of great benefit. Follow the natural guidelines to hormone replacement, given at the end of this chapter, especially if your ovaries were also removed.

Hysterectomy Operations

The indications for having a hysterectomy have been discussed under each specific disease. Several types of hysterectomy are available. The options best for you depend on whether your problem is benign or malignant,

the size of your uterus, whether you have had previous abdominal surgery, your overall medical condition, and your wishes. After hysterectomy, of course, you will not be able to become pregnant, and will no longer have periods.

Total Abdominal Hysterectomy or Simple Hysterectomy

Total abdominal hysterectomy (TAH) or simple hysterectomy removes only the uterus, and is the most common type of hysterectomy. (See Figure 19.3.) The operation is usually performed under general anesthesia. Once you are asleep, a catheter is placed in your bladder. A four- to eight-inch incision can be made in your midline, from your navel to pubis, or crosswise just at the pubis hairline. This latter *"Pfannensteil"* or "bikini" incision is much less obvious.

Your surgeon then pulls up the uterus and cuts the two ligaments connecting it to the abdominal wall. The fallopian tubes are divided near their attachments to the body of the uterus. The vagina is separated very close to where it joins the cervix. After the uterus is removed, the opening in the back of the vagina is closed with stitches. In the rarely performed *subtotal hysterectomy*, the cervix is not removed. The incision is repaired with stitches, clips, or skin tapes. This operation usually take one to two hours.

You awake in the recovery room and, after an hour or so, are transferred to your room. Pain can be controlled with an epidural catheter, or intravenous or intramuscular injections. The following day, you should be ready to eat and can switch to pain pills. The bladder catheter can be removed in a day or two. Most likely, you can be discharged after two to four days.

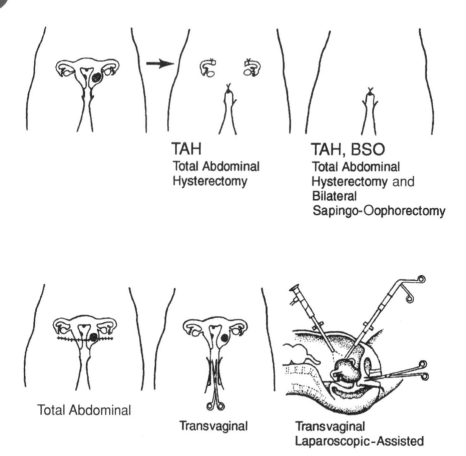

TAH
Total Abdominal
Hysterectomy

TAH, BSO
Total Abdominal
Hysterectomy and
Bilateral
Sapingo-Oophorectomy

Total Abdominal

Transvaginal

Transvaginal
Laparoscopic-Assisted

Fig. 19.3 Types of hysterectomies and surgical approaches

You need to see your surgeon again in a week, to ensure you are healing well. Be certain to report any increased pain, fever, or unusual vaginal discharge. Some vaginal blood spotting is usual for a week or so, followed by a brownish discharge for a few weeks. Use a sanitary pad, not tampons, and don't douche. If you are premenopausal, you may continue to have your usual premenstrual symptoms, though without periods. Your ovaries still produce hormones and release eggs, which are reabsorbed, until menopause. After six or eight weeks, you should be fully healed and able to resume sexual intercourse. Sensations should be unchanged for both you and your partner, and no restrictions are necessary. If the condition for which you required the hysterectomy caused pelvic pain, your sex life should be better.

Total Abdominal Hysterectomy and Bilateral Sapingo-Oophorectomy

Total abdominal hysterectomy and bilateral sapingo-oophorectomy (TAH-BSO) removes both of your fallopian tubes and ovaries with your uterus. It may be recommended if both are diseased, to decrease your risk of ovarian cancer if you are post-menopausal, since risk increases with age, or if you have a type of cancer that may be stimulated by female hormones produced by the ovaries. If you are premenopausal, just one ovary may be removed if it is diseased, or to decrease your risk of ovarian cancer. If you are premenopausal and both your ovaries are removed, after the operation your female hormone levels will decrease, you will no longer have premenstrual symptoms. and you will experience menopause. You may have hot flashes and mood swings. Discuss taking hormonal replacement therapy with your doctor.

Transvaginal Hysterectomy

This procedure can be performed through the vagina if your uterus is small and you have benign disease, or if you have very early cervical or endometrial cancer. No scar can be seen. Although it is usually technically possible to remove the fallopian tubes and ovaries as well, they are not often taken out through this approach.

You can choose general or spinal anesthesia. You lie on the operating table with your feet up in stirrups. Retracting instruments are placed into the vagina, giving your surgeon working space and a good view of the cervix. The tissue between the cervix and back of the vagina is divided. Your uterus is freed from all its attachments to the tubes, ovaries, and abdominal wall, and then pulled out through the vagina. Finally, the opening in the back of the vagina is closed with absorbable stitches, which do not need to be removed. A gauze pack may be placed in the vagina. If you choose this approach, you recover more

quickly, are able to take fluids on the evening of surgery, and can be discharged in two or three days. The rest of the recovery period is similar to total abdominal hysterectomy.

Laparoscopic-Assisted Hysterectomy

This procedure has recently been developed so that a TAH-BSO can be done using the transvaginal approach. Gynecologists have used the laparoscope for more than twenty-five years (in fact, laparoscopic gall bladder surgery was first perfected by gynecologists). You are under general anesthesia for this operation.

While watching on a TV monitor, your surgeon divides the tissues connecting the tubes, ovaries, and uterus to your abdominal wall. The attachment of the cervix to the back of the vagina is disconnected from below, then the whole works removed through the vagina. The vaginal opening is closed with absorbable stitches and the abdominal port incisions with skin tapes. Postoperative recovery is similar to transvaginal hysterectomy. You may be discharged in one to three days and, in some cases, may have your operation as an outpatient procedure. A 1995 study of over 3,000 patients who had this procedure found a lower rate of complications than with standard vaginal or abdominal hysterectomy.[59, 60]

Radical Hysterectomy

This operation is performed for advanced stages of cervical, uterine, vaginal, and ovarian cancer. It is the same as TAH-BSO, except that more of the vagina, tissues adjacent to the uterus, fallopian tubes, and ovaries, and pelvic and abdominal lymph nodes are removed. (See Figure 19.4.) Postoperative recovery is quite similar.

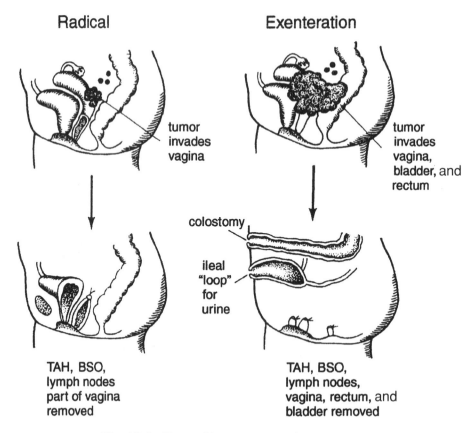

Radical

tumor invades vagina

TAH, BSO, lymph nodes part of vagina removed

Exenteration

tumor invades vagina, bladder, and rectum

colostomy

ileal "loop" for urine

TAH, BSO, lymph nodes, vagina, rectum, and bladder removed

Fig. 19.4 Types of hysterectomies for cancer

Pelvic Exenteration

This extensive procedure may be necessary if a malignant tumor invades the neighboring bladder and/or rectum. This is similar to radical hysterectomy, with the addition of removal of the rectum (posterior exenteration), bladder (anterior exenteration), or both (complete pelvic exenteration). If the rectum is removed, you will need a permanent colostomy (see page 446). If the bladder is removed, you must have an ileal conduit. Your surgeon makes a seven-inch tube out of a piece of your small intestine. The ureters from your kidneys are sewn into one end, and the other end

brought through your abdominal wall to make a permanent ileostomy. Urine is then collected in a plastic bag, held in place over the stoma. Postoperative recovery is more prolonged, since you have to learn how to care for the colostomy and/or ileostomy. Likelihood of complications is also increased.

Complications of Hysterectomy

The mortality rate of hysterectomy is less than 1 per 1,000 for benign disease and less than 1 in 50 when it is done for cancer, with serious complications in 2 to 5 percent, and minor ones in about 20 percent. Such complications include infection in the pelvis or abdominal incision, excessive bleeding requiring blood transfusion, urinary tract infection, injury to nearby organs such as bowel, bladder, ureters, and rectum, blood clots or phlebitis, and bowel obstruction from scar tissue. Complications are lower for transvaginal than transabdominal hysterectomy, and the newer laparoscopic approaches may prove to be even safer.[61]

Recovering from hysterectomy, especially if both your ovaries were removed, can be very stressful. Emotional swings, discomfort, and a change in your body image can make you feel depressed. Understand that this is a normal transition and be easy on yourself. You may have heard that a hysterectomy will cause you to gain weight, decrease your desire for sex, change your femininity, and other myths.

The relationship between hysterectomy and sexual function remains uncertain as various studies have shown conflicting evidence for both improvement and deterioration. A 1999 prospective study reported in the *Journal of the American Medical Association* interviewed 1,101 women from the Maryland Women's Health Study, both before and twenty-four months after hysterectomy for benign conditions. The researchers found substantial improvements in sexual function in terms of increased libido, increased frequency of sexual activity, decreased pain with intercourse, increased frequency and strength of orgasm, and decreased vaginal dryness. For each sexual functioning problem they found the rate of relief was more than 60 percent whereas the rate of its new development was less than 10 percent.[62]

The discrepancy between studies, some of which show improvement in sexual functioning and some of which do not, may be partly explainable by the consideration of different categories of orgasms: those composed of clitoral sensations and those that include sensations coming from the uterus.

The presence of abnormal bleeding, uncomfortable fibroids, a prolapsed uterus, fear of pregnancy, or other condition may have led to the hysterectomy. When the problem was eliminated, an improvement in sexual function and orgasm may have followed, leading to the outcome of the studies showing sexual benefit after hysterectomy.

However, once the uterus is removed, having an orgasm that includes the rhythmic contractions of the uterus is not possible. Some women do become aware of this change, while for others, the overriding relief of symptoms may take precedence.

In order for you to choose wisely, you thus need to consider all of the ramifications of your uterine removal, then weigh these against your current sexual function and satisfaction.

Other prospective studies of sexual function have found improvement or no change after hysterectomy. A study by A. Coppen and colleagues published in the *Lancet* followed sixty premenopausal women before and after hysterectomy for benign disease. They found "no evidence that this group of patients showed depression or sexual difficulties related to the hysterectomy. In comparison with their baseline gynecological condition, they showed improved mood and vigor and unimpaired sexual activity."[63]

No evidence suggests that the operation increases psychological distress or psychiatric symptoms. In fact, the opposite has been found to be true.[64, 65] Use this as a time to become closer to family and friends.

Ovarian Cysts and Benign Tumors

Each month during your childbearing years, a cystlike follicle forms around an egg in one of your ovaries. As the egg matures, the follicle enlarges and finally ruptures, releasing the egg. After ovulation, the empty follicle is called the corpus luteum. If the egg is not fertilized, the corpus luteum usually shrinks and disappears. However, if the corpus luteum persists, it can form into a fluid-filled *functional cyst*. This is a fairly common occurrence; such cysts usually do not cause symptoms, and disappear spontaneously after a few menstrual cycles. This type of cyst does not form after menopause.

The ovary can form other types of benign cysts and masses. *Dermoid cysts* and *dermoid tumors* are thought to grow from unfertilized eggs within the ovary, and can form growths containing different kinds of tissue, including hair, skin, and even teeth. *Cystenadenomas* are cysts that contain fluid produced by a glandular cell lining. If the lining becomes thickened, a tumor mass develops. *Endometriosis* can form "cysts" and benign tumor masses (*endometriomas)* on the ovaries. *Polycystic ovarian syndrome* is a condition where the ovaries form large numbers of follicular cysts and a tough outer covering, which causes infertility by preventing an egg from breaking through and being released.

Ovarian cysts and benign tumors can become surprisingly large, up to a foot or more in diameter, causing symptoms of pelvic pain, pressure, abdominal or pelvic swelling, menstrual irregularities, frequent urination, and discomfort during intercourse. Sudden, severe pain can develop if one ruptures or bleeds into the abdominal cavity, commonly causing confusion with acute appendicitis. Also, a cyst can twist upon itself, shutting off its own blood supply or that of the ovary (*torsion*), thus causing severe pain. Rarely, cysts can become infected, causing pain, fever, and systemic illness.

Ovarian cysts and masses may be found during a pelvic or abdominal exam or on a sonogram, which can determine whether they are cystic or solid. Laparoscopy or open surgery may be necessary to determine whether such masses harbor a malignancy.

Your treatment choices depend on your age, the size and characteristics of the mass on a sonogram, the presence of symptoms, and your desire to retain fertility. Cysts rarely contain cancer before age 50. Solid masses are more likely to be malignant than simple cysts that contain a single fluid-filled space.

Alternative Medicine Approaches to Ovarian Cysts and Benign Tumors

If you are premenopausal, don't have symptoms, and the simple fluid-filled cyst measures less than 4 centimeters and has a thin wall, you can choose to observe it for a few menstrual cycles. You have a 70 percent chance it will disappear without any treatment. If you are postmenopausal and the simple cyst is less than 5 centimeters, it is also safe to have it watched closely. If the cyst enlarges or develops changes suspicious for cancer, you should have surgery.

If you develop one cyst, you are likely to develop more in the future. Therefore, if treatment of the first cyst needs surgery, you should observe the following guidelines to prevent another.

Quit Smoking

A study at Group Health Cooperative in Seattle found that women who smoked had twice the risk of developing functional ovarian cysts as those who did not.[66]

A complex combination of local, hormonal, nervous system, and stress-related factors may explain this. Higher carbon dioxide levels in the blood of smokers, along with lowered oxygen levels, may interfere with ovarian repair mechanisms. The nicotine in even one cigarette causes your small blood vessels to constrict, further effecting local maintenance systems.

You can use the powerful alternative medicine approaches to help you quit smoking for good. See Chapter 2 for tips.

Change Your Diet

Alterations in how the body can effect tissue repair may be achieved by changes in the diet. Follow the guidelines for a whole-foods, low-fat, high-fiber diet given in Chapter 2. Particularly avoid caffeine, alcohol, dairy products, sugar and other concentrated sweets, and chocolate.

Take Supplements

Adding vitamin E (the D-alpha type), at a dose of 400 IU three times daily, acts to promote the formation of certain prostaglandins, specifically the ones that help reduce inflammation. Taking vitamin E may thus help to quell the underlying process of cyst formation.

Add Herbal Preparations

The herbs gelsemium, phytolacca, and bryonia, as part of "Turska's Formula," have been used to treat the underlying hormonal imbalance leading to cyst formation.[67] Take 25 drops, three times daily.

Use Additional Alternative Medicine Approaches

Utilizing acupuncture, chiropractic, homeopathy, and hypnosis may provide additional healing capabilities. The most often recommended homeopathic remedies are aconite, apis (for right-sided cysts), and colocinthus (for left-sided cysts), though these approaches should be individualized by a practitioner experienced in homeopathy. Magnetic therapy, using a diathermy machine or individual magnets taped over the cyst-forming area, has been anecdotally indicated to be of some use. Also recommended is castor oil, rubbed into the skin of the lower abdominal wall over the ovary, then topped with a hot water bottle for an hour or so each night for a month or two.

Practice Visualization

First, do the deep relaxation, as given in Chapter 2. Then, for example, imagine your ovary as a small velvet purse, containing many beautiful pearl-like pink eggs, but with one larger yellow egg that does not belong there. Gently remove it, and picture the ovary as perfectly healthy. Hold these images in your mind, while at the same time feeling them within your body.

Conventional Medicine Approaches to Ovarian Cysts and Benign Tumors

Cysts can be treated with a trial of nonsurgical techniques. Following are two to consider.

Birth Control Pills

Hormones may be successful in shrinking ovarian cysts. A few months of birth control pills can be tried, under the direction of your doctor. Since these pills prevent ovulation, functional cysts are very rare in women using oral contraceptives.

Cyst Aspiration

Using sonographic guidance, a long needle can be passed through the abdominal skin or through the vagina into the cyst and the fluid removed. This can be considered if you are a young woman or are postmenopausal with a simple cyst of less than 5 centimeters. However, many authorities feel aspiration should not be performed, since the results are unreliable, and if the cyst contains tumor cells, they can leak out the needle hole and spread within the abdomen.

Surgical Approaches to Ovarian Cysts and Benign Tumors

If you are premenopausal and your cyst or mass is large, causes significant symptoms, does not go away after a few menstrual cycles, or has characteristics suspicious for cancer on an ultrasound, you should have surgery. If you are postmenopausal, it is wisest to have it removed unless it is small, shrinks on observation, and does not have any suspicious characteristics. The cyst or mass can simply be cut out of the ovary or the whole ovary removed using the following techniques.

Cyst Excision

If your cyst or mass is small and benign, and you wish to retain your ovaries, a simple excision, with ovary preservation, can usually be performed. The cyst is "shelled out" along with a small amount of adjacent, normal ovarian tissue. This operation can usually be performed or assisted through a laparoscope, giving you a smaller incision and quicker recovery.

Oophorectomy

If you don't wish to retain fertility, or are postmenopausal, one or both ovaries (plus or minus the fallopian tubes) can be removed, usually through the laparoscope. If suspicion of malignancy is present, a laparoscopic approach is not recommended, because an adequate cancer operation cannot be performed using this technique. (For a discussion of oophorectomy, see page 519.)

If you are found to have a cyst or mass that contains a malignancy, you should be treated for cancer of the ovary. Because of this possibility, you should discuss your treatment wishes before undergoing any diagnostic laparoscopy or open surgical procedure.

OVARIAN CYSTS AND BENIGN TUMORS SUMMARY

Prevention

Diet and Supplements

• Follow a low-fat, high-fiber diet.
• Avoid caffeine, alcohol, refined sugar, and dairy products.
• Vitamin E, D-alpha, 400 IU, 3 times daily.

Lifestyle

• Don't smoke.
• Maintain optimum weight.

Alternative Medicine Approaches

• Follow the preventive guidelines, above.
• Turska's Formula, consisting of the herbs

gelsemium, phytolacca, and bryonia, 25 drops, 3 times daily.

- Use acupuncture, chiropractic, osteopathic, homeopathy.
- Magnets, castor oil packs (under supervision only).
- Practice visualization.

Conventional Medicine Approaches

- Birth control pills.
- Cyst aspiration.

Surgical Approaches

- Cyst excision.
- Oophorectomy.

Ovarian Cancer

Cancer of the ovary affects 1 in 70 women, is the fourth leading cause of cancer mortality in women, and is responsible for more deaths than cervical and uterine cancer combined—about 23,300 new cases and 13,900 deaths will occur in 2002.[68] Your chances of developing ovarian cancer are decreased if you have had at least one child, have breast-fed, used birth control pills (40 to 50 percent decreased risk, the longer the better), have had your fallopian tubes tied or had a hysterectomy, and follow a low-fat diet. Your risk is increased if you have a family history of breast or ovarian cancer (10 percent of all women with ovarian cancer have a hereditary predisposition), if you have had endometrial, colon, or breast cancer, or if you have used fertility drugs or been exposed to vaginal talcum powder. In the United States, rates for African-American women are 40 percent lower than for white women. Incidence increases with age, beginning to rise steeply at age 35 and peaking at age 72.

Ovarian cancer is dangerous because it causes no symptoms in its early stages, is difficult to feel during a pelvic exam, and no good screening tests are available for the general population. Although the cure rate can be as high as 80 percent when the tumor is found still confined to the ovary, only 25 percent are treated before spread, and your overall chance of cure is less than 40 percent. (See Table 19.3.) In its later stages, ovarian cancer causes abdominal swelling with fluid, pelvic pain, interference with urination and passing stool, pain on intercourse, nausea and vomiting, increased gas and indigestion, weight loss, and vaginal bleeding.

Unfortunately, at this time no technique is suitable for routine screening for ovarian cancer. A yearly pelvic exam is the only present recommendation. Your doctor should feel your vagina, rectum, and lower abdomen for abnormal growths. However, even experienced examiners may miss ovarian masses. Pap smears, highly accurate in cervical cancer, are only positive in 10 to 30 percent of ovarian cancer cases. A blood test for ovarian cancer called CA 125 may be recommended if a suspicion of ovarian cancer exists, but it is not sufficiently reliable to be used for general screening.

If you have any symptoms suggestive of ovarian cancer, you should have an abdominal or transvaginal sonogram. Because many women are found to have ovarian abnormalities on a sonogram, 5 to 10 percent of all women undergo a surgical laparoscopy or open surgery to determine its nature. However, only 10 to 20 percent of these prove to have cancer. You do not need surgical exploration unless your sonogram shows an ovarian abnormality that has suspicious characteristics, or if such a mass enlarges or persists on follow-up exams. Biopsy of a suspicious area must remove the entire ovary, rather than just a piece of it, because partial removal could allow tumor cells to leak out through the biopsy incision and spread in the abdomen. If cancer is found, further surgical treatment can usually be performed during the same operation.

Two general types of cancer of the ovary are found. The rarer (less than 5 percent of all cases) arises in the egg-producing, or *germ*, cells. These tumors occur in girls and younger women. The common type of ovarian cancer, called *epithelial cancer*, arises in the cells lining the ovary, usually in older, post-menopausal women.

Treatment recommendations and prognosis are determined by your tumor cell characteristics (*clear cell* and *mucinous* are worse than other types), stage, age, and overall health. Staging requires a surgical laparoscopy or open surgery, which biopsies lymph nodes, surfaces of the inside of the abdomen, and looks for any tumor cells found in peritoneal washings (saline fluid is collected and analyzed after it is used to irrigate the inside of the abdomen, thereby picking up any loose tumor cells).

The staging and treatment outline for the rare germ cell tumor is similar for that for epithelial cancer. In some cases, simply removing the involved ovary followed by chemotherapy may preserve fertility in these young women.

Alternative Medicine Approaches to Ovarian Cancer

Fortunately, you can act to help prevent, and perhaps fight, ovarian cancer. Following are several good methods to use.

Change Your Diet

Here is another disease that may be prevented by a low-fat, high-fiber, whole-foods, vegetarian diet. Even once you have developed this disorder, you may improve your chances of recovery, and prevent recurrence, by adopting the dietary guidelines given in Chapter 2.[70]

Take Supplements

Vitamins C and E, along with selenium, may act as aids to immune system functioning. Follow the supplement guidelines given in Chapter 2.

TABLE 19.3.
Prognosis of Ovarian Cancer[69]

	Percent of Patients Surviving 5 Years	Percent of Patients in This Stage
All Patients	52.1%	
Not Staged	27.2%	6%
By Stage		
Localized to ovary	95.1%	26%
Lymph node spread	80.5%	10%
Distant spread	29.4%	59%

Avoid Talc

Women who use talc to dust their perineal or vaginal area or their sanitary napkins have double the risk for ovarian cancer.[71] Although the full dynamics of causation are as yet not fully clear, the reason for this connection may be that small particles of talc may move up the vagina, into the uterus, and out of the fallopian tubes, where they can then land on your ovaries and become a source of irritation that may lead to the formation of a tumor. Talc particles have been identified in the ovaries of women with ovarian cancer. Further research is needed, but meanwhile, it is prudent to avoid any hygiene product labelled with the words "talc" or "talcum powder."

Practice Visualization

First, practice deep relaxation, given in Chapter 2. Then image your ovary as a beautiful small egg-containing purse, in which a marble has mistakenly been placed. Remove the marble, and see the purse clear and radiant. Picture this in your mind, and feel it happening within your body.

Join a Support Group

Joining a support group, shown to double life expectancy in breast cancer patients, may also be of benefit for this cancer. Please refer to the section on alternative approaches to breast cancer treatment, pages 201–12.

Conventional Medicine Approaches to Ovarian Cancer

Conventional medicine treatments for local or metastatic cancer of the ovary may provide benefit in addition to surgical treatment or when an operation is inappropriate. Radiation and/or chemotherapy may be tried.

Since this is a difficult cancer to treat, especially when it has spread, newer drug and radiation treatments and combinations are constantly being tested, so you should check with your doctor and other sources, such as the Internet, for the latest reported data and recommendations.

Following are the usual treatment guidelines for conventional medical approaches.

Radiation Treatment

X-ray treatment can be added to surgery and chemotherapy in an attempt to increase chances for survival, although its usage is controversial because of its small benefit and increased chance for complications. It can be given by external beam or, in some cases, as a liquid radioactive isotope infused directly into the abdominal cavity through a catheter.

Chemotherapy

Since surgery and radiation provide only local treatment, chemotherapy is recommended for later stages of ovarian cancer. These drugs travel throughout the body to kill tumor cells that may have spread outside the pelvic area. Such therapy is most effective after as much tumor as possible has been surgically removed. Recent advances using different drugs and combinations have benefited many women. Drugs can be given intravenously, by mouth, or directly into the abdominal cavity through a catheter. Intensive chemotherapy and bone marrow transplant are now being studied.

Surgical Approaches to Ovarian Cancer

Surgery is recommended as the first treatment for most women with ovarian cancer. If the tumor is caught early, when localized to the ovary (24 percent of all cases), simply removing it with the ovary may allow continued fertility, if the other ovary is normal. If the cell characteristics are favorable, no further X-ray or chemotherapy is necessary. For later stages, however, oophorectomy is just a preliminary step to remove as much of the tumor as possible (*debulking*), reducing the amount of cancer so your body's immune system and follow-up chemotherapy and/or radiotherapy can be more effective. This operation must include total abdominal hysterectomy, removal of both tubes and ovaries, pelvic and abdominal lymph nodes, omentum (the thin, fatty layer hanging off the colon, which tends to attract tumor cells), and as much other intra-abdominal tumor spread as can be safely taken out. (See Figure 19.5.)

A "second look" operation after primary treatment to look for and remove any remaining cancer is controversial in most cases.

Since surgery for ovarian cancer can be complicated, it is best performed by a surgeon who specializes in gynecological cancer surgery. This recommendation includes any initial surgical diagnostic evaluation, if treatment is planned during the same operation.

If you are premenopausal and both ovaries have been removed, symptoms of menopause begin soon after surgery. (For a discussion of oophorectomy, see page 519.)

Ovarian Cancer Follow-Up

After your primary treatment for ovarian cancer, you will need to have regular pelvic and abdominal exams, blood tests including CA 125 (a tumor marker substance produced by ovarian tumors), chest X-rays, and CAT scans. If recurrent tumor is discovered, you may still have a chance for cure with further surgery and chemotherapy.

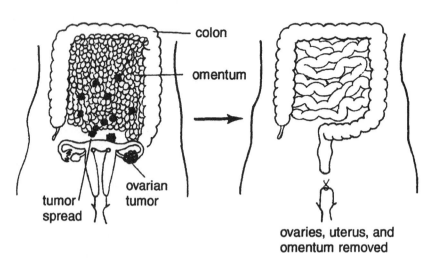

Fig. 19.5 Procedures involved in ovarian cancer surgery

OVARIAN CANCER SUMMARY

Prevention

Diet and Supplements

- Follow a low-fat, high-fiber, vegetarian diet.
- Eat foods high in phytoestrogens, such as soy.
- Vitamin C, 1,000–2,000 mg, 2–3 times daily.
- Vitamin E, D-alpha, 400 IU 1–3 times daily.
- Take selenium, 200 mcg daily.

Lifestyle

- Avoid talc use.
- Maintain optimum weight.
- Practice daily yoga and stress management.

Alternative Medicine Approaches

- Follow the preventive guidelines, above.
- Practice visualization.
- Join a weekly support group.

Conventional Medicine Approaches

- Radiation.
- Chemotherapy.

Surgical Approaches

- Oophorectomy.
- Hysterectomy, oophorectomy, and debulking.

Prophylactic Oophorectomy to Prevent Ovarian Cancer

Alternative Medicine Approaches

Linda's story is typical. Like so many people, she just followed her doctor's recommendation, when she needed a hysterectomy, that "As long as we are in there, we might as well take out your ovaries too, since they might become cancerous later." So her two perfectly normal ovaries were removed, and she was placed on hormone replacement therapy (HRT). Unfortunately, her hot flashes remained severe despite the hormones, and she gained twenty-five pounds she was unable to shed. Eight years later, despite continuing the HRT, which had by now given her an increased risk for breast cancer, she was still suffering from hot flashes and night sweats.

Just as the uterus needs an advocate, the ovaries also need to have one, and fast. They are not just a source of future problems, which have no function. They can't simply be replaced by a pill, which in turn dramatically and unacceptably increases risk for breast cancer (see page 196).

The ovaries serve to provide small amounts of estrogen and progesterone for as long as twenty-five years after menopause.[72] They also secrete testosterone, normally present in small amounts in all women, which acts to support sexual desire. Surgical removal of the ovaries leads to a much more difficult menopause.[73]

Just to prevent the very small risk that you may develop a problem with your ovaries in the future, it is not worth making yourself sick for many years, and increasing your risk of breast cancer, should you want to try to ameliorate your symptoms with HRT. You can decrease your risk for further problems with your ovaries by adopting the lifestyle changes associated with each disorder, generally including a shift to a high-fiber, low-fat diet, and taking the supplements given in Chapter 2, along with the daily stress-management practice presented there.

Conventional Medicine Approaches

Should the ovaries be removed when you are having abdominal surgery for another problem, even if they have *no* disease? After age 40, 5 percent of all women will need an operation because of some ovarian problem—benign or malignant. Because it eliminates a potential source of malignancy, and the increased surgical risk of taking them out at the same time as another operation is minimal, many surgeons and gynecologists have favored this action. However, when the consequent problems of premature menopause are considered, along with the possible harmful effects of hormone replacement treatment, it may not be an appropriate move. If you are already postmenopausal, and your ovaries have therefore lost most of their original ovarian function, it only makes sense to have them routinely removed at the time of hysterectomy or other surgery if you have an increased risk for ovarian cancer. Even after menopause, the ovaries continue to function, albeit less prominently.

Ten percent of all women with ovarian cancer have a positive family history for this disease. Most of these test positive for mutation in the BRCA I or BRCA II genes that increase risk for breast and ovarian cancer. If two or more sisters in two successive generations of your family have had ovarian cancer, you have a 40 percent risk of developing the disease and should probably have your ovaries removed after age 35 or completing your family. This can easily be done laparoscopically in day surgery. Recently, as for women in general, it has been shown that by preventing ovulation, oral contraceptive pills can decrease the risk by about 50 percent for women in these families.[74] This may be a favorable alternative for some premenopausal women.

Oophorectomy and Salpingectomy Operations

Removal of part or all of one ovary for benign problems such as cysts, benign tumors, or endometriosis can usually be done laparoscopically. Generally, this is an outpatient procedure performed under general anesthesia. A TV camera and instrument port are passed through a small incision in your belly button. The abdomen is inflated with CO_2. The camera is used to image the pelvic area as your surgeon operates while watching on a TV monitor. Secondary one-quarter-inch incisions may be used to pass in other instruments.

The ovary is pulled up out of the pelvis with a grasping instrument. The artery and vein supplying the ovary are tied off and divided. If part of the ovary can be saved, the benign problem is "shelled out" like a pea from its pod, along with a small margin of normal tissue. Bleeding points can be stitched or cauterized. Most often, when the other ovary is normal, the whole diseased ovary is removed. The attachment to the uterus is cut, then the ovary removed through the naval incision. The incisions are closed with stitches or skin tapes.

Postoperatively, you may have some incision soreness and bruising. Your discomfort can be controlled with pain pills. You should be able to eat that evening, and have full recovery in a week or so.

If both of your ovaries are to be removed, your uterus and tubes are often taken also, since this prevents future cancers, although you may choose to keep them. For benign problems, an up-and-down abdominal incision from your pubis to navel, side-to-side "bikini" incision, or in some cases, even a laparoscopically assisted transvaginal approach can be chosen. If your operation is for ovarian cancer, a midline incision from just above the pubis to above your navel is usually selected, since it provides better access to the upper abdomen to remove the omentum and lymph nodes and search for cancer spread. The details of these operations, postoperative recovery, and complications are similar to TAH-BSO, as described on page 538.

CHAPTER 20

MALE REPRODUCTIVE SYSTEM

For me it was like war. First thing you do is learn about the enemy.
General Norman Schwarzkopf,
on discovering that he had prostate cancer

Unless we talk to each other fairly frankly, we don't learn much . . . Some of the things that we read about don't return as quickly as advertised.
Senator Bob Dole,
speaking about his own recovery
from prostate cancer surgery

You never really appreciate bladder control until it's gone.
From the movie *The Paper*

From infancy, because of the presence of a penis and testicles, boys are differentiated from girls. Sometimes this contrast is noted in utero by ultrasound, leading to the formation of expectations even before the birth of the child. Higher levels of the male hormone testosterone further separate the sexes. However, whether the behavioral differences between the sexes are due to nature versus nurture is still being hotly debated.

Unlike women with their monthly cycles, men—once past puberty—are usually continuously fertile. The constant production of sperm is difficult to interrupt, and is one of the reasons why so few choices are at present available for male birth control. Also unlike women, whose ovaries at birth contain all the eggs they will ever produce, men generally continue to make sperm throughout their lives.

Currently, life expectancy for men in the United States is seven years less than that for women. This may partly be due to dietary, stress, and other lifestyle factors, but some evidence indicates that simply the act of delaying medical attention may contribute to the discrepancy. Although male self-exam and screening are no more uncomfortable than female self-exam and screening, male compliance is much worse.

For most men, it is just not compatible with a strong self-image to allow anyone to know they don't feel well or notice something amiss, or even to take time for regular checkups, especially the notorious yearly rectal exam. Men's tendency to delay after symptoms develop urgently needs to change, since we are all the losers by this stoic tradition.

Denial and avoidance, while true for all of men's health problems, is especially so in the arena of the male sexual parts. A little known fact is that prostate cancer is almost as common and causes nearly the same number of deaths in men as does breast cancer in women, a much more familiar and discussed disease. Only recently, with the alarmingly increased incidence of prostate cancer discovered through the use of the PSA blood test for screening, have public figures begun to discuss their own illnesses, and encourage education and research in this previously private area of suffering.

Fortunately, you can act preventively to avoid male surgical disorders and, even once they are present, choose new and effective alternative medicine approaches to assist your return to health.

Structure and Function of the Male Reproductive System

The male reproductive system consists of the external genitalia, the *penis* and *scrotum*, and an elaborate internal system. (See Figure 20.1.) The two *testis* or *testicles* sit within tough white capsules that in turn are enclosed within the *scrotum*, the loose sack of skin that hangs below the penis. With the onset of puberty the testicles increase in size and become mature organs that perform two important functions. The *leydig cells* of the testicles produce the male hormone *testosterone*, which helps determine typical male characteristics such as facial hair, muscularity, and behavior. The elaborately coiled *seminiferous* tubules contain the *germinal cells*, in varying stages of development, which mature to become sperm. These tubules converge together to form the *epididymus*, a structure that can be felt as a sort of comma on the back and top of the testis. This forms into a larger duct called the *vas deferens* (site of sterilizing vasectomy), which passes out of the scrotum, through the abdominal wall, and then circles around to pass into the *prostate*, where it joins the *urethra* from the bladder, which then finally empties out through the penis.

The prostate is a doughnut-shaped gland wrapped around the urethra at the base of the bladder. Though quite small in the child, weighing only a few grams, it enlarges under the influence of adolescent hormonal increases to weigh about an ounce in the adult, becoming the size of a chestnut. The prostate secretes most of the nutritious, alkaline fluid in which the sperm swim. This fluid's alkalinity aids fertilization by counteracting acids in the urethra and vagina, which impede sperm function.

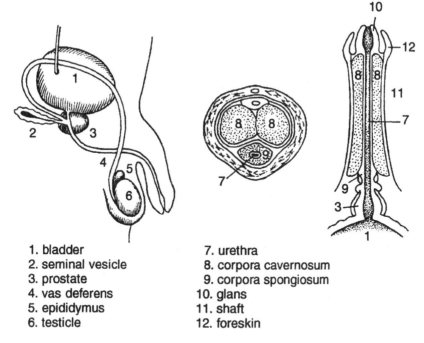

1. bladder
2. seminal vesicle
3. prostate
4. vas deferens
5. epididymus
6. testicle

7. urethra
8. corpora cavernosum
9. corpora spongiosum
10. glans
11. shaft
12. foreskin

Fig. 20.1   The anatomy of the male reproductive system

Near the prostate, joining each vas, are two small sacklike outpouchings called the *seminal vesicles*. These glands produce a sticky white fluid that is mixed with sperm from the testes and the prostatic secretions during orgasm to form *semen*.

The penis functions for both elimination of urine and sexual reproduction. Its urethra connects the bladder to the outside world, and also delivers sperm to the vagina. The *glans* is the highly sensitive tip that is covered by the retractable *foreskin* at birth. The *shaft* is composed of two bundles of a unique type of expandable tissue rich in blood vessels, the *corpora cavernosum*, and a spongy tube, the *corpus spongiosum*.

Erection and ejaculation are very complex processes involving elements of both con-scious and unconscious brain activity, along with nerve reflexes responsive to tactile stimulation. Erection begins when these processes cause a dilation of small arteries leading into the spongy chambers of the shaft of the penis. This increased blood flow causes the corpora cavernosa and corpus spongiosum to fill with blood, thereby increasing their length and diameter and compressing veins leading away from them. Since outflow is blocked, the blood is entrapped. During male orgasm, semen is discharged as the vas, prostate, and seminal vesicle muscles contract. Afterward, the vein constriction relaxes, allowing blood to flow out of the penis.

How Disorders of the Male Reproductive System Are Diagnosed

Unlike in the female, much of the male reproductive tract is external and self-exam is easy. You should regularly, at least monthly, examine your testicles, becoming familiar with their size, shape, and consistency, and learn to identify your epididymus and vas as well. Stony hard or persistently tender areas can thus be readily found. Sensitive areas, ulcerations or growths, inability to retract the foreskin, urethral discharge, or blood in urine or semen all should be reported to your doctor. Some of the following tests should be done routinely and others only when you have symptoms.

History

The male urological evaluation begins with detailed questions regarding your general medical history. Your doctor should especially be informed if you have had a severe case of mumps, which can destroy the ability to make sperm, have thyroid disease or diabetes, or take medications that may cause erectile dysfunction or infertility.

The questions then narrow in on your urinary tract and function. Your doctor will ask about frequency of urination, if you have to get up at night to urinate, the force of your urinary stream, whether you have to bear down to empty your bladder, and if you have any burning or pain on urination. A past history of sexually transmitted disease or penile discharge is important. Reproductive history questions include whether your family has any history of genetic disorders or problems with fertility. Your own sexual desires, ability to achieve and maintain erection and ejacula-tion, and any problems with fertility complete your sexual history.

Physical Exam

Your doctor should examine and feel your penis, testicles, epididymus, and vas. The size and consistency of your prostate can be assessed by your doctor inserting a rubber-gloved finger into your rectum, where a normal gland is felt as a small, rubbery chestnut.

Culture of Urethra

If you have a penile discharge, it should be cultured to check for sexually transmitted diseases or other type of infection. Often the specimen can be collected after a rectal exam, using prostate massage to express some secretions.

Urinalysis

A urine specimen may show evidence of epididymus, bladder, or prostate infection, irritation, or tumor. It can be analyzed for the type of organism that may be causing an infection, for bleeding from anywhere in the urinary tract, and for abnormal cells that may be shed by a polyp or tumor.

Blood Tests

Routine blood tests screen for underlying general medical problems. Specific urological blood tests include prostate specific antigen (PSA) and prostate alkaline phosphatase (PAP), both of which can be elevated if you have prostate cancer. Decreased blood levels of male sex hormones sometimes correlate with lack of development of male sex characteristics and problems with erection, ejaculation, or fertility.

Sperm Tests

This test is part of an infertility evaluation. You give a fresh semen specimen to be analyzed for the number of sperm (sperm count), their size and shape, and their swimming movements. After masturbation or intercourse, the sample is collected in a clean glass container or condom. It is then kept warm, and should be examined as soon as possible, within a few hours at most.

Residual Urine and Cystometrics

An enlarged prostate can interfere with complete bladder emptying. These two office tests take only a few minutes, and give an indication of its severity. The amount of urine left in the bladder after urination is called *residual urine*. Your doctor can measure this with a painless bladder scan device that uses sound waves. Or a catheter can be into your bladder through your penis after you empty your bladder. *Cystometrics* can be done at the same time. After your bladder is filled with fluid, the catheter is hooked up to a simple recording device, to measure pressure in your bladder over time, as the bladder empties itself. You may experience some mild discomfort associated with the catheter insertion.

Cystoscopy

This test is usually performed in outpatient surgery. Local anesthesia jelly is inserted into your penis. You lie on your back on an operating table with your feet up in stirrups. Your doctor introduces a lighted tube through the penis into your bladder, for a direct view of your urethra, prostate, and bladder. Biopsies can be taken. Cystoscopy is rather uncomfortable, though it usually only takes ten to

twenty minutes. Afterward, you may have some burning on urination for a few days. Complications are rare, including significant bleeding, infection, acute inability to urinate afterward, and perforation of the urethra or bladder.

Intravenous Pyelogram and Cystourethrogram

These are X-ray tests that show the urinary system. In the intravenous pyelogram (*IVP*), after dye is injected into a vein, it concentrates and "lights up" the kidneys, the ureter tubes that connect the kidneys to the bladder, and the bladder. The *cystourethrogram* is a functional test that shows the bladder and urethra as you void. How fast and how completely you empty your bladder and the pressures generated are measured. These tests can identify prostatic enlargement and obstruction, urethral strictures or narrowings, as well as other bladder, kidney, and ureteral problems.

Complications are uncommon, but may include an allergic reaction to the dye that causes a skin rash or itching. Severe, life-threatening reactions causing difficulty breathing and shock occur very rarely. If you are allergic to iodine or shellfish, you are at increased risk and should notify your doctor.

Sonogram

In this test, a sound wave probe is used to pick up harmless sound waves as they bounce off various parts of your anatomy. A computer constructs a picture from reflected waves. This is usually the first and best test for testicle problems such as tumor or cyst, or for finding a testicle not located in the scrotum. A special probe can be placed in the rectum to get a close look at the prostate, to find enlargement and tumor. A probe passed over the skin of your abdomen can see your kidneys.

CAT and MRI Scans

These expensive tests are used mostly to detect a suspected, but otherwise undetectable, small tumor of the testicle or prostate or to find cancer that may have spread out from the original site to lymph nodes or other areas of your body. You lay inside the MRI scanner as a powerful magnet changes the orientation of your cell atom components. Abnormal cells look different than normal cells on X-ray–type images reconstructed by a computer. Likewise, for a CAT scan, you lay inside a spinning arm that takes multiple X-ray images, which a computer reassembles to produce cross sections of your anatomy. Abnormal growths and changes can be seen.

Bone Scan

This test is most useful in prostate cancer to determine if the cancer involves bone, the most common site of spread. You are given an intravenous radioactive tracer formulated to be picked up by bone cells. Abnormal areas of increased or decreased activity indicating cancer spread may show up as you lay under a nuclear camera.

Biopsy

Tissue can be easily taken from an abnormal area on the penis by direct biopsy using local anesthesia. If malignancy is suspected in a testicle, it is usually not biopsied but removed entirely, because it has been shown that cutting directly into a testicular tumor increases its risk of spread. A testicular biopsy may be used to determine if a problem with sperm production is present. This can be performed under local anesthesia, by taking a core of tissue with a special needle or a small wedge of tissue using a scalpel.

A tissue sample from an abnormal area of the prostate can usually be taken in your doctor's office, using a special needle introduced through the rectum. Anesthesia is not necessary. Alternatively, using local anesthesia, the needle can be inserted through the skin in the space between your scrotum and anus, then aimed to the right spot in the prostate, using sonogram guidance. These procedures may cause some soreness and blood in the urine for a few days, but complications are rare (2 percent).

Benign Prostate Enlargement (Hypertrophy)

Harold Macmillan, former British prime minister, developed difficulty urinating at age 69, and assumed he had cancer. "Of course I'm finished," he announced to his press secretary. "I shall probably die." He resigned even before he sought medical help. He then deeply regretted his decision, when it was found he simply was suffering from benign prostate enlargement. He lived for 23 more years and died at the age of 92.[1]

Unlike Macmillan, President Ronald Reagan, who had his first partial prostate removal at age 55, chose to have the rest of his prostate removed while he was in office, at age 75, and uneventfully continued as president.

Disorders of the prostate are very common, and may lead you to consider surgery.

Prostate enlargement, present in the majority of older men in the United States, can cause problems with urination and urinary infection.

By age 40, half of all the men in Western countries have the beginnings of *benign prostate hypertrophy* (enlargement), called *BPH* for short; by 80 years of age, 80 percent are affected. Luckily, less that half of the men with BPH have symptoms, and only 30 percent need surgery. The cause of BPH is presumed to be related to years of prostate stimulation by male hormones. As the body ages, increased conversion of testosterone to its potent metabolic breakdown product, *dihydrotestosterone (DHT)*, and other sex hormone changes, increase the concentration of DHT in the prostate and decrease its removal, thereby stimulating excessive multiplication of prostate cells.[2] Diet may also influence this conversion. An enlarged BPH gland is otherwise normal, and does not cause cancer.

As your prostate enlarges, it can squeeze in upon the region where the urethra passes through the gland. Onset of symptoms is generally gradual. Slight difficulty is noticed in starting or stopping your urinary stream. As enlargement continues, further constriction causes the need to strain to start and continue your urine stream, decreased stream size and force, interruption of flow, and incomplete emptying of the bladder. As a consequence, you may have a very frequent need to urinate, especially distressing when it interferes with a good night's sleep. Bladder wall muscles first become thick, strong, and sensitive, causing spasm and urgency to pass urine immediately, and dribbling when you don't. Later, the muscles may thin out and the bladder may stretch to an enormous size. Complete blockage can occur, and you may suddenly become completely unable to urinate (urinary retention).

Blood may be found in the urine, caused by infection due to bacteria proliferating in the stagnant urine, or from straining at urination. At times, bleeding can be massive, requiring immediate treatment. Bladder stones can form in this setting, causing continuing infection and bladder outlet obstruction. Prostate, bladder, and kidney infections can cause severe pain and systemic illness. Left untreated, chronic urinary blockage causes increased pressure and permanent damage to the kidneys.

Your doctor usually diagnoses BPH by your history, finger rectal exam, and a urinalysis that may show blood or infection. However, the size of the gland found on rectal exam does not always correlate with the degree of symptoms, since it is the internal impingement upon your urethra that determines problems with urination. Still, the more invasive and expensive tests such as urine flow studies and cystoscopy are unnecessary unless your symptoms suggest you need surgery. You should have a cystoscopy if you have blood in your urine, to rule out a bladder tumor, or to determine the best operation when surgery is necessary.

Alternative Medicine Approaches to Benign Prostate Enlargement

Douglas, a 65-year-old pilot with a history of prostate infections, had ended his first marriage a number of years before and was just recently involved in a new serious relationship, but found difficulty achieving and maintaining an erection. His doctor's examination revealed a significantly swollen prostate. He elected to try alternative medicine approaches, including a shift in diet, the addition of supplements and herbs, homeopathy, and a daily yoga program. Within a few weeks, his symptoms had improved. He felt better than ever in his life, had normal erections, and his prostate returned to its normal size.

———————————

Enlargement of the prostate can be a miserable affliction. Waking up in the middle of the night and having difficulty with urination are not simply consequences of aging you should just have to live with.

However, the prostate is not a "gland for no reason," as has been traditionally asserted by Western doctors. Especially if you are older or have medical problems, surgery can be dangerous, producing unpleasant after-effects, such as the inability to control urine, or complete sexual dysfunction. Given *no treatment at all,* 20 percent of all patients who have symptoms from BPH improve, and 33 percent do not get any worse.

Think very carefully before you choose surgery. Even with the most limited kind of operation, the death rate is as high as one in 56, 5 to 10 percent of the patients become impotent, and one in five needs another follow-up operation.

Alternative medicine offers some new hope for prevention and treatment of BPH without these risks, as well as acting to improve the quality of the rest of your life. A trial period of the following approaches seems worthwhile, before you choose an operation to relieve your symptoms.

Change Your Diet

Your eating habits may play a role in the hormonal imbalances that cause the prostate to enlarge. BPH is increased in persons who eat a high-fat diet. As noted, in the United States, 50 percent of all males have the begin-

nings of BPH by age 40: this is the highest rate in the world. In China, where consumption of meats and fats is much lower, only 5 percent are affected by this age. Increased conversion of testosterone to DHT, caused by the high-fat diet, may account for the increased incidence of this disease in the West. Especially important to avoid are red meats, butter, and all hydrogenated oils, including margarine and mayonnaise.

Some studies have also indicated that BPH is more common in coffee drinkers, and in those who eat refined white sugar. Both of these substances also affect fat metabolism, which in turn affects your DHT production. It seems prudent to avoid these harmful dietary elements to achieve prevention.

The constipation commonly associated with a low-fiber diet may play a role in this disease. Persons in countries where BPH is uncommon have an average of two to three bowel movements per day; the U.S. average is one or fewer.

Since prostatectomy can be quite painful, if you have symptoms from BPH, try changing to the whole-foods, low-fat, high-fiber, caffeine-free, vegetarian diet, given in Chapter 2. Add foods rich in zinc and vitamin E such as tahini; kelp; sesame, sunflower, pumpkin, and squash seeds; and almonds. Many persons with BPH respond very well to this simple alternative medicine approach. It may not only help treat your BPH, but reduce your risk for cancer of the prostate as well.

Take Supplements

Supplemental zinc has been documented to reverse prostate enlargement and to reduce symptoms in the majority of patients. This effect is most likely due to zinc's influence upon testosterone metabolism, sugar metabolism, and wound healing.[3] Zinc inhibits the enzyme that converts testosterone to DHT.[4] Doses range from 50 to 300 mg three times per day. Doses of zinc higher than 150 mg per day should not be taken for more than a few months, unless you are monitored by your doctor. You can also eat pumpkin and sunflower seeds, at least two handfuls of each per day, since these foods are high in zinc. Avoid refined sugar since it has been shown to reduce body zinc levels.

In one study, essential fatty acids helped reduce residual urine retention.[5] You can take flaxseed oil, one tablespoon per day, added to your food. The antioxidant selenium was shown to inhibit the adverse effects of cadmium, which in animals causes prostate swelling. You can take 200 mcg daily. The antioxidant vitamin E, 400 to 800 IU daily, may also be beneficial.

Some authorities recommend the amino acids glycine, L-alanine, and L-glutamic acid, which when taken daily may affect DHT conversion rates.[6] Initially, dosage is 250 mg of each, three times daily, and after you receive relief, a maintenance dose of 125 mg of each, three times daily.

Use Herbal Remedies

The herbal preparation saw palmetto (Serenoa repens) is extracted from the berry of a dwarf palm tree native to the Southeastern United States, naturally high in fatty acids and sterols. It inhibits conversion of testosterone to DHT, prevents its binding to cells, blocks uptake of DHT into the cell nucleus, and also inhibits another enzyme that may affect prostate growth. Thus, it has been termed a multisite inhibitor, whereas the drug finasteride (Proscar) acts at only one site. Saw palmetto has been found to reduce nighttime

urination, increase urinary flow, and reduce post-voiding urine in the bladder. A 1998 study reported in the *Journal of the American Medical Association* analyzed eighteen randomized controlled trials that compared saw palmetto with placebo or finasteride. Saw palmetto was found as effective in improving urologic symptoms and urine flow measurements as finasteride and was associated with fewer adverse side effects, including erectile dysfunction.[7] This herb has been widely used in France, which has a long history of herbal medicine use. Rare side effects are limited to headache and stomach upset. Dosage is individual; begin with one 80 mg capsule or a dropperful of the liquid extract, two to three times daily, increasing up to three capsules or droppersful, three times daily, if needed.

The powdered tree bark *Pygeum africanum*, 50 mg two times per day, is similar though slightly weaker in effect. When combined with the amino acids glycine, L-alanine, and glutamic acid, it provided superior results in one study.[8] The herb stinging nettle, 300 mg daily, helped relieve symptoms in several studies.[9]

Flower pollen, sold at health food stores as *bee pollen*, has long been used in Europe to alleviate the symptoms associated with prostatic enlargement. Research has supported its ability to help prevent residual urine in the bladder.[10]

You can begin with one of these herbs, then add the others, as needed.

Use Homeopathy, Acupuncture, and Hypnosis

Acupuncture has been found to relieve the symptoms of nighttime urinary frequency and incontinence.[11] Homeopathy and hypnosis seem to offer promise for treatment of prostate enlargement, though they have not yet been researched. The most common homeopathics used are sabal serrulata, causticum, argentum nitricum, or sulfur, though this avenue of treatment works best when individualized by an experienced homeopathic practitioner.

Drink Less Fluid Before Bedtime

You can decrease your need to wake up to urinate by avoiding fluids close to bedtime—especially alcohol and caffeine-containing beverages. Be sure to urinate just before going to bed.

Practice Yoga Daily

Yoga acts to increase circulation to the prostate area, which may assist in both prevention and treatment of disorders. Directions for specific postures are contained in Chapter 2. The most important pose is the shoulder stand, ten to fifteen minutes twice daily. (See Figure 20.2.) Spinal twist, butterfly, and supine butterfly positions should be added, twice a day.

Practice Stress Management

Stress can contribute to prostate stimulation by increasing prolactin secretion. Prolactin increases DHT concentration in the prostate.[12] Follow the guidelines for stress reduction in Chapter 2.

Exercise Regularly

Active exercise may help ensure the health of the prostate by increasing its circulation, so that the gland can more effectively maintain and repair its function. Aerobic exercise increases local supplies of oxygen, removes carbon dioxide, and improves lymph flow. In addition, it helps to normalize testosterone levels, thought to be at the root of benign prostate enlargement.

Further research on the exact effects of exercise on the prostate is needed. However, by exercising regularly—considered to be one hour three to five times a week, or at least half an hour daily—not only may you help your prostate win its battle with hypertrophy, but you may help prevent prostate cancer as well: although one out of three Americans develops cancer, only one out of seven regular exercisers does.

Practice Visualization

First, practice deep relaxation, given in Chapter 2. Then, for example, imagine your prostate as a large sponge filled with too much water. Picture it shrinking to a chestnut-sized shape. While you image this in your mind, feel it happening within your body. Repeat three to five times daily.

Don't Use Decongestants

Decongestants, many available over-the-counter, may have the side effect of making urination difficult. Along with other ingredients, they may contain the active ingredient pseudoephedrine hydrochloride, a drug that constricts the small blood vessels and may contribute to the retaining of urine in your bladder and problems with starting or stopping your urinary stream. It is therefore prudent to avoid them altogether. You may choose to try the herbal remedy nettles, available from your local health food store. Take one to two capsules when needed.

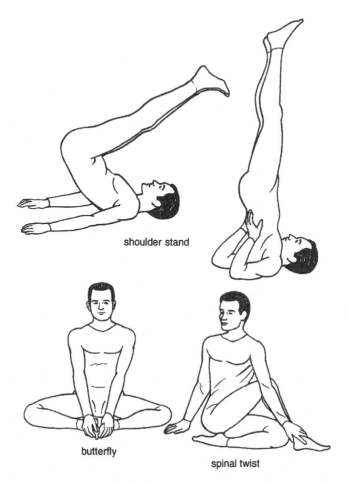

shoulder stand

butterfly

spinal twist

Fig. 20.2 Yoga postures for prostate health

Do Supervised "Watchful Waiting"

Surgery can be delayed or avoided altogether if your kidney function has not been impaired and your symptoms are not too severe, even if you do have intermittent bladder retention. If infection is present, it must be treated, and retention can be relieved by the insertion of a catheter when needed.

If you have more significant symptoms, they may improve after six to eight weeks of the above program, combined with the lifestyle and exercise program given in Chapter 2. Relief of symptoms, however, is not enough; kidney damage can still silently develop. You should continue to be supervised by your doctor, so that he or she can monitor the alternative medicine program's effectiveness and check for any hidden problems.

Conventional Medicine Approach to Benign Prostate Enlargement

The drug finasteride (Depocar, Proscar) prevents the conversion of testosterone to DHT, thereby shrinking prostate enlargement in some people. It shrinks the prostate 20 percent, on average, for 50 percent of all users, and improves urine flow in 30 percent. Its effects take from three to six months to be evident, and your symptoms may reappear if it is stopped. However, it doesn't decrease the need for future surgery and may have the side effects of decreased interest in sex, and difficulties with erection and ejaculation. A recent VA study found Proscar to be no more effective than a placebo.[13] As noted above, the herb saw palmetto has performed better in controlled clinical trials, and is much cheaper: Proscar costs on average about $65 per month, versus $21 for saw palmetto.

Alpha-blocking drugs such as prazocin (Minipress) and terazosin (Hytrin) relax muscles surrounding the urethra, making urination easier, and have been found to reduce symptoms in 50 to 70 percent of all users. However, you may have the side effects of headache, decreased blood pressure, and dizziness. These medications also don't reduce the need for future surgery.

Surgical Approaches to Benign Prostate Enlargement

The decision to have surgery for BPH can be easy if you are having severe difficulty with urination, frequent bladder infections, bladder stones, unrelieved discomfort, significant bleeding, or kidney damage. On the other hand, if you are having symptoms without any urinary tract or medical illness, deciding can be very difficult. You need to ask yourself how much your life is being affected by your symptoms. Are you losing sleep from constant nighttime urination? Are you embarrassed by having to leave meetings, the theater, or other events to relieve yourself? Does your problem interrupt your daily activities or stop you from doing things that you enjoy? Do you have pelvic discomfort? Most of us would like to be relieved of burdens such as these.

You must also consider that, although surgery has the best results in terms of treating BPH, there are real risks, including permanent problems with urinary continence, erection, and ejaculation, which can make your life much worse. You need a frank discussion with your doctor and partner before deciding on a course of treatment. If your symptoms do not require surgery, you should first try the alternative medicine approaches.

If you decide to have surgery, you may choose among the following methods of treatment, each with its advantages and disadvantages.

Minimally Invasive Surgical Techniques

You may ask about the following alternative procedures as a first line of treatment. Although results are probably not as long-lasting as those with transurethral resection of the prostate, or TURP (see page 565), they can be done under local anesthesia, with or without sedation, in day surgery. Postoperative catheterization is not routine and, if necessary, is usually not prolonged. Troublesome side effects are rare and convalescence is much quicker than with TURP.

Balloon Dilation

Strictly speaking, balloon dilation is not really a surgical procedure, though it is an invasive one. This treatment can be performed under local anesthesia in your doctor's office or outpatient surgery. A balloon-tipped catheter is passed through the penis into the bladder, and the balloon placed in the urethra, where it is compressed by the prostate. The balloon is then forcefully dilated, thereby stretching the encasing prostate. As you can imagine, since no prostate tissue is removed, the beneficial effect, if any, is usually short-lived. Complications can include temporary inability to urinate afterward, bleeding, infection, and urethral perforation.

Prostate Stents

These devices are now available to keep the urethra open after a balloon dilation. An expandable metal tube is carried on top of the balloon, then employed as the balloon is inflated. The rigidity of the metal holds the stent open. Since this procedure is very new, its results and complications are not yet well delineated.

Transurethral Incision of the Prostate

Transurethal incision of the prostate (TUIP) also does not remove any prostate tissue. It is similar to TURP, described below, except that rather than removing prostate tissue, cuts are made into it, relieving the constricting pressure on the urethra. It can be used only on smaller glands, and its effect is likely to be short-lived. The risks, however, are less than that of prostatectomy.

Transurethral Needle Ablation and Microwave Thermotherapy

The obstructing prostate tissue can also be treated by using a device introduced through the penis and inserted into or localized next to prostate tissue.

In the needle ablation technique, needles are inserted through the urethra into the pros-

tate. Low-energy radio-frequency waves create heat that acts to coagulate and destroy prostate tissue in a controlled fashion. A 1998 randomized study at seven medical centers across the United States compared needle ablation with TURP one year later. Needle ablation was effective in reducing symptoms and increasing urinary flow, although not quite as good as TURP. However, it was as good as TURP in enhancing quality of life and produced no changes in sexual function, whereas TURP resulted in retrograde ejaculation (38.2 percent) and erectile dysfunction (12.7 percent).[14]

Microwave thermotherapy, commonly used in Europe, uses a microwave antenna-probe placed within the urethra next to the prostate. High-energy microwaves generate heat deep in the prostatic tissue, causing cell death. The best treatment designs are still being worked out. So far, long-term results have not been great and side effect problems seem higher than with other "minimally invasive" techniques.

Transurethral Resection of the Prostate

Transurethral resection of the prostate (TURP) is the most commonly performed and simplest way to remove the constricting part of the prostate. In this procedure, a lighted scope is passed through the penis to the narrow area. Instruments are passed through this scope to cut out part of the gland, to widely open the channel. The cutting is done with electrified cautery that removes tissue and simultaneously seals blood vessels. TURP is usually successful, the results lasting for several years. However, with scarring and regrowth of prostate tissue, symptoms recur in 5 to 15 percent of all patients. If they do, another TURP is usually possible.

Instead of using electrocautery, a laser attached to a telescope (visual laser ablation of the prostate, or VLAP) or guided by ultrasound (transurethral ultrasound-guided laser-induced prostatectomy, or TULIP) can be used to vaporize the tissue and enlarge the channel. Laser cuts the operative time from an hour or so to ten to fifteen minutes, and allows you to have outpatient surgery or leave the hospital the next day. Another similar method called transurethral electrovaporization of the prostate (TVP) uses a special roller device to boil tissue away while simultaneously coagulating the surface left behind. Claimed benefits include minimal bleeding, fewer complications, and a quicker recovery than standard TURP.

Open Prostatectomy

This procedure is reserved for those whose glands are too large for the transurethral route, where the operative time and amount of blood loss would be excessive. The whole gland is removed through one of two possible approaches. Suprapubic prostatectomy uses an incision in the lower abdominal wall above the pubic bone, while a perineal prostatectomy is performed through an incision between the scrotum and anus.

In 10 percent of all prostatectomies for BPH, cancer is unexpectedly found.

BENIGN PROSTATE ENLARGEMENT SUMMARY

Prevention

Diet and Supplements

- Follow a low-fat, high-fiber diet.
- Avoid coffee and white sugar.

- Eat protective foods—tahini; kelp; sesame, sunflower, pumpkin, and squash seeds; and almonds.

Lifestyle

- Exercise regularly: 1 hour, 3–5 times weekly.
- Drink less fluid before bedtime.
- Don't use decongestants.
- Practice stress reduction.
- Do yoga postures, especially the inverted ones.

Alternative Medicine Approaches

- Follow preventive guidelines, above.
- Supplements—vitamin E, 400 IU, 1–2 times daily; zinc, 50 mg, 3 times daily; selenium, 200 mcg daily; essential fatty acids, 500 mg daily; amino acids—glycine, L-alanine, and L-glutamic acid, 250 mg, 3 times daily.
- Herbal remedies—saw palmetto, 500 mg daily; *pygeum africanum,* 50 mg, 2 times daily; stinging nettle, 300 mg daily; bee pollen 450 mg, 2–3 times daily.
- Use homeopathy, acupuncture, and hypnosis.
- Practice visualization.
- Do supervised "watchful waiting."

Conventional Medicine Approaches

- Prostate shrinking drugs—finasteride (Depocar, Proscar).
- Muscle relaxing drugs—prazocin (Minipress), terazocin (Hytrin).

Surgical Approaches

- Balloon dilation, prostate stent, transurethral incision of the prostate.
- Transurethral needle ablation and microwave thermotherapy.

- Transurethral resection of the prostate.
- Open prostatectomy—retropubic, perineal.

Prostate Cancer

Prostate cancer is the fourth most common cause of cancer death in the United States, lagging only behind lung, colorectal, and breast cancer. We are in the midst of an alarming epidemic. In the two decades prior to 1996, it had been diagnosed at a rate increase of almost 5 percent per year, due at least in part to widespread use of the prostate specific antigen (PSA) blood test. In 2002, an estimated 189,000 new cases will be detected, and 30,200 deaths will occur.[15] New York City Mayor Rudolph Giuliani, age 55, chose to withdraw from the U.S. Senate race partly to focus on his treatment for this disease found by a routine PSA. He then publicly recommended this screening test for all men.

One in every six American men must confront this disease sometime during his lifetime, a disease rate higher than the one in eight for women developing breast cancer. Excluding skin cancer, it is the most common malignancy in men, and one of every three cancer deaths in men above age 50 is due to this disease.

Prostate cancer is usually very slow-growing, producing no symptoms in its early stages. In fact, autopsies reveal that up to one-half of all men have this cancer, although most did not have symptoms and were not even diagnosed before their death from other conditions. Although early cancer is readily curable, one-third of all patients have cancer that has already spread outside of the prostate at the time of their diagnosis. (See Table 20.1.)

The older you are, the greater your risk for prostate cancer. Eighty percent of these cancers are diagnosed in men older than 65, and 80 percent of all 80-year-olds are found to have some cancerous cells in their prostates. However, it can also affect younger men: rock star Frank Zappa died at age 52, and entrepreneur Michael Milken was diagnosed at age 46.

Genetics may be responsible for 5 to 10 percent of these cancers. Your risk is three times higher if you have a family member who developed it. African-American men have the highest incidence in the world, almost twice that of white males, with more than two times the death rate.

Your risk for prostate cancer is increased if you live in a Western country. It is rare in Asia, Africa, and South America. This may be partially explained by the typical high-fat diet, which when compared to one low in fat, increases your risk by 30 percent.[16] Increased fat may interfere with circulation, or trigger abnormal hormonal effects. The higher your fat intake, the higher your risk for this disease.[17] Beef consumption seems to convey the highest risk.[18] Higher fiber may be protective by its effects on hormone levels.[19]

Coffee intake has also been correlated with cancer of the prostate. In a 1957 English study, the inhabitants of twenty countries were compared in terms of the average number of cups of coffee drunk per day. Increasing risk correlated with increasing coffee consumption.[20] Chronic prostate irritation may account for this association.

Environmental and industrial exposure to certain chemicals has been associated with increased risk. Cadmium, electroplating compounds, and those used in the rubber industry are suspected.

Though the mechanism is unknown, very high or very low levels of sexual activity seem to slightly increase your risk. Studies are unclear regarding any increased risk from having had multiple sexual partners, a sexually transmitted disease, or a vasectomy, or having an enlarged prostate (BPH).

Prostate cancer is usually a slow-growing tumor arising in an otherwise normal prostate, though it can also develop in one with BPH. It usually begins in the outer part of the gland, away from the urethra, and therefore doesn't cause early obstructive symptoms. As the tumor enlarges, it can cause symptoms similar to those of BPH—changes in the urinary pattern, blood in urine and semen, and painful ejaculation. Once it affects the urinary stream, it may already have spread beyond the confines of the gland itself, or through the lymph or blood vessels. The disease is often diagnosed when persistent back pain results from metastasis to the bony vertebrae or when spread to the lungs, hips, pelvis, ribs, or liver causes symptoms.

Fortunately, you can take action to prevent this cancer, or help slow its growth once it is present. The more fat in your diet—especially from red meat—the higher your risk of this cancer becoming fatal.[21] Alternative medicine approaches offer strong hope that you can avoid this cancer by a shift to a low-fat, high-fiber, vegetarian diet.

Establishing a Diagnosis of Prostate Cancer

Prostate cancer is difficult to find early in its course, as it is often a tiny hard lesion hidden deep within the rubbery prostate gland. The blood tests for prostate specific antigen (PSA) and prostate alkaline phosphatase (PAP) can be used to detect very early cancer spread. They can also be used to judge the success of treatment. However, their use for screening is controversial, as BPH can also elevate the antigens that these tests detect, and there are many false positives. There have been no randomized trials that show that detection of prostate cancers by PSA decreases the cancer complication and death rates. Transrectal ultrasound screening exams have also been advocated by some as a noninvasive way to find early cancers. So far, however, this test has not been shown to be a cost-effective way to find them.

A very important issue is that screening tests can now find very slow-growing tumors that would not threaten your health during your lifetime, and finding them could lead to complications from risky diagnostic workup and treatment: that is, the treatment may be worse than the disease. At present, this hotly debated issue is one of the most controversial in medicine. As many as 50 percent of all men have this cancer discovered after death from other diseases, and they may have had it for years, without having had any problems caused by it. In addition, as of now, evidence does not show that screening rectal exams, PSA, PAP, and transrectal ultrasound decrease mortality or increase life expectancy.

Given the uncertainty about the net benefit of early detection and treatment of prostate cancer, in 1997, the American College of Physicians issued a general recommendation against the routine use of screening tests, stating, "Available evidence does not justify the common but arbitrary policy of annual digital rectal examination and PSA measurement for men who are older than 50 years of age.... [R]ather than screening all men for prostate cancer as a matter of routine, physicians should describe the potential benefits and known harms of screening, diagnosis, and treatment; listen to the patient's concerns; and then individualize the decision to screen."[22]

Nevertheless, we, along with the National Cancer Institute, recommend that all males should have their prostates examined by rectal exam once a year after age 40. No medical organization now recommends yearly PSA screening. The American Cancer Society and the American Urological Association, which endorsed screening in the past, now recommend *offering* PSA testing after age 50 to men who have a life expectancy greater than ten years. In summary, by being screened, your risk of dying from prostate cancer may be decreased but your risk of complications from treatment that may alter your quality of life is increased. You should make this decision in consultation with your family and doctor based on your personal risks and objectives. New and better screening tests are on the horizon, aimed at finding early aggressive cancers that should be treated early on. Discuss the latest screening information with your doctor.

If either the rectal exam or the PSA test suggests cancer, a transrectal ultrasound test with possible biopsy should be done. Once cancer is proven by prostate needle biopsy, you need studies to determine prognosis and best treatment options. The characteristics of the tumor cells themselves are important, and determine the *grade* of disease. The Gleason Score is determined from cell characteristics and patterns that indicate the aggressiveness of the tumor. Very well-differentiated tumor cells, or those that look close to normal and form a more normal growth pattern, those that reproduce slowly, and those that have a normal number of chromosomes, are considered low grade, with a better prognosis.

Men with a Gleason Score of 2 to 4 face a low risk of death from prostate cancer within fifteen years. On the other hand, men with a Gleason Score of 7 to 10 face a high risk of death when treated conservatively. Tests to determine the extent or *stage* of the tumor may include a transrectal ultrasound or MRI that shows tumor size, extracapsular extension, and local invasion. Chest X-ray, abdominal and pelvic CAT scans, bone scan, and blood tests can be used to look for distant tumor spread.

The goals of treatment are to relieve symptoms and to cure or control the cancer, depending on your stage when it is found. Current treatment cannot cure distant spread, but may slow tumor growth and relieve symptoms for many years. Your best treatment op-

TABLE 20.1.
Prognosis of Prostate Cancer[23]

	Percent of Patients Surviving 5 Years	Percent of Patients in This Stage
All Patients	96.2% (10 yr—68.0%, 15 yr—52.0%)	
Not Staged	87.7%	11%
By Stage		
Localized to prostate	100.0%	83%
Lymph node spread	100.0%	83%
Distant spread	33.0%	6%

tions depend on your age, general medical condition, symptoms, Gleason Score and stage, PSA levels, tumor volume, and your desires regarding potential benefits versus side effects.

Controversy exists regarding staging, and the most appropriate treatment for each stage. In many cases, no treatment at all may be best. If you are not having symptoms and your tumor is growing slowly, and if you don't wish to take the risk that treatment might cause impotence and urinary incontinence, you may choose to wait for symptoms to develop before considering your options. Delaying treatment may be especially prudent if you are elderly or have significant medical problems; you may never develop symptoms, and can avoid the significant complications and side effects of treatment. In the early stages, when the cancer is still confined to the prostate, the cure rates of surgery, radiation therapy, and hormonal therapy are similar. Make sure you get several opinions from a urologic surgeon, cancer specialist, and radiotherapist.

Alternative Medicine Approaches to Prostate Cancer

Michael Milken, the 46-year-old Wall Street celebrity, decided to take a PSA test when a close friend died of prostate cancer. Surprisingly, his level was abnormal and his disease was found to already be present in the local lymph nodes. It was too widespread to be cured by surgery. He chose to be treated with radiation and hormone therapy, then devoted much of his time and money to research and education about this disease, starting CaP Cure, the second largest prostate cancer research foundation, after the National Cancer Institute. He supplemented the treatment of his disease with oral antitestosterone hormone therapy, as well as began eating a vegetarian, low-fat, high-fiber, soy-based, whole-foods diet. As of seven years after his metastatic diagnosis, he remained in complete remission, with a normal PSA, continuing with an active life and having his progress closely monitored.

Dean Ornish, M.D., has conducted research on a lifestyle program, similar to that applied to heart disease, to see if it could be utilized to reverse prostate cancer. Results after three years showed that all of the patients had lowered their PSA levels, while the control group had experienced increased test results.

Rates of symptomatic prostate cancer can almost certainly be decreased, since vegetarians have a lower incidence.[24] As noted above, impressive evidence has shown that risk for this cancer in the United States is increased owing to the prevalent high-fat, meat-based diet. Fats in the diet influence the production of hormones, particularly the conversion of testosterone to DHT, which in turn can induce abnormal cell growth. This cancer is quite rare in populations that eat little red meat, such as the Japanese,[25] but if they adopt a Western diet, their incidence then becomes the same as Americans in general.

Once you have developed this cancer, changes in diet may slow its growth or prevent recurrence; research on animals placed on a low-fat diet after the onset of their tumors showed a slower growth rate than those maintained on a high-fat diet.[26] Since so many of these cancers are slow-growing, and the side effects of surgery can include impotence or incontinence, making a decision to have surgery is a critical and currently very difficult one. At this point, it is not clear how many small tumors of the prostate will simply stay that way, although tumor cell grade gives some indication if yours is one of the ones that will spread.

A rock and a hard place this is: to decide to live with cancer in your prostate that may never bother you, versus choosing surgery or another conventional treatment path that may damage you. Perhaps the safest avenue is to discuss your options with several authorities, both conventional and alternative medicine, then ask yourself which approach feels most satisfying and safe to *you*.

Jesse A. Stoff, M.D., has reported on a series of cases of varying stages of prostate cancer in his book *The Prostate Miracle*. In it, he outlines a combined approach of vitamins, herbs, and other supplements that have helped reverse this disease.

Following is a brief summary of the currently most promising research-based alternative medicine approaches.

Change Your Diet

You can reduce your risk of prostate cancer if you give dietary change a chance. The total amount of fat in the diet is contributory. Red meat consumption puts you most at risk, due to its high fat content and carcinogens created by the grilling process; its per capita consumption is most directly correlated with prostate cancer incidence. In one study, those patients eating red meat were 2.6 times as likely to develop this cancer than those who did not eat red meat.[27] Fats from fish, dairy, or vegetables were not correlated with metastatic illness, though the more fat you eat, the more at risk you are. Vegetarian diets generally keep the daily fat intake to 20 grams or less.

If you already have prostate cancer, a low-fat diet with lots of fresh fruits and vegetables, along with eliminating coffee and other sources of caffeine, may help prolong your life; as noted, animal studies have shown slower growth, and anecdotal evidence in humans has indicated benefit from switching to this diet.[28]

Avoiding refined sugar in your diet may also help prevent this cancer; its intake has been associated with a higher incidence.[29]

Eating chicken and eggs may also be contributory. In addition to their high fat content, a carcinogen, the avian lukosis virus, is found in these hosts, and contributes to their own high cancer rate. Exposure to this virus, which may not be killed by cooking, is felt by some researchers to induce cancer in humans.[30] Further research is needed to establish such a link.

Adding soy to your diet may provide extra protection against cancers in general, including prostate; initial animal research indicates that those fed a soy-based diet had fewer tumors.[31] Another food found helpful is tomatoes: the consumption of tomato-based foods ten times per week reduced risk for prostate cancer by 46 percent.[32] This effect may be due to an associated lower fat intake, as well as the vitamin C and antioxidant carotenoid and lycopene content of tomatoes. Raw and cooked tomatoes were effective, although tomato paste gave higher protection. Other sources of lycopene, such as purple grapes, may also prove helpful. Also, each day, choose foods from the cruciferous family, known to be associated with reduced cancer rates: cabbage, Brussels sprouts, broccoli, and cauliflower. One study found that if you eat at least three half-cup servings of these each week you can decrease your risk by 41 percent.[33]

Follow the general guidelines for a whole-foods, low-fat, high-fiber diet, given in Chapter 2.

Take Supplements

A general supplementation program may help your immune system resist this cancer. Prostate cancer patients have been found to have low levels of zinc, selenium, and vitamin A in their blood. [34] Individual supplements of zinc, vitamin C, and vitamin E may be protective.[35] Selenium supplements have been found to reduce the risk of prostate cancer by 63 percent in one study.[36] Trials are currently under way to ascertain if a vitamin A derivative may be effective in prevention. Follow the supplement guidelines given in Chapter 2.

Use Herbal Preparations

The herbs saw palmetto and pygeum africanum act to block testosterone conversion to DHT, and so may be beneficial in slowing progression of this disease.

The use of garlic in the diet is inversely related to cancer rates.[37] For a more complete consideration of herbal adjuncts that may affect immune function, see *Choices in Healing*, by Dr. Michael Lerner, and *Beating Cancer with Nutrition*, by Patrick Quillin. Also useful may be *Alternative Medicine* and *Cancer*, compiled by the Burton Goldberg group. These and other cancer references are listed in the Resources section of this book. See also Chapter 2.

A combination of eight Chinese herbs called PC-SPES was found to reduce tumor volume in a study conducted by the University of California Medical Center in San Francisco. It did give some side effects, such as loss of libido and breast enlargement, but seemed to be effective in those who had failed

hormone treatment. For further information, the researcher can be contacted by e-mail at tom.burton@ wsj.com.

Maintain Your Optimum Weight

Prostate cancer is two and a half times more common in overweight men.[38] Follow the low-fat, high-fiber diet given in Chapter 2, along with a daily exercise regimen, to achieve your optimum weight.

Limit Your Sexual Partners

Although studies are conflicting, the higher your number of sexual partners, the more you might be at risk for this disease. It also might be correlated with venereal disease.[39] It's best to play it safe.

Do Yoga and Stretching Exercises Daily

Make certain you do the yoga postures in Figure 20.1 and add yoga stretching exercises to increase local circulation, bringing the best of your body's resources to bear at the point of pathology to fight the tumor. These are described in Chapter 2.

Sunbathe in Moderation and Spend Time Outdoors

Prostate cancer is more common in northern climates, and vitamin D may have anticancer effects. Of course, you will need to keep your sun exposure moderate, to prevent skin cancer.

Avoid Vasectomy

Although still controversial, several studies have indicated a higher risk for prostate cancer after vasectomy.[40] Other studies have indicated no association. To avoid this potential risk, you may wish to choose to use a diaphragm or condoms, or tubal ligation, as your form of birth control.

Practice Visualization

Initially, do deep relaxation, as described in Chapter 2. Then, for example, imagine your prostate as a small loaf of bread, with some marbles representing tumor areas. Remove the marbles, and scan to make certain none are to be found anywhere else in your body. Leave a special maintenance crew to regularly inspect your body, to eliminate them in the future. Picture this in your mind's eye, while feeling it within your body. Repeat three to five times daily.

Join a Support Group

As discussed more fully in Chapter 2, joining a weekly support group of men with cancer may be helpful, as it has been shown to significantly increase life expectancy in women with breast cancer.[41]

Senator Bob Dole discovered he had prostate cancer when routine screening detected an increased PSA level. He had his prostate removed surgically, then founded a national support group, called Us Too. See "Resources" on page 721 for details.

Conventional Medicine Approaches to Prostate Cancer

Radiotherapy and hormone therapy have a well-proven role in the treatment of prostate cancer and are likely to be an alternative to surgery for your disease. Chemotherapy and immunotherapy are more experimental at this point but may be considered depending on your stage.

Radiotherapy

Radiation can be utilized to damage and kill cancer cells. The most common technique employs *external beam* radiation. Radiation can also be delivered by *implants* or *seeds*. These are radioactive isotopes that can be temporarily or permanently inserted directly into the tumor.

Radiation treatment can be chosen in early-stage tumors for cure and later-stage tumors to slow growth and relieve symptoms. Results are equal to surgical radical prostatectomy (see page 574), and there may be lower rates of incontinence, erectile dysfunction, and death.[42] If the tumor has spread to the bone, it may relieve pain and prevent fractures.

Hormone Treatment

The prostate needs the male hormone testosterone to function; this hormone also stimulates prostate cancer. Hormone therapy is aimed at reducing your circulating testosterone, or counteracting its effects. This treatment is usually recommended in later stages, when cure is not possible. However, most patients have a good response, and this approach may dramatically slow growth for many years.

Most testosterone is produced in the testicles and some in the adrenal glands. The effect of testosterone can be blocked by giving drugs that act like female hormones or eliminated by removing the testicles and blocking that produced by the adrenals.

Removing the testicles is a better choice than these drugs for some men, since it is a one-time treatment, and avoids the drugs' cardiac risks. However, this treatment method can cause hot flashes, loss of interest in sex, impotence, and psychological depression.

Drug Treatments

Chemotherapy using powerful drugs can be used to attempt to kill or slow growth of the rapidly dividing prostate cancer. Immunotherapy is another drug-based approach, using "biological" or immunotherapy drugs to boost your immune system's natural defenses against cancer cells.

Experimental trials using chemotherapy and immunotherapy are now under way. So far, there has been no demonstrated advantage or improvement in survival. If other forms of treatment have failed, you might consider one of these trials. Although you have no guarantee that you may be helped, and you may experience risky side effects, you will make a contribution to science and may be among the first to receive benefits from a new treatment.

Surgical Approaches to Prostate Cancer

In general, prostatectomy or removing the prostate is most suitable for patients who are in good health and have no evidence of tumor spread outside the gland. Newer "nerve-sparing" techniques, which limit damage to nerves near the prostate, may decrease the side effects of incontinence and impotence.

Before deciding if prostatectomy is a good treatment option, a *staging pelvic lymph node* evaluation may be recommended. This is often performed while you are under anesthesia, before proceeding with the prostatectomy. It can be done through the use of a laparoscope or a larger "open" incision, with equally reliable results. If a tumor is found in lymph nodes, the prostatectomy is canceled, and another form of treatment that more effectively addresses the spreading cancer can be initiated.

Radical prostatectomy removes the pros-

tate and some of the tissue around it. One of two approaches can be used. In the *retropubic* approach, an incision is made above the pubic bone and carried down in front of the bladder to the prostate. The pelvic lymph node operation can be completed through this same incision, proceeding with prostatectomy only if there has been no spread. In the *perineal* approach, the gland is removed through an incision made between the scrotum and the anus. A separate laparoscopic or open incision is needed to assess lymph nodes. After the prostate is removed, the bladder neck is sewn to the urethra.

If you are able to have radical prostatectomy for localized disease, your chances of cure is 70 percent. See page 578 for a description of prostatectomy and possible complications. For a discussion of retropubic and perineal prostatectomy, see page 576.

If your tumor has progressed beyond cure, urinary obstruction symptoms can be relieved by a *transurethral resection of the prostate* to remove blocking tissue. For a discussion of this procedure, see page 575.

Prostate cancer cells are stimulated by testosterone, produced mostly by the testicles. If your cancer has spread beyond the prostate, *orchiectomy*, the removal of both your testicles, may be recommended to eliminate this hormone stimulation, thereby slowing the cancer's growth. This effect may last for years.

Cryosurgery, where a freezing probe is inserted into the prostate tumor to kill the cells, is a new experimental approach that may have some application in the future.

Prostate Cancer Follow-Up

If you have no symptoms from your prostate cancer and have chosen to delay any treatment until they develop, you will need frequent check-ups. If you have already had treatment, you also need regular tests to ensure you have been cured, or the tumor has been held in check. Periodic physical exams, PSA and PAP blood tests, and X-rays, CAT scans, and bone scans are all needed to monitor your status.

PROSTATE CANCER SUMMARY

Prevention

Diet and Supplements

- Follow a low-fat, vegetarian diet.
- Avoid refined sugar, chicken, eggs.
- Eat foods from cruciferous family daily.
- Eat 5 servings of tomato sauce weekly.
- Replace meat and dairy with soy.
- Eat garlic.
- Selenium, 200 mcg daily.
- Vitamin C, vitamin E.
- Vitamin A, 10,000 IU daily.
- Zinc, 50 mg daily.

Lifestyle

- Follow screening guidelines for rectal exam; consider PSA.
- Practice daily yoga, especially the inverted poses.
- Maintain optimum weight.
- Limit sexual partners.
- Sunbathe (moderately) and spend time outdoors.
- Avoid vasectomy (controversial).

Alternative Medicine Approaches

- Follow the guidelines for prevention, above.
- Saw palmetto, 100 mg, 3 times daily.
- *Pygeum africanum*, 50-100 mcg, 2 times daily.
- Practice visualization.
- Join a support group.

Conventional Medicine Approaches

- Radiotherapy.
- Hormone treatment.
- Chemotherapy.
- Immunotherapy.

Surgical Approaches

- Radical prostatectomy—retropubic, perineal.
- Staging pelvic lymph node evaluation.
- Orchiectomy.
- Cryosurgery.

Specific Prostate Operations

The following procedures have already been discussed in the sections on treatment of prostate enlargement and prostate cancer. Less invasive surgical procedures are explained in detail in the prostate enlargement section. Here we take a closer look at the two most commonly recommended prostate operations.

Transurethral Resection of the Prostate

This procedure, commonly known as TURP, is most often used to treat BPH when it is causing constriction of the urethra as it passes through the prostate from the bladder to the penis. It can also be used to alleviate obstructive symptoms caused by prostate cancer. This operation is so safe and simple that it can be recommended to all but the most medically debilitated.

You are admitted to the hospital on the morning of surgery. The operation is usually performed under spinal or general anesthesia. You lie on your back with your feet up in stirrups. Your doctor inserts a long, narrow instrument into your penis, up the urethra, to the level of the prostate. (See Figure 20.3.) It carries a viewing lens and a channel for cutting instruments and electrocautery. Your doctor then cuts out sections of the internal part of the gland as it is viewed through the lens. After the channel is enlarged sufficiently, a rubber catheter (Foley) is placed through the penis into the bladder, to drain urine and help with the control of bleeding. The catheter's balloon tip holds it in the bladder postoperatively.

A "two-way" catheter may be necessary to flush out blood clots and prevent the catheter from becoming blocked. It has channels for both drainage and irrigation fluid, which may need to be continuous. It can be changed to a single-channel catheter after a day or two.

You will need the urinary catheter for a few days, along with some pain medication. The cut area of your prostate heals in a week or so. Most likely, you will be discharged in three or four days. Since postoperative straining might initiate bleeding, it is especially important that you avoid constipation—here is a good time to include whole bran in your food and eat a low-fat, high-fiber diet. Early walking can also help. You can return to work in two weeks or so.

The mortality rate of this operation is less than 1 percent. One-third of men will experi-

ence retrograde ejaculation. This occurs when semen is discharged back into the bladder, rather than out the penis. This is experienced as a "dry orgasm" that doesn't need to affect sexual pleasure. However, you may not be able to father children without sperm recovery techniques. About 5 to 10 percent experience erectile dysfunction.

Recently, TURP has been performed using a laser instrument instead of electrocautery, with the advantage of less bleeding. Some patients can be sent home the same day. Postoperative recovery is similar.

Retropubic and Perineal Prostatectomy

It may be necessary to remove all of the prostate if it is quite large or contains cancer. The operations described in this section take two to three hours to complete. Because blood loss can be considerable, it is advisable to donate two units of your own blood in the weeks before your operation.

You are admitted on the morning of surgery. General or spinal anesthesia can be used. The prostate gland can be removed through incisions in the abdomen or perineum. For the *retropubic* approach, you are on your back on the operating table. Your surgeon makes an incision just above the pubic bone that continues down in front of your bladder to the prostate, where it is cut out, including the part of the urethra that goes through the gland. A Foley catheter with a balloon tip is inserted through the penis and fed in through the bladder neck, thereby joining the cut ends of the urethra, which are then stitched together over the catheter. A soft drain is placed next to the urethra and brought out through the incision or a separate small abdominal incision.

For the *perineal* approach you will be on your back with your feet up in stirrups. The

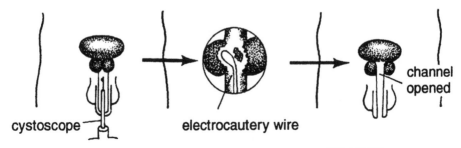

Transurethral Resection of the Prostate (TURP)

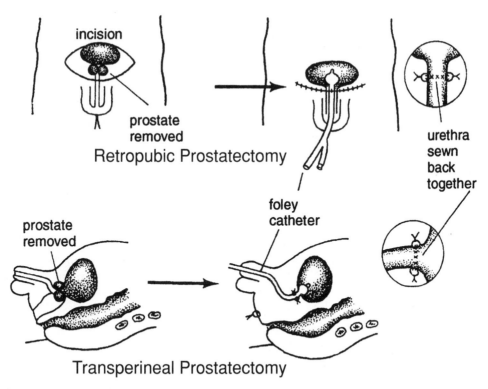

Fig. 20.3 Procedures involved in prostate operations

incision is made between the scrotum and anus. The rest of the operation is similar to the retropubic approach.

If you have prostate cancer, you may need a *radical prostatectomy*, which is similar to prostatectomy for BPH, except that some of the tissues adjacent to the prostate are also removed, to ensure that tumor that may have broken through the prostate capsule is also removed. A *pelvic lymph node dissection* adds removal of lymph nodes that drain the prostate gland to look for evidence of cancer spread. It can be combined with radical prostatectomy when done through the retropubic approach, but a separate abdominal incision must be made if the prostatectomy is performed through the perineum. This can be done laparoscopically.

You will wake up in the recovery room with a catheter in your bladder, which will be left in place for five to ten days. The incision drain catheter is taken out after a few days. Twice as much hospital and recovery time are needed for "open" operations as for TURP. You can go home after four or five days. You should see your doctor after a week or so to check your incision and to ensure that you can urinate satisfactorily after the catheter is removed. It may take several weeks or months before you can fully control urine flow.

Complications of Prostate Surgery

Prostatectomy carries a 0.5 to 2 percent risk of mortality, and an 8 percent chance for cardiovascular complications, with these figures increased after 75 years of age. Statistically, risks of TURP are actually higher than the open procedures but this may be due to use of this procedure on patients who are older and in poorer overall medical health. The TURP is probably safer for the average patient.[43]

Excessive bleeding occurs after 5 percent of TURPs and 2 percent of open prostatectomies.

All of these treatments carry a risk for incontinence. TURP carries a risk for severe incontinence, requiring a permanent catheter and urine-collecting leg bag or urinary pads in 1 to 2 percent of all patients. The rate is 10 to 30 percent after radical prostatectomy. Urinary stricture can occur when scarring shrinks down the urinary passage (3 percent).

Retrograde ejaculation occurs after 40 to 70 percent of all cases. Postoperative impotence can occur after TURP but is much more common after open prostatectomy. After radical prostatectomy 20 to 85 percent of all patients have erectile dysfunction and 35 to 60 percent are impotent. In one national Medicare study, 60 percent reported no erections since surgery.[44]

Recently "nerve-sparing" prostatectomy has been developed in an attempt to avoid injury of nerves near the prostate which are involved in urinary and sexual function, thereby avoiding incontinence and impotence. At this point there seems to be maintenance of potency in 50 to 70 percent of the patients receiving this procedure.

A 2000 report to the American Society for Therapeutic Radiology and Oncology compared all the modalities for treating localized prostate cancer in terms of preserving erectile function. A meta-analysis of eighty-six studies involving 9,991 patients with normal pretreatment erectile function found that one year after treatment 76 percent of these patients were able to maintain the ability after radiotherapy seed implants, 67 percent after standard external beam radiotherapy, 58 percent after a combination of seed implants and external radiation, 58 percent after nerve-sparing radical prostatectomy, 30 percent after standard radical prostatectomy, with the worst results—only 14 percent—after cryotherapy (freezing the tumor with low-temperature probes).[45] These results may be helpful in making your treatment decisions.

Erectile Dysfunction

Viagra has taken over the title as the fastest money-maker in U.S. drug history—2.9 million prescriptions were given in the first three months! Its popularity, the many ways that have been figured out to get the drug without a prescription, its usage even by those without erectile dysfunction (ED), and the myriad of jokes told by all ages and varieties of people in all sorts of settings indicate the present pervasive public concern with the quality of sexual function. It may be that this new and "easy" way to deal with ED will lead to a more comfortable discussion of the problem both in public and between partners suffering from its effects. Media exposure and pronouncements by public figures such as Bob Dole give evidence to this other beneficial effect of Viagra.

The National Institutes of Health defines erectile dysfunction (ED), as the "inability to achieve an erect penis sufficient for satisfactory sexual performance." Sexual desire and the ability to ejaculate and have orgasm may still be present.

The incidence of erectile dysfunction is unknown. It is poorly understood by both the general public and health professionals. Questionnaires are subjective and unreliable, and objective data is poor. Estimates suggest that 5 percent of all men are affected at age 40, and 15 to 25 percent after age 65. In total, 20 to 30 million men in the United States have erectile dysfunction.[46]

Of all the components of male sexual function—desire, ability to achieve a satisfactory erection, ability to attain orgasm, ejaculation, and fertility—erectile dysfunction causes the severest problems with self-esteem and interpersonal relations in the family and, by extension, at work. Advertisements spread misinformation and false expectations of what "normal" is supposed to be. There are lots of reasons and opportunities for misery.

Erection involves a complex interaction between psychic function, hormones, nervous system sensation and reflexes, and blood supply. Problems can occur at any level. Usually, a combination of factors contributes.

A psychic block to erection can be caused by chronic stress, sexual inhibitions, performance anxiety, and fear of pregnancy or sexually transmitted disease. Lack of education about sex and poor sexual technique should not be overlooked. Poor personal relationships may be the most important factor. Nerve sensation and reflex pathways may be damaged. Pelvic surgery (prostate, rectum, bladder, or vascular operations) or X-ray treatment may interrupt nerve response. Neurologic and psychiatric diseases such as spinal cord injury, Alzheimer's disease, alcoholism, or depression may be responsible.

Inadequate production of the male hormone testosterone or increased female hormone levels can decrease sex drive and interfere with performance. Alcohol intake, smoking, and side effects of medication (especially diuretics, beta-blockers, stomach acid blockers, sedatives, antidepressants, and antihypertensives) may decrease erectile ability.

Arterial blood vessels may be unable to supply enough blood to fill the spongy chambers of the shaft of the penis or enough pressure to attain satisfactory rigidity. The venous outflow vessels may not be compressed against the thick fibrous sheath surrounding the spongy shaft to keep blood trapped within the penis, maintaining rigidity.

Erectile dysfunction increases with age. Most likely this is true because general medical problems such as increased cholesterol, hypertension, vascular disease, and other chronic diseases are increased with aging. Diabetics are especially at risk, with rates as high as 35 to 50 percent.

After your diagnostic workup, your doctor can usually determine if the cause of erectile dysfunction is psychological or a physical problem of hormonal, vascular, or neurologic origin, or a combination of these. About 80 percent of erectile dysfunction is due to organic disease and 20 percent to psychological disturbance. Unfortunately, even if underlying abnormalities can be found, treatment aimed at the problem cannot guarantee successful erections. Treatment programs often include a combination of medical, psychological, and behavioral recommendations.

How Erectile Dysfunction Is Diagnosed

The cause or combination of factors that may contribute to your predicament can be determined by a careful history, physical exam, and, if necessary, a series of increasingly complex tests.

History

Determining the cause or causes of erectile dysfunction begins with a medical history searching for symptoms of the problems listed above. Your doctor will want to know what drugs you may be taking and your usual level of alcohol intake, if any. Questions will be asked about your psychosocial history and personal relationships. A detailed sexual history answers questions about your expectations, techniques, and performance. A psychological test may be helpful.

Physical Exam

The physical exam checks your general condition and focuses in on your breasts, distribution of body hair, testicles, penis, and prostate. Circulation is checked by feeling for pulses in your groin and penis. Nerve function is checked by testing sensation and the bulbocavernosis reflex, where your anus contracts when the penile glans is squeezed.

Tests

Simple blood tests may reveal underlying medical disease or abnormal testerostone levels. More sophisticated tests may be required if the cause is in doubt. Nerve conduction tests determine whether a neurologic problem is present. A noninvasive duplex Doppler sound wave test may be requested to look at vascular function. Occasionally, an invasive arteriogram may be necessary to accurately evaluate pelvic and penile blood vessels, especially if reconstructive vascular surgery is a consideration. The penile blood pressure can be measured directly by using a special blood pressure cuff. A blood vessel–relaxing drug can be injected directly into your penis to determine if the blood supply is adequate (see page 584).

You may have a test to determine whether you have normal erections during sleep. A healthy man has several lasting fifteen to forty-five minutes every night. It is performed with a strain gauge attached to your penis, then connected to a recording device or with a simple penile cuff that pulls apart during erection. Alternatively, your partner can stay awake and record the frequency and degree of erections. If you do have erections, problems with hormones, nerves, and blood supply are unlikely; therefore, psychological factors are probably the cause of dysfunction.

Alternative Medicine Approaches to Erectile Dysfunction

Alternative medicine offers much hope for erectile dysfunction, in terms of both prevention and treatment. In addition, changes you embark upon with these measures may help prevent other diseases as well.

These measures are therefore recommended for everyone suffering from this disorder, and especially for persons who cannot safely take Viagra but who still wish to avoid a painful and not necessarily successful surgical procedure.

Following are the most important and promising alternative medicine solutions to erectile dysfunction.

Change Your Diet

Since inadequate circulation may be at the root of the impotence associated with aging, a trial of a low-fat, high-fiber diet may be beneficial. Many patients in the Dean Ornish Heart Disease Reversal Project have noted marked improvement in sexual function within a short time of beginning the program.

Quit Smoking

Smoking causes constriction of blood vessels leading into the penis and contracts penile muscle, causing blood to leak from its veins and thereby interfering with erection.[47] Quitting smoking can lead to a dramatic improvement in circulation. Men who smoke are 50

percent more likely to suffer from erectile dysfunction.[48] Smoking can also contribute to infertility. A sperm of a man smoking one pack of cigarettes a day is only half as likely to penetrate and fertilize the female's egg.[49] Recommendations to help you stop are given in Chapter 2.

Eliminate Alcohol and Certain Drugs

A drink or two of alcohol can improve erection by increasing blood vessel flow and decreasing anxiety. However, larger amounts can cause problems through sedation, decreased libido, and temporary erectile dysfunction. Chronic alcohol abuse decreases testicular function and causes neuropathy that may effect penile nerves.[50] Many prescription drugs, especially beta-blockers used to control hypertension, cimetadine (Tagamet) for stomach acid control, and antidepressants can contribute; as many as 25 percent of all cases of erectile dysfunction may be traced to drug side effects. Ask your doctor about changing medications if one you are taking may be suspect.

Take Supplements

Vitamin E, 400 IU once daily, and the herbs coryanthe, ginseng, and ginkgo biloba are suggested to assist in reversal of age-related impotence. One study showed ginkgo restored potency in 50 percent of its users after a trial of six months.[51] Begin with one capsule, increasing up to six, as needed.

Yohimbine is derived from the bark of the yohim tree. It acts on brain centers to enhance libido and erection. A 1998 meta-analysis of seven placebo-controlled studies showed that yohimbine can improve erectile function. It worked particularly well for psychological causes. Serious reactions were rare and reversible.[52]

Practice Stress Management and Yoga Daily

Stress is notorious for interfering with sexual function, and everyone probably needs regular stress management for optimum health in this area. In addition, the gentle stretching of yoga has been shown to improve local blood and lymph circulation, helping to reverse circulatory impairment. Follow the stress management and yoga guidelines in Chapter 2.

Exercise Regularly

Sedentary men are at high risk for ED. Although too much exercise may actually decrease sexual desire, regular moderate exercise not only improves circulation, but enhances the feeling of well-being so helpful to an optimal sexual functioning. A study from the Harvard School of Public Health investigating the sexual activity of 2,000 male health professionals aged 51 to 87 reported that those who exercised vigorously for twenty to thirty minutes a day were half as likely to have problems with ED as those with the lowest level of exercise. They also found that as waist size increased, so did ED.[53]

Add Massage and Aromatherapy

Mutual massage, especially with sensually stimulating oils such as the fragrance of apple pie, cinnamon, sandalwood, jasmine, lavender, rose, or ylang-ylang, will help you relax, encourage gentle communication, and get your juices flowing. Stress can play a significant role in impotence at any age; anything that helps you relax may have a psychophysi-

ological impact, affecting nerve transmission and hormone output.

In addition, both the nose and penis contain erectile tissue that becomes engorged during sexual arousal. Aromatic stimulation of the nasal tissue may help, via a sympathetic connection, to stimulate the penile area. In addition, aromatic memories may assist in this process. Clinical research has indicated that apple pie and lavender are extremely sexual stimulant smells for men, while licorice and lavender are the most effective for women.

Practice Visualization

First, practice deep relaxation, as given in Chapter 2. Then imagine your penis is perfectly erect, with a beautiful bone inside, encased in velvet. Picture this in your mind, while feeling it within your body. Repeat three to five times daily.

Obtain Counseling

These techniques focus on understanding psychological factors that may be contributing to erectile dysfunction, increasing communication with your partner, and decreasing performance anxiety, guilt, and inhibitory attitudes toward sex. Both partners should be actively involved. The average couple seeking help for ED has not had intercourse for from two to five years. Courage, sympathy, and understanding are necessary when reestablishing this intimacy after a period of frustration, even when Viagra or other treatment options hold much promise for success.

Conventional Medicine Approaches to Erectile Dysfunction

There are a number of nonsurgical approaches for erectile dysfunction that has not improved after a trial of alternative approaches. Following are several to consider.

Treat Medical Conditions

Decreased production of the hormone testosterone or increased levels of the hormone prolactin inhibit libido and erectile function. Specific therapy may be all that is necessary. There are many other chronic medical conditions that may be contributing to erectile dysfunction, as described above. Ensure that you are doing your best to minimize the effects of any health problems you have.

Viagra

In March 1998, the Food and Drug Administration approved sildenafil (Viagra) as the first oral medicine treatment of erectile dysfunction. It has become wildly popular with accounts of incredible recovery of sexual prowess, even in octogenarians. It is now considered the treatment of choice for most patients and has eclipsed all other forms of therapy, at least for an initial trial. It has little effect on libido. Taken about an hour before anticipated sexual activity, it acts by increasing the penile response to sexual stimulation and arousal. Viagra works by potentiating cyclic GMP, an enzyme that is increased during arousal, which relaxes arterial smooth muscle cells and thereby allows more blood flow into the penis. However, without arousal, cyclic GMP is not increased and Viagra won't work. Therefore, the role of the partner is also emphasized.

Several studies have documented excellent results with Viagra. A summary of twenty-one clinical trials involving over 3,000 men with organic or combined organic and psychogenic associated ED was discussed in the *New*

England Journal of Medicine in 2000. It concluded that Viagra was associated with a significantly higher number of erections, rates of penile rigidity, orgasmic function, and overall sexual satisfaction than placebo.[54] Goldstein et al., in the *New England Journal of Medicine,* described their results in two double-blind studies of 532 men with organic, psychogenic, and mixed causes of sexual dysfunction. They found successful intercourse followed 69 percent of attempts after use of Viagra versus only 22 percent after taking a placebo pill. The men receiving Viagra had 5.9 successful attempts per month compared to 1.5 taking a placebo. It also provides more "staying power," increasing self-confidence and decreasing performance anxiety. Side effects included headache, flushing, and upset stomach in 6 to 18 percent of the users.[55] Bladder inflammation has been reported in partners. A study funded by the manufacturer found that only 2 percent of the patients discontinued Viagra because of side effects.

There have been severe cardiovascular complications, including death, reported in men using Viagra. You should not take Viagra if you are taking a nitrate-containing drug as is commonly prescribed for angina or heart pain. A severe drop in blood pressure can occur. Also, it may be dangerous if you have a risk for certain types of cardiac rhythm disturbances. Even without Viagra the risk of a heart attack increases by 2.5 times in the two hours after sexual activity.[56] Many physicians advise taking and passing a cardiac stress test before trying Viagra. You must discuss your personal health history with your doctor. Because of the short time length of the clinical trials, the long-term safety of Viagra is still unknown.

Insurance coverage for Viagra ($10 a dose) is now a very hot topic among Medicaid,

Medicare, VA, and insurance providers. Many companies are balking at the projected huge increase in costs for unselectively covering the explosion in prescriptions for this drug. The VA has predicted Viagra could account for more than one-fifth of its total pharmaceutical budget and, so far, has not provided coverage.

Uprima

Apomorphine (Uprima) is another drug that may soon be available in the United States. It acts on brain centers involved in the erection response, rather than on the penis itself. Its advantage is that it acts within fifteen to twenty minutes, much more quickly than Viagra—increasing the "spontaneity" of sexual activity. Its major drawback is that is causes nausea in 18 to 22 percent of all users. At the more effective dose level, it has also caused a drop in blood pressure in 3 to 6 percent and fainting in 1 to 2 percent, such that its safety is questionable at this point.[57]

Vacuum/Constriction Device

First patented in 1917, this device is now widely available. In this method, the penis is placed in a plastic cylinder connected to a handheld vacuum pump. The suction has the effect of pulling blood into the penis, producing erection. A constriction band is then placed at the penis's base to prevent blood outflow until after intercourse. Due to decreased arterial inflow, usage should be limited to thirty minutes. A certain amount of dexterity is necessary. Side effects in some patients include bruising, interference with ejaculation (12 percent), and initial pain and discomfort from the constricting band (41 percent).

The success rate is about 90 percent, regardless of the cause of erectile dysfunction. However, since this method may interfere with spontaneity of lovemaking and ejaculation, the dropout rate is high (only 26 percent are still using it after one to three years). This is a very good method to start with as, compared with other methods, it is the least expensive ($150 to $450 per device), least invasive, and safest, and does not interfere with any other treatment approach.

Intracavernosal Injections

This approach utilizes injection of a penile artery smooth muscle relaxant—papaverine, phentolamine, the prostaglandin alprostadil (Caverjet), or a mixture of these—directly into the penile spongy tissue using a syringe and tiny needle. This relaxes and enlarges small arteries, mimicking the normal physiology of erection by increasing arterial blood inflow, engorging the spongy corpora cavernosum that then compress the venous outflow, trapping the blood in the penis. A major study using alprostadil found this technique is successful in producing a usable erection after 94 percent of all injections. Depending on drug and dosage, it can be sustained for an hour or more. Orgasm and ejaculation are unaffected. Sexual activity is rated as satisfactory by men and their partners after 86 percent of all injections.[58]

Side effects of alprostadil injections include prolonged erections that can be painful and become dangerous in a few percent of the patients. This occurs with less than 1 percent of all injections after the optimum dosage is titrated for each individual. If you have an erection lasting more than four hours, you need to see your doctor immediately. Other possible effects are testicular and scrotal pain and swelling, penile fibrotic complications (2 percent), and temporary low blood pressure. Fifty percent of men experience pain at times, but only after eleven percent of the injections.[59] As too frequent usage is more likely to cause penile fibrosis, its usage should be restricted to two times a week. In those who have intercourse infrequently, this method is preferable to the more invasive penile implant surgery. Its high dropout rate (38 to 80 percent) reflects its cost of $5 to $25 per dose, slight pain, and cumbersome usage.

Intraurethral Pellets

The Muse system is a promising approach that may make the injection technique obsolete. It uses a small semisolid pellet inserted into the urethra using a disposable plastic applicator just prior to intercourse. The pellet contains alprostadil, the penile artery muscle relaxant described above, which is absorbed across the urethra directly into the spongy chambers of the shaft. The increased blood flow produces an erection in five to ten minutes that lasts for thirty to sixty minutes, depending on the dose that is selected by each individual. It can be used twice per day. Initially, there may be some mild discomfort with insertion. Possible side effects include mild penile pain (after 11 to 41 percent of all insertions), minor bleeding (5 percent), dizziness (2 percent), and vaginal itching and burning in female partners. Prolonged erection and penile fibrosis are very rare. A 1997 report by Harlin in the *New England Journal of Medicine* found that this method will produce an erection sufficient for intercourse in 66 percent of all users, regardless of the cause of the erectile dysfunction. In these men, successful

intercourse follows 70 percent of all insertions.[60] The dropout rates vary from 4 to 82 percent, the reasons being disappointing results and cost. Results are not as good for older patients with multiple medical problems. Major advantages over the needle injection technique are that it is less invasive and intrusive and avoids the risk of penile fibrosis. The cost is $25 per dose.

Combining an adjustable penile constriction band to the base of the penis to block venous blood outflow with MUSE has been reported to increase the rate of satisfactory successful intercourse to over 80 percent.[61]

Surgical Approaches to Erectile Dysfunction

A few episodes of impotence are not an indication for surgery; but if you have sustained, unremitting difficulty in achieving or maintaining erections, and the alternative and conventional medicine recommendations suggested are not satisfactory, several operations are now available.

Vascular Surgery

Abnormalities of blood flow into or out of the penis are felt to be the most common organic causes of erectile dysfunction.[62] If you have a problem with blood supply, where the blood pressure in the penile arteries is significantly decreased, as measured by a small blood pressure cuff, a vascular operation to bring more blood to the arteries may be helpful. If you qualify for this type of surgery, you have a 31 to 80 percent chance that an operation will restore or improve your potency.[63] The results are better in younger men with localized arterial blockages.

Prior to surgery, an angiogram will have

demonstrated the site of arterial blockage. In one operation, done under general anesthesia, an incision is made in the lower abdomen. The blocked artery is exposed at the back of the pelvis and the block removed or bypassed to increase blood flow and pressure to the penile arteries. Another operation, using microsurgical techniques, connects an artery from the abdominal wall directly to a penile artery or vein. A successful result will be soon apparent.

A surgical procedure to restrict venous outflow from the penis may be helpful if a "venous leak" is demonstrated by specialized X-ray tests and nighttime erection testing. With this problem, the arterial supply is satisfactory but there is an inability to keep blood trapped in the penis to sustain erection. The operation ties off veins leading away from the penis, increasing resistance to outflow. If you qualify for this operation, there is up to a 74 percent change for a good short-term result, but as new venous connections develop, success falls to 24 percent at two years.[64]

Vascular procedures cost from $10,000 to $15,000. For a discussion of vascular surgery, see Chapter 9.

Prosthetic Implants

Various types of silicone prosthetic devices can be inserted into the shaft of the penis to give it rigidity. The least expensive, *semirigid* or *malleable rods,* give a permanent erection that is folded out of the way when not in use. The malleable type is more easily concealed. There are one-, two-, and three-piece *inflatable hydraulic* prostheses. The one-piece, self-contained model can be made firm by squeezing the reservoir in the head of the penis and made soft by bending the shaft, but does not change size and can't be made as

rigid as the others. It feels more natural than the semirigid rods.

The two-piece inflatable consists of a collapsible penile implant connected by a soft plastic tube to a pump-reservoir filled with fluid that is placed in the scrotum. The three-piece model has a scrotal pump connected to a separate fluid reservoir placed under the skin of the lower abdomen. The pump is manually squeezed to force fluid into the implant as needed. A valve is manipulated to move the fluid back to the reservoir, deflating the prosthesis and penis. The costlier three-piece device has the advantages of a smaller, less noticeable scrotal pump and its reservoir can contain more fluid, so that the erection can be larger and firmer and the flaccid state more natural appearing. Prices range from $8,000 to $15,000.

These operations can be outpatient procedures or you may be hospitalized for a day or two. They can be performed using local, spinal, or general anesthesia, depending on the complexity of the implant and your wishes. A bladder catheter is inserted. Your surgeon makes incisions in the penis, scrotum, and lower abdomen, depending on the type of prosthesis. The two rods or inflatable cylinders are inserted into the corpora cavernosa. If you have a two- or three-piece inflatable model, the pump and reservoir are then connected and tested. The incisions are closed with stitches or skin tapes. The operation takes one to three hours, depending on the type of implant chosen. With the inflatable implant, after surgery the penis is kept upward on the abdomen for the first several weeks, until a fibrous capsule forms around the silicone. With the rigid and malleable models, the penis is bent downward.

After surgery there will be some swelling and bruising. You may have burning with urination until swelling resolves. Discomfort may last for six to eight weeks. Pain pills should be adequate. Occasionally, prolonged pain indicates that too long a prosthesis was used and a revision may be necessary. You should see your doctor several times to ensure successful healing and for instructions in prosthesis usage. The inflatable prostheses are kept deflated for the first month, then can be tested cautiously. You should wait four to six weeks before beginning intercourse.

All of these devices have a significant rate of mechanical failure (4 percent) and local complications including discomfort, infection, and erosion through the skin. Also, silicone particles can migrate, with uncertain medical effects. The more complex inflatable prostheses are more complicated to implant and more subject to mechanical failure. Recently, however, only 2 percent of patients have required removal of the prosthesis.

After prosthesis implantation, sex drive, sensation, and ability to have orgasm and ejaculate should be unchanged. Patient and partner satisfaction is high, since little interference with intercourse takes place. Ninety-five to 99 percent of penile implants remain usable at one year after surgery. Patient satisfaction is 90 percent. Because these procedures are the most invasive, they should probably not be chosen unless the other approaches have failed. However, a 2000 study from Tulane University found that despite the availability of new oral medications such as Viagra, the number of protheses placed remained stable over ten years because a significant portion of ED patients do not respond to oral medications.[65]

ERECTILE DYSFUNCTION SUMMARY

Prevention

Diet and Supplements

- Follow a low-fat, high-fiber diet.
- Vitamin C, 1,000–2,000 mg, 1–3 times daily.
- Vitamin E, D-alpha, 400 IU daily.
- Zinc, 50 mg.

Lifestyle

- Don't smoke.
- Avoid alcohol.
- Avoid drugs.
- Exercise, 1 hour, 3–5 times weekly.
- Practice yoga daily, especially the inverted postures.
- Practice stress management.

Alternative Medicine Approaches

- Follow the preventive guidelines, above.
- Herbs: coryanthe, gingko biloba, 500 mg, 1–3 times daily; ginseng, 500 mg, 1–3 times daily; yohimbe 15–30 mg daily (this must be used only with supervision, due to its side effects).
- Try massage and aromatherapy.
- Practice hypnosis and visualization.
- Seek counseling and behavioral treatment.

Conventional Medicine Approaches

- Drug therapy—sildenafil (Viagra), apomorphine (Uprima).

- Vacuum/constriction device.
- Intracavernosal injections—papaverine, phentolamine, prostaglandin alprostadil (Caverjet).
- Intraurethral pellets alprostadil (Muse).

Surgical Medicine Approaches

- Vascular surgery—arterial, venous.
- Prosthetic implants—malleable, inflatable.

CHAPTER 21

THYROID

. . . think of the human body as a hotel switchboard lit up by a constant stream of room-service orders and complaint calls: "Can you lower the temperature of the room?" "Would you send up a couple of cheeseburgers please?" The mediators of this ceaseless biological babble—the messengers rushing from cell to cell to satisfy all requests—are powerful molecules called hormones.

"On Health," *Newsweek*[1]

Your endocrine system produces and regulates your hormones. It consists of highly specialized cells arranged in different ways. The word "hormone" derives from the Greek "to set in motion." Your hormones, complex proteins released directly into your bloodstream, act like messengers, telling their "target tissues" to undergo changes or otherwise function in different ways. They help regulate virtually all aspects of your body's function, including circulation, growth and development, sexual maturation and activity, menstrual cycles, pregnancy, nursing, digestion, cell nutrition and metabolism, body chemistry, blood pressure, and preparation for "fight or flight."

Hormone levels are continuously regulated by other hormones, blood constituents, or nerves, so that an extremely complex relationship of stimulation and suppression takes place. When this balance system is functioning harmoniously, a steady state of bodily functioning is achieved. When one or more hormones is produced in too little or too large amounts, the associated or opposing hormones then become unbalanced, giving you wide variety of resulting signs and symptoms.

You can take action to help protect and adjust your hormone activity. Lifestyle factors such as stress, smoking, and dietary choices all can contribute to destabilizing the body's natural internal harmony, affecting hormone levels. The brain's interaction with the glandular system is very complex and only beginning to be understood. Undoubtedly, however, higher centers in your brain, related to your emotions, can contribute to endocrine disturbances and be enlisted in their resolution. The field of psychoneuroendocrinology has begun to systematically investigate these links. Yoga, acupuncture, biofeedback, and other alternative medicine tools have been documented to assist in prevention and treatment of some endocrine disorders.

Identifiable large clusters of hormone-producing cells are called glands, such as the familiar pituitary, thyroid, parathyroid, pancreas, adrenal, ovary, and testicle. Some hormones are produced by cells scattered in other organs such as the intestine and kidneys. In this chapter, we will discuss the common disorders of the thyroid gland.

How Your Thyroid Gland Works

The butterfly-shaped *thyroid gland* is located at the base of your neck, in front and on the sides of the trachea or windpipe. (See Figure 21.1.) It normally weighs less than an ounce and is usually unnoticed and difficult to feel, unless enlarged or nodular.

The thyroid gland plays a major role in the regulation of your metabolism by manufacturing and secreting thyroid hormone, which affects the speed of cellular function. Thyroid hormone affects the processes of uptake of

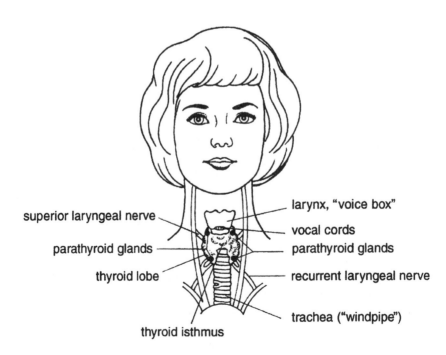

superior laryngeal nerve

parathyroid glands

thyroid lobe

thyroid isthmus

larynx, "voice box"

vocal cords

parathyroid glands

recurrent laryngeal nerve

trachea ("windpipe")

Fig. 21.1 The location of the thyroid

nutritional substances, conversion of these into energy, and elimination of waste products by the cells. Too much hormone causes hyperactivity of the body's tissues and organs, while too little slows them down.

The thyroid gland makes its hormone by first trapping circulating iodine that has been absorbed into the bloodstream from the intestines. Rate of release is governed by the pituitary hormone called thyroid stimulating hormone (TSH). Your brain's hypothalamus is in intimate association with the pituitary and secretes neurohormones directly into the pituitary's blood circulation, stimulating the pituitary to release TSH. One area of the hypothalamus is sensitive to circulating thyroid hormone levels. If the thyroid hormone level is too high, it will decrease its pituitary stimulation, thereby decreasing TSH release. If the thyroid hormone is too low, stimulation occurs, so that a delicate "thermostatic" feedback mechanism controls the rate of activity of cellular and organ function. Disease can result from malfunction at any point.

How Thyroid Disease Is Diagnosed

Diseases of the thyroid are second only to diabetes among endocrine disorders, affecting 3 to 5 percent of our population. Once you have developed signs and symptoms, most problems can be readily identified. Tests required for diagnosis are widely available, though they are often expensive.

History

Your doctor should ask a series of questions about any symptoms you may have which might reflect over- or underproduction of thyroid hormone. General symptoms include appetite changes, weight gain or loss, intolerance to cold or heat, problems sleeping, and overall energy level. Many different systems can be affected. Gastrointestinal effects can cause nausea, vomiting, and constipation. You may feel heart palpitations. There may be disturbances in your menstrual cycle or fertility. Neurologic symptoms include nervousness, tremor, mood swings, apathy, a progressive decline in mental ability, confusion, and psychosis. There can be changes in your skin with increased sweating or dryness, scaling, and loss of hair. Visual disturbances may occur. Some thyroid problems can cause symptoms in the neck including pain, shortness of breath, difficulty in swallowing, or a change in your voice. As you can see, the possibilities are almost endless.

If you have noticed any changes in your appearance such as loss or thinning of hair, eyes becoming more prominent or "bugging out," leg swelling, or other changes, be sure to report them.

Your doctor should also ask about any prescription, over-the-counter, or recreational drugs you may be taking. They can affect thyroid function, both increasing or decreasing hormone levels and activity.

Your family history of thyroid disease is important, as well as where you have lived, and if you've ever received radiation to your neck area. Report any other medical problems, especially kidney, liver, or heart disease.

Physical Exam

Your doctor should start with a thorough physical examination of all your body systems because of the widespread effects of thyroid disease. Your thyroid especially should be carefully examined, and checked for tenderness, enlargement, irregularity in consistency, nodules, and enlarged lymph nodes.

Blood Tests

A *thyroid hormone level* blood test determines whether your gland is producing thyroid hormone at increased, normal, or decreased rates. *TSH assay* tells how much of this hormone is being produced by your pituitary.

Iodine-131 uptake is another test for thyroid function. A small dose of radioactive iodine, called I-131, is injected into your bloodstream. The thyroid gland picks it up, then incorporates it into thyroid hormone. Its level is measured by blood samples at predetermined time intervals. If the thyroid gland is hyperfunctioning, it will take up the I-131 more rapidly than normal; if hypofunctioning, less rapidly.

Thyroid antibodies can be found if the thyroid is being mistakenly attacked by your immune system.

Radioactive Isotope Thyroid Scan

This test measures the activity of the thyroid and reflects the anatomy of functioning tissue. Radioactive iodine or technetium is injected into your bloodstream and is then taken up by the thyroid. You lie on a special table while the isotope camera scans back and forth over your neck obtaining a "picture" of the trapped radioactivity. This scan reveals overactive "hot" or underactive "cold" areas, as well as size and shape of the gland. Abnormal collections of thyroid tissue in areas other than the normal gland location, a result of congenital abnormalities or thyroid cancer spread, can also be identified.

Whenever possible, this scan and the Iodine-131 uptake test should not be repeated, since they do give you some radiation exposure.

Thyroid Sonogram

This painless test can distinguish whether a thyroid nodule is solid or cystic, which may have a bearing on recommendation for surgery. You lay on a table while an ultrasonic probe is passed over your neck, picking up sound waves as they bounce off your thyroid and adjacent tissues. The sonogram cannot in itself determine whether a nodule is benign or malignant.

Needle Biopsy

This test can be easily and safely performed, and is almost always used in evaluation of nodules when malignancy is a consideration. A sonogram can be used to direct needle biopsy to nodules not able to be felt clearly. After skin preparation with an antiseptic and local anesthesia, your doctor uses a small needle to remove cells. Two or more specimens are taken. One of two techniques can be employed. *Fine needle aspiration* sucks out some cells through a very thin needle, with the cells then analyzed microscopically in the same way as the familiar Pap smear. *Core needle biopsy* uses a larger, cutting needle that removes a solid piece of thyroid tissue for microscopic analysis. The latter technique is more accurate, but hazards such as bleeding are increased. After the biopsy you may have some minor soreness and bruising for a few days.

This test is falsely negative or misses cancer in less than 5 percent of all biopsies. Needle biopsy has decreased the rate of thyroid surgery by 25 percent and increased the rate of cancer found in surgical specimens from 15 to more than 30 percent.

Hyperthyroidism

Hyperthyroidism, also called Grave's disease, develops when the thyroid gland produces too much thyroid hormone. Usually, it results from abnormal antibodies attaching to the TSH receptor on thyroid cells, resulting in an overstimulation of the gland. The body's immune system may be faulty in making these antibodies, or it may be responding normally to defects in the thyroid cells.

Genetic factors, as well as stress, may play a role in its development. Less commonly, benign thyroid tumors can cause hyperthyroidism, by producing thyroid hormone in excessive amounts. In both cases, the thyroid's activity cannot be suppressed by the usual feedback mechanism.

Excess thyroid hormone induces hyperactivity of specific organs, causing the symptoms of hyperthyroidism that you may experience. Your heart beats faster and is more subject to abnormal rhythms. You may feel palpitations. Gastrointestinal disturbance and diarrhea are common, with sweating, fever, and intolerance to heat typical. Increased appetite and thirst are experienced, since the cells' demands are increased when they are forced to function at abnormally rapid rates. Even so, weight loss often accompanies hyperthyroidism, since nutrition cannot keep up with metabolic demand, and muscular weakness and easy fatigability follow. Shaking tremors, nervousness, insomnia, anxiety, and psychiatric disorders reflect stress on the nervous system. *Exopthalmus* is the term for when the eyes "bug out" as a consequence of hyperthyroidism's effects upon the soft tissue of the eye socket. The hair becomes very fine, the skin moist, warm, and thin. Menstrual disturbances such as irregular and excessive bleeding usually develop.

If you have some or all of the symptoms mentioned above, a diagnosis of hyperthyroidism is suspected by specific findings on physical examination. The thyroid is usually diffusely enlarged, although occasionally a localized "toxic" nodule or hyperfunctioning benign tumor is the cause of the hyperthyroidism. The diagnosis is confirmed by high blood levels of thyroid hormone and rapid uptake of the I-131 isotope.

Down through the ages, hyperthyroidism has caused disease, insanity, and death. The infamous "asylums" were populated by many individuals with this malady. Only in the last century has the nature of hyperthyroidism been understood and very effective treatment become available.

Historically, therapy began with surgical removal of the gland, then very hazardous, since the thyroid overactivity was not controlled before surgery. Mortality was high, with frequent surgical complications. Damage involving the parathyroid glands and nerves to the larynx, or voice box, was common. Thyroid surgery is now quite safe, using sophisticated methods of preoperative preparation to counteract the hyperactivity, along with carefully worked out surgical techniques. However, current treatment of hyperthyroidism is usually nonsurgical.

Without treatment, symptoms of hyperthyroidism regress in about one-third of persons, and one-third remain hyperthyroid. The remaining third progress and would eventually die, usually of "thyroid storm" and congestive heart failure.

The conventional medical approach consists of measures to block the release of thyroid hormone, prevent its manufacture, and counteract its systemic effects. Radioactive iodine destroys functioning thyroid tissue, and surgery removes most or all of the gland. The best treatment depends on the severity of the disease, your age, desires about pregnancy, and prediction of success of each treatment depending on your individual case. Radioactive iodine is recommended for almost all adult patients.

Your feelings toward the various types of available treatment options will influence your choice of therapy. Many persons have strong feelings about radiotherapy, fear of surgery, or aversion to taking medications on a long-term basis. An alternative medicine program must be monitored by your doctor.

Alternative Medicine Approaches to Hyperthyroidism

―――――――――――――――――――

Marjorie, an advertising executive, was feeling overwhelmed by her stressful Madison Avenue job. She first noticed her hair falling out in larger than usual amounts, followed by severe fatigue, which she tried to avoid by simply drinking more coffee and caffeinated diet drinks. When she could no longer easily climb the stairs to her first-floor office, she went to see her doctor, who found she was suffering from Grave's disease–induced hyperthyroidism. She was recommended for surgery, but sought out a second opinion, which suggested one or two year's trial of medication. Finally, she sought a third, alternative medicine approach, and was placed on the program given below, emphasizing a caffeine-free diet, with plenty of exercise, relaxation, and yoga. After only six months, she was able to taper off her antithyroid medications, had no further signs of her disease, and felt better than she had in years.

―――――――――――――――――――

You must undertake alternative medicine approaches to Grave's disease only under your doctor's careful supervision, to make certain you avoid any complications of hyperthyroidism, such as its effects upon your eyes, and to check that you are indeed making progress in its control.

One important reason to consider at least a trial of alternative medicine methods is that a major disadvantage of the surgery and radiation treatment approaches is their risk of causing hypothyroidism. You would then most likely be required to take thyroid replacement therapy—usually a brand of thyroid hormone called Synthroid—for the rest of your life. Taking such external hormone replacement has been associated with decreased bone density in the hips,[2] arrhythmias in the heart, and possibly heart disease.[3]

Following are the alternative medicine approaches currently most promising in reversal of this disorder.

Practice Stress Management and Yoga Daily

A number of researchers have found a link between stressful events and the onset of Grave's disease. Dr. K. N. Udupa analyzed 800 cases and found a strong association. He then intervened with daily yoga postures, and showed that this disease could be reversed by such a regimen.[4] If your symptoms are mild, a trial of combined conventional and alternative medicine approaches can be instituted before radioactive iodine therapy or surgery are contemplated. These simple methods are virtually free of side effects, and may help you avoid surgery or radiation, and then having to take replacement thyroid medication for the rest of your life. Regular practice of the poses outlined in Chapter 2, especially emphasizing the shoulder stand, should be practiced daily. The shoulder stand should be held for gradually increasing periods, working up to fifteen minutes twice a day.

Yoga may have an effect in as little as a few weeks, but before it takes hold, the usual conventional medications such as propranolol (Inderal and Lopressor) and propylthiouracil (see page 596) should be used to gain control of your symptoms. *It is not safe* to use alternative medicine approaches without taking these antithyroid medications, since your disease may not come under immediate control.

Because they tend to increase your stress levels, caffeine and other stimulants should be replaced by herb teas. Chamomile is a soothing herb tea that is a good substitute.

Practice Visualization

Follow the guidelines for visualization given in Chapter 2. You may wish to imagine your thyroid gland as a butterfly that has become overly active. Gently stroke its wings, sing it a lullaby, and tell it that both it and the centers in the brain and cells affecting its function can relax. As you hold this image in your mind, feel the equivalent effects within your body.

Change Your Diet

Broccoli-hater George Bush's diet may have had something to do with the onset of his hyperthyroidism. Certain vegetables—broccoli, cabbage, cauliflower, Brussels sprouts, kale, collard greens, mustard greens, and other members of the mustard family—have been found to act as natural inhibitors of thyroid function. Their absence in the diet may aggravate the underlying immunity problem at the cause of this disease.

Use Homeopathy and Acupuncture

Homeopathy was used as an adjunct to treatment in one Japanese study, where homeopathic formulations were given to patients after their conventional antithyroid treatment was discontinued. They were found to have reduced numbers of recurrences of their hyperthyroidism and lowered blood levels of autoantibodies.[5] Another study found acupuncture to be successful in treatment, allowing patients to stop medication.[6] Consult an experienced homeopathic or acupuncture practitioner. A few weeks to months may be needed for successful treatment. Meanwhile, you must be treated by the conventional medications in order to avoid worsening of your disease.

Quit Smoking

An association has been found between cigarette smoking and risk for developing Grave's disease.[7] See Chapter 2 for tips on how to quit smoking.

Conventional Medicine Approaches to Hyperthyroidism

Medications that decrease thyroid hormone production, or limit its effects, and radiation that destroys hormone-producing cells are by far the most common treatments for hyperthyroidism. However, after drug treatment is discontinued, more than 50 percent of patients have recurrence of symptoms, requiring another form of treatment. Radiation is easy and effective but may not be best for you. Following are the conventional medicine approaches from which to choose.

Drug Treatments

Antithyroid drugs such as propylthiouracil (PTU) and methimazole (Tapazol) are the mainstay in conventional medical treatment of younger patients. These drugs prevent manufacture of thyroid hormone within the gland. If you take these medications, you must also take supplemental thyroid hormone tablets to prevent hypothyroidism. Propranolol (Inderal) is a "beta-blocking" drug that blocks some of the systemic effects of thyroid hormone and thus controls symptoms in about 90 percent of all users. Lithium sometimes has been given to effectively reduce thyroid function, and has fewer side effects than PTU and Inderal. These drugs can have significant, unacceptable side effects.

After drug treatment is discontinued, more than 50 percent of all patients have a recurrence of symptoms, requiring another form of treatment.

Radioactive Iodine Treatment

Destruction of thyroid tissue by radioactive iodine is now the treatment of choice for hyperthyroidism. A radioactive iodine isotope is mixed with water, then taken orally. It is absorbed from the intestine, carried to the thyroid through the bloodstream, and selectively concentrated within the thyroid cells. There the concentrated radioactivity destroys these cells without injury to other tissue, making it, indeed, a "magic bullet."

Radioactive iodine can be given in larger doses to completely destroy thyroid function and more rapidly relieve symptoms, or in smaller doses in an attempt to leave you with normal thyroid function and avoid posttreatment hypothyroidism. Symptoms of hyperthyroidism are usually gone after two to three months.

Treatment is successful in 90 percent of the cases after one dose of isotope, and failures are rare, although a second dose may be necessary. Cure of hyperthyroidism is permanent, and other advantages include treatment that is quick, easy, one-third to one-half the cost of surgery or continuing medication, and with no discomfort, scarring, or hospitalization.

Some endocrinologists do not advise this treatment for younger patients. It should not be used if you are pregnant, or likely to become pregnant within the next six months, because of possible genetic mutation induced by radiation.

The effects of the radioactive iodine are cumulative over time, as the radiation-damaged thyroid cells eventually die. Ten years after treatment, you have a 40 to 70 percent chance you will be hypothyroid, and this increases by 2 to 3 percent each year thereafter. Therefore, most specialists recommend you take lifelong thyroid replacement medication to avoid the insidious effects of hypothyroidism, which may not be immediately recognizable.

Surgical Approach to Hyperthyroidism

Surgical treatment of hyperthyroidism removes all or almost all of the gland (or half of it, in the rare case of the "toxic nodule"), leaving a remnant of each lobe to protect the blood supply of the parathyroid glands and act as some insurance against hypothyroidism, should you stop taking replacement hormone pills. Twenty-five percent of all patients become hypothyroid and need to take thyroid replacement pills for the rest of their lives. Five percent have recurrent hyperthyroidism because too much of the gland has been left behind.

Because of the fear of complications,

surgery is infrequently used to treat hyperthyroidism in the United States. Its advantages are that the effect of treatment is quick, prolonged therapy is unnecessary, and you avoid the possible risks of radioactive iodine treatment. Surgery should be considered if you are a younger patient unable or unwilling to rigidly follow a medical treatment regimen, pregnant, or unable to tolerate antithyroid drugs, or if you refuse radioactive iodine treatment. Also, if your gland is large, causing pressure symptoms, surgery may be the best form of therapy for you, for mechanical and cosmetic reasons. Radioactive iodine does not shrink the gland to a significant extent.

If your hyperthyroidism is caused by a "toxic nodule," surgeons would argue that removing the nodule, along with its lobe, is better than medications or radioactive iodine. Unlike the other treatment options, the tissue can be examined completely for malignancy, no X-ray exposure takes place, much less problem with hypothyroidism develops afterward, and the problem is rapidly solved.

Of course, surgery may have complications that can be quite devastating (see page 594). Although such problems are rare in experienced hands, the overall complication rate is higher for surgery for hyperthyroidism than for other types of thyroid disease. Also, as the incidence of thyroid surgery has decreased, experienced thyroid surgeons are harder to find.

HYPERTHYROIDISM SUMMARY

Prevention

Diet and Supplements

- Follow a low-fat, high-fiber diet.
- Add broccoli, cabbage, Brussels sprouts, kale, collard greens, and mustard greens to your diet.

Lifestyle

- Don't smoke.
- Practice daily yoga, especially the shoulder stand.
- Practice stress management.

Alternative Medicine Approaches

- Follow the preventive guidelines, above.
- Use acupuncture, hypnosis, homeopathy.
- Practice visualization.

Conventional Medicine Approaches

- Antithyroid medication—propylthiouracil (PTU) and methimazole (Tapazol).
- "Beta-blocking" drugs—propranolol (Inderal).
- Lithium.
- Radioactive iodine.

Surgical Approaches

- Thyroid lobectomy—for "toxic" nodule only.
- Subtotal thyroidectomy.
- Total thyroidectomy.

Goiter

As many as one in ten of the elderly may suffer from goiter, which is a diffuse enlargement of the thyroid gland. It develops when a normal-sized thyroid is unable to make sufficient thyroid hormone to shut off the pituitary's production of thyroid-stimulating hormone (TSH). A goiter can grow when the thyroid is not supplied with enough iodine to make thyroid hormone, when "goitrogenic" substances interfere with hormone manufacture, or when a genetic defect prevents normal hormone formation. The gland then enlarges until it is able to produce sufficient thyroid hormone to turn down TSH stimulation.

Goiter is the most common glandular problem in the world. The most common cause is a lack of iodine in the diet, most often in developing areas as in Africa. Such endemic goiter is now uncommon in the United States, because iodine is routinely added to table salt. In developed countries an immunologic mistake causing antibodies to attack the thyroid (Hashimoto's thyroiditis) is the most common cause of goiter. "Goitrogenic" foods such as vegetables of the cabbage family, turnips, and soy milk contain substances that can lead to decreased thyroid hormone manufacture, especially when associated with inadequate iodine intake from the diet. Drugs such as lithium and certain asthma medications can have a similar goiter-inducing effect.

If you have a goiter, you are not likely to be hypothyroid. The enlarged gland usually manages to produce enough thyroid hormone to keep your body's cells and organs running at a normal rate. You may have symptoms, however, if your gland enlarges enough to press against your windpipe, the trachea, in which case you may experience coughing, wheezing, or a sense of shortness of breath. Pressure against the esophagus can create swallowing difficulty. A large, obvious swelling may be of cosmetic concern.

Alternative Medicine Approaches to Goiter

The initial approach to treatment of goiter is assurance of adequate iodine in your diet and avoidance of goitrogenic foods and medication. Surgery can be considered if your enlarged thyroid is causing you difficulty in breathing or swallowing, local discomfort, or if you are unhappy with the way it looks. Surgical treatment is not urgent, so you can safely give the following recommendations a trial.

Practice Stress Management and Yoga Daily

Alternative medicine treatments for goiter shown to be effective include yoga postures. The shoulder stand, especially, helps to rebalance thyroid activity. It should be held for increasing lengths of time, gradually up to fifteen minutes twice daily.

Change Your Diet

Insufficient dietary intake of iodine, necessary for your thyroid to make thyroid hormone, is a major cause of goiter. The amounts of iodine needed are quite low, and by watching your diet, you can ensure that you get enough. Fish and other seafoods contain iodine. If you do not eat these items, you can eat kelp or seaweed regularly, or take a kelp supplement or multivitamin pill containing iodine. The Japanese suffer from thyroid diseases only very rarely. They usually eat up to one-third of their diets from sea-based food items such as fish, kelp, and other seaweeds. However, if they adopt a Western diet, they develop similar rates of thyroid illness.

Iodine is added to table salt. The problem with relying on table salt to provide your iodine requirements is that long-term intake of sodium chloride in large amounts may be associated with high blood pressure. Make certain you do not take too much iodine, which would suppress your thyroid; no more than six kelp capsules per day is recommended. One study showed decrease in goiter size in children supplemented with iodized poppy-seed oil.[8]

Avoid excess consumption of goitrogenic cruciferous vegetables such as cabbage, broccoli, or cauliflower, which inhibit thyroid function.

Take Supplements

Vitamins A, B-complex, C, and E; minerals zinc, copper, chromium, and selenium; and the amino acid tyrosine may all play a role in proper thyroid function, though no specific research has documented their effectiveness in treating goiter. You may wish to follow the supplement guidelines given in Chapter 2.

Use Homeopathy and Hypnosis

Both of these modalities have shown anecdotal promise in the treatment of this disease. Further research is needed. Meanwhile, since side effects are absent, an experienced homeopath or hypnotist can customize a remedy or treatment plan appropriate for you. Information on both of these modalities can be found in the Resources section of this book.

Practice Visualization

Follow the guidelines given for visualization in Chapter 2. You may wish to use the following specific visualization: See your thyroid as a slightly enlarged inflatable pillow.

Gently remove some of the air, making it normal size again. Visualize this final result at the same time as feeling it take place within your neck.

Conventional Medicine Approaches to Goiter

Supplemental thyroid hormone medication (Synthroid) turns down the pituitary's TSH stimulation. This regimen may be sufficient to prevent further enlargement and may cause some shrinkage. However, enough shrinkage to relieve established pressure symptoms or cosmetic concerns may not occur. Radioactive iodine treatment is not very effective in producing shrinkage. Large doses are required and not recommended.

Surgical Approaches to Goiter

Surgery is necessary in a few cases to relieve symptoms, improve cosmetic appearance, and whenever it is a possibility that the gland may harbor a malignancy. There are two surgical options. *Subtotal thyroidectomy* removes most of the gland, leaving enough behind to protect the blood supply to the parathyroid glands and the nerves to the voice box. Thyroid hormone supplementation is then prescribed postoperatively to suppress stimulation of the remaining thyroid tissue to prevent recurrent enlargement. *Total thyroidectomy* removes all of the gland and is best if obstructive symptoms are prominent. It eliminates the possibility of recurrence, but has a higher complication rate. You must take thyroid replacement hormone pills afterward. For a discussion of the thyroid operations, see page 604.

GOITER SUMMARY

Prevention

Diet and Supplements

- Follow a low-fat, high-fiber diet.
- Eat foods containing iodine: seaweed, kelp, fish.
- Avoid excess broccoli, cabbage, cauliflower, kale, mustard greens.
- Follow the supplement guidelines given in Chapter 2.

Lifestyle

- Practice daily yoga postures, especially the shoulder stand.
- Practice stress management.

Alternative Medicine Approaches

- Follow the preventive guidelines, above.
- Vitamins A, B-complex, C, E; minerals zinc, copper, chromium, selenium; amino acid tyrosine.
- Use acupuncture, hypnosis, homeopathy.
- Practice visualization.

Conventional Medicine Approach

- Thyroid hormone medication (Synthroid).

Surgical Approaches

- Subtotal thyroidectomy.
- Total thyroidectomy.

Thyroid Cancer

Thyroid cancer can occur at any age, with a peak incidence in the twenties and thirties. There will be an estimated 20,700 new cases diagnosed in 2002 and 1,300 deaths.[9] More women than men develop this cancer, in a three-to-one ratio. The cause of thyroid cancer is unknown, though one known predisposing risk factor is prior X-ray exposure to the region of your head and neck.

These cancers are usually found as a single thyroid nodule that does not pick up isotope on a thyroid scan, thereby being seen as a blank or "cold" area. Roughly 10 to 20 percent of all cold nodules are malignant. This percentage is higher in males and in the age groups under age 21 and over age 60. If you have had a history of X-ray therapy in the vicinity of the neck, your nodule is more likely to be malignant. If the nodule is hard, gritty, or fixed to the underlying tissue, or there are enlarged lymph nodes near the thyroid, the possibility of malignancy is increased. Only 5 percent of all thyroid cancers cause local symptoms, but if your nodule causes pain, swallowing difficulty, or voice change, malignancy is more likely.

Cancerous nodules are also those more likely to have been noted recently and to be growing rapidly. If a nodule enlarges during an attempt at thyroid suppression, it is more suspicious. Surgical reports in the medical literature report that anywhere from 20 to 60 percent of all specimens show malignancy.

The several different cell types of thyroid cancer are grouped into *well-differentiated* (papillary, follicular, and medullary) and *undifferentiated* categories. The clinical course and prognosis are quite different for the various types. In general, the benign natural history of well-differentiated thyroid cancer is illustrated by the fact that rigorous microscopic examination of "normal" thyroid glands picks up tiny islands of cancer in 5 to 15 percent of the overall population. Thus, up to 40 million unsuspecting Americans have thyroid cancer that never becomes evident or causes a problem.

Papillary cancer (80 percent of all cases) is almost always slow growing and unaggressive, and is the cancer with the best prognosis. If you had to have a cancer, other than skin cancer, this is the type you would pick. With proper treatment, 95 percent of all patients live a normal life span, even if spread to local lymph glands has already occurred. (See Table 21.1.) Follicular cancer (10 percent of the cases) is also relatively benign, though less so than papillary.

Medullary cancer (5 percent of the cases) does not actually involve the thyroid hormone–producing cells, but arises from "parafollicular" cells, of different origin, though in close approximation with the usual thyroid cells. These cells produce the hormone thyrocalcitonin, which helps regulate calcium balance. Medullary cancer is usually well differentiated, and takes two forms. The "familial type," which runs in families, is more aggressive than the more common "sporadic type."

Undifferentiated thyroid cancer (1 percent of the cases) is one of the worst types of malignancies. Most patients succumb within a matter of months, and cures are very rare. This type of cancer usually develops from a long-standing preexisting well-differentiated tumor.

Alternative Medicine Approaches to Thyroid Cancer

Alternative medicine lifestyle approaches may be utilized to help prevent and possibly to treat thyroid cancer and to avoid recurrence. Although you should have any tumor removed surgically, by instituting the following changes, you can assist your body in preventing a return of your disease.

Exercise Regularly

Prevention plays a role in this disease. Persons who exercised during college were found to have a lower incidence.[11] Once you have developed this cancer, adopting an active exercise program may help prevent its recurrence.

TABLE **21.1.**
Prognosis of Thyroid Cancer[10]

	Percent of Patients Surviving 5 Years	Percent of Patients in This Stage
All Patients	95.2%	
Not Staged	81.9%	4%
By Stage		
Localized to thyroid	99.3%	63%
Lymph node spread	94.1%	28%
Distant spread	41.7%	4%

Limit X-ray Exposure to Your Neck

Make certain to limit X-ray exposure to your head and neck, thereby averting a major risk factor, which begins above a total dose of 100 rads. You can simply request that a lead shield be placed over your neck at the time you receive any X-rays, such as a mammogram, and keep a running record of how much exposure you have endured.

Change Your Lifestyle

Surgery should be chosen if you have a good chance of cure by this method. An alternative medicine program may be used for follow-up after surgical removal of your primary tumor, to prevent its recurrence. Following the low-fat, high-fiber, vegetarian diet; stress reduction, yoga; and visualization described in Chapter 2 may be beneficial. Homeopathy, acupuncture, and qi gong may be utilized as well, and some success has been anecdotally reported, although further research is needed. Aromatherapy has been found helpful in reducing the stress associated with cancer.[12] If you have an inoperable tumor, an alternative medicine program may be helpful. Refer to Resources on page 721.

Practice Visualization

You may wish to try this specific visualization: Imagine your tumor as a small mushroom growing on the side of a mound of bread. Your white cells surround it and gobble it all up. Feel this also taking place within your body. See the final result as free of any cancer cells, then place your white cells in strategic positions to prevent any recurrence.

Conventional Medicine Approaches to Thyroid Cancer

Surgery is the primary treatment for thyroid cancer. However, thyroid medication and radioactive iodine isotope I-131 treatment can be used as adjuncts after surgery and are advised for most high-risk patients. Thyroid medication suppresses TSH, which may have a stimulatory effect on tumor tissue and is usually recommended for all patients. I-131 concentrates in thyroid cancer tissue and may destroy any tumor cells that have been left behind in the neck or that have already spread elsewhere in the body. These treatments have been shown to decrease recurrence rates and improve survival in differentiated cancer. At this point, adding radioactive iodine is controversial if you already are in a low-risk group and have an excellent prognosis. You need to discuss the latest recommendations with your doctor.

Surgical Approaches to Thyroid Cancer

While there is no dispute that surgery is justified, controversy remains about just how much thyroid and adjacent tissue to remove. A major concern, on the one hand, is that well-differentiated thyroid cancer usually pursues a benign course, though not invariably so. On the other hand, aggressive surgery can cause complications that may be worse than the disease your surgeon is trying to cure. If it were not for the danger of permanent damage to the vocal cords (up to 14 percent) and parathyroid glands (up to 11 percent), more common after removing the whole gland, most practitioners would favor such surgery. Many experienced surgeons, however, report complication rates of less than 1 to 3 percent.

The minimum operation should include

complete removal of the lobe containing the tumor, along with the isthmus, the area of thyroid tissue in front of the trachea that connects the two lobes. Simply removing the lump is not acceptable because of the high rate of tumor recurrence and because this is no safer than removing the whole lobe.

The controversy boils down to "how much is enough surgery?" The aggressive position argues that all patients with thyroid cancer should have all of their thyroid tissue removed because it decreases the chance for a local recurrence and increases the effectiveness of postoperative blood tests, scans for diagnosis, and radioactive iodine treatment of any cancer spread. The opposite, conservative opinion is that removing only the thyroid lobe containing the tumor and any suspicious-looking lymph glands is sufficient and decreases the chances for a complication, decreases the operative time, and, since the opposite lobe is left behind, may avoid hypothyroidism if you fail to take postoperative thyroid medication. Little evidence suggests that either position is best, since no randomized studies comparing the two approaches has ever been done, and at present, most surgeons favor a middle ground that is closer to the conservative position.

However, there is a subpopulation of patients with differentiated tumors who do not do as well as the rest of the patients. Many risk-criteria formats have been devised that attempt to separate those patients at lower risk from those at higher risk who might do better with more extensive surgery. For example, the AMES criteria, formulated by Dr. Blake Cady of the New England Deaconess Hospital in Boston, identifies the following as low risk factors for death from thyroid cancer: women 50 years of age and younger and men 40 years of age and younger without evidence of distant metastasis. Older patients are included in this low-risk group if they have tumors less than 5 centimeters and papillary cancer without gross invasion outside the thyroid itself or follicular cancer without invasion into the thin tissue layer covering the thyroid (capsule) or into thyroid blood vessels. Any distant spread puts you in the high-risk group. Using these criteria, Dr. Cady found a 98 percent fifteen-year survival for patients at low risk and 47 percent for high-risk patients.[13]

Although in low-risk patients the Mayo Clinic has demonstrated a threefold increase in local tumor recurrence and lymph node spread when the surgery was limited to one lobe only, there has been no demonstrated improvement in survival in low-risk patients who have had more extensive surgery removing most or all of both lobes.[14]

An operation that removes most or all of the thyroid gland and adjacent lymph nodes has been shown to reduce recurrence rate as well as increase survival if you are in the high-risk group or have a medullary or undifferentiated cell type, or if your neck has previously been treated with radiation. Also, most thyroid surgeons would advise this operation if you have a follicular cell type.

You will need to talk over your specific risk factors with your surgeon as well as his or her philosophy and experience. For a discussion of the specific thyroid operations, see page 604.

After surgery, patients with well-differentiated thyroid cancer are usually placed on lifelong thyroid medication, both to ensure against hypothyroidism and to suppress stimulation of any remaining normal or cancerous thyroid tissue.

THYROID CANCER SUMMARY

Prevention

Diet and Supplements

- Follow a low-fat, high-fiber, whole-foods diet, to optimize immune function.
- Follow the supplement guide given in Chapter 2.

Lifestyle

- Exercise 1 hour, 3–5 times weekly.
- Limit X-ray exposure to your neck.
- Practice yoga daily, especially the shoulder stand.
- Practice stress management.

Alternative Medicine Approaches

- Follow the preventive measures, above.
- Use hypnosis, acupuncture, aromatherapy, qi gong.
- Practice visualization.

Conventional Medicine Approaches

- Suppression—thyroid hormone medication (Synthroid)—after surgery.
- Radioactive iodine isotope I-131—after surgery.

Surgical Approaches

- Thyroid lobectomy.
- Subtotal thyroidectomy.
- Total thyroidectomy.

Specific Thyroid Operations

In the late nineteenth century, Dr. Theodor Kocher of Switzerland, one of the pioneers of surgery, developed modern techniques that reduced the mortality from thyroid operations from about 50 percent to less than 1 percent, a miraculous accomplishment considering the lack of modern anesthesia, drugs, and intensive care units. For this work, in 1909, he received the first Nobel Prize awarded to a surgeon.

Thyroid surgery is a favorite operation for surgeons because of its challenge: it requires meticulous techniques in a small critical area of anatomy. The aim is to remove the appropriate amount of thyroid tissue, while at the same time avoiding damage to your parathyroid glands and the nerves of your voice box (larynx).

You are admitted to the hospital on the morning of surgery. The operation is done under general anesthesia. After you are asleep, a tube is placed down your windpipe to ensure that your breathing is protected—the operation is performed just on top of your upper airway. A "low collar," gently curved, three-inch incision is placed within one of your skin folds. Skin flaps are elevated to expose the thyroid. During the procedure, your surgeon identifies and protects nerves that control your voice box and avoids damage to the parathyroid glands, which regulate calcium levels.

The three types of operation are *total thyroidectomy,* in which all thyroid tissue is removed, *subtotal thyroidectomy,* where a small amount of tissue is left behind to manufacture thyroid hormone and to protect the blood supply to the parathyroid glands, and *lobectomy with isthmusectomy,* which removes one lobe and the isthmus, the bridge of tissue connecting to the other lobe. (See Figure 21.2.) After the tissue is removed, the incision is closed with stitches, staples, or skin tapes.

Postoperatively, you may experience some neck stiffness because of the extended position required by this surgery. The slight hoarseness from the endotracheal tube rubbing on your vocal cords should disappear in a few days. You may have some neck swelling and bruising. If you have a lobectomy, everything went extremely well, and you are fine after several hours of observation, you may be discharged the evening of your surgery if your surgeon thinks it safe. More likely, you will be discharged in one or two days. If concern for your parathyroid function develops, a longer stay, with blood tests to measure calcium levels, may be necessary.

Stitches or staples, if any, are removed in two or three days. You can resume your normal activities as soon as comfort allows. After a year or so, most incisions are inconspicuous. If desired, your scar may be hidden by a scarf, necklace, or high collar.

The mortality rate from thyroid surgery is 1 in 1,000 cases. Hemorrhage, while rare, is always a worry, since even a relatively small amount of bleeding may compress the windpipe, causing asphyxiation. Some surgeons routinely put a drain in the incision to avoid this hazard. Infection of the incision is very rare because of the neck's excellent blood supply.

During surgery, the main complications your surgeon has to guard against involve the laryngeal nerves and parathyroid glands. Permanent damage, although rare, can be quite disabling. The worry is enhanced by the fact that there is some normal anatomical variation in the position and number of nerve trunks. Likewise, the parathyroid glands may vary in number and position and are hard to distinguish from lymph glands, thyroid nodules, and lumps of fat.

Two sets of nerves pass to the larynx or voice box. The two *recurrent* laryngeal nerves control the opening of the vocal cords. Damage to one nerve causes hoarseness. Damage to both may cause a life-threatening airway obstruction. Temporary damage due

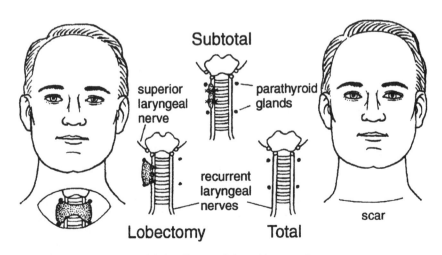

Fig. 21.2 Types of thyroid operations

to stretching or squeezing is seen in 3 to 4 percent of all cases. Permanent damage occurs in 0.5 percent. Damage to both nerves is extremely rare, found only during surgery on both lobes. However, fear of this damage is a major reason many surgeons favor a more conservative approach to treating thyroid cancer.

The two *superior* laryngeal nerves help control the strength and timbre of your voice. Damage may not even be noticed by some persons. Others may note an easy fatigability of voice and, especially, inability to sing or sustain high notes. Damage is not a threat to life.

Parathyroid gland complications that occur during thyroid surgery may be temporary or permanent. The parathyroid glands are responsible for calcium balance.

The complication rates for the various types of thyroidectomy vary widely in the surgical literature. Reports documenting permanent recurrent laryngeal nerve injury vary from 0 to 14 percent and permanent hypoparathyroidism from 1.2 to 11 percent. Your risk depends on your type of disease, age, underlying medical condition, and neck size; the extent of the surgery; and whether the procedure is an initial or secondary neck operation. However, by far the most important factor is the skill and experience of your surgeon.

A study of 5,860 patients undergoing thyroid surgery in Maryland from 1991 to 1996 in 52 hospitals involving 658 surgeons looked at the complication rates of "high-volume" (about 15 to 20 cases per year) compared with "low-volume" surgeons (less than 1 case per year). Although it found that the statewide average was only 0.8 percent nerve injury and 0.3 percent hypoparathyroidism, there was a significant pattern of association between increasing surgeon volume and improved outcomes. The high-volume surgeons had one-third fewer complications for benign conditions and two-thirds fewer complications for cancer surgery than the low-volume surgeons.[15]

CHAPTER 22

BACK, NECK, AND JOINTS

The Back

Mac, an active 55-year-old house painter, had suffered from back pain off and on for years. Finally, he had agonized enough, and sought a surgical solution. He consulted a total of five different specialists, all of whom recommended surgery for his protruding disk. However, his last consultant, an internist, said to him, "Listen, Mac, if you just lose twenty-five pounds, you may be able to save yourself from an operation." Mac went on an eating plan similar to the one discussed in Chapter 2, eliminating added fats from his diet and increasing his fiber intake. He easily lost the twenty-five pounds, and his back pain disappeared. He was still happily thinner, free of pain, and painting houses ten years later.

"Oh, my aching back!" is an all too common cliché for many of us. As many as 60 to 80 percent of all Americans are disabled by back or neck pain for at least a brief period at some point during their lives. This epidemic is becoming more frequent, with a cost of up to $100 billion each year in healthcare expenses and absenteeism. Every day, about 31 million Americans, 14 percent of the population, suffer from some degree of back pain, which, next to colds, is the most common cause of lost workdays.[1]

As humans, our upright posture places our backs at risk for the effects of gravity. We are literally "propped up" for a fall: if our backs are not regularly flexed and exercised, the muscles, cartilages, and disks can become weak, and a sudden twist while

607

lifting groceries, for example, can result in the nucleus of the disk becoming displaced and irritating a nerve. Sitting for long periods of time in chairs—including in whatever position you are sitting while reading this book—chronically puts pressure on the lower two disks of the back, as well as the disks at the base of the neck.

Perhaps you have wondered whether or not a surgical fix could help resolve your back pain. Author Fred Setterberg, writing about his own struggle with back discomfort, which began one day while he was emptying the garbage, stated: "At least two-thirds of people with lower back pain get better within 30 days, regardless of treatment. . . . One month! I wasn't about to surrender my back, the flexible pole around which flagged my very being, for an entire month. Impatiently, I wanted action."[2]

But is an operation the answer for you? Since up to 98 percent of all back pain patients have been found to be better in two months without surgery,[3] you may be able to use alternative medicine to help you get through this period, and thereby avoid surgery.

What if you are discovered to have an abnormal disk? Interestingly, such findings may just be coincidental. A study of MRI back exams on volunteers who had never had back complaints found that two-thirds of them had some abnormality and one-quarter had herniated disks.[4] Bad disks are so common you can't simply assume that this is the cause for your discomfort, even if you have tested positive for one.

Indeed, the vast majority of people with back pain—up to 85 to 98 percent—are not found to have a specific cause.[5] If you have back discomfort, it is *most* likely simply because you do not exercise enough, don't stretch regularly, and suffer from the effects of

stress, which chronically tightens your muscles. Dr. John Basmajian, a biofeedback researcher at Atlanta's Emory Medical Center, has stated, "Back pain is just a tension headache that has slipped down the back."[6] Dr. Charles Steiner, a New Jersey osteopath, has found that all but 2 percent of low back pain is caused by muscular spasm, which can be relieved by manipulation treatment.[7] Another study showed that only 1.4 percent of all patients with back pain consulting a family doctor actually had disk disease.[8]

Given these statistics, even though surgery to relieve back pain may be an enormous blessing to some people, many investigators feel it is currently overutilized, with rates fifteen times as high in some parts of the country as in others.[9] Each year in the United States, more than 200,000 operations are performed to remove part of one or more vertebrae. As many as one out of six of these patients requires another back operation within one year, and 10 percent are left with a "failed back syndrome"—where surgery didn't help, and they end up in *more* pain even after a series of operations.[10] Most investigations looking at why failures occur with surgery conclude that an operation was not really indicated in the first place.

We both therefore recommend, since so many patients complain of side effects after back surgery, that you try a program of alternative medicine approaches to treat your back pain before you choose surgery. Even if your pain moves down the back of your leg (called *sciatica*, seen in only 1.5 percent of all patients with acute back pain), or is accompanied by numbness or tingling and therefore may be due to pressure of a slipped disk or bone spur on your back's nerve roots, you may be able to avoid an operation by first trying the alternative regimen given on page 613.

A simple program of stretches, exercise, and dietary change usually quickly brings excellent relief, along with significant benefits to the rest of your life as well.

How Your Back Works

Sometimes the spine is called the "lifebone." Its bony structure is comprised of a stack of bones call *vertebrae.* Seven vertebrae are located in the neck (cervical), twelve in the chest (thoracic), five in the low back (lumbar), five in the pelvis (sacral), and four in the tail bone (coccygeal), giving you a grand total of thirty-three. (See Figure 22.1.)

Each vertebra has a rounded *body* in front, and two backward-projecting *lamina,* which meet in the middle to form a bony arch. These lamina have cartilage-covered *articular processes* above and below, which connect to neighboring articular processes, forming your back's joints.

Between each of your neck, chest, and low back vertebrae sit the twenty-three shock-absorbing soft cartilages, the *vertebral disks.* Each disk is made up of an outer, tough fibrous layer *(annulus)* and an inner, softer gel-like substance *(nucleus);* your disks thus resemble jelly doughnuts. The vertebrae of your sacrum and tailbone are fused together, so that they do not contain any disks. The elasticity of the disks and the lamina articular processes work together to allow your vertebrae to move upon themselves.

This whole "stack of blocks and cushions" is kept in place by ever-serving ligaments attaching the vertebrae together, as well as by the back muscles, which are linked to bony extensions projecting off the lamina (the *transverse* and *spinous processes*). The only part of your vertebra you can easily feel is the

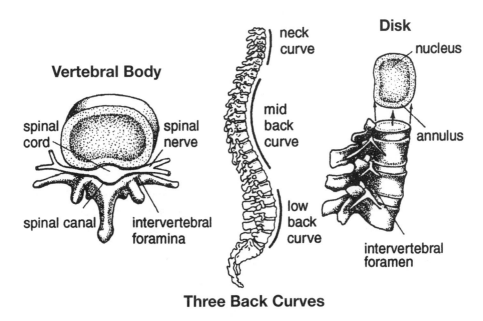

Vertebral Body

spinal cord

spinal nerve

spinal canal

intervertebral foramina

neck curve

mid back curve

low back curve

Three Back Curves

Disk

nucleus

annulus

intervertebral foramen

Fig. 22.1 The anatomy of the back

spinous process, which forms the ridge of your backbone.

A normal alignment of bones, cartilages, and muscles allows for flexibility, so you can bend forward and backward, twist side-to-side, and carry out your daily activities with ease. When seen from the side, your spine should have three natural, gentle curves: the neck forward, the thoracic spine backward, and the low back forward; your ears, shoulders, and hips should be in a straight line. When seen from the front, your ears, shoulders, and hips should be parallel with each other and level with the ground. These relationships ensure even distribution of weight and muscle pull on your vertebrae, making you least vulnerable to discomfort and injury.

A very important duty of your vertebral column is to protect your spinal cord and its nerve branches. The cord lies safely within the *vertebral canal,* formed by the bony circle of the vertebral body and its lamina. Nerves branch off the cord at each level. The lamina of adjacent vertebrae form a bony circle called the *intervertebral foramen,* through which these nerves exit to your skin, muscles, and organs.

Back Problems

When the natural curves of your spine are changed by chronically incorrect posture, aging, injury, or disease, you may develop back discomfort. The postural strain resulting from inappropriate work habits or body use is the most common cause of back pain. Lifting primarily using your back muscles, or while leaning or twisting, causes undue strain on those muscles attaching to your vertebrae. You then may experience muscle spasm, stiff-ness, aching, or limitation of comfortable movement.

Chronic distortion of your back's natural curves in turn increases pressure on your disks and articular surfaces, causing them to flatten, wear out faster, or even suddenly break down. Collapsed disks allow your vertebrae to slip back and forth on each other, and your spine to become unstable. The ligaments and fibrous part of the disk can then be stretched or torn, giving you severe pain.

A "slipped" disk does not actually slip, but rather, the inner substance presses against the fibrous outer ring, creating a bulge into the spinal canal. (See Figure 22.2.) A "ruptured" or "herniated" disk occurs whenever the inner gel squeezes out through a hole in the outer ring. With associated loss of water, the displaced substance begins to harden, and can pinch one or more nerves emerging between the vertebrae, or even press on the spinal cord itself. Pressure on these nerves causes pain, numbness, and tingling in your back or down into your arms and legs, and can also lead to bowel and bladder disturbances. Ninety-five percent of such slipped or ruptured disks occur in the "lumbar" region, the low-back part of your spine.

Simply the "normal" wear and tear of aging leaves you at risk for arthritis, deformities, and bone spurs that can create pain whenever the vertebrae move against each other. *Spinal stenosis* develops when the spinal canal is narrowed by these processes. Your spinal cord and its nerves can be squeezed and irritated, causing symptoms similar to a bulging disk. If not corrected, permanent damage may result.

Decreased calcification of the bones (osteoporosis) results in excessively brittle bones subject to compression fractures; broken bones

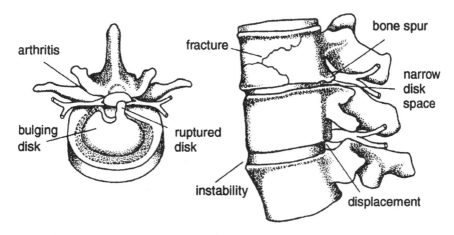

Fig. 22.2 Types of vertebral and disk problems

are a very common source of back pain and nerve irritation in women after menopause, so you should be checked for this and act preventively, by adopting the alternative medicine changes given on page 613.

How Back Problems Are Diagnosed

In addition to chronic back strain and disk disease, various other disorders such as arthritis, infection, and, rarely, tumors can cause back and neck pain, so you need a full evaluation before embarking on any course of treatment.

History

A careful history is the first step in diagnosing your back problem. You should be asked about your symptoms of pain and its pattern, weakness in any muscles, presence of numbness and tingling, and if you have any difficulties with bladder and bowel control and sexual function. Your doctor should know about your exercise habits, job requirements at work, and any previous injury. It is especially important to tell your doctor what triggers and what relieves your symptoms. Report any known medical problems and any medicines you are taking.

Physical Exam

The physical exam should include evaluation of your posture while you sit, lie, stand, walk, bend, twist, and perform other movements. The alignment of your three natural spinal curves should be evaluated. Office testing should also include you moving your arms and legs into certain positions to check their flexibility and range of motion, and to see if this causes discomfort. One of the most useful tests is the "straight leg raising test." You lie flat on your back, while your doctor raises each of your legs, with the knee straight; pain in your leg from this maneuver may indicate disk protrusion.

Your doctor should also test your reflexes and strength in various muscles, as well as check for decreased or absent sensation to pin prick, vibration, heat and cold, and light touch. These simple tests can pick up early nerve damage.

X-Rays

Routine back X-rays show the alignment and the spacing between your vertebrae. If narrowing is found, it indicates flattened disks. X-rays also show vertebral fractures, bone spurs, arthritis, and osteoporosis. Since your disks themselves do not show up on routine X-rays, some authorities suggest skipping these extra sources of radiation, at an average cost of $100 or more, and moving right into the CAT scan or MRI if your symptoms are suggestive of a disk problem needing surgery.

However, only if you are contemplating an operation, or your doctor suspects other sources for your pain, should you have those tests.

CAT Scan

For this study, you lay inside a spinning arm that takes multiple X-ray images that a computer reassembles to produce cross sections of your anatomy. With some units, three-dimensional images can be constructed. This study shows the bony anatomy most clearly.

MRI Scan

Here you lay inside an MRI scanner as a powerful magnet changes the orientation of your cell atom components. If you have metal in your body (an artificial joint or a pacemaker, for example), you cannot have this test. The MRI best reveals subtleties in the soft tissue: disks, muscles, ligaments, and nerves.

Bone Scan

You are given an intravenous radioactive tracer formulated to be picked up by bone cells. As you lay under a nuclear camera, this intravenous radioactive isotope test lights up areas of increased bone-tissue activity, which can be caused by fractures, arthritis, infection, or cancer deposits.

Nerve Conduction Tests, Electromyelogram, and Nerve Block

These studies, most often performed by neurologists, test transmission velocity of nerve impulses and your muscles' reactions. They detect damage caused by pressure on the nerves from slipped or ruptured disks, bone spurs, spinal stenosis, or tumors. In nerve conduction tests, two needles are placed through your skin into or next to the nerve to be tested. The distance between them is measured. A small electrical current is then passed through the first needle and picked up by a second while it is connected to a recording device. The strength of the impulse and time it took to arrive are registered. Many different nerves are tested and one arm or leg is compared to the other. Diseased nerves show low electrical impulses and prolonged conduction times. These tests can take an hour or more, and may be quite uncomfortable, though complications are very rare.

An electromyelogram (EMG) is similar to the nerve conduction test, except that a specific muscle's response to electrical stimulation is recorded. Degree of damage can be measured.

In a nerve block test, a nerve is deadened by injecting an anesthetic to see if your pain is eliminated, thereby determining if that particular nerve is, or is not, the source of your symptoms.

Myelogram

This is an invasive test, not recommended unless the other noninvasive tests have been unable to adequately define your problem. Dye that shows up on X-ray is injected directly into your spinal canal. It can show spinal stenosis (narrowing of the spinal canal), protruding disks, or other diseases that cause pressure on the spinal cord and its roots. This test is sometimes combined with a CAT scan, to give your doctor more clear definition of your tissues.

A myelogram is an outpatient procedure. You lie on your side while your doctor uses a local anesthetic to deaden the skin overlying the joint space between two of your vertebrae. A long, thin needle is passed into your spinal canal. The dye is then injected and travels up and down, outlining on X-ray the disks, spinal canal, foramina, spinal cord, and nerve roots. Abnormal bulging and narrowing can thus be seen.

The procedure takes about one hour. The most common problem is headache, which may last for several days or longer. Very rarely, this test itself can *cause* chronic back pain, owing to a reaction to the dye used.[11]

Psychological Testing

If your symptoms are unusually resistant to treatment, psychological testing may be useful. These tests, usually interviews or questionnaires such as the Minnesota Multiphasic Personality Inventory (MMPI) administered by a psychologist, may help determine if chronic stress, depression, or other psychological problems may be playing a role.

Alternative Medicine Approaches to Back Problems

Lucy, *a 59-year-old research chemist, began to experience low back pain, related to the unremitting long hours sitting still in front of a microscope. She began the program given below. She especially found that the yoga stretching, performed very simply and easefully, as a method sometimes termed "gentle yoga," immediately began to relieve her pain. With just a few classes, not only did her back discomfort disappear, but she felt generally much healthier as well.*

"Use them or lose them" applies to the health of your pivotal back and abdominal muscles, and the program given below acts to influence both the availability of nutrients for repair work to your muscles, ligaments, disks, and bones, and their circulation. "Low-back pain is largely a social problem. It's as much due to the way we live as anything else," stated Dr. Kenneth Casey, a pain researcher at the University of Michigan.[12] Orthopedic surgeon Dr. William Donaldson has concluded that the most effective steps you can take to relieve back pain are the ones that only you yourself can take.[13]

Once you have back surgery, you are never anatomically the same. As noted, your problems could also well be made *worse* by this surgery. As one experienced surgeon said, "The last surgery I would ever have is back surgery. My good friend went in to that operation walking and has been unable to walk since."[14] Many people think to themselves, "I'll just take the surgery and get back to work." But this just may not be true for you.

"Your back has never been at greater risk, because you have far more opportunities than your ancestors for damaging yourself with treatment. The wrong choices in back therapy are no more than a phone call away from you. And we're not talking about quackery: these are well-intentioned procedures administered by well-intentioned practitioners," wrote Dr. Edward Tarlov, of Boston's prestigious Lahey Clinic.[15]

As noted, *most* herniated disks tend to shrink over time and heal naturally on their own, within about six weeks, *without* surgery. In prospective studies of patients even with nerve root compression, only 3 to 4 percent required surgery. Interestingly, regardless of the treatment used, 90 percent of all patients complaining of acute low back pain have been found to be free of pain within four weeks.[16]

In addition, unfortunately, treatment of back pain by laminectomy, described on page 623, is simply not always successful in relieving your back discomfort. In a number of studies, only 30 to 60 percent of the laminectomies provided a complete cure, as defined by full relief of pain.[17] A controlled, prospective study comparing exercise with surgery for confirmed disk hernia that had caused sciatica found no difference in pain relief after four and ten years' follow-up.[18] In 10 percent[19] of these surgical patients, the pain was actually made worse. If you are one of the failures, not only are you still in pain, but now you also must live with a stiff back for the rest of your life.

If you have a bad back, you may benefit most by a daily short "back workout" regimen. Even if you do choose to undergo an operation, you may help yourself during your recovery, and prevent further problems, by practicing the following principles, yoga stretches, and back exercises every day.

Adopt Better Posture Habits

Gravity itself is not the problem; poor posture habits, placing pressure on your vulnerable disks, can lead to an unhealthy spine. For ideal posture, which places the least amount of strain on your back, your spine's three natural curves should be preserved. *The low back should be tucked forward, and the upper back arched slightly.* Each segment should sit easily on the next, in alignment with the plumb line of gravity. Watch yourself from the side in the mirror, and see what it takes to put your ears, shoulders, and hips into a straight line.

The cultural support of fashionable high heels may also put you at risk for falling "low" with back pain. Heels on shoes are really a cultural anachronism, developed simply to prevent the foot from coming out of the stirrup while riding horses, and act to throw your back forward and cause the pelvis to tilt backward, the opposite of ideal posture, increasing strain. See if you can find shoes with little or no heel, and make your own personal contribution to creating cultural fashion statements that are healthier.

If your work requires you to be upright for long periods of time on a hard surface, find a compressible mat to stand on, and keep your knees slightly bent.

Sitting puts twice the pressure on your disks as does standing, and four times that of lying down. Sitting with your low back straight, pelvis tucked under, upper back slightly arched, neck squarely over the shoulders, not leaning forward, is the optimum position for preventing back strain and pain. When at home or at work, find a comfortable chair that supports your low back's natural curve. You can use a special low-back cushion, and take it with you when you are away from home or at work, or use a rolled-up towel or sheet if nothing else is available.

Drivers of Japanese or Swedish cars have been found to have a lower rate of ruptured disks than those who drive cars with less "anatomically correct" back support.[20] You can supplement any car seat with your own back pillow. A rolled towel placed in your low back may suffice. Some people prefer a special neck or back pillow, available at stores that sell orthopedic supplies.

If you normally sit for long periods of time, change your position frequently, and stand whenever possible. Take breaks and walk around as often as you can.

Even the position in which you sleep can affect your back. The worst posture is lying on your stomach, which creates a swayback arrangement. Try sleeping on your back or side, with both knees and hips bent; it may help to place one or two pillows under your knees. Since a soft bed allows your spine to sag as your back muscles relax during sleep, use a firm mattress. One study compared persons sleeping on conventional mattresses (500 springs), orthopedic mattresses (720 springs), waterbeds, and waterbeds combined with foam, and found those sleeping on the orthopedic mattress reported the least amount of back pain. Waterbeds came in second.[21] If you have a neck problem, try a special pillow that gives your neck slight traction while you sleep.

Practice Careful Bending and Lifting

When you bend over, don't keep your knees straight, since this puts too much pressure on your back ligaments and the front part of your vertebrae and disks. Even lifting a lightweight object from the wrong position can precipitate back strain and disk disease. First, squat down, keeping the object as close as you can to your body, and use your leg muscles, not your back muscles, to raise the weight. Lift only by first bending your knees, and never from a twisted position.

Maintain Your Optimum Weight

This may be all that is needed to relieve your back problem. In addition to simply making your back have to carry more pounds, excess weight pulls your body forward, placing chronic strain on it. Therefore, weight loss alone may greatly alleviate back pain, even that caused by a protruding disk. Follow the basic high-fiber, low-fat diet suggestions in Chapter 2.

If you have a "potbelly," so common in middle age, it is especially problematic for your back. The normal tone of the abdominal muscles, which decrease the work of the back muscles in holding you up, is gone. You should make an effort to reduce any excess abdominal weight, and act to strengthen your abdominal muscles by adding sit-ups to your exercise routine.

A protruding belly is not just a benign sign of aging, or a result of overeating, but may be associated with excess cortisol production, caused by stress. Follow the stress reduction program below and in Chapter 2. An enlarged abdomen can also be a warning signal for higher cholesterol levels or liver dysfunction.

One study determined that 70 percent of all back problems were associated with excess weight.[22] "Ten pounds of extra weight on the abdomen is equal to 100 pounds of weight at the disk," states Dr. Ronald Taylor, from the Troy-Beaumont in Detroit.[23] Therefore, even if you are only ten or fifteen pounds overweight, it can increase your chances for back pain. Follow the dietary guidelines given in Chapter 2, to help you keep the excess pounds off for good.

Quit Smoking

Scientific studies comparing twins who smoke with those who don't have found an increased incidence of disk disease in those who smoke. Smoking is also a major factor in osteoporosis. Nicotine interferes with the elasticity of your tissues, reduces blood flow to your vertebra, and has been found to decrease your strength, coordination, and balance, making you more likely to injure your bones and muscles.[24] See Chapter 2 for help in quitting smoking.

Prevent Osteoporosis

Osteoporosis makes your bones weak and more at risk for fractures, bone spurs, and instability. This problem is most likely to develop in women after menopause or removal of their ovaries, when estrogen is no longer produced. You are even more at risk if you are white or Asian, slender with small bones, smoke, take cortisone, or follow a diet low in calcium or high in alcohol or caffeine. Since it increases your risk for breast cancer, I do not recommend taking estrogen replacement medication to prevent osteoporosis. Instead, try adopting a vegetarian diet, exercising regularly, and taking supplemental calcium and vitamin D tablets. The recommended dosages are 1,000 mg calcium, 500 mg vitamin C, and 400 IU of vitamin D daily.

Wear a Corset or Body Brace

To support your back and help with its alignment, the new lighter Velcro and nylon braces we see all the folks at the discount warehouses sporting are effective in relieving pain. However, since you need to maintain the strength of your back and neck muscles to prevent future injury, such back or neck braces should be used only as temporary solutions, whenever you have acute pain or during times when you are lifting heavy objects, or are subject to injury during exercise. Don't wear a back belt in its tight position all day long, but only as needed.

Exercise Regularly

Regular exercise both prevents and is one of the best treatments for low back pain. Your back and abdominal muscles support your spine's three natural curves. *Weakness* and *poor flexibility* of these muscles increase the possibility of a disk protruding from its normal position, resulting in enough back pain to lead you to consider surgery. *Injury to the back occurs ten times as often if you are not exercising regularly.*[25]

Even once your disk has degenerated, your pain may be relieved by making the tissues that surround it stronger and more supportive. In one study, 81 percent of the back patients showed improvement after a six-week exercise training program, including those who had previously undergone back surgery.[26] A 1991 Danish study demonstrated that as little as an hour a week made a difference, and gave relief even to those with sciatica and X-ray-documented disk disease.[27] In one study, exercise in which the back was bent slightly backward was found to relieve the pressure on the disk enough to allow healing.[28]

Half sit-ups and sit-ups on an incline are especially helpful for chronic low back pain, because they gradually strengthen your abdominal muscles. Such sit-ups, performed on a slant board, have been found in one study to be all that is needed to relieve chronic low back pain.[29] In another study of sixty-six patients, Dr. Ernest Johnson, a researcher at Ohio State University, found that 80 percent were able to achieve good to excellent relief of pain with one or two daily sit-up sessions. He states about surgery, "As for [spinal] fusion, it's like killing a fly on the windowpane with a sledgehammer. The fly is dead, but you've also broken the glass."[30] Start with 5 sit-ups per day, supporting the feet, and then work up to 100 or so per day. Pelvic tilts may also be helpful. You may want to use a corset-style back supporter at the outset. If you have trouble doing sit-ups, the *Tony Little Ab Isolator* (See "Resources") is particularly helpful.

Regular fast walking is highly recommended; make certain to keep your back straight and your low back tucked under, with your abdominal muscles kept tight. Find a comfortable pair of cushioned shoes.

Swimming is one of the *best* exercises for the relief of back pain, because it relieves you of the pull of your body weight, and in the buoyant state, you can increase the strength of your back muscles without straining your back itself. You can also more easily practice your yoga stretches while in the water, especially if you are in significant pain.

Exercise also relieves back discomfort by increasing your body's natural painkillers, the *endorphins* and *enkephalins.* Any gentle exercise, except that which feels straining to your back, is recommended, generally for one hour, three to five times per week.

You should begin any exercise session with a period of warm-up movements, to soften your disks and stretch your back ligaments and muscles, making them less vulnerable to stress and strain. Avoid sudden, violent movements, especially in the morning, and balance your active exercise with the basic yoga routine given below and discussed more fully in Chapter 2.

Practice Yoga Daily

A daily routine of gentle yoga stretches increases circulation, reduces stress, and is especially suited to help prevent and reverse back difficulties. Significantly, the spaces between the vertebrae, where the disks are located, are systematically stretched, providing increased access for nutrients and removal of waste products—and waist products too—thus ensuring optimum repair of your cartilages. Yoga also acts to give you a deep massage, to help rebalance your muscles and correctly align your spine.

If you have a ruptured disk, you may be able to relieve the pressure on it by gently extending your back, thereby saving yourself from an operation. In one study of 32 patients who went on to require surgery, 30 could not extend their backs more than 5 to 10 degrees, while a 30-degree extension was found in 34 of 35 patients who did not eventually need an operation.[31] *In general, never sit or stand for long periods of time without stretching!*

Yoga is especially helpful for the relief of acute and chronic stress. Emotional stress has been shown to correlate with the degree of severity of back pain, and lack of response to treatment.[32] Dr. John Sarno, in his book *Mind Over Back Pain,* asserts that tension in the back muscles due to emotional stress is the main cause of back pain and even disk problems. He notes, "A combination of further patient observation and a search of the medical literature suggested to me that tension affected the circulation of blood to the involved areas and that when muscles and their associated nerves were deprived of their normal supply of blood, the result was pain in the back and/or limbs. Specifically, a reduction in local blood supply resulted in reduced oxygen to the muscles and nerves, which appeared to be the direct cause of muscle and nerve pain." He cites a report in which electron microscopic studies of the back muscles of patients suffering from back pain showed oxygen deprivation.[33] Whenever you are tense, your body diverts blood away from your back muscles and disks to your arms and legs, in preparation for "fight or flight."

Studies have demonstrated the special efficacy of yoga training for the relief of back pain.[34] The gentle stretches help release stress-related tension, providing improved circulation to both prevent and repair back problems. Particularly useful in the beginning for treatment of disk problems are the half forward bend, back release, knee to chin, child pose, and the yoga seal. Additional yoga stretches, along with the other yoga and stress management practices, as given in Chapter 2, may also be beneficial; just make certain never to strain, and do the backward-bending poses especially gently, since they increase disk pressure. Alternate nostril breathing, followed by visualization, may be especially helpful. For best results, sessions should be conducted twice daily.

The deep relaxation yoga exercise, presented in Chapter 2, is especially helpful therapeutically. Relaxation training has been found to relieve pain in 88 percent of all patients with documented disk disease.[35] Another study showed that patients responded better to treatment if they were taught relaxation exercises.[36] You will also need to address the stress in your life, by learning to take relaxation breaks, or other necessary changes in life and lifestyle.

Maintain Your Activity Level; Rest Only When Necessary

Change has taken place in the traditional recommendation for rest in the treatment of low back pain. Bed rest simply contributes to muscle weakness. A number of recent studies have indicated that maintaining a normal activity level is better for both acute and chronic back pain than resting in bed.[37] Sit up, walk, and stretch as tolerated, just making certain not to strain. Try to go about your regular routines.

However, if you have tried to maintain normal activity without resolution of your pain, before you give yourself over to surgery for a dislocated disk, you may try spending some time lying *flat on your back* in bed, in a position of comfort with your spine's three natural curves aligned, and see if your pain can then be relieved. Lying on your side or sitting increases pressure on the disk, and so must be avoided during this healing time. Such rest alone can often be enough to eliminate persistent back pain, even from a ruptured disk. "Surgery provides only symptomatic relief for low back pain, but bed rest can be curative," asserts Dr. Earnest Johnson, chairman of the Department of Physical Medicine, Ohio State University. He conducted a study of 150 patients with disk disease, in which treatment consisted of rest, exercise—gradual introduction of sit-ups after three to four weeks—and a back corset; only five of these patients ultimately needed surgery.[38]

For severe problems, continuous flat rest in bed may have to be prolonged from a few days to two weeks. Strained muscles can be repaired, and the disk may even ease back into place. Don't rest completely in bed for longer than two weeks, however, since you would then start to lose too much muscle tone and begin to demineralize your bones—and so find it harder to return to health. Most authorities now prefer complete bed rest of no longer than twenty-four to forty-eight hours, so see if you can move about some after this period of time without worsening your pain.

Practice Tai Chi and Qi Gong

These Chinese exercises, with their graceful, gently swaying movements, may help greatly to relieve the underlying tension at the root of your back pain. Further investigation of these modalities, for specific treatment of acute and chronic back problems, is needed.

Use Ice and Heat; Avoid Medication

Ice packs can markedly reduce pain, and are especially important in the first twenty-four to seventy-two hours after injury. Alternating ice and heat every two hours seems to provide the best pain relief, and also acts to increase local circulation of the nutrients that encourage tissue repair. Hot baths can restore your soul, as well as relieve spasm in your back muscles. Try adding arnica oil (see below) to the bath water. One study showed that patients taking less medication actually had diminished pain,[39] and another found that patients receiving no medication did best.[40]

Use Chiropractic and Osteopathy

A number of studies have documented the benefit of chiropractic adjustments for relief of back pain. One investigation showed chiropractic effective for treating acute back pain.[41] A prospective controlled study showed that chiropractic relieved chronic low back pain more quickly and effectively, when compared to physiotherapy.[42] Another showed that its benefits continued through three years of follow-up.[43] Especially if your disk is bulging owing to weakness in the posterior ligament behind it, chiropractic manipulation may be able to correct your problem, helping you avoid surgery. To avoid the rare possibility of injury, seek out a recommended chiropractor.

Osteopathic adjustments are similar to chiropractic, though the techniques differ somewhat; these manipulations also may provide excellent results. The specific technique termed "cranio-sacral" is an osteopathic variant that may be of benefit.

Add Massage, Rolfing, and the Alexander Technique

Massage can provide great relief to tense back muscles, helping them become relaxed enough to maintain proper position and receive optimum nutrition. In one study, massage even beat out acupuncture and self-care for chronic low back pain, in a randomized clinical trial conducted by the University of Washington at Seattle.[44]

Rolfing is a type of deep massage pioneered by Ida Rolf. Experience has refined this system, which is no longer as painful as when it was first introduced. "Before and after" photos of the postural changes it can create are impressive, and pain relief may be significant after only a few sessions. This modality has been found particularly beneficial to treat any contributory scoliosis, and to help avoid the painful necessity for surgical insertion of a rod to prevent permanent curvature of the spine.

The Alexander Technique utilizes awareness of the physical posture, in combination with gentle stretching. Originated by Nicholas Alexander, who was suffering from back problems himself, it is available from trained practitioners in most major cities. To find a Rolfer or Alexander practitioner near you, see "Resources."

Use Acupuncture

Numerous studies have shown the benefits of acupuncture for relief of low back pain, both acute and chronic.[45] A 1998 meta-analysis of nine studies found acupuncture more than twice as successful in improving symptoms for any type of back pain compared to various other interventions.[46]

Use Magnets

Initial case reports are promising for the use of magnets as an effective treatment of back pain; further investigation is needed. Magnetic pads are available to specifically apply to the back (see "Resources"). Apply the magnet to the point of your maximum pain or, in the case of sciatica, over your low back. Leave on until you are free of pain. You may also find relief by utilizing other magnetic devices, such as magnetic shoe insoles or a magnetic mattress. You can reapply the magnets as needed, for any recurrence of your symptoms. See Chapter 2 for further discussion of magnetic therapy.

Use Biofeedback

Dr. John Basmajian, at Emery Medical Center in Atlanta, has shown that biofeedback augmented relaxation can help in the treatment of low back pain.[47] He uses an electromyographic (EMG) test, which measures the strength of the tension in your muscles, to give feedback of the degree of back muscle tension. He then teaches patients to consciously relax tense areas, in one-hour sessions two or three times a week for six weeks.

Use Herbal Remedies, Homeopathy, and Supplements

The herb comfrey, known as "the bruise plant" in the American Indian tradition, may help you find relief for chronic back problems. You can begin treatment as soon as your injury occurs, and it will appreciably decrease pain, swelling, and bruising. A "comfrey pack" is first made by boiling a cup of the dried herb in enough water to make a moistened bundle; then this is applied directly to the skin over the painful area. Place a hot water bottle over this, and leave in place for an hour or so. Repeat as needed. Do not ingest the fresh herb internally, but alkaloid-free comfrey, specially formulated for internal use, is now available, and one dropperful can be taken every few hours. Arnica is another herb that can similarly provide pain relief when applied externally; it shouldn't be taken internally.

The most commonly utilized homeopathic remedies are arnica (for acute back pain), calcarea carbonica and calcarea phosphorica, hypericum (for nerve injury), and symphytum. See Chapter 2 for a more in-depth discussion of homeopathy.

Supplemental calcium and magnesium are often very helpful in the relief of back pain. Take 500 to 1,000 mg of calcium citrate, once daily at bedtime, and magnesium—sometimes called "nature's tranquilizer"—100–200 mg three times daily and at bedtime. Vitamin C, B complex, and manganese may also be added. See Chapter 2 for further details on these supplements.

Seek Counseling; Join a Support Group

As noted, stress may play a major role in the onset of back and neck problems. One study showed that one-third of the patients with low back pain were found to suffer from measurable psychological problems.[48]

Even accidents often do not happen "by accident." Situations that injure the spine, such as automobile, skiing, or lifting accidents, often occur within a setting of emotional distress. Also, stress-related fatigue increases the risk of back injury. Follow the full program given in Chapter 2 for complete stress management recommendations and for help with stress-related psychological problems.

Chronic fear or depression may lead to habitual postures that themselves may cause back pain. "Burden-bearing thoughts" may pathologically increase the curvature in the upper back; a condition termed *kyphosis,* can develop, characterized by flattened, misshapen disks in your neck and low back. A fearful animal assumes an arched position, tilting the pelvis backward, shortening the back, and increasing its *lumbar lordosis,* the opposite of the optimum curvature for the low back. The sum result of these postural shifts increases structural stress on your disks.

Orthopedic surgeon Dr. Vert Mooney, from the University of Texas Southwestern Medical School, has stated, "Pain is not a separate entity. It's connected with the patient's whole lifestyle—his rewards, relationships, and feelings of worth."[49] In a follow-up study of 177 patients who simply became more aware of the relationship of their emotional tension to their back pain, and who then practiced remembering to "stay loose," Dr. John Sarno found that 76 percent showed improvement.[50]

This does not mean that your back pain is merely psychosomatic, or "all in your head." "We have never found a case in the several thousand that have been referred to our center [where] the pain actually was all in their head," reported Renee Steele-Rosornoff, of the University of Miami Department of Neurological Surgery.[51] The mind-body connection activates structural components in your body that cause the pain. Such tension can best be relieved by exercise, stretching and breathing, and general stress reduction.

Practice Visualization

One visualization you may wish to apply to reduce your back's tension is to imagine "breathing into your heels." First, use the deep relaxation techniques in Chapter 2. Then "see" your breath in your mind's eye traveling all the way into your heels. Another image is to see your spine as a tower of light wooden blocks with soft doughnuts between each. Imagine each doughnut and block in perfect position, and ease the jelly back into the center of the doughnuts. Hold this picture, and at the same time, feel it happening within your body. You may also imagine your spine as the Eiffel Tower. Each level is beautifully aligned with a soft cushion between, and the view from the top is magnificent!

Conventional Medicine Approaches to Back Problems

In addition to rest and braces, the following are the standard conventional medicine treatments.

Physical Therapy

A combination of massage, guided exercise, gentle manipulation, hot and cold treatment, and ultrasound applications may be utilized. One study found that patients with back pain managed by physical therapists were more satisfied with their care than by patients managed by physicians.[52]

Drug Treatments

Muscle relaxants (Valium, Robaxin, Flexeril, Parafon Forte, Soma), antiinflammatory agents (aspirin, Motrin, Advil, ibuprofen,

Alleve), and stronger pain medications (Percocet, Tylenol #3, Vicodin) all may be used during episodes of acute back pain. Muscle relaxants do not actually relax your muscles, but simply sedate you. However, because of their addictive potential and significant side effects, you should not use these medications for chronic problems.

The gout medication colchicine has been found to be beneficial, even in cases where surgery has failed to relieve the back pain. One researcher followed 6,000 patients over thirty years, using intravenous injections once or twice a week, combined with daily pill intake, and 92 percent had sufficient relief of pain to return to work.[53]

Trigger-Point Therapy

A "trigger point" is a localized area which when pressed upon produces shooting pain. It is usually a hard area of bunched muscle. The spasm and fluid retention at this location can be relieved by injection of the anesthetic lidocaine, followed by multiple needle insertions to release fluid buildup.

Nerve Injections and Transcutaneous Nerve Stimulation

Anesthetics, sometimes combined with steroids, can be injected directly into sore muscles and ligaments, near the disks, and into the space next to the spinal canal (epidural space), anesthetizing the nerves as they leave the spinal canal. These procedures may relieve pain temporarily, or even on a long-term basis. Dr. Kenneth Scholz of the Texas Tech University School of Medicine found that when epidural injections were used, 75 percent of the patients with documented disk disease were still pain-free at one year.[54]

A transcutaneous nerve stimulator (TENS) machine can provide pain relief by generating minute electrical shocks through a skin electrode. However, recent studies have found this method to have only the pain-relieving capacity of a placebo, and it does nothing to address your underlying problem.

Surgical Approaches to Back Problems

It was the NFL football season opener, and the San Francisco 49ers were playing Tampa Bay. As legendary quarterback Joe Montana, age 30, described it: "I was running to my left, and I threw back to my right. No one hit me, but as I twisted my body to release the ball, I felt something snap."[55] The immediate pain and numbness were so significant, he could not raise his legs or even stand.

Operated on just a week after sustaining what was found to be a ruptured disk, he and his surgeon chose simply to have one-third of the disk removed, relieving the pressure on the nerves causing the numbness and pain. He chose not to have a fusion, so that his back could maintain its flexibility, and he could recover more quickly. He was jogging within two weeks of his surgery, and returned to the starting lineup two months later, winning the game, and continued on to play championship football for ten more years without further incident or pain.

The key to whether you will have a successful back operation is being certain you are one of those most likely to be helped by surgery. If your radiological picture and other tests *correspond with your signs and symptoms*, and if your problem is quite severe, especially if it involves muscle weakness, bowel or bladder dysfunction, or you do not respond to alternative and conventional nonsurgical measures, you may be a good candidate for surgical relief.

Studies have also shown that success is more likely if you are well motivated to get back to work, do not have to do heavy manual labor, have no financial incentive (e.g., pending lawsuit), and are psychologically well adjusted. Overall, results are not as good if you are a woman, have psychosocial problems, have been out of work for more than three months, or have degenerative changes on X-rays.[56]

The American Neurological Association and the American Academy of Orthopedic Surgeons have established strict criterion for the selection of patients undergoing surgery. These include:

1. Failure to improve after four or more weeks of nonsurgical treatment.
2. A myelogram or CAT scan showing nerve compression corresponding to the area of your symptoms and abnormal physical exam.
3. Radiating pain, loss of sensation, muscle weakness, and/or decreased reflexes in the area of your body that the nerve supplies.

Other considerations favoring surgery are if you have problems with bladder or bowel function, increasing weakness with evidence of nerve damage, and recurrent incapacitating periods of pain.

If you pass these selection criteria, you need to choose an orthopedic surgeon or a neurosurgeon to discuss back surgery. Surgeons from both of these specialties perform the same types of procedures, but you should try to locate a surgeon who does more than 100 back operations per year. If you can, find out his or her reputation as well, by asking other doctors or nurses familiar with this surgeon's work.

Several different techniques are available for your operation, depending on the location and extent of your disease.

Laminectomy and Laminotomy

These are the most common procedures used to treat a slipped or bulging disk, or bone that is pressing on the spinal cord or its nerves.

You are admitted to the hospital on the morning of surgery. Spinal or general anesthesia is necessary. After you are anesthetized, you lie facedown on the operating table. A two- to four-inch incision is made in the middle of your back, centered over the area of the bulging disk, where the spinal canal is narrowed, or where your nerve is pinched as it passes out of the spinal canal. Your muscles are separated to expose the lamina of your vertebra.

In *laminotomy*, typically, one-third to one-half of one of the lamina of each of two adjacent vertebrae are removed, using bone-biting instruments. (See Figure 22.3.) Exactly how much bone is taken out depends on the size of the space between your bone segments, and the size and location of the disk bulging or bone pressing on your nerve. A relatively large incision is needed to give adequate exposure, so that your surgeon can clearly see your spinal cord and nerves, to avoid damaging them.

Laminectomy is similar to laminotomy, except that all of the lamina is removed to get better exposure. The offending disk or bone is taken out piecemeal, with several different sizes and shapes of biting instruments.

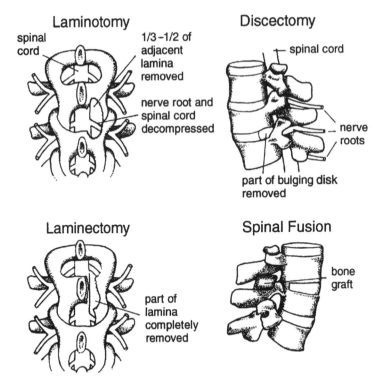

Fig. 22.3 Types of back operations

Your incision is closed with stitches or skin tapes. The operation may take from one to five hours, depending on the procedure and the amount of material which must be removed to free the nerve. You may be discharged the next day but, typically, would spend a few days in the hospital.

Microdiscectomy

This operation is very similar to laminotomy except that the material pressing on the nerve is removed through a smaller, one- to two-inch incision, with less trauma to your surrounding tissue. A main goal is to maintain your spinal stability. The surgeon uses small "microsurgical" instruments, viewing the diseased area through an operating microscope.

This procedure can be performed in less than an hour, and you can be discharged in two or three days. The advantage is that your postoperative pain may be less, and your recovery more rapid. However, this type of surgery cannot be chosen if you have a narrow or abnormal spinal canal.

Percutaneous Discectomy

In *percutaneous discectomy,* a one-eighth-inch-diameter needle is passed into the space between two vertebrae. Using specially designed instruments passed through the needle, fragments of the disk are removed by suction, laser, or tiny forceps while your surgeon watches on a television screen. Use of a computer and robot arm to make incisions more precise is being investigated. The idea is to remove the bulging part of the disk while avoiding damage of neighboring tissue. Bone is not removed. This procedure is somewhat controversial, and can be done only if your amount of disease is small. Long-term results are not yet known. However, major complications are rare, and this approach can even be performed with you as an outpatient, under local anesthesia.

Spinal Fusion

If your spine is unstable or would be after laminectomy, your operation may be followed by fusion of two or more of your adjacent vertebrae.

Spinal fusion is similar to laminectomy, except that small pieces of bone graft material, taken from one of your hips, or alternatively, chemically sterilized, freeze-dried bone obtained from a bone bank, are placed into the space between the vertebral bodies and/or across the lamina, so that once these pieces grow together, your vertebrae become fused. Metal rods, screwed-in plates, "cages" packed with bone graft pieces, and wires are also sometimes used to accomplish this goal. These operations can take from three to eight hours to complete. The end result of spinal fusion is that your spine becomes rigid where it once could bend.

Postoperatively, bed rest is usually required for several days, to allow the bone grafts time to "knit." You may have a sore hip as well as a sore back.

Fusion has not been found to improve your chances for pain relief, and 10 percent of the time, the fusion does not "take," meaning the joint remains movable. Most doctors do not recommend fusion unless your particular operation would leave your spine unstable.

After back surgery, you need a period of bed rest. Continuous ice packs may be applied, to relieve muscle spasm and reduce the necessity for pain medication. You may need a urinary catheter, an intravenous line for pain medication, and a small plastic drain in your incision to collect secretions and blood into a suction bulb. These can be removed in a day or two. Most likely, you will be able to eat the day after surgery, and can then be switched to oral pain pills and muscle relaxant medication. However, it is not uncommon for your intestines to undergo a short period of reflex paralysis, where they do not move gas and food normally. If so, you may become nauseated, distended with gas, and vomit, and therefore need a nasal stomach tube for a few days.

You should get out of bed and become active as soon as possible, being carefully supervised by your doctor, physical therapist, and/or rehabilitation specialist. You can progress from sitting to standing to walking, then to various exercises to increase flexibility and strength. Your rehab team will show you the best ways to get up from bed, climb stairs, and dress yourself, to limit strain on your back. You should be able to go home in two to seven days.

After hospital discharge, you may be visited in your home by a physical therapist and later make trips to a physical therapy center. You should see your doctor regularly to ensure good healing, determine your progress and the effects of the surgery, and to obtain advice regarding when you can return to driving, work, and other activities. Be sure to discuss when it is safe to resume sex, along with the most comfortable positions, and speak up if any exercises or activities increase your pain or other symptoms.

As quarterback Joe Montana wrote about

his own recovery from his laminectomy: "I had to learn to walk again after the operation. . . . The therapist came to my house every morning, made me walk, made me exercise, no matter how much I complained. . . . I never worked so hard in my life. It was unbelievable."[57] His efforts paid off—he missed only eight games before he was back in action.

Depending on your problem and type of surgery, you may have restrictions on your activities for up to nine months, which is the time it takes for full bone healing. Your limitations may include avoiding bending in certain ways, heavy lifting, and contact sports. If your spine is or was unstable, a back brace may be necessary for a period of time.

Devices that help you avoid certain awkward movements and keep you steady may be very beneficial. Get a high toilet seat, which makes it easier to get up. Likewise, avoid soft, low easy chairs and mattresses. You can rent or purchase reaching devices, to retrieve objects from the floor or shelves. Railings can be added to your tub, or in other areas in your home or work where you might be unsteady.

You should follow the alternative medicine program beginning on page 613, especially the yoga stretching, to help you return to maximum back function and freedom from pain after your operation.

In patients who are properly selected for surgery, good to excellent results are obtained in 70 to 90 percent. Ten to 20 percent may have little or no improvement, and for the few patients made even worse after surgery, it is usually due to residual disk material at the operated site, another bulging disk, an unstable spine, scar tissue in the operative site, or a piece of bone irritating a nerve. Repeat surgery may be an appropriate recommendation in 10 percent. The chance that a second operation will cure your problem is about the same as for the first operation, but after that, subsequent operations have only a 10 percent chance of a good result.

Laminectomy has a mortality rate of 1 to 3 per 1,000 operations. Complications occur in about 5 percent, and include those associated with the anesthesia, blood loss with need for transfusion (autodonation in the weeks before surgery is often recommended, especially if a fusion is anticipated), incision infection, temporary or permanent nerve root injury (less than 1 in 100), and damage to major blood vessels in front of the spine (less than 1 in 1,000). Recurrent disk herniation occurs in 1 to 5 percent.

BACK PROBLEMS SUMMARY

Prevention

Lifestyle

- Exercise regularly: 1 hour, 3–5 times weekly.
- Practice yoga daily.
- Maintain good posture habits.
- Be careful in bending and lifting.
- Maintain proper weight.
- Practice stress management.
- Don't smoke.
- Prevent osteoporosis.

Alternative Medicine Approaches

- Herbal remedies—comfrey and arnica packs; alkaloid-free comfrey, one dropperful every few hours.
- Supplements—calcium citrate, 500–1,000

mg at bedtime; magnesium, 100–200 mg, 3 times daily and at bedtime; vitamin B complex, 50 mg daily; vitamin C, 1,000–2,000 mg daily; manganese, 10 mg daily.
- Homeopathy—arnica, calcarea carbonica and calcarea phosphorica, hypericum, and symphytum.
- Maintenance of activity level; rest only when necessary.
- Ice and heat.
- Tai chi and qi gong.
- Chiropractic and osteopathic treatment.
- Massage, Rolfing, and the Alexander Technique.
- Acupuncture.
- Biofeedback.
- Magnets.
- Psychological counseling, support group.
- Visualization.

Conventional Medicine Approaches

- Rest.
- Corset or body brace.
- Physical therapy.
- Medications—muscle relaxants, antiinflammatories, pain pills, colchicine.
- Trigger-point therapy.
- Nerve injections and TENS.

Surgical Approaches

- Laminectomy and laminotomy.
- Microdiscectomy.
- Percutaneous discectomy.
- Spinal fusion.

The Neck

John, *an energetic 28-year-old, was vacationing in the Caribbean. He rented a motor scooter and went whizzing around the island. Unfortunately, he slipped on a turn, breaking his neck. Surgery, including fusion, was necessary to stabilize the broken vertebrae, and he was left with partial paralysis in his leg and arm. His surgeon told him, "Well, just get a cane, and learn to live with it." However, soon after his injury, he began using alternative medicine approaches. He took homeopathic* hypericum *for nerve injury and* arnica *for soft tissue injury, in high potencies. He worked with a gentle massage therapist, to release and relax the injured area. He took the herbs comfrey and burdock, and B vitamins, to rebuild his nerves. He had sessions with a cranio-sacral osteopath, as well as a physical therapist. He then became almost fully recovered, with normal walking ability, and used his experience to become active in the healing field himself.*

Pain in your neck region can be very disabling, where even a simple turn to look to the side, up, or down can be excruciating. Whiplash, a forceful twist, or a direct blow can injure the neck's structures, causing muscle strain, dislocation, and fracture, and result in neurologic damage and chronic pain. Luckily, most of the time neck pain is not due to problems with bones or nerves, but is caused by chronic strain, acute sprain, or simple injury to the muscles that support your ten-pound head. As with the back, postural problems often underlie neck pain.

How Your Neck Works

The cervical spine has seven vertebrae, between which are disks that normally provide flexibility and a shock-absorbing, cushioning effect. Degenerating, flattened disks lose their height and elasticity, decreasing your neck's ease of movement, and allowing the vertebrae to rub on each other, causing stiffness and pain. This may even give you a headache.

The vertebral lamina form a large central spinal canal through which runs the spinal cord; spinal nerves branch off between each pair of vertebrae. (For a discussion of the spine, see "How Your Back Works" on page 609.) These nerves then pass through small bony canals (called foramina) on each side, to supply muscles and provide sensation.

Neck Problems

Trauma, arthritis, bone spurs, ligament thickening, and bulging disks can narrow your spinal canal and foramina, thereby impinging on your nerve roots (the part of the nerve as it takes off from the spinal cord and travels through the foramina). This can cause pain, affect sensation, and weaken muscles in your neck, hands, arms, and shoulders. Your muscles may then shrink in size, and you may lose coordination or develop clumsiness in using your hands. If pressure develops on the spinal cord itself, the muscles and sensation in the lower half of your body can also be affected, causing instability in walking, as well as bowel or bladder problems.

Radiculopathy is the medical term used to describe such symptoms, caused by pressure on your spinal nerve roots. The part of the body to which the nerve provides sensation and muscle control is affected, giving your doctor clues as to what portion of your neck is the basis of the problem. Nerve root pain may be sharp, but more commonly is a constant, dull ache, increased by certain neck positions or movements.

If your symptoms are acute, the cause is usually a diseased disk. Chronic problems are more commonly due to degenerative bony changes, which have narrowed your spinal canal and foramina, a condition termed *spondylosis*. Some degree of spondylosis is very common; nearly everyone has it after age 70. However, most persons with typical X-ray findings do not have symptoms.

Some persons have relatively large spinal canals and foramina and, therefore, can tolerate significant changes in their disks and bones without developing symptoms, while others have narrow canals, so that even small disturbances can produce severe discomfort, such as the athlete who becomes symptomatic with seemingly minor trauma.

How Neck Problems Are Diagnosed

The diagnosis of neck problems should include a careful history of your symptoms, a physical exam, and simple X-rays. More sophisticated tests may be necessary.

History

A careful history is the first step in diagnosing your neck problem. You should be asked about your symptoms of pain and its pattern, weakness in any muscles, and presence of numbness and tingling, particularly involving your arms. Report any difficulties with bladder or bowel control and sexual function. Your doctor should know about your exercise habits, job requirements at work, and any previous injury. It is especially important to tell your doctor what triggers and what relieves your symptoms. Report any known medical problems and any medicines you are taking.

Physical Exam

Your doctor should test your neck mobility, reflexes, and strength in various muscles, as well as check for decreased or absent sensation to pinprick, vibration, heat and cold, and light touch. These simple tests can pick up early nerve damage.

X-Rays

Several types of X-rays and scans may be necessary if surgery is being considered. The simplest is the plain X-ray, taken with your neck bent forward and backward. It shows curvature, alignment, disk space height, and bony changes of arthritis, spurs, bone collapse, and unstable or hypermobile joints.

CAT Scan

For this study, you lay inside a spinning arm that takes multiple X-ray images that a computer reassembles to produce cross sections of your anatomy. This is the best way to see the bony architecture, including your spinal canal and nerve outlet size and shape. The CAT scan may be combined with a myelogram to define the relationship of the bones and disks with the spinal cord and nerves. It can show spinal stenosis (narrowing of the spinal canal), protruding disks, or other diseases that cause pressure on the spinal cord and its roots. However, myelography is an invasive exam, requiring injection of contrast material into your spinal canal, and should be avoided whenever possible.

MRI Scan

Here you lay inside the MRI scanner as a powerful magnet changes the orientation of your cell atom components. Tissue images are constructed by a computer. This noninvasive study is the best way to localize and evaluate soft tissue changes—i.e., those within your disks, spinal cord, and nerves themselves. This test has nearly replaced all the other studies in many medical centers. If you have metal in your body (an artificial joint or pacemaker, for example) you cannot have this test.

Nerve Conduction and Electromyelogram

These tests play an important role in diagnosing neck problems. These studies, most often performed by neurologists, test transmission velocity of nerve impulses and your muscles' reactions. They detect damage caused by pressure on the nerves from slipped or ruptured disks, bone spurs, spinal stenosis, or tumors. In nerve conduction tests, two needles are placed through your skin into or next to the nerve to be tested. The distance between them is measured. A small electrical current is then passed through the first needle and picked up by a second while it is connected to a recording device. The strength of the impulse and the time it took to arrive are registered. Many different nerves are tested, and one arm is compared to the other. Diseased nerves show low electrical impulses and prolonged conduction times. These tests can take an hour or more and may be quite uncomfortable, though complications are very rare.

An electromyelogram (EMG) is similar to the nerve conduction test, except that a specific muscle's response to electrical stimulation is recorded. Degree of damage can be measured.

Alternative Medicine Approaches to Neck Problems

Jayn, an active 35-year-old mother of two young boys, flew over the handlebars of her bicycle to avoid a traffic accident. Fortunately, the automobile missed her, but unfortunately, she twisted her neck as she hit the curb. After months in a collar, medications, and physical therapy, she was still miserable and restricted in her daily activities. Her surgeon husband recommended she see a chiropractor, who applied some manipulations which relieved her discomfort. She was then able to bicycle and even ski without neck pain.

Alternative medicine treatment of neck problems is very similar to that of the back. I especially recommend chiropractic or osteopathic manipulative therapy. Very rarely, these approaches have exacerbated patients' problems, so make certain you have a practitioner who is experienced and recommended. In addition, try the following alternative medicine approaches to prevent and treat neck problems.

Use a Neck Collar and Neck Pillow

These simple devices allow your neck muscles to rest and relax, which increases the flow of nutrients to them and to your disks, and allows your neck region to accomplish more repair work. You can now obtain versions with supportive foam and embedded magnets to further increase circulation. Information for obtaining them is found in the Resources section of this book.

Use Gentle Traction

Special traction devices for the neck that attach to the ceiling or door jamb can give your neck relief from the effects of bad posture and the splinting that comes from pain. Simple to install, they can be utilized several times per day to help you relax and to remind your body to maintain proper posture. They are available at most large pharmacies or medical supply stores.

Use Neck Roll Exercises

Very gentle neck rolls and stretches, derived from yoga, may help to release tension and assist you in realigning your posture. Simply begin by slowly rolling your head in a circular fashion, going only as far as is completely comfortable—about half as far as you *can* go. Repeat in the opposite direction. Try to do these movements every one to two hours during the day, making certain not to strain yourself. Gradually, your neck flexibility will improve and the local circulation of nutrients will be increased, assisting your neck's repair work.

Use Acupuncture

Several studies have shown the benefit of acupuncture in the relief of neck pain.[58] When compared with standard physiotherapy, acupuncture was found to be better at restoring range of motion: 87 percent in the acupuncture group improved, compared to 54 percent in the physiotherapy group.[59]

Conventional Medicine Approaches to Neck Problems

Many people obtain relief from neck pain using conventional medicine approaches. The following are among the most successful.

Immobilization

As for back pain, rest and traction are to be discouraged. A neck collar may be useful to relieve acute pain and to allow you to move around and take care of yourself, go to work, and perform other necessities, but should be limited to only a few days. It prevents some of the more useful treatments that require movement and exercise.

Mobilization and Manipulation

Mobilization involves gentle manual movements to improve joint function. Manipulation is an aggressive and rapid bending or twisting of the neck aimed at increasing movement in one or more joints. These treatments seem to work better than muscle relaxants, bed rest, and other usual medical care.[60] Early mobilization has been shown to be superior to immobilization if you have a more severe "whiplash" type of injury.[61]

Physiotherapy and Physical Treatments

Massage, hot and cold treatments, electrotherapy, short-wave diathermy, ultrasound applications, and home exercise are all popular forms of physical therapy. However, they may be not much better than placebo.

Drug Treatments

Opium-based pain medications such as Percocet, Tylenol #3, and Vicodin may be necessary to get you through the acute pain phase, but should not be used for longer periods due to their addictive potential. The NSAIDs aspirin, Motrin, Advil, and Alleve may be beneficial in reducing inflammation and swelling, and help provide pain relief. They should be used only for short periods, since they have a potential for significant bleeding and gastrointestinal, liver, kidney, and neurologic side effects. The muscle relaxants Valium, Robaxin, Flexeril, Parafon Forte, and Soma have been shown to work better than placebos.

Antidepressants are sometimes prescribed, but their effect hasn't been well studied.

Steroid Injections

Steroids can be injected around the neck nerve roots when radiating pain (radiculopathy) is significant. One study found excellent results in patients who otherwise might have had surgery.[62]

Surgical Approaches to Neck Problems

Neck pain in itself is not an indication for surgery. However, if you have sudden and severe loss of muscle function, you should consider urgent surgery. If your symptoms are more chronic, a trial of nonsurgical treatment is indicated, with rest, collar, traction, physical therapy, medication, and alternative medicine approaches. These should continue as long as you are improving. However, your pain may decrease even when ongoing nerve damage and increasing weakness are present, so you need to be closely followed by your doctor during this period. If your symptoms persist or increase in severity, you should investigate surgery. Especially if you have significant muscle weakness, the earlier a decompression procedure can be performed, the more likely it will be successful in reversing your deficits.

For surgery to be indicated, a specific cause-and-effect relationship between the findings on tests and your symptoms should be present. "Prophylactic" operations are not justified if a herniated disk found on X-rays does not produce symptoms or signs of nerve damage in this area.

Those who eventually undergo surgery typically fall into two groups—younger patients with acute herniated disks, and older patients with arthritic changes narrowing their bony canals.

Laminoforaminotomy

This is the most common operation for radiculopathy caused by a disk or narrow foramina pressing on a nerve. It can be accomplished via an incision placed on the front or back of your neck.

The *posterior approach* is most commonly used in simple cases. After general anesthesia, your neck is prepped with an antibacterial solution. You are positioned either facedown, on your side on the operating table, or sitting in an operating chair. A one-and-one-half- to two-inch incision is made in the middle or just off to the side of the back of your neck. To gain exposure to the nerves, disk, and spinal canal, usually one-half of the lamina above and one-third of the lamina below the compressed nerve root is removed. The nerve root is then freed up, by removal of the compressing bone or disk with tiny biting instruments or drills.

In the *anterior approach* you lie on your back. A one- to three-inch incision is made off to the side of the front of your neck, at your collar level. The muscles and other tissues are separated to expose the disk and adjacent vertebrae. The part of the disk or bone spur compressing your nerves or spinal cord is removed with tiny biting instruments.

Neck Fusion

Fusion may be added to laminoforaminotomy. It immobilizes the joint, so that part of your neck will not bend forward, backward,

side-to-side, or twist. Although unnecessary in most cases, fusion of adjacent neck vertebrae is indicated to protect against further discomfort and nerve damage if instability is present, a lot of bone has to be removed, a vertebral body fracture or compression is present, a previous laminectomy has failed, or an abnormal neck alignment is found. Neck fusion naturally develops in 50 percent of anterior laminoforaminotomies, and in 95 percent when grafts are placed.

Bone for the graft material is usually taken from the prominent part of your hip bone at the belt line. Alternatively, chemically sterilized, freeze-dried bone can be obtained from a bone bank. In an anterior fusion, bits of bone are wedged into the space between the vertebral bodies. If more than two vertebrae need to be stabilized, metal plates and screws are added. In posterior fusion, wires and pieces of bone hold the lamina together.

After the bony work is completed, to prevent fluid buildup, a drain may be placed, brought through your skin, and connected to a soft plastic collection bulb. Your incision is closed with stitches, staples, or skin tapes. A neck brace or collar is usually placed before you wake up from anesthesia.

You should be out of bed the day of your operation, and active as soon as possible. In the early postoperative period, concentrate on maintaining good posture, holding your head erect, minimizing your neck's motion, and moving cautiously. A collar or brace eases neck discomfort. If you have had a fusion, the bone graft harvest spot will be sore for a week or two. Pain pills can usually manage any pain.

Drain tubes can be removed in a day or two, and stitches or staples a few days later. You should be home after one to four days, and back to work in two to four weeks. You should see your doctor for several follow-up visits, to ensure that your operation has accomplished its objectives. Immediately report any increasing pain, muscle weakness, or change in sensation. When you are told it is safe, you can begin exercises to strengthen the muscles and range of motion of your neck. Heavy labor is usually permissible after six weeks.

How long you should wear a brace or collar depends on your particular operation, postoperative discomfort, and your doctor's recommendations. If you had a simple laminoforaminotomy, this period may be only a few days, weeks, or not at all. If you underwent a fusion, your neck needs to be immobilized for an extended period, to allow the vertebrae and graft material to "knit" solidly together. You start with a rigid neck brace, then gradually progress to a soft collar. The collar can usually be removed after four to six weeks. Your healing process is monitored on X-rays, and should be completed in three months. After a fusion heals, you may have mild limitation of your neck's range of motion.

Good results are obtained in 95 percent of cases of laminoforaminotomy and neck fusion. Significant symptoms of neck or nerve pain persist in only 5 percent. Complications include incision infection in 1 to 2 percent, nerve damage in less than 1 percent, and rarely, with the anterior approach, swallowing difficulty or hoarseness. After the fusion operation, the vertebrae fail to heal solidly together in 5 percent of all patients, but less than half of these need more surgery. Complications of fusion specific to the donor site such as pelvic bone infection, fracture, and adjacent nerve damage are rare.

NECK PROBLEMS SUMMARY

Prevention

Diet and Supplements

- Follow a low-fat, high-fiber diet.
- Follow the dietary guidelines for back problems on page 615.

Lifestyle

- Practice daily yoga postures.
- Use a neck pillow.
- Do neck roll exercises.

Alternative Medicine Approaches

- Follow the guidelines for prevention, above.
- Use acupuncture, chiropractic, osteopathy, Rolfing massage, and magnets.
- Practice visualization.

Conventional Medicine Approaches

- Immobilization—rest, traction, neck collar.
- Mobilization and manipulation.
- Physiotherapy and physical treatments.
- Medications—pain medications, NSAIDs, muscle relaxers, antidepressants.
- Steroid injections.

Surgical Approaches

- Laminoforaminotomy.
- Neck fusion.

The Knee

The knee is not simply a hinge connecting your thigh and lower leg bones. It is much more complex, made up of many strong components, allowing it to bend forward, backward, and slightly from side to side, as well as permitting the bones to twist inward and outward on themselves to a small degree. Your knee must both support your body weight while you engage in normal activities and accommodate the sometimes severe stresses of work and recreation.

The advent of the arthroscope has dramatically changed knee operations. Gone are the days when normal structures had to be divided and the whole knee joint opened to gain access to the damaged part. Most operations within the knee joint can now be performed using a tiny camera and instruments inserted through one-quarter- to one-half-inch incisions, while your surgeon watches on a TV monitor. Simple injuries to your knee's menisci and ligaments, commonly caused by sudden twisting or turning too far while skiing or playing tennis, can be easily repaired as an outpatient. New techniques have replaced the prolonged casting and months of recuperation associated with the old methods. Now you can be up and walking in a few days.

If the smooth surfaces of the bones of the joint break down beyond simple repair, the whole knee joint can be safely and reliably replaced using carefully researched methods and high-tech materials.

However, you may be able to avoid even such new, improved knee surgery by the use of alternative medicine approaches.

How Your Knee Works

The bones of the thigh (femur) and lower leg (tibia) are connected by four major liga-ments (anterior and posterior cruciate, medial and lateral collateral), the tough fibrous joint capsule that surrounds the joint, and the muscles that attach both above and below the joint. (See Figure 22.4.) Where the ends of these bones press on each other, the articular cartilages and the medial and lateral menisci supply cushioning. The joint is lubricated by a small amount of fluid supplied by the synovium. The kneecap (patella) connects the tendon of the strong quadriceps muscle of the front part of the thigh to the lower leg bone just below the knee. It provides smooth muscle pull across the joint as you straighten or bend your knee.

How Knee Injuries Are Diagnosed

If you have an injury to your knee, you should have it evaluated. An untreated injury of one knee structure will often lead to further injury in others. Early nonsurgical treatment may help you avoid the need for surgery down the road.

History

Your history should begin with questions about your overall health, especially to determine if you have any medical problems that predispose you to bone or joint disease, such as gout or rheumatoid arthritis. Your usual level of activity and knee stresses during recreation may help your doctor determine what is wrong, and help plan the treatment best for you. Your doctor needs to know what makes your symptoms worse and what you have done to relieve them, such as take over-the-counter antiinflammatory medications (ibuprofen, Motrin, Advil, Alleve).

If you have had an injury, how you were hurt is a clue to which structures may be involved. Tell your doctor exactly what you

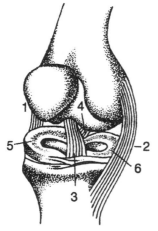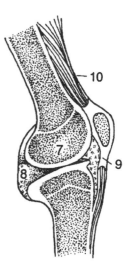

1. lateral collateral ligament
2. medial collateral ligament
3. anterior cruciate ligament
4. posterior cruciate ligament
5. lateral meniscus
6. medial meniscus

7. cartilage
8. synovium
9. kneecap tendon
10. muscle tendon

Fig. 22.4   The anatomy of the knee

were doing at the time, the position your knee was in when it was struck or twisted, and whether you felt it buckle, pop, or "give out."

Physical Exam

Your doctor should watch how you walk and sit down, and feel around the knee for areas of swelling or tenderness. Your knee is bent, straightened, and moved in many different directions to determine limitation of the normal range of motion or ways in which it moves too far, indicating joint "laxity" from stretched or torn ligaments. Pain, grating sensations, and lack of smooth movements are noted. Since differences are very important, both knees are tested.

X-Rays

X-rays are usually the simplest first test. They can show any problems with your bones, such as fracture, narrowed joint space, or the irregular bony joint surfaces characteristic of arthritis.

Arthrogram

In this test, a dye is injected directly into your joint through a small needle. The inside of the joint with its ligaments, menisci, and cartilage surfaces is then outlined on plain X-ray or CAT scan. Any irregularity or torn areas may be seen.

MRI Scan

This is the best noninvasive test for showing the "soft tissues" of cartilage, menisci, and ligaments, which are not seen on plain X-rays. In this test a large magnet is put around your knee, which creates an electric field, causing these tissues to appear on a film similar to an X-ray. The entire joint structure is seen, not just its surfaces.

Arthroscopy

This is the best way to diagnose joint problems. It is usually an outpatient procedure.

For arthroscopy, you lie on your back on the operating table. You can have general, spinal, or local anesthesia with intravenous sedation. After skin preparation with an antiseptic solution, your surgeon makes one or more small one-quarter-inch incisions over your knee joint. A hollow needle is placed into the joint space, then a tiny camera introduced through it, to relay the image of the inside of your joint onto a television monitor. Ligaments, menisci, and joint surface cartilage can be clearly seen. If surgical repair is indicated, it can usually be performed at the same time, though larger incisions and a short hospital stay may then be necessary.

After arthroscopy, your knee is usually a bit sore and swollen for a few days. An Ace bandage or a brace may be helpful, depending on your underlying knee problem.

Knee Meniscus Injury

The *medial meniscus* is a quarter-moon-shaped cartilage, about three-eighths-inch thick on its outer edge, tapering to one-eighth inch on its inner edge. It is positioned on the inner side of the knee, between the femur and tibia. The similar *lateral meniscus* is on the outer side of the joint.

Menisci play several important roles in healthy knee function. Their concave surfaces help stabilize the joint by providing a "cup" for the bones to sit in. They act as shock absorbers and compress when a load is placed on the joint, taking some of the pressure off the cartilages of the bones and thereby reducing their wear and tear. By moving with joint motion, they help distribute the small amount of joint fluid that lubricates the joint surfaces. Normally well supplied with blood, they are pushed and squeezed during joint motion, so that their nutriments are spread to the other less-vascular joint cartilages.

Menisci are usually injured when a sudden twisting force is placed on the joint, such as when a football player or skier makes a sharp change of direction. Repetitive stress such as squatting can also cause degenerative damage.

The rough surface of a torn meniscus causes joint irritation, swelling, fluid accumulation, and pain. You may feel a "pop" as the irregular fragment catches between the bones. Many types and degrees of tear can occur, some of them healing with rest and time, while others need to be surgically repaired whenever possible. If meniscus function is lost, your bone cartilages wear out much more rapidly, causing painful knee arthritis.

Recommendation for treatment depends on the severity of your symptoms, the type and degree of meniscus damage, associated injuries of other knee structures, and the demands of your job, recreation, and lifestyle. In general, nonsurgical treatment is worth a try, unless your diagnosed injury is unlikely to heal on its own or is severe enough to place you at risk for further damage.

Alternative Medicine Approaches to Knee Meniscus Injury

Once a meniscus has been removed, you are at increased risk for degenerative arthritis.

Unless you are playing a highly competitive sport, if you have only slight damage to your knee meniscus, you may do best to simply protect your knee with a brace and do physical therapy.

Usually these problems are healed quite effectively by a period of rest, along with protecting your joint with a brace. Following is the specific program.

Use an Ice Pack

Ice acts to reduce inflammation, swelling, and pain. You can apply an ice pack, placed around your knee, for twenty to thirty minutes three to four times a day. After two days postinjury, you can alternate ice and heat to stimulate circulation, which aids in the healing process. You can then also see which modality or combination of modalities gives you the best pain relief.

Elevate Your Leg

Whenever you are resting, keep your leg elevated above your heart level. This will decrease swelling and allow the veins and lymph in your leg to drain. Local circulation will be improved, which will aid in your body's intrinsic repair work.

Rest

After any acute injury, for as long as you are experiencing pain, rest your knee using crutches, then graduate to an Ace bandage or knee brace. Be careful not to overdo any exercise or lifting, wearing a knee brace whenever you might be likely to strain your knee. Further rest is needed if you still feel any pain.

Take Supplements

Flaxseed oil and glucosamine sulfate have been indicated to reduce inflammation. Start with 1 tablespoon of the oil two to three times daily, and 500 mg of glucosamine, three times daily. You can also try rubbing the flaxseed oil or castor on your knee at night.

Exercise Regularly

Simple exercises that strengthen the muscles surrounding your knee will give the knee better support. This will take some of the burden off the weakened meniscus.

Practice Yoga and Relaxation Daily

Keeping your knees flexible, by the gentle stretching of yoga, may help prevent any injury caused by sudden twisting. Slowly stretch your quadriceps, hamstrings, and calf muscles. You should feel a gentle pull, but not an ache or pain.

Conventional Medicine Approaches to Knee Meniscus Injury

If you have an acute meniscus injury, you will likely need to rest, elevate your leg, and use measures to reduce pain and swelling and protect your knee. After this phase subsides and you are comfortable enough to begin a rehabilitation program, you may consider the following approaches.

Ice Packs and Heating Pads

Ice cold packs can reduce pain and swelling. Don't put ice against your bare skin for more than five minutes. Heat can be beneficial after the initial pain disappears. It may help relieve stiffness. Use a warm heating pad or hot water bottle for about twenty minutes several times a day.

Drug Treatments

You may find benefit from the short-term use of nonsteroidal antiinflammatory medication (Motrin, Advil, Alleve) that decrease the body's inflammatory response to injury. This will reduce knee swelling and fluid within the joint. The stronger pain medications (Percocet, Tylenol #3, Vicodin) may help you through episodes of acute pain. Glucosamine sulfate may be indicated if you also have arthritis in the knee.

Crutches and Braces

These protect your knee, particularly if it is unstable and tends to lock. Braces also keep it warm. Increased comfort and confidence will allow you to be more active in a rehabilitation program.

Physical Therapy

Range-of-motion and knee-strengthening exercises under the supervision of a physical therapist are keys to a structured rehabilitation. You can do most of this at home with the aid of inexpensive physical-therapy ropes, pulleys, straps, and weights.

Joint Injection

Your doctor can inject your knee joint with cortisone and anesthetics to decrease pain and swelling. This way, you may be able to participate in a more vigorous rehab plan.

Surgical Approach to Knee Meniscus Injury

The importance of the menisci is now more fully appreciated. Previously, surgeons were much more likely to totally remove a damaged one. Studies subsequently showed that this caused a narrowing of the joint space, accelerated wear on the bone articular cartilages, and increased risk for arthritis. Now surgeons have many techniques to repair cartilage, or remove only the part that is irreparably damaged. Most repairs can be performed through or assisted by the arthroscope, giving you smaller incisions and much quicker recovery.

You are admitted the morning of surgery. You lie on your back on the operating table. General, spinal, or local anesthesia with sedation can be used. The operation can be done open through a two- to three-inch incision, exclusively through the arthroscope with tiny incisions, or using a combination of both ("arthroscopic-assisted"), depending on the type of meniscus injury and your need for repair of other damaged knee structures. Your surgeon will use small instruments to smooth the ragged edges of the torn or frayed meniscus and stitches to repair any splits or cracks. (See Figure 22.5.) Irreparable fragments are removed, with an emphasis on saving as much as possible, to maintain your joint spacing.

Your incisions are closed with stitches or skin tapes. A dressing followed by a soft elastic bandage and brace or splint are usually placed before you leave the operating room. Most patients go home a few hours after surgery.

For the first few days you should rest and elevate your leg and apply ice packs for twenty to thirty minutes, three or four times a day. This relieves pain and swelling. Pain pills and antiinflammatory medications can manage discomfort. Keep your ankle and toes moving to prevent stagnant blood from clotting in your calf veins. Crutches or a cane may help you minimize weight bearing on the affected leg.

You should see your doctor in a week or so, to ensure your incision has healed satisfac-

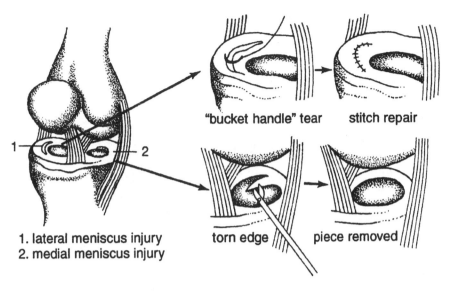

"bucket handle" tear   stitch repair

1. lateral meniscus injury
2. medial meniscus injury

torn edge   piece removed

Fig. 22.5 Types of knee meniscus operations

torily, and then regularly, until you have achieved your full rehabilitative potential.

Postoperative recommendations for physical therapy and rehabilitation are varied, depending on the degree of meniscus damage and associated injury. They will involve a period of immobilization and restrictions on range of joint motion and weight bearing. Activity can be gradually resumed during a period of physical therapy emphasizing exercises that increase range of joint motion, flexibility, and strength in the muscles that help support your knee. Most likely, you will be able to return to full activity in six to eight weeks, although you may need a brace for demanding sports such as football and skiing.

Risks of meniscus surgery include damage to the nerves, artery, and vein passing through the back of your knee. Your incision can become infected. The repair itself may weaken or another tear occur. Scar tissue can form in the joint giving you a stiff knee. Further sur-

gery is required for a complication in 4 percent of cases.

Knee Ligament Injury

The four knee ligaments act both to support your knee during its normal movements and brace it against abnormal motion. Torn ligaments cause a wobbly knee. Commonly, if the force was substantial, more than one ligament is injured. Tears may be partial or complete.

The *anterior cruciate ligament (ACL)* is a strong ropelike structure running through the middle of your knee joint, connecting the back of the femur to the front of the tibia. It prevents the tibia from sliding forward or rotating on the femur. This ligament is the one most frequently injured, usually having been torn by a twist during a quick turn or direct blow. The *posterior cruciate ligament (PCL)* connects the front of the femur to the back of the tibia, bracing the tibia against sliding backward on the femur. It is most often injured during direct athletic trauma or an automobile accident.

The *medial collateral ligament (MCL)* connects the femur and tibia on the inner side of your knee, restraining it from bending inward. It is most often torn by a direct blow to the outer side of the joint. The *lateral collateral ligament (LCL)* connects the femur and tibia on the outer side of the joint, bracing your knee against buckling outward. A tear is usually associated with cruciate ligament injuries.

Alternative Medicine Approaches to Knee Ligament Injury

The natural history of a knee without an ACL is unknown. No studies show that restructuring the ACL prevents arthritis. In fact, when the ACL is reconstructed, a higher rate of degenerative joint changes may follow than if it were not reconstructed, due to the newly changed interface dynamics. Only the most disabling injuries should therefore be surgically repaired. Especially if you have other injuries, damage to your MCL or PCL is usually best treated nonoperatively.

As with knee meniscus injury, if you do not place great demands upon your knee, you may do best by simply protecting it with a brace and doing regular physical therapy. Often, conventional physical therapy is all that is needed.

Following are the most promising alternative medicine approaches to knee ligament injury.

Use an Ice Pack or Alternating Ice and Heat

Applying an ice pack alone or alternating it with a heating pad for twenty to thirty min-

utes, three to four times a day, should help to increase local circulation of blood and lymph to assist in healing. In addition, it may provide enough pain relief that you do not need surgical correction.

Elevate Your Leg

When you have an opportunity, elevate your leg using cushions so that it sits above your heart level. This will help the blood and lymph to drain from your leg, increasing their circulation and thus helping their ability to assist healing. Try to elevate your leg two to three times daily, for at least twenty minutes each time.

Rest

Resting your knee, using a bandage, a knee brace, and crutches as needed, may give your knee adequate opportunity to heal itself. By this nonstep alone, you may be able to avert an operation.

Take Supplements

Flaxseed oil and glucosamine sulfate with chondroitin have been shown to reduce inflammation. Start with 1 tablespoon of flaxseed oil two to three times daily and 500 to 1,000 mg of glucosamine with chondroitin three times daily. You can also try rubbing flaxseed or castor oil on your knee at night. Also promising are taking 5 to 10 gm of methylsulfonylmethane, more popularly known as MSM, two to three times daily and 1 gm of bromelain two times daily.

Exercise

Strengthening the muscles surrounding your knee gives you better support while taking some of the burden off your ligament.

Regular exercise is needed, but in small amounts, increasing your workout time according to your individual tolerance. Begin after any acute inflammation has subsided, usually twenty-four to forty-eight hours postinjury.

Practice Yoga Daily

By keeping your knees flexible, the gentle stretching of yoga may help prevent injury caused by sudden twisting. Slowly stretch your quadriceps, hamstrings, and calf muscles. You should feel a gentle pull, but not an ache or pain. Yoga practice helps increase local blood and lymph flow, and thus may help in healing your ligament enough to avert surgery.

Try Acupuncture, Chiropractic, and Osteopathy

Acupuncture has been shown to be an effective treatment for ligament injury.[63] Chiropractic and osteopathic treatments may also be helpful.

Conventional Medicine Approaches to Knee Ligament Injury

Torn collateral ligaments and partially torn anterior cruciate ligament tears can be treated with ice packs and a sleeve-type brace to reduce pain and swelling. The acronym is RICE—rest, ice, compression, and elevation. Most will go on to heal with braces, exercise, and a structured rehabilitation.

Ice Packs and Heating Pads

Ice cold packs can reduce pain and swelling. Use for no more than twenty minutes at any one time. Don't put ice against your bare skin for more than five minutes.

Heat can be beneficial after the initial pain disappears. It may help relieve stiffness. Use a warm heating pad or hot water bottle for about twenty minutes several times a day.

Drug Treatments

You may find benefit from the short-term use of nonsteroidal antiinflammatory medication (Motrin, Advil, ibuprofen, Alleve) that decrease the body's inflammatory response to injury. This will reduce knee swelling and fluid within the joint. The stronger pain medications (Percocet, Tylenol #3, Vicodin) may help you through episodes of acute pain.

Crutches and Braces

These are prescribed to protect your knee from whatever movements would stress the healing ligament. They also keep your knee warm. Increased comfort and confidence will allow you to be more active in a rehabilitation program.

Physical Therapy

Controlled range-of-motion and knee-strengthening exercises under the supervision of a physical therapist are keys to a structured rehabilitation. You can do most of this at home with the aid of inexpensive physical therapy ropes, pulleys, straps, and weights.

Ultrasound and Electrical Stimulation

These treatments may help decrease pain and possibly speed healing.

Surgical Approaches to Knee Ligament Injury

In general, recommendation for treatment of a knee ligament problem depends on your degree of injury, associated ligament and/or meniscus injury, and your desired level of activity. Many people do not place much stress on their knees and are able to carry out their normal activities without ligament repair or knee reconstruction. For them, a period of rehabilitation is all that is necessary. However, if you choose not to have your ligament surgically repaired, it can lead to damage of other joint structures, a permanently unstable knee, and increased likelihood of knee arthritis.

Minor injuries, such as incomplete ligament tears, generally heal with a period of rest, protection, and physical therapy. Injuries should be surgically repaired if they are severe or when pain or instability persists after a trial of alternative and conventional nonsurgical treatment. Your ability to perform the activities of daily living, job requirements, recreational activities, potential for further joint damage, and risks of surgery must be factored into the decision. Also, you should be willing and able to commit yourself to a lengthy, and at times demanding, postoperative rehabilitation program.

Surgery is usually delayed until the acute swelling, inflammation, and pain have subsided, since operating too early can lead to an increased risk of permanent joint stiffness. Usually this means surgery is postponed for at least three to four weeks after the damage occurred. During the initial period, you are treated with ice, rest, elevation, and antiinflammatory medication.

Most ligament repairs are now performed through the arthroscope, or with an arthroscopic assist, on an outpatient basis, or with just an overnight stay. General, regional, or local anesthesia, with intravenous sedation, can be chosen. After anesthesia, your leg is prepped with an antibacterial solution from your toes to your groin. A small incision is made in the front part of your knee, and a tiny TV camera inserted, while your surgeon watches on a TV monitor. Degree of ligament damage and associated meniscus injury is determined.

Anterior Cruciate Ligament Repair

Most patients older than 40 years of age with ACL injuries are treated nonoperatively because of a high rate of fibrosis across the joint and subsequent loss of motion. However, good results have recently been reported in patients between the ages of 40 and 60 who are active and wish to continue to participate in sports activities.[64] If the ACL must be replaced, a graft is taken from part of your strong kneecap or hamstring tendon. Small holes are drilled in the front of your tibia and the back of your femur. (See Figure 22.6.) The graft is then inserted through the hole in the tibia, across the joint space, and its end brought out through the hole in the femur. After carefully adjusting the tension to equal that in the normal ACL, the graft is fixed in place with screws into your bones.

Posterior Cruciate Ligament Repair

A PCL injury commonly detaches a small piece of bone from the tibia. If so, a second incision must be made over the fracture site, to reattach the piece of bone with a screw. When necessary, the tendon itself can be replaced with a graft, similar to ACL repair.

Medial and Lateral Collateral Ligament Repair

Usually, the MCL and LCL are repaired when there are other ligament and/or meniscus injuries. These ligaments cannot be seen through an arthroscope, so a two- to three-

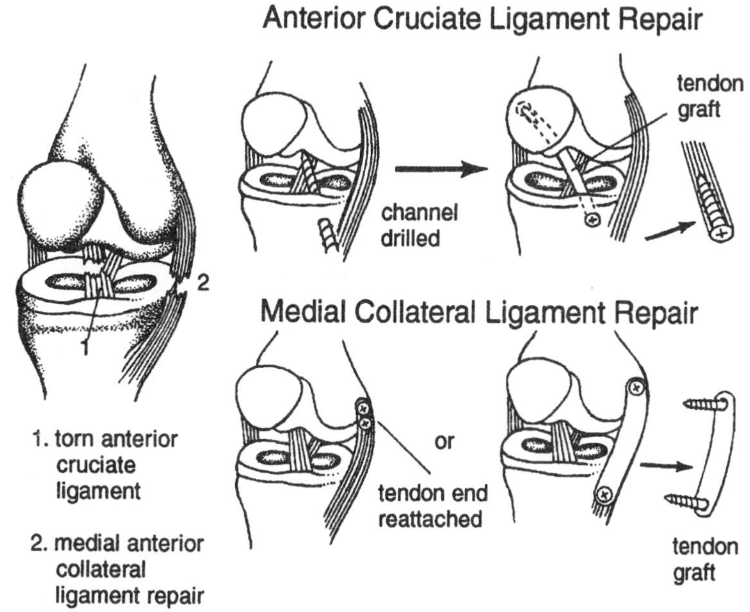

Anterior Cruciate Ligament Repair

tendon graft

channel drilled

2

Medial Collateral Ligament Repair

or

tendon end reattached

tendon graft

1. torn anterior cruciate ligament

2. medial anterior collateral ligament repair

Fig. 22.6 Types of knee ligament operations

inch incision running down the inside or outside of your knee is necessary. A torn ligament is repaired with stitches, or if its end is detached, it is stapled or screwed back down on the bone. If the injury is beyond repair, a tendon graft can be used.

After ligament repair is completed, a soft plastic drain may be placed into the joint space to remove blood and joint fluid. It may be left to drain into the bandage or connected to a suction device. The skin is closed with stitches, staples, or skin tapes. A soft dressing covers the wound followed by a brace or splint to restrict your joint's range of motion.

For the next few days, you need to elevate your leg and place ice on your knee. Most likely, you will be given antiinflammatory medication to help minimize swelling. You should slowly bend the joint, and do simple exercises, prescribed by your doctor or physical therapist. You may be given an automatic continuous passive motion machine to bend your knee, slowly increasing its range of motion and preventing joint stiffness.

You should see your doctor in two or three days to remove your drain and staples or stitches, if any. You then need to be seen on a regular basis, until you have achieved your full rehabilitative potential.

Postoperative recommendations for physical therapy and rehabilitation are varied, depending on degree of ligament damage, associated injury, and type of repair. Your activities can be gradually resumed during this period of physical therapy, with emphasis on exercises to increase range of joint motion, flexibility, and strength in the muscles that help support your knee. You should then continue these exercises indefinitely, to protect your knee for a lifetime. You can first begin weight bearing on crutches, then progress to a walker or cane.

Most likely, you will be able to return to full activity in nine to twelve weeks, although a brace may be necessary for any strenuous activities.

Risks of ligament surgery include damage to the nerves, artery, and vein passing through the back of your knee. The ligament repair may weaken, or if a graft has been used, it can stretch or tear. Incision infection can develop, or scar tissue can form in the joint, giving you a stiff knee. Further surgery may be required for such a complication.

KNEE MENISCUS AND KNEE LIGAMENT INJURY SUMMARY

Prevention

Diet and Supplements

• Follow a low-fat, high-fiber diet.

Lifestyle

• Practice daily yoga postures.
• Exercise 1 hour, 3–5 times weekly.

Alternative Medicine Approaches

• Follow the preventive guidelines, above.
• Bromelain, 500 mg, 3 times daily.
• Flaxseed oil, 1 tablespoon, 2–3 times daily.
• Glucosamine sulfate, 500 mg, 3 times daily.

Conventional Medicine Approaches

• Ice pack.
• Elevate leg.
• Rest, protection, and physical therapy.

• Antiinflammatory medication—aspirin, Tylenol; nonsteroidal—ibuprofen (Motrin, Advil, Alleve), piroxicam (Feldene), rofecoxib (Vioxx).
• Pain medication—codeine derivatives (Percocet, Tylenol #3, Vicodin).

Surgical Approaches

• Repair and reconstruction—arthroscopic, arthroscopic-assisted, or open.

Knee Joint Cartilage and Bone Damage

Total knee replacement is performed more than 180,000 times each year in the United States.[65] Severely painful degenerative arthritis of the knee joint is the usual indication for this seemingly drastic surgery, which removes the ends of the femur and tibia, substituting them with metal and plastic replacement parts.

Arthritis of the knee is caused by a long period of wear and tear on the normally smooth cartilages that cushion the ends of your femur (thigh) and tibia (lower leg) bones. Breakdown of the cartilages and menisci allows the bony ends to rub and grate against each other, producing such irregular surfaces that pain, joint swelling, and loss of joint motion follow. This process is accelerated by direct trauma and damage to the joint's menisci and ligaments by athletics, strenuous daily activities and work requirements, obesity, and accidents. If you have rheumatoid arthritis, and your knee remains swollen and painful, you may also need a knee replacement. Occasionally, tuberculosis or a bone tumor can destroy the joint enough to warrant replacement.

Alternative Medicine Approaches to Knee Joint Cartilage and Bone Damage

Once you have your knee surgically replaced, you give up the chance for full range of motion in that knee. Knee replacement is not recommended for younger patients, who tend to be more affected by the restrictions of knee movement following this surgery, and are more subject to complications. Especially if you are young, it is recommended that you follow an alternative medicine approach first.

Change Your Diet

Following a vegetarian diet may help treat any underlying arthritis. Both osteoarthritis and rheumatoid arthritis are rare in populations that follow a low-fat, high-fiber vegetarian diet, but are very common in Western cultures. The reason may be that fats in the bloodstream interfere with local circulation in your joints and affect the joints' ability to repair themselves. In addition, such a diet may also affect your intestinal lining, allowing whole proteins to cross into the bloodstream, where they may act as foreign invaders and cause inflammatory reactions. Follow the dietary guidelines given in Chapter 2.

Take Supplements

Adding calcium and magnesium supplements may give you relief from pain. Try 1,000 mg of calcium citrate at bedtime, combined with 500 mg of magnesium. Some people also benefit from additional calcium and magnesium during the day, 250 mg of calcium and 100 mg of magnesium.

Studies have indicated that evening primrose oil or fish oil may effect pain relief in persons with arthritis. Further research is needed.

Rest and Support Your Knee

Resting your knee or using a bandage or knee brace may be all that is needed to assist your knee in self-repair. Rest will allow your knee to focus on its restoration and avoid further injury. Keep the knee above the level of your heart whenever possible to encourage drainage of veins and lymph and to promote optimum circulation.

Maintain Your Optimum Weight

If you are overweight, this alone can overwhelm the ability of your knee to repair itself properly. Follow the nutritional guidelines and stress-management advice given in Chapter 2, and join a support group to help maintain these changes. Knee replacement is especially problematic if you are overweight, so you will need to change your eating habits anyway to help assure success from an operation.

Exercise Regularly and Do Physical Therapy

Exercise, both in general and that specific to the knee, may assist the body to repair itself more effectively. Also, increasing the strength in the muscles around the knee may prevent or delay the progression of arthritis, a benefit that no conventional drugs can achieve. In addition to active exercise for an hour, three to five times per week—swimming is especially helpful—add a series of weight-bearing exercises to strengthen the muscles that support the knee.

Practice Yoga and Relaxation Daily

Doing gentle yoga stretches increases the availability of nutrients to the tissues for proper repair, and removes waste products.

Learning deep relaxation and meditation produces a shift in blood flow, again making your body more able to effect repair. Follow the guidelines given in Chapter 2.

Use Acupuncture, Massage, Chiropractic, and Osteopathy

Acupuncture, massage, chiropractic, and osteopathy also act by improving nutrient availability via an increase in local and systemic circulation. They may give you relatively rapid pain relief, as discussed more fully in Chapter 2. Although no specific research has thus far documented their degree of success in the treatment of knee pain, anecdotal reports are promising and future research seems warranted.

Use Natural Topicals

Flaxseed and castor oils have been reported to provide relief.[66] Rub either oil on your knee four times daily. Other traditions suggest peanut oil may also give the same benefit.

Conventional Medicine Approaches to Knee Joint Cartilage and Bone Damage

There is no proven way to prevent progression of the osteoarthritis other than weight reduction and knee muscle strengthening. Conventional treatment falls into the category of symptom relief. Any underlying disease such as rheumatoid arthritis should be treated. In addition to education, rest and joint protection when necessary, supervised exercise, and physical therapy, you can try the following conventional approaches.

Pain Medications

Because of low potential for harmful side effects, it is generally recommended that pain

relievers be tried before antiinflammatories. Acetaminophen (Tylenol) is a pain reliever widely used because of its safety. Stronger codeine-family drugs should be used only for short periods because of their side effects and addictive potential. Glucosamine and chondroitin sulfate are intermediate compounds the body uses in protein synthesis. Over-the-counter tablets have been shown to help relieve pain, but so far haven't shown any effect on the progression of the arthritis.

Antiinflammatory Medications

The non-steroidal antiinflammatory drugs (NSAIDs) decrease inflammation and swelling, and may also help provide pain relief. There are a great many types of NSAIDs. The salicylates include aspirin, which is the most commonly prescribed medication to treat degenerative arthritis. Others are the proprionic acids ibuprofin (Motrin, Advil), naproxen (Naprosyn, Alleve) and oxaprozin (Daypro); the oxicam piroxicam (Feldene); the heteroarylacetic acid diclofenac (Volteren); the indoacetic acids indomethacin (Indocin) and sulindac (Clinoril); and the napthyalkanone nabumetone (Reladin). These should not be used for extended periods, since they have a potential for significant bleeding and gastrointestinal, liver, kidney, and neurologic side effects, and may in fact contribute to joint breakdown. If one type of NSAID doesn't seem to be working, you can try another, as an individual's response to each type may be quite variable. You can use NSAIDs with pain medication, as they have different mechanisms of action, but do not use two different types of NSAIDs concurrently, as the risk of toxity is increased.

Most NSAIDs inhibit both cyclooxygenase types 1 and 2. COX-1 is an enzyme found in all tissues. COX-2 is another form of the enzyme found in large quantities in areas of inflammation. It may be that the toxity of NSAIDs is mostly due to its effect on COX-1, while its beneficial effect in arthritis is due to inhibition of COX-2. Recently, the selective COX-2 inhibitors celecoxib (Celebrex) and rofecoxib (Vioxx) have been used to treat osteoarthritis with some evidence for decreased gastrointestinal and bleeding side effects.

Topical Applications

NSAIDs can also be applied as a gel with proven pain relief effects. If this works for you, the possible systemic toxic effects can be avoided.[67] Capsaicin (Zostrix) is a compound found in hot peppers. It can be applied in a gel or cream. It diffuses through your skin and acts by decreasing a substance involved in the pain process. It is much safer than drug treatments and has been shown to help decrease pain from knee osteoarthritis.[68] It can be rubbed on the area three to four times per day. Local skin irritation and burning decreases with time. Don't let your hands contact your eyes or mouth until thoroughly cleansed with soap and water.

Joint Injection

Injections of cortisone compounds into the painful joint may reduce inflammation, giving temporary pain relief and allowing you to be more active. The effect may last from a few days to a month.[69] However, these injections do not halt progression of your disease and should not be used more than three times a year.

Hyaluronic acid (Synvisc, Hyalgan) can also be injected and has been found to be helpful.[70] These injections are given weekly for three to five weeks.

Physical Aids

Braces, knee taping, shoe inserts, walkers, and canes have been shown to have a beneficial effect by redistributing your weight or supporting your joint. These can help you be more comfortable with your exercise program.

Surgical Approach to Knee Joint Cartilage and Bone Damage

If your knee pain and loss of joint motion are severe enough to affect your ability to carry out the activities necessary for your daily living, and your problems are not sufficiently relieved by an alternative and conventional medicine treatment program, you should consider a total knee replacement. Modern techniques and prosthetic devices designed to recreate this joint's complex normal movements have made the outcome very reliable, with 90 percent satisfactory results at ten years.

Preoperative preparation is very important in joint replacement surgery. Since you are likely to need blood transfusion, donate two pints of your own blood in the weeks prior to your operation. Do leg exercises to strengthen your muscles for the increased burden necessary during your period of rehabilitation. Make sure that you do not have any skin sores or other infections that might increase your risk for infection of your prosthetic knee.

You are admitted the morning of surgery. General or regional anesthesia may be chosen. Your leg is prepped with a antiseptic solution, and a tourniquet applied to your thigh, to decrease bleeding and create a clearer operative field. To minimize your risk of infection, you are given intravenous antibiotics.

An eight- to ten-inch incision is made, running down the front of your knee. After the joint and the ends of the femur and tibia are exposed, your surgeon removes what is left of the cartilages, then reshapes the ends of the bones so that the prosthetic components fit securely. (See Figure 22.7.) Measurements are taken, and components selected for shape and thickness, so that after they are in place, your leg is normally aligned and your muscle ligaments under proper tension. Screws, stems, or pegs that fit into the bone then attach the components. In some types, the bond is further strengthened by cement, while others have a porous surface into which the bone grows. If the undersurface of your kneecap is irregular, it can be replaced with a smooth plastic component. A soft plastic drain, to minimize fluid collection and swelling, is left in the joint space, with a second small incision connecting it to a bulb collector. The incision is closed with stitches or staples and wrapped with a soft bandage. A brace or splint is then applied. This operation takes two to three hours.

You will spend an hour in the recovery room. Postoperative pain can be controlled with intravenous or epidural medication. After a few days you can switch to pain pills. The drain is removed before you go home.

Your first few days after surgery should be spent in the hospital, so that the beginning of your rehabilitation can be closely monitored. You may be given a passive motion machine set to slowly move your joint to preset degrees. You can begin limited walking before going home. Weight bearing is progressively increased with the help of a walker, crutches, and then a cane. Most patients are discharged after four to six days.

Your rehabilitation program continues at home, usually under the watchful eye of a visiting physical therapist. You will need to work on knee flexibility, range of motion, and strengthening the muscles of the thigh and calf that support the knee. Two or three months may be needed to achieve your maximum function. The prosthetic joint is de-

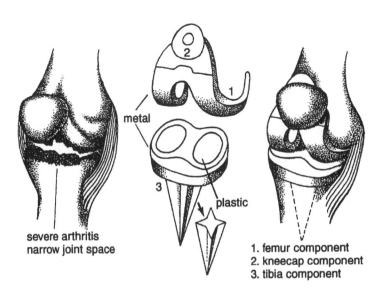

severe arthritis
narrow joint space

metal

plastic

1. femur component
2. kneecap component
3. tibia component

Fig. 22.7 Total knee replacement

signed for normal daily activities, but should not be bent beyond 90 degrees, so you must give up kneeling, squats, pushing forward in a chair, and most vigorous sports. These restrictions should be well worth your increase in mobility and relief of daily pain.

Complications specific to total knee replacement include prosthetic loosening—almost always the lower leg component, bone fracture, bone loss due to poor blood supply, dislocation of the prosthetic joint, and damage to the nerves, artery, and vein passing behind the knee. Also, blood clots can develop in the deep veins of the leg (thrombosis) with possible subsequent migration to the lungs (1 percent). The risk of joint infection is 0.5 to 2 percent. Poor results occur in 5 percent of the cases. Most problems happen in the first six years, few thereafter. Failure is most often due to infection so that you should receive antibiotics if you have dental work or a colonoscopy and must not delay treatment for any sort of skin or other infection. If your prosthesis needs to be replaced, you have a 90 percent chance for a successful outcome.

KNEE JOINT CARTILAGE AND BONE DAMAGE SUMMARY

Prevention

Diet and Supplements

- Follow a low-fat, high-fiber, vegetarian diet.

Lifestyle

- Maintain optimum weight.

- Exercise regularly: 1 hour, 3–5 times weekly.
- Practice yoga daily.

Alternative Medicine Approaches

- Follow the preventive guidelines, above.
- Calcium citrate, 250 mg during the day, 1,000 mg at night.
- Magnesium, 100 mg during the day, 500 mg at night.
- Evening primrose oil or fish oil.
- Flaxseed oil, castor oil, or peanut oil, rubbed in 4 times daily.
- Use acupuncture, chiropractic, osteopathy, hypnosis, magnets.
- Practice visualization.

Conventional Medicine Approaches

- Rest, protection, and physical therapy.
- Physical aids—braces, taping, walker, cane, shoe insert.
- Pain medication—Tylenol; codeine derivatives Percocet, Tylenol #3, Vicodin.
- Antiinflammatories—aspirin, ibuprofen (Motrin, Advil, Alleve), piroxicam (Feldene), rofecoxib (Vioxx).
- Topical applications—NSAIDs, capsaicin. Zostrix.
- Joint injection—cortisone.

Surgical Approach

- Total knee replacement.

The Hip

More than 238,000 total hip replacements are performed in the United States each year for hip fracture or advanced arthritis.[71] This is a common operation in the elderly; two-thirds of these patients are more than 65 years of age. Because of the greater risk of osteoporosis and fracture, women need hip replacement more often than men. With modern techniques, you are quickly up, walking, and out of the hospital—whereas just a few years ago, the disability of a very painful hip made independent living almost impossible.

How Your Hip Works

Your hip is a "ball and socket" joint that allows your thigh to move forward, backward, inward, and outward, as well as twist clockwise and counterclockwise. The "head" of the femur (thigh bone) fits into the socket of pelvic bone. (See Figure 22.8.) The joint is held together by strong muscles and ligaments connecting the femur with the pelvis. The cartilages covering and cushioning the bony weight-bearing surfaces are critically important to smooth, painfree movement.

Hip Joint Damage

The normal wear and tear of aging can destroy the hip joint's smooth surfaces, allowing your bones to grate against each other, causing jagged contact points that further the grinding process. The result is a narrowed joint with flattened, irregular surfaces, loss of joint range of movement, and pain on weight bearing and walking. This outcome, termed *osteoarthritis,* or more simply *arthritis,* is the major indication for total hip replacement.

Other diseases that can cause a painful, dysfunctional hip are rheumatoid arthritis, traumatic arthritis caused by a major injury to the joint, some types of bone fractures that would be difficult to simply "pin" back together, bone tumors, and injury to the blood supply of the femur top, causing its cells to die and the bone to disintegrate.

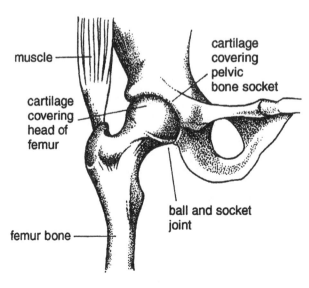

Fig. 22.8 The anatomy of the hip

How Hip Joint Damage Is Diagnosed

The diagnosis of hip disease is straight forward and involves the following elements.

History

Your doctor should ask you questions about your overall health, especially to determine if you have any problems that predispose you to bone or joint disease such as gout or rheumatoid arthritis. Coexisting medical problems such as heart, kidney, or lung disease are more important than your age in determining your risk for hip surgery.

Tell your doctor what makes your symptoms worse, and what you have been able to do to relieve them. Detail how often you require pain pills or antiinflammatory medications (Motrin, Advil, ibuprofen, Alleve), how much time you have lost from work, or, if retired, how often you have had to miss out on activities that you would like to do. If you feel unstable when walking, or have fallen, you should convey this information. Your lifestyle, recreational desires, and especially your ability to perform necessary activities for daily living (ADLs) will help plan the treatment that is best for you.

Physical Exam

Your doctor will watch how you walk, sit down, and get up from a chair. Your hip will be moved in many different directions to determine any limitation in normal range of motion. Pain, grating sensations, and lack of smooth movements are noted. Since differences are important, both hips are tested.

X-Rays

This is usually the only test necessary. It will show the narrowed joint space and irregular bony surfaces of arthritis. Other problems with the bones such as fracture and tumor can also be seen.

CAT and MRI Scans

These scans may sometimes be helpful in diagnosing unusual joint problems such as bone and cartilage tumors, but are not necessary in the usual case of degenerative arthritis. For a CAT scan you lay inside a spinning arm that takes multiple X-ray images that a computer reassembles to produce cross sections of your thigh, hip, and pelvis anatomy. For the MRI you lay inside a scanner as a powerful magnet changes the orientation of your cell atom components. X-ray type images are constructed by a computer. The soft tissue structures of cartilage and muscle are most clearly seen.

Alternative Medicine Approaches to Hip Joint Damage

―――――――――――

Isobel was a joyful 84-year-old former schoolteacher who now devoted her time to tutoring Hispanic children who were having difficulties reading English. Her abundant zest for life had always included indulging in lots of rich fatty foods; she was markedly overweight and had developed significant osteoarthritis in her hips, despite regular swimming and dancing.

Her pain had begun to interfere with these favorite activities, so she decided to try a hip replacement operation in order to continue with her exuberant life. Unfortunately, perhaps partly because of her obesity, she was one of those whom surgery did not help. She did not heal well from her operation and ended up having to use a walker and then a wheelchair for the rest of her life.

―――――――――――

Although it can be a boon to your overall functioning, hip replacement does have its limitations, and rarely, some people do not function as well as they expect after their surgery. You may, therefore, want to try one of these other avenues of treatment first, before deciding in favor of surgery.

Change Your Diet

Dietary changes may help alleviate any underlying arthritis. Red meats, dairy products, refined sugar, fats, salt, and caffeine intake has all been associated with this disease.[72] Eliminating nightshade vegetables (tomatoes, potatoes, eggplant, and peppers) may be helpful.[73] Follow the nutritional guidelines given in Chapter 2.

Take Supplements

Glucosamine sulfate is available in health food stores, and is being used by many people who report benefit, though further research is needed. Methionine, an amino acid, in a double-blind study, proved more effective than ibuprofen in relieving pain from osteoarthritis.[74] Calcium and magnesium supplements may assist in improving any underlying arthritis. Take 1,000 mg of calcium, and 500 mg of magnesium at bedtime.

Vitamin E, 600 IU per day, was found to be effective in helping relieve arthritic pain and inflammation.[75] Vitamin C and pantothenic acid may help with cartilage repair; take 1,000 mg of each, three times daily. Take 2 capsules of evening primrose oil, three times daily, for its antioxidant activity. Fish oil, one to two capsules, three times daily, may also be of help.

According to a 1997 National Health and Nutrition Examination Survey Study, an estimated 26 million to 38 million U.S. adults

have osteoporosis or are at risk for osteoporosis in the hip. Vitamin D is required for efficient absorption of dietary calcium and for normal mineralization of bone. Vitamin D deficiency contributes to osteoporosis and has been found in 50 percent of all women with devastating and life-threatening hip fractures.[76] This deficiency is preventable by vitamin D supplementation and sun exposure. The 1997 Dietary Reference Intake guidelines from the National Institutes of Health recommend 400 IU of supplemental vitamin D daily for individuals from age 51 through 70 years and 600 IU daily for those older than 70. Supplements of about 800 IU of vitamin D per day and calcium may be necessary to attenuate bone loss in the winter. Follow these guidelines to reduce your fracture risk and facilitate fracture healing if it has already occurred.

Maintain Your Optimum Weight

Excess weight is strongly associated with increased risk of arthritis of the hip, and weight loss itself may help reverse this problem. If you are overweight, reducing your weight decreases the stress on your hip and increases the nutrient supply to the joint, assisting in recovery. Since in order to help yourself heal and ensure ultimate success of the operation you will need to make an effort to achieve and maintain your optimum weight, even if you decide to have surgery, you may wish to give weight loss a trial before embarking upon hip replacement surgery. See Chapter 2 for dietary and stress-management guidelines to help you.

Use Walking and Balancing Aids

A cane and handrails near your toilet and bathtub can make your daily activities easier.

Get a raised toilet seat and don't sit in low, soft chairs. Avoid activities which cause hip discomfort.

Exercise Regularly and Try Physical Therapy

A remarkable study of young patients suffering from rheumatoid arthritis of the hips, severe enough to show up on an X-ray, found that an intervention of simply swimming one hour daily, combined with one aspirin per day, resulted in significant X-ray improvement one year later.[77]

Practice Yoga Daily

Do one hour daily of the combined yoga stretches and relaxation exercises, to improve circulation and repair activity in your hip region. Follow the guidelines given in Chapter 2.

Use Acupuncture, Massage, Chiropractic, and Osteopathy

Anecdotally, many people have found relief from pain through these modalities. Even if a joint has broken down with arthritic changes, a shift in energy flow and circulation offered by these treatments may help the joint rebuild itself enough to leave you free of significant impairment. Further research is needed.

Practice Visualization

First use deep relaxation, given in Chapter 2. Then imagine your thigh bone as a baseball bat, and your hip socket as a glove. Picture them with an easeful, smooth junction, well oiled with Neetsfoot oil. Hold this image in your mind, while feeling it within your body. Repeat several times daily.

Conventional Medicine Approaches to Hip Joint Damage

There is no proven way to prevent progression of osteoarthritis other than weight reduction and muscle strengthening. Conventional treatment falls into the category of symptom relief. Any underlying disease such as rheumatoid arthritis should be treated. In addition to education, rest and joint protection when necessary, supervised exercise and physical therapy, the following conventional approaches are recommended.

Exercise

Although you may have to limit activities that cause discomfort, becoming less active will decrease your muscle and bone strength and have adverse effects on your overall health. Studies show that if you attempt to be as active as possible, you will not accelerate the deterioration of your hip joint and you will do best. Avoid any activities such as jogging that aggravate your pain. Swimming is the best form of exercise, as it allows you to use your joint without full weight bearing. Riding a bike is also great if you have good balance. If you need to, take some pain medication before you exercise.

Pain Medications

Because of low potential for harmful side effects, it is generally recommended that pain relievers be tried before antiinflammatories. Acetaminophen (Tylenol) is a pain reliever widely used because of its safety. Stronger codeine family drugs should be used only for short periods because of their side effects and addictive potential. Glucosamine and chondroitin sulfate are intermediate compounds the body uses in protein synthesis. They may possibly be protective by repairing cartilage and decelerating the degenerative process.[78] Over-the-counter tablets have been shown to help relieve pain but so far haven't been scientifically proven to have any effect on the progression of arthritis.

Antiinflammatory Medications

The nonsteroidal antiinflammatory drugs (NSAIDs) decrease inflammation and swelling and may also help provide pain relief. There are a great many types of NSAIDs. The salicylates include aspirin, which is the most commonly prescribed medication to treat degenerative arthritis. Others are the proprionic acids ibuprofin (Motrin, Advil), naproxen (Naprosyn, Alleve), and oxaprozin (Daypro); the oxicam piroxicam (Feldene); the heteroarylacetic acid diclofenac (Volteren); the indoacetic acids indomethacin (Indocin) and sulindac (Clinoril); and the napthyalkanone nabumetone (Reladin). These should not be used for extended periods, since they have a potential for significant bleeding and gastrointestinal, liver, kidney, and neurologic side effects, and may in fact contribute to joint breakdown. If one type of NSAID doesn't seem to be working, you can try another, as an individual's response to each type may be quite variable. You can use NSAIDs with pain medication, as they have different mechanisms of action, but do not use two different types of NSAIDs concurrently, as the risk of toxity is increased.

Most NSAIDs inhibit both cyclooxygenase types 1 and 2. COX-1 is an enzyme found in all tissues. COX-2 is another form of the enzyme found in large quantities in areas of inflammation. It may be that the toxity of NSAIDs is mostly due to its effect on COX-1, while its beneficial effect in arthritis is due to

inhibition of COX-2. Recently, the selective COX-2 inhibitors celecoxib (Celebrex) and rofecoxib (Vioxx) are being used to treat osteoarthritis with some evidence for decreased gastrointestinal and bleeding side effects.

Topical Applications

NSAIDs can also be applied as a gel with proven pain relief effects. If this works for you, the possible systemic toxic effects can be avoided.[79] Capsaicin (Zostrix) is a compound found in hot peppers. It can be applied in a gel or cream. It diffuses through your skin and acts by decreasing a substance involved in the pain process. It is much safer than drug treatments and has been shown to help decrease pain from osteoarthritis.[80] It can be rubbed on the area three to four times per day. Local skin irritation and burning decreases with time. Don't let your hands contact your eyes or mouth until thoroughly cleansed with soap and water.

Physical Aids

Shoe inserts, walkers, and canes have been shown to have a beneficial effect by weight redistribution. These can help you be more active and comfortable with your exercise program.

Surgical Approach to Hip Joint Damage

Jack McLanahan, the authors' father, now 82 years old, had always led a very active and optimistic life. In his seventies, the family legacy of bad hips, and a history of pole-vaulting into a sawdust heap in college, finally caught up with him. Like his father before him, he struggled along with canes, but finally the constant discomfort became so intense and his joie de vivre *so constricted, he decided to choose hip replacement. The first hospitalization was a totally new experience, and at times the pain and adversity were discouraging. After a few weeks of rehab, all was well, and eight months later, he decided to have the second hip also replaced. Knowing what to expect, the second hospitalization went much more smoothly. Jack was able to move freely and painlessly, and wondered why he had waited so long.*

The world's first total hip replacement was done in 1962. An enormous amount of research has perfected techniques and developed high-tech metal, plastic, and ceramic materials for replacement components, with cement, screws, pegs, and surfaces that permit bony ingrowth to fix them in place. The state of the art is such that a National Institutes of Health Consensus Conference in 1994 concluded that total hip replacement offers "immediate and substantial improvement in the patient's functional status, and overall health-related quality of life." Results are good to excellent in 90 percent of all cases.[81] Data suggest that these outcomes hold up over time, and that fewer than 10 percent have to be revised.[82]

However, a guaranteed perfect hip is not yet available. While your new hip can be considered a "good" hip, it is not a "normal" hip. Significant restrictions in range of motion follow. Unless you are Bo Jackson, the professional baseball player who returned to the big leagues with an artificial hip, some of your activities may be limited. The younger you are, the more likely a revision may be necessary (10 to 30 percent after ten years). If you are vigorous or obese, you have a higher risk of your new hip components loosening, creating

a need for further surgery. Because total hip replacement components wear out over an extended period of time, if you are younger than age 55, you should consider nonsurgical treatment or another form of surgery, such as hip fusion.

Since arthritis tends to affect both hips, 20 to 40 percent of all patients require replacement of both hips. The procedures are usually staged several months apart, the second operation following a period of rehabilitation after the worst side has been replaced.

You should get yourself into your best possible physical condition before this operation, and lose as much excess weight as possible. This puts less stress on your new joint, lessening its likelihood of loosening. Exercise to build strength in the muscles around your hip helps them carry the load. Stop smoking, to lessen your chances of a lung complication and increase the blood and oxygen supply to the healing tissue. See Chapter 2 for help in how to quit. For this operation, most patients require blood transfusions. In the weeks before your surgery, you can donate two pints of your own blood, to avoid the major risks of transfusion.

You are admitted the morning of surgery. Hip replacement can be performed using general or spinal anesthesia. You are positioned on your side, and your whole leg, hip, and buttock prepped with an antiseptic solution. An incision infection might doom the success of this operation, so you are therefore given intravenous antibiotics. Some "total joint" operating rooms are set up with "laminar flow" air circulating systems, so that only filtered air passes over the operating table. Only your surgeon, anesthesiologist, and nurses are permitted in the operating room.

Without measures to thin your blood, you would have a very high risk of clot formation in your legs or pelvis (venous thrombosis) during this particular operation. Such clots could migrate to your lungs (pulmonary embolism). Therefore, you are given anticoagulants in the operative period and for a few days afterward, until you are up and around. This can increase the blood loss during the operation, but has been proven to dramatically reduce the severe risk associated with blood clots, and so is now standard procedure.

A ten- to twelve-inch skin incision is made laterally over your hip. The muscles are separated, and the femur and pelvic bones exposed by opening the joint capsule. The head and part of the neck of the femur are then cut out. The remaining cartilage of the pelvic part of the joint is removed, and the bony socket enlarged and shaped to accept the prosthetic component. (See Figure 22.9.) This new socket is usually made out of high-density polyethylene, within a metal hemisphere, to give it strength. The pelvic component is most often fixed in place with screws or pegs, and later, by bony ingrowth.

The soft bone of the canal inside the remaining neck and upper third of the femur is removed, and a femoral component chosen to fit within the new socket, so that your leg is held in proper length and position. The femoral component is made out of alloys of titanium and cobalt. The weight-bearing surface is either highly polished or covered with a layer of ceramic, to ensure smooth joint motion. Bone cement is then mixed into a putty-like consistency and packed into the cavity. The femoral component is placed into this cement-lined space and held in place for twelve to fifteen minutes, while the cement hardens. A drain is placed, passed through the skin, and connected to a soft plastic collection bulb. Your incision is closed with stitches, staples, or skin tapes.

You stay in the recovery room for about an hour, with your knees separated by pillows or a special brace. Pain can be controlled by an epidural catheter or intravenous pain medication. You may be wearing plastic automatic compression stockings, which squeeze your legs to prevent sluggish blood flow in your veins, helping prevent blood clots.

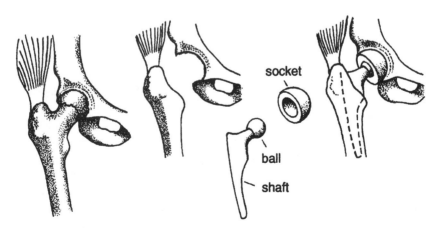

Fig. 22.9 Total hip replacement

You generally stay in the hospital for four or five days. This is a time of closely supervised physical therapy and learning how to live with and protect your new hip. You can be out of bed the next day and begin progressive weight bearing using a walker, crutches, and finally, a cane. Strengthening exercises concentrate on the muscles of your leg and hip. To avoid dislocating the new joint, you should not bend forward beyond 90 degrees, internally rotate your leg, or cross your legs. You will be shown safe ways to sit, get out of a chair, bend over, climb stairs, and so forth. Your drain and skin stitches or staples can be removed before you go home.

Rehabilitation continues at home, usually with the help of a visiting physical therapist. It is very important you build strong muscles, since weakness is the major risk for a fall, which could dislocate your hip or cause other injury. It is important to keep your hips higher than your knees. You should have your toilet seat raised, and not sit in soft, low chairs. Get a "grabber" to pick up things, to avoid bending your hip more than 90 degrees. To help with balance and stability, you should install tub bars and handrails around the house.

You should see your doctor several times over the following months. After a successful initial outcome is assured, you should see your doctor in a year, and then at least once every five years. If you sense that something is changing in your hip, notify your doctor immediately. Follow-up exams and X-rays can detect developing problems, which can be repaired before a more severe complication, such as a fracture, develops.

Unfortunately, some restrictions on your lifestyle are the price you pay for now having painfree activities of daily living. Your new hip will have a satisfactory range of motion for normal activities, but not the extended range of motion of a normal hip. It is subject to wear and tear, which can be accelerated by vigorous work or recreation. Nonstressful recreation—golf, swimming, bowling, even bicycle riding (don't fall off)—is okay, but tennis, skiing, horseback riding, and demanding physical work can increase the risk of displacement, component loosening, and premature joint wear.

The overall mortality risk of total hip replacement is 1 percent. Serious complications occur in 5 percent. These include significant bleeding (less than 4 percent); damage to the nerve, artery, or vein around the hip and thigh; femur fracture; deep vein blood clots (less than 15 percent), blood clots traveling to the lungs, and infection in the new joint (less than 1 percent at one year).

Long-term failure of the joint is most often caused by component-loosening *osteolysis*— reabsorption of bone that occurs when an inflammation reaction to the particulate matter from the prostheses and cement develops. This happens in less than 5 percent at ten years for the cemented pelvic bone component, and less than 2 percent at five years for the noncemented type. Fracture of the femur occurs in 1 to 3 percent of the cases. Your joint may have to be revised if you develop fracture, dislocation, or infection. A revision operation, much more difficult than the first operation, is followed by a 10 to 20 percent failure rate.

HIP JOINT DAMAGE SUMMARY

Prevention

Diet and Supplements

- Follow a low-fat, high-fiber, vegetarian diet.
- Avoid caffeine, red meats, dairy products, refined sugar, fats, salt, flour.
- Take vitamin D, 400–800 IU daily.

Lifestyle

- Maintain optimum weight.
- Exercise 1 hour, 3–5 times weekly.
- Practice yoga daily.
- Practice stress management.

Alternative Medicine Approaches

- Follow the preventive guidelines, above.
- Try eliminating nightshade foods, such as potatoes, eggplant, tomatoes, peppers, or other foods such as dairy products, to which you may be sensitive.
- Vitamin E, D-alpha, 600 IU daily.
- Vitamin C, 1,000 mg 3 times daily.
- Pantothenic acid, 1,000 mg 1–3 times daily.
- Evening primrose oil, 500 mg 3 times daily, or flaxseed oil, 1 tablespoon 1–3 times daily, or fish oil, 1–3 capsules daily.
- Glucosamine sulfate, 500 mg 3 times daily.
- Methionine, 1,000 mg daily.
- Calcium citrate, 1,000 mg, with magnesium, 500 mg.
- Use acupuncture, chiropractic, osteopathy, Rolfing and other forms of massage, hypnosis, homeopathy, magnets.
- Practice visualization.

Conventional Medicine Approaches

- Rest, protection, and physical therapy.
- Exercise.
- Pain medication—Tylenol; codeine derivatives Percocet, Tylenol #3, Vicodin.
- Antiinflammatory medications—aspirin, Tylenol; nonsteroidal (Motrin, Advil, ibuprofen, Alleve), piroxicam (Feldene), rofecoxib (Vioxx).
- Topical applications—NSAIDs, capsaicin, Zostrix.
- Physical aids—walkers, cane, shoe insert.

Surgical Approach

- Total hip replacement.

The Wrist

Lysieng, a refugee from Cambodia, got a job sewing goose down parkas. She worked eight-hour days at a warehouse factory sewing machine, then brought home piecework to complete at home, so she could further provide for her family. She developed such discomfort and weakness in both hands that she could not keep up with the demands of her boss. Braces did not help. Her insurance covered surgical procedures on both wrists, and she soon returned to work.

Our wrists are beautifully complex joints that help us achieve the remarkable variety of creative endeavors we enjoy as humans. Chronic pain in the wrist can therefore be more than annoying, and if it is due to entrapment of one of the wrist's nerves, termed *carpal tunnel syndrome (CTS)*, you may wonder if surgery might be the only answer.

Carpal tunnel syndrome is very common, affecting as many as 1 percent of the U.S. population, and is more common in women after age 50. Rheumatoid arthritis, gout, diabetes, hypothyroidism, the last three months of pregnancy, birth control pills, and excessive alcohol consumption all increase your risk for this problem.

You can act to avoid an operation by first trying alternative methods. If you do choose surgery, you can choose endoscopic repair, which will lessen your pain and recovery time.

How Your Wrist Works

The carpal tunnel is the narrow passageway between the wrist bones and the tough *transverse carpal ligament* that holds the tendons and nerves against the front of the wrist bones as they cross into your hand. These tendons flex the fingers when you make a fist or grasp objects. The *median nerve* runs through this tunnel. It provides sensation to the thumb, index, and middle fingers; to the thumb-side half of the ring finger; and to some small muscles in the thumb.

Carpal Tunnel Syndrome

Carpal tunnel syndrome develops when the median nerve is compressed within the carpal tunnel. Compression irritates the nerve, causing numbness, tingling, and pain in your thumb and first three fingers (the little finger is not affected). Pain may radiate from your wrist up your arm. These symptoms are typically first worse at night and may wake you with a feeling that your hand is asleep. Swelling of your wrist and hand can develop later. As the median nerve also controls some muscles of the thumb, weakness and poor coordination may lead to difficulty in holding a cup of tea or accomplishing fine motor tasks, such as fastening your buttons.

CTS can be precipitated by anything that causes swelling and increased pressure in the carpal tunnel such as arthritis, cysts, wrist fracture or other injury, and arm swelling from whatever cause. Most commonly, it is brought on by the repetitive use of the hand and fingers during work or sports. A study of all surgical cases of the adult population of the island of Montreal found that 55 percent of the cases in women and 76 percent of the cases in men were attributable to work-related activity.[83] Rapid, continuous flexing of your wrist back and forth, or holding it in a bent or gripping position for too long a time, typically while typing, sewing, driving, bicycling, rowing, weight lifting, or working with vibrating tools, may cause inflammation and swelling in the tendons. Using a computer mouse for hours, without relief of position, has led to a recent increase in this disorder. Since the rigid carpal tunnel cannot stretch, the nerve is compressed and irritated to the point it cannot function normally.

How Carpal Tunnel Syndrome Is Diagnosed

Diagnosis of CTS may be easy, but if the picture is not exactly typical, more sophisticated tests may be necessary.

History

The diagnosis of CTS is suggested by typical symptoms and a history of repetitive activity, such as may be required by your job or leisure-time activities. However, anything that causes swelling of the hand or forearm such as trauma, edema, infection, and tumors may be the cause. Also, medical conditions such as pregnancy, diabetes, thyroid dysfunction, and rheumatoid arthritis may be associated. Typical symptoms include tingling, numbness, and pain in the thumb, index, and middle fingers. There may be some pain in the inside part of your forearm. Often these symptoms are worse at night. You may tend to drop small objects. If holding your wrist in its maximum flexion (cocked forward) position for 60 seconds increases numbness or tingling, you probably have CTS.

Physical Exam

Your doctor should test sensation and strength in your fingers. There may be a mild atrophy or shrinking of the muscles on the thumb side of your hand. Tapping over the wrist with a finger may reproduce the symptoms. In most cases, no further complicated tests are necessary.

Nerve Conduction Tests

When the diagnosis is not obvious, nerve conduction velocity studies can be useful. For this test, a small needle is placed next to a proximal site of your nerve, and nerve impulse velocities are recorded at the wrist after nerve stimulation. Slow velocity indicates the presence of nerve damage.

Alternative Medicine Approaches to Carpal Tunnel Syndrome

Carpal tunnel syndrome is a condition that may go away on its own, and since it usually responds to alternative medicine approaches, you not only avoid an operation, but also

may act to prevent other health problems related to your lifestyle. Following are the most promising alternative medicine approaches to carpal tunnel syndrome.

Avoid Repetitive Activity; Modify Your Wrist Position

First, if possible, stop the activity that caused your CTS. If this relieves your symptoms, resume your necessary activities gradually. If you must do repetitive activity such as type, drive, or play the piano, keep your wrist as straight as possible. Never hold your wrist in one position for a long period, or flex it repeatedly, without taking frequent breaks to gently release its tension.

Use a Wrist Splint

The simple measure of a special carpal tunnel wrist splint, which is designed to hold your wrist straight or slightly extended, is often enough to relieve the pressure on the nerve so that your wrist can heal. The splint is usually made of plastic that is heat formed to the contour of the front of your hand and wrist. Velcro bands hold it snugly and comfortably in place.

The splint is especially helpful at night when your wrist tends to assume a bent, compressing position. At first you may also need to wear it during the day. It can take as long as six to eight weeks to have its full effect, but you are usually able to stop wearing the splint after two or three months. You should continue to wear it whenever your wrist is at risk, such as during your favorite sports.

Practice Special Exercises

Gently stretch your fingers. Flex, extend, and rotate your wrist joint. Slowly do these exercises for five minutes, four times a day.

Take Supplements

CTS has been shown to be alleviated by the addition of vitamin B_6 to the diet, as little at 50 mg daily being enough to eliminate symptoms, usually within one to three months.[84] This regimen is especially helpful for those whose problem may have developed due to excess alcohol use or late pregnancy, conditions that are known to lead to B_6 deficiency. Since larger doses of B_6 may have side effects, try higher doses, if needed, only under your doctor's supervision.

Practice Stress Management and Yoga Daily

Stress causes tightening of muscles, which may precipitate this problem. Follow the guidelines given in Chapter 2, especially emphasizing deep relaxation several times per day, and gentle flexing and releasing of your wrist area.

A 1998 study reported in the *Journal of the American Medical Association* compared a yoga program with wrist splinting for management of CTS. The yoga program consisted of a series of eleven yoga postures designed to strengthen, stretch, and balance each joint in the upper body along with relaxation twice weekly for eight weeks. The yoga program was found to be significantly more effective than splinting or no treatment in relieving pain and increasing grip strength.[85]

Use Physical Therapy, Massage, Rolfing, Chiropractic and Osteopathy

Physical therapy, massage, Rolfing, chiropractic and osteopathy all have anecdotally reported success with treatment of CTS by reducing the tension in the ligaments and fascia that make up the carpal tunnel or by relieving any contributory problems in nerve transmission located in the elbow or neck. The therapies themselves consist of direct physical manipulation and are discussed more fully in Chapter 2. More than one session may be necessary for you to experience symptom relief. Further research is needed.

Try Hot and Cold Treatments

You can immerse your hand and wrist in hot water (three minutes) alternating with ice water (thirty seconds). This increases local circulation, providing more nutrients to the irritated nerve. Cold or warm compresses may also be helpful. Try each for twenty minutes, three times per day.

Use Acupuncture

Acupuncture has been found to be highly successful in treating CTS.[86] This method can often give you immediate partial or complete relief of your pain, although more than one treatment session may be needed for your full recovery. See Chapter 2 for a more complete discussion of how acupuncture may act to eliminate discomfort and accelerate your body's tissue repair and healing mechanisms.

Practice Visualization

Do deep relaxation, given in Chapter 2. Then, for example, imagine your wrist's main nerve as a train track headed toward a narrow tunnel. First widen the tunnel, by making the roof higher and the sides farther apart. Then see a train passing easily through, joyfully echoing its distant whistle. Picture this and, at the same time, feel it happening within your body. Repeat several times per day.

Conventional Medicine Approaches to Carpal Tunnel Syndrome

In addition to splints, physical therapy, and avoiding activities that cause symptoms, the following conventional medicine measures are recommended.

Drug Treatments

Aspirin or nonsteroidal antiinflammatory drugs (Motrin, Advil, ibuprofen, Alleve) may be useful in short-term treatment to reduce wrist inflammation and pressure on the nerve. But, do not take them for more than a few months, owing to their significant side effects.

Cortisone Injections

Injections of a corticosteroid directly into the carpal tunnel decreases the inflammation and may also give temporary relief, giving enough time for the wrist splint and vitamin B_6 to work. Injections may give relief for as long as a year, in about 40 percent of the cases.

Surgical Approach to Carpal Tunnel Syndrome

I *(David) had an experience with CTS in both hands after I rushed to complete a backyard fence to keep my German shorthaired pointer from annoying the neighborhood. This required digging fifteen or twenty post holes in very hard ground, using a post hole digger. The repetitive ramming caused my wrists to swell, and gave me typical CTS symptoms. They weren't severe enough that I couldn't operate, but it was painful at night. Being somewhat macho, I ignored it, but when it was still bothering me after two months, I got*

a bit nervous. Not the least bit interested in surgery, I took the vitamin pills my sister recommends. The symptoms gradually receded, although I still get mild tingling when I hold a surgical retractor or carve wood for extended periods of time.

You should first undertake a dedicated trial of alternative medicine approaches to treat your CTS before considering surgery. However, if your symptoms persist, if the numbness and tingling are frequent and severe, limiting your ability to work and carry out your usual activities, if the muscles in your hand begin to shrink or lose their strength, or if you have sensation loss, you should have an operation.

Surgical treatment of CTS, called *carpal tunnel release,* is quite simple, and is performed on an outpatient basis. You can choose local, arm block, or general anesthesia. A tourniquet is usually placed on your upper arm so that your surgeon has a clear, bloodless field in which to see the delicate nerve structures. In the classical approach, your surgeon begins with a very small one- to two-inch incision located in the middle, lower portion of the palm of your hand. The restricting tunnel is opened by cutting the tough transverse carpal ligament that overlies the median nerve, releasing its compression. (See Figure 22.10.) Care is taken to avoid damaging any branches of the underlying nerve. Your skin incision is closed with stitches and a dressing applied, followed by a wrist splint. You can ask if your doctor can use an endoscope, a small operating tube inserted into the wrist through a one-quarter-inch incision, but since the view is less wide, you face an increased risk for complications.

Postoperatively, you should see your doc-

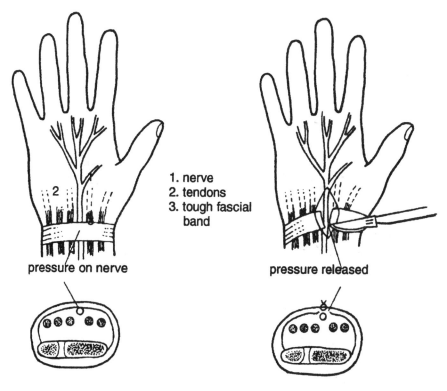

1. nerve
2. tendons
3. tough fascial
   band

pressure on nerve

pressure released

Fig. 22.10 Procedures involved in carpal tunnel surgery

tor in several office visits to remove stitches, if any, and ensure a good result. You should wear the splint continuously for a week or two and then at night, until your symptoms are gone. You can resume activity when it is comfortable, but try to avoid those that may have caused the problem. Avoid heavy lifting or demanding usage of the wrist for a month or two. Follow the preventive measures, described above.

Bleeding, wound infection, excessive scarring, and prolonged wrist tenderness are possible complications. A degree of pain, numbness, and weakness may persist in as many as 10 percent of all cases if the nerve was already permanently damaged or if there was accidental injury during the operation.

CARPAL TUNNEL SYNDROME SUMMARY

Prevention

Diet and Supplements

• Follow a low-fat, high-fiber diet.

Lifestyle

• Avoid repetitive activity; modify wrist position.
• Practice yoga daily.

- Practice special wrist exercises.
- Practice stress management.

Alternative Medicine Approaches

- Follow the preventive guidelines, above.
- Vitamin B_6, 50 mg daily.
- Special wrist exercises.
- Hot and cold treatments.
- Use acupuncture, chiropractic, osteopathy, Rolfing, massage, magnets.
- Practice visualization.

Conventional Medicine Approaches

- Splints, physical therapy.

- Pain medication—Tylenol, codeine derivatives (Percocet, Tylenol #3, Vicodin).
- Antiinflammatory medication—aspirin, Tylenol; nonsteroidal (Motrin, Advil, ibuprofin, Alleve), piroxicam (Feldene), rofecoxib (Vioxx).
- Cortisone injections.

Surgical Approach

- Carpal tunnel release.

CHAPTER 23

OTHER SURGICAL DISORDERS

Robert, a 65-year-old architect, had managed to let his body get out of shape. By giving up jogging, spending most of his time working, and eating junk foods to keep himself company, he had developed a significant potbelly, which greatly annoyed him when he looked at himself sideways in the mirror. He decided to have liposuction, aiming to return toward the washboard effect of his youth. The results were not what he had expected: he developed new, hard furrows, experienced changes in nerve sensation, and some of his skin developed a pocked, grapefruit-like appearance. His feelings about the surgery were mixed: He appreciated that he could now fit into smaller clothes, but disliked the overall feel and look of his altered body.

Everyone wants to look good and feel satisfied with his or her body. If nature hasn't given you exactly what you'd like, you may be considering turning to surgery to fix yourself. Cosmetic plastic surgery is a booming field continuing to grow in popularity: Over a million people each year in the United States now choose to have some sort of elective plastic surgery operation. Reconstructive plastic surgery, to correct deformities induced by disease or other surgeries, is also becoming more routine and successful.

You can now choose from a number of safe, reliable operative options; we will provide information so you can decide what is best for you among these new choices. Alternative medicine also offers fresh hope that you may be able to improve your appearance without having to undergo the rigors of an operation. Many alternative approaches also have the advantage of giving you a chance to deepen your peace of mind and overall enjoyment of life, from the inside out. Whether or not you choose surgery, you may still want to make these changes anyway, to prevent further problems and other disorders as well.

"Plastic" surgery derives its name from the Greek word *plastesis,* which means "to shape." Within the last few decades, techniques and choices have blossomed. Safer and more effective than ever, plastic surgery can often provide quick relief to significant suffering. However, it may not change any underlying self-image issues, which you should address before you choose an operation.

Sometimes, the results of plastic surgery may be quite different from what you expected: You may have new wrinkles and scars, or final effects that can appear unnatural. On the other hand, many patients experience as much satisfaction from plastic surgery as they had hoped for. You may feel pushed to take action—clearly the media and a culture that values physical beauty so highly *(form* over *content* in many cases) place excruciating pressure for action on anyone whose appearance is outside an almost impossibly narrow expectation. In this chapter, we give you a variety of choices for looking better and for feeling good at the same time.

Excess Body Fat

A layer of fat lies just under your skin in all the regions of your body. Very thin in some areas, such as the fingers, eyelids, and ears, it is typically distributed and stored in much thicker layers on your buttocks, hips, thighs, and abdomen.

As an adult, you have a fixed number of fat cells. You don't add more when you take on or lose weight: you just add to the size of the cells you have, making them larger or smaller, as the fat is stored or burned off. Too much body fat can be harmful, as most of the chapters in this book point out. Here, we focus on your aesthetic choices.

The fat stored in your body has several important roles to play for your self-protection. It stores energy for prolonged periods of vigorous activity; it has twice as many calories per ounce as protein or carbohydrates, the other body reserves that can release fuel for your body's work and vital processes. Fat protects against periods of starvation, when breaking down muscle protein for energy would be damaging. By its cushioning effect, it also helps protect your body, as well as serving as an insulator, to assist in regulating body temperature.

Fat has a cultural role to play. It helps determine our body size and shape. Typical male and female distribution patterns help define the "angular" male from the "curvaceous" female. Various societies have differing standards as to what constitutes the most desirable, or beautiful, appearance. These expectations very much help define the way we want to look, how we perceive ourselves, and how others see us. In the United States, advertisements constantly show us images of what it defines as beautiful and induce us to spend vast amounts of money on various diets, exercise machines, and body toners, and ultimately, in increasing numbers, to turn to surgery for help.

Alternative Medicine Approaches to Excess Body Fat

When I (Sandy) reached menopause, I started putting on weight. It is usual to add ten to fifteen pounds at this time, just as prepubescent girls chub up before their first periods. Our bodies anticipate the possible future stresses of aging by layering reserves of energy around the adrenals.

However, I discovered that by paying more attention to my diet and exercise habits, I could take off the excess weight, at the same time preventing other illnesses, and treat my underlying adrenal exhaustion, the root of the problem in the first place. I designed the guidelines given in Chapter 2 for diet, exercise, and stress reduction based on my own experience and that of witnessing the success of my patients.

Fat is fat. Just vacuuming it off your thighs or stomach does not prevent it from building up in your arteries, thereby leading to problems with blood circulation. Excess fat also increases your risk for cancer by affecting your hormones and immune system.

Excess abdominal fat has been found to be strongly associated with an increased risk for heart disease. You can take the accumulation in this area as a great impetus for diet and exercise changes, to help shrink your abdominal problem while at the same time protecting your heart.

You will need to make lifestyle changes *anyway,* to protect yourself from future illness, as well as help the quality of your life now. Try the following ones first, before choosing the risks of the suction tube or the knife.

Change Your Diet

The very *best* way to get rid of unwanted fat is to change your diet and exercise habits. A low-fat diet makes weight loss much more easily attainable than other types of diet, and has become much simpler to stick to, now that no-fat varieties of favorite foods are widely available. See the guidelines given in Chapter 2.

Exercise Regularly

Although so-called "spot reducing" has not been found to be effective in changing your body's shape, general aerobic exercise can help burn off any of your overall excess body fat, which will have the result of optimizing your form. Strength-building exercises can help you develop muscles; the more muscles you have, the more fat you are capable of metabolizing. Exercising aerobically (meaning you work up a sweat) three to five times a week, alternated with weight lifting two times a week, is recommended. Please see Chapter 2 for more information on exercise.

Practice Stress Management and Yoga Daily

By following the stress-management and yoga guidelines given in Chapter 2, you may be able to avoid the unnecessary scarring, lumpiness, bagging skin, and large plastic surgery bills associated with choosing an operative solution to your problem. Yoga acts to tone each muscle group in your body systematically, which may help to change your body's configuration. This practice also leaves you in a more relaxed state, which may enable you to more easily make peace with whatever shape you are able to achieve. Other stress management activities, such as aromatherapy and music, may similarly prove helpful. Please see Chapter 2 for details.

Practice Visualization

First, practice deep relaxation, given in Chapter 2. Next, image your fat cells, located in the target areas, to be like ice cubes on a hot stove. Picture them melting away, while feeling this happen within your body. Repeat this technique three to five times daily.

Join a Support Group

Support groups can help you stick to an optimum lifestyle regimen, to see what you can achieve in arriving at a desirable body shape. In addition, they can help you rethink your quest for the media's standard of beauty and aid you in working on accepting your body as it is. Especially for those who prefer to share their experiences, joining a support group can help reduce stress and achieve optimum weight. See Chapter 2 and the Resources section of this book for further information about support groups.

Watch for New Research

A newer, nonoperative option, using external ultrasound to eliminate fat cells, has shown promise in European usage, and may help you avoid the side effects and risk for the conventional liposuction approach. Further research is needed.

Surgical Approaches to Excess Body Fat

The two common techniques to eliminate excess body fat surgically are sucking it out through tiny skin incisions (liposuction) and cutting it out, usually along with excess overlying skin (abdominoplasty).

Liposuction

What American adult hasn't at least once dreamed of having just a tad of fat here and there—"Presto!"—vacuumed away. *Suction-assisted lipectomy,* commonly known as *liposuction,* was developed in France and introduced in the United States in 1982. It gives you the option of "body sculpturing," and is now the most common type of cosmetic surgery in the United States.

If you picture your fat as cheese, after lipo-suction it becomes Swiss cheese. Your overlying skin then presses down on the operated area, to create a newer, smaller you. However, this is only a method to define or refine body contours and remove spot areas resistant to diet and exercise programs, and does not work as a method for overall weight reduction.

The best results from liposuction are on people under age 40, near ideal body weight, whose skin is still elastic enough to contract effectively. Wrinkles, age spots, stretch marks, acne, or other skin problems can't be corrected by this method. It also does not cure *cellulite,* which is caused by surface indentations rather than subcutaneous fat. If you are older, you are more likely to develop postoperative wrinkling, lumpiness, and dimpling as a *result* of the liposuction.

Almost any area of your body can be altered by liposuction, including your chest, breasts, stomach, buttocks, hips, thighs, knees, and even ankles. Fat can be removed from your face—lips, neck, chin, cheeks, and jowls—often in association with other facial cosmetic surgery. The results on the arms are not as successful, since skin elasticity is less there. Today, liposuction procedures are most commonly done on the legs. Lipomas can also be treated by this method; they are discussed in Chapter 5.

Prior to your surgery, you and your surgeon must have a clear understanding of the goals of the operation. You should go over photos of pre- and postoperative results of other patients. A computer simulation using photos of your own body can be especially helpful. It is a good idea to donate some of your own blood in the weeks before your operation if a large blood loss is anticipated, though with modern techniques, transfusion is rarely necessary. You shouldn't use aspirin or other antiinflammatory medications for two weeks preoperatively, as they increase bleeding and bruising.

The standard liposuction operation is usually quick and simple. It can be performed in a doctor's office surgical suite or an outpatient surgery operating room. The type of anesthesia varies, depending on the amount of tissue to be removed and the locations treated. General anesthesia may be your best choice if a large area or several different areas are to be done; spinal or epidural anesthesia is commonly used for areas below the waist, and local can be chosen for smaller areas anywhere on the body.

After anesthesia and skin preparation, small one-quarter- to one-half-inch incisions are made in areas where they can be hidden, such as natural skin creases, the navel, or hair lines. Next, a blunt-nosed vacuum tube called a cannula is repeatedly passed through the incisions to create a number of small tunnels underneath your skin. (See Figure 23.1.) The blunt tip pushes aside skin nerves, blood vessels, and fibers that attach the skin to the un-

derlying tissue. High suction pulls out the fat, which is then collected into a plastic container. Up to 2,000 cc, or five pounds, about 25 percent of which is blood, can be removed in one session. Attempting to remove more would increase the danger of losing too much body fluid and blood, and could cause shock.

Tumescent liposuction is a newer technique where, before suctioning, your surgeon injects large volumes of saline fluid containing anesthetic and bicarbonate to relieve pain, and epinephrine to constrict blood vessels, decrease bleeding, and prolong the effects of the anesthetic. Tiny suction tubes, from 1.5 to 2.5 millimeters in diameter, are passed through very small incisions to remove the fat. Stitches are unnecessary. Excess anesthetic fluid and serum is allowed to leak out over the few days after surgery, preventing its buildup in your tissues, and thereby decreasing bruising, soreness, and swelling.

Proponents of this technique claim that it gives less pain, and local anesthesia without sedation is all that is necessary, thereby making it safer, minimizing blood loss, giving

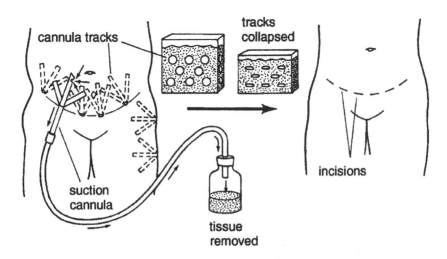

Fig. 23.1 Procedures involved in liposuction

fewer postoperative surface irregularities, and making prolonged postoperative use of compression garments unnecessary. Recovery is much quicker than by the older technique. The anesthetic injection technique can also be used for other types of plastic surgery including abdominoplasty, reconstruction flaps, face lifts, hair transplant, and dermabrasion.

A new liposuction technique, *ultrasound-assisted liposuction,* uses high-frequency ultrasound waves to liquefy fat, which is then sucked out by standard liposuction probes. Damage to arteries, veins, and ligaments that support the skin is minimized, allowing the skin to shrink and contour more smoothly.

The usual liposuction operation takes one or two hours per area treated. After your surgeon determines that the preoperative goals have been met, the incisions are left open, to drain into gauze dressings, or closed with stitches or skin tapes. You are then tightly bandaged with an elastic compression garment, which helps collapse the newly created tunnels and keeps swelling to a minimum. You can go home after a couple of hours of observation.

Postoperatively, you may experience significant bruising and swelling, along with some discomfort and aching, though surprisingly you should have little pain. You may not even need pain pills. You may tire easily for a few days, until your body restores its fluid balance. Drink plenty of liquids. You may have some numbness in the skin overlying the treated areas, lasting up to several months. You should wear the compression garment for two to six weeks, and avoid any activities that might traumatize or pull on the operative area for several weeks. You should be able to see effects from the procedure in two or three weeks, after the operative swelling subsides, but the final results may not be apparent for three to six months.

If your skin is not sufficiently elastic to contract, it may ultimately be a bit loose, and wrinkling, indentations, or dimpling may be permanent. It is best to choose a "conservative" procedure—that is, it is better to remove too little, and follow this with a minor corrective procedure, rather than too much, which is much more difficult to correct.

Most patients feel very satisfied with their liposuction results. The changes in contour in the liposuction area should be lasting. Remaining fat cells don't reproduce; they just enlarge or shrink with weight changes. But your proportions should remain the same. The whole process may be just the incentive you need to stick to a lifetime program of diet and exercise to maintain your ideal body weight.

Complications of liposuction are rare. Deaths have been reported, but the mortality rate is less than 1 in 50,000 cases.[1] Blood clots, or blood collections requiring treatment occur in 1 percent, and the infection risk is less than 1 percent. The complications of skin loss, requiring a skin graft, or excess scarring, are rare.

Abdominoplasty ("Tummy Tuck")

One of the favorite places your body stores fat is in the lower abdominal wall—the area of "middle-aged spread" and the proverbial "spare tire." Many adults seem to store a disproportionate amount of fat here and develop a *pannus,* the term for a large flap overhanging the belt and pubic area. As it becomes more overhanging and subject to the effects of gravity, this tissue collects fluid and swells even more. The stretched skin and moist areas in the deep fat folds are more prone to irritation, rashes, infections, and ulcers. Aside from aesthetic considerations that might lead you to want to remove this extra fat, at times, if you develop an infection, emergency surgery may be needed.

Small-to-medium-size areas of excess lower abdominal fat can be removed, using local anesthesia, in day surgery. Even a huge lower abdominal pannus can be safely thus excised. The larger the area taken off, however, the more likely the need for general anesthesia and a short hospital stay.

Often a "tummy tuck" is part of a general body "sculpting," using liposuction or other plastic surgical techniques for other areas where reshaping is desired. Other procedures may be performed at the same time as this abdominal operation, or may best be conducted at another session. As in liposuction surgery, you and your surgeon need to clearly agree upon the objectives of your operation.

Before you are given anesthesia, your surgeon marks the outlines of the area to be removed. Usually a large transverse ellipse is laid out, so that the scar is placed within your natural skin fold at the pubic hairline. (See Figure 23.2.) After anesthesia, your abdomen is prepped with an antibacterial solution. The incisions are carried down to the abdominal muscles, and the excess tissue removed. Your surgeon then makes "skin flaps" by separating the remaining skin and underlying fat from their attachments, so that they can be pulled together. In some cases, the navel is either removed or transplanted to a more normal position. If removed, it can be recreated by plastic surgery or tattoo, after your healing is complete.

With the larger procedures, at least two soft plastic drains are necessary to remove

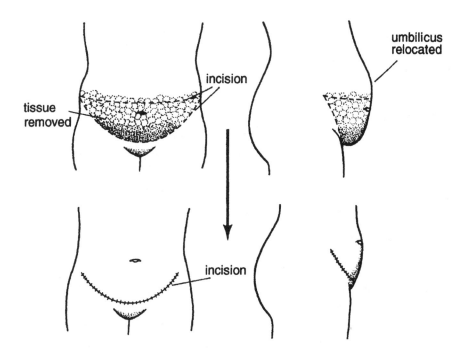

Fig. 23.2 Procedures involved in abdominoplasty or the "tummy tuck"

serum, so that it doesn't collect under the flaps, thereby lifting them off the underlying tissues. These drains are brought out through small incisions below the wound. The incision is then closed with stitches, staples, or skin tapes. A Velcro abdominal binder may be recommended to help decrease drainage and provide comfort. After recovering from anesthesia, you either go home or stay in the hospital for one to three days.

You will need to see your doctor after a few days, to ensure your wound is healing well. The drains usually stay in until drainage is less than a few tablespoons per day, though they are rarely left in more than five to seven days. You may have some soreness that can usually be managed by pain pills. Bruising disappears after a week or two. The results of the abdominoplasty are immediate, and may be dramatic, if your pannus was large. A whole new wardrobe may be necessary. Your confidence and self-image can be markedly improved.

Complications include seroma or serum collection under the flaps, which can be treated by a few office needle aspirations. Incision infection occurs in about 5 percent of all cases. Occasionally, loss of part of the skin flap or transplanted navel may require further surgery.

Facial Cosmetic Problems

A wrinkle in time: Should you put yours to the knife? One of the most popular of plastic surgeries, the "face-lift" aims to reduce the effects of aging on your face. If you suffer from a neck that has started to resemble a turkey's, a surgical procedure can not only tighten your sagging skin, but also the muscle beneath it.

Separate maneuvers can lift your forehead and eyebrows, affecting a dramatic "opening" of your eyes.

Skin doesn't shrink—it must be removed or pulled up to tighten it. Unfortunately, time is relentless, and stretching continues even if you have an operation. Face-lifts last an average of five to ten years, and then you may look similar to how you looked before. However, alternative approaches offer new hope to help you improve your appearance without resorting to the scalpel to do it, or if you do have cosmetic surgery, to retain its effects longer into the future.

Your Face's Aging Process

As you age, your skull becomes smaller and its bones thinner, and your nose and chin change their shapes slightly, so that their angularity is lost. Your skin and facial muscles also tend to loosen from your underlying bony structure.

As your fibrous connections weaken, your facial tissue may then hang from those points with stronger attachments to bony ridges, like Roman drapes. As your muscles weaken, gravity contributes further to this process, and your face, eyebrows, and the skin beneath your chin may begin to droop. Your skin loses its tautness and smoothness, and becomes progressively thinner, less elastic, and drier, while loss of your underlying fat provides less of a cushion beneath it. Fat may be redistributed around your eyes, chin, and neck, adding to your overall sagging appearance.

The aging process occurs at different rates in different people. Factors that affect its progression include heredity, weight fluctuations, and lifestyle choices. Excessive exposure to sunlight accelerates the above skin changes and contributes to wrinkling. Smoking is a major cause of premature aging. The multitude of fine wrinkles of a "cigarette smoker's face" are the result of years of nicotine affecting your small capillaries, causing them to constrict and restricting the blood supply to your skin.

Alternative Medicine Approaches to Facial Cosmetic Problems

You may be happy with what plastic surgery can do to your face, but you do face (pun intended) some risk by choosing the operative path. Meditation, acupuncture, and other measures may help relieve worry-related wrinkles, or if they do persist, you might think of yourself as following in the lineage of Mother Teresa, who despite plenty of them, still was generally considered very beautiful.

I (Sandy) witnessed as a good friend of mine went through a cosmetic surgery nightmare. Her husband had received an eye lift because his sagging tissue had interfered with his vision. So she decided to have her eyes done, just for fun. After the surgery, she could not close either eye effectively and was relegated to wearing dark glasses, using eye drops, and being in pain. A second procedure, which included a face-lift to free up more tissue for her eyes to close, did help one eye to close, but it dislodged her mouth, making normal symmetrical smiling impossible, and left her with an almost unrecognizable, masklike appearance. Further surgery is still needed, but may not be able to fully correct all of her new problems.

Although such a scenario is rare, I would recommend you first try alternative medicine methods, to see if you can achieve a satisfying outcome without putting yourself at risk.

Rather than choosing to cover up the effects of aging, alternative medicine approaches aim to change your biochemistry, to prevent the accumulation of free radicals, to forestall, and even reverse, the aging process throughout your body via changes in lifestyle. Making these adjustments can also help you avoid other, more serious, problems and illnesses.

The masklike appearance that can follow classical face-lifts may actually make you appear older, since your subtle flexibility of expression is lost, especially after time passes. Since even successful face-lifts often must be repeated, usually within ten years or so when their effectiveness is lost, increasingly ineffective results may follow. Here are the most promising alternative medicine methods to help you avoid having to undergo facial plastic surgery.

Quit Smoking

Smoking is the most common cause of unacceptable facial aging. Follow the guidelines for quitting smoking given in Chapter 2.

Avoid Excessive Sun Exposure

Moderate sun exposure may protect you against colon and prostate cancer, but excess sun ages your skin. The most important action is to avoid sunburn, but any level of tanning causes your skin to be damaged.

Change Your Diet

A whole-foods, low-fat, high-fiber diet is naturally high in antioxidants and low in the factors that generate free radicals. Follow the guidelines given in Chapter 2.

Take Supplements

The antioxidants found in vegetables act to clear your body of harmful free radicals.

Vitamins A and B$_6$, beta-carotene, lecithin, and kelp are particularly thought to be helpful in maintaining your skin's elasticity and health. Levels are given in Chapter 2.

Use Natural Topicals; Take Saunas or Steam Baths

The use of mud is an ancient tradition now employed at many spas to keep the skin supple and free of wrinkles. Some actresses, such as Candice Bergen, have been reported to make use of this on a daily basis. If you have oily skin, you can use mud masks daily without adverse effects; if your skin is dry, use them less often and in conjunction with a moisturizer. Saunas and steam baths draw increased blood supply, and thereby more nutrients, to your skin, so that it can maintain its health more optimally.

The herb witch hazel acts as a toner, to tighten skin temporarily. Similarly, seaweed applications give an absorbable nutritional supply to the skin, helping it to do optimum maintenance and repair.

Fine wrinkles and minor blemishes may be improved by topical applications of vitamins A and C, glycolic acid, and salicylic acid. Look for these preparations in your local health food store.

Practice Yoga Daily

This route is now well known to Hollywood, and many others in the public eye. It increases circulation and restedness, so that you both feel and appear more refreshed and youthful. Follow the guidelines in Chapter 2.

Use Massage, Acupressure, and Acupuncture

These act by reducing the tension of underlying face muscles that can contribute to wrinkling. They also act to promote circulation of nutrients so that the skin can maintain its health more easily and eliminate waste-product buildup from your lymph channels. Several videos, including Lindsay Wagner's *New Beauty: The Acupressure Face Lift,* detail how to practice your own facial massage, or you can visit an acupressure or acupuncture practitioner. You can also try a thorough type of massage known as zone therapy.

In addition, by reducing fatigue and helping you sleep better, massage may help your face appear more youthful, eliminating a "tired " look.

Surgical Approaches to Facial Cosmetic Problems

Surgical "rejuvenation" of the face addresses the eyelids, forehead, cheeks, and chin as well as the neck. Surgery seeks to redefine aesthetic landmarks such as the chin, cheekbones, and eyebrows, which have been distorted by the aging process and any abnormal fatty deposits in the cheeks, neck, and around the eyes. Many techniques are available and can be combined to achieve this goal. Your surgeon may remove excess sagging skin, lift or reposition tissue that may have drooped, and "sculpt" fat by surgical excision or liposuction, to give you a more pleasing contour.

Unfortunately, these procedures do not eliminate creases associated with deep wrinkles, rough skin texture, age spots, blemishes, discolorations, scars, and moles. They can be covered by makeup, or plastic surgery "resurfacing" can be added later, using chemical "skin peel," dermabrasion (akin to sandpapering), laser, tattooing, and other techniques.

Safe injectable filling materials such as collagen and your own fat have been developed to raise any deeper wrinkles, scars, and other depressed areas. These can also be used to augment lip lines and enhance other normally prominent features. Unfortunately, such effects are often temporary, since the material is ultimately absorbed, making retreatment necessary. Implants using nonabsorbable materials are being developed and may lead to a more permanent solution.

Face-Lift

As with all cosmetic surgery, you and your surgeon must have realistic goals for your operation. A face-lift cannot achieve "perfection," and won't make you look like a teenager again, so your expectation must be for improvement only, with some residual aging elements still present. Though plastic surgery can make a person look younger or rested, trying for too much change can lead to an unnatural facial expression and a stiff, frozen appearance, which may be much less pleasing and more uncomfortable than before the surgery. Such changes are then difficult to correct. Drawings and computerized simulations of your face can be very helpful in selecting your best options.

Face-lift surgery is usually performed in an outpatient setting, or in your doctor's office operating suite. Local anesthesia with sedation is most commonly used. Longer or more complicated operations involving bony tissue are best performed under general anesthesia in a hospital setting.

You lie on your back on the operating table. After skin preparation, the anesthetic is injected at several points, to block the main nerves of sensation to your face.

Your doctor begins by making an incision in the hair line of the temple. It is carried down in front of your ear, then curves around the ear lobe and back behind the hair line of the neck. (See Figure 23.3.) Newer procedures

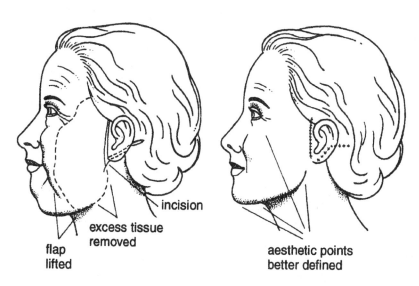

incision

excess tissue removed

flap lifted

aesthetic points better defined

Fig. 23.3 Face-lift procedure and outcome

using an endoscope reduce the size of the necessary incisions, causing less external scarring. The skin, fat, and muscles of the face are freed from their underlying attachments. Excessive fat in the neck, cheeks, chin, and eyelids is eliminated, to reshape these areas. Separate, small incisions placed in natural skin folds may be necessary. Occasionally, prominent bone surfaces may be flattened, or implants of bone, cartilage, or plastic material added, to accentuate the aesthetic landmarks of your cheekbones and chin, resulting in a more pleasing effect.

After completing work on the underlying layers, your surgeon pulls the skin back and up, removing the extra portion, then reattaches the tightened skin and muscle to the underling bony structures. The incision is closed with fine stitches or skin tapes. This operation can take two to three hours or more, depending on the necessary procedures.

Afterward, you may have some soreness, which can usually be controlled with pain pills. Swelling and bruising may be apparent for two weeks. Your skin may seem too tight, and have a sense of numbness, for several weeks. Your scars should be inconspicuous. In the first few months, they may be pink and somewhat thickened, and can be hidden with makeup. Later, as the scars mature, they usually become thinner and white. If you develop abnormal thickening in your scars, they can be injected with steroids. It may take up to six months for you to see the final results of your face-lift.

Complications of face-lift surgery include excessive bleeding or blood clots, in 4 to 15 percent of all cases.[2] A clot can usually be removed through the incision, or aspirated by needle or suction tube. Rarely, a return to the operating room is necessary, to control active bleeding. Incision infection is very unusual,

since the blood supply to your face is so extensive. It is possible to "slough," to lose small areas of skin on your incision edges, usually the result of too much tension. Such areas are usually treated with dressing changes, until healing occurs naturally. Occasionally, further corrective surgery is necessary, if excessive scars develop at these sites.

Commonly, hair is lost when skin flaps are made underneath hair-bearing areas of the temple or scalp, and though the loss can be permanent, it usually takes four to six months to regrow. Damage to facial nerves, which give sensation to the ear and cheek, is usually transient. Rarely, injury to nerves of the muscles involved in facial expression, the corner of the mouth, or eyelids (0.4 to 2.6 percent) causes a poor cosmetic result, and danger to the eye.[3] A neuroma, caused when a nerve is trapped in scar tissue, can cause shooting, burning pain, but is rarely permanent.

Blepharoplasty (Eyelid Surgery)

The bulging beneath your upper and lower eyelids accompanying aging is usually caused by loss of tissue strength, which allows the normal fat around your eye to bulge, in addition to loss of skin elasticity and drooping of your eyebrows. All of this can make you look older and more tired. In extreme cases, puffy skin folds can interfere with your vision. Surgical reduction of this fat, and removal of extra skin, offers you the possibility of a smoother, more youthful eye appearance.

Eyelid surgery, called *blepharoplasty,* is relatively easy, and can be performed as an outpatient or in your doctor's office under local anesthesia. Many different types of surgeons do these operations—plastic surgeons, ophthalmologists, and ear, nose, and throat specialists. If you are considering this procedure, make certain you consult a well-trained and experienced eyelid surgeon, since significant problems, which can threaten your eye, may be created by inexperience and sloppy technique.

Since the most common blepharoplasty complications are linked to bleeding, you should discontinue aspirin and any other medications that may interfere with blood clotting, for at least ten days before your operation.

You lie on your back on the operating table. Anesthetic is injected to block the nerves that give sensation to your eyelids. For the lower lids, the incision is made under the eyelash or inside the lid itself. (See Figure 23.4.) For the upper lid, it is placed in the skin crease. Such incisions should be unnoticeable. Excess fat and skin is trimmed away, and fine stitches used to close.

After the operation, you can expect very little pain, and it's unlikely you will need strong pain pills. You may have some swelling and bruising, which can be kept to a minimum by using ice packs for the first two days.

Complications include *ectropion,* where the lid is pulled out, down, and away from the eyeball, causing a dry eye, which can result in irritation, and even blindness, if not relieved. If you already have a tendency for dry eyes, you should avoid surgery on your lower lids.

Nasal Disorders

Discriminating smell and taste is your nose's most apparent function. Less obvious are its humidifying, warming, and filtering actions, of each inspired breath. A nose of any external shape can perform these duties as long as the flow of air is not obstructed. In this section, we will discuss nasal airway obstruction disorders.

How Your Nose Works

Your nose is composed of the *nasal bones,* the *cartilaginous* and *bony septum,* and several thin paired *cartilages,* providing its structure. Draped on these like a tent are your skin and a thin layer of subcutaneous fat. The two elliptical external openings, or *nares,* are separated by the *collumella.* The two *ala* are the

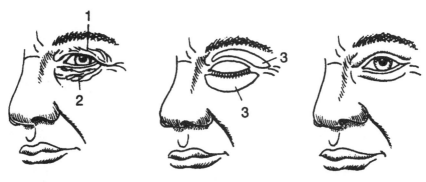

1. overhanging upper lid   3. tissue removed
2. baggy lower lid

Fig. 23.4   Blephoroplasty procedure and outcome

lower lateral flared edges that join the upper lip. The *maxillary, cribiform,* and *cavernous sinuses* empty into the two nasal air passageways. These sinuses, hollow cavities located in the bones of your face, act to decrease the weight of your head. They are lined by cells that secrete a thin fluid.

Alternative Medicine Approaches to Nasal Disorders

Unless your septum is severely deviated or giving you significant symptoms, you can simply choose to live with it, avoiding the risks of an operation. Septum deviation itself does not mean you must have correction; many individuals have a slight asymmetry, and many others live quite asymptomatically, comfortably, and peacefully with significant variations of alignment.

If your septum deviation may be giving you symptoms, you can take action via alternative medicine approaches to help yourself back to wellness without surgical intervention. Following are the most promising alternative medicine solutions for symptomatic nasal septum deviation.

Change Your Diet

Allergies to certain foods may cause your nasal passages to become swollen, making you symptomatic. The reaction may be to the food itself or may be due to the absorption of foreign substances from your digestive tract, a process termed "leaky gut syndrome." You may find benefit from switching to a vegetarian diet or embark on a trial of eliminating dairy, wheat, fruit juices, dried fruits, and refined sugar to see if your breathing is improved enough to live comfortably with your deviated septum. See Chapter 2 for basic dietary guidelines.

Practice Yoga Daily

By relaxing the entire body, you shift your blood flow from the "fight-or-flight" mode into a "relaxation response." This allows your nasal tissues to receive improved circulation, so that they can focus on repair work. The yoga breathing exercises strengthen local resistance in these tissues and may help you to breathe better through both nostrils. Developing a daily practice routine is best. See Chapter 2 for further details.

Take Supplements

The herb *nettles,* one to two capsules two to three times daily, can greatly help relieve nasal congestion if it is due to allergies. You can also add vitamin C, 1,000 mg one to three times daily.

Surgical Approach to Nasal Disorders

The most common cause of nasal airway obstruction occurs when the septum in your nose is deviated to one side, usually as a result of trauma. Obstruction can also happen when allergies cause your nose tissue to swell, and by congenital malformation, nasal polyps, or tumor.

Significant problems can result. Your sense of smell and taste can be decreased. Your sinuses may not be able to drain properly, causing irritation of your nasal lining tissues, chronic sinusitis, headaches, and generalized illness. Nasal discharge and sniffling may be disagreeable. If you must mouth-breathe, it can give you smelly breath, a sore throat, hoarseness, snoring, and restless sleep. Asthma and bronchitis can be exacerbated.

An obstructing deviated septum can be relieved by an operation called a *septoplasty.* Preoperatively, your doctor should take a careful history, including questions about your sense of smell, history of sinus infections, headaches, and problems with sleep. The minimum physical exam includes looking in your nose with a nasal speculum or a flexible nasal endoscope, so your doctor can have a clearer view of your airway passages and sinus openings.

If you have a nasal infection or sinusitis, it must be treated before you have your operation. Septoplasty is an outpatient procedure. Anesthesia is usually accomplished by a combination of topical local anesthetics applied to your nasal tissues, small amounts of local injections, and IV sedation. You may also choose general anesthesia.

Incisions are made inside your nose, then the lining tissue lifted off the underlying septum on one side, so that the cartilage and bone can be directly seen. Deformed bone, cartilage, and any other excess tissue is removed, to enlarge the air passageways, then the septum straightened and replaced in the midline. Other steps can be added, to change the size and shape of your nose, if needed, for a best cosmetic result. The operation is then termed a *septorhinoplasty*. Dissolvable stitches are used to close the incisions.

Septoplasty can take one to two hours, or even longer, depending on the complexity of the procedure. A light gauze internal dressing may be placed, along with a specially molded plastic external splint, to keep your nose in position and minimize swelling. Usually the packing is removed before you go home.

Postoperatively, you may experience some pain and aching, which can usually be relieved by pain pills. You must not blow your nose until given permission. You can dab with a Kleenex instead. Stuffiness can be relieved by decongestants. Keep your splint and any dressings dry. You should avoid smiling, laughing, and any other extreme facial expressions. Your splint is carefully removed by your doctor on a follow-up office visit, after a few days to a week. Be gentle when you wash your face. You should not wear glasses that rest on your nose, and refrain from vigorous activities, especially those which might traumatize your nose, for at least a month. You can apply makeup as soon as the splint is removed, to cover any discoloration. Swelling and bruising may take a week or two to resolve. The final outcome is not generally apparent for several weeks.

As complications are more likely with radical than conservative procedures, fairly often a minor "fine-tuning" revision of one area or another is required to achieve the desired results.

Complications of septoplasty include chronic nasal obstruction caused by internal distortion, swelling, or reabsorption of cartilage and graft materials, if used, and collapse of the nose's framework when air is breathed in. Occasionally, excess scarring needs to be treated with cortisone injections. Smoking, use of constricting nasal sprays, and some immune problems can interfere with blood supply. Incision infection is rare, unless your blood supply is impaired.

FACIAL COSMETIC PROBLEMS SUMMARY

Prevention

Diet and Supplements

- Follow a low-fat, high-fiber diet.
- Vitamin A, 10,000 IU daily.

- Vitamin C, 2,000 mg, 2–3 times daily.
- Vitamin E, D-alpha, 400 IU, 1–3 times daily.
- Vitamin B_6, 50 mg daily.
- Lecithin, 1,200 mg, 1–3 times daily.
- Kelp, 1 capsule daily.

Lifestyle

- Don't smoke.
- Avoid excessive sun exposure.
- Maintain optimum weight.
- Exercise 1 hour, 3–5 times weekly.
- Practice yoga daily.
- Practice stress management.

Alternative Medicine Approaches

- Follow the preventive guidelines, above.
- Saunas or steam baths.
- Seaweed and/or mud masks.
- Alpha-hydoxy, and/or vitamin C masks.
- Vitamin A, vitamin C, glycolic acid, and salicylic acid, topical applications.
- Massage, acupuncture.

Surgical Approaches

- Face lift.
- Sculpting fat, liposuction.
- Resurfacing—chemical "skin peel," derm-abrasion (akin to sandpapering), laser, tattooing.
- Injectable filling materials—fat, collagen, plastics.

Thinning Hair and Baldness

One-third of all American men develop a drastic recession of the hairline or become bald. More than 60 percent are affected to some extent. More than 50,000 hair trans-plants are performed yearly in the United States, and the numbers are climbing. However, these procedures are generally rather expensive, ranging from $4,000 to $25,000, and may not achieve the anticipated results.

The typical head has 100,000 hairs. Hair from different areas may be of different color, thickness, length, and shape, and grow at different rates. Hair pattern and tendency to baldness is strongly influenced by your genes. Hair loss most commonly occurs on the top and front of your scalp.

Alternative Medicine Approaches to Thinning Hair and Baldness

---

John, a Florida resident, flew to New York for treatment, and spent $6,000 for a transplant of 300 hair micrografts. Six months later, with his scalp still tender, his resulting hair was patchy and looked like beard stubble. He stated, "People were looking at my hair instead of me. I kept trying to be optimistic, but the hair never grew in. This is not something you want to go through. It's a shock to the system."[4]

You may think that having more hair will increase your confidence, improve your love life, or help you be successful at work. Certainly, our society moves us in that direction. But should you put your health at risk, even minimally, for something so external? We don't get to take our hair with us after we leave our bodies. I think, however, we can carry with us the amount of love we create in our lives, which is generated by loving others, not getting them to love us.

For example, before I (Sandy) began my current male relationship, I dated a number of men. I was attracted most to what their values were, and whether or not they had hair did not enter into this. I think most women feel the way I do, and I want to let men become aware of that fact, so they do not feel as much pressure to conform to a culturally unhelpful and potentially unhealthy tradition and push.

In addition to often not being cosmetically satisfactory, surgical treatment of baldness may leave you with uncomfortable scarring.

Joining the Hair Club for Men may also not be an entirely side-effect-free option. The average price of a good toupee is $2,000 to $3,000, and wearing it constantly may cause scalp irritation.

Perhaps our culture simply needs to embrace the inherent beauty in bold baldness. Think of the Tibetan monks, or Hindu swamis, who intentionally choose to be bald. The following alternative medicine approaches, however, do offer some hope of restoring hair growth through nonsurgical means.

Change Your Diet

Male pattern baldness may be worsened by dietary insufficiencies. Follow the dietary program guidelines given in Chapter 2.

Take Supplements

The most commonly advocated supplement is the B vitamin biotin, 1,000 to 3,000 mcg three times daily. It may take six months to see the difference. Adding B-complex, C, and the other vitamins and supplements listed in Chapter 2 may also be helpful.

Practice Stress Management

Male pattern baldness may be worsened by stress. Follow the stress management program guidelines given in Chapter 2.

Practice Yoga Daily

All of the practices together work to reduce stress, as well as increase circulation to your scalp. The shoulder stand and headstand postures most directly increase circulation to the scalp, and so should be practiced twice daily, gradually increasing the time spent up to ten to fifteen minutes.

Practice Visualization

First, practice deep relaxation, given in Chapter 2. Then, imagine your scalp as a beautiful lawn. See new, thick grass forming there, and feel it happening. Repeat this three to five times daily.

Conventional Medicine Approaches to Thinning Hair and Baldness

Drugs taken internally or applied topically can increase hair growth and may provide enough improvement that you will lose any interest in surgery.

Propecia

The balding scalp contains an increased concentration of 5 alpha-dihydrotestosterone (DHT), a breakdown product of testosterone. Finisteride (Propecia) pills act to block conversion of testosterone to DHT, decreasing blood and scalp DHT concentrations. Somehow this effect enhances hair growth in men genetically predisposed to baldness. Studies have shown a significant increase in hair growth for such men at three months with an increasing effect for up to two years. Between 66 and 80 percent will respond with decreased rate of hair loss, increased hair counts, and hair regrowth. This effect is maintained with continuous treatment for at least three years. Side effects include a slight decrease in sexual function, without a significant difference in overall satisfaction with sex life.

Rogaine

Recently, the topical preparation minoxidil (*Rogaine*) has become available over the counter. Its effectiveness requires continuous use, and it is satisfactory for only one-third of all users. If it is going to work, you should see results in two to four months of twice daily application. The hair it restores is initially thinner and finer, like peach fuzz, but after continued use should look like the rest of your hair. Its effects are not lasting, so it must by applied continuously to maintain your hair regrowth. Side effects include scalp itching and irritation. Rogaine may cause facial hair growth in women, and may be harmful during pregnancy or breast-feeding.

Hairpieces

You can wear a wig or toupee made from synthetic material or real human hair. Human hair can be recolored and "permed," whereas synthetics can't. Synthetics have less maintenance but tend to get fuzzy while human hair doesn't. You can get a hairpiece "off the shelf" or, for more expense, have one custom made to the exact specifications and shape of your head. Prices can range from several hundreds to thousands of dollars.

The hairpiece can be attached to your scalp with double sided tape and clips for short-term (daily) use. For extended wear (four to six weeks) it can be attached by bonding adhesives or cable weaving into your own hair. These pieces last from six months to two years depending on whether you use them for short-term or extended periods where they are more subject to trauma from showering and sleeping on them. Daily-wear systems last longer. Scalp irritation may occur with the various bonding methods.

Surgical Approaches to Thinning Hair and Baldness

Mike, *an internist, married and had several children later in life. As the hair on his head disappeared, he began to feel self-conscious. He underwent many sessions of transplants, along with ribbing from his children, who referred to him as "Boris" (Karloff), before his forehead finally was filled in enough to appear almost natural. After a bit of coloring, he does appear much younger.*

Richard, *another internist, lost all of his hair when he underwent cancer chemotherapy, and it never grew back. He, on the other hand, is very comfortable with his appearance, and although he has to spend money for hats in the winter, he saves on haircuts.*

A hair transplant for treating male pattern baldness takes hair from areas that do not thin, such as at the back of your neck and above your ears, and moves them to the bald areas on the front and top of your scalp. Why doesn't the transplanted hair fall out just like the old? The explanation is termed "donor site dominance." That is, the hair acts like it did in its original site, despite being moved to the new location. However, if too much graft material is taken from any one area, it too will look thin. If it is placed too uniformly, a noticeably abnormal hairline can be the result. Transplanted hair can also develop a bristle quality, making it difficult to comb or shape properly.

Multiple transplant sessions are necessary to achieve a satisfactory result. Most of the grafts are placed on the forehead and front of the scalp. A natural-appearing hairline can usually be recreated if enough grafts are placed.

Hair transplants are performed in your doctor's office. Micrografting is the most common technique. It can be accomplished with you lying or sitting in a special chair. Ice may be applied before surgery, to decrease bleeding. After injecting local anesthesia, your surgeon removes the grafts utilizing a tiny cookie-cutter-type punch. Each graft contains two to fifteen individual hairs. The same punch is used to remove corresponding pieces of bare skin in the bald area.

Alternatively, holes can be created by various-sized dilators, without skin removal. The grafts are then pushed down into the tiny pockets created at the new site.

Each session takes one to three hours, depending on the number of grafts performed. The micrograft incision sites are so small that stitch closure is unnecessary. A scab forms, and healing takes a few days. After your surgery is completed, you may need to wear a compression garment for one day.

Other hair-grafting techniques are also available. Special two- or three-bladed scalpels can be employed, to remove 2.5 mm strips of hair. These strips can then be cut up into grafts of various sizes and shapes (round, square, mini, micro, or slits of tissue). The donor site, usually at the back of your head, is closed with stitches. Your scar should be inconspicuous.

Flap movement is a method applicable to cover a small bald spot or scar caused by a burn or other trauma. Here, the bald area is simply cut out, and the hair-bearing scalp edges stitched together. The result is immediate. However, this approach is appropriate only for small areas, and for locations where the incision scar can be hidden. A combination of techniques may give you the best result.

After surgery, your scalp may be sore for a week or so. Six weeks later, the grafted hair may fall out, though about three months after that a new hair should appear, then grow at a rate of one-quarter to one-half inch per month.

Complications include the graft being rejected or "popping out," infection, bruising, and eye swelling. You may experience some scalp numbness for two or three months.

THINNING HAIR AND BALDNESS SUMMARY

Prevention

Diet and Supplements

- Follow a low-fat, high-fiber, whole-foods diet.
- Avoid caffeine.
- Multivitamin daily.
- Biotin, 1,000 mcg, 3 times daily.
- Vitamin C, 1,000–2,000 mg, 3 times daily.

Lifestyle

- Practice daily yoga especially the inverted poses.
- Practice stress management.

Alternative Medicine Approaches

- Follow the guidelines for prevention, above.

• Practice visualization.

Conventional Medicine Approaches

• Finisteride (Propecia) pills.
• Minoxidil (Rogaine) topical.
• Hairpiece.

Surgical Approaches

• Hair transplant—micrografting, strip harvesting, flap movement.

Tonsil and Adenoid Disorders

Jamaille, a 10-year-old girl who had excelled in school, began to suffer increasingly frequent bouts of sore throat, fever, and swollen tonsils. Repeated treatment with antibiotics did not seem to eliminate these attacks, and she began to fall behind in her schoolwork. Her mother then sought alternative medicine care, which included eliminating dairy products and adding vitamins C and E. No further episodes occurred, and Jamaille was soon back at the head of her class.

Your tonsils and adenoids help to develop your immunity to foreign bacterial and viral invaders. They are particularly active and important in the first few years of your life. These tissues provide a defensive line against harmful organisms that might have been breathed in or taken in to the mouth—for example, as when a baby sucks on a toy a puppy has been playing with.

Surgery on the tonsils and adenoids has been largely abandoned by most major medical centers, yet as many as 400,000 of these operations are still performed each year in the United States, and these procedures continue to be the second most common operation performed upon children after appendectomy. Many adults also subject themselves to these surgeries. You can take alternative measures to help ensure that you won't be faced with the need to make a decision about surgery.

How Your Tonsils and Adenoids Work

Your tonsils can been seen as two upholstered three-quarter-inch buttons of reddish pink tissue on the sides of your throat in the rear portion, at the level of the base of your tongue. (See Figure 23.5.) Your adenoids are a thickened mat of tissue in the air passageways behind your nose, above the back of your soft palate. The eustachian tubes connect your middle ears with the back of your throat, providing a means to equalize pressure in these areas and prevent fluid collection.

Waldeyer's ring refers to the sum total of the lymph tissue encircling the back of your throat, consisting of your tonsils, adenoids, tissue at the base of your tongue, and the back wall of your throat. This ring is a component of your body's lymphatic defense system, which also includes your spleen, thymus, other smaller areas of lymph tissue concentration, and lymph glands scattered throughout your body.

Your lymphatic ring cells trap and analyze various pathologic bugs, the first step in producing the specific antibodies that are necessary to kill them. The resulting antibodies circulate in your bloodstream for extended periods of time, sometimes for life, helping to overcome and prevent future infections caused by these organisms. However, after age three, no solid evidence suggests that removing these tissues has any deleterious effect

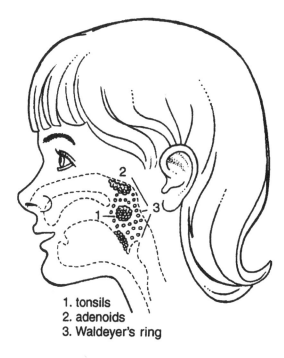

1. tonsils
2. adenoids
3. Waldeyer's ring

Fig. 23.5 The location of the tonsils and adenoids

on immunity, since by this time other lymphatic system areas are well developed.

Unfortunately, the defenses of the tonsils and adenoids may be weakened, overcome, and infected by virulent organisms, and instead of a protective area, they then can become "nests" for these organisms, and a site of frequent acute infection or chronic low-grade infection. Recurrent sore throat from "strep" infection is a classic example. Rarely, an abscess may even develop, causing severe pain and high fever, and requiring immediate treatment. Enlarged tonsils can cause a sense of throat dryness, annoying irritation, and even interfere with swallowing. Bad-smelling breath may be offensive to others. Chronically infected adenoids may also enlarge, producing blockage of nasal passageways, problems with runny nose, obstructed

breathing, and snoring. Sleep disturbances can lead to daytime sleepiness, behavioral problems, difficulty keeping up in school, and accidents. Speech and dental problems can also result.

How Tonsil and Adenoid Disorders Are Diagnosed

Evaluation to determine if your symptoms are due to tonsil and adenoid disorders, their extent, and what the options are for treatment requires a careful history, physical exam, and likely some other testing.

History

Evaluation of problems linked to your tonsils and adenoids should begin with you informing your doctor about your history of ear, nose, and throat problems. Have you had more than four sore throats a year? Do you snore such that you wake yourself or others up? Do you hold your breath or stop breathing when you sleep? Do you have problems with your hearing, frequent earaches, or ear infections?

Physical Exam

A complete ear, nose, and throat physical exam should include your doctor looking into your mouth and throat with a light source and tongue blade. The adenoid area cannot be seen without the aid of a small mirror angled upward at the back of your throat or via a special flexible viewing scope. Nasal passageways can be viewed with a simple speculum or flexible scope. Your ears and eardrums can be examined with the familiar otoscope. Lastly, your doctor should feel all around your neck for enlarged lymph nodes, frequently found with chronic tonsil or adenoid infections.

Lab Tests

Swab bacterial cultures can be taken from your tonsils and adenoids to look for streptococcus, or "strep," a bacteria that can cause tonsillitis as well as heart and kidney damage. Other cultures can be performed looking for unusual organisms and even viruses, but this expense is seldom necessary.

X-Rays and Scans

Plain X-rays, occasionally special X-rays, and rarely, CAT or MRI scans may be necessary to determine the size and shape of your facial bones, sinuses, and adenoids, and to look for abnormal soft tissue in your airway passages.

Hearing Tests

Inflammation in the back of your throat can interfere with normal hearing. Simple hearing tests should be conducted initially and can be followed with more sophisticated tests if abnormalities are found.

Sleep Pattern Tests

Snoring and difficulty breathing can keep you from restful sleep. If you feel tired much of the day, special tests can evaluate if you have an abnormal sleep pattern.

Alternative Medicine Approaches to Tonsil and Adenoid Disorders

Faced with a child who is frequently sick and who also has large, swollen tonsils at the back of their throat, it is difficult not to want to take drastic action. However, even though removing the tonsils after the age of three does not cause further immune problems that we now know about, removing them may put your child at risk for the unnecessary complications of surgery and still not solve the underlying immune problem that caused the tonsils to be swollen in the first place. Swollen tonsils are simply a fire alarm to a deeper problem; cutting out the fire alarm without putting out the fire does not make sense.

Studies have shown that simply removing your child's tonsils if he or she has frequent ear infections, sore throats, coughs, colds, sinus problems, or even bronchitis will *not* prevent or even reduce them in the future. Even though parents tend to overestimate the number and severity of sore throats in their child, in several randomized studies of the effects of tonsillectomy, at two-year follow-up, no significant difference in the number of moderate or severe throat infections was found after the tonsils were removed, though mild episodes were less frequent.[5] However, operative complications and side effects such as severe bleeding or induced infection outweigh even this slight benefit. Removal of the adenoids, however, may diminish the number of these infections.

Resistance to infection is dependent upon the overall status of your immune system, and even severe infections of the tonsils and adenoids are often amenable to alternative medicine approaches. Following are the most important alternative medicine approaches for maintaining optimum tonsil health and avoiding an operation.

Change Your Child's Diet, and Your Own

Eliminating dairy products may be all that is necessary for prevention of tonsil and adenoid problems, both in children and adults. You may substitute soy-based formulas and other soy foods. Also useful is a trial of eliminating sugar, dried fruit, chocolate, and fruit juice from the diet, all of which act to elevate blood sugar even in normal persons, thereby lowering white cell function and decreasing your immunity.

Take Supplements

Try the addition of the vitamins, herbs, and homeopathic agents that enhance the immune system, given in Chapter 2. In particular, try vitamins A and C, and zinc. (Modify the dosages for pediatric use.)

Especially helpful to relieve sore throat pain is powdered vitamin C, in the form of ascorbic acid crystals. Place one teaspoon in a half-cup of water, and sip it. Spiced herb tea or hot water with lemon may also be soothing.

Chewing on fresh garlic can also help, as can the immune-stimulating herbs echinacea, 500 mg three times daily, if the root of the problems is infection, and nettles, 500 mg three times daily, if allergy plays a role.

Try Steam Treatments

Steam treatments can be created by bringing a large covered pot of water to a boil, taking it off the burner, putting a towel over your head, taking the lid off, and inhaling the steam for ten minutes or so, then lying back down and placing the warm moist towel over your face for a while. This can give you significant relief, especially before bed. This treatment draws your blood supply to the area that needs assistance, increasing local white cell concentration and nutrition, and thereby improving its ability to repair itself.

You may also find benefit by regularly visiting a sauna or steam bath. Gargling with hot salt water may also help.

Practice Stress Management

A specific program to enhance immune function should be undertaken before considering tonsillectomy or adenoidectomy. Since diet, exercise, and stress management all impact on the immune system, follow all the guidelines given in Chapter 2.

Conventional Medicine Approach to Tonsil and Adenoid Disorders

Although most infections of the tonsils are viral, a common cause is the streptococcus bacterium. White spots on your tonsils do not necessarily mean you have a streptococcus infection, or that you need to have your tonsils removed, but you should be tested for its presence, and may be treated with antibiotics if it persists.

Surgical Approaches to Tonsil and Adenoid Disorders

If you have severe symptoms caused by chronic infection or swelling in your tonsils and/or adenoids, removing them may be helpful. However, most doctors agree that surgery should *not* be performed unless you are still having significant problems after a year's treatment consisting of antibiotics for acute flare-ups, therapy for any allergies that may have been causing swelling in these passageways, along with the other alternative medicine approaches given on page 689.

You must distinguish between problems associated with tonsil infection, and those created by enlarged adenoids. The typical childhood problems of frequent colds, runny nose, sinusitis, allergic sniffles, earaches, and fevers are usually not caused by the tonsils, and tonsillectomy will not decrease the frequency of these problems. Surgery is indicated only if a direct relationship can be established between your enlarged or chronically infected tonsils and your symptoms, and other treatment is unsuccessful. The frequency of throat infections generated by the tonsils can be decreased by surgery, but episodes tend to subside anyway as the child grows older, when the tonsils typically shrink in size.

At this point, no good criteria exist to identify just who would benefit the most from tonsillectomy, so it is best to be conservative. However, if your child's infections are severe, with a lot of time lost from school, removal of the tonsils may be worthwhile.

Tonsillectomy should rarely be recommended before three years of age. This tissue is still important in the immune system development, and waiting often allows your child to outgrow such problems. If your child typically has more than four to six sore throats per year, with pain, fever, chills, time lost from school, and especially with recurrent strep infection, surgery can be chosen. If chronic swelling of the tonsils causes problems with talking or swallowing, removing them can be especially useful.

Enlarged adenoids can block the nasal passages, causing chronic mouth breathing, snoring, and a "nasal" tone to speech. Sense of smell and taste can be decreased. If your child is having problems getting a good night's sleep, surgery may be helpful. Also, some evidence suggests that prolonged mouth breathing in young children may lead to structural changes, including a longer, narrower face with an elongated or receding jaw, and poor teeth alignment. Blockage of adequate breathing through the nose is the most common reason for removing the adenoids.

Recurrent ear infections, with fluid collections caused by swollen adenoids blocking the eustachian tubes, can be relieved by removal of the adenoids, and may prevent hearing loss and further ear infections. However, a study from the University of Pittsburgh concluded that removing the adenoids and/or tonsils should not be the first surgical treatment as the beneficial effect is limited and short-term in children whose only problems is recurrent otitis media. The risks, complications, and cost outweighed any advantages.[6] A simpler first surgical treatment is to place a temporary tiny drainage tube (tympanostomy) through the eardrum.

Another rare reason to remove tonsils or adenoids, especially in adults, is to eliminate the possibility that the enlarged tissue contains a tumor.

Surgery can extract the tonsils or adenoids, or both together, depending on the kinds of problems present. You should delay the operation until your child is in the best possible medical condition. Surgery in the presence of an acute tonsil or adenoid infection is riskier and rarely done, unless an abscess needs to be drained. Your child should not take aspirin or other antiinflammatory medications, which can prolong bleeding, for at least two weeks before the operation.

You and your child's doctor should discuss as many of the details of the experience as possible with your child, emphasizing that this will make him or her feel much better, even if it is scary, and that a short period of postoperative throat discomfort may have to be endured. If a playmate has been through the experience, perhaps they can provide some cocounseling.

Tonsillectomy and adenoidectomy are usually outpatient surgery procedures. Since they are done under general anesthesia and the protective gag reflex is blocked, your child cannot eat or drink anything for at least eight hours before the operation, to avoid the breathing of stomach contents into the lungs.

After your child is asleep, a retractor is placed to keep the jaws separated and tongue out of the way. Your surgeon removes the tonsils by simply separating them gently from their bases, using blunt, finger dissection. A hot or cold wire loop or sharper instruments can be employed. The adenoids are removed by loops, or sharp scraping instruments. Bleeding is controlled by stitches and electrocautery.

After monitoring in the recovery room, your child can generally be released home six to ten hours after the procedure, when control of bleeding is assured and breathing is satisfactory. Sometimes an overnight stay may be necessary.

You can expect a sore throat, smelly breath, and perhaps some ear pain for a week or so. Any discomfort can usually be controlled by pain pills, gargling with an anesthetic mouth wash, or other means, as recommended in the alternative medicine section, below. A small amount of bleeding may also develop. Your doctor should see your child in a week or so, to ensure adequate healing and to check that the surgery was successful in accomplishing its objectives.

The risk of these operations is quite small. Although the major complication rate is 1.5 percent and is mostly limited to excessive bleeding, deaths are essentially zero (1 in 16,000), and these very rare fatalities are usually caused by the anesthetic, significant bleeding, or cardiac arrest.[7]

TONSIL AND ADENOID PROBLEMS SUMMARY

Prevention

Diet and Supplements

- Follow a low-fat, high-fiber diet.
- Vitamin A, 5,000 IU daily.
- Vitamin C, 1,000–2,000 mg 2–3 times daily.
- Vitamin E, D-alpha, 200 IU daily.
- Zinc, 50 mg daily.

Lifestyle

- Practice yoga daily.
- Practice stress management.

Alternative Medicine Approaches

- Follow the preventive guidelines, above.
- Follow a dairy-free diet; also try elimination of refined sugar, wheat, dried fruit, chocolate, fruit juices.

- Echinacea, 500 mg, 3 times daily, for 3 weeks.
- Garlic oil capsules, 500 mg, 1–2 times daily.
- Hot saltwater gargle.
- Steam treatments, sauna, steam bath.
- Use chiropractic, osteopathy, homeopathy, acupuncture, hypnosis, aromatherapy (especially eupcalytus).
- Practice visualization.

Conventional Medicine Approach

- Antibiotics when appropriate.

Surgical Approaches

- Tonsillectomy.
- Adenoidectomy.

Cataracts

A *cataract* is a cloudy area in the lens of your eye. It causes visual changes, making it harder for you to see clearly, by blocking some of the light passing through it from reaching the retina in the back of your eye. "Cataract" means "waterfall," and describes the common distortion, an appearance that looks like water falling in front of your eyes.

Your chances for having to decide about this operation are very great. After reaching age 70, up to 70 percent of us have some decreased vision caused by cataracts. Over 1.35 million cataract extractions are performed each year in the United States; it is the most common operation conducted on Americans after age 65.[8] Many seniors just attribute their decreased vision to "aging," not realizing that they have this problem. Though at any one time only 5 percent of such vision distur-

bances are significant enough actually to require surgical correction, untreated cataracts are still the leading cause of impaired vision and legal blindness in the United States.

The first recorded cataract removal operation was performed 3,000 years ago in India. Currently, advances in surgical technique using intraocular plastic lenses to replace the damaged natural lens makes the postoperation visual rehabilitation much easier, and you no longer need to wear thick glasses or contact lenses afterward. However, is this surgery really necessary? This problem may be preventable, even reversible, through alternative medicine approaches. Newer research is very promising that a combined vitamin program may help you avoid surgery in this delicate area.[9]

How Your Eyes Work

To understand eye function, it is helpful to follow rays of light as they bounce off an object you are viewing, return to your eye, and go through it, reaching its light-sensitive layer.

The cornea is your eye's clear outer layer. (See Figure 23.6.) Light rays are slightly bent as they pass through it into the anterior chamber of the eye, then pass through the pupil, the opening in your colored iris that contracts to admit fewer light rays in bright settings or dilates to let in more when it is dim. Light then passes through your eye's posterior chamber, where it encounters the clear, soft lens, the only transparent organ in your body.

Shaped like a small egg, one-eighth-inch thick, the lens has three parts. The outer layer is a clear sac, the capsular bag. Next, the cortex is found; it surrounds a central nucleus. The lens has no blood supply of its own; the salty fluid of the aqueous humor diffuses nutrients to it. Fibers connect a circular ciliary

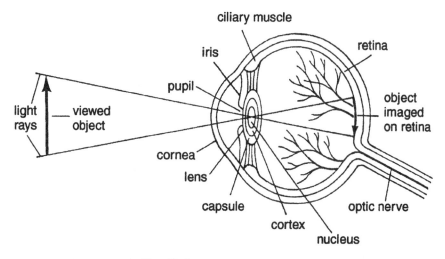

Fig. 23.6 Anatomy of the eye

muscle to the lens, and as this muscle contracts and relaxes, the shape and thickness of your lens changes, thereby bending the light rays as they pass through. As you look at objects at different distances, your lens accommodates to bend the incoming light rays, becoming thicker for near objects and thinner for distant ones.

After light rays pass through your lens, they travel through the *vitreous humor,* and are focused on the light-sensitive *retina,* the inside lining of your eyeball. Your retina translates the light's energy into electrical signals, which are carried to your brain via the optic nerve. Your brain interprets the signals, immediately recreating for your consciousness the image of the object you are looking at.

The proteins and minerals within your lens can clump together, shifting from egg-white clear to fried-egg opaque, creating the cloudiness responsible for your inability to see well. Your lens then increases in weight, size, and density. Light rays can only be poorly focused, and the retina receives a blurred image. Most people have cataracts in both eyes, although the cataracts may progressively block vision at different rates. It usually takes from five to ten years for them to reach "maturity," where they may interfere with enough vision to bring you to consider surgery.

The causes of cataracts include:

- Environmental factors, such as exposure to large amounts of sunlight, other sources of ultraviolet radiation, and X-rays.
- Lifestyle choices, such as diet, smoking, and alcohol.
- Side effects of medication, such as cortisone.
- Medical problems, such as diabetes, high triglyceride levels,[10] and German measles exposure in the uterus.
- Other concurrent eye problems such as iritis, glaucoma, tumor, and congenital eye anomaly.
- Penetrating or blunt eye trauma.

The alternative medicine approaches of dietary change, supplements, and herbs may help prevent, or even possibly reverse, early cataracts, as shown by both in vitro and in vivo research.[11]

Your first symptoms of cataract may be a slight blurring of vision, inability to read fine print, reduced perception of colors, or a halo effect seen around lights. You may need brighter light for reading or may experience difficulty driving at night. The increased density in the central part of your lens makes its focusing power stronger, increasing *myopia*—difficulty with far vision—causing you to need frequent eyeglass prescription changes. Double vision in one or both eyes may occur.

Cataracts do not cause pain; if you experience any pain, you need to be tested for other problems. Cataract onset is gradual, so if you experience any sudden changes in vision, you need immediate further investigation.

How Cataracts Are Diagnosed

Diagnosing cataracts is generally very easy. Usually, a history and eye exam are all that are necessary.

History

Tell your doctor about your visual acuity (ability to see fine detail)—how long you have worn glasses, the need for prescription changes, and how well you can see at present. Are you having problems seeing well enough to carry out your daily chores, reading, watching television, or driving a car? Do you have a problem distinguishing colors? Do you ever see double or things floating across your visual fields, or have eye pain?

Eye Exam

Your eyes are examined to look for a cataract or other causes of poor vision. First, you should read the familiar Snellen eye chart,

to determine your visual acuity. When your eyes are examined, a whitening of your pupil may be seen, a sign of an advanced cataract. Early cataracts are undetectable without special instruments.

Eye drops are placed on your eyes to dilate your pupils. This allows a wide view of your lens, along with the retina at the back of your eyeball. Your doctor uses the light and magnifying lens of a handheld ophthalmoscope to see the various parts of the eye. A slit-lamp is a more complicated stationary magnifying instrument that gives a closer look. After your sensitive cornea has been numbed by anesthetic eye drops, an internal pressure reading instrument should be pressed against your eye, to check for the high pressures found in glaucoma.

Ultrasound Eye Scan

An ultrasound scan of your eye may be recommended, to determine the size and shape of your eyeball, thereby helping your doctor select the focusing power for a new lens implant. Other more specialized and expensive testing is rarely necessary, since little evidence suggests that these tests are useful for most patients with cataracts.

Alternative Medicine Approaches to Cataracts

A cataract presents little danger to your eyes. The deterioration of your vision is usually quite slow, and delaying surgery does not cause future eye problems. However, cataracts aren't generally known to improve spontaneously without your taking some action.

Traditional cultures have sought to treat cataracts by placing various substances onto or in the eye, including ox dung and honey, but modern alternative medicine approaches focus mainly on prevention, and now, excitingly, possible reversal, using a combined program of dietary change, supplements, and herbs. You may be able to protect yourself from the formation of cataracts, slow their growth, or even reverse their development, by practicing the following alternative measures.

Wear Sunglasses

There is a strong link shown between chronic excessive exposure to bright sunlight, which may alter eye proteins, and cataract formation. Those living in sunbelt states in the United States have higher rates. *Even persons exposed to continuous fluorescent lighting have increased risk*. You may consider wearing slightly tinted glasses if you must be constantly exposed to fluorescent lights.

Change Your Diet

A link has been found between diets low in vitamins A,[12] C,[13] riboflavin,[14] and selenium[15] and the formation of cataracts. To help in prevention, slowing of growth, and possible reversal of early cataracts, choose five to seven servings of fresh fruits and vegetables each day, especially those high in these nutrients, such as tomatoes, carrots, squash, and dark green leaves like kale.

The association of cataract development with the presence of harmful free-radical forms of oxygen created when food decays means that you should be careful to avoid rancid foods. Since cataracts are more common in diabetics, intake of refined sugar may increase your risk. Consuming milk products, especially by adults who are lactose intolerant, is being considered as a possible cause of cataract formation.[16] The mechanism may be an effect of the milk proteins upon the pro-teins of the eye, or through high levels of galactose antagonizing the function of vitamin B_2. Follow the dietary guidelines given in Chapter 2.

Maintain Your Optimum Weight

A Harvard study found that obese men have a 50 percent higher risk of developing cataracts compared with average-weight men. This may be related to increased blood sugar levels.[17] See Chapter 2 for optimum dietary information, which can help you achieve and maintain your best weight.

Take Supplements

The lens contains one of the highest concentrations of vitamin C in your body. Vitamin C is an antioxidant, which helps to rid the body of free radicals, including those that form in the eye when it is exposed to sunlight. Damage to lens proteins by free radicals appears to be the major cause of cataracts associated with aging. Thus taking a supplement of vitamin C complex, 1,000 mg three times daily, may assist in prevention and reversal of early cataracts.

Animal tests exposing the lens to free radicals found that cataracts were prevented by supplemental vitamin C.[18] Human studies have shown that vitamin C, 1,000 mg per day, stops cataract progression.[19] Initial research by Wilmington, Delaware, ophthalmologist Dr. Robert Abel has, importantly, demonstrated reversal of cataracts, with over 400 patients using the addition of beta-carotene and vitamin C. In one published study, 60 to 90 percent of the patients who had early cataracts showed vision improvement with the addition of these supplements.

In his book *Healing Through Nutrition: A Natural Approach to Treating 50 Common*

Illnesses with Diet and Nutrients, Melvin Werbach reports, "Four hundred and fifty patients with early (incipient) cataracts received vitamin C along with vitamin A. Though similar patients had previously required surgery after about four years, only a small group of supplemented patients required surgery at that time. The cataracts of some did not progress over 11 years of follow-up."[20]

Vitamin E, 400 IU daily, may also act to scavenge detrimental free radicals; animal studies show that vitamin E can prevent experimentally induced cataracts.[21] Take 400 IU daily.

Low blood levels of zinc may also increase risk, and improvement of vision and possible reversal has been associated with zinc supplementation, 30 mg daily.[22] Since decreased amounts of the free-radical-scavenging mineral selenium have been discovered in the eyes of cataract formers, supplementation with 200 mcg daily may be beneficial. Deficiencies of the B vitamins B_1, B_2, inositol, and pantothenic acid may also be associated with this disease. Take the amounts for these and other supplements listed in Chapter 2.

Use Herbs

The Chinese and Japanese have used combination herbal preparations for the prevention and treatment of cataracts, and some success has been reported, especially during the early stages.[23] A combination of eight herbs, called *hachimijiogan*, is available from health food stores, though its efficacy has not yet been established through double-blind studies. You can take 150 to 300 mg per day.

Quit Smoking

Smoking is associated with increased risk for cataract formation. A prospective study of 20,907 male physicians in the Physicians' Health Study found a 36 percent decreased risk in those who had never smoked. If you smoke, the sooner you quit the better off you are.[24] You can follow the guidelines for quitting given in Chapter 2.

Practice Yoga Eye Exercises Daily

Although no research has of yet investigated this connection, exercise to your eye muscles may be able to improve nutrient distribution, helping assure maintenance of the health of your lens. The eye movements consist of back and forth, up and down, and circular exercises, performed gently. They should be practiced on a daily basis. Books and tapes offering instructions are listed in the Resources section at the back of this book.

Avoid Steroid Use

Steroid medications such as cortisone can contribute to cataract formation. Whenever possible, choose another medication or natural approach to limit the use of this class of drugs.

Conventional Medicine Approaches to Cataracts

Cataract surgery is almost never an emergency. You can take as long as you want to gather information and consider alternatives.

Wait for Significant Symptoms

You should not choose cataract surgery simply to prevent possible worse vision in the future. How you are seeing now is what is important. If your enjoyment of life is not affected, and you can function well with corrective eyeglasses, you do not need an operation. Also, if you have severe general medical problems, surgery may be unwise.

Get a New Pair of Glasses, Use Visual Aids, and Optimize Viewing Conditions

Cataracts cause increasing nearsightedness, which in its early stages can usually be dramatically improved with a new glasses prescription. Make certain your prescription is up-to-date; it may change faster than it used to as you age. You may need bifocals or trifocals. You can first use a reader's magnifying glass for small print. Good illumination is also essential for best vision. Eye drops, to slightly dilate your pupils, let in more light through a larger area of your lens, and may be temporarily helpful, though they will also increase glare.

Surgical Approaches to Cataracts

Visual needs vary widely. When deciding whether to have surgery, consider the degree to which your visual problems are interfering with your ability to carry out your necessary daily functions and the activities important for your enjoyment of life, such as sewing, reading, and watching television or movies. Also, does your present level of vision present a hazard, making injury more likely? If you must drive a car, can you do it safely? If you drive a car, in most states, you need to pass an eye test to get a driver's license. Are you in a safe home or work environment, with help available should an accident happen? If you have double vision or a big discrepancy in the acuity of your two eyes, you may especially wish to choose cataract surgery.

Two other circumstances indicate you should have your cataracts removed surgically as soon as possible. If you also have other eye disorders, the presence of cataracts can interfere with your doctor seeing and treating these more dangerous eye diseases, such as those affecting the retina. Rarely,

cataracts can even cause glaucoma, which can lead to blindness if untreated.

In general, though, age is no obstacle to cataract surgery. If your functional abilities and enjoyment of life are impaired because of poor eyesight from cataracts, you should strongly consider surgery however old you are. Improved vision is possible in the vast majority of patients, but be certain to get a clear understanding from your doctor just how much improvement you can expect in your specific case. You must decide if the expected degree of improvement is worth the small risks and expense.

With the newer surgical techniques, you do not have to wait until your cataract has fully "matured," as in the past, but can choose to have surgery whenever your visual difficulties prove significant to you. The most common surgical approach is to correct one eye at a time, removing your more diseased lens first, substituting it with a clear plastic lens. After you have recovered successfully, and can see well out of the first eye, the other can be fixed.

Cataract surgery is usually performed in an outpatient facility or in a well-equipped doctor's office. Good monitoring of blood pressure, heart function, and oxygen levels must be available. An intravenous line is started, in case medication is necessary.

Local anesthesia is most commonly used, often with intravenous sedation. However, if you are very nervous or can't keep still because of tremor or other problems, general anesthesia may be best.

After you are positioned on the operating table, your doctor places eye drops under your eyelids to numb the external tissues. A needle is then used to inject anesthetic around your eyeball. A soft weight may be placed on the eye for ten minutes, to help spread the anesthetic. The eye and lid muscles are paralyzed, keeping things perfectly still. An eyelid retractor keeps your upper and lower lids separated. The only sensation you may have is pressure on your forehead.

Using an operating microscope, your doctor makes a minute incision at the edge of your cornea, just above your iris, after which a small piece of the front of your lens capsule is removed, so the cataract can be reached. (See Figure 23.7.)

Three methods can be used to remove the nucleus of the lens, which contains the largest part of the cataract. The rarely chosen *intracapsular extraction* takes out the entire lens, including the nucleus and the anterior and posterior capsules. An *extracapsular extraction* removes the anterior capsule, nucleus, and cortex, and is the most common method used today. Your lens is simply expressed or pulled out, leaving the back half of the capsule intact. *Phacoemulsification* uses a smaller 3.5-millimeter corneal incision. A tiny ultrasound probe *(not* laser) is inserted and placed

next to the lens, which is then softened and emulsified via sound vibrations. After being liquefied, it is sucked out through a small needle.

Your new plastic lens is put in the empty space previously occupied by the extracted lens. It is held in place by the remaining capsule, along with two looped threads extending from the edges of your new lens. The cornea incision may need to be repaired with tiny absorbable stitches. A soft dressing and eye patch are placed at the end of the procedure.

Cataract surgery usually takes thirty to forty minutes. After the operation is finished, you can go home in the company of your family or a friend. Someone should stay with you until you can see well enough to take care of your needs. Your postoperative pain should be minimal.

You will need to see your doctor frequently after your operation. The next day, you should be seen so you can have your eye patch removed, and your eye inspected to ensure that things are okay. Visual acuity and

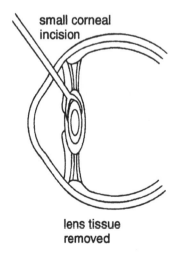

small corneal incision

lens tissue removed

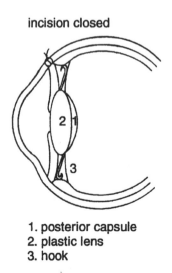

incision closed

1. posterior capsule
2. plastic lens
3. hook

Fig. 23.7 Procedures involved in cataract surgery

eye pressure should be checked at each visit. You may be asked to use antibiotic and anti-inflammatory eye drops to lessen the risk of infection and eye swelling. Avoid getting soap and water into your eye.

You may be more comfortable wearing a patch or dark glasses for a while, but these are not usually necessary. If you can see well out of your other eye, you can drive soon after surgery. In the first month, you should avoid any straining, such as in heavy lifting, bending, or coughing from cigarettes, all of which increase pressure inside your eye. Some doctors recommend protecting your eye with a metal shield at night for several weeks.

Healing is complete in four to six weeks, though it may take six to twelve weeks for your eye to fully recover its optimum sight. You may have some difficulty judging distances accurately, until you get used to your new visual ability, usually between 20/40 and 20/20.[25] *Multifocal intraocular lenses* can give you reading as well as distant vision, so that you may not need to use glasses at all. If you still need glasses to get your best distance and close-up vision, they should be fitted after six to eight weeks. If, for some reason, a new lens couldn't be placed, after recovery from the operation, you can use special cataract contact lenses, or thick cataract glasses instead.

Success rate is 95 percent in otherwise reasonably good eyes. Mortality is virtually zero. You may develop a small degree of astigmatism (localized blurriness) after surgery, its size depending on the length of your incision. Rare serious complications include hemorrhage, *hyphema* (blood leaking into the eye, causing cloudiness), infection, iris damage, fragments of the lens lost into the vitreous humor and causing cloudy vision, incision separation, dislocation of the lens, eyeball in-

flammation, glaucoma, retinal detachment causing areas of blindness, damage to eyelid nerves causing drooping, complete blindness, and, extremely rarely, loss of the eye.

Your cataract can't return because the lens was removed, though you may develop a *posterior capsular opacification,* where the remaining lens capsule becomes cloudy, causing the same visual problems as a cataract. This problem is rare in the first six months after surgery, but increases to 25 percent within two years. About one-half of all patients eventually get it to some extent. If the degree of your symptoms warrant, you can be easily treated by another simple procedure. Your surgeon uses a neodymium-yttrium-aluminum-garnet (ND-YAG) laser to make a small hole in the posterior capsule, so that light can pass through. This painless outpatient treatment then increases your visual acuity. Complications are rare, including transient glaucoma, damage to the lens, retinal swelling, and retinal detachment.

CATARACTS SUMMARY

Prevention

Diet and Supplements

- Follow a low-fat, high-fiber diet.
- Avoid refined sugar and flour.
- Vitamin A, 10,000 IU daily.
- Vitamin C, 1,000 mg, 3 times daily.
- Vitamin E, D-alpha, 400 IU daily.
- Multi-B vitamins, 50 mg daily.
- Selenium, 200 mcg daily.
- Zinc, 50 mg daily.

- Magnesium, 250–500 mg daily.
- Quercetin, 400 mg 2–3 times daily.
- Alpha-lipoic acid, 600 mg daily.
- Bilberry, 250–500 mg daily.

Lifestyle

- Don't smoke.
- Wear sunglasses.
- Maintain optimum weight.
- Avoid steroid use.
- Practice yoga eye exercises daily.

Alternative Medicine Approaches

- Follow the preventive guidelines, above.
- Vitamin C complex, 1,000 mg 3 times daily: Beta-carotene, 25,000 IU daily.
- Chinese herbal combination *hachimijio-gan*, 150–300 mg daily.

Conventional Medicine Approaches

- Wait for significant symptoms.
- Get a new pair of glasses, use visual aids, and optimize viewing conditions.

Surgical Approaches

Cataract extraction

- Intracapsular lens extraction.
- Extracapsular lens extraction.
- Phacoemulsification.

Plastic replacement lens

- Unifocal.
- Multifocal.

Kidney Stones

---

*C*eleste, a 35-year-old laboratory technician, although a recent vegetarian, still loved cheese, ice cream, and cappuccino with lots of whipped cream. While driving home after an especially long working day during which she was too busy even to drink water, she developed sudden severe pain in the left midback. Tests revealed a stone in the upper part of her ureter, but with only partially blocked urine flow. She elected to try alternative medicine, and spent the next day drinking copious amounts of barley water and eating watermelon. The pain diminished, but was still present. She visited an acupuncturist, whose treatment gave immediate relief to her pain, and the stone passed within a few hours. She then chose to avoid caffeine and dairy products, and always carry a bottle of spring water in her purse.

Your kidneys are fist-sized, bean-shaped organs located behind your upper abdomen, under your diaphragm. They perform the very vital function of filtering your blood, removing unwanted chemicals and harmful waste products of cellular metabolism, which then pass out with the urine. You can easily live with only one normal kidney, but need machine dialysis if both fail. The kidneys are also intimately involved with other body processes, including fluid and mineral balance, blood pressure regulation, and maintenance of red blood cell production.

The kidneys make urine from blood filtered through their *nephrons*. (See Figure 23.8.) This urine then passes into your urine-collecting system. Each kidney subunit, or *calyx,* has its own collecting apparatus, which empties into a funnel-shaped *kidney pelvis.* From each of these kidney pelvises, your urine moves into an attached *ureter.* Your right and left ureters are long, one-quarter-inch tubes that travel behind the abdominal cavity, then circle around the side of your lower abdomen and pelvis to connect with and pass urine into your *bladder.* The rest, as they say, is water under the bridge.

Kidney stones have plagued humans throughout recorded history. The incidence has been increasing, *fivefold in the last fifty years.* Your chances of having a stone are one in three if you are a man, and one in five if a woman. Stones are most common in the 20- to 50-year age range. They develop most frequently in hot, dry climates, which tend to cause dehydration. The states bordering the Gulf of Mexico have the highest incidence, and this area of the southeast United States is therefore called the "Stone Belt." Excess intake of meats, fats, and salt, in combination with inadequate fluid intake (less than eight glasses per day) during the summer in this area seem to be the precipitating factors.

Seventy-five percent of all kidney stones are composed of calcium oxalate, a hard salt compound. Other types of stones include those made predominately of uric acid and the mineral combination struvenite.

A diet high in oxalates such as spinach and including tea is also associated with increased risk for stones. Other dietary factors such as high intake of purines from consumption of animal products, alcohol, and caffeine also increase your risk. Stones can be caused by taking too much calcium or vitamin D supplements, or by lithium medication.

Twenty percent of all stones are associated with an identifiable underlying medical problem, including those diseases which increase

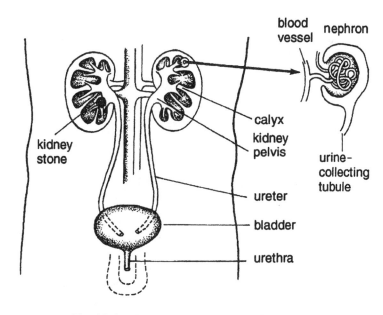

Fig. 23.8 Anatomy and location of the kidney

calcium and oxalate content of the urine, such as hyperparathyroidism, kidney disease, sarcoidosis, and intestinal disorders. Other predisposing medical problems include frequent kidney infections, gout, and, rarely, various genetic metabolic disorders.

Persons who have higher rates of calcium absorption from the intestine, high urinary calcium and oxalate excretion, alkaline urine, and low volumes of urine output are more prone to stones. More than half of all stone patients excrete high levels of calcium in the urine, sometimes for unknown reasons. Genetics may play a role in your risk.

Normally, urine is saturated with calcium, oxalate, uric acid, and phosphates, but they stay in solution due to both the urine's acid-base balance and the presence of substances which protect against crystallization. The abovementioned risk factors and anything else that increases debris in your urine can cause these ions in solution to precipitate, forming a solid, small seed. If it is not immediately washed away with the urine, such a seed can attach itself to any kidney surface, other debris, or crystals, and then grow in size, forming a stone.

Stones vary in size, shape, and color. Most appear as small, round, black, brown, or tan specks or grains of sand. They can grow to become larger than an egg. Stones which are angular and sharp are likely to cause more pain and bleeding. "Stag horn" stones stay in the kidney, growing to fill the kidney pelvis and taking the shape of a stag's antler with a rough surface like coral.

About 80 percent of all kidney stones simply pass on their own, usually with your urine within forty-eight hours. However, the best approach is prevention, and alternative medicine offers strategies both for prevention, as well as for treatment, to assist the swift passage of any stones you may develop. Since if you have one stone, you have a 60 percent chance you will form another within ten years, you should adopt alternative measures in any case.

Kidney stones are a common cause of pain, but they rarely cause kidney failure or death. Your symptoms depend on the size and shape of the stone and where it is located. Stones are usually formed in the kidneys, and then move down your ureter. Staghorn stones can grow silently, until they completely fill and block your kidney pelvis.

Stones can pass without causing any symptoms. Typically, "renal colic" is a severe pain that has a sudden onset, as the stone blocks the kidney outlet or moves into your very sensitive ureter. The pain begins in your flank, and radiates down around the lower abdomen into your groin area. You can't get comfortable. The discomfort may first come in waves, intensifying over a fifteen- to thirty-minute period, to then become steady and excruciating. Finally, the pain may suddenly vanish, as the stone stops moving or is passed into your bladder. An attack may be accompanied by nausea and vomiting. You may notice blood in your urine, burning and frequency with urination, or urinary retention. If you also have an accompanying infection, you may develop fever and chills.

Stones may also give you no symptoms and yet cause recurrent infections, obstruction to urine flow, increased pressure and swelling in your kidney, or kidney damage, so they always require careful treatment and monitoring. Do not attempt the alternative medicine approaches given below without a doctor's supervision.

How Kidney Stones Are Diagnosed

The diagnosis of kidney stones involves the search for their presence and determination of the specific type that you may have. The steps include a good history, physical exam, blood and urine tests, X-rays, scans, and stone composition lab analysis.

History

The search for evidence of kidney stones should begin by your giving your doctor a careful history of any urinary tract symptoms such as burning, urgency, and noticeable blood in the urine. Report any history of urinary infections. Your doctor needs to know about your usual diet and fluid intake, and medications. Medical problems often associated with these stones include gout, bowel absorption problems, previous intestinal surgery, and parathyroid disease. Family history of stones may be a tip-off.

Physical Exam

Your doctor should perform a general physical exam with special care to feel your abdomen, sides, and back beneath your ribs. Enlarged or tender kidneys may be associated with stones anywhere in the urinary tract.

Laboratory Tests

Blood tests can screen for elevated blood cystine levels, calcium, uric acid, and other stone-related chemicals. Urine analysis can look for crystals, red and white blood cells, and for evidence of infection.

X-Rays and Scans

Stones can usually be seen on plain X-rays, IVP (an X-ray where you are given an intravenous dye that "lights up" your kidneys, ureters, and bladder), or sonogram. Limited CAT scan without contrast dye may be the best test to show tiny calcified stones passing in the ureter.

Other Tests

The diagnosis of kidney stones is usually quite easy, based on the typical history and the above simple tests. Stones may be recovered from strained urine. If you have recurrent or enlarging stones, or if the stones are in a child, a twenty-four-hour urine collection can be examined for stone-related chemicals and crystals. Tests in which you take in increased levels of stone-related chemicals can show if your kidneys process them abnormally. Once a stone is passed, it can be analyzed, so that your doctor can tailor preventive advice to your specific needs.

Alternative Medicine Approaches to Kidney Stones

The agony of passing a kidney stone is one of the worst on the Richter scale of bodily pain, and without preventive measures, about half of the people who have one episode will have to endure another within ten years.

I know. I (Sandy) had two bouts of kidney stones, before I changed my lifestyle. The first time, the stone passed after three days of intense suffering; the second episode was immediately arrested by one acupuncture treatment.

Previous views of the dietary causes of kidney stone formation placed the blame on foods high in oxalates, such as spinach. Poor Popeye! Newer understanding places responsibility more on his side-kick Wimpy, who scarfed hamburgers at every opportunity.

Alternative medicine treatment of kidney

stones has traditionally included a full range of methods: Over 4,000 years ago, the Egyptians were recorded to have used herbs to assist in stone passage. Happily, operations on the kidneys for stones have largely been replaced by lithotripsy, and only 5 percent of all stones now require a full operation for their removal.

Your kidney stone may be a warning signal of other risks. By choosing to treat your kidney stone with alternative medicine approaches, you can also act to prevent many other dietary-related diseases, such as heart disease and the major cancers.

Since 80 percent of all kidney stones pass on their own, it is difficult to sort out exactly what effects alternative medicine treatments have on the elimination of stones, which might have gone through on their own without treatment, but it seems reasonable to use their assistance to aim for passage of a stone before you rush to either lithotripsy or surgical treatment. However, you must be monitored by your doctor, to avoid damage to your kidney.

Following are the most significant alternative medicine approaches for the prevention and treatment of kidney stones.

Change Your Diet

Most kidney stones are preventable. A diet high in meat, eggs, and dairy products is the root cause of this prevalent problem. Animal protein in the diet causes the body to excrete more calcium in the urine, to buffer the presence of the excess amino acids in your bloodstream. Meat also contains purine, which is changed to uric acid in the urine, favoring stone formation. Vegetarians have a lower risk for kidney stones.[26] Changing to a low-fat, vegetarian diet, free of dairy, may be all

you need to do to prevent new stones from forming.

Even a vegetarian diet can be too high in fat. Excess fat in the diet may itself be an independent risk factor.[27] Follow the guidelines for the optimum low-fat diet given in Chapter 2, to prevent this disorder along with many other common Western diseases.

Adequate fiber in your diet is important too: it acts to bind calcium in your digestive tract, and thus prevent increased amounts from reaching your bloodstream and ultimately your urinary tract.[28] Even if you eat meat, consuming more fresh fruits and vegetables will decrease your risk for stone formation.[29] Most Americans eat much too little fiber; make certain to follow the guideline for fiber intake—20 to 40 grams per day—given in Chapter 2.

Avoid ingestion of refined sugar, since it has been shown to increase urinary calcium levels.[30] Alcohol can also elevate your risk for calcium stone formation.[31] Infection in the upper urinary tract is felt to contribute to the precipitation of stones. Avoiding alcohol and sugar can also reduce your risks for infection-related stones, since both of these substances diminish your white cell activity.

If you are at risk for developing stones, you should avoid milk products fortified with vitamin D. Vitamin D accelerates calcium absorption from the intestines, and increases its concentration in your urine.

Ninety-nine percent of your body's calcium is stored in your bones. You need dietary sources of calcium to maintain their health. Dietary calcium was originally felt to contribute to the risk of kidney stones, but recently this thinking has been reversed, since it was found that persons eating a diet higher in calcium actually were at a lower risk for stones.[32] Dietary calcium reduces urinary excretion of oxalate. The problem with dairy products is not the calcium, but the protein. Your body needs calcium, but you should obtain it from sources such as spinach, broccoli, and other dark green vegetables, which provide adequate calcium in a substratum lower in protein.

Oxalate in the diet—found in high concentrations in foods such as beans, spinach, rhubarb, okra, wheat germ, peanuts, and chocolate—was for a long time erroneously felt to contribute to stone formation, but newer nutritional wisdom has shown that although stones may be artificially induced in animals by the ingestion of oxalate, dietary sources do not act in this manner in the majority of stone formers.[33] Feel free to eat both beans and spinach even if you have a history of kidney stones; these foods are now felt to actually be protective.

Take Some Supplements; Limit Others

Taking magnesium citrate, 250 mg one to three times daily, may relax the muscles of your urinary tract enough to pass a stone, and prevent a new one from forming. If you are in the middle of an attack, start with 500 mg as an initial dose.

Magnesium deficiency in animal studies has been linked to stone formation. Magnesium acts to prevent the precipitation of calcium in the urine, and regular supplementation is proven to prevent recurrence of stones.[34] Taking magnesium in the citrate form has the additional advantage of increasing urinary citrate, also felt to help in stone prevention.

Deficiencies of vitamin B_6, glutamic acid, and vitamin K have also been implicated in kidney stone formation. Restoring normal levels prevents future stones. Take at least 500

mg of B_6 three times daily (take this along with equal amounts of B_1, and B_2), but only for a few weeks; rarely, excess B_6 can cause nerve damage if continued for long periods. Also take 300 mg of glutamate, (also called L-glutamate or glutamic acid) 200 mcg of vitamin K, and 99 mg of potassium, in addition to green leafy vegetables, which may act preventively.

Citrate is decreased in the urine of many stone formers. Citrates form soluble complexes with calcium and also make overly acidic urine more alkaline, ensuring the solubility of calcium compounds, inhibiting stone formation. Supplementation has been shown to decrease recurrent stones.[35] Citrates can be taken as potassium citrate (150 mg per day), sodium citrate (1,500 mg per day), magnesium citrate (450 mg per day), or calcium citrate (1,500 mg per day).

Excess use of supplemental (not dietary) calcium, more than 2,000 mg per day, may act to precipitate stones. Taking your daily calcium supplement in its citrate form has the advantage of giving you a higher concentration of urinary citrate.

Taking too many antacids containing calcium may increase your risk for stones. See Chapter 11 for alternative medicine approaches to heartburn treatment that do not employ such antacids.

The belief that vitamin C might contribute to kidney stone formation has been found to be untrue in repeated studies, even when this vitamin is taken in high doses.[36]

Keep Your Urine Relatively Acidic

A urinary pH of 5.5 to 6.6, slightly acidic, helps to prevent the infection associated with stone formation. If your urine is too alkaline, it favors infections, though if it is too acid, it can also contribute to crystal precipitation. Excess meats, dairy, and stress can all contribute to an unhealthy pH.

Drink Lots of Fluids, Especially Barley Water

Drinking plenty of fluids can help a stone pass on its own. The water in which barley has been boiled has a mucilaginous quality and a high magnesium-calcium ratio, and so has been found to be especially helpful in passing a stone. Eating watermelon may also help, for similar reasons. You should produce at least one and one-half to two quarts of urine per day.

Another combination often recommended is zucchini and green bean broth: Chop the vegetables, boil them for ten minutes or so, then blend them and drink plenty of the resulting thin soup. This soup is high in magnesium and relatively alkaline, and so reduces the amount of calcium in your urine.

Water that is "soft" contains more calcium, and so may increase the risk of stone formation. In addition, copper in pipes may contribute to higher cadmium levels in the urine, known to favor stone growth. Therefore especially avoid drinking water from old pipes; in general, use spring water.

Avoid Caffeine

Any source of caffeine—coffee, tea, cola, chocolate—acts to dehydrate you and increase the amount of calcium in your urine. If you have a tendency to form stones, you increase your risk by taking these substances, which also have other negative effects. Follow the guidelines given in Chapter 2 to find substitutes.

Maintain Your Optimum Weight

Excess weight may itself contribute to the formation of stones, by stressing your urinary tract with increased calcium excretion.[37] Follow the dietary and lifestyle advice in Chapter 2 to achieve your optimum weight.

Practice Visualization

First, do deep relaxation, given in Chapter 2. Then imagine your kidneys as a glistening waterfall. See the stone falling out of its position, down into the pool below. Hold this image in your mind, while feeling it happen within your body. Repeat this process three to five times daily.

Conventional Medicine Approaches to Kidney Stones

If you have a known medical disease associated with stone formation, as is the case in 20 percent of patients, it should be treated first by means of lifestyle and dietary changes and medications. If these noninvasive approaches don't work, you can try lithotripsy.

Conventional management of kidney and ureteral stones depends on your symptoms and the medical problems they may be creating, as well as their cause, composition, size, and position.

Stones that block urine flow, are associated with recurrent kidney infections, or cause painful symptoms need to be eliminated or removed as soon as possible.

Fluid Intake

No drug treatment is currently available to dissolve stones, but medical intervention can limit their growth and prevent new ones from forming. The primary goal is to increase fluid intake and urine volume, thereby decreasing the concentration of substances likely to precipitate out as crystals. An achievable goal is to double your urine output to more than two quarts per day.

Most stones less than 5 millimeters in diameter will pass spontaneously. If they are not giving you symptoms, they should not be treated by invasive methods. You simply are advised to drink lots of water, twelve 8-ounce glasses per day, since this dilutes the stone-forming chemicals and flushes them out, and avoid dehydration and dehydrating liquids such as coffee and alcohol. You should strain your urine, to collect the stone, so that its composition can be analyzed. Knowing the type of stone will help you determine a specific program to prevent another one from developing.

Dietary Restrictions and Medications

If you have calcium oxalate stones, you should decrease your dietary intake of calcium to less than 1 gram per day and increase your sodium intake. Cellulose phosphate citrate supplements bind calcium in the gut, so it will not be absorbed. The thiazide diuretics chlorothiazide (Diuril) and hydrochlorothiazide (HydroDiuril) will decrease calcium concentration in the urine.

Uric acid stones form when increased uric acid is present in the urine. If you have this type of stone, you should especially decrease your dietary animal protein, particularly organ meats such as liver, heart, kidneys, and pancreas, which are high in uric acid. If your urine is acidic, you are more likely to precipitate a uric acid crystal. Avoiding animal products keeps your urine more alkaline. You can also take bicarbonate or citrate to alkalize your urine, to lessen this tendency. The drug allopurinol increases urinary output of uric acid, and so may cause you to form stones.

Cystine stones are associated with a genetic disorder. They are treated by acidifying your urine, increasing urine output by increasing fluid intake, decreasing intake of foods high in methionine such as fish, and taking medications to decrease urinary cystine.

Urinary Infection Treatment

Stones caused by infection occur when organisms in your urinary system split urea into insoluble compounds. You first must be treated to clear out these bugs, and then all of your stones should be removed.

Extracorporeal Shock Wave Lithotripsy

If your stone is greater than 7 millimeters, it has little chance of passing spontaneously. *Extracorporeal shock wave lithotripsy (ESWL)*, referred to simply as lithotripsy, was introduced in the United States in 1984. It is capable of treating most stones smaller than 2 centimeters in size. Stones larger than that are usually treated with a combination of lithotripsy and percutaneous nephrolithotomy (see below).

Lithotripsy is an outpatient procedure. The high-tech lithotripsy machine is very expensive, so it may be placed in a trailer and shared by several different institutions. You may be given some sedation, but anesthesia is not usually necessary. You lie on a water cushion, or in a water bath, with the machine pressed against your flank. Your stone is localized on a sonogram, and then high-energy shock waves focused on it. Since water and your soft tissues are the same density, the shock waves don't meet a change in density until they reach the hard stone, at which point their energy is released, shattering it into fragments. Multiple pulses of shock waves are usually necessary. The whole procedure generally takes an hour or so.

After lithotripsy, you should strain your urine, to catch the stone fragments so they can be analyzed. You may have some blood in your urine for a few days, and some discomfort, as stone fragments pass over the next weeks to months. If large fragments remain, the procedure may need to be repeated.

In combination with lithotripsy, a ureteral stent may be passed from your bladder to your kidney, to ensure that stone fragments do not block urine flow in your ureter. The success rate of lithotripsy is about 80 percent without a ureteral stent and 90 percent if a stent is used. If a ureteral stone can be pushed back up into your kidney, the success rate of lithotripsy then approaches 100 percent.

Lithotripsy has fewer complications than percutaneous nephrolithotomy. However, its long-term side effects are less certain. Magnetic resonance images show that lithotripsy carries some risk of damage to your kidneys and resulting high blood pressure, though generally this is only temporary. Also, stone fragments left behind may not all pass, giving you residual problems. For all of these reasons, lithotripsy is therefore not usually recommended for children.

Surgical Approaches to Kidney Stones

If your stones do not pass on their own and are not suitable for lithotripsy, you may need a surgical approach to treat them.

Cystoscopy

Cystoscopy is an outpatient procedure. You lie on a special table with your feet up in stirrups. Local anesthetic jelly is placed into your urethra and sedation usually given, although spinal or general anesthesia may be used. The cystoscope, a lighted scope which can be passed into your bladder, allows your doctor to watch through a magnifying lens or on a TV screen. Special instruments are passed through a channel in the cystoscope, then on into the ureter containing the stone. Most stones in the lower third of the ureter can be grabbed with a wire basket, dissolved using an infusion of chemicals, or, by use of a laser, physically broken into fragments small enough to pass spontaneously. Dye can be introduced, and X-rays then taken of your urinary tract.

If your stone is stuck in your upper ureter, it can often be pushed up into your kidney pelvis, where it can later be broken into small fragments by lithotripsy. If the stone can't be budged, your surgeon can pass a plastic tube (stent) from your bladder to your kidney, allowing urine to pass around the stone. The stone can then be treated by lithotripsy or removed by percutaneous nephrolithotomy.

You can go home right after the procedure. You may have some mild urethral soreness and urinary frequency, burning with urination, or some blood in your urine for a day or two.

The success rate of cystoscopic removal of suitable ureteral stones is 98 percent. Rare complications include a hole being made in the ureter, in 3 percent.

Percutaneous Nephrolithotomy

If your stone is greater than 2 centimeters, or greater than 1 centimeter in the lower pole of your kidney, this procedure may be recommended. You need to be hospitalized for a few days, and usually general anesthesia is chosen. After you are asleep, your doctor uses a sonogram to locate the stone. A small skin incision is made, and a metal catheter maneuvered into the kidney. A shock wave probe or crushing instrument fragments the stone, which is then extracted through the catheter. A small drain, left to drain urine, can be removed after a few days.

The success rate of percutaneous nephrolithotomy is about 80 percent. Complications include bleeding, kidney damage, prolonged drainage of urine through the incision, and incision infection.

Open Nephrolithotomy

If your stones can't be reached by any other method, you may then need to have this more invasive procedure. It is necessary in less than 5 percent of all kidney stone patients. If you have a staghorn stone, complex kidney or ureteral anatomy, or complete urine obstruction, you are more likely to require it.

You are admitted the morning of the procedure. General anesthesia is usually necessary. After you are asleep, you are rolled on your side, and an incision made over your kidney, starting between your ribs and hipbone, and carried across your flank. Your muscles are separated, exposing your kidney and ureter. The kidney pelvis or ureter is then opened, and the stone extracted. If you have a staghorn stone, a large kidney incision may be needed. A drain is placed, to prevent accumulation of urine in your incision, and a catheter put in your bladder, to avoid increased urinary tract pressure, allowing your incision to heal more rapidly. The flank incision is closed with stitches, staples, or skin tapes.

Postoperatively, if you have some incision pain, it can be treated by intravenous or intramuscular injections. After a day or two, pain pills may suffice. Some blood may be present in your urine for a few days. The drain can be removed after four or five days, and you can usually be discharged home in four to seven days. A week after you are discharged, you need to see your doctor, to ensure no urinary tract blockage has developed, and have your incision checked to see that it is healing well. You should be able to return to work in three or four weeks.

Complications include death in less than 1 percent of the cases, but bleeding, incision infection, and persistent drainage of urine out of the wound occur in about 15 percent.

KIDNEY STONES SUMMARY

Prevention

Diet and Supplements

- Follow a low-fat, high-fiber diet.
- Substitute soy for dairy products, especially cheese.
- Eat green leafy vegetables.
- Drink 8–10 large glasses of water daily.
- Magnesium, 250 mg, 1–3 times daily.
- Vitamin B_6, 50 mg daily.
- Glutamate, 300 mg daily.
- Vitamin K, 200 mcg daily.
- Potassium, 99 mg daily.
- Avoid caffeine, citrates, alcohol, antacids.

Lifestyle

- Exercise 1 hour, 3–5 times weekly.
- Practice daily yoga postures, especially the spinal twist.
- Practice stress management.
- Maintain optimum weight.

Alternative Medicine Approaches

- Follow the guidelines for prevention, above.
- Magnesium citrate, 500 mg.
- Drink barley water, and eat watermelon.
- Aloe juice or gel, 1 tablespoon, 1–3 times daily.
- Vitamins B_6, B_1, B_2, 500 mg, 3 times daily, under supervision.
- Potassium citrate, 150 mg, daily; sodium citrate, 1,500 mg, daily; magnesium citrate, 450 mg, daily; or calcium citrate, 1,500 mg, daily.
- Herb teas: marshmallow, chamomile, madder root, cleavers, buchu, uva ursi, wood betony, khella, and/or cough grass.
- Use acupuncture, hypnosis, homeopathy.
- Practice visualization.

Conventional Medicine Approaches

- Increase fluid intake so urine output is more than 2 quarts per day.
- Medications and dietary restrictions—depending on type of stone.
- Treat urinary infection.
- Extracorporeal shock wave lithotripsy.

Surgical Approaches

- Cystoscopy and stone removal.
- Percutaneous nephrolithotomy.
- Open nephrolithotomy.

CHAPTER 24

AN INTEGRATED APPROACH TO YOUR OPERATION

Dr. Mehmet Oz, a cardiac surgeon at Columbia-Presbyterian Medical Center in New York City and chief of its Complementary Care Center, helped pioneer the integrative approach to surgery. Since the creation of the center's program in 1994, he and his co-workers researched many of the alternative medicine modalities discussed in this book, for application to surgical patients, including music therapy, hypnosis, massage and reflexology, guided imagery, yoga, meditation, aromatherapy, therapeutic touch, and nutrition modification.

About 40 percent of the nearly 1,400 cardiac care patients treated at Columbia each year have chosen to use the center's services. In one randomized trial, Dr. Oz studied the effects of self-hypnosis in patients undergoing coronary bypass, finding that those who chose to use self-hypnosis tapes were more relaxed after surgery and required significantly less pain medication.[1]

In this chapter, we will briefly summarize for you how to apply the information given in this book to create an integrated approach to your individual operation. This chapter is designed to be a quick reference, one you can use as an easy checklist, with simple guidelines for you to follow before, during, and after your surgery.

You can develop an alternative medicine aspect to integrate with any operation. Most surgeons, if you simply explain what you would like to do and why, are now willing to accommodate these ideas. Although they have been taught to focus mainly on the technical aspects of their craft, a vision of the whole patient has always been part of many surgeons' "bedside manner."

Some of the alternative medicine approaches, such as acupuncture or aromatherapy, may still seem strange to your particular surgeon or hospital, but since scientific rationale for many of these options is now available, you may be able to introduce them to these newer avenues for assisting your body to heal. Once the province of a few separate centers, the alternative medicine movement is now more and more frequently and routinely integrated right alongside mainstream medical thinking.

As explained in Chapter 2, if you and your doctor do pay attention to mind-body and other alternative influences, it may affect your body's abilities to withstand the stress of an operation, and you can come through surgery more successfully. The chief of surgery at Wilmington Hospital in Delaware, Dr. Gerald Lemole, was one of the country's first surgeons to begin giving postoperative dietary recommendations, vitamins, and other supplements to all of his patients. As he stated in his book *An Integrated Approach to Cardiac Care,* which summarizes the use of these and other alternative medicine methods in the cardiac setting, "Ideally, only therapies that have been scientifically shown to be effective should be incorporated into an integrative practice. However, some modalities are difficult to prove by classical methods, and they shouldn't be rejected out of hand, even though they may seem ineffective or counter to our current philosophies of practice. We should be conversant with alternative, complementary and integrative therapies to best treat our patients."[2]

One survey showed that, already, 51 percent of all surgical patients were found to be taking some form of herbs, vitamins, supplements, or homeopathic medicines directly prior to their operations, and that 70 percent did not tell their surgeons what they were tak-

ing.[3] However, some herbs and supplements may interact with your anesthesia, blood clotting, and other aspects of your operation, so you need to inform your doctor completely about what you are doing.

Getting Ready for Surgery: A Program of Diet, Supplements, and Stress Management

Whether your operation is elective or an emergency, you can act to help yourself through surgery. If you have time, read through the Preface, Introduction, and Chapters 1 through 4 of this book, along with the section dealing with your specific disorder.

Following are the most important preparatory steps you can take toward creating an integrated approach to your surgery. They are divided into categories, but since they act in varying ways, they may best be applied together.

Prepare Yourself

If possible, spend at least two weeks to a month preparing yourself for your surgery. Read Chapters 1 through 4 and 24, and especially follow the guidelines for diet, relaxation, and visualization. Even if your operation must be performed as an emergency, you can still utilize these approaches postsurgically.

Follow a Good Diet; Take Supplements

The basic diet, with the addition of the super shakes two or three times per day, acts to increase your stores of protein and other nutrients, and enhance your immune system functioning, so you may better endure the rigors of surgery. The vitamin, mineral, and herbal supplement program should be followed, at the increased amounts indicated.

If you drink coffee or tea, consider quitting. They tend to make you more nervous, and you will most likely have to be without them for some time before and after your operation anyway. If you quit suddenly, you may suffer from a withdrawal headache, so taper off, and use the substitutes given in Chapter 2.

The following supplements and herbs can interfere with your surgical care, so they should be stopped at least two weeks prior to your operation, and not restarted until two weeks afterward, unless you are otherwise instructed by your doctor:

- Those that may affect blood clotting—alfalfa, capsicum, celery, chamomile, fenugreek, feverfew, fish oil, garlic, ginger, gingko, ginseng and a number of other Chinese herbs, horseradish, kava kava, licorice, passionflower, red clover, vitamin E.
- Those that have sedative effects and that might interfere with your anesthesia—celery, chamomile, ginseng, goldenseal, hops, kava kava, marijuana, passionflower, St. John's wort, valerian.
- Those that may effect your blood pressure or have cardiac effects—black cohosh, capsicum, celery, ephedra, fenugreek, garlic, ginseng, goldenseal, hawthorn, horseradish, licorice, lobelia, St. John's wort.
- Those that can affect your mineral (electrolyte) balance—aloe, artichoke, celery, dandelion, licorice.[4]
- Immune-oriented herbs such as echinacea, although safe to continue, should be limited to a total of three weeks.

Practice Stress Management and Yoga Daily; Have Massages

Two sessions per day of the yoga postures, and three or more of yoga breathing, deep relaxation, and meditation are the best plan. In addition to the information given in Chapter 2, tapes and videos are listed in "Resources" on pages 729–30 to assist you with this training. If you are having difficulty making progress in relaxation, access to a biofeedback machine can help. You may visit a biofeedback center, or purchase a small machine for home use. Familiarize yourself with the other stress management approaches given in Chapter 2, such as laughter, and apply them where appropriate as well.

Massage can both provide immediate relaxation, and encourage optimum circulation, which will help you physically to heal.

Access Your Spiritual Side

Contemplating surgery is very stressful, even if you are looking forward to the relief it will provide. You can use this opportunity to get in touch with your conscious essence, the spiritual part of yourself. It can help create a framework of peacefulness to greatly diminish your stress. Most hospitals have chaplaincy services, which can provide extra support. See "Resources" for this and other sources for help in accomplishing this.

Two particularly helpful books were written by three-time near-death survivor Dannion Brinkley: *Saved by the Light* and *At Peace in the Light,* listed in "Resources." They intriguingly describe how he transformed his illnesses and surgeries into occasions for deepening his spiritual understanding and connection, and can help you be inspired on your healing path.

Practice Visualization and Imagery

Visualization and imagery is best practiced three to five times per day, after you have completed deep relaxation. You may benefit from drawing pictures of yourself easily coming through your operation, and then meditating upon them, or making pictures of what you "see" during visualization, then analyzing them for ways to improve this process. The more often you do the visualization and imagery, the more likely it is to work.

Choose or Make a Music and Suggestion Tape

Try out various music tapes, to find which ones help you feel most positive and relaxed. A number of ready-made tapes are listed in the Resources section of this book. You may even wish to make your own tape for use the night before, during, and after surgery, on which you tell yourself you will stay relaxed, and that your body will "help out" during the operation, as discussed below. You can make suggestions to yourself: for example, that you will awake easily from anesthesia and feel refreshed, without pain or nausea, alert, appropriately hungry, thirsty, and healthy.

Use Homeopathy

Here are the homeopathic remedies to be taken before surgery:

- For prevention of pain and bruising—*arnica 30C,* 3 pellets, 4 times daily for two days.
- For prevention of bleeding and infection—*ferrum phosphoricum* 30C, 3 pellets, 4 times daily for two days.
- For anxiety—*arsenicum album 30C,* 3 pellets, 4 times daily, or *Gelsemium*, 30C, 3 pellets, 4 times daily.
- For fear of death—*aconitum, 30C,* one time only; repeat as needed.

Ask for a Private Room

If you can afford it, ask for a private room. This allows you to focus on your healing techniques, and you can decorate it in a way comforting to you. If this is too expensive, strive to make your own space uniquely cozy to you, without interfering with your roommate(s).

Talk to Your Surgeon and Anesthesiologist About Your Plans

Using these mind-body and alternative practices may result in your needing less preoperative medication to relax, and perhaps less anesthesia during your operation, so inform whoever is giving you the anesthetic that you may need less medication. As noted, especially make certain to inform both your anesthesiologist and surgeon about any herbs, supplements, or homeopathic remedies you are taking.

Just Before Anesthesia, Perform Deep Relaxation

Right before your anesthesia is administered, do deep relaxation as explained in Chapter 2. This technique involves first tightening your muscles, letting their tension go, and then using your mind to scan your body and make certain it is fully relaxed. With practice, this process can be accomplished in just a few minutes. Make certain to tell your surgeon what you are doing, since you may need less than the usual amount of anesthesia.

Follow your relaxation exercise with conscious visualization, imagery, or affirmations to yourself such as "I am sailing easily through this surgery," or "I am coming through surgery well and see myself fully recovered." Please see Chapter 2 for further details on these methods of helping yourself to relax and heal.

During Surgery: What Your Surgeon Can Do

If you have time beforehand, or even sometimes in an emergency situation, you can ask your surgeon to perform certain actions that may help you feel comfortable, relax, enlist the assistance of the mind-body connection, and help ensure a good outcome. You can also take action yourself, via tapes, to enlist your mind and body to help during the procedure. These actions are discussed in more detail in Chapters 2 and 4 of this book.

Following are the most important steps to take to develop an integrated approach during your operation.

Ask Your Surgeon and Operating Team to Help

Enlist the support of your surgeon and anesthesiologist, so that they and others in the operating room do not make negative comments while you are anesthetized. Studies, as presented earlier in this book, have shown that your unconscious mind reacts to this input. You may wish to discuss with your surgeon ways in which he or she can even make *encouraging* comments to you and "ask" your body to help during the operation. You may wish to confer about the music to be played over the operating room's speakers.

Use Music and Affirmation Tapes

You may wish to use guided imagery or music tapes played to you individually, through a personal cassette player with earphones, during your operation. Ready-made choices are listed in "Resources," or you can make your own. Affirmations such as "My body is helping the surgeon to accomplish the task," and "My body is reacting well to the procedure" can be used. Halfway through the operation, you can ask your surgeon to stop, take your headphones off, and read aloud to you, "Your operation is going nicely. When it is over, you will heal well, with a minimal amount of discomfort," or something similar. He or she can also ask you to help out in any appropriate way, whenever it is needed, during your procedure; even if you are asleep, your subconscious mind will hear this input, and your body can respond.

After Surgery

Have an Assistant

An integrated approach may be especially useful in the recovery room, and for the first few days after your operation, to enhance your convalescence. Try to have a friend or family member help you during this time. Disorientation and shaking chills are common and may be reduced by the presence of a familiar face. See Chapter 4 for a further discussion about this period.

Create a Soothing Environment

Music and imagery tapes can be played throughout your recovery, through a cassette player, using headphones. Uplifting pictures can even be brought into the recovery room. Soft music especially can make a significant difference. Decorating your room with inspiring pictures and wearing comfortable pajamas can affect your mind, and thus your immune system. Getting into regular clothes soon may be very helpful.

Practice Yoga

After your surgery, as soon as you feel awake, you can try alternate nostril breathing and deep relaxation; follow these by visualization and imagery. Make certain not to strain; just do whatever feels totally easy and comfortable. These two practices can be gently performed anytime, by anyone. Very easy stretching can be added gradually during the next few days, taking care not to affect the area of your incision. Meditation can be extremely relaxing and helpful. See the yoga stretching and recovery exercises given in Chapter 2.

Choose a Healthy Diet

Diet at this time is very important, and should be discussed with your doctor. The best approach, even once you can begin to eat, is usually to consume only liquids for a day or two, using the Superdrinks. This allows your body to focus its blood supply on healing your incision and fighting infection, rather than digesting food, and yet you will be receiving the nutrients you need for your optimum recovery. Someone can bring them in to you during this time; occasionally, a hospital can prepare them for you. Avoid caffeine and foods made with refined sugar, since these are known to depress immune function. After a few days, adopt the diet outlined in Chapter 2.

Take Supplements

Until you can eat, you can request that your doctor add vitamins to your intravenous fluids. Then continue the supplement program given in Chapter 2. Take the herbs echinacea, two capsules three times daily; astragalus, one capsule two times daily; *blue-green algae*, three capsules two times daily; and immune-stimulating mushrooms, two capsules two times daily, to activate your immune system.

Make Friends with Your Nurses

Nurses are often more emotionally accessible than doctors and sometimes know more about small details of comfort, pain relief, and even appropriate drug use than the shifting population of doctors, especially the new interns. For example, when our 90-year-old father was in the hospital, the intern recommended a type of medication that can cause hallucinations in his age group. A savvy nurse quietly pointed this out, the medication was stopped, and Dad quickly became his wisecracking self again.

Act to Minimize Your Scar

After your stitches are removed, apply calendula ointment, three times daily. You may also apply aloe vera gel, and puncture a vitamins A and D capsule and apply it topically. Each of these has a different effect to reduce scarring. Use of a magnet machine, where available, or individual magnets, by accelerating local lymph flow and bringing increased nutrients to your incision site, as discussed in Chapter 2, may also act to minimize your scarring.[5] Castor oil may also be applied, three times daily, with benefit, especially for keloid (very large, thick) scars.[6]

WARNING: Vitamin E may be applied topically three times daily once your scar has fully formed, to help soften it, but should *not* be used while the scar is forming, as it has been shown to delay healing.[7]

Use Homeopathy

To assist your healing process, you may add homeopathic preparations, following the guidelines given in Chapter 2. Use the remedies specific for your problem, as given in that chapter, as well as these:

> For bruising or pain—Arnica 200C, repeated as needed (good to use in any case).
> If any nerves were cut—Hypericum 200C, repeated as needed.
> For bleeding—Arnica 200C; if this fails, try Phosphorus 200C.
> For weakness or fever—Cinchona 30C; repeat as needed.
> For wound infection—Topical Calendula and Hypericum, four times daily.

These remedies may be repeated, as needed, or given in higher potencies, as discussed in Chapter 2.

Apply a Comfrey Poultice

In areas away from your incision, this can help relieve pain, swelling, and bruising. Once your stitches have been removed, you may apply a compress of the herb comfrey. Follow the directions given in Chapter 2.

Give Yourself Time to Heal

Surgery may end up being much easier and satisfying than you had anticipated. Many people say afterward they wish they hadn't delayed it, since it turned out to be so easy, and they needn't have been so concerned about its difficulty.

Others, however, are surprised by the length of time it takes to fully recover. Your best course is to be prepared to take it easy. Don't be in a hurry to recover. Surgery is always a challenge for the body, so give it time to focus on repair. Don't try to immediately resume your usual life, and don't deny that you have gone through something. Instead, focus on embracing relaxation, rather than jumping right back into action. Honor the limits of your own body; you are best advised to go slow, and notice carefully what is best for you.

Our mother, for example, who underwent a cardiac ablation procedure, in which a wire is inserted in the groin and moved into the heart to correct an arrhythmia, came home the next day and immediately jumped up to make dinner. Her heart, irritated by the operation, began to beat irregularly again, and another trip to the hospital was needed. Bed rest then corrected the problem, which might have been avoided if she had taken adequate time to rest in the first place.

Use Alternative Medicine for Infections

If you develop an infection and it does not respond to conventional approaches, see the advice in Chapter 5 for skin infections. You may initiate a trial of calendula ointment, comfrey cream, or even sugar or honey (applied to the skin), all of which have antibacterial effects, with your physician's supervision. Apply three times daily.

Use Acupuncture, Chiropractic, Osteopathy, and Massage

Massage has special importance postsurgically. A study conducted at the University of

Virginia Medical Center showed that patients given massage before and after surgery had less need for pain medication, and were discharged, on average, two days sooner.[8] As noted earlier, Chicago plastic surgeon Dr. Craig Bradley uses a Shiatsu therapist to massage his patients after their operations, and has found their return to function more rapid, less painful, and more complete. He also mentally "talks" to the tissue to secure its cooperation before rearranging it, and believes that this makes a difference in the results he sees.

Every scar necessarily cuts across an acupuncture meridian, affecting your body's subtle energy flow. An acupuncturist can assist in reversing this effect, and help restore you to good health. Your positioning during the operation may also have affected your spinal alignment, so that chiropractic and/or osteopathic realignment may help in your recovery.

Preventing Future Recurrence

Once you have come through your surgery, you will still need to address the underlying issues that led to your problem in the first place. These factors often include multiple aspects of lifestyle. Review Chapters 1 through 4 of this book, as well as the section dealing with your specific disease. You may also wish to consult with a healthcare provider familiar with alternative medicine, to learn about all the options you can take to prevent further illness in this or other systems of your body and to obtain support in accomplishing this.

Following are the most important alternative medicine steps you can take to help prevent future recurrences.

Use Your Operation as an Opportunity for Personal Transformation

A surgical illness can be a time of individual change, in which you can deepen your experience of life, and begin to become more in touch with your spiritual self. The shock of diagnosis, going through the difficulties of treatment, and the slow return to health can be a time of great opportunity for personal growth.

After your operation, ask yourself several questions, directed at preventing future disease. What changes do you need to make, to prevent the return of this problem? Is there any psychological meaning to this disorder? Was there anything that you "gained" from having the illness? Can you obtain these benefits by other means? Can you now accomplish some "lifestyle surgery" that will prevent a need for further operations? Since some studies estimate that as much as 80 percent of all illness may be stress-related, stress management techniques may be very important to prevent any further problems.

Change Your Lifestyle

One of the most effective ways to change your lifestyle—your diet, exercise habits, attitudes of mind, and reactions to stress—is to put *new habits* into action, and then gradually the detrimental ones tend to leave. For example, if you need to quit smoking, you can begin by focusing on adding the yoga breathing exercises and relaxation to your daily schedule, and you may find it much simpler to quit.

Join a Support Group

For many reasons, you will likely do better if you join a support group, where you can be helped to make necessary changes in attitude and lifestyle, which encourage wellness and enhance immune function. As discussed, some studies have shown a doubling of survival rates for participants.

Examples of Integrative Surgery

We began this book with the story of Bruce Hart. He pioneered how to put alternative medicine and surgery together, to create an "integral medicine" approach to your operation, with excellent results. His is an excellent example of how conventional and alternative approaches to surgery can *complement* each other.

He had first simply noticed some abdominal distress. His doctor recommended a CAT scan, which showed his stomach to be in good shape, but revealed a suspicious mass located in his right kidney. The consulting surgeon suggested an operation, to remove this probable cancer. The surgery was scheduled for three weeks later.

Bruce read through the initial manuscript of this book and chose to combine conventional and alternative methods to help treat his disease. He interviewed three different urological surgeons, then selected the one with whom he felt most humanly comfortable and connected. He asked his surgeon to add some alternative medicine practices to his routine, and although somewhat skeptical, his doctor agreed to do so.

Before his operation, Bruce began preparing himself. He drank 20 ounces daily of a mix of fresh carrot, red cabbage, and spinach juice; he practiced yoga stretching, breathing, relaxation, and meditation twice daily, and used a hypnosis tape prepared especially for him by a hypnotherapist. The tape induced him to enter a trancelike state, spoke to him

of the power and wisdom of his body to heal, and directed him to control bleeding, whenever necessary, during the operation, then to resume the flow of blood appropriately afterward, to aid in his healing.

Bruce designed and made a unique four-hour audiotape to be played during his surgery; it was a combination of music and suggestions, to please his own sense of enjoyment, and create a certain atmosphere in the operating room. It began with the calming sounds of Eastern chanting—*Om Shanti,* meaning "*Om* peace"—then continued with Native American chants, Duke Ellington, and, finally, Van Morrison. He requested the tape be played to the entire operating room, rather than through personal headphones, so everyone else would also be calm, and his surgeon agreed to do this. The boom box on which it would run was admitted to the operating room as an "unsterilized specimen." The music was also played in the recovery room.

He requested no shaving, and his surgeon, although somewhat amused and doubtful, agreed. He gave his surgeon two cards on which were written affirmations. One, to be read halfway through the operation, went: "Bruce, the operation is going nicely. When it is over, you will heal well, with minimal discomfort." Another, to be read only if Bruce began to bleed significantly, would have been: "Bruce, you seem to be bleeding more than we would like. Please control and stop the bleeding."

The results of the operation were outstandingly positive. Although he had put aside a quart of his own blood, he needed none during the five-hour operation. His first words upon awakening were, "What a neat room!" responding to the single room a friend had donated to him. Even though he had needed an entire rib removed, he experienced no significant postoperative pain, and went home after three days. Two weeks later, because he was favoring his incision site, with his walking affected, he had a Tibetan Chua Kah massage (reputedly favored by Kubla Khan), and afterward was immediately walking normally again.

His surgeon, residents, and interns' reactions were also significant. The students could hardly believe it when their "hip" chief surgeon, more flexible than they themselves might have been, stopped in the middle of the operation to read the affirmation card. (He didn't need to read the one about bleeding, since no excess bleeding occurred.) He reported, "I felt like I was talking to myself, but it was good for me to hear it."

Pathology showed Bruce's tumor had been a rare papillary cancer of the kidney, thought to be genetically related, and more common in those of northeastern European Jewish descent. Bruce was soon back at work, feeling wonderful—especially knowing that his early and supremely successful encounter with the scalpel had prevented the spread of this potentially fatal cancer, and thereby likely saved his life. He then continued to practice his yoga routine daily and to explore other dietary and relaxation alternatives, to prevent recurrence of his illness as well as enhance the quality of his life.

Such integrated surgical practice is now becoming more widespread. For example, one cardiac surgeon in Wisconsin even employed a specific music therapist to consult with all of his patients, to help them choose just the right tapes of music they loved best to listen to before and after their surgery. The anesthesiologist himself then played the music to them, while they were under anesthetic, through a portable cassette player. Cardiac surgeon Dr. Mehmet Oz, mentioned above, has also developed a unique tradition of music in the oper-

ating room: he uses "opening music," usually marches; "operating music," such as Bach; and "closing music," like Beethoven. Both his patients and fellow healthcare providers have been enthusiastic in their appreciation of the resulting changes in ambiance.

Many hospitals also now offer relaxation tapes, and some have a closed circuit television channel that teaches wellness and shows relaxation videos.

Beyond the Scalpel

The process toward a more balanced vision of surgery, which will give you new choices, is only beginning. The new approaches of diet, relaxation, mental training such as visualization and meditation, and therapies such as acupuncture and hypnosis have only relatively recently begun to be scientifically investigated, and may have special value in the surgical setting.

You can *empower* yourself by taking an active role in your own operation. Once you are going through the surgery, you can then more easily "go with the flow," and consciously give yourself time for the process of healing that surgery offers. Use this book like a friend, choosing those suggestions most comfortable to you.

Optimally, you can take the best from the alternative and complementary traditions, and combine them with the best from current Western surgical information. Your operation, which at first seemed an extreme solution, may not only be lifesaving, but also becoming life-uplifting. If you can discover positive insights from your illness and its form of treatment, you place yourself right on the proper sort of cutting edge, beyond the scalpel.

FOR FURTHER INFORMATION

Organizations

Academy for Guided Imagery
  PO Box 2070
  Mill Valley, CA 94942
  Phone: 800-726-2070

American Association of Naturopathic
  Physicians
  2366 Eastlake Avenue East
  Suite 322
  Seattle, WA 98102
  Phone: 206-323-7610
  Web Site: www.naturopathic.org

American Board of Chelation Therapy
  407B North Wells Street
  Chicago, IL 60610
  Phone: 800-356-2228

American Board of Medical Specialties
  1007 Church Street
  Suite 404
  Evanston, IL 60201
  Phone: 847-491-9091

American Botanical Council
  PO Box 201660
  Austin, TX 78720
  Phone: 512-331-8868

American Cancer Society
  1599 Clinton Road, Northeast
  Atlanta, GA 30329-4251
  Phone: 800-ACS-2345
  Fax: 404-325-2217
  Web Site: www.cancer.org

American Chiropractic Association
  1701 Clarendon Boulevard
  Arlington, VA 22209
  Phone: 800-986-4636
  Fax: 703-243-2593
  Web Site: www.amerchiro.org
  E-mail: amerchiro@aol.com

American Heart Association
  7272 Greenville Avenue
  Dallas, TX 75231
  Phone: 800-AHA-USA
  Web Site: www.americanheart.org

American Holistic Medical Association
6728 Old McLean Village Drive
McLean, VA 22101
Phone: 703-556-9728 or 703-556-9245
E-mail: holistmed@aol.com

American Holistic Nurses' Association
4101 Lake Boone Trail
Suite 201
Raleigh, NC 27607
Phone: 919-787-5181

American Lung Association
1740 Broadway
New York, NY 10019
Web Site: www.lungusa.org

American Massage Therapy Association
820 Davis Street
Suite 100
Evanston, IL 60201-4444
Phone: 847-864-0123
Fax: 847-864-1178
Web Site: www.amtamassage.org

Ayurvedic Institute
11311 Menaul Northeast
Suite A
Albuquerque, NM 87112
Phone: 505-291-9698

Herb Research Foundation
1007 Pearl Street
Suite 200
Boulder, CO 80302
Phone: 303-449-2265

Humor Project
110 Spring Street
Saratoga Springs, NY 12866-3397
Phone: 518-587-8770

International Association of Yoga Therapists
PO Box 2418
Sebastopol, CA 95473
Phone: 707-928-9898
Web Site: www.iayt.org

International Foundation for Homeopathy
2366 Eastlake Avenue East
Suite 329
Seattle, WA 98102
Phone: 206-324-8230

International Institute of Reflexology
PO Box 12462
St. Petersburg, FL 33733
Phone: 813-343-4811

Joint Commission on Accreditation of
Healthcare Organizations
One Renaissance Boulevard
Oakbrook Terrace, IL 60181
Web Site: www.jcaho.org

National Acupuncture and Oriental
Medicine Alliance
PO Box 77511
Seattle, WA 98177-0531
Phone: 206-524-3511
Fax: 206-728-4841
E-mail: 76143.2061@compuserve.com

National Alliance of Breast Cancer
Organizations
9 East 37th Street
Tenth Floor
New York, NY 10016
Phone: 212-719-0154
Fax: 212-689-1213
E-mail: nabcoinfo@aol.com

National Cancer Institute
Phone: 800-4-CANCER

National Cancer Institute's Office of
  Alternative Medicine
  6120 Executive Boulevard
  Suite 450
  Bethesda, MD 20892
  Phone: 301-402-2466

National Center for Homeopathy
  801 North Fairfax Street
  Suite 306
  Alexandria, VA 22314
  Phone: 703-548-7790
  Fax: 703-548-7792
  Web Site: www.homeopathic.org

National Coalition for Cancer Survivorship
  1010 Wayne Avenue
  Fifth Floor
  Silver Spring, MD 20910
  Phone: 301-650-8868

National Comprehensive Cancer Network
  Phone: 888-909-6226
  Web Site: www.nccn.org

National Women's Health Network
  1325 G Street, Northwest
  Washington, DC 20005
  Phone: 202-347-1140

North American Society of Teachers of the
  Alexander Technique
  PO Box 517
  Urbana, IL 61801
  Phone: 800-473-0620

Rolf Institute of Structural Integration
  205 Canyon Boulevard
  Boulder, CO 80302
  Phone: 303-449-5903 or 800-530-8875
  Fax: 303-449-5978
  E-mail: rolfinst@aol.com

Support Groups

Exceptional Cancer Patients, Inc. (Bernie
  Siegel)
  300 Plaza Middlesex
  Middletown, CT 06457
  Phone: 860-343-5950
  Web Site: www.hmt.com/cyp/nonprof/ecap

Reach to Recovery International
  3, Rue du Conseil-General
  1205 Geneva
  Switzerland
  Web Site: www.cope.uicc.org/breast/rri/
  rri.html

United Ostomy Association
  19772 MacArthur Boulevard
  Suite 200
  Irvine, CA 92612-2405
  Phone: 800-826-0826
  Web Site: www.uoa.org

Us Too
  5003 Fairview Avenue
  Downers Grove, IL 60515
  Phone: 800-808-7866
  Web Site: ustoo.com

Provider Referrals

Alternative Medicine Providers

American Association of Naturopathic
  Physicians
  2366 Eastlake Avenue East
  Suite 322
  Seattle, WA 98102
  Phone: 206-328-8510
  Web Site: www.naturopathic.org

American Holistic Health Association
  PO Box 17400
  Anaheim, CA 92817-7400
  Phone: 714-779-6152
  Web Site: www.ahha.org/ahhasearch.htm

Acupuncture Providers

American Association of Acupuncture and
  Oriental Medicine
  4101 Lake Boone Trail
  Suite 201
  Raleigh, NC 27607
  Phone: 919-787-5181

National Commission for the Certification of
  Acupuncturists
  PO Box 97075
  Washington, DC 20090-7075
  Phone: 202-232-1404

Chiropractic Providers

American Chiropractic Association
  1701 Clarendon Boulevard
  Arlington, VA 22209
  Phone: 800-986-4636
  Fax: 703-243-2593
  Web Site: www.amerchiro.org
  E-mail: amerchiro@aol.com

Homeopathy Providers

National Center for Homeopathy
  801 North Fairfax Street
  Suite 306
  Alexandria, VA 22314
  Phone: 703-548-7790
  Fax: 703-548-7792
  Web Site: www.homeopathic.org

Hypnotherapy Providers

American Society of Clinical Hypnosis
  2200 East Devon Avenue
  Suite 291
  Des Plaines, IL 60018
  Web Site: www.asch.net

Society for Clinical and Experimental
  Hypnosis
  3905 Vincennes Road
  Suite 304
  Indianapolis, IN 46268

Massage Therapy Providers

American Massage Therapy Association
  820 Davis Street
  Suite 100
  Evanston, IL 60201-4444
  Phone: 847-864-0123
  Fax: 847-864-1178
  Web Site: www.amtamassage.org

Music Therapy Providers

American Association of Music Therapy
  8455 Colesville Road
  Suite 1000
  Silver Spring, MD 20910
  Phone: 301-589-3300
  Fax: 301-589-5175
  Web Site: www.musictherapy.org

Osteopathy Providers

American Osteopathic Association
  142 East Ontario Street
  Chicago, IL 60611
  Phone: 800-621-1773
  Fax: 312-202-8200
  Web Site: aoa-net.org

Qi Gong Providers

Qi Gong Association of America
 27133 Forest Springs Lane
 Corvallis, OR 97330
 Web Site: www.qi.org

Yoga Providers

International Association of Yoga Therapists
 PO Box 2418
 Sebastopol, CA 95473
 Phone: 707-928-9898
 Web Site: www.iayt.org

Integrative Health Services

Integrative Healthcare Programs

Preventive Medicine Research Institute
 Phone: 415-332-2525
 Web Site: www.pmri.org

Integrative Health Retreats

Integral Yoga
 Phone: 800-858-YOGA
 Web Site: www.yogaville.org

Integrative Hospice Care

Compassion in Action
 Phone: 310-473-1941
 Web Site: www.lightbrigade.com

Integrative Hospital Care

The Planetree Project
 Phone: 415-522-3873
 Web Site: www.planetree.org

Books

General Medicine

Gray, H. *Gray's Anatomy.* New York: Churchill Livingstone, 1995.

Netter, F. *The CIBA Collection of Medical Illustrations.* Summit, NJ: CIBA-Geigy, 1948–2001.

Physicians' Desk Reference. Montvale, NJ: Medical Economics Co., 2001.

Physicians' Desk Reference for Nonprescription Drugs and Dietary Supplements. Montvale, NJ: Medical Economics Co., 2001.

Rakel, R., and E. Bope. *Conn's Current Therapy.* Philadelphia, PA: Saunders, 2001.

Tierney, L. *Current Medical Diagnosis and Treatment.* Stamford, CT: Lange, 2000.

Alternative Medicine

The Alternative Advisor: The Complete Guide to Natural Therapies and Alternative Treatments. Richmond, VA: Time-Life Books, 1997.

Alternative Medicine: Expanding Medical Horizons: A Report to the National Institutes of Health on Alternative Medical Systems and Practices in the United States. Washington, DC: Health and Human Services Department, Public Health Service, National Institutes of Health, Office of Alternative Medicine, 1994.

Barney, P. *Doctor's Guide to Natural Medicine.* Pleasant Grove, UT: Woodland Publishing, 1998.

Bernard, N. A. *Comprehensive Manual for Wellness and Self Care: A Consumer*

Reference. New York: Times Books/Henry Holt, 2001.

Bhat, N. *How to Reverse and Prevent Heart Disease and Cancer.* Np: Healthworld, 1995.

Bratman, S. *The Alternative Medicine Ratings Guide: An Expert Panel Ranks the Best Treatments for Over 80 Conditions.* Rocklin, CA: Prima Publishing, 1998.

Bratman, S. *The Alternative Medicine Sourcebook: A Realistic Evaluation of Alternative Healing Methods.* Los Angeles: Lowell House, 1997.

Bricklin, M. *The Practical Encyclopedia of Natural Healing.* Emmaus, PA: Rodale Press, 1976.

Brody, J., editor. *New York Times Guide to Alternative Health.* New York: Henry Holt, 2001.

Burton Goldberg Group. *Alternative Medicine: The Definitive Guide.* Tiburon, CA: Future Medicine Publishing, 1998.

Chopra, D. *Quantum Healing: Exploring the Frontiers of Mind/Body Medicine.* New York: Bantam Books, 1989.

Clark, S. *What Really Works: The Insider's Guide to Natural Health: What's Best and Where to Find It.* London: Thorsons, 2001.

Cohen, K. *The Way of Qi Gong.* New York: Random House, 1999.

Courteney, H. *What's the Alternative?* London: Macmillan, 1996.

DerMarderosian, A., editor. *The Review of Natural Products.* St. Louis, MO: Facts and Comparisons Publishing Group, 2001.

Diamond, W. J., et al. *An Alternative Medicine Definitive Guide to Cancer: Alterna-tive Medicine.* Tiburon, CA: Future Medicine Publishing, 1997.

Fugh-Berman, A. *Alternative Medicine: What Works.* Baltimore, MD: Williams & Wilkins, 1997.

Gaby, A. *Preventing and Reversing Osteoporosis.* Rocklin, CA: Prima Publishing, 1994.

Gaynor, M., and J. Hickey. *Dr. Gaynor's Cancer Prevention Program.* New York: Kensington Books, 1999.

Golan, R. *Optimal Wellness.* New York: Ballantine Books, 1995.

Gordon, J. S. *Manifesto for a New Medicine: Your Guide to Healing Partnerships and the Wise Use of Alternative Therapies.* Reading, MA: Addison-Wesley Publishing, 1997.

Haas, R. *Permanent Remissions.* New York: Pocket Books, 1997.

Heimlich, J. *What Your Doctor Won't Tell You.* New York: HarperPerennial, 1990.

Lemole, G. M. *An Integrative Approach to Cardiac Care.* Np: Medtronic, 2000.

Lemole, G. M. *The Healing Diet.* New York: William Morrow, 2001.

Lerner, M. *Choices in Healing: Integrating the Best of Conventional and Complementary Approaches in Cancer.* Cambridge, MA: MIT Press, 1994.

Liberman, J., et al. *Light Years Ahead.* Berkeley, CA: Celestial Arts, 1996.

Lockie, A., and N. Geddes. *DK Natural Health Complete Guide to Homeopathy.* New York: Dorling Kindersley, 2000.

Murphy, G. P., L. B. Morris, and D. Lange. *Informed Decisions: The Complete Book of Cancer Diagnosis, Treatment, and Recovery.* New York: Viking Press, 1997.

Murray, M. *Menopause.* Rocklin, CA: Prima Publishing, 1994.

Murray, M., and J. Pizzorno. *Encyclopedia of Natural Medicine,* Second Edition. Rocklin, CA: Prima Publishing, 1998.

Murray, M., and J. Pizzorno, editors. *The Textbook of Natural Medicine.* London: Churchill Livingstone, 1999.

Null, G. *The Complete Encyclopedia of Natural Healing.* New York: Kensington Books, 1998.

Ornish, D. *Dr. Dean Ornish's Program for Reversing Heart Disease.* New York: Random House, 1990.

Ornish, D. *Stress, Diet, and Your Heart.* New York: Holt, Reinhart and Winston, 1983.

Oz, M. *Healing from the Heart: A Leading Surgeon Explores the Power of Complementary Medicine.* New York: Dutton, 1998.

Page, L. *Healthy Healing: A Guide to Self-Healing for Everyone.* Miami, FL: Quality Books, 2000.

Pearsall, P. *The Heart's Code: Tapping the Wisdom and Power of Our Heart's Energy.* New York: Broadway Books, 1998.

Pearsall, P. *Superimmunity: Master Your Emotions and Improve Your Health.* New York: McGraw-Hill, 1986.

Peterson, C. *Mind/Body Partnership in the Treatment of Cancer Patients.* Orlando, FL: Moonlight Press, 1994.

Phalen, P. *Integrative Medicine: Achieving Wellness Through the Best of Eastern and Western Medical Practices.* Boston: Journey Editions, 1998.

Pinckney, N. *The Healthy Heart Handbook.* Deerfield Beach, FL: Health Communications, 1994.

Pizzorno, J. *Total Wellness: Improve Your Health by Understanding the Body's Healing Systems.* Rocklin, CA: Prima Publishing, 1996.

Philpott, W. *Magnet Therapy: An Alternative Medicine Definitive Guide.* Tiburon, CA: Alternative Medicine Publishing, 2000.

Pressman, A., and D. Shelley, editors. *The Patient's Essential Guide to Conventional and Complementary Treatments for More Than 300 Common Disorders.* New York: St. Martin's Press, 2000.

Reilly, H. *The Edgar Cayce Handbook for Health Through Drugless Therapy.* New York: Macmillan, 1975.

Rennaker, M., editor. *Understanding Cancer.* Palo Alto, CA: Bull Publishing, 1988.

Robbins, J. *Reclaiming Our Health.* Tiburon, CA: H. J. Dramer, 1996.

Rondberg, T. *Chiropractic First: The Fastest Growing Healthcare Choice Before Drugs or Surgery.* Chandler, AZ: Chiropractic Journal, 1996.

Simonton, C., et al. *Getting Well Again: A Step-by-Step, Self-Help Guide to Overcoming Cancer for Patients and Their Families.* Los Angeles: JP Tarcher, 1978.

Sobel, D., and R. Ornstein. *The Healthy Mind Healthy Body Handbook.* Los Altos, CA: DRX, 1996.

Spencer, J. W., and J. J. Jacobs, editors. *Complementary Medicine: An Evidence-*

Based Approach. St. Louis, MO: Mosby-Year Books, 1998.

Stengler, M. *The Natural Physician.* Burnaby, BC, Canada: Alive Books, 1997.

Stengler, M. *The Natural Physician's Healing Therapies: Proven Remedies That Medical Doctors Don't Know.* Upper Saddle River, NJ: Prentice-Hall, 2001.

Sullivan, K., and C. N. Shealy. *The Complete Family Guide to Natural Home Remedies.* Rockport, MA: Element, 1997.

Weil, A. *Eight Weeks to Optimum Health: A Proven Program for Taking Full Advantage of Your Body's Natural Healing Power.* New York: Alfred A. Knopf, 1997.

Weil, A. *Health and Healing.* Boston, MA: Houghton Mifflin, 1998.

Weil, A. *Spontaneous Healing: How to Discover and Enhance Your Body's Natural Ability to Maintain and Heal Itself.* New York: Ballantine Books, 2000.

Whitaker, J. *Whitaker's Guide to Natural Healing.* Rocklin, CA: Prima Publishing, 1995.

Exercise

Bailey, Covert. *The New Fit or Fat.* Boston, MA: Houghton Mifflin, 1991.

Cooper, Kenneth. *The New Aerobics.* Philadelphia, PA: Lippincott, 1970.

Cooper, Kenneth. *The New Aerobics for Women.* New York: Bantam Books, 1988.

Winfrey, O., and B. Greene. *Make the Connection.* New York: Hyperion, 1996.

Herbs and Natural Medicine

Chevallier, A. *Encyclopedia of Medicinal Plants.* New York: DK Publications, 1996.

Duke, J. *The Green Pharmacy.* Emmaus, PA: Rodale Press, 1997.

Graedon, J. *The Peoples Pharmacy Guide to Home and Herbal Remedies.* New York: St. Martin's Press, 1999.

Israel, R. *The Natural Pharmacy Product Guide.* Garden City Park, NY: Avery Publishing Group, 1991.

Lininger, S., et al. *The Natural Pharmacy: Complete Home Reference to Natural Medicine.* Rocklin, CA: Prima Publishing, 1998.

Mobrey, D. *The Scientific Validation of Herbal Medicine.* New Canaan, CT: Keats, 1986.

Murray, M. T. *Natural Alternatives to Over-the-Counter and Prescription Drugs.* New York: William Morrow & Co., 1994.

Physicians' Desk Reference for Herbal Medicine. Montvale, NJ: Medical Economics Co., 2001.

Polunin, M. *The Natural Pharmacy: An Illustrated Guide to Natural Medicine.* New York: Collier Books, 1992.

Werbach, M., and M. T. Murray. *Botanical Influences on Illness.* Tarzana, CA: Third Line Press, 1994.

Meditation, Mind-Body Connection, and Visualization

Acterberg, J. *Imagery in Healing: Shamanism and Modern Medicine.* Boston, MA: New Science Library, 1985.

Adler, R., editor. *Psychoneuroimmunology.* New York: Academic Press, 1981.

Bolen, J. *Close to the Bone: Life-Threatening Illness and the Search for Meaning.* New York: Scribner, 1996.

Borysenko, J. *Minding the Body, Mending the Mind.* Reading, MA: Addison-Wesley, 1987.

Gawain, S. *Creative Visualization.* San Rafael, CA: New World Library, 1955.

Gerber, R. *Vibrational Medicine: New Choices for Healing.* Santa Fe, NM: Bear & Co., 1988.

Goleman, D., and J. Gurin, editors. *Mind/Body Medicine: How to Use Your Mind for Better Health.* Yonkers, NY: Consumers Reports Books, 1993.

Lynch, J. J. *The Broken Heart: The Medical Consequences of Loneliness.* New York: Basic Books, 1977.

Norris, P., et al. *I Choose Life: The Dynamics of Visualization and Biofeedback.* Walpole, NH: Stillpoint Publishing, 1987.

Ornish, D. *Love and Survival: The Scientific Basis for the Healing Power of Intimacy.* New York: HarperCollins, 1998.

Ornstein, R., and D. Sobel. *The Healing Brain: Breakthrough Discoveries About How the Brain Keeps Us Healthy.* New York: Simon & Schuster, 1987.

Rossman, M. *Guided Imagery for Self Healing.* Tiburon, CA: H. J. Kramer, 2000.

Siegel, B. *Love, Medicine, and Miracles: Lessons Learned About Self-Healing from a Surgeon's Experience with Exceptional Patients.* New York: HarperPerennial, 1990.

Siegel, B. *Peace, Love, and Healing: Body/Mind Communication and the Path to Self-Healing: An Exploration.* New York: Perennial Library, 1990.

Nutrition

Arnot, S. *The Breast Cancer Prevention Diet: The Powerful Foods, Supplements, and Drugs That Can Save Your Life.* Boston, MA: Little, Brown, 1998.

Balch, J. F., and P. Balch. *Prescription for Nutritional Healing,* Third Edition. New York: Avery, 2001.

Barnard, N. *Eat Right, Live Longer.* New York: Harmony Books, 1995.

Barnard, N. *Food for Life: How the New Four Food Groups Can Save Your Life.* New York: Harmony Books, 1993.

Carper, J. *Food—Your Miracle Medicine: How Food Can Prevent and Cure Over 100 Symptoms and Problems.* New York: HarperCollins, 1998.

Cherniske, S. *Caffeine Blues: Wake Up to the Hidden Dangers of America's #1 Drug.* New York: Warner Books, 1998.

Lemole, G. M. *The Healing Diet: A Total Health Program to Purify Your Lymph System and Reduce the Risk of Heart Disease, Arthritis, and Cancer.* New York: William Morrow, 2001.

McDougall, J., and M. McDougall. *The McDougall Plan for Super Health and Life-Long Weight Loss.* Piscataway, NJ: New Century Publishers, 1983.

Nolfi, K. *Raw Food Treatment of Cancer.* Brushton, NY: Teach Services, 1995.

Null, G. *The Complete Guide to Health and Nutrition.* New York: Delacorte Press, 1984.

Ornish, D. *Eat More, Weigh Less.* New York: Quill, 2001.

Ornish, D. *Everyday Cooking with Dr. Dean Ornish.* New York: HarperCollins, 1996.

Parachin, V. *365 Good Reasons to Be a Vegetarian.* Garden City Park, NY: Avery Publishing Group, 1998.

Parham, B. *What's Wrong with Eating Meat?* Denver, CO: Ananda Marga Publications, 1979.

Quillin, P. *Beating Cancer with Nutrition.* Tulsa, OK: Nutrition Times Press, 1994.

Quillin, P. *Healing Nutrients: The People's Guide to Using Common Nutrients That Will Help You Feel Better Than You Ever Thought Possible.* New York: Vintage Books, 1989.

Satchidananda, S., et al. *The Healthy Vegetarian.* Buckingham, VA: Integral Yoga Publications, 1987.

Walford, R. *Maximum Life Span.* New York: Norton, 1983.

Weil, A. *Eating Well for Optimum Health: The Essential Guide to Bringing Health and Pleasure Back to Eating.* New York: Quill, 2001.

Yeager, S., et al. *The Complete Book of Alternative Nutrition: Powerful New Ways to Use Foods, Supplements, Herbs and Special Diets to Prevent and Cure Disease.* Emmaus, PA: Rodale Press, 1997.

Spirituality and Inspiration

Barks, C., editor. *The Essential Rumi.* San Francisco, CA: Harper, 1995.

Brinkley, D. *At Peace in the Light.* New York: HarperCollins, 1995.

Brinkley, D. *Saved by the Light.* New York: HarperCollins, 1995.

Dossey, L. *Healing Words.* San Francisco, CA: Harper, 1993.

Satchidananda, S. *The Golden Present.* Buckingham, VA: Integral Yoga Publications, 1987.

Satchidananda, S. *To Know Your Self.* Buckingham, VA: Integral Yoga Publications, 1998.

Siegel, B. *Love, Medicine, and Miracles: Lessons Learned About Self-Healing from a Surgeon's Experience with Exceptional Patients.* New York: HarperPerennial, 1990.

Surgery

Alvord, L. *The Scalpel and the Silver Bear.* New York: Bantam Books, 1999.

Austin, S. *Breast Cancer.* Rocklin, CA: Prima Publishing, 1994.

Baker, R. *Successful Surgery: A Doctor's Mind-Body Guide to Help You Through Surgery.* New York: Pocket Books, 1996.

Bunker, J. P., editor. *Costs, Risks, and Benefits of Surgery.* New York: Oxford University Press, 1977.

Cameron, J. L. *Current Surgical Therapy.* St. Louis, MO: Mosby, 1998.

Christian, R., et al. *Surgery and Its Alternatives.* Emmaus, PA: Rodale Press, 1980.

Deardorff, W., and J. L. Reeves. *Preparing for Surgery.* Oakland, CA: New Harbinger Publications, 1997.

Hirshberg, C., and M. Barasch. *Remarkable Recovery.* New York: Riverhead Books, 1995.

Huddleston, P. *Prepare for Surgery, Heal Faster: A Guide of Mind-Body Techniques.* Cambridge, MA: Angel River Press, 1996.

Hufnagel, V. *No More Hysterectomies.* New York: New American Library, 1988.

Inlander, C. B. *Good Operations Bad Operations: The People's Medical Society's Guide to Surgery.* New York: Viking, 1993.

Lawrence, P. *Essentials of Surgery.* Philadelphia, PA: Lippincott, Williams, and Wilkins, 1999.

Love, S. *Dr. Susan Love's Breast Book.* Reading, MA: Addison-Wesley, 1995.

McDougall, J. *McDougall's Medicine: A Challenging Second Opinion.* Piscataway, NJ: New Century Publishers, 1985.

Millman, M. *The Unkindest Cut.* New York: William Morrow, 1977.

Nolan, W. *Surgeon Under the Knife.* Geoghegan, NY: Coward, McCann, 1976.

Schneider, R. *When to Say No to Surgery: How to Evaluate the Most Often Performed Operations.* Englewood Cliffs, NJ: Prentice-Hall, 1982.

Schwarz, Z., et al. *Principles of Surgery.* New York: McGraw-Hill, 1999.

Selzer, R. *Mortal Lessons: Notes on the Art of Surgery.* San Diego, CA: Harcourt Press, 1996.

Wilmore, D. W., et al., *ACS Surgery: Principles and Practice.* New York: WebMD Corporation, 2002.

Yoga Practices

Satchidananda, S. *Integral Yoga Hatha.* Buckingham, VA: Integral Yoga Publications, 1995.

Sivananda Yoga Vedanta Centew. *Yoga Mind and Body.* New York: Dorling Kindersley, 1996.

Periodicals

Alternative Medicine Magazine (800-333-HEAL)

Alternative Therapies in Health and Medicine (800-345-8112)

American Health

Berkeley Wellness Letter (www.wellness letter.com)

Harvard Health Letter (www.health. harvard.edu/abouthealth.shtml)

Herbal Gram (512-331-8868)

Medical Self Care

Natural Health Magazine (www.natural healthmagazine.org)

New Age Journal (888-815-6180)

Nutrition Action Health Letter (www. cspimet.org/hah)

Audiotapes

McLanahan, S. *Surgery Instruction Tape: Deep Relaxation.* Buckingham, VA: Shakticom, 2001. Available by calling 800-476-1347.

McLanahan, S. *Surgery Instruction Tape: 5-Minute Deep Relaxation*. Buckingham, VA: Shakticom, 2001. Available by calling 800-476-1347.

McLanahan, S. *Surgery Instruction Tape: The Healing Power of Yoga*. Buckingham, VA: Shakticom, 2001. Available by calling 800-476-1347.

McLanahan, S. *Surgery Instruction Tape: Yoga Class*. Buckingham, VA: Shakticom, 2001. Available by calling 800-476-1347.

Satchidananda, S. *Guided Relaxation*. Buckingham, VA: Shakticom, nd. Available by calling 800-476-1347.

Satchidananda, S. *Guided Visualization*. Buckingham, VA: Shakticom, nd. Available by calling 800-476-1347.

Siegel, B. *Getting Ready: Preparing for Surgery, Chemotherapy, and Other Treatments*. Carlsbad, CA: Hay House, 1999.

Weil, A. *Meditation for Optimum Health: How to Use Mindfulness and Breathing to Heal Your Body and Refresh Your Mind*. Louisville, CO: Sounds True, 2001.

Videotapes

Hart, B., and C. Hart. *Question of Faith*. Np: Worldvision, nd.

Kumar, Dhanajaya. *Healing Science of Yoga*. Series of tapes for 62 different diseases. Falls Church, VA: Yoga System, nd.

McLanahan, S. *Health, Yoga, Anatomy*. Buckingham, VA: Shakticom, nd. Available by calling 800-476-1347.

Satchidananda, S. *Yoga with a Master*. Buckingham, VA: Shakticom, nd. Available by calling 800-476-1347.

CD-Roms

The Family Doctor. Milwaukee, WI: CMC Books, 1996.

Mayo Clinic Family Health. Osseo, MN: IVI Publishing, 1996.

Web Sites

Due to the rapidly expanding and changing nature of the Internet, it is impossible to list all possible resources. A search based on key words will identify sources of information, materials, referrals to practitioners, and support groups. Bear in mind that it is very easy to publish on the Internet, and there are no controls or peer-reviews. Some information on commercial sites, identified by a ".com" extension, is simply advertising.

American Botanical Council
www.herbalgram.org

American Cancer Society
www.cancer.org

American Holistic Health Association
www.ahha.org

American Medical Association
www.ama~assn.org

Ask Dr. Weil
www.drweil.com

Association of Cancer Online Resources
www.acor.org

Breast-Cancer Answers
www.medsch.wisc.edu/bca

Cancer Care
www.cancercare.org

Cancer Guide
www.cancerguide.org

Centers for Disease Control
www.cdc.gov

FACT: Focus on Alternative and
Complementary Therapies
www.exeter.ac.uk/FACT/

Fact Sheets on Alternative Medicine
www.cpmcnet.columbia.edu/dept/rosenthal

FDA Guide to Choosing Medical
Treatments
www.fda.gov/oashi/aids/fdaguide.html

Medicine On Line
www.meds.com

National Alliance of Breast Cancer
Organizations
www.nabco.org

National Cancer Institute
www.nci.nih.gov

National Comprehensive Cancer Network
www.nccn.org

National Library of Medicine
www.nlm.nih.gov

NIH National Center for Complementary
and Alternative Medicine
www.nccam.nih.gov

Oxford Health Plans
www.oxhp.com

Planetree Programs
www.planetree.org

Quackwatch
www.quackwatch.com

University of Texas Center for Alternative
Medicine Research in Cancer
www.sph.uth.tmc.edu/utcam/default.htm

Y-Me National Breast Cancer
Organization
www.yme.org

Publisher's Resource List

We recommend purchasing supplements from reliable sources. There are many products available in outlet stores, discount stores and bargain shops. It is virtually impossible to determine if these products are effective or even safe. We suggest obtaining supplements from health food stores, top ranked mail-order houses and your doctor's office.

The companies and products listed here are, we believe, among the best in their respective fields. However, there are so many fine health food stores who take pride in the products they offer to the public that we cannot list them all. Use your judgment to determine if your local store deserves your patronage. Check for clean and orderly aisles, friendly and knowledgeable personnel.

Note: The authors and Kensington Publishing Corp. receive no financial or other compensation for these listings. The commentary is supplied by the publisher.

Carlson® Laboratories
1-800-323-4141
www.carlsonlabs.com

Source Naturals®
1-800-815-2333
www.sourcenaturals.com

Healthy Origins®
Lyc-O-Mato™
1-888-228-6650
www.healthyorigins.com

Carotec, Inc.
1-800-522-4279
www.carotec.com

Jarrow Formulas™
1-800-726-0886
www.jarrow.com

Here are some examples of first rate mail-order houses:

N.E.E.D.S

1-800-634-1380

www.needs.com

This organization stocks quality supplements from every important manufacturer. Call them for a catalog or check their web site. They also carry a variety of many other products, including environmental.

Wilner Chemists

1-800-633-1106

www.willner.com

They are the oldest and largest nutritionally oriented pharmacy in the United States. They offer a large selection of nutritional, herbal and homeopathic supplements. Catalog available or check their web site. This pharmacy is one of the very few who will do special compounding of special medications that your doctor may require.

Carotec, Inc.

1-800-522-4279

www.carotec.com

This company manufactures their own privately branded line of supplements. All of their products are made with superior and safe ingredients. They have an interesting catalog that explains how each of their supplements are made and what ingredients they use.

There are firms that specialize in distributing supplements to offices of MDs homeopaths, NDs, chiropractors, and other health professionals.

We are listing one of the very best:

Moss Nutrition

1-800-851-5444

www.mossnutrition.com

This organization supplies quality nutritional supplements exclusively to healthcare professionals throughout the United States.

Having been in existence for ten years, Moss Nutrition has developed contacts with many quality health practitioners of various types throughout the country. If you would like the name of a practitioner in your area who can serve your needs and provide you with these quality supplements, please feel free to call them at the above number.

Supplements

We are discovering that because of the depleted nutritive values of food available today, supplements are extremely important for human health.

Vitamin A

Source Naturals®

Active A™

Each tablet contains 15,000 IU of vitamin A (beta-carotene) and 10,000 IU of vitamin A (palminate), yielding 25,000 IU of total vitamin A activity.

Moss Nutrition

Bio-AE-Mulsion

This is an emulsified form of vitamin A. Because the emulsification process creates such a small particle size, the vitamin A in the product requires little or no liver metabolism. This, plus the fact that Bio-AE-Mulsion is provided in a liquid form, makes it ideal for use with children. Each drop contains 12,500 IU of vitamin A palminate.

Vitamins A and D

Carlson®

Vitamins A and D_3

Each softgel contains 10,000 IU of natural source vitamin A and 400 IU of natural source vitamin D_3 from fish liver oil.

Source Naturals®
Vitamin A Palminate
Each tablet contains 10,000 IUs (vitamin A palminate).

Vitamin B Complex

Available from the following companies:

Carlson®
B-Compleet™
Provides all the B vitamins plus vitamin C in a balanced formulation. Available in tablets.

Carotec
Bio B-Complex
Each capsule contains 25 milligrams of each of the "macro" B vitamins (B_1, B_2, B_6) plus pantothenic acid; 25 micrograms of B_{12} and D biotin; 200 micrograms of folic acid; 80 mg of Bioperine®, an ingredient that makes the B vitamins and other nutrients better absorbed and metabolized.

Source Naturals®
Coenzymate™ B Complex
Contains coenzymes along with a full range of B vitamins and CoQ10. Available in orange or peppermint flavored tablets that are taken sublingually (under the tongue) for direct absorption into the bloodstream.

Source Naturals®
Broccoli Sprouts
This product contains a key component of broccoli called sulforaphane, which is believed to stimulate enzymes in the body that play a role in detoxification. Each tablet provides the daily equivalent of 4.5 oz of fresh broccoli.

Vitamin C

Available from the following companies:

Carlson®
Mild-C Chewable
Buffered form of chewable vitamin C that is nonacidic and gentle to the teeth. Each orange and tangerine flavored tablet supplies 250 mg of vitamin C and 28 mg of calcium.

Mild-C™
Vitamin C crystals. A buffered form of vitamin C. Very gentle for both stomach and teeth. Each teaspoon contains 3,600 mg vitamin C and 400 mg calcium.
Suggestion: Use no more than ⅛ teaspoon to start with and increase gradually.

Source Naturals®
Wellness C-1000™
Each tablet contains 1,000 mg of vitamin C and several sources of bioflavonoids and alpha-lipoic acid.

Carotec
Vitamin C with grape seed contains 500 mg vitamin C and 50 mg of Masquelier's OPC of grape seed. Very high in polyphenols.

Vitamin D

Available from the following companies:

Moss Nutrition
1-800-851-5444
Bio-D-Mulsion
An oil in water emulsion in which vitamin D has been dispersed. Each drop supplies 400 IU of emulsified vitamin D. If you wish to have your dentist or physician inquire about this product, they can call Moss Nutrition.

Carlson®
Vitamin D$_3$

Natural source vitamin D$_3$ from fish liver oil. Available in 400 IU and 1,000 IU softgels.

DIM™

A new and important supplement that has been shown to support the body in healthy estrogen metabolism and hormone regulation. Contains BioResponse DIM™, a formulation of pure dietary indole from cruciferous vegetables such as broccoli. Available from the following companies:

Allergy Research Group
1-800-545-9960

Moss Nutrition
1-800-851-5444

Vitamin E

Available from the following companies:

Carotec
Vitamin E

Each softgel contains 200 IU alpha tocopherol, 75 mg gamma tocopherol, 28 mg delta tocopherol, and 1 mg beta tocopherol.

Carlson®
E-Gems® Plus

Each softgel contains vitamin E derived from soybean oil, supplying alpha tocopherol plus mixed tocopherols. Available in three strengths: 200 IU, 400 IU, and 800 IU.

Source Naturals®
Vitamin E with mixed tocopherols
Fat-soluble antioxidant 400 IUs in softgels.

Calcium

There has been a huge amount of study and debate relating to which supplements containing calcium are best absorbed by the body. A new invention using a patented formulation known as BioCalth™ ensures that more calcium is delivered to the bones and collagen of your body. This product ensures that more calcium is made bioavailable and efficiently absorbed. This is an important addition to any diet for individuals who want to improve the balance between bone formation and resorption. BioCalth™ inhibits bone and collagen loss, and it has demonstrated the ability to regenerate collagen tissue. This is important for the prevention and mitigation of osteoporosis, rickets and other degenerative joint diseases. It will improve bone strength, joint flexibility, and generally can help build bone mass. Its beneficial effects of both preventative and treatment measures play a positive role in reducing the risk of bone fractures (very important for an aging population). BioCalth™ improves joint function and reduces the symptoms associated with bone disease. Also effective for pain, cramps, and weakness in limbs and the body. For further information on this product please contact the following:

Giantceutical Inc
1870 Wright Avenue
La Verne, CA 91750
1-888-275-1717
www.giantceutical.com

Coenzyme Q10

Available from the following:

Carlson®
Co-Q10
   Available in 10 mg, 30 mg, 50 mg, 100 mg and 200 mg softgels.

Carotec
Co-Q10
   Each softgel contains 100 mg coenzyme Q10 with 50 mg palm tocotrienols and 200 mg of virgin coconut oil as the carrier.

Source Naturals®
Coenzyme Q10
   Available in 30 mg and 100 mg softgels.

Glutathione

   An antioxidant essential for functioning of the immune system. Necessary for bodily health. Available from the following companies:

Carlson® Laboratories
Glutathione Booster™
   Provides the body with the nutrients needed to elevate or maintain healthy glutathione and glutathione peroxidase levels. Each capsule contains vitamins C and E, riboflavin (vitamin B_2), selenium, n-acetyl cysteine, milk thistle extract (silymarin), garlic, alpha lipoic, L-glutamine, L-glycine, asparagus concentrate, and glutathione.

Source Naturals®
L-Glutathione
   Composed of the amino acids L-cysteine, L-glutamic acid, and L-glycine. Available in 50 mg tablets.

Chem-Defense™
   Molybdenum/glutathione complex. Helps to remove toxins from the body. Each orange-flavored tablet contains 1.6 mg of riboflavin (as 2.25 mg flavin mononucleotide Coenzymated™), 120 mcg of molybdenum (as molybdenum aspartate citrate), and 50 mg of glutathione. Taken sublingually (under the tongue) for direct absorption into the bloodstream.

Green Tea Extract

   Science has shown that Asiatic people derive health benefits from drinking five to ten cups of green tea daily. As this may be impractical for most people, Green Tea Extract is a wonderful way to accomplish the same thing.

Source Naturals®
Green Tea Extract
   Contains antioxidants known as polyphenols. Each tablet contains 100 mg of polyphenols.

Carotec, Inc.
Green Tea Phytomicrosphere.
   Each capsule contains 350 mg of Green Tea Extract and 50 mg of catechins.

Lutein

Carlson® Laboratories
Lutein plus kale
   This lutein is derived from kale and a variety of other plants. It contains 15 mg lutein and a base of 100 mg kale. It is available in capsule form.

Lutein
   This product contains 6 mg of lutein, 264 mg of zeaxanthoin and vitamin E. Available in softgels.

Jarrow Formulas™
1-800-726-08886
www.jarrow.com
Lutein

A powerful antioxidant carotenoid. Combination of lutein/zeaxanthoin 20 mg. Available in health food stores or call N.E.E.D.S. at 1-800-634-1380.

Source Naturals®
Lutein

Antioxidant carotenoid with 6 mg of lutein per capsule.

Lycopene

Available from the following company:

Healthy Origins®
P.O. Box 12615
Pittsburgh, PA 15241-0615
1-888-228-6650
www.healthyorigins.com

Lyc-O-Mato Clinical Trio™

An antioxidant combination. Two capsules contain "clinical strength" dosages of lycopene, 30 mg.; selenium, 200 mcg; and natural vitamin E, 400 IU (with 100% mixed tocopherols including d-alpha, beta, gamma, and delta tocopherols) in a base of olive oil.

Lyc-O-Mato Plus

Lycopene/selenium combination. Two capsules contain: lycopene, 30 mg. and selenium, 200 mcg. This non-GMO product contains no genetically modified organisms in a base of olive oil.

Lyc-O-Mato (with olive oil)

Contains "clinical strength" lycopene 15mg per softgel capsule. This is an improved formula that replaces the soybean oil with olive oil. A non-GMO product, it contains no genetically modified organisms.

Clinical studies show that olive oil when added to lycopene enhances the absorption of the lycopene.

Multi-vitamins/Minerals

Carlson® Laboratories
Super 2 Daily™

A comprehensive vitamin and mineral combination in softgel form

Source Naturals®
Life Force™ Multiple

Provides nutritional support especially for the liver and the immune system. Available in tablet form with iron and without iron.

These two multivitamins are available in health food stores or call N.E.E.D.S. at 1-800-634-1380.

Multi-Mineral Complex

Source Naturals®
Life Minerals

A comprehensive formulation of necessary life minerals, including boron and cilica in tablet form.

Carotec
Trace Sea Minerals

Phytomicrosphere complex in a capsule form.

Plant Sterols and Sterolins

Extensive clinical research shows that plant sterols and sterolins help regulate immune function and reduce effects of environmental toxins. Available from:

Moducare
1-877-297-7332
www.moducare.com

Probiotics

For a healthy colon and digestion. Available from the following companies:

Garden of Life
1-800-622-8986
www.gardenoflifeusa.com or
www.gardenoflife.cc

Primal Defense™

A natural whole-food, certified-organic probiotic blend of homeostatic soil organisms. Contains fourteen different non-dairy probiotic strains, including lactabacillus acidophilus, lactabacillus bulgarus, lactabacillus plantarum in 900 mg caplets. Also available in powder form. Available in health food stores or call N.E.E.D.S. at 1-800-634-1380.

Source Naturals®
Freeze stabilized acidophilus powder

Ten billion cells per gram; ¼ teaspoon with meals.

Quercetin

Quercetin has been found in various studies to be active against cancer cells.

Allergy Research Group
1-800-545-9960
Quercetin 300

Contains 300 mg of quercetin, 75 mg vitamin C, and 70 IU vitamin E in capsule form.

Source Naturals®
Activated Quercetin Biolflavonoid Complex

It contains 1,000 mg quercetin, 300 mg bromelain (pineapple enzyme), and 600 mg vitamin C. Available in tablet form.

Carlson® Laboratories
Rutin

A natural source of quercetin containing 250 mg quercetin and 500 mg rutin. Available in tablet form.

Selenium

Available from the following company:

Healthy Origins®
Seleno Excell

Each tablet contains 200 mcg of selenium in the organically bound form. Seleno Excell was used in the Nutritional Prevention of Cancer Study conducted at the University of Arizona by Larry C. Clark, M.P.H., Ph.D.

Silicon (Silica)

Silicon is a trace mineral required for healthy bone, skin, hair, and nails. Regulates calcium deposition in bones.

Jarrow Formulas™
Biosil

Biologically active silicon (silica). Available in liquid silicon concentrate. Available in health food stores or from N.E.E.D.S. 1-800-634-1380.

Transfer Factor

This product is derived from bovine colostrum that has been found to play a role in immune function. It is actually a protein fraction of colostrum, which appears to be effective in facilitating immunity. Available from the following company.

Moss Nutrition
1-800-851-5444
www.mossnutrition.com

Zinc

Available from the following companies:

Carotec
Chelated zinc aspartate
Each tablet supplies 9.9 mg elemental zinc.

Source Naturals®
OptiZinc®
Each tablet contains 30 mg of zinc (from 150 mg of OptiZinc® zinc monomethionine).

Specialty Vitamins

Kosher and vegeterian

Freeda Vitamins
36 East 41 Street
New York, NY 10017
1-800-777-3737
www.freedavitamins.com
For those with special needs, all their supplements are kosher, 100% vegetarian, sugar-free, yeast-free, gluten-free, salt-free, free of artificial colors, flavors, and lactose-free. This line also caters to diabetics, Muslims who require Halal certification and Feingold dieters. This organization has been manufacturing high-quality vitamins for over seventy years. Also available in health food stores.

Herbs

Even more so than supplements, it is important that herbs be purchased only from those companies who take pride and care in the way they grow and manufacture their herbal compounds. There are a number of very good herbal companies, but because of space limitation we will list only a few of the very best. You can find these fine products in your local health food store. You can also contact the companies and ask for a store near you that distributes their products.

Herbalist and Alchemist
1-800-611-8235
www.herbalist-alchemist.com
H & A was founded by herbalist David Winston, AHG, and provides some of the highest-quality herbal tinctures and herbal products available in the United States.

They have over three hundred herbal products formulated in tinctures. Their formulated tinctures and herbs are mostly organic or wildcrafted. They are one of the very few herbal companies that will check every batch of herbs for impurities and inferior parts of the plant. They also have audiotapes available for information about how to use herbs correctly for various body functions.

Planetary Formulas
1-800-606-6226
www.planetherbs.com
Planetary Formulas makes numerous products combining Western, Chinese, and Ayurvedic herbs. Dr. Michael Tierra, OMD, L.Ac., is one of the foremost authorities on herbal medicine in North America and has had a clinical practice for thirty years. He is the product formulator for Planetary Formulas and is an internationally recognized authority on the world's herbal traditions. Planetary Formulas carries a wide range of herbs and herbal formulas in tablets and tinctures extracted with alcohol. They also carry for children a line of herbs with glycerin added to neutralize any alcohol taste.

Gaia Herbs

1-800-831-7780

www.gaiaherbs.com

Founded by Ric Scalzo, Gaia uses mostly certified organic and ecologically wildcrafted herbs that are specifically selected and formulated to work synergistically within the body. This company also has a full line of herbs in capsules and liquid phytocaps—a revolutionary new delivery system for liquid herbal extracts. All phytocaps are vegetable based and alcohol-free.

Mail Order for Herbs

N.E.E.D.S.

1-800-634-1380

www.needs.com

If you can't find the herbal supplement you are looking for in your local health food store, try calling N.E.E.D.S. They carry virtually all of the top herbal lines and will supply a catalog upon request.

Herbal Combinations for Prostate Cancer

Combining herbs can sometimes be extremely effective and even dramatic.

Epilobium

A very effective anticancer herb in a liquefied, whole-herb preparation providing the herb's full spectrum of beneficial components. This herb is found extensively in Germany and other European countries for use primarily against cancer. Epilobium is derived from a small-flowered willow herb to be used as a dietary supplement. Take five to ten drops two times a day on an empty stomach. Also used as an antiinflammatory and helps to control incontinence in both men and women. There

have been many studies around the world showing the effect of this herb against cancer. It is available from:

Beachwood Canyon, Naturally, Ltd.

1-888-803-5333

www.bcm4life.com

Olive Leaf Extract

Seagate (also known as First Fishery)

1-888-505-4283

www.seagateproducts.com

As we enter a new millennium, antibiotics are no longer seen as a risk-free panacea. Their rampant overuse has created resistant strains of bacteria that are not so easy to treat. Antibiotics have also been found to have serious side effects such as allergic reactions, colitis, and yeast overgrowth. The olive leaf and its extract have been used for thousands of years against almost all pathological micro-organisms, including fungi, bacteria, viruses, parasites, and other microscopic organisms. There has been increasing interest in the use of natural antimicrobial products in recent years as a result of the increasing awareness of the public to the side effects of pharmaceutical drugs and their reduced ability to combat the evolving mutant strains of these micro-organisms.

Olive leaf extract has been used safely for thousands of years by people along the Mediterranean Sea. This is a natural plant product. The only known side effect that has been noted from the use of olive leaf extract is the possibility of a Herxheimer reaction, which is the rapid die-off of a large number of harmful fungi that suddenly release toxins; then this may trigger an immune response, similar to an allergic or flulike reaction, for a few days. If this reaction is experienced and becomes too uncomfortable, the level of use of the extract can be reduced or stopped until the reaction disappears. Some doctors believe that a Herxheimer reaction is an excellent response for an antifungal treatment.

For therapeutic use, take 4 to 9 capsules per day. As a natural antimicrobial health food supplement, for most applications (other than fungal disorders) the suggested use is 3 capsules three times per day for a week to ten days. For antifungal support, the suggested use is 2 capsules three times per day for up to six months; or in more severe cases, up to twelve months. Olive leaf extract is available in fine health food stores.

Herbal Advice

If you require the services of a master herbalist for herbal advice relating to any of the medical conditions listed in this book, this person is knowledgeable in Western, Chinese and Ayurvedic herbal modalities.

Chrysalis Natural Medicine Clinic
Alan Keith Tillotson, Ph.D., A.H.G.—
    Medical Herbalist
Naixin Hu Tillotson, O.M.D., La.C.—
    Chinese Medicine
1008 Milltown Road
Wilmington, DE 19808 USA
Phone: 302-994-0565 Fax: 302-995-0653
E-mail: AlanT3@aol.com

The Chrysalis Natural Medicine Clinic consultants are highly trained in prescribing herbal medicine treatments for serious or difficult to treat diseases. Phone consultations or office visits are available. Chrysalis maintains a large pharmacy of over 1,000 herbal medicines and nutrients available by mail to any location in the world.

Herbal Cautionary Note

Dr. Sandra McLanahan has already reminded us within this book that certain herbs may cause adverse responses and complications during surgery when anesthesia is used. Dr. McLanahan wishes to thank Stanley Meyerson of N.E.E.D.S. for sending a recent study showing that feverfew, ginseng, gingko biloba, ginger, ephedra, and garlic, as well as St. John's wort, valerian, and kava kava taken before surgery or used by the patient right after surgery, can impair and may adversely effect bleeding, blood pressure, and poor clotting. Usage of these herbs must be stopped within two weeks of surgery.

In this special resource section, we have selected foods, teas, and oils, which are mostly organic and of the highest quality.

ORGANIC FOOD

Flaxseeds

Living Tree Community Foods
1-800-260-5534
www.livingtreecommunity.com

Organic Golden Flax

Golden flaxseeds are larger and softer than the dark brown flaxseeds. They have a mild nutty flavor that is really delicious mixed in food. This flaxseed has about 3½ times as much omega-3 fatty acids as omega-6 fatty acids. It is also the richest known source of potassium, magnesium, and boron. To maintain a fresh supply grind daily in a coffee grinder.

Omega Nutrition
1-800-661-3529

www.omeganutrition.com
Flax of Life—Cold Milled Organic Flaxseeds

Certified organic flaxseeds, vacuum packed in a lined, resealable foil bag to retain freshness. Flaxseed is a terrific source of the essential oil omega-3.

Flax of Life—Whole Organic Flaxseeds
Certified organic flaxseeds

Organic Beans

Dried organic beans
There are a wide variety available including Aduki domestic, blackeye peas, black turtle, chickpeas, kidney beans, pinto beans, navy beans, mung beans, green lentils, red lentils, split peas, and baby limas. Available from:

Natural Lifestyle
1-800-752-2775
www.natural-lifestyle.com

Organic Culinary Herbs

A wonderful assortment of certified organic culinary herbs that are nonirradiated, unfumigated, and packed in glass spice jars. Includes basil leaves, bay leaves, cayenne pepper, garlic powder, ginger root, tumeric root, and many others. Available from:

Natural Lifestyle.
1-800-752-2775
www.natural-lifestyle.com

Teas (Green)

Try switching from coffee to green tea and enjoy the benefits of antioxidants and less caffeine. There is an amino acid in green tea (*Camellia sinensis*) that balances caffeine's effects and delivers a sense of relaxation.

Maitake Products, Inc.
1-800-747-7418
www.maitake.com
Mai Green™Tea

Contains organically grown maitake mushroom and premier Japanese green tea (matcha) leaves. Low in caffeine. Available in tea bags.

Rishi Tea
866-747-4483 (866-RISHI TEA)
www.rishi-tea.com

Rishi imports premium loose-leaf teas directly from tea gardens in Asia. An integral component of tea quality is its purity. Rishi offers more than two dozen certified organic teas, including ten green tea varietals. While the positive health benefits of regular consumption of green tea are now well documented, this company sells only high quality loose tea. Usually this will deliver a more potent and healthful drink, which is superior to tea packed in tea bags.

Rooibos Tea

Rooibos is an herb that has been used in South Africa for centuries and has been shown to have very high levels of vitamins and minerals. Rooibos has a mildly sweet flavor and earthy aroma, as well as some potential health benefits. It contains calcium, iron, zinc, vitamin C, and several other important minerals. Rooibos is naturally caffeine-free and is believed to relieve insomnia, cramps, constipation, skin irritations, and allergic symptoms. Recent research has also shown that it has higher antioxidant concentrations than green tea. This is organically grown and in loose-leaf form.

Available from Rishi Tea.
Rooibos Tea is also available in tea bags and is organic. It is available from:

Wisdom of the Ancients®
1-800-899-9908
www.wisdomherbs.com

Pu-erh Tea

Even less known, but certainly worthy of investigation is Pu-erh tea. Pu-erh imparts a warming energy and the Chinese believe it cleanses the blood and tonifies the body. More than any other tea in China, Pu-erh is prized for its medicinal properties.

Available from Rishi Tea.

Negata Green Sencha Tea

Negata organic Japanese green tea is made from the season's first young leaves, hand harvested at their peak of flavor, steamed and dried—mildly stimulating. Green Sencha is available in both bulk tea and in Sencha Haiku tea bags.

Available from:

Natural Lifestyle
1-800-752-2775
www.natural-lifestyle.com

Tea Filter Bags

Loose tea suffers from a stigma of being too complicated to prepare. In fact, loose tea is about as simple as it gets: pouring hot water on tea leaves. Standard tea bags are easy enough, but quality and flavor are sacrificed and as the tea in tea bags is a product for mass production, it often contains pesticides and herbicides.

The main sticking point for many people when brewing loose tea is having some sort of implement with which to infuse the tea. Teapots are ideal, but if you want something even more convenient, check out the tea filter bags that **Rishi Tea** uses. It's simple—you spoon the tea leaves into the bag, place the bag in the cup and pour the water on it. In effect, you make your own tea bag. The filter bags are made of all-natural biodegradable hemp fiber and are designed to let the tea leaves expand. Tea balls and clamps, on the other hand, prevent the tea leaves from steeping properly and can introduce heavy metals into tea. A wonderful way to brew loose tea.

Tea Press

Another unique method and very easy to use, a tea press, produces a rich full-bodied tea made with a heat-resistant tempered glass carafe and a permanent stainless steel filter.

Available from:

Natural Lifestyle
1-800-752-2775
www.natural-lifestyle.com

Triple Leaf Tea, Inc.
1-800-552-7448
maryanne@tripleleaf-tea.com
www.tripleleaf-tea.com

Effective, authentic, traditional Chinese green, naturally decaffeinated green, medicinal and diet teas, made with authentic Chinese herbs and traditional herbal formulas, packaged in convenient tea bag form. All teas are GMO-free.

Triple Leaf Tea's **Decaf Green Tea** and **Decaf Green Tea** blends uses a natural solvent-free carbon dioxide decaffeination process that researchers have found maintains almost all of green tea's beneficial antioxidants, including EGCG, while leaving no chemical residue. Other decaffeination methods use either a chemical solvent, ethyl acetate, which researchers have found removes much of the antioxidants, or water, which also is likely to deplete the antioxidants, since they are extremely water-soluble.

If you drink a lot of green tea and don't want the caffeine, this is the ideal tea to use.

Decaf Green Tea with Ginseng:
Naturally decaffeinated green tea leaves, honeysuckle flower, chrysanthemum flower, dandelion root, mulberry leaf, peppermint leaf, astragalus root, Siberian ginseng root (*Ekleutherococcus senticosus*), American ginseng root (*Panax quinquefolius*), Asian ginseng root (*Panax ginseng*), jiaogulan (*Gynostemma pentaphyllum*), licorice root.

Ginkgo and Decaf Green Tea
Ginkgo biloba leaf, naturally decaffeinated green tea leaves, eucommia leaf, Ho Shou Wu (*fo ti*) root, Poria cocos mushroom, astragalus root, Siberian ginseng root (*Eleutherococcus senticosus*), American ginseng root (*Panax quinquefolius*), Asian ginseng root (*Panax ginseng*), licorice root.

American Ginseng Herbal Tea
Made from 100 percent American ginseng root, this tea has the maximum amount of this beneficial adaptogenic herb. It is used to help build the body's vitality, strength, and resistance to mental and physical stress, and to help support the healthy function of the immune system. Prized by Chinese herbalists for long-term use, it was considered beneficial for fatigue and recovery from illness.

Jasmine Green Tea
Made from jasmine flowers combined with green tea, creating a delicious aromatic tea. Jasmine was traditionally used for its calming, relaxing, and warming properties, for brightening the mood, and as a soothing digestive tea.

100 percent ginger root tea is a delicious and spicy tea bag that supplies a terrific boost at any time. Also available: 100 percent American ginseng root tea, to support balance, health and well-being.

Detox Tea
A very gentle way to detox in a tea bag. Includes red clover, dandelion root, licorice root, peppermint leaf, ginger root, rhubarb root, burdock root, and other ingredients.

All the above is available from Triple Leaf Tea, Inc.

Pau d' arco
A legendary tea from the Paraguayan rain forest which is antiinflammatory and works well against fungal, bacterial, and yeast problems. Comes in both tea bags and bulk.
Available from:

Wisdom of the Ancients
l-800-899-9908
www.wisdomherbs.com

Grains

Available from the following companies:

Lundberg Family Farms
530-882-4550 (ext. 319)
www.lundberg.com
Grower and marketer of organic rice and rice products. They have an amazing variety of rices, rice cakes, etc. Reliable quality. Also available in health food stores or order from Natural Lifestyle at 1-800-752-2775.

Organic Whole Grains
Natural Chef Organization whole grains
High quality grains that include whole oats, spelt, barley, buckwheat, and many others. It is available from:

Natural Lifestyle
1-800-752-2775
www.natural-lifestyle.com

Green Drinks—Powdered

Available from the following companies:

Garden of Life
1-800-622-8986
www.gardenoflifeuse.com

Super Green Formula
Over forty-five nutrient dense super foods equivalent to five to ten servings of vegetables. Contains ninety antioxidants plus one hundred minerals and vitamins. Available in both powdered form and capsules.

Wakunaga of America
1-800-421-2998
www.kyolic.com

Kyo-Greens®
A combination of organically grown barley and wheat grasses, kelp, chlorella, and brown rice. Two teaspoons provide the nutrients of a serving of deep green leafy vegetables. This company also markets one of the most highly rated garlic products available.

Garlic Extract, Aged

Wakunaga of America
1-800-421-2998
www.kyolic.com
Kyolic®Aged Garlic Extract (AGE)
The most scientifically researched garlic product in the world (over 220 studies). As mentioned earlier in this book, the use of garlic in the diet is inversely related to cancer rates. Available in capsules as well as in liquid form (that can be added to food).

Mushrooms

Shiitake Mushrooms
High grade shiitakes in various forms. Shiitakes' medicinal capabilities are being used worldwide. This mushroom may be helpful in illnesses such as heart disease, cancer, and AIDS. Available from:

Natural Lifestyles
1-800-752-2775
www.natural-lifestyle.com

Nuts, Nut Butters, and Seeds—Organic

Available from the following company:

Living Tree Community Foods
1-800-260-5534
www.livingtreecommunity.com
Organically grown nuts and nut butters, including almonds (many varieties), macadamia nuts, pine nuts, pumpkin seeds, sunflower seeds, walnut quarters, raw almond butter, raw macadamia nut butter, and raw cashew butter. A delicious new combination, which they aptly named Milk of Paradise is a combination of organic macadamia and cashew spread. Their quality is really terrific. They also stock raw honey, raw tahini, organic cranberries, and a variety of dried fruits. Plus they carry dates that have not been processed with sugar and are delicious. They make their organic nut butters in small batches so that they are always fresh when shipped. Available in health food stores as well as mail order.

Omega Nutrition
1-800-661-3529
www.omeganutrition.com
Pumpkin Seed Butter
A delicious, highly nutritious spread made from grade A pumpkin seeds.

Oils

Available in bottles and in gel capsules. Recommended from the following companies:

Omega Nutrition
1-800-661-3529
www.omeganutrition.com
Essential Balance Jr. (for children)

Omega's proprietary blend of five fresh-pressed oils scientifically blended in the evolutionary 1:1 omega-3/omega-6 ratio. Contains certified organic flax, sunflower, sesame, pumpkin, and borage oils. Also contains gamma-linolenic acid (GLA) and omega-6 fatty acids. Formulated with a natural butterscotch flavoring that kids will love.

Fish Oil

Carlson Laboratories
1-800-323-4141
www.carlsonlabs.com
Norwegian Cod Liver Oil

Bottled in liquid form. This product is an effective blend of omega-3 and other essential fatty acids, as well as vitamin E. Available in natural and lemon-flavored. Can be mixed into food.

Super-DHA™

Each softgel contains 1,000 mg of a special blend of fish body oils, including menhaden sardines, which are high in DHA (Docosahexaenoic acid) and EPA (Eicosapentaenoic acid). This product is unique because it supplies as much as 500 mg of DHA and 200 mg of EPA.

Super Omega-3 Fish Oils

Contains a special concentrate of fish body oils, from deep coldwater fish, including mackerel and sardines, which are especially rich in EPA and DHA. Each softgel provides 570 mg of total omega-3 fatty acids consisting of EPA (Eicosapentaenoic acid), DHA (Docosahexaenoic acid), and ALA (Alpha-Liolenic acid).

DHA Essential Fatty Acids—Omega-3

DHA, an essential fatty acid necessary for life, is available in a non-fish, micro-algae form (for those who don't want to use fish products). Look for a product called **Neuromins® DHA** (in softgel form). Two of the very best companies distributing Neuromins are:

Source Naturals®
1-800-815-2333

Carotec, Inc.
1-800-522-4279

Neuromins® DHA is available at health food stores.

Flaxseed Oil

Unrefined and certified organic, grown without pesticides or artificial fertilizers and processed using Omega's exclusive Omegaflo® process. Also available from Omega Nutrition.

Olive Oil

Made from unrefined, extra-virgin olives that are fresh-pressed and Omegaflo® bottled.

Also available from Omega Nutrition.

Living Tree Community Foods
1-800-323-5534
www.livingtreecommunity.com

Living Tree has a raw organic olive oil that is not pressed. It's centrifuged at 75 degrees Fahrenheit, room temperature.

Most poultry and fish available in this country today are loaded with unhealthy food colorings, antibiotics, hormones, and many other additives the human body was not meant to absorb. For total body health it is important to use food products that are free of toxic substances. Natural products will taste even better than the products that are loaded with all kinds of artificial additives.

Poultry

Available from the following company:

Sheltons Poultry, Inc.
1-800-541-1833
www.sheltons.com

Free-range chickens and turkeys with no added antibiotics. The taste quality of these natural products is far superior to products that are laced with all sorts of additives and hormones. Available in natural foods stores. Noted health expert, Andrew Weil, M.D., cautions people to avoid eating poultry and meat with added antibiotics, which has been linked to drug-resistant strains of disease-causing bacteria. This company also has a wide array of other products including sausage, liver, and many other items from organically raised turkeys and chickens. Call them for their extensive catalog.

Available in some health food stores.

Organic Chicken Broth

A wonderful all-natural organic chicken broth with no preservatives or chemicals added. Contains organic chicken broth concentrate, sea salt, organic chicken fat, organic onion powder and organic celery seeds. Available in cans in regular and also in fat free/sodium free.

Seafood

Seafood Direct
1-800-732-1836
www.seafooddirect.com

This company is a wonderful source for wild-caught salmon. Most of the salmon available in restaurants and stores are farm-raised. Usually this means medications such as antibiotics and hormones have been added to the feed, as well as synthetic coloring. Wild-caught salmon has none of these problems and has a high level of omega-3 fatty acids and much less fat than farm-raised salmon. It tastes better as well. Their line includes wild Alaskan salmon, king salmon, and sockeye salmon. Alaskan-caught king crab, crab, and Alaskan cod are also available. They come in frozen filets and steaks. Also in jars and cans. An excellent canned salmon and canned solid white albacore tuna, which is caught with hook and line to guarantee quality, are also available. Again there are no added preservatives. Available in some health food and gourmet stores.

Stevia

Wisdom of the Ancients®
1-800-899-9908
www.wisdomherbs.com

Natural sweetener made from whole leaf Stevia (*Stevia rebaudiana Bertoni*) 6:1 concentrated extract. Available in concentrated tablets, liquid, and as a tea. Hundreds of scientific studies have been conducted on Stevia's effectiveness as a nutritional addition to the diet.

Wine—Organic

Frey Vineyards
1-800-760-3739
or call their distributor to find a local store that carries this brand.

Organic Vintages
877-ORGANIC

If you enjoy an occasional glass of wine, we strongly suggest avoidance of pesticides and other chemicals. Frey Vineyards is a fine and reliable certified organic wine company. They do not add sulfites to their wine.

Dental Products

There is a holistic connection between the health of your teeth and gums and your whole body. This is especially true for diabetics, who need to be vigilant about their teeth and gums because they have a tendency to develop periodontal disease. Woodstock Natural Products are formulated by a holistic dentist and contain soothing and healing herbs, with no alcohol, sugar, or harsh chemicals. These products have been clinically proven to kill germs that cause gum disease. In a study published in the *Journal of Clinical Dentistry* in 1998, researchers at the New York University College of Dentistry in New York City found that The Natural Dentist toothpaste removed plaque more effectively than the leading commercial brand. The same group also found that The Natural Dentist mouth rinse killed more germs than the leading commercial brand.

Woodstock Natural Products, Inc.
The Natural Dentist™
1-800-615-6895
Toothpaste: mint, cinnamon, and fluoride-free mint
Mouth rinse: mint, cinnamon, and cherry flavored
Available in health food stores.

Desert Essence®
1-800-476-8647
www.desertessence.com
Oral Care Collection

A complete line of antiseptic and cleansing oral care products using tea tree oil for deep cleaning and disinfecting of teeth and gums. All products are animal and eco-friendly and made without artificial colors, sweeteners, or harsh abrasives.

Tea Tree Oil Dental Floss: creates a germ-free mouth and cleans between teeth.
Tea Tree Oil Dental Tape: provides same benefits as floss with a wider ribbon.
Tea Tree Oil Dental Pics: cleans between teeth with antiseptic power.
Tea Tree Oil Breath Freshener: contains natural and organic essential oils.

Environment

Environmentally Safe Toxin Free Cleansers
Toxic chemicals can play a very significant role in causing a variety of illnesses.

There are many dangerous and toxic chemicals that can migrate into the human body. An easy way to keep some of them away is to avoid commercial brands of cleansers. There are several excellent companies that market effective cleansers that do not contain harmful chemicals. Here are two of the very best:

Earth Friendly Products
1-800-335-3267 (ext. 10)
www.ecos.com

ECOS®
A toxic free liquid or powder washing machine cleanser.

Stain & Odor Remover

An effective non-polluting 100 percent biodegradable cleanser for removing all sorts of stains and dirt. This product will work on carpets, fabrics, clothing, laundry, wood floors, and other surfaces.

The Wave Automatic Machine Dishwashing Powder. (Also available in gel form.)

A very effective non-toxic cleanser. Chlorine free and phosphate free.

Earth Friendly Products also has a variety of other products including window cleaner, all purpose cleansers, and even a drain opener and maintainer made with enzymes. Available in health food stores.

Allens Naturally
1-800-352-8971
www.allensnaturally.com

All of the cleansing products at this company are free of perfume and dyes, are biodegradable and very powerful. They have a long list of natural cleansers ranging from dishwasher and washing machine cleansers, as well as glass and several all-purpose cleansers. Available in health food stores or can be obtained from N.E.E.D.S at 1-800-634-1380.

Environmental Products for Air and Water

Mail Order

N.E.E.D.S
1-800-634-1380
www.needs.com

An excellent resource for top-notch environmental products. Call them for a full listing of their products.

Aireox Home Purifer (Model 45)

Removes mold spores, pollen dust, formaldehyde, and more.

Aireox Car Air Purifier (Model 22)

An unusual purifier for the car.

Elite Shower Filter and Massager

For removing chlorine, heavy metals and bacteria. The amount of chlorine that can penetrate the skin while taking a shower is substantial. Chlorine is a toxin, which can cause damage to body tissues.

Water Filters

N.E.E.D.S. carries a variety of high-quality water filters.

Environmental Pressure Cooker

SILIT Pressure Cooker

Most cooking appliances use an aluminum cooking surface. This metal is very inexpensive for the manufacturer, but the user must beware, aluminum can cause toxic reactions in the human body. More expensive appliances will use stainless steel. However, there are several other metals within stainless steel. One of which is nickel, which again, when absorbed by the body can set off toxic reactions.

An ideal cooking surface is enamel. This is much like glassware, but is not breakable and has no known toxic materials. A wonderful new pressure cooker using an enamel surface is now available. This sophisticated device has new controls, which automatically controls steam to avoid burns, while at the same time retaining all the natural flavors and nutrients within food. This superb cooker enhances the taste with aromatic steam because of its patented hermetically sealed system. It will cook most everything safely and much quicker than most cooking systems. Available from:

Natural Lifestyle
1-800-752-2775
www.natural-lifestyle.com

Water

Water is the forgotten element in our daily lives. We forget, or do not realize, that the human body can survive for weeks without food. But this is not the reality of water. Without water, our survival time is limited to at best a few days. We usually have at our disposal municipal supplied water, which may be subject to contamination. Or we can carefully choose bottled water, which is now a multibillion dollar industry. There are dozens of brands available, some of which are no more than processed water, obtained from regular municipal water supplies.

Making a choice: Consider the source. The best water will be obtained from protected spring waters that are contaminant free and bottled under stringent quality control procedures at the natural source. Ideally, this water would be available in pure glass bottles or containers, which unlike some plastic bottles will not leak dangerous chemi-

cals into the body. Additionally, water should be sodium free, contain important minerals and hopefully be slightly alkaline rather than acidic.

One of the very best having all of these qualifications is the following:

Mountain Valley Spring Water
1-800-643-1501
www.mountainvalleyspring.com

This water company has been bottling and distributing their pure, delicious spring water since 1871. They are one of the few bottled waters that still offer their product in glass.

Purified Water

It is often thought that distilled drinking water is the purest of all water. But, distilled has no minerals for the body's use. Now a new and improved water is even purer than distilled or even reverse osmosis water. This product has less than 0.4 PPM or 25 times less dissolved solids than either distilled or reverse osmosis. It is available from:

Penta™ Purified Drinking Water
1-800-531-5088
www.hydrateforlife.com

NOTES

Introduction

1. Clawson, TA, et al., "The hypnotic control of blood flow and pain: the cure of warts and the potential for the use of hypnosis in the treatment of cancer," *American Journal of Clinical Hypnosis,* v. 17, n. 3, 1975, pp.160–69.

2. Schneider, Robert, *When to Say No to Surgery,* Prentice-Hall, 1982, p. viii.

3. *Newsweek,* 12/13/74, p. 47.

4. "HHS Watchdog asks forced second opinions," *American Medical News,* 4/15/83, p. 12.

5. Easterday, CL, et al., "Hysterectomy in the U.S.," *Obstetrics and Gynecology,* v. 62, n. 2, 7/83, pp. 203–12.

6. Eisenberg, DM, et al., "Unconventional medicine in the United States," *New England Journal of Medicine,* v. 328, n. 4, 1/28/93, pp. 246–52.

7. Colt, George, "The Healing Revolution," *Life,* 9/96, p. 39.

8. Anderson, EA, "Preoperative preparation for cardiac surgery facilitates recovery, reduces psychological distress, and reduces the incidence of acute postoperative hypertension," *Journal of Consulting and Clinical Psychology,* v. 55, n. 4, 1987, pp. 513–20; also Egbert, LD, et al., "Reduction of postoperative pain by encouragement and instruction of patients," *New England Journal of Medicine,* v. 270, 10/64, pp. 825–27.

9. Millman, Marcia, *The Unkindest Cut,* William Morrow, 1978.

10. Bennet, H, et al., "Non-verbal response to intraoperative conversation," *British Journal of Anesthesia,* v. 57, 1985, pp. 174–79.

Chapter 1

1. Nixon, Peter, unpublished research.

2. Austin, John, "Why patients use alternative medicine: results of a national study," *Journal of the American Medical Association,* v. 280, 1998, pp. 1604–9.

3. Burg, MA, et al., "Personal use of alternative medicine therapies by health science center faculty," *Journal of the American Medical Association,* v. 280, 1998, p. 1563.

4. Scheirer, Michael, et al., as reported in *New York Times*, 2/3/87.

5. Lynch, JJ, *The Broken Heart: The Medical Consequences of Loneliness*, Basic Books, 1977.

6. *A.M.A. Medical News*, 10/17/86, p. 50

7. Erickson, M, "Hypnosis in painful terminal illness," *American Journal of Clinical Hypnosis*, v. 1, 1959, pp. 117–21; and Erickson, M, "The interpersonal hypnotic technique for symptom correction and pain control," *American Journal of Clinical Hypnosis*, v. 8, 1966, pp. 198–209.

8. "Helping the dying to live—through hypnosis," *Journal of the American Medical Association*, v. 249, n. 3, 1/21/83, p. 322.

Chapter 2

1. "Hypnotherapy can reduce anxiety, pain of child in medical care," *Family Practice News*, v. 14, n. 21, Nov. 1–14, 1984, p. 56.

2. Cooper, RA, "Tension free dentistry with tension free patients," *Journal of the American Institute of Hypnosis*, v. 116, n. 5, 1975, pp. 227–29.

3. Morse, DR, "Use of a meditative state for hypnotic induction in the practice of endodontics, and oral surgery," *Oral Medicine, Oral Pathology*, v. 41, 1976, pp. 664–72.

4. Monro, Robin, et al., "Yoga research: a bibliography of scientific studies on yoga," Yoga Biomedical Trust, P.O. Box 140, Cambridge, U.K.

5. Udupa, KN, *Disorders of Stress and Their Management by Yoga*, Banares Hindu University Press, 1978, p. 83–93.

6. Agras, W, "Behavioral approaches to the treatment of essential hypertension," *International Journal of Obesity*, v. 5, n. 1, 1981, pp. 173–81.

7. Kuvalayananda, Swami, "Cecal constipation," *Yoga Mimamsa*, v. 1, n. 1, 2, 1924–25, pp. 42–47, 114–25, 201–14; and Parandekar, MN, "Notes on constipation, its causes and cure," *Yoga Mimamsa*, v. 4, n. 4, 1933, pp. 332–37.

8. Meares, A, "What can the cancer patient expect from intensive meditation," *Australian Family Physician*, v. 9, 1980, pp. 322–25.

9. Patel, C, et al., "Controlled trial of biofeedback-aided behavioral methods in reducing mild hypertension," *British Medical Journal*, v. 282, 1981, pp. 2005–8.

10. Mandle, CI, et al., "Relaxation response in femoral angiography," *Radiology*, v. 174, n. 3, pt. 1, 3/90, pp. 737–39.

11. Desiraju, T, et al, "Study of EEG spectra and autonomic parameters of pranayama practitioners," *Indian Journal of Physiology and Pharmacology*, v. 26, n. 5, 1982, pp. 88–89.

12. Monro, Robin, et al., op cit.

13. Benson, H, "The physiology of meditation," *Scientific American*, v. 22, 1972, pp. 84–90.

14. Levine, J, "Pain, placebos, and endorphins," in *The Healing Brain*, Institute for the Advancement of Human Knowledge, Los Altos, California, 1981.

15. Benson, H, et al., "Decreased premature ventricular contractions through use of the relaxation response in patients with stable ischaemic heart disease," *Lancet*, v. 2, n. 7931, 8/75, pp. 380–82.

16. Humor's Healing Powers," *Medical Tribune*, 5/15/89.

17. Rosch, P, personal communication.

18. Acterberg, J, *Imagery in Healing: Shamanism and Modern Medicine*, New Science Library, 1985.

19. Bridge, R, et al., "Relaxation and imagery in the treatment of breast cancer," *British Medical Journal*, v. 297, n. 6657, 11/88, pp. 1169–72.

20. Norris, P, et al., *I Choose Life*, Stillpoint Publishing, 1987.

21. Evans, C, et al., "Improved recovery and reduced postoperative stay after therapeutic sug-

gestions during general anaesthesia," *Lancet*, v. 2, n. 8609, 8/27/88, pp. 491–93.

22. Acolet, D, et al., "Changes in plasma cortisol and catecholamine concentrations in response to massage in pre-term infants," *Archives of Disease in Childhood*, v. 68, 1993, pp. 29–31.

23. Menard, M, "The effect of therapeutic massage on post-surgical outcomes," doctoral thesis, University of Virginia, 1995.

24. Joachim, G, "The effects of two stress management techniques on feelings of well-being in patients with inflammatory bowel disease," *Nursing Papers*, v. 15, 1983, pp. 5–18.

25. Balke, B, et al., "The effects of massage treatment on exercise fatigue," *Clinical Sports Medicine*, v. 1, 1989, pp. 189–96.

26. Kreiger, D, "Relationship of touch with the intent to help or heal subjects' in-vivo hemoglobin values," paper presented to the American Nursing Association, Kansas City, Missouri, 3/21/73.

27. Stevenson, C, "The psychophysiological effects of aromatherapy following cardiac surgery," *Complementary Therapies in Medicine*, v. 2, 1994, pp. 27–35.

28. Dale, A, et al., "The role of lavender oil in relieving personal discomfort following childbirth: a blind randomized clinical trial," *Journal of Advanced Nursing*, v. 19, 1994, pp. 89–96.

29. Guillemain, J, et al., "Neurodepressive effects of the essential oil of lavandula augustifolia," *Annales Pharmaceutiques Françaises*, v. 47, 1989, pp. 337–43.

30. Allen, K, and Blascovich, J, "Effects of music on cardiovascular reactivity among surgeons," *Journal of the American Medical Association*, v. 272, n. 11, 9/21/94, pp. 882–84.

31. Bonny, H, and McCarron, N, "Music as an adjunct to anaesthesia in operative procedures," *Journal of the American Association of Nurse Anesthetists*, 2/84, pp. 55–57.

32. Manson, JE, et al., "A prospective study of walking as compared to vigorous exercise in prevention of coronary disease in women," *New England Journal of Medicine*, v. 341, n. 9, 9/26/99.

33. Hakin, AA, et al., "Effects of walking on mortality among nonsmoking retired men" *New England Journal of Medicine*, v. 338, n. 2, 1998.

34. Spiegel, D, et al., "Effect of psychosocial treatment on survival of patients with metastatic breast cancer," *Lancet*, v. 2, n. 8668, 10/14/89, pp. 888–91.

35. Forester, B, et al., *The American Journal of Psychiatry*, v. 150, 1993, pp. 1700–6.

36. Skelly, Flora J, "Cancer and the mind," *American Medical News*, June 17, 1991.

37. Ibid.

38. Skelly, op. cit.

39. "Research is showing healthful benefits of laughter," *Family Practice News*, 5/15/92, p. 52.

40. Humor's Healing Powers," *Medical Tribune*, 5/15/89.

41. Ibid.

42. Unpublished data; contact www.edencare.com.

43. Zmuda, A, et al, "Experimental atherosclerosis in rabbits," *Prostaglandins*, v. 14, 1977, pp. 1035–41.

44. Adolph, Jonathan, *San Francisco Examiner Magazine*, March/April 1991.

45. "Humor's Healing Powers," op. cit.

46. Dossey, L, *Healing Words*, Harper, San Francisco, 1993.

47. Ibid.

48. Byrd, RC, "Positive therapeutic effects of intercessory prayer in a coronary care unit," *Southern Medical Journal*, v. 81, 7/88, pp. 826–69.

49. Dossey, op. cit.

50. Hankin, JH, et al., "Diet and breast cancer: a review," *American Journal of Clinical Nutrition*, v. 31, 1978, p. 2005.

51. *Diet, Nutrition and Cancer,* National Academy Press, 1982; and Lerner, M, *Choices in Healing,* M.I.T. Press, 1994.

52. Plotnick, G, et al., "Effect of antioxidant vitamins on the transcient impairment of endothelium-dependent brachial artery vasoactivity following a single high-fat meal," *Journal of the American Medical Association,* v. 278, n. 20, 11/26/97, pp. 1682–6.

53. Leakey, Richard, *People of the Lake,* Avon, 1978, p. 96.

54. Ringdorf, VM, et al., "Vitamin C and human wound healing," *Oral Surgery,* v. 53, n. 3, 1982, pp. 231–6.

55. Godfirnon, Manu, O.M.D., unpublished research.

56. Birch, S, et al., *Acupuncture Efficacy: A Summary of Controlled Clinical Trials,* The National Academy of Acupuncture and Oriental Medicine, 7/96.

57. Fox, EJ, et al., "Transcutaneous electrical stimulation and acupuncture: comparison of treatment for low-back pain, *Pain,* v. 2, 1976, pp. 141–48.

58. Coan, RM, et al., "The acupuncture treatment of neck pain: a randomized controlled study," *American Journal of Chinese Medicine,* v. 9, 1982, pp. 326–32.

59. Tsuei, JJ, et al., "Induction of labour by acupuncture and electrical stimulation," *Obstetrics and Gynaecology,* v. 43, 1974, pp. 337–42.

60. *Advances in Acupuncture and Acupuncture Anesthesia,* The People's Medical Publishing House, 1979.

61. Birch, S, et al., *Acupuncture Efficacy: A Summary of Controlled Clinical Trials,* The National Academy of Acupuncture and Oriental Medicine, 7/96.

62. Christensen, P, "Electro-acupuncture and post-operative pain," *British Journal of Anesthesia,* v. 62, 1989, pp. 258–62.

63. Knapman, J, "Controlling emesis after chemotherapy," *Nursing Standard,* v. 7, 1993, pp. 38–39.

64. Huang, X, "The treatment of 114 cases of chemotherapeutic leucopenia by cone moxibustion," *Journal of Chinese Medicine,* v. 44, 1994, pp. 22–23.

65. Schneider, et al., "Health promotion with a traditional system of natural health care," *Journal of Social Behavior and Personality,* v. 5, n. 3, 1990, pp. 1–27.

66. Miller, N, "Learning of visceral and glandular responses," *Science,* v. 163, 1969, pp. 434–45.

67. Schwartz, MS, *Biofeedback—A Practitioner's Guide,* Guilford Press, 1987.

68. Patel, C, et al., "Controlled trial of biofeedback-aided behavioral methods in reducing mild hypertension," *British Medical Journal,* v. 282, 1981, pp. 2005–8.

69. Fahrion, S, et al., "Biobehavioral treatment of essential hypertension: a group outcome study," *Biofeedback Self Regulation,* v. 11, 1991, pp. 257–77.

70. Basmajian, JV, et al., "Biofeedback treatment of foot-drop after stroke compared with standard rehabilitation technique: effects on voluntary control and strength," *Archives of Physical Medicine and Rehabilitation,* v. 56, 1975, pp. 231–36; and Basmajian, JV, "Biofeedback: the clinical tool behind the catchword," *Modern Medicine,* 10/1/1976.

71. Altmaier, EM, et al., "The effectiveness of psychological interventions for the rehabilitation of low-back pain: a randomized controlled trial evaluation," *Pain,* v. 49, 1981, pp. 329–35.

72. Sharpless, S, "Susceptibility of spinal roots to compression block," in Goldstein, M, *The Research Status of Spinal Manipulation,* Government Printing Office, nd.

73. Brennan, PC, et al., "Enhanced phagocytic cell respiratory burst induced by spinal manipulation: potential role of substance p," *Journal of Manipu-*

lative *Physiology and Therapy,* v. 14, 1991, pp. 399–408.

74. *Canadian Family Physician,* March 1995.

75. "Some M.D.'s back chiropractic," *Medical Tribune,* 6/28/90, p. 16.

76. Personal communication.

77. *New York Times,* 1/9/85.

78. Bowers, KS, *Hypnosis for the Seriously Curious,* Brooks/Cole Publishing, 1976.

79. Ewin, DM, "Condyloma acuminatum: successful treatment of four cases by hypnosis," *American Journal of Clinical Hypnosis,* v. 17, 1974, pp. 73–78.

80. Jabush, MA, "A case of chronic recurring multiple boils treated with hypnotherapy," *Psychiatric Quarterly,* v. 43, 1969, pp. 448–55.

81. Lenox, J, "Effect of hypnotic analgesia on verbal report and cardiovascular responses to ischemic pain," *Journal of Abnormal Psychology,* v. 7, 1970, pp. 199–206.

82. Clawson, TA, et al., "The hypnotic control of blood flow and pain: the cure of warts and the potential for the use of hypnosis in the treatment of cancer," *American Journal of Clinical Hypnosis,* v. 17, 1975, p. 1609.

83. Erickson, MH, "Hypnosis in painful terminal illness," *American Journal of Clinical Hypnosis,* v. 1, 1959, pp. 117–21.

84. "Hypnosis gains legitimacy, respect, in diverse clinical specialties," *Journal of the American Medical Association,* v. 249, n. 3, 1/21/83, pp. 319–23.

85. Ibid, p. 320.

86. Bowers, op. cit.

87. Santiesteban, A. Joseph, et al., "Post-surgical effect of pulsed shortwave therapy," *Journal of the American Podiatric Medical Association,* v. 75, n. 6, 6/1985, pp. 306–9.

88. "Device may ease osteoarthritis," *Medical Tribune,* 2/11/93, p. 12.

89. Walford, Roy, *Maximum Life Span,* Avon, 1983.

90. Ibid.

Chapter 3

1. "Second Opinion Elective Surgery Consultation Program; Prepared Testimony," U.S. House of Representatives, as cited in Christian, R, et al., *Surgery and Its Alternatives,* Rodale Press, 1980, p. 28.

2. Berger, Stuart, *What Your Doctor Didn't Learn in Medical School,* William Morrow, 1988, p. 84.

3. Christian, R, et al., op. cit., p. 55.

4. Ibid.

5. Andrews, Edson, "Moon talk: the cyclic periodicity of postoperative hemorrhage," *Journal of the Florida Medical Association,* v. 46, n. 11, 1960, p. 1366.

6. Rhyne, WP, "Spontaneous hemorrhage," *Journal of the Medical Association of Georgia,* v. 55, n. 12, 1966, pp. 505–6.

7. Hackler, T, "That ol' devil moon," *Milwaukee Journal, Sunday Magazine,* March 18, 1979, p. 52.

8. Hagen, A, and Hrushesky, W, "Menstrual timing of breast cancer surgery," *The American Journal of Surgery,* v. 173, n. 3, 1998, pp. 245–61.

9. Begg, C, et al., "Impact of hospital volume on operative mortality for major cancer surgery," *Journal of the American Medical Association,* v. 280, 1998, pp. 1747–51.

10. Dodley, RA, et al., "Selective referral to high-volume hospitals: estimating potentially avoidable deaths" *Journal of the American Medical Association,* v. 283, n. 9, 3/1/00.

11. Begg, et al., op. cit.

12. Himmelstein, DU, et al., "Quality of care in investor-owned vs not-for-profit HMOs," *Journal of the American Medical Association,* v. 282, n. 2, 7/14/99.

Chapter 4

1. Nolen, W, *A Surgeon Under the Knife,* Coward, McCann, Geoghegan, 1976.

2. Janik, Carol, Carnegie-Mellon research team, unpublished research.

3. Wilson, LM, "Intensive care delerium," *Archives of Internal Medicine,* v. 130, 1972, pp. 225–26.

4. Peterson, R, et al., "The effects of furniture arrangement on the behavior of geriatric patients," *Behavioral Therapy,* v. 8, 1977, pp. 464–67.

5. Melin, L, et al., "The effects of rearranging ward routines on communication and eating behaviors of psychogeriatric patients," *Journal of Applied Behavioral Analysis,* v. 14, 1981, pp. 47–51.

6. Harris, CS, et al., "A comparison of the effects of hard rock and easy listening on the frequency of observed inappropriate behaviors: control of environmental antecedents in a large public area," *Journal of Music Therapy,* v. 29, 1992, pp. 6–17.

7. Baker, CF, "Discomfort to environmental noise: heart rate response of SICU patients, *Critical Care Nursing Quarterly,* v. 15, n. 2, 8/15/92, pp. 75–90.

8. Greer, Steven, King's College, England, as noted in Lerner, Michael, *Choices in Healing,* MIT Press, 1994, p. 339.

9. Ulrich, Roger S., "View through a window may influence recovery from surgery," *Science,* v. 224, n. 4647, 4/27/84, pp. 420–21.

10. Ulrich, Roger S, "Natural versus urban scenes: some psychophysiological effects," *Environment and Behavior,* v. 18, n. 5, 1981, pp. 523–56.

11. Kulik, et al., research at University of California at San Diego, as reported in "Surgery: safety in hindsight," *American Health,* 9/86, p. 22.

12. Egbert, LD, et al., "The value of the preoperative visit by an anesthesiologist," *Journal of the American Medical Association,* v. 185, 1963, pp. 553–55.

13. Egbert, LD, et al., "The value of the preoperative visit by an anesthesiologist," *Journal of the American Medical Association,* v. 185, 1963, pp. 553–55.

14. "Epidural increases risks of chronic back pain, Cesarean section," *Family Practice News,* 9/15/94, p. 14.

15. "General anesthesia in Cesareans 'major cause' of maternal death," *Family Practice News,* v. 20, n. 19.

16. Goldsmith, M, "As better training and machines improve safety, speed becomes focus of newest anesthetic drugs," *Journal of the American Medical Association,* v. 267, n. 12, 1/25/92, pp. 1576–78.

17. *Medical Tribune,* v. 28, n. 2, 1/14/87, p. 1.

18. Katz, J, "A survey of anesthetic choice among anesthesiologists," *Anesthesia and Analgesia,* v. 52, n. 3, 5/6/73, pp. 373–75.

19. Zharkin, N, "Acupuncture in obstetrics," *Journal of Chinese Medicine,* v. 33, 1990, pp. 10–13.

20. "Hypnosis: up-and-coming anesthesia alternative," *Cortlandt Forum,* 4/93.

21. Lang, EV, et al., "Adjunctive non-pharmacological analgesia for invasive medical procedures: a randomized trial" *Lancet,* v. 355, 4/29/00, pp. 1486–90.

22. "Hypnosis: up-and-coming anesthesia alternative," op. cit.

23. Werbel, E, *One Surgeon's Experience with Hypnosis,* Pageant Press, 1965.

24. August, Ralph V, *Hypnosis in Obstetrics,* McGraw Hill, 1961.

25. Ibid.

26. Selzer, Richard, *Confessions of a Knife,* Simon & Schuster, 1979, pp. 15–21.

27. Frank, S, et al., "Perioperative maintenance of normothermia reduces the incidence of morbid cardiac events, *Journal of the American Medical Association,* v. 277, n. 14, 4/9/97, pp. 1127–34.

28. Melling, AC, et al., "Effects of preoperative warming on the incidence of wound infection after clean surgery: a randomized study," *Lancet,* v. 358, 9/01, pp. 876–80.

29. Allen, K, et al., "Effects of music on cardiovascular reactivity among surgeons," *Journal of the American Medical Association,* v. 272, 1994, pp. 882–84.

30. Ornstein, R, and Sobel, D, *Healthy Pleasures,* Addison-Wesley, 1989.

31. Bennet, HL, et al., "Non-verbal response to intraoperative conversation," *British Journal of Anesthesiology,* v. 57, 1985, pp. 174–79.

32. Bennett, H, "Behavioral anesthesia," *Advances,* v. 2, n. 4, fall 1985, pp. 11–21.

33. Woodham, A, et al., *Encyclopedia of Healing Therapies,* Dorling Kindersley, 1997, p. 231.

34. Albertini, H, et al., "Homeopathic treatment of dental neuralgia using arnica and hypericum: a summary of 60 observations," *Journal of the American Institute of Homeopathy,* v. 78, 9/85, pp. 126–28.

35. Christensen, PA, et al., "Electroacupuncture and postoperative pain," *British Journal of Anesthesia,* v. 62, 1989, pp. 258–62; also Martelete, M, et al., "Comparative study of the analgesic effect of transcutaneous nerve stimulation (TNS), electroacupuncture (EA) and meperidine in the treatment of postoperative pain," *Acupuncture Electro-Therapeutic Research Journal,* v. 10, 1985, pp. 183–93.

36. Lao, Lixing, "Placebo-controlled clinical acupuncture study on postoperative oral surgery pain," presented at the Sixth Meeting of the Alternative Medicine Program Advisory Council, National Institutes of Health, June 13–14, 1996.

37. Menard, M, "The effect of therapeutic massage on post-surgical outcomes," doctoral thesis, University of Virginia, August 1995.

38. Mills, W, et al., "The transcendental meditation technique and acute experimental pain," *Psychosomatic Medicine,* v. 43, n. 2, 1981, pp. 157–64.

39. Sutcliff, JP, "'Credulous' and 'skeptical' views of hypnotic phenomena: experiments on esthesia, hallucination, and delusion," *Journal of Abnormal Psychology,* v. 76, 1970, pp. 260–66.

40. Blanfield, RP, et al., "Taped therapeutic suggestions and taped music as adjuncts in the care of coronary-artery-bypass patients," *American Journal of Clinical Hypnosis,* v. 37, n. 5, 1995, pp. 32–42.

41. Loesin, RG, et al., "The effect of music on the pain of selected postoperative patients," *ANOPHI Papers,* 1979, pp. 1–10.

42. Menegazzi, JJ, et al., "A randomized controlled trial of the use of music during laceration repair," *Annals of Emergency Medicine,* v. 20, 1991, pp. 348–50.

43. Moss, VA, "Music and the surgical patient; the effect of music on anxiety," *American Organization of Registered Nurses Journal,* v. 48, n. 1, 1988, pp. 64–69.

44. Geden, E, et al., "Effects of music and imagery on physiologic and self-report of analogued labor pain," *Nursing Research,* v. 38, n. 1, 1–2/89, pp. 37–41.

45. Williamson, J, "The effects of ocean sounds on sleep after coronary artery bypass graft surgery," *American Journal of Critical Care,* v. 1, 1992, pp. 91–97.

46. Seltzer, S, et al., "Perspectives in the control of chronic pain by nutritional manipulation," *Pain,* v. 11, n. 2, 10/81, pp. 141–48.

47. Sharma, VD, et al., "Antibacterial property of

allium sativum linn: in vivo and in vitro studies," *Indian Journal of Experimental Biology*, v. 15, n. 6, 1977, pp. 466–68.

Chapter 5

1. Reilly, Harold, et al., *The Edgar Cayce Handbook for Health Through Drugless Therapy*, Macmillan, 1975, p. 312.

2. "Wrinkle cream found helpful against cancer," *Hippocrates*, 9/93, p. 24.

3. Bollag, W, et al., "Vitamin A acid in benign and malignant epithelial tumours of the skin," *Acta Dermato-Venereologica*, supp. 74, 1/27/75, pp. 163–66.

4. Stahelin, HB, et al., *Journal of the National Cancer Institute*, v. 73, 11/84, p. 1463.

5. Ahser, R, "Respectable hypnosis," *British Medical Journal*, v. 1, 1956, pp. 309–13.

6. Frank, SB, "Dietary fat may be associated with excess sebum production," in *Acne Vulgaris*, Charles C Thomas, 1971, pp. 66–72.

7. Kaufman, WF, "The diet and acne," *Archives of Dermatology*, v. 119, n. 4, 1983, p. 276.

8. McGarey, William, *The Oil That Heals*, A.R.E. Press, 1993, p. 217.

9. Hubler, WR, "Unsaturated fatty acids in acne," *Archives of Dermatology*, v. 79, 1959, p. 644.

10. Bowers, Kenneth, *Hypnosis for the Seriously Curious*, Brooks/Cole Publishing, 1976, p. 141.

11. Duchateau, J, et al., "Influence of oral zinc supplementation on the lymphocyte response to mitogens of normal subjects," *American Journal of Clinical Nutrition*, v. 34, 1981, pp. 72–74.

12. Holman, D, Western Australia Health Department, Epidemiology Branch.

13. "Low-fat diet may cut keratosis rate," *Medical Tribune*, 3/19/94.

14. Quillin, Patrick, *Healing Nutrients*, Vintage Books, 1987, p. 136.

15. Keane, Maureen, et al., *What to Eat If You Have Cancer*, Contemporary Books, 1996, p. 169.

16. Belman, S, "Onion and garlic oil inhibit tumor growth," *Carcinogenesis*, v. 4, n. 8, 1983, p. 1063.

17. Ahser, R, op. cit.

18. McGarey, William, *The Oil That Heals*, A.R.E. Press, 1993, p. 217.

19. "Acne drug seen as cancer blocker," *Medical World News*, 12/12/88.

20. Ibid.

21. Adler, Psychoneuroimmunology, Academic Press, 1981.

22. Simonton, Carl, *Getting Well Again*, Bantam Books, 1980.

23. "Interferon shows promise in basal cell carcinoma," *Family Practice News*, 10/15/92.

24. Jemal, A, et al., "Cancer statistics, 2002," *CA: A Cancer Journal for Clinicians (2002)*, v. 52, n. 1, pp. 23–47.

25. Stern, R, "Malignant melanoma in patients treated for psoriasis with Methaxsalen (psoralen) and ultraviolet radiation (PUVA). The PUVA follow-up study," *New England Journal of Medicine*, v. 336, n. 15, 4/10/97, pp. 1041–45.

26. Ries, LAG, et al., eds., *SEER Cancer Statistics Review, 1973–1998*, National Cancer Institute, 2001.

27. "Vitamin B_6 for melanoma?," *Medical World News*, 2/11/85; Reynolds, Robert D, "Vitamin B_6 deficiency and carcinogenesis," in Poirier, LA, et al., eds, *Essential Nutrients in Carcinogenesis*, 1985, pp. 339–45.

28. Hanck, "Vitamin C and cancer," in Tryfiates and Prasad, eds, *Nutrition, Growth and Cancer*, p. 310.

29. Page, Linda, *Healthy Healing*, Healthy Healing Publications, 1997, pp. 132–33.

30. Mobrey, Daniel, *The Scientific Validation of Herbal Medicine*, Cormorant Books, 1986.

31. Greer, et al., *Psychological Concomitants of Cancer,* p. 568.

32. Fawzy, IF, et al., "Malignant melanoma: effects of early structured psychiatric intervention, coping, and affective state on recurrence and survival six years later," *Archives of General Psychiatry,* v. 50, 9/93.

33. Simonton, Carl, *Getting Well Again,* Bantam Books, 1980.

34. Kirkwood, J, et al., "Interferon alfa-2b adjuvant therapy of high-risk resected cutaneous melanoma: the Eastern Cooperative Oncology Group Trial EST 1684," *Journal of Clinical Oncology,* v. 17, 1996, pp. 7–17.

35. Kirkwood, JM, et al., "Preliminary analysis of the E1690/S9111/C9190 intergroup postoperative adjuvant trial of high- and low-dose IFN-2b (HDI and LDI) in high risk primary or lymph node metastatic melanoma," *Proceeding of the American Society of Clinical Oncologists,* v. 18, abstract 2072, 1998.

36. Holder, WD, et al., "Effectiveness of positron emission tomography for the dectection of melanoma metastasis," *Annals of Surgery,* v. 227, n. 5, 5/1998, pp. 764–71.

Chapter 6

1. Mennella, JA, Transfer of alcohol to human milk—effects on flavor and the infant's behavior," *New England Journal of Medicine,* v. 325, n. 14, 1992, p. 981.

2. Mennella, JA, and Beauchamp, GK, "Smoking and the flavor of breast milk," *New England Journal of Medicine,* v. 339, n. 21, p. 1559.

3. Unpublished research.

4. Willard, RD, "Breast enlargement through visual imagery and hypnosis," *American Journal of Clinical Hypnosis,* v. 19, n. 4, 1977, p. 195.

5. Gabriel, S, et al., "Complications leading to

surgery after breast implantation," *New England Journal of Medicine,* v. 336, 3/97, pp. 677–82.

6. Noone, RB, "A review of the possible health implications of silicone breast implants," *Cancer,* v. 79, n. 9, 5/97, pp. 1747–56.

7. Janowsky, EC, et al., "Meta-analysis of the relation between silicone breast implants and the risk of connective-tissue diseases" *New England Journal of Medicine,* v. 342, n. 11, 3/16/00.

8. Sanchez-Guerrero, J, et al., "Silicone breast implants and the risk of connective tissue diseases and symptoms," *New England Journal of Medicine,* v. 332, n. 25, 6/95, pp. 1666–70.

9. Ferguson, JH, "Silicone breast implants and neurologic disorders," Report of the Practice Committee of the American Academy of Neurology, *Neurology,* v. 48, 3/97, pp. 1504–7.

10. Foster, RS, et al., "Clinical breast examination and breast self-examination: past and present effect on breast cancer survival," *Cancer,* v. 69, n. 7, 4/92, pp. 1992–98.

11. Antman, K, and Shea, S, "Screening mammography under age 50," *Journal of the American Medical Association,* v. 281, n. 16, 4/28/99, pp. 1505–11.

12. "Health United States 1994," National Center for Health Statistics, Hyattsville, MD: Public Health Service, 1995, p. 4.

13. Freer, Timothy, as reported at the Radiology Society of America annual meeting, Chicago, 11/29/00.

14. Elmore, JG, et al., "Ten-year risk of false-positive screening mammograms and clinical breast exams," *New England Journal of Medicine,* v. 338, n. 16, 1998, pp. 1089–96.

15. Fletcher, SW, et al., "Report of the International Workshop on Screening for Breast Cancer," *Journal of the National Cancer Institute,* v. 85, 1993, pp. 1644–56.

16. Smart, CR, et al., "Benefit of mammography screening in women ages 40 to 49: current evi-

dence from randomized controlled trials," *Cancer,* v. 75, n. 7, 4/1/95, pp. 1619–26.

17. Sickles, EA, "Probably benign breast lesions: when should follow-up be recommended and what is the optimal follow-up protocol?," *Radiology,* v. 213, 1999, pp. 11–14.

18. Velanovich, V, et al., "Comparison of mammographically guided breast biopsy techniques," *Annals of Surgery,* v. 229, n. 5, 1999, pp. 625–33.

19. Smith, DN, et al., "Large-core needle biopsy of non-palpable breast cancers: the impact on subsequent surgical excisions," *Archives of Surgery,* v. 132, 1997, pp. 256–59.

20. Parker, S, et al., "Percutaneous large-core breast biopsy: a multi-institutional study," *Radiology,* v. 193, n. 2, 11/94, pp. 359–64.

21. Bundred, NJ, et al., "Smoking and periductal mastitis," *British Medical Journal,* v. 307, 1993, pp. 772–73.

22. Minton, JP, et al., "Clinical and biochemical studies on methylxanthine-related fibrocystic breast disease," *Surgery,* v. 90, 1981, p. 299.

23. Sharma, AK, et al., "Cyclical mastalgia—is it a manifestation of aberration in lipid metabolism?" *Indian Journal of Physiology and Pharmacology,* v. 38, 1994, pp. 267–71.

24. Abrams, AA, "Use of vitamin E in chronic cystic mastitis," *New England Journal of Medicine,* v. 272, n. 1065, 1960, p. 1080.

25. London, RS, et al., "Endocrine parameters and alpha-tocopherol therapy of patients with mammary dysplasia," *Cancer Research,* v. 41, 1981, p. 3811.

26. Abraham, G, et al., "Effect of vitamin B_6 on premenstrual symptomatology in women with premenstrual tension syndrome: A double-blind crossover study," *Infertility,* v. 3, n. 2, 1980, pp. 155–65.

27. Pashby, NL, et al., "A clinical trial of evening primrose oil in mastalgia," *British Journal of Surgery,* v. 68, 1981, p. 801.

28. "Medical Care News," *Prevention Magazine,* 11/87, p. 21.

29. "My Turn: A scar I did not want to hide," *Newsweek,* 3/21/94, p. 16.

30. Jemal, A, et al., "Cancer Statistics, 2002," *CA: A Cancer Journal for Clinicians (2002),* v. 52, n. 1, pp. 23–47.

31. "Health United States 1994," op. cit., p. 3.

32. Gregorio, DI, "Dietary fat consumption and survival among women with breast cancer," *Journal of the National Cancer Institute,* v. 75, n. 1, 1986, pp. 37–41.

33. Wingo, PA, et al., "Age-specific differences in the relationship between oral contraceptive use and breast cancer," *Obstetrics and Gynecology,* v. 78, 1991, pp. 161–70.

34. Neugut, AI, and Jacobson, JS, "The limitations of breast cancer screening for first-degree relatives of breast cancer patients," *American Journal of Public Health,* v. 85, 1995, pp. 832–34.

35. Frost, MH, "Long-term satisfaction and psychological and social function following bilateral prophylactic mastectomy," *Journal of the American Medical Association,* v. 284, n. 3, 7/19/00.

36. Lewis, M, et al., "Breast cancer risk and residence near industry or traffic in Nassau and Suffolk Counties, Long Island, New York," *Archives of Environmental Health,* v. 51, n. 4, 7/96, pp. 255–65.

37. "Local physicist suspects link between radon, breast cancer," *The Maryland Gazette,* 11/9/94, p. A18.

38. Schatzkin, A, et al., "The dietary fat–breast cancer hypothesis is alive," *Journal of the American Medical Association,* v. 261, n. 22, 6/89, pp. 3284–87.

39. Hill, DK, et al., "Lessons learned from 500 cases of lymphatic mapping for breast cancer," *Annals of Surgery*, v. 229, n. 4, 1999, pp. 528–35.

40. Cox, CE, "Guidelines for sentinel node bopsy and lymphatic mapping of patients with breast cancer," *Annals of Surgery*, v. 227, n. 5, 1998, pp. 645–53.

41. Ries, LAG, et al., eds., *SEER Cancer Statistics Review, 1973–1998*, National Cancer Institute, 2001.

42. Hunter, DJ, et al., "Cohort studies of fat intake and the risk of breast cancer—a pooled alalysis," *New England Journal of Medicine*, v. 334, n. 6, 6/96, pp. 356–61.

43. Austin, Steven, et al., *Breast Cancer*, Prima Publishing, 1994.

44. Schatzkin, loc. cit.; *Diet, Nutrition and Cancer*, National Academy Press, 1982, p. 17.

45. Carroll, KK, et al., "Dietary fat and mammary cancer," *Canadian Medical Association Journal*, v. 98, 1968, pp. 590–93.

46. Howe, GR, et al., "A cohort study of fat intake and risk of breast cancer," *Journal of the National Cancer Institute*, v. 83, n. 5, 3/91, pp. 336–40.

47. Howe, GR, et al., "Dietary factors and risk of breast cancer: combined analysis of 12 case-controlled studies," *Journal of the National Cancer Institute*, v. 82, n. 7, 4/90, pp. 561–69.

48. Phillips, RL, "Role of life-style and dietary habits among Seventh-Day Adventists," *Cancer Research*, v. 35, 1975, pp. 3513–22.

49. Wynder, EL, et al., "A rationale for dietary intervention in the treatment of post-menopausal breast cancer patients," *Nutrition and Cancer*, v. 3, n. 4, 1982, pp. 195–99.

50. Gregorio, DI, "Dietary fat consumption and survival among women with breast cancer," *Journal of the National Cancer Institute*, v. 75, n. 1, 1986, pp. 37–41.

51. "Low-fat, high-fiber diet improves post-breast cancer immune function," *Family Practice News*, 2/1/95.

52. Rohan, TE, et al., "Dietary fiber, vitamins A, C, and E and risk of breast cancer: a cohort study," *Cancer Causes Control*, v. 4, n. 1, 1/93, pp. 29–37.

53. Rose, D, of the American Health Foundation, Valhalla, NY, as reported in *Redbook*, 4/92, p. 27.

54. Lee, HP, "Dietary effects of breast-cancer risk in Singapore," *Lancet*, v. 337, 1991, pp. 1197–1200.

55. Messina, M, et al., "The role of soy products in reducing risk of cancer," *Journal of the National Cancer Institute*, v. 83, 1992, pp. 1233.

56. Adlercreutz, H, et al., "Dietary phytoestrogens and the menopause in Japan," *Lancet*, v. 339, 1992, p. 1233.

57. Howe, GR, et al., "Dietary factors and risk of breast cancer: combined analysis of 12 case-controlled studies," *Journal of the National Cancer Institute*, v. 82, n. 7, 4/90, pp. 561–69.

58. Willett, W, and Hunter, D, "Vitamin A and cancers of the breast, large bowel, and prostate: epidemiologic evidence," *Nutrition Review*, v. 52, n. 2, pt 2, 2/94, pp. S53–59.

59. "Eggs implicated in breast cancer," *Medical Tribune*, 3/11/91, p. 24.

60. Horowitz, Len, unpublished data.

61. Longnecker, MP, "Alcoholic beverage consumption in relation to risk of breast cancer: meta-analysis and review, *Cancer Causes Control*, v. 5, 1994, pp. 73–82.

62. Friedenreich, CM, et al., "A cohort study of alcohol consumption and risk of breast cancer," *Cancer Causes and Control*, v. 4, n. 1, 1993, pp. 29–37.

63. "Even social drinking may raise lifetime risk of breast cancer," *Family Practice News*, 12/1/93, p. 12.

64. Lubin, JH, et al., Breast cancer following high dietary fat and protein consumption," *American Journal of Epidemiology*, v. 114, 1981, p. 422.

65. Wolff, MS, et al., "Blood levels of organochlorine residues and risk of breast cancer," *Journal of the National Cancer Institute*, v. 85, n. 8, 4/93, pp. 648–52.

66. Falck, F, et al., "Pesticides and polychlorinated biphenyl residues in human breast lipids and their relation to breast cancer," *Archives of Environmental Health*, v. 47, 1992, pp. 143–46.

67. Lewis, MEL, et al., "Breast cancer risk and residence near industry or traffic in Nassau and Suffolk Counties, Long Island, New York," *Archives of Environmental Health*, v. 51, n. 4, 7/96, pp. 255–65.

68. Rohan, TE, et al., "A population-based case-control study of diet and breast cancer in Australia," *American Journal of Epidemiology*, v. 128, 1988, pp. 478–79; and Graham, S, et al., "Diet in the epidemiology of breast cancer," *American Journal of Epidemiology*, v. 116, 1982, pp. 68–75.

69. Greenwald, Peter, "Principles of cancer prevention: diet and nutrition," in DeVita, Vincent, ed, *Cancer: Principles and Practice of Oncology*, Lippincott, 1989, p.169.

70. Lerner, Michael, *Choices in Healing*, MIT Press, 1994.

71. Kandil, OM, "Garlic and the immune system in humans: its effect on natural killer cells," *Federal Proceedings*, v. 46, n. 3, 1987, p. 441.

72. Lin, X, et al., "Dietary garlic powder sulte in vivo formation of DNA adducts induced by N-nitroso compounds in liver and mammary tissues," *Federation of American Society for Experimental Biology Journal*, v. 6, 1992, p. A1392.

73. "Lavender, orange oils tried for cancer," *Medical Tribune*, 6/10/93, p. 13.

74. Silverstein, P, "Smoking and wound healing," *American Journal of Medicine*, v. 93, suppl. 1A, 7/92, pp. 22S–24S.

75. Cooper, CL, ed, *Stress and Breast Cancer*, Wiley, 1988.

76. Meares, A, "What can the cancer patient expect from intensive meditation," *Australian Family Physician*, v. 9, 1980, p. 32205.

77. Brown, Daniel, et al., *Hypnosis and Behavioral Medicine*, Lawrence Erlbaum, 1987, p. 137.

78. Greer, S, et al., "Psychological attributes of women who develop breast cancer: a controlled study," *Journal of Psychosomatic Research*, v. 19, 1975, pp.147–53.

79. Mitchell, E, et al., "Principles of combining biomodulators with cytotoxic agents in vivo," *Seminars in Oncology*, v. 19, n. 2, suppl. 4, 4/92, pp. 51–56.

80. Kiecolt, Jancie, et al., "Stress and immune function in humans," in Ader, Robert, et al., *Psychoneuroimmunology*, pp. 789–90.

81. Simonton, OC, et al., "Psychological intervention in the treatment of cancer," *Psychosomatics*, v. 21. 1980, pp. 226–33.

82. Spiegel, David, et al., "Effect of psychosocial treatment on survival of patients with metastatic breast cancer," *Lancet*, v. 2, n. 8668, 10/14/89, pp. 888–91.

83. Spiegel, D, et al., "Effects of medical and psychotherapeutic treatment on the survival of women with metastatic breast cancer," *Journal of American Cancer Society*, v. 80, n. 2, 7/97, pp. 225–30.

84. Greer, S, "Psychological response to cancer and survival," *Psycological Medicine*, v. 21, 1991, pp. 43–49.

85. *Physical Activity and Health: A Report of the Surgeon General*, U.S. Department of Health and Human Services, Centers for Disease Control and Prevention, Atlanta, GA, p. 124.

86. Frisch, R, et al., "Lower prevalence of breast cancer and cancers of the reproductive system among former college athletes compared to non-athletes, *British Journal of Cancer,* v. 52, 1985, pp. 885–91.

87. Bernstein, I, et al., "Physical exercise and reduced risk of breast cancer in young women," *Journal of the National Cancer Institute,* v. 86, 1996, pp. 1403–8.

88. "Physical activity and risk of breast cancer," *New England Journal of Medicine,* v. 336, n. 18, 5/1/97.

89. Bastarrachea, J, et al., "Obesity as an adverse prognostic factor for patients receiving adjuvant chemotherapy for breast cancer," *Annals of Internal Medicine,* v. 120, n. 1, 1994, pp. 18–25.

90. deWaard, F., "Breast cancer incidence and nutritional status with particular reference to body weight and height," *Cancer Research,* v. 35, 1975, pp. 3351–56.

91. Newcomb, PA, et al., "Lactation and a reduced risk of premenopausal breast cancer" *New England Journal of Medicine,* v. 330, 1994, pp. 81–87.

92. Daling, JR, et al., "Risk of breast cancer among young women: relationship to induced abortion," *Journal of the National Cancer Institute,* v. 86, n. 21, 11/94, pp. 1569–70.

93. Rookus, MA, and van Leeuwen, FE, "Induced abortion and risk for breast cancer: reporting (recall) bias in a Dutch case-control study," *Journal of the National Cancer Institute,* v. 88, n. 23, 11/96, pp. 1759–64.

94. Collaborative Group on Hormonal Factors in Breast Cancer, "Breast cancer and hormonal contraceptives: collaborative reanalysis of individual data on 53,297 women with breast cancer and 100,239 women without breast cancer from 54 epidemiological studies, *Lancet,* v. 347, 6/11/96, pp. 1713–27.

95. Grabeck, DM, et al., "Risk of breast cancer with oral contraceptive use in women with a family history of breast cancer," *Journal of the American Medical Association,* v. 284, n. 14, 10/11/00.

96. Colditz, GA, et al., "The use of estrogens and progestins and the risk of breast cancer in postmenopausal women," *New England Journal of Medicine,* v. 332, n. 24, 6/15/95, pp. 1589–93.

97. Colditz, GA, et al., "Use of estrogen plus progestin is associated with greater increase in breast cancer risk than estrogen alone," *American Journal of Epidemiology,* v. 1998, n. 147 (suppl), p. 64S.

98. Colditz, GA, et al., *New England Journal of Medicine,* v. 333, n. 20, 11/16/95, p. 1358, in response to correspondence regarding their article: "The use of estrogens and progestins and the risk of breast cancer in postmenopausal women," *New England Journal of Medicine,* v. 332, n. 24, 6/15/95, pp. 1589–93.

99. Singer, S, and Grismaijer, S, *Dressed to Kill,* Avery Publishing Group, 1995.

100. Hseih, C, and Tricholopoulos, D, "Breast size, handedness and breast cancer risk," *European Journal of Cancer,* v. 27, n. 2, 1991, pp. 131–35.

101. *Newsweek,* 2/21/94, p. 15.

102. Austin, Steven, et al., *Breast Cancer,* Prima Publishing, 1994.

103. "The Hodgkin's–breast cancer relationship," *Coping,* (1–2/95), p.16.

104. "Vena, JE, "Electric blankets appear to increase risk of breast cancer," *American Family Physician,* 10/90, p. 1065.

105. CancerNet, from the National Cancer Institute, 6/97.

106. "Badwe, RA, et al., "Timing of surgery during menstrual cycle and survival of premenopausal women with operable breast cancer," *Lancet,* v. 337, 5/25/91, pp. 1261–64.

107. Fisher, B, et al., "Eight-year results of a randomized clinical trial comparing total mastectomy and lumpectomy with or without irradiation in the treatment of breast cancer," *New England Journal of Medicine,* v. 320, 1989, pp. 822–28.

108. Fisher, B, et al., "Significance of ipsilateral breast tumor recurrence after lumpectomy," *Lancet,* v. 338, 1991, pp. 327–31.

109. Fisher, B, et al., "Reanalysis and results after 12 years of follow-up in a randomized clinical trial comparing total mastectomy with lumpectomy with or without irradiation in the treatment of breast cancer," *New England Journal of Medicine,* v. 333, n. 22, 1995, pp. 1456–61.

110. Nemoto, T, et al., "Factors affecting recurrence in lumpectomy without irradiation for breast cancer," *Cancer,* v. 67, 1991, pp. 2079–82.

111. Frykberg, E, and Bland, K, "Management of in situ and minimally invasive breast carcinoma," *World Journal of Surgery,* v. 18, n. 1, 1–2/94, pp. 45–57.

112. Hetelekidis, S, et al., "Management of Ductal Carcinoma in Situ," *CA: A Cancer Journal for Clinicians,* v. 45, n. 4, 7–8/95, pp. 244–53.

113. Silverstein, MD, et al., "Influence of margin width on local control of ductal carcinoma in situ of the breast," *New England Journal of Medicine,* v. 340, n. 19, 1999.

114. Silverstein, MJ, et al., Axillary lymph node dissection for T1a breast carcinoma: is it indicated?" *Cancer,* v. 73, 1994, pp. 664–67.

115. Maibenco, D, et al., "Axillary lymph node metastases associated with small invasive breast carcinomas," *Cancer,* v. 85, 1999, pp. 1530–36.

116. Greco, M, et al., "Breast cancer patients treated without axillary surgery: clinical implications and biologic analysis," *Annals of Surgery,* v. 232, n. 1, 7/00, pp. 1–7.

117. Cox, CE, "Guidelines for sentinel node biopsy and lymphatic mapping of patients with breast cancer," *Annals of Surgery,* v. 227, n. 5, 5/1998, pp. 645–53.

118. Cody, HS III, et al., "Credentialing for breast lymphatic mapping: how many cases are enough?," *Annals of Surgery,* v. 229, n. 5, 1999, pp. 723–28.

119. Guiliano, AE, et al., "Improved staging of breast cancer with sentinel lymphadenectomy," *Annals of Surgery,* v. 223, 1995, pp. 394–401.

120. Krag, D, et al., "The sentinel node in breast cancer: a multicenter validation study," *New England Journal of Medicine,* v. 33, 1998, pp. 941–46.

121. Smith, IC, "Staging of the axilla in breast cancer: accurate *in vivo* assessment using Positive Emission Tomography with 2–(fluoro-18)-fluoro-2-deoxy-D-glucose," *Annals of Surgery,* v. 228, n. 2, 1998, pp. 220–27.

122. The Early Breast Cancer Trialists' Collaborative Group: "Effects of radiotherapy and surgery in early breast cancer: an overview of the randomized trials," *New England Journal of Medicine,* v. 333, n. 22, 1995, pp. 1444–55.

123. Maunsell, E, "Arm problems and psychological distress after surgery for breast cancer," *Canadian Journal of Surgery,* v. 36, 1993, p. 315.

124. Kroll, SS, et al., "Risk of recurrence after treatment of early breast cancer with skin-sparing mastectomy," *Annals of Surgical Oncology,* v. 4, 1997, pp. 193–97.

125. Roses, DF, et al., "Complications of level 1 and 2 axillary dissection in the treatment of carcinoma of the breast," *Annals of Surgery,* v. 230, n. 2, 9/99, pp. 194–201.

126. Krag, D, et al., "The sentinel node in breast cancer: a multicenter validation study," *New England Journal of Medicine,* v. 339, n. 14, 10/1998 pp. 941–46.

127. Carlson, GW, "Skin sparing mastectomy: anatomic and technical considerations," *American Surgeon,* v. 62, n. 2, 2/96, pp. 151–55.

128. Gabriel, S, et al., "Complications leading to surgery after breast implantation," *New England Journal of Medicine,* v. 336, 3/97, pp. 677–82.

129. Noone, RB, "A review of the possible health implications of silicone breast implants," *Cancer,* v. 79, n. 9, 5/97, pp. 1747–56.

130. Silverstein, P, "Smoking and wound healing," *American Journal of Medicine,* v. 93 (suppl 1A), 7/92, pp. 22–24S.

131. Consensus Development Panel—Consenus statement: "Treatment of early-stage breast cancer," *Journal of the National Cancer Institute,* monograph #11, Washington, D.C, Government Printing Office, 1992, pp. 1–5.

132. Fallowfield, IJ, "Psychosocial and sexual impact of diagnosis and treatment of breast cancer," *British Medical Bulletin,* v. 47, 1991, pp. 388–99.

133. Schover, LR, "The impact of breast cancer on sexuality, body image, and intimate relationships," *Cancer,* v. 41, 1991, pp. 112–20.

134. Fisher, B, et al., "Significance of ipsilateral breast tumor recurrence after lumpectomy," *Lancet,* v. 328, 1991, pp. 327–31.

135. McGuire, W, and Clark, G, "Prognostic factors and treatment decisions in axillary-node-negative breast cancer," *New England Journal of Medicine,* v. 326, n. 26, 6/25/92, pp. 1756–60.

136. Ibid.

137. McDonald, CC, and Steward, HG, "Fatal myocardial infarction in the Scottish adjuvant tamoxifen trial," *British Journal of Medicine,* v. 303, 1991, pp. 435–37.

138. Fisher, B, et al., "Tamoxifen for the prevention of breast cancer: report of the National Surgical Adjuvant Breast and Bowel Project P-1 Study," *Journal of the National Cancer Institute,* v. 90, 1998, pp. 1371–88.

139. Consensus Development Panel—Consensus statement, op. cit.

140. Hellman, S., "Stopping metastases at their source," editorial, *New England Journal of Medicine,* v. 337, n. 14, 1997.

141. Mick, R, et al., "Diverse prognosis in metastatic cancer: Who should be offered alternative initial therapies?," *Breast Cancer Research and Treatment,* v. 13, 1989, pp. 33–38.

142. Wong, K, and Henderson, I, "Management of metastatic breast cancer," *World Journal of Surgery,* v. 18, n. 1, 1/2/94, pp. 98–111.

143. Stadtmauer, EA, et al., "Conventional-dose chemotherapy compared with high-dose chemotherapy plus autologous stem-cell transplantation for metastatic breast cancer," *New England Journal of Medicine,* v. 342, n. 15, 4/13/00.

144. Broet, P, et al., "Contralateral breast cancer: annual incidence and risk parameters," *Journal of Clinical Oncology,* v. 13, n. 7, 1995, pp. 1578–83.

Chapter 7

1. Anderson, W, and Light, W, "Invasive Diagnostic Procedures," in George, RB, et al., eds, *Chest Medicine,* 3d ed, Williams & Wilkins, 1995.

2. Ibid.

3. Ibid.

4. Ibid.

5. Ibid.

6. Bauman, MH, et al., "Management of spontaneous pneumothorax: an American College of Chest Physicians delphi consensus statement," *Chest,* v. 119, 2001, pp. 590–602.

7. Jemal, A, et al., "Cancer statistics, 2002," *CA: A Cancer Journal for Clinicians (2002),* v. 52, n. 1, pp. 23–47.

8. Ries, LAG, et al., eds., *SEER Cancer Statistics Review, 1973–1998,* National Cancer Institute, 2001.

9. Lerner, Michael, *Choices in Cancer,* MIT Press, 1994, p. 383.

10. Matthay, R, and Carter, D, "Lung neo plasms," in George, et al., op. cit.

11. Henschke, CI, et at., "Early Lung Cancer Action Project: overall design and findings from baseline screening," *Lancet,* v. l354, n. 9173, 7/10/99.

12. *SEER Cancer Statistics Review,* op. cit.

13. Shekelle, RB, et al., "Dietary vitamin A and risk of cancer in the Western Electric Study," *Lancet,* v. 2, n. 8257, 11/28/81, pp. 1186–90.

14. Watson, RR, et al., "Cancer prevention by retenoids: role of immunological modification," *Nutrition Research,* v. 5, 1985, pp. 663–75.

15. Quillin, Patrick, *Beating Cancer with Nutrition,* Nutrition Times Press, 1990.

16. Woodson, K, et al., "Serum a-tocopherol and subsequent risk of lung cancer among male smokers," *Journal of the National Cancer Institute,* v. 91, n. 20, 10/20/99.

17. Alavanja, M, et al., "Estimating the effect of dietary fat on the risk of lung cancer in nonsmoking women," *Lung Cancer,* v. 14 (suppl 1), 3/96, pp. S63–75.

18. Lerner, Michael, op cit.

19. Wagner, H, "Radiotherapeutic management of stage I and II lung cancer," In Pass, M, et al., eds, *Lung Cancer: Principles and Practice,* Lippincott-Raven, 1996.

20. Wagner, H, "Carcinoma of the lung," in Rakel, R, ed, *Conn's Current Therapy,* Saunders, 1997.

21. Warren, WH, and Faber, LP, "Segmentectomy versus lobectomy in patients with stage I pulmonary carcinoma. Five year survival and patterns of intrathoracic recurrence," *Journal of Thoracic and Cardiovascular Surgery,* v. 107, n. 4, 4/1994 pp. 1087–93.

Chapter 8

1. "Get slim and protect your heart the way Regis and Joy do," *Women's World,* May 27, 1997, pp. 20–22.

2. "Monitoring health care in america," National Center for Health Statistics, 3/96.

3. Tu, JV, et al., "Use of cardiac procedures and outcomes in elderly patients with myocardial infarction in the United States and Canada," *New England Journal of Medicine,* v. 336, 1997, pp. 1500–5.

4. Lange, R, "Use and overuse of angiography and revascularization for acute coronary syndromes," editorial, *New England Journal of Medicine,* v. 338, n. 25, 6/1998.

5. Ornish, Dean, *Dr. Dean Ornish's Program for Reversing Heart Disease,* Ballantine, 1990.

6. Ornish, Dean, McLanahan, S, et al., "Can lifestyle changes reverse coronary heart disease: the lifestyle heart trial," *Lancet,* v. 336, n. 8708, 7/21/90, pp. 129–33.

7. Ornish, Dean, op. cit., p. 268.

8. Ibid.

9. Gould, KL, et al., "Short-term cholesterol lowering decreases size and severity of perfusion abnormalities by positron emission tomography after dipyridamole in patients with coronary artery disease—a potential marker of healing endothelium," *Circulation,* v. 89, 1994, pp. 1530–38.

10. Ornish, D, et al., "Intensive lifestyle changes for reversal of coronary heart disease," *Journal of the American Medical Association,* v. 280, n. 23, 1998, pp. 2001–07.

11. Ornish, Dean, McLanahan, S, et al., "Can lifestyle changes reverse coronary heart disease: the lifestyle heart trial," *Lancet,* v. 336, n. 8708, 1990, pp. 129–33.

12. Gould, KL, Ornish, D, et al., "Changes in my-

ocardial perfusion abnormalities by positron emission tomography after long-term, intense risk factor modification," *Journal of the American Medical Association*, v. 274, n. 11, 9/20/95, pp. 894–901.

13. Ornish, D, "Avoiding revascularization with lifestyle changes: the Multicenter Lifestyle Demonstration Project," *American Journal of Cardiology*, v. 82, 11/98, pp. 72T–76T.

14. Taylor, AE, et al., "Environmental tobacco smoke and cardiovascular disease," *Circulation*, v. 86, 1992, pp. 1–4.

15. Steenland, K, et al., "Environmental tobacco smoke and coronary heart disease in the American Cancer Society CPD-II Cohort," *Circulation*, v. 94, 1996, pp. 622–28.

16. Dobson, AJ, et al., "How soon after quitting smoking does risk of heart attack decline?," *Journal of Clinical Epidemiology*, v. 44, 1991, pp. 1247–53.

17. Ornish, op. cit., p. 268.

18. Ibid., pp. 263–64.

19. Watts, GF, et al., "Nutrient intake and progression of coronary artery disease," *American Journal of Cardiology*, v. 73, n. 5, 1994, pp. 328–32.

20. deLongeril, M, et al., "Mediterranean alpha-linolenic acid-rich diet in secondary prevention of coronary heart disease," *Lancet*, v. 343, n. 8911, 6/11/94, pp. 1454–59.

21. Daviglus, ML, et al., "Fish consumption and the 30-year risk of fatal myocardial infarction," *New England Journal of Medicine*, v. 336, 4/96, pp. 1046–53.

22. Kromhout, D, "Fish consumption and sudden cardiac death," *Journal of the American Medical Association*, v. 279, pp. 119–24.

23. Wolk, A, "Long-term intake of dietary fiber and decreased risk of coronary heart disease among women," *Journal of the American Medical Association*, v. 1281, n. 21, 6/2/00.

24. Kritchevsky, D, et al., "Influence of an eggplant (*Solanum melongena*) preparation on cholesterol metabolism in rats," *Experimentelle Pathologie*, v. 10, n. 3–4, 1975, pp. 180–83.

25. Sacks, FM, McLanahan, S, et al., "Effect of ingestion of meat on plasma cholesterol of vegetarians," *Journal of the American Medical Association*, v. 246, n. 6, 1981, pp. 640–41.

26. He, J, et al., "Dietary odium intake and subsequent risk of cardiovascular disease in overweight adults," *Journal of the American Medical Association*, v. 1282, n. 21, 12/1/99.

27. Story, JA, "Dietary carbohydrates and atherosclerosis," *Federation Proceedings*, v. 41, 9/82, p. 2797.

28. Bieri, J, et al., "Medical uses of vitamin E," *New England Journal of Medicine*, v. 308, n. 18, 5/5/83, p. 1063.

29. Rimm, EB, et al., "Folate and vitamin B_6 from diet and supplements in relation to risk of coronary heart disease among women," *Journal of the American Medical Association*, v. 279, 1998, pp. 359–64.

30. Oakley, GP, Jr, "Eat right and take a multivitamin," *New England Journal of Medicine*, v. 338, n. 15, 1998, pp. 1060–61.

31. McCully, K, "In reply to letter to the editor," *Journal of the American Medical Association*, v. 280, n. 5, 1998, p. 418.

32. Lawson, L, "Effect of garlic on serum lipids," letter to the editor, *Journal of the American Medical Association*, v. 280, 11/1998 pp. 1563–64.

33. Novakova, V, et al., "The effect of vitamin C deficiency on the aorta of the guinea pig," *Atherosclerosis*, v. 43, 1982, p. 139.

34. Kosolcharcen, P, et al., "Improved exercise tolerance after administration of carnitine,"

Current Therapeutic Research Clinical and Experimental, v. 30, 1981, p. 753.

35. Schroeder, HA, "Cadmium, chromium, and cardiovascular disease," *Circulation,* v. 35, 1967, p. 570; also, Abraham, AS, et al., "The action of chromium on serum lipids and on atherosclerosis in cholesterol-fed rabbits," *Atherosclerosis,* v. 42, 2/82, p. 185.

36. Shamberger, RJ, et al., "Epidemiological studies on selenium and heart disease," *Federal Proceedings,* v. 35, 1976, p. 578.

37. Rimm, E, et al., "Review of moderate alcohol consumption and reduced risk of coronary heart disease: is the effect due to beer, wine, or spirits?," *British Medical Journal,* v. 312, 3/23/96, pp. 731–36.

38. Stefanick, ML, et al., "Effects of diet and exercise in men and postmenopausal women with low levels of LDL cholesterol and high levels of LDL cholesterol," *New England Journal of Medicine,* v. 339, n. 1, 7/1998, p. 12.

39. Manson, JE, et al., "A prospective study of walking as compared with vigorous exercise in the prevention of coronary heart disease in women," *New England Journal of Medicine,* v. 341, n. 9, 9/26/99.

40. Rosch, Paul, research of American Institute of Stress, Yonkers, NY.

41. Scherwitz, L, et al., "Type A behavior, self-involvement, and behavior-type assessment in the Multiple Risk Factor Intervention Trial (MRFIT) structured interviews," *Journal of Behavioral Medicine,* v. 10, n. 2, 1987, pp. 173–95.

42. Kaplan, JR, et al., "Social stress and atherosclerosis in normocholesterolemic monkeys," *Science,* v. 220, n. 4598, 1983, pp. 733–35.

43. Ornish, op. cit.

44. Ornish, op. cit., p. 13.

45. Nerem, RM, et al., "Social environment as a factor in diet-induced atherosclerosis," *Science,* v. 208, 1980, p. 1475.

46. Ornish, p. 13.

47. Iribarren, C, et al., "Association of hostility with coronary artery calcification in young adults: the CARDIA Study," *Journal of the American Medical Association,* v. 283, n. 19, 5/17/00.

48. Ornish, op. cit.

49. Scherwitz, L, et al., "Self-involvement, and coronary heart disease incidence in the Multiple Risk Factor Intervention Trial," *Psychosomatic Medicine,* v. 48, n. 3–4, 3–4/86, pp. 187–99.

50. Clarke, NE, et al., "Treatment of angina pectoris with disodium ethylene diamine tetraacetic acid," *American Journal of Medical Science,* v. 232, 1956, pp. 654–66.

51. Scandinavian Simvastatin Survival Study Group, "Randomized trial of cholesterol-lowering in 4444 patients with coronary heart disease: the Scandinavian Simvastatin Survival Study, *Lancet,* v. 344, 1994, pp. 1383–89.

52. Sachs, FM, et al., "The effect of pravastatin on coronary events after myocardial infarction in patients with average cholesterol levels," *New England Journal of Medicine,* v. 335, 1996, p. 1001.

53. Shepherd, J, et al., "West of Scotland coronary prevention study," *New England Journal of Medicine,* v. 333, 1995, p. 1301–7.

54. Downs, JR, et al., "Primary prevention of acute coronary events with lovastatin in men and women with average cholesterol levels: Results of AFCAPS/TexCAPS," *Journal of the American Medical Association,* v. 279, 1998, pp. 1615–22.

55. Rubins, HB, et al., "Gemfibrozil for the secondary prevention of coronary heart disease in men with low levels of high-density lipoprotein cholesterol," *New England Journal of Medicine,* v. 341, n. 6, 8/5/99, pp. 410–18.

56. National Cholesterol Education Project, "Second report of the expert panel on detection, evaluation, and treatment of high blood cholesterol in adults," *National Institute of Health,* 9/93.

57. Steering Committee of the Physicians' Health Study Research Group, "Final report on the aspirin component of the ongoing Physicians' Health Study," *New England Journal of Medicine,* v. 321, n. 3, 1989, pp. 129–35.

58. Antiplatelet Trialists' Collaboration, "Collaborative overview of randomized trials of antiplatelet therapy," *British Medical Journal,* v. 308, n. 6921, 1994, pp. 81–106.

59. Hong, MK, et al., "Effects of estrogen replacement therapy on serum lipid values and angiographically defined coronary artery disease in postmenopausal women," *American Journal of Cardiology,* v. 69, n. 3, 1992, pp. 176–78.

60. Grady, D, et al., "Hormone therapy to prevent disease and prolong life in postmenopausal women," *Annals of Internal Medicine,* v. 117, n. 12, 12/15/92, pp. 1016–37.

61. Herrington, DM, et al., "Effects of estrogen replacement on the progression of coronary-artery atherosclerosis," *New England Journal of Medicine,* v. 343, n. 8, 8/24/00.

62. Hulley, S, et al., "Randomized trial of estrogen plus progestin for secondary prevention of coronary heart disease in postmenopausal women," *Journal of the American Medical Association,* v. 280, 1998, pp. 605–13.

63. Murray, MT, *Menopause: How You Can Benefit from Diet, Vitamins, Minerals, Herbs, Exercise, and Other Natural Methods (Getting Well Naturally),* Pima Publications, 1994.

64. Lincoff, MA, "Stent scrutiny," editorial in *Journal of the American Medical Association,* v. 284, n. 14, 10/11/00.

65. Suwaidi, JA, "Coronary artery stents," *Journal of the American Medical Association,* v. 284, n. 14, 10/11/00.

66. Jacobs, JK, "Coronary stents—have they fulfilled their promise?," *editorial, New England Journal of Medicine,* v. 341, n. 26, 12/23/99.

67. Lincoff, op. cit.

68. Jacobs, op. cit.

69. Zijlstra, F, et al., "Long-term benefit of primary angioplasty as compared with thrombolytic therapy for acute myocardial infarction," *New England Journal of Medicine,* v. 341, n. 19, 11/4/99.

70. George, BS, et al., "Multicenter investigation of coronary stenting to treat acute or threatened closure after percutaneous transluminal coronary angioplasty: clinical and angiographic outcomes," *Journal of the American College of Cardiology,* v. 22, n. 1, 6/93, pp. 135–43.

71. Ellis, SG, et al., "Relation of operator volume and experience to procedural outcome in percutaneous coronary revascularization at hospitals with high interventional volumes," *Circulation,* v. 95, 1997, pp. 2479–84.

72. Jollis, JG, et al., "Relationship between physician angioplasty volume and outcome in 97,000 elderly Americans," *Circulation,* v. 95, n. 11, 6/3/97, pp. 2485–91.

73. Teirstein, PS, "Credentialing for coronary interventions: practice makes perfect," editorial, *Circulation,* v. 95, n. 11, 6/3/97, pp. 2467–70.

74. Lincoff, op. cit.

75. Greenfield, LJ, ed., *Surgery: Scientific Principles and Practice,* 2d ed., Lippincott-Raven, 1996, p. 1548.

76. Ibid., p. 1543.

77. National Heart, Lung, and Blood Institute, Clinical Alert: Bypass Over Angioplasty for Patients with Diabetes, 1995.

78. American Heart Association, "Heart and stroke A–Z guide."

79. Garratt, KN, "Percutaneous revascularization strategies," *Postgraduate Medicine,* v. 99, n. 2, 1996, pp. 125–37.

80. Gersh, BJ, et al., "Percutaneous transluminal coronary angioplasty or coronary bypass surgery in management of chronic angina pectoris," *International Journal of Cardiology,* v. 40, n. 2, 1993, pp. 81–88.

81. Yusuf, S, et al., "Effect of coronary artery bypass graft surgery on survival: overview of 10 year results from randomized trials by the Coronary Artery Bypass Graft Surgery Trialists' Collaboration," *Lancet,* v. 344, n. 8922, 8/27/94, pp. 563–70.

82. Ornish, D., *Dr. Dean Ornish's Program for Reversing Heart Disease,* Ballantine, 1990.

83. Hannan, EL, et al., "Coronary artery bypass surgery: the relationship between inhospital mortality rate and surgical volume after controlling for clinical risk factors," *Medical Care,* v. 29, n. 11, 1991, pp. 1094–107.

84. Greenfield, LJ, ed., *Surgery: Scientific Principles and Practice,* 2d ed. Lippincott-Raven, 1996, p. 1548.

85. Savage, MP, et al., "Stent placement compared with balloon angioplasty for obstructed coronary bypass grafts," *New England Journal of Medicine,* v. 337, n. 11, 1997.

86. Greenfield, op. cit., p. 1546.

87. Ibid., p. 1548.

88. Ibid.

89. Kwon, K, et al., "Complete myocardial revascularization on the beating heart," *American Journal of Surgery,* v. 178, n. 6, 12/1999 pp. 501–4.

90. Information presented by Brack Hattler, M.D., at the Pacific Northwest Cardiovascular Symposium in Seattle, as reported by Warren King, in the *Seattle Times,* 7/1/97.

91. Verrier, E, "Cardiac surgery," *Journal of the American College of Surgeons,"* v. 188, n. 2, 1999, pp. 104–10.

Chapter 9

1. Rutherford, R, ed., *Vascular Surgery,* Saunders, 1995.

2. Blankenhorn, D, et al., "Reversal of atherosis and sclerosis, the two components of atherosclerosis," *Circulation,* v. 79, 1989, pp. 1–5.

3. Markus, R, et al., "Influence of lifestyle modification on atherosclerotic progression determined by ultrasonic change in the common carotid intima-medisa thickness," *American Journal of Clinical Nutrition,* v. 65, n. 4, 4/97, pp. 1000–4.

4. Haeger, K, "Long-time treatment of intermittent claudication with vitamin E," *American Journal of Clinical Nutrition,* v. 27, 1974, p. 1179.

5. Patel, CH, "Reduction of serum cholesterol and blood pressure in hypertensive patients by behavior modification," *Journal of the Royal College of General Practitioners,* v. 26, 1976, pp. 211–15.

6. Dawson, DL, et al., "Cilostazol has beneficial effects in treatment of intermittent claudication: results from a multicenter randomized, prospective, double-blind trial," *Circulation,* v. 98, 1998, n. 7, pp. 678–86.

7. Golledge, J, et al., "Outcome of femoro-popliteal angioplasty," *Annals of Surgery,* v. 229, n. 1, 1/1999, pp. 146–53.

8. Antiplatelet Trialists' Collaboration, "Collaborative overview of randomized trials of antiplatelet therapy—II: maintenance of vascular graft or arterial patency by antiplatelet therapy," *British Medical Journal,* v. 308, 1994, pp. 159–68.

9. Becquemin, JP, "Effect of ticlopidine on the long-term patency of saphenous-vein bypass grafts in the legs," *New England Journal of Medicine,* v. 337, 1997, pp. 1726–31.

10. Camerota, A, and Rutherford, R, "Graft thrombosis and thromboembolic complication," in Rutherford, R, ed., *Vascular Surgery,* Saunders, 1995.

11. Robicsek, F, et al., "The effect of continued

cigarette smoking on the patency of synthetic vascular grafts in Leriche syndrome," *Journal of Cardiovascular and Thoracic Surgery,* v. 70, n. 1, 1975, pp. 107–13; Wiseman, S, et al., "Influence of smoking and plasma factors on patency of femoralpopliteal vein grafts," *British Medical Journal,* v. 299, n. 6700, 1989, pp. 643–46; and Wiseman, S, et al., "The influence of smoking and plasma factors on prosthetic graft patency," *European Journal of Vascular Surgery,* v. 4, n. 1, 1990, pp. 57–61.

12. Ameli, FM, et al., "The effect of postoperative smoking on femorapopliteal bypass grafts," *Annals of Vascular Surgery,* v. 3, n. 1, 1989, pp. 20–25.

13. Ernst, C, "Abdominal aortic aneurysm," *New England Journal of Medicine,* v. 328, n. 16, 4/24/93, pp. 1167–72.

14. "Infrarenal aortic aneurysms," in Rutherford, R, ed., *Vascular Surgery,* 4th ed., Saunders, 1995.

15. Nicholls, SC, et al., "Rupture in small abdominal aortic aneurysms," *Journal of Vascular Surgery,* v. 28, n. 5, 1998, pp. 884–88.

16. Makaroun, M, et al., "The experience of an academic medical center with endovascular treatment of aortic abdominal aneurysms," *American Journal of Surgery,* v. 176, n. 2, 8/1998 pp. 198–202.

17. Brewster, DC, et al., "Initial experience with endovascular aneurysm repair: comparison of early results with outcome of conventional repair," *Journal of Vascular Surgery,* v. 27, 1998, pp. 992–1005.

18. Zarins, CK, et al., "AneuRx stent graft versus open surgical repair of abdominal aortic aneurysms: a multicenter prospective clinical trial," *Journal of Vascular Surgery,* v. 29, 1999, pp. 292–305.

19. Moore, WS, et al., "Abdominal aortic aneurysm: a 6-year comparison of endovascular versus transabdominal repair," *Annals of Surgery,* v. 230, n. 3, 9/99.

20. Zarins, CK, et al., "Aneurysm rupture after endovascular repair using the AneuRx stent graft," *Journal of Vascular Surgery,* v. 31, n. 5, 5/00.

21. Gorelick, PB, et al., "A review of guidelines and a multidisciplinary consensus statement from the National Stroke Association," *Journal of the American Medical Association,* v. 281, n. 12, 1999, pp. 1112–20.

22. Ibid.

23. Ibid.

24. Collins, R, et al., "Blood pressure, stroke, and coronary artery disease. Part 2, Short-term reductions in blood pressure: Overview in randomized drug trials in their epidemiological context," *Lancet,* v. 335, 1990, pp. 827–38.

25. Blankenhorn, DH, et al., "Angiographic trials of lipid-lowering therapy," *Arteriosclerosis,* v. 1, 1981, pp. 242–49.

26. Liu, S, et al., "Whole grain consumption and risk of ischemic stroke in women: a prospective study," *Journal of the American Medical Association,* v. 284, n. 12, 9/27/00.

27. Joshipura, KJ, "Fruit and vegetable intake in relation to risk of "schemic stroke," *Journal of the American Medical Association,* v. 282, n. 13, 10/6/99.

28. Lorenz, R, "The problem with intensive therapy," *Diabetes Care,* v. 21, 1998, pp. 2021–22.

29. Steiner, M, "Effect of alpha-tocopherol administration on platelet function in man," *Thrombosis and Haemostasis,* v. 49, n. 2, 4/28/83, pp. 73–77.

30. Shamberger, R, et al., "Selenium and heart disease," in Hemphill, DD, ed., *Trace Substances in Environmental Health—IX.* University of Missouri, 1975, pp. 15–22.

31. *American Journal of Clinical Nutrition,* v. 39, 1984, p. 677.

32. Black, KL, et al., "Eicosapentaenoic acid: effect on brain prostaglandins, cerebral blood flow

and edema in ischemic gerbils," *Stroke*, v. 15, n. 1, 1–2/84, pp. 65–69.

33. Selhub, J, et al., "Association between plasma homocysteine concentrations and extracranial carotid artery stenosis," *New England Journal of Medicine*, v. 332, 1995, pp. 286–91.

34. Kleijnen, J, et al., "Drug profiles—gingko biloba," *Lancet*, v. 340, 1993, pp. 1136–39.

35. Keli, S, et al., "Dietary flavonoids, antioxidant vitamins, and incidence of stroke: the Zutphen study," *Archives of Internal Medicine*, v. 156, n. 6, 3/25/96, pp. 637–42.

36. Gorelick, op. cit.

37. Hu, FB, et al., "Physical activity and risk of stroke in women," *Journal of the American Medical Association*, v. 283, n. 22, 6/14/00.

38. Berger, K, "Light-to-moderate alcohol consumption and the risk of stroke among US male physicians," *New England Journal of Medicine*, v. 341, n. 21, 11/18/99.

39. Klatsky, AL, "Alcohol use and subsequent cerebrovascular disease hospitalizations," *Stroke*, v. 20, n. 6, 6/89, pp. 741–46.

40. Gorelick, op. cit.

41. Bonita, R, et al., "Cigarette smoking and risk of premature stroke in men and women," *British Medical Journal*, v. 293, 1986, pp. 6–8.

42. Wolf, PA, et al., "Cigarette smoking as a risk factor for stroke," *Journal of the American Medical Association*, v. 259, 1988, pp. 1025–29.

43. Kawachi, I, et al., "Smoking cessation and decreased risk of stroke in women," *Journal of the American Medical Association*, v. 269, 1993, pp. 232–36.

44. Denson, KW, et al., "Passive smoking and an increased risk of acute stroke," *Tobacco Control*, 9/00.

45. Gillum, LA, "Ischemic stroke with oral contraceptives: A meta-analysis," *Journal of the American Medical Association*, v. 284, n. 1, 7/5/00.

46. Everson, E, Results of a study presented at the American Heart Association 70th Scientific Session in Orlando, Florida, November 1998.

47. *Advances in Acupuncture and Acupuncture Anesthesia*, The People's Medical Publishing House, 1980.

48. Gorelick, op. cit.

49. Ibid.

50. Antiplatelet Trialists' Collaboration, "Collaborative overview of randomized trials of antiplatelet therapy—I: Prevention of death, myocardial infarction, and stroke by prolonged antiplatelet therapy in various categories of patients," *British Medical Journal*, v. 308, n. 6921, 1994, pp. 81–106.

51. CAPRIE Steering Committee, "A randomized trial of clopidigrel versus aspirin in patients at risk of ischemic events," *Lancet*, v. 348, 1996, pp. 1329–39.

52. Gorelick, op. cit.

53. White, HD, "Prevastatin therapy and the risk of stroke," *New England Journal of Medicine*, v. 343, n. 5, 8/3/00.

54. Naylor, AR, et al.,"Randomized study of carotid angioplasty and stenting versus endarterectomy: a stopped trial," *Journal of Vascular Surgery*, v. 28, n. 2, 1998, pp. 326–34.

55. North American Symptomatic Carotid Endarterectomy Trial Collaborators, "Beneficial effects of carotid endarterectomy in symptomatic patients with high-grade carotid stenosis," *New England Journal of Medicine*, v. 325, 1991, pp. 445–53; "Benefit of carotid endarterectomy for patients with high-grade stenosis of the internal carotid artery," National Institutes of Neurological Disorders and Stroke, 2/26/91.

56. North American Symptomatic Carotid Endarterectomy Trial Collaborators, "Prevention

of functional impairment by endarterectomy for symptomatic high-grade carotid stenosis," *Journal of the American Medical Association,* v. 271, n. 16, 4/27/94, pp. 1256–59.

57. Barnett, HJM, "Benefit of carotid endarterectomy in patients with symptomatic moderate or severe stenosis," *New England Journal of Medicine,* v. 339, 1998, pp. 1414–25.

58. Executive Committee for the Asymptomatic Carotid Atherosclerosis Study, "Endarterectomy for asymptomatic carotid artery stenosis," *Journal of the American Medical Association,* v. 273, 1995, pp. 1421–28.

59. Biller, J, et al., "Guidelines for carotid endarterectomy: a statement for healthcare professionals from a Special Writing Group of the Stroke Council, American Heart Association," *Circulation,* v. 97, 1998, pp. 501–9.

60. Wennberg, DE, et al., "Variation in carotid endarterectomy mortality in the Medicare population: trial hospitals, volume, and patient characteristics," *Journal of the American Medical Association,* v. 279, 1998, pp. 1278–81.

Chapter 10

1. Burkitt, Denis, *Don't Forget Fibre in Your Diet,* Martin Dunitz Publishing, 1979, p. 63.

2. Latto, C, et al., "Diverticular Disease and Varicose Veins," *Lancet,* v. 1, n. 812, 5/19/73, pp. 1089–90.

3. Burkitt, op. cit.

4. Pointel, JP, et al., "Titrated extract of centella asiatica (TECA) in the treatment of venous insufficiency of the lower limbs," *Angiology,* v. 38, 1987, pp. 46–50.

5. Pizzorno, JE, and Murray, MT, *Textbook of Natural Medicine,* Bastyr University Press, 1987.

6. Pittler, M, and Ernst, E, "Horse-chestnut seed extract for chronic venous insufficiency," *Archives of Dermatology,* v. 134, 1998, pp. 1356–60.

7. Seligman, B, "Oral bromelains as adjuncts in the treatment of acute thrombophlebitis," *Angiology,* v. 20, 1969, pp. 22–26.

8. Visudhiphan, S, et al., "The relationship between high fibrinolytic activity and daily capsicum ingestion in Thais," *American Journal of Clinical Nutrition,* v. 35, 1982, pp. 1552–58.

9. Trowell, H, et al., *Dietary Fibre, Fibre-Depleted Foods and Disease,* Academic Press, 1985.

Chapter 11

1. Young, H, and Keeffe, E, "Complications of gastrointestinal endoscopy," in Sleisenger & Fordtran, eds., *Gastrointestinal and Liver Disease,* 6th ed., Saunders, 1998.

2. Lagergren, et al., "Symptomatic gastroesophageal reflux as a risk factor for esophageal adenocarcinoma," *New England Journal of Medicine,* v. 340, n. 11, 1999.

3. Sampliner, RE, "Adenocarcinoma of the esophagus and gastric cardia: is there progress in the face of increasing cancer incidence?," *Annals of Internal Medicine,* v. 130, 1999, pp. 67–69.

4. Burkitt, Denis, et al., "Low-residue diets and hiatus hernia," *Lancet,* v. 2, n. 1973, p. 128.

5. Luthe, W, *Autogenic Therapy,* v. II, 1969, p. 14.

6. Ibid., p. 16.

7. Korr, IM, *Neurobiological Mechanisms in Manipulative Treatment,* Plenum Press, 1979.

8. Zatta, P, et al., "Alzheimer dementia and the aluminum hypothesis," *Medical Hypothesis,* v. 26, 1988, pp. 139–42.

9. Whitaker, Julian, *Dr. Whitaker's Guide to Natural Healing,* Prima Publishing, 1995, p. 68.

10 Kuipers, EJ, et al., "Atrophic gastritis and helicobacter pylori infection in patients with reflux esophagitis treated with omeprazole or fundoplica-

tion," *New England Journal of Medicine,* v. 334, n. 16, 4/18/96, pp. 1018–22.

11. Trus, TL, "Improvement in quality of life measures after laparoscopic antireflux surgery," *Annals of Surgery,* v. 229, n. 3, 1999, pp. 331–36.

12. Jemal, A, et al., "Cancer statistics, 2002," *CA: A Cancer Journal for Clinicians (2002),* v. 52, n. 1, pp. 23–47.

13. Cohen, S, "Heartburn—a serious symptom," *New England Journal of Medicine,* v. 340, n. 12, 1999.

14. Gao, Y, et al., "Reduced risk of esophageal cancer associated with green tea consumption," *Journal National Cancer Institute,* v. 86, n. 11, 6/1/94, pp. 855–58.

15. Ries, LAG, et al., eds, *SEER Cancer Statistics Review, 1973–1998,* National Cancer Institute, 2001.

16. Cooper, JS, et al., "Long-term follow-up of a prospective randomized trial (RTOG 85– 01)," *Journal of the American Medical Association,* v. 281, 1999, pp. 1623–27.

Chapter 12

1. "The enigma of endoscopy: Does it really improve the outcome?," *Modern Medicine,* May 1983, p. 11.

2. Talley, NJ, et al., "AGA technical review: evaluation of dyspepsia," *Gastroenterology,* v. 114, 1998, pp. 582–92.

3. McQuaid, K, "Dyspepsia," in Sleisenger and Fordtran, et al., *Gastrointestinal and Liver Disease: Pathophysiology/Diagnosis/Management,* 6th ed, v. 1, Saunders, 1998, pp. 105–17.

4. Young, H, and Keeffe, E, "Complications of Gastrointestinal Endoscopy," in Sleisenger & Fordtran, pp. 301–9.

5. Levenstein, S, et al., "Stress and peptic ulcer disease," *Journal of the American Medical Association,* v. 281, n. 1, 1/6/99, pp. 10–11.

6. "Understanding ulcer helps patients cope," *Medical World News,* 6/13/83.

7. Sontag, S, et al., "Cimetidine, cigarette smoking, and recurrence of duodenal ulcer," *New England Journal of Medicine,* v. 311, n. 11, 9/13/84, pp. 689–93.

8. Rynding, A, et al., "Prophylactic effect of dietary fibre in duodenal ulcer disease, *Lancet,* v. 2, n. 1982, p. 736.

9. "Findings document role of stress in development of duodenal ulcers," *Family Practice News,* 7/15/92.

10. Levenstein, S, et al., "Psychologic predictors of duodenal ulcer healing," *Journal of Clinical Gastroenterology,* v. 22, 1996, pp. 84–89.

11. Luthe, *Autogenic Therapy,* v. II, 1969, p. 14.

12. Ibid.

13. Desai, BP, et al., "Effect of madhya nauli on stomach acidity," *Yoga Mimamsa,* v. 223–24, 1983–84, pp. 110–17.

14. Levenstein, S, et al., "Psychologic predictors of peptic ulcer incidence in the Alameda County Study," *Journal of Clinical Gastroenterology,* v. 24, 1997, pp. 140–46.

15. Chernow, MS, et al., "Prevention of stress ulcers," *American Journal of Surgery,* v. 122, 1971, p. 674.

16. Patty, I, et al., "Controlled trial of vitamin A in gastric ulcer," *Lancet,* v. 2, n. 8303, 10/16/82, p. 876.

17. Chernow, MS, et al., "Stress ulcer: a preventable disease," *Journal of Trauma,* v. 12, 1972, p. 831.

18. Lindenbaum, ES, et al., "Effects of pyridoxine on mice after immobilization stress," *Nutrition Metabolism,* v. 17, 1974, p. 368.

19. Naunyn-Schmiedeberg's *Archives of Pharmacology,* v. 313, 1980, p. 238.

20. Dubey, SS, et al., "Ascorbic acid, dehydroascorbic acid, glutathione and histamine in peptic

ulcer," *Indian Journal of Medical Research,* v. 76, 1982, pp. 859–62.

21. Kangas, JA, et al., "Effect of vitamin E on the development of stress-produced gastric ulceration in the rat," *American Journal of Clinical Nutrition,* v. 25, n. 9, 9/25/72, pp. 864–66.

22. Frommer, DJ, "The healing of gastric ulcers by zinc sulfate," *Medical Journal of Australia,* v. 2, 1975, p. 793.

23. Mowrey, Daniel, *The Scientific Validation of Herbal Medicine,* Cormorant Books, 1986.

24. Szelenyi, I, et al., "Pharmacological experiments with compounds of chamomile—III: experimental studies of the ulcer protective effect of chamomile," *Plant Medica,* v. 35, n. 3, 3/79, pp. 218–27.

25. Zatta, P, et al., "Alzheimer dementia and the aluminum hypothesis," *Medical Hypothesis,* v. 26, 1988, pp. 139–42.

26. Kuipers, EJ, et al., "Atrophic gastritis and helicobacter pylori infection in patients with reflux esophagitis treated with omeprazole or fundoplication," *New England Journal of Medicine,* v. 334, n. 16, 4/18/96, pp. 1018–22; and Hansson, L, et al., "The risk of stomach cancer in patients with gastric or duodenal ulcer disease," *New England Journal of Medicine,* v. 335, n. 4, 7/25/96, pp. 242–49.

27. Vanderhurst, RW, et al., "Prevention of ulcer recurrence after eradication of helicobacter pylori: a prospective long-term follow-up study," *Gastroenterology,* v. 113: 1997, pp. 1082–86.

28. Lau, JY, et al., "Endoscopic retreatment compared with surgery in patients with recurrent bleeding after initial endoscopic control of bleeding ulcers," *New England Journal of Medicine,* v. 340, n. 11, 1999.

29. Donovan, AJ, et al., "Perforated duodenal ulcer: an alternative therapeutic plan," *Archives of Surgery,* v. 133, n. 11, 1998 pp. 1166–71.

30. Ng, EKW, et al., "Eradication of Helicobacter pylori prevents recurrence of ulcer after simple closure of duodenal ulcer perforation: randomized controlled trial," *Annals of Surgery,* v. 231, n. 2, 2/00.

31. Sanderson, CR, et al., "Serum pyridoxal in patients with active peptic ulceration," *Gut,* v. 16, 1975, p. 177.

32. Frommer, op. cit.

33. Jemal, A, et al., "Cancer statistics, 2002," *CA: A Cancer Journal for Clinicians (2002),* v. 52, n. 1, pp. 23–47.

34. Ries, LAG, et al., eds, *SEER Cancer Statistics Review,* 1973–1998, National Cancer Institute, 2001.

35. Adachi, Y, et al., "Quality of life after laparoscope-assisted Billroth I gastrectomy," *Annals of Surgery,* v. 229, n. 1, 1999, pp. 49–54.

Chapter 13

1. Roslyn, JJ, et al., "Open cholecystectomy: a contemporary analysis of 42,474 patients," *Annals of Surgery,* v. 218, 1993, p. 129.

2. McSherry, CK, et al., "The natural history of diagnosed gallstone disease in symptomatic and asymptomatic patients," *Annals of Surgery,* v. 202, 1985, p. 59.

3. "Treatment usually unnecessary for 'silent' gallstones," *Journal of the American Medical Association,* v. 245, n. 23, 6/19/81, p. 2383.

4. Mann, J, *Journal of the American Medical Association,* v. 255, 2/66, p. 666.

5. Trowell, H, et al., *Dietary Fibre, Fibre-depleted Foods and Disease,* Academic Press, 1985.

6. Nervi, F, et al., "Influence of legume intake on biliary lipids and cholesterol saturation in young Chilean men," *Gastroenterology,* v. 96, 1989, pp. 825–30.

7. Breneman, JC, "Allergy elimination diet as the most effective gallbladder diet," *Annuals of Allergy,* v. 26, 1968, p. 83.

8. Tuzhilin, SA, et al., "The treatment of patients with gallstones by lecithin," *American Journal of Gastroenterology,* v. 65, 1976, p. 1231.

9. Tooli, J, et al., "Gallstone dissolution in man using cholic acid and lecithin," *Lancet,* v. 2, 1975, p. 1124.

10. Ginter, E, *World Review of Nutrition and Dietetics,* v. 33, 1979, p. 104.

11. Bordia, A, et al., "Effects of the essential oils of garlic and onion on alimentary hyperlipidemia," *Atherosclerosis,* v. 21, 1975, pp. 15–19.

12. Bennion, L, and Grundy, S, "Effects of obesity and caloric intake on biliary lipidmetabolism in man," *Journal of Clinical Investigation,* v. 56, n. 4, 10/75, pp. 966–1011.

13. Canfield, AJ, et al., "Biliary dyskinesia: A study of more than 200 patients and review of the literature," *Journal of Gastrointestinal Surgery,* v. 2, n. 5, 9–10/1998, pp. 443–8.

14. Keulemans, Y, et al., "Laparoscopic cholecystectomy: day-care versus clinical observation," *Annals of Surgery,* v. 228, n. 6, 1998, pp. 734–40.

Chapter 14

1. Tanimura, H, et al., *Annals of the New York Academy of Sciences,* v. 393, 9/82, p. 214.

2. Frey, CF, et al., "Pancreatic resection for chronic pancreatitis," *Surgical Clinics of North America,* 1989, p. 499.

3. Jemal, A, et al., "Cancer statistics, 2002," *CA: A Cancer Journal for Clinicians (2002),* v. 52, n. 1, pp. 23–47.

4. Renneker, Mark, *Understanding Cancer,* Bull Publishing, 1988, p. 179.

5. Boing, H, et al., "Regional nutritional pattern and cancer mortality in the Federal Republic of Germany," *Nutrition and Cancer,* v. 7, n. 3, 1985, pp. 121–30.

6. Ibid.

7. Gold, EB, et al., "Diet and other risk factors for cancer of the pancreas," *Cancer,* v. 55, n. 2, 1985, pp. 460–67.

8. Block, Gladys, "Epidemiological data on the role of ascorbic acid in cancer prevention," National Institutes of Health, 9/90.

9. Page, Linda, *Healthy Healing,* Healthy Healing Publications, 1997, p. 182.

10. Renneker, loc. cit.

11. Ibid.

12. Ibid.

13. Ibid.

14. Ries, LAG, et al., eds., *SEER Cancer Statistics Review, 1973–1998,* National Cancer Institute, 2001.

15. Hirschberg, C, et al., *Remarkable Recovery: What Extraordinary Healings Tell Us About Getting Well and Staying Well,* Putnam, 1995.

16. Renneker, loc. cit.

17. Quillin, Patrick, *Beating Cancer with Nutrition,* The Nutrition Times Press, 1994, p. 54.

18. Page, loc. cit.

19. Lerner, Michael, *Choices in Healing,* MIT Press, 1994, p. 600.

20. Huguier, M, and Mason, NP, "Treatment of cancer of the exocrine pancreas," *American Journal of Surgery,* v. 177, n. 3, 3/1999, pp. 257–65.

21. Ibid.

22. Jimenez, RE, et al., "Impact of laparoscopic staging in the treatment of pancreatic cancer," *Archives of Surgery,* v. 135, n. 4, 4/00.

Chapter 15

1. Parham, Vistara, *What's Wrong with Eating Meat?,* Sisters Universal Publishing, 1979, p. 17.

2. Burkitt, DP, et al., "Dietary fiber and disease,"

Journal of the American Medical Association, v. 229, 1976, pp. 1068–78.

3. Hague, A, et al., "Apoptosis in colorectal tumor cells: induction by the short chain fatty acids butyrate, propionate, and acetate and by the bile salt deoxycholate," *International Journal of Cancer*, v. 60, 1995, pp. 400–6.

4. Mandel, JS, et al., "Reducing mortality from colorectal cancer by screening for fecal occult blood: Minnesota Colon Cancer Control Study," *New England Journal of Medicine*, v. 328, n. 19, 5/13/93, pp. 1365–71.

5. Selby, JV, et al., "A case-control study of screening sigmoidoscopy and mortality from colorectal cancer," *New England Journal of Medicine*, v. 326, 1992, pp. 653–57.

6. Young, H, and Keeffe, E, "Complications of gastrointestinal endoscopy," in Sleisenger & Fordtran, eds, *Gastrointestinal and Liver Disease*, 6th ed., Saunders, 1998.

7. Tomeo, CA, et al., "Harvard report on cancer prevention: v. 3: prevention of colon cancer in the United States," *Cancer Causes Control*, v. 10, 1999, pp. 167–80.

8. Podolsky, DK, "Going the distance: the case for true colorectal-cancer screening," *New England Journal of Medicine,* v. 343, n. 3, 7/00.

9. Ozik, LA, et al., "Pathogenesis, diagnosis, and treatment of diverticular disease of the colon," *The Gastroenterologist*, v. 2, n. 4, 2/94, pp. 299–310.

10. Burkitt, DP, et al., "Dietary fiber and disease," *Journal of the American Medical Association*, v. 229, 1976, pp. 1068–78.

11. Ozik, et al., op. cit.

12. Ferzoco, LB, et al., "Acute diverticulitis," *New England Journal of Medicine*, v. 338, n. 21, 1998, pp. 1521–26.

13. Findlay, JM, et al., "Effects of unprocessed bran on colon function in normal subjects and in diverticular disease," *Lancet*, v. 1, n. 849, 2/2/74, pp. 146–49; and Brodribb, AJ, "Treatment of symptomatic diverticular disease with high-fiber diet," *Lancet*, v. 1, n. 8013, 3/26/77, pp. 664–66.

14. Aldoori, WH, et al., "Prospective study of physical activity and the risk of symptomatic diverticular disease," *Gut*, v. 36, 2/95, pp. 276–82.

15. Parks, TG, "Natural history of diverticular disease of the colon: a review of 521 cases," *British Medical Journal*, v. 4, 1969, pp. 639–42.

16. Grimes, D, "Refined carbohydrate, smooth muscle spasm and disease of the colon," *Lancet*, v. 1, 1975, p. 395.

17. Bernstein, J, et al., "Depression of lymphocyte transformation following oral glucose ingestion," *American Journal of Clinical Nutrition*, v. 30, 1977, p. 613.

18. "Fast food and sugar linked to Crohn's," *Medical Tribune*, 2/27/92.

19. Heaton, KW, et al., "Treatment of Crohn's disease with an unrefined-carbohydrate, fibre-rich diet," *British Medical Journal*, v. 279, 1979, pp. 762–64.

20. Siegel, J, "Inflammatory bowel disease: another possible facet of the allergic diathesis," *Annals of Allergy*, v. 47, 1981, p. 92.

21. Elsborg, L, et al., "Folate deficiency in chronic inflammatory bowel disease," *Scandinavian Journal of Gastroenterology*, v. 14, 1979, p. 1019.

22. Dvorak, AM, "Vitamin A in Crohn's disease," *Lancet*, v. 1, 1980, p. 1303.

23. Solomons, NW, et al., "Zinc deficiency in Crohn's disease," *Digestion*, v. 16, 1977, p. 87.

24. McClain, CJ, et al., "Zinc-deficiency-induced retinal dysfunction in Crohn's disease," *Digestive Diseases Science*, v. 28, 1977, p. 33.

25. Gerson, CD, et al., "Ascorbic acid deficiency and fistula formation in regional enteritis," *Gastroenterology*, v. 67, 1974, p. 428.

26. Aslan, A, and Triadafilopoulos, G, "Fish oil fatty acid supplementation in active ulcerative colitis: a double-blind, placebo-controlled, crossover study," *American Journal of Gastroenterology*, v. 87, n. 4, 1992, pp. 432–37.

27. Belluzzi, A, et al., "Effect of an enteric-coated fish-oil preparation on relapses in Crohn's disease," *New England Journal of Medicine*, v. 334, n. 24, 6/13/96, pp. 1557–60.

28. Verzame, PG, et al., "Effect of certain chamomile compounds," *Acta Pharmaceutica Hungarica*, v. 49, n. 1, 1979, pp. 13–20.

29. Mobrey, Daniel, *The Scientific Validation of Herbal Medicine*, Cormorant Books, 1986, p. 255.

30. Engel, GL, "Studies of ulcerative colitis. III: The nature of the psychologic processes," *American Journal of Medicine*, v. 19, 1955, p. 231.

31. Russel, MG, et al., "Inflammatory bowel disease: is there any relation between smoking status and disease presentation?" *Inflammatory Bowel Disease*, v. 4, 1998, pp. 182–86.

32. Micozzi, M, ed., *Fundamentals of Complementary and Alternative Medicine*, Churchill Livingstone, 1996, p. 209.

33. Blickston, SJ, "Treatment of Crohn's disease at the turn of the century," *New England Journal of Medicine*, v. 339, n. 6, 1998.

34. Thirlby, R, et al., "Effect of surgery on health-related quality of life in patients with inflammatory bowel disease," *Archives of Surgery*, v. 133, 1998, pp. 826–32.

35. Ekbom, A, et al., "Ulcerative colitis and colon cancer: a population based study," *New England Journal of Medicine*, v. 323, 11/90, pp. 1228–33.

36. Mannes, GA, et al., "Relation between the frequency of colorectal adenoma and the serum cholesterol level," *New England Journal of Medicine*, v. 315, 1986, pp. 1634–38.

37. Baron, M, et al., "Calcium supplements for the prevention of colorectal adenomas," *New England Journal of Medicine*, v. 340, 1999, pp. 101–7.

38. Nelson, RL, "Diet and adenomatous polyp risk," *Seminars of Colon and Rectal Surgery*, v. 2, 1991, pp. 262–68.

39. "Vitamin C and E after polyps surgery," in Bricklin, Mark, ed, *Natural Healing and Nutrition*, Rodale Press, 1989, p. 18.

40. Giovannucci, E, et al., "A prospective study of cigarette smoking and risk of colorectal adenoma and colorectal cancer in US men," *Journal of the National Cancer Institute*, v. 86, n. 3, 2/2/94, pp. 183–91.

41. Cope, GF, et al., "Alcohol consumption in patients with colorectal adenomatous polyps," *Gut*, v. 32, n. 1, 1991, pp. 70–72.

42. Bond, J, for the Practice Parameters Committee of the American College of Gastroenterology, "Polyp guideline: diagnosis, treatment, and surveillance for patients with non-familial colorectal polyps," *Annals of Internal Medicine*, v. 119, n. 8, 10/15/93, pp. 836–43.

43. Selby, et al., op. cit.

44. Winawer, S, et al., "Reduction in colorectal cancer incidence following colonoscopic polypectomy: report from the National Polyp Study," *Gastroenterology*, v. 100, 1991, p. A410.

45. Jemal, A, et al., "Cancer statistics, 2002," *CA: A Cancer Journal for Clinicians (2002)*, v. 52, n. 1, pp. 23–47.

46. Giovannucci, E, "Tobacco, colorectal cancer, and adenomas: a review of the evidence," *Journal of the National Cancer Institute*, v. 88, n. 23, 12/96, pp. 1717–30.

47. Chao, A, et al., "Cigarette smoking and colorectal cancer mortality in the Cancer Prevention Study II," Journal of the National Cancer Institute, v. 92, n. 23, 12/6/00.

48. Gilbertson, VA, "Proctosigmoidoscopy and polypectomy in reducing the incidence of rectal cancer, *Cancer*, v. 34, 1974, pp. 936–39.

49. Winawer, SJ, et al., "Prevention of colorectal

cancer by coloscopic polypectomy," *New England Journal of Medicine,* v. 329, 1993, pp. 1977–81.

50. Ries, LAG, et al., eds., *SEER Cancer Statistics Review, 1973–1998,* National Cancer Institute, 2001.

51. "Diet as medicine," *Self,* 9/89, p. 230.

52. "High-fat, calorie diet linked to colon cancer" (reporting on the research of Saxon Graham at the State University of New York, Buffalo), *Modern Medicine,* v. 56, 11/88, p. 23.

53. Willett, WC, et al., "Relation of meat, fat, and fiber intake to the risk of colon cancer in a prospective study among women," *New England Journal of Medicine,* v. 323, 1990, pp. 1664–71.

54. Arbman, G, et al., "Nutrition plays role in preventing colon cancer," *Cancer,* v. 69, 1992, pp. 2042–48.

55. Reddy, B, et al., "Biochemical epidemiology of colon cancer: effects of types of dietary fiber on fecal mutagens, acid, and neutral sterols in healthy subjects," *Cancer Research:* v. 49, 1989, pp. 4629–35.

56. Alberts, DS, et al., "Lack of effect of a high-fiber cereal supplement on the recurrence of colorectal adenomas," *New England Journal of Medicine,* v. 342, n. 16, 4/00.

57. Schatzkin, A, et al., "Lack of effect of a low-fat, high-fiber diet on the recurrence of colorectal adenomas," *New England Journal of Medicine,* v. 342, n. 16, 4/00.

58. Reddy, BS, et al., "Metabolic epidemiology of large bowel cancer: fecal bulk and constituents of high risk North American and low-risk Finnish population, *Cancer,* v. 42, 1979, pp. 2832–38.

59. Howe, GR, et al., "Dietary intake of fiber and decreased risk of cancers of the colon and rectum: evidence from the combined analysis of 13 case-controlled studies," *Journal of the National Cancer Institute,* v. 84, n. 24, 12/92, pp. 1887–96.

60. Griffin, PM, et al., "Adenocarcinoma of the colon and rectum in persons under 40 years old," *Gastroenterology,* v. 100, 1991, pp. 1033–40.

61. Goldin, BR, et al., "The effect of milk and lactobacillus feeding on human intestinal bacterial activity," *American Journal of Clinical Nutrition,* v. 39, 1984, pp. 756–61.

62. Alberts, DS, et al., "Effects of dietary wheat bran fiber on rectal epithelial cell proliferation in patients with resection for colorectal cancers," *Journal of the National Cancer Institute,* v. 82, n. 15, 8/90, pp. 1280–85.

63. The American Cancer Society 1996 Advisory Committee on Diet, Nutrition, and Cancer Prevention, "Guidelines on diet, nutrition, and cancer prevention: reducing the risk of cancer with healthy food choices and physical activity," *CA: A Cancer Journal for Clinicians,* 1996, v. 46, pp. 325–41.

64. "Diet, nutrition, and the prevention of cancer: a global perspective," World Cancer Research Fund/American Institute for Cancer Research, Washington D.C., 1997.

65. Arbman, et al., op. cit.

66. Reichel, H, et al., "The role of the vitamin D endocrine system in health and disease," *New England Journal of Medicine,* v. 320, 1989, pp. 980–91.

67. Schrauzer, GN, et al., "Cancer mortality correlation studies—III: statistical associations with dietary selenium intakes," *Bioinorganic Chemistry,* v. 7, n. 1, 1977, pp. 23–31.

68. Nelson, RL, "Diet and adenomatous polyp risk," *Seminars of Colon and Rectal Surgery,* v. 2, 1991, pp. 262–68.

69. Chao, A, et al., "Cigarette smoking and colorectal cancer mortality in the Cancer Prevention Study II," *Journal of the National Cancer Institute,* v. 92, n. 23, 12/6/00.

70. Arbman, et al., op. cit.

71. Kune, S, et al., "Case-control study of alco-

holic beverages as etiological factors: the Melbourne colorectal cancer study," *Nutrition & Cancer*, v. 9, 1987, pp. 43–56.

72. U.S. Department of Health and Human Services, *Physical Activity and Health: A Report of the Surgeon General*, Atlanta, 1996.

73. Garabrant, D, et al., "Job activity and colon cancer risk," *American Journal of Epidemiology*, v. 119, n. 6, 1984, pp.1005–14.

74. Giovanni, E, et al., "Aspirin and the risk of colorectal cancer in women," *New England Journal of Medicine*, v. 333, n. 10, 9/95, pp. 609–14.

75. Giovanni, E, et al., "Aspirin use and the risk of colorectal cancer and adenoma in male health professionals," *Annals of Internal Medicine*, v. 121, n. 4, 8/94, pp. 241–46.

76. Thun, MJ, et al., "Aspirin use and reduced risk of fatal colon cancer," *New England Journal of Medicine*, v. 325, 1991, pp. 1593–96.

77. Nanda, K, et al., "Hormone replacement therapy and the risk of colorectal cancer: a meta-analysis," *Obstetrics and Gynecology*, v. 93, n. 5, 1999, pp. 880–88.

78. Camma, C, et al., "Preoperative radiotherapy for resectable rectal cancer," *Journal of the American Medical Association*, v. 284, n. 8, 8/00.

79. "Cancernet" from the National Cancer Institute, PDQ information for health professionals, "Colon cancer," 6/97.

80. Porter, PA, et al., "Surgeon-related factors and outcome in rectal cancer," *Annals of Surgery*, v. 227, n. 2, 1998, pp. 157–67.

81. Heald, RJ, et al., "Rectal cancer: the Basingstoke experience of total mesorectal excision, 1978–1997," *Archives of Surgery*, v. 133, 1998, pp. 894–99.

82. Brodsky, JT, et al., "Variables correlated with the risk of lymph node metastases in early rectal cancer," *Cancer*, v. 69, n. 2, 1992, pp. 322–26.

83. Graham, RA, et al., "Local excision of rectal carcinoma," *The American Journal of Surgery*, v. 160, 9/90, pp. 308–12.

84. Goldberg, RM, et al., "Surgery for recurrent colon cancer: strategies for detecting resectable recurrence and success rate after resection," *Annals of Internal Medicine*, v. 129, 1998, pp. 27–35.

85. Olsen, KO, et al., "Reduced female fertility after ileal-anal pouch anastomosis," *Diseases of Colon and Rectum*, v. 41, 1998, pp. A43–A44.

86. Kohler, LW, et al., "Quality of life after proctocolectomy," *Gastroenterology*, v. 101, 1991, pp. 679–84.

Chapter 16

1. Rao, PM, et al., "Effect of computed tomography of the appendix on treatment of patients and use of hospital resources," *New England Journal of Medicine*, v. 338, 1998, pp. 141–46.

2. Burkitt, DP, et al., *Refined Carbohydrate Foods and Disease*, Academic Press, 1975, p. 87.

3. Rao, PM, et al., "Effect of computed tomography of the appendix on treatment of patients and use of hospital resources," *New England Journal of Medicine*, v. 338, 1998, pp. 141–46.

4. Chung, RS, et al., "A meta-analysis of randomized controlled trials of laparoscopic versus conventional appendectomy," *American Journal of Surgery*, v. 177, n. 3, 1999, pp. 250–56.

Chapter 17

1. Burkitt, Denis, *Don't Forget Fibre in Your Diet*, Arco Publishers, 1984.

2. Moesgaard, F, et al., "High-fiber diet reduces bleeding and pain in patients with hemorrhoids," *Diseases of Colon and Rectum*, v. 25, 1982, pp. 454–56.

3. Arabi, T, et al., "Trial of high fibre diet or local treatment for patients with hemorrhoids," *Gut*, v. 19, 1978, p. A987.

4. Craven, JL, "The use of bulk evacuation in patients with hemorrhoids," *British Journal of Surgery*, v. 65, 1978, pp. 291–92.

5. Moore, GS, "Fungicidal and fungistatic effects of an aqueous garlic extract on medically important yeast-like fungi, *Mycologia*, v. 69, pp. 341–48.

6. Geissler, C, et al., *American Journal of Clinical Nutrition*, v. 39, 3/84, p. 478.

7. *Current Therapeutic Research*, August 1963.

8. Shute, William, *Vitamin E for Healthy and Ailing Hearts*, Pyramid House, 1969.

9. Aprahamiam, M, et al., *American Journal of Clinical Nutrition*, 1985, pp. 578–79.

10. Parandekar, MN, "Notes on constipation: its causes and cure," *Yoga Mimamsa*, v. 4, n. 4, 1933, pp. 332–37.

11. Pdus, Emrika, *Emotions and Your Health*, Rodale Press, 1992, p. 516.

12. Goleman, Daniel, *Mind Body Medicine: How to Use Your Mind for Better Health*, Consumer Reports Books, 1993.

13. Samuels, Mike, et al., *Seeing with the Mind's Eye*, Random House, 1975, p. 225.

14. *Medical Letter on Drugs and Therapeutics*, v. 18, 12/3/76.

15. Lund, JN, and Scholefield, JH, "A randomised, prospective, double-blind, placebo-controlled trial of glyceryl trinitrate ointment in treatment of anal fissure," *Lancet*, v. 349, 1997, pp. 11–14.

16. Maria, G, et al., "A comparison of botulinum toxin and saline for treatment of chronic anal fissure," *New England Journal of Medicine*, v. 338, n. 4, 1998.

17. Brisinda, G, et al., "A comparison of injections of botulinum toxin and topical nitroglycerin ointment for the treatment of chronic anal fissure," *New England Journal of Medicine*, v. 341, n. 2, 7/99.

18. Wiley, DJ, and Beutner, K, "Genital warts," *Clinical Evidence*, v. 4, 12/2000, pp. 910–20.

19. Park, JJ, et al., "Repair of chronic anorectal fistulae using commercial fibrin sealant," *Archives of Surgery*, v. 135, n. 2, 2/00.

Chapter 18

1. Bricklin, Mark, *The Practical Encyclopedia of Natural Healing*, Rodale Press, 1976, p. 279.

2. Neuhauser, D, in Barker, et al., eds, *Costs, Risks, and Benefits in Surgery*, Oxford University Press, 1977, pp. 223–39.

3. Personal communication to Sandra.

4. McLanahan, DJ, et al., "Retrorectus prosthetic mesh repair of midline abdominal hernia," *American Journal of Surgery*, v. 173, n. 5, 1997, pp. 445–49.

5. Heniford, BT, et al., "Laparoscopic ventral and incisional hernia repair in 407 patients," *Journal of the American College of Surgeons*, v. 190, n. 6, 6/00.

6. McGregor, DB, et al., "The unilateral pediatric inguinal hernia: should the contralateral side be explored?" *Journal of Pediatric Surgery*, v. 15, 1980, pp. 313–37.

Chapter 19

1. "Utilization of hysterectomies under scrutiny," *American Medical News*, 8/24–31, 1990, p. 5.

2. Skakkeback, N, Research conducted at the University of Copenhagen, presented at the World Health Organization meetings, 1990.

3. Hufnagel, Vicki, *No More Hysterectomies*, Penguin, 1988.

4. Hufnagel, op. cit.

5. Ibid.

6. Taymor, ML, et al., "The etiological role of chronic iron deficiency in production of menorrhagia," *Journal of the American Medical Association*, v. 187, 1964, p. 323.

7. Lithgow, DM, et al., "Vitamin A in the treat-

ment of menorrhagia," *South African Medical Journal,* v. 51, 1977, p. 191; and Samuels, AJ, "Studies in patients with functional menorrhagia. The antihemorrhagic effect of the adequate repletion of iron stores," *Israel Journal of Medical Science,* v. 1, 7/1965 p. 851.

8. Cohen, JD, et al., "Functional menorrhagia: Treatment with bioflavonoids and vitamin C," *Current Therapeutic Research,* v. 2, 1960, p. 539.

9. Butler, EB, et al., "Vitamin E in the treatment of dysmenorrhea," *Lancet,* v. 1, 1955, p. 844.

10. Gubner, et al., "Vitamin K therapy in menorrhagia," *Southern Medical Journal,* v. 37, 1944, pp. 556–58.

11. Steinberg, A, et al., "Role of oxalic acid and certain related dicarboxylic acids in the control of hemorrhage," *Annals of Oto-Rhinology and Laryngoscopy,* v. 49, 1940, pp. 1008–21.

12. Harada, M, et al., "Effect of Japanese angelica root and peony root on uterine contraction in the rabbit in situ," *J.Pharmacobiodyn,* v. 7, n. 5, 1984, pp. 304–11

13. Priest, AW, et al., *Herbal Medication,* Fowler, 1982.

14. Pousset, JL, "Antihemolytic action of an extract of carica papaya bark," *Dakar Medicine,* v. 24, n. 3, 1979, pp. 255–62.

15. Ellingwood, R, *American Materia Medica, Therapeutics and Pharmacognosy,* Eclectic Medical Publications, 1983, p. 391.

16. Stoffer, SS, "Menstrual disorders and mild thyroid insufficiency: Intriguing cases suggesting an association," *Postgraduate Medicine,* v. 72, n. 2, 1982, p. 75.

17. Hufnagel, op. cit.

18. Neinstein, LS, "Menstrual dysfunction in pathophysiologic states," *Western Journal of Medicine,* v. 143, 10/85, pp. 476–84.

19. Carlson, KJ, et al., "Current Concepts: Indi-cations for Hysterectomy," *New England Journal of Medicine,* v. 328, n. 12, 3/93, pp. 856–60.

20. Gambone, JC, and DeCherney, AH, "Editorial," *New England Journal of Medicine,* v. 337, n. 4, 7/97, pp. 269–70.

21. Olive, DL, "Medical treatment: alternatives to Danazol," pp. 189–211, in Schenken, RS, ed, *Endometriosis: Contemporary Concepts in Clinical Management,* Lippincott, 1989.

22. Lu, PY, and Ory, SJ, "Endometriosis: current management," *Mayo Clinic Proceedings,* v. 70, 1995, pp. 453–63.

23. Bayer, SR, et al., "Efficacy of Danazol treatment for minimal endometriosis in infertile women: a prospective randomized study," *Journal of Reproductive Medicine,* v. 33, n. 2, 2/88, pp. 179–83.

24. Lu, and Ory, op. cit.

25. Vancaille, T, and Schenken. RS, "Endoscopic surgery," in Schenken, RS, ed, *Endometriosis: Current Concepts in Clinical Management,* Philadelphia: Lippincott, 1989, pp. 249–66.

26. Gordts, S, et al., "Microsurgery of endometriosis in infertile patients," *Fertility and Sterility,* v. 42, 1984, pp. 520–25.

27. Lu, and Ory, op. cit.

28. Marcoux, S, et al., "Laparoscopic surgery in infertile women with minimal or mild endometriosis," *New England Journal of Medicine,* v. 337, n. 4, 7/97, pp. 217–22.

29. Olive, DL, and Schwartz, LB, "Endometriosis," *New England Journal of Medicine,* v. 328, 1993, pp. 1759–69.

30. Golan, R., *Optimal Wellness,* Ballantine Books, 1995, p. 365.

31. Ibid.

32. Dasgupta, PR, et al., "Vitamin E (alpha tocopherol) in the management of menorrhagia associated with the use of intrauterine contraceptive

devices," *International Journal of Fertility,* v. 28, 1983, pp. 55–56.

33. Cohen, et al., op. cit.

34. Schumann, E, "Newer concepts of blood coagulation and control of hemorrhage," *American Journal of Obstetrics and Gynecology,* v. 38, 1939, pp. 1002–7.

35. Moghissi, KS, "Hormonal therapy before surgical treatment for uterine leiomyomas," *Surgery, Gynecology, and Obstetrics,* v. 172, n. 6, 1991, pp. 497–502.

36. Vedantham, S, et al., "Uterine artery embolization for fibroids: Considerations in patient selection and clinical follow-up," from the Departments of Radiological Sciences and Obstetrics and Gynecology, UCLA Medical Center, Los Angles, (based on 120 procedures), 1998.

37. Lacey, CG, "Benign disorders of the uterine corpus," in Pernoll, ML, ed, *Current Obstetric and Gynecologic Diagnosis and Treatment,* 7th ed, Appleton & Lange, 1992, pp. 647–53.

38. Carlson, et al., op. cit.

39. Lacey, op. cit.

40. Stovall, TG, et al., "Hysterectomy for chronic pelvic pain of presumed uterine etiology," *Obstetrics & Gynecology,* v. 75, 1990, pp. 676–79.

41. Jemal, A, et al., "Cancer statistics, 2002," *CA: A Cancer Journal for Clinicians (2002),* v. 52, n. 1, pp. 23–47.

42. Ries, LAG, et al., eds, *SEER Cancer Statistics Review, 1973–1998,* National Cancer Institute, 2001.

43. Butterworth Jr., CE, et al., "Folate-induced regression of cervical intraepithelial neoplasia (CIN) in users of oral contraceptive agents (OCA), *American Journal of Clinical Nutrition,* v. 33, 1980, p. 926.

44. Clarke, E, et al., "Cervical dysplasia: association with sexual behavior, smoking, and oral contraceptive use," *American Journal of Obstetrics and Gynecology,* v. 51, 1985, pp. 612–26.

45. Marshall, J, et al., "Diet and smoking in the epidemiology of cancer of the cervix," *Journal of the National Cancer Institute,* v. 70, n. 5, 5/83, pp. 847–51.

46. Ibid.

47. Romey, SL, et al., "Retinoids and the prevention of cervical dysplasia," *American Journal of Obstetrics and Gynecology,* v. 141, 1981, p. 890.

48. DeWys, WD, "The chemoprevention program of the National Cancer Institute," in Meykens Jr., Frank, et al., *Vitamins and Cancer: Human Cancer Prevention by Vitamins and Micronutrients,* Humana, 1986, pp. 301–10.

49. "Vitamin C may help prevent cervical dysplasia," *Family Practice News,* 3/1–14/83, p. 26.

50. Whitehead, N, et al., "Megaloblastic changes in the cervical epithelium association with oral contraceptive therapy and reversal with folic acid," *Journal of the American Medical Association,* v. 226, 1973, pp. 1421–24.

51. Goldberg, Burton, Group, *Alternative Medicine,* Future Medicine Publishing, 1993, p. 833.

52. Thomas, G, "Improved treatment for cervical cancer—concurrent chemotherapy and radiotherapy," *New England Journal of Medicine,* v. 340, n. 15, 1999.

53. Jemal, et al., op. cit.

54. Quillin, P, *Beating Cancer with Nutrition,* The Nutrition Times Press, 1994, p. 7.

55. *SEER Cancer Statistics Review,* op. cit.

56. Siddle, N, and Whitehead, M, "The effect of hysterectomy on the age at ovarian failure: identification of a subgroup of women with premature loss of ovarian function and literature review," *Fertility and Sterility,* v. 47, n. 1, 1987, pp. 94– 100.

57. Brown, JS, et al., "Hysterectomy and urinary incontinence: a systematic review," *Lancet,* v. 356, n. 9229, 8/00.

58. Hufnagel, Vicki, op. cit., p. 43.

59. Rhodes, JC, et al., "Hysterectomy and sexual functioning," *Journal of the American Medical Association,* v. 282, n. 20, 11/99.

60. Garry, R., and Phillips, G, "How safe is the laparoscopic approach to hysterectomy?" *Gynecologic Endoscopy,* v. 4, 1995, pp. 77–78.

61. Carlson, et al., op. cit.

62. Rhodes, et al., op. cit.

63. Coppen, A, et al., "Hysterectomy, hormones, and behavior: a prospective study," *Lancet,* v. 1, 1981, pp. 126–28.

64. Ryan, MM, et al., "Psychological aspects of hysterectomy: a prospective study," *British Journal of Psychiatry,* v. 154, 4/89, pp. 516–22.

65. Martin, RL, et al., "Psychiatric status after hysterectomy: a one year prospective follow-up," *Journal of the American Medical Association,* v. 244, n. 4, 1980, pp. 350–53.

66. Holt, VL, et al., "Cigarette smoking and functional ovarian cysts," *American Journal of Epidemiology,* v. 139, n. 8, 4/94, pp. 781–86.

67. Golan, op. cit., p. 400.

68. Jemal, et al., op. cit.

69. *SEER Cancer Statistics Review, 1973–1993,* op. cit.

70. *Diet, Nutrition, and Cancer,* National Academy Press, 1982, pp. 17–19.

71. "Ovarian cancer risk double in women who talc perineum," *Family Practice News,* v. 12, n. 24, 12/15–31/82, p. 4.

72. Narod, SA, et al., "Oral contraceptives and the risk of hereditary ovarian cancer," *New England Journal of Medicine,* v. 339, n. 7, 1998.

73. Hufnagel, op. cit.

74. Ibid.

Chapter 20

1. Carlson, Robert, *American Health,* 10/92, p. 59.

2. Horton, R, "Benign prostatic hyperplasia: a disorder of androgen metabolism in the male," *Journal of the American Geriatric Society,* v. 32, 1984, pp. 380–85.

3. Fahim, M, et al., "Zinc treatment for the reduction of hyperplasia of the prostate," *Federation Proceedings,* v. 35, 1976, p. 361.

4. Leake A, et al.,"The effect of zinc on the 5-alpha-reduction of testosterone on the hyperplastic human prostate gland," *Journal of Steroid Biochemistry,* v. 20, 1984, pp. 651–55.

5. Hart, JP, et al., "Vitamin F in the treatment of prostatic hyperplasia," Report Number 1, Lee Foundation for Nutritional Research, Milwaukee, WI, 1941.

6. Dumrau, F, "Benign prostatic hyperplasia: amino acid therapy for symptomatic relief," *American Journal of Gerontology,* v. 10, 1962, pp. 426–30.

7. Wilt, TJ, et al., "Saw palmetto extracts for treatment of benign prostatic hyperplasia," *Journal of the American Medical Association,* v. 240, 1998, pp. 1601–3.

8. Menendez, FH, et al., "Use of amino acids as a combination in the treatment of prostatic hypertrophy," *Archives of Experimental Urology,* v. 41, n. 7, 1988, pp. 495–99.

9. Belaiche, et al., "Clinical studies on the palliative treatment of prostatic adenoma with extract of urtica root," *Phytotherapy Research,* v. 5, 1991, pp. 267–69.

10. Buck, AC, et al., "Treatment of outflow tract obstruction due to benign prostatic hyperplasia with the pollen extract, Cernilton: a double-blind, placebo-controlled study," *British Journal of Urology,* v. 66, n. 4, 1990, pp. 398–404.

11. Ellis, N, et al., "The effect of acupuncture on nocturnal urinary frequency and incontinence in the elderly," *Complementary Medicine Research,* v. 4, 1990, pp. 16–17.

12. Corenblum, B, and Whitaker, M, "Inhibition of stress-induced hyperprolactinemia," *British Medical Journal,* v. 275, 1977, p. 1328.

13. Lepor, H, "A Department of Veterans Affairs Cooperative randomized placebo controlled clinical trial of the safety and efficacy of terazosin/finasteride monotherapy and terazosin/finasteride combination therapy in men with clinical BPH," *Journal of Urology,* v. 155, n. 5, 5/96, p. 587A.

14. Bruskewitz, MM, et al., "A prospective randomized 1-year clinical trial comparing transurethral needle ablation to transurethral resection of the prostate for the treatment of symptomatic benign prostatic hyperplasia," *Journal of Urology,* v. 159, 1998, pp. 1588–94.

15. Jemal, A, et al., "Cancer statistics, 2002," *CA: A Cancer Journal for Clinicians (2002),* v. 52, n. 1, pp. 23–47.

16. Kolonel, LN, "Nutrient intake in relation to cancer incidence in Hawaii," *British Journal of Cancer,* v. 44, 1981, pp. 332–39.

17. Giovannucci, Edward, Harvard research reported in "Dietary fat intake found to speed progression of prostate cancer," *Medical Tribune,* 10/21/93.

18. Howell, MA, "Factor analysis of international cancer mortality data and *per capita* food consumption," *British Journal of Cancer,* v. 29, 1974, pp. 328–36.

19. Howie, GJ, et al., "Dietary and hormonal interrelationships among vegetarian Seventh-Day Adventists and nonvegetarian men," *American Journal of Clinical Nutrition,* v. 42, n. 1, 7/85, pp. 127–34.

20. Stocks, P, "Cancer incidence in North Wales and Liverpool region in relation to habits and environment," *British Empire Cancer Campaign, Thirty Fifth Annual Report, Supplement to Part II,* Cancer Research Campaign, London, 1957, p. 156.

21. Blair, A, et al., "Geographic patterns of prostate cancer in the United States," *Journal of the National Cancer Institute,* v. 61, 1978, pp. 1379–84.

22. American College of Physicians—Coley, C, et al., "Screening for prostate cancer: part III," *Annals of Internal Medicine,* v. 126, n. 6, 3/15/97, pp. 480–84.

23. Ries, LAG, et al., eds, *SEER Cancer Statistics Review, 1973–1998,* National Cancer Institute, 2001.

24. Hirayama, T, "Epidemiology of prostate cancer with special reference to the role of diet," *National Cancer Institute Monograph,* v. 53, 1979, pp. 149–54.

25. Renneker, Mark, *Understanding Cancer,* Bull Publishing, 1988, p. 148.

26. Jaroff, Leon, "The Man's Cancer," *Time* magazine, 4/1/96, p. 65.

27. Stocks, op. cit.

28. Sattilaro, Anthony, *Recalled by Life,* Avon Books, 1982.

29. Martin, W, "Treatment of prostate and breast cancer," *Townsend Letter for Doctors,* 5/90.

30. Gibbons, D, *Family Practice News,* 2/1/92, p. 7.

31. Messina, M, "The role of soy products in reducing risk of cancer," *Journal of the National Cancer Institute,* v. 83, n. 8, 1991, pp. 541–46.

32. Giovannucci, E, "Intake of carotenoids and retinol in relation to prostate cancer," *Journal of the National Cancer Institute,* v. 87, n. 23, 1995, pp. 1767–76.

33. Cohen, JH, "Fruit and vegetable intakes and prostate cancer risk," *Journal of the National Cancer Institute,* v. l92, n. 1, 1/00.

34. Whelen, P, et al., "Zinc, vitamin A, and prostate cancer," *British Journal of Urology*, v. 55, n. 5, 1983, pp. 525–28.

35. Kristal, KR, et al., "Vitamin and mineral supplement use is associated with reduced risk of prostate cancer," *Cancer Epidemiology Biomarkers and Prevention*, v. 18, n. 10, 10/99.

36. Clark, LC, et al., "Decreased incidence of prostate cancer with selenium supplementation: results of a double-blind cancer prevention trial," *British Journal of Urology*, v. 81, n. 5, 5/98.

37. Lau, B, et al., "Allium sativum (garlic) and cancer prevention," *Nutrition Research*, v. 10, 1990, pp. 937–48; also Dorant, E, et al., "Garlic and its significance for the prevention of cancer in humans: a critical review, *British Journal of Cancer*, v. 67, 1993, pp. 424–29; and Dausch, JG, et al., "Garlic: a review of its relationship to malignant disease," *Preventive Medicine*, v. 19, 1990, pp. 346–61.

38. Morgan, Brian, *Nutrition Prescription*, Crown Books, 1993, p. 273.

39. Renneker, Mark, *Understanding Cancer*, Bull Publishing, 1988.

40. Giovannucci, Edward, "A prospective cohort study of vasectomy and prostate cancer in U.S. men," *Journal of the American Medical Association*, v. 269, n. 7, 2/17/92, pp. 873–77.

41. Spiegel, David, "A psychosocial intervention and survival time of patients with metastatic breast cancer," *Advances*, v. 7, n. 3, summer 1991, pp. 10–19.

42. Nicolaou, N, presented at the American Society for Therapeutic Radiology and Oncology, Los Angeles, 10/30/96.

43. Concato, J, et al., "Problems of comorbidity in mortality after prostatectomy," *Journal of the American Medical Association* v. 267, 1992, pp. 1077–82.

44. Fowler, FJ, et al., Patient-reported complications and follow-up treatment after radical prostatectomy—the National Medicare experience: 1988–1990 (updated June 1993), *Urology*, v. 42, n. 6, 1993, p. 6229.

45. Robinson, J, et al., "Erectile function of men following brachytherapy compared with other treatments for localized prostate carcinoma," *International Journal of Radiation Oncology, Biology, and Physics*, v. 48, n. 3, 2000.

46. NIH Consensus Development Panel on Impotence, *Journal of the American Medical Association*, v. 270, 1993, pp. 83–90.

47. Juenemann, KP, et al., "The effect of cigarette smoking on penile erection," *Journal of Urology* v. 138, 1987, pp. 438–41.

48. Research from the Centers for Disease Control and Prevention, 12/94.

49. Research from the Medical College of South Carolina at Charleston, 1994.

50. Miller, NS, and Gold, MS, "The human sexual response and alcohol and drugs," *Journal of Substance Abuse Treatment*, v. 15, 1988, pp. 171–77.

51. Sikora, R, et al., "Gingko biloba extract in the therapy of erectile dysfunction," *Journal of Urology*, v. 141, 1989, p. 188A.

52. Ernst, E, and Pittler, MH, "Yohimbine for erectile dysfunction: a systematic review and meta-analysis of randomized clinical trials," *Journal of Urology* v. 159, n. 2, 2/98, pp. 433–36.

53. Rimm, Eric, report to a meeting of the American Urological Association in June 2000.

54. Lue, TF, "Erectile Dysfunction," editorial, *New England Journal of Medicine*, v. 342, n. 24, 6/00.

55. Goldstein, I, et al., "Oral sildenafil in the treatment of erectile dysfunction," *New England Journal of Medicine*, v. 338, 1998, pp. 1397–1404.

56. Muller, JE, et al., "Triggering myocardial infarction by sexual activity: low risk and prevention by regular physical exertion," *Journal of the*

American Medical Association, v. 275, 1996, pp. 1405–9.

57. Wolfe, SM, Director, Public Citizen, Letter to Dr. Janet Wookcock, Director for Drug Evaluation and Research, FDA, 6/5/00.

58. Linet, O, et al., "Efficacy and safety of intracavernosal alprostadil in men with erectile dysfunction," *New England Journal of Medicine,* v. 334, n. 14, 1996, p. 8737.

59. Ibid.

60. Harin, PN, et al., "Treatment of erectile dysfunction with transurethral alprostadil," *New England Journal of Medicine,* v. 336, n. 1, 1/97, pp. 1–7.

61. Lewis, RL, MUSE-ACTIS Study Group report at the 93rd Meeting of the American Urology Association, San Diego, 1998.

62. Krane, RJ, "Impotence," *New England Journal of Medicine,* v. 321, n. 24, 12/14/89, pp. 1648–59.

63. Cookson, MS, "Analysis of microsurgical penile revascularization results by etiology of impotence," *Journal of Urology,* v. 149, 5/93, pp. 1308–12.

64. Freedman, AL, et al., "Long-term results of penile vein ligation for impotence from venous leakage," *Journal of Urology,* v. 149, 5/93, p. 13013.

65. Stanley, GE, et al., "Penile prosthetic trends in the era of effective oral erectogenic agents," *Southern Medical Journal 2000,* v. 93, n. 12, pp. 1153–56.

Chapter 21

1. "On Health," *Newsweek,* spring 1987, p. 18.

2. Paul, T, et al., "Long-term L-thyroxine therapy is associated with decreased hip bone density in premenopausal women," *Journal of the American Medical Association,"* v. 259, n. 21, 6/3/88, pp. 3137–41.

3. *Family Practice News,* 6/15/83, p. 14.

4. Udupa, KN, *Disorders of Stress and Their Management by Yoga,* Benares Hindu University Press, 1978, pp. 144ff.

5. Hashizume, K, et al., "Administration of thyroxine in treated Grave's disease: effects on the level of antibodies to TSH receptors and on the risk of recurrence of hyperthyroidism," *New England Journal of Medicine,* v. 324, n. 14, 4/1991, p. 947.

6. Rui, Li, "Clinical observation on treating exopthalmic thyroidismus with acupuncture," in *Advances in Acupuncture and Acupuncture Anaesthesia,* The People's Medical Publishing House, 1980, p. 85.

7. Prummel, Mark, "Smoking and risk of Grave's disease," *Journal of the American Medical Association,* v. 269, n. 4, 1/27/93, pp. 497–82.

8. Bautista, A, et al., "The effects of oral iodized oil on intelligence, thyroid status, and somatic growth in school-age children from an area of endemic goiter," *American Journal of Clinical Nutrition,* v. 35, n. 1, 1/82, pp. 127–34.

9. Greenlee, RT, et al., "Cancer statistics, 2001," *CA: A Cancer Journal for Clinicians (2001),* v. 51, n. 1, pp. 15–36.

10. Ries, LAG, et al., eds, *SEER Cancer Statistics Review, 1973–1998,* National Cancer Institute, 2001.

11. Frisch, RE, et al., "Lower prevalence of non–reproductive system cancers among former college athletes," *Medicine and Science in Sports and Exercise,* v. 21, n. 3, 1989, pp. 250–53.

12. Horrigan, C, "Complementing cancer care," *International Journal of Aromatherapy,* v. 3, n. 4, 1991, pp. 15–17.

13. Sanders, LE, and Cady, B, "Differentiated thyroid cancer," *Archives of Surgery,* v. 133, 1998, pp. 419–25.

14. Hay, ID, et al., "Unilateral total lobectomy: is it sufficient surgical treatment for patients with

AMES low-risk papillary thyroid carcinoma?" *Surgery,* v. 124, n. 6, 12/1998, pp. 958–64.

15. Sosa, JA, et al., "The importance of surgeon experience for clinical and economic outcomes from thyroidectomy," *Annals of Surgery,* v. 228, n. 3, 1998, pp. 320–30.

Chapter 22

1. Shields, CB, et al., "Low back pain," *American Family Practice,* p. 173, 3/86.

2. Setterberg, F, "How I got my back up," *Hippocrates,* 3–4/1990, pp. 36–45.

3. Jensen, MC, et al., "Magnetic resonance imaging of the lumbar spine in people without back pain," *New England Journal of Medicine,* v. 331, 1994, pp. 69–73.

4. Ibid.

5. "Back pain relief depends on whom you ask," *Medical Tribune,* 9/9/93, p. 2.

6. *Time,* 7/14/80, p. 35.

7. "Back pain relief depends on whom you ask," op. cit.

8. Barton, JE, et al., "Low back pain in the primary care setting," *The Journal of Family Practice,* v. 3, n. 4, 1978, pp. 363–66.

9. Volinn, E, et al., "Theories of back pain and health care utilization," *Neurosurgical Clinics of North America,* v. 2, 1991, pp. 739–48; and Taylor, VM, et al., "Low back pain hospitalization: recent United States trends and regional variations," *Spine,* v. 19, 1994, pp. 1207–12.

10. Fisher, W., III, "Selection of patients for surgery," *Neurosurgery Clinics of North America,* v. 4, n. 1, 1/93, pp. 35–44.

11. "Pantopaque may cause low-back pain," *American Family Physician,* 4/78, p. 271.

12. *Time,* op. cit., p. 31.

13. Donaldson, Norman, et al., *The Book of Back Care,* Random House, 1982.

14. Personal communication to Sandra.

15. Tarlov, E, et al., *Back Attack,* Little Brown, 1985, as quoted in "A primer for students—and sufferers—of back pain," *Medical Tribune,* 10/16/85, p. 29.

16. Federal practice guidelines from the Agency for Health Care Policy and Research, as reported in "Less is more in managing acute low back problems," *Family Practice News,* v. 25, n. 6, 3/15/95, p. 1.

17. Roukoz, S, et al., "Critical study of 200 surgically treated lumbar disk hernias," *Annals de Chirurgie,* v. 44, n. 1, 1990, pp. 44–48; and Tarlov, et al., op. cit.

18. Saal, JA, et al., "Nonoperative treatment of herniated lumbar intervertebral disc with radiculopathy: an outcome study," *Spine,* v. 14, 1989, pp. 431–37.

19. Wiltse, LL, "Surgery for intervertebral disk disease of the lumbar spine," *Clinical Orthopaedics and Related Research,* 11–12/77, pp. 22–45.

20. Unpublished research conducted at Columbia University School of Public Health.

21. "What's the best kind of bed for a bad back?" *Hippocrates,* 2/92, p. 92.

22. Barton, et al., op. cit.

23. *Time,* 7/14/80, p. 33.

24. *Medical World News,* 3/1/82, p. 29.

25. Klein, A, et al., "Put an end to back pain," *American Health,* 9/93, pp. 48–53.

26. Krause, H, et al., "Evaluation of an exercise program for back pain," *American Family Physician,* v. 28, n. 3, 1983, pp. 153–58.

27. Klein, et al., op. cit.

28. "Flexibility may predict need for back surgery," *Modern Medicine,* 1/83, p. 47.

29. "Sit-ups alone found to end back pain," *Medical World News,* 1/24/83.

30. *Time*, p. 34.

31. "Flexibility," op. cit.

32. Jarvikoski, A, "Symptoms of psychological distress and treatment effects with low-back pain patients," *Pain*, v. 25, n. 3, 6/86, pp. 345–55.

33. Sarno, J, *Mind over Back Pain*, Berkeley Books, 1986.

34. Ananthanarayanan, TV, et al., "Physiological benefits in Hatha Yoga training," *Yoga Review*, v. 3, n. 1, 1983, pp. 9–24.

35. Sarno, J, *Healing Back Pain*, Warner, 1991.

36. Jarvikoski, op. cit.

37. Maimivaara, A, et al., "The treatment of acute low back pain—bed rest, exercises, or ordinary activity," *New England Journal of Medicine*, v. 332, 1995, pp. 351–55.

38. "Bed rest said to be curative treatment for low back pain," *Family Practice News*, v. 5, n. 14.

39. Von Karff, M, et al., "Effects of practice style in managing back pain," *Annals of Internal Medicine*, v. 121, 1994, pp. 187–95.

40. Change, WD, et al., "Functional approach to treatment of back pain in primary care: a preliminary report," *Chung Hua l Hsueh Tsa Chih*, Taipei, v. 53, 1994, pp. 338–45.

41. Shekelle, P, "Spinal manipulation for low back pain," *Annnals of Internal Medicine*, v. 117, n. 7, 10/92, pp. 590–98.

42. Koes, BW, et al., "Randomized clinical trial of manipulative therapy and physiotherapy for persistent back and neck complaints: results of one year follow-up," *British Medical Journal*, v. 304, n. 6827, 3/92, pp. 601–5.

43. Meade, TW, "Low back pain of mechanical origin: randomized comparison of chiropractic and hospital outpatient treatment," *British Medical Journal*, v. 300, n. 6737, 6/90, pp. 1431–37.

44. Cherkin, D, "A comparison of physical therapy, chiropractic manipulation, and provisions of an educational booklet for the treatment of patients with low back pain," *New England Journal of Medicine*, v. 339, n. 15, 1998, pp. 1021–29.

45. Laitinen, J, "Acupuncture and transcutaneous electric stimulation in the treatment of chronic sacrolubalgia and ischialgia," *American Journal of Chinese Medicine*, v. 4, 1976, pp. 169–75; and Coan, RM, et al., "The acupuncture treatment of low back pain: a randomized controlled study," *American Journal of Chinese Medicine*, v. 8, 1980, p. 1819.

46. Ernst, E, and White, AR, "Acupuncture for back pain: a meta-analysis of randomized controlled trials," *Archives of Internal Medicine*, v. 158, 1998, pp. 2235–41.

47. "Some 'back pain' is termed treatable behavior," *Medical Tribune*, n. 12, 1980, p. 9.

48. Barton, et al., op. cit.

49. "Patients diagram their pain and orthopedist moves in with drugs, surgery, counseling," *Medical Tribune*, 4/1/81.

50. Sarno, *Healing Back Pain*, op. cit.

51. "Surgery held rarely appropriate for low back pain," *Family Practice News*, 5/15–31/89, p. 46.

52. Overman, SS, et al., "Physical therapy care for low back pain," *Physical Therapy*, v. 68, n. 2, 2/88, pp. 199–207.

53. Rask, MR, *Journal of Neurologic and Orthopedic Medicine and Surgery*, v. 10, 1989, p. 291.

54. "Epidural shots for back pain held often obviating surgery," *Medical Tribune*, 11/24/82, p. 3.

55. Montana, Joe, et al., *Montana*, Turner Publishing, 1995, p. 67.

56. Weber, H, "Lumbar disc herniation, a controlled, prospective study with ten years of observation," *Spine*, v. 8, n. 2, 3/83, pp. 131–40.

57. Montana, et al., *Montana,* Turner Publishing, 1995.

58. Coan, RM, et al., "The acupuncture treatment of neck pain: a randomized controlled study," *American Journal of Chinese Medicine,* v. 9, 1982, pp. 326–32.

59. Loy, TT, "Treatment of cervical spondylosis, electroacupuncture versus physiotherapy," *Medical Journal of Australia,* v. 2, 1983, pp. 32–34.

60. Hurwitz, EL, et al., "Manipulation and mobilization of the cervical spine. A systematic review of the literature," *Spine,* v. 21, n. 15, 8/1/96, pp. 1746–59.

61. Rosenfeld, M, et al., "Early intervention in whiplash-associated disorders: a comparison of two treatment protocols," *Spine,* v. 25, n. 14, 7/00, pp. 1782–87.

62. Bush, K, and Hillier, S, "Outcome of cervical radiculopathy treated with periradicular/epidural corticosteroid injections: a prospective study with independent clinical review," *European Spine Journal,* v. 5, n. 5, 1996, pp. 319–25.

63. Wang, LQ, et al., "Clinical analysis and experimental observation on acupuncture and moxibustion treatment of patellar tendon terminal disease in athletes," *Journal of Traditional Chinese Medicine,* v. 5, 1985, pp. 162–66.

64. Plancher, KD, et al., "Reconstruction of the anterior cruciate ligament in patients who are at least forty years old, a long-term follow up and outcome study," *Journal of Bone and Joint Surgery,* v. 80A, n. 2, 1998, pp. 184–97.

65. American Academy of Orthopedic Surgeons, 1992 statistics.

66. McGarey, William, *The Oil That Heals,* A.R.E. Press, 1993, pp. 202–4.

67. Moore, RA, et al., "Quantative systematic review of topically applied non-steroidal anti-inflammatory drugs," *British Medical Journal,* v. 316, 1998, pp. 333–38.

68. Deal, CL, et al., "Treatment of arthritis with topical capsaicin: a double-blind trial," *Clinical Therapy,* v. 13, 1991, pp. 383–95.

69. Ravaud, et al., "Effects of joint lavage and steroid injection in patients with osteoarthritis of the knee: results of a multicenter, randomized, controlled trial," *Arthritis and Rheumatology,* v. 42, 1999, pp. 475–82.

70. Huskisson, EC, and Donnelly, S, "Hyaluronic acid in the treatment of osteoarthritis of the knee," *Rheumatology,* v. 38, 1999, pp. 602–7.

71. American Academy of Orthopedic Surgeons, op. cit.

72. Sobel, D, *Arthritis: What Works,* St. Martin's Press, 1989.

73. Childers, NF, et al., *The Nightshades and Health,* Somerville, NJ: Horticulture Publications, 1973.

74. Marcolongo, R, "Doule-blind multicentre study of the activity of S-adenosyl-methionine in hip osteoarthritis," *Current Therapeutic Research,* v. 37, 1985, pp. 82–94.

75. Machtey, I, et al., "Tocopherol in osteoarthritis: a controlled pilot study, *Journal of the American Geriatrics Society,* v. 26, 1978, pp. 328–30.

76. LeBoff, MS, et al., "Occult vitamin D deficiency in postmenopausal women with acute hip fracture," *Journal of the American Medical Association,* v. 281, 1999, pp. 1505–11.

77. "Healing of hip joint may avoid surgery in juvenile arthritis," *Medical Tribune,* 8/4/76, p. 3.

78. Brief, AA, et al., "Perspective on modern orthopedics use of glucosamine and chondroitin sulfate in the management of osteoarthritis," *Journal of the American Academy of Orthopedic Surgeons,* v. 9, n. 2, 2001, pp. 71–78.

79. Moore, RA, et al., "Quantative systematic review of topically aplied non-steroidal anti-inflammatory drugs, *British Medical Journal,* v. 316, 1998, pp. 333–38.

80. Deal, CL, et al., "Treatment of arthritis with topical capsaicin: a double-blind trial," *Clinical Therapy,* v. 13, 1991, pp. 383–95.

81. Harris, W, and Sledge, C, "Total hip and knee replacement," *New England Journal of Medicine,* v. 323, n. 11, 8/13/90, pp. 725–31.

82. NIH Consensus Development Conference on Total Hip Replacement, *Journal of the American Medical Association,* v. 273, n. 24, 6/28/95, pp. 1950–56.

83. Rossignol, M, et al., "Carpal tunnel syndrome: what is attributable to work? The Montreal Study," *Occupational and Environmental Medicine,* v. 54, 7/1997, pp. 519–23.

84. Ellis, JM, et al., "Clinical results of a cross-over treatment with pyridoxine and placebo of the carpal tunnel syndrome," *American Journal of Clinical Nutrition,* v. 32, 1979. p. 2040; and Ellis, J, "Response of vitamin B$_6$ deficiency and the carpel tunnel syndrome to pridoxine," *Proceedings of the National Academy of Sciences,* 12/82, pp. 7494–98.

85. Garfinkel, MS, et al., "Yoga-based intervention for carpal tunnel syndrome," *Journal of the American Medical Association,* v. 280, 1998, pp. 1601– 3.

86. Chen, GS, "The effect of accupuncture treatment on carpal tunnel syndrome," *American Journal of Accupuncture,* v. 18, 1990, pp. 5–9.

Chapter 23

1. Berggren, RB, "Liposuction: what it will and won't do," *Postgraduate Medicine,* v. 87, n. 6, 5/90, pp. 187–88, 193–95.

2. Fuleihan, NS, et al., "The facelift and ancillary procedures," *Journal of Dermatologic Surgery and Oncology,* v. 16, 1990, pp. 975– 87.

3. Ibid.

4. *The Philadelphia Inquirer,* 10/22/95, p. 3.

5. *Family Practice News,* 8/1/92, p. 10.

6. Paradise, JL, et al., "Adenoidectomy and adenotonsilectomy for recurrent otitis media: parallel randomized clinical trials in children not previously treated with tympanostomy tubes," *Journal of the American Medical Association* v. 282, n. 10, 9/99.

7. Pratt, L, "Tonsillectomy and adenoidectomy: mortality and morbidity," *Transactions of the American Academy of Ophthalomology and Otolaryngology,* v. 74, 1970, p. 1114.

8. American College of Ophthalmology web site: www.eyenet.org.

9. Werbach, Melvyn, *Healing Through Nutrition: A Natural Approach to Treating 50 Common Illnesses with Diet and Nutrients,* HarperCollins, 1993, p. 69.

10. Ibid.

11. "The nutritional origins of cataracts," *Nutrition Reviews,* v. 42, n. 11, 1984.

12. Atkinson, D, "Malnutrition as an etiological factor in senile cataract," *Eye, Ear, Nose and Throat Monthly,* v. 31, 1952, pp. 79–83.

13. Bellows, J, "Biochemistry of lens: some studies on vitamin C and lens," *Achives of Opthalmology,* v. 16, 1936, p. 58.

14. Skalka, HW, et al., "Riboflavin deficiency and cataract formation," *Metabolic and Pediatric Opthalmology,* v. 5, n. 1, 1981, pp. 17–20.

15. Swanson, A, et al., "Elemental analysis in normal and cataractous human lens tissue," *Biochemical and Biophysical Research Communications,* v. 45, 1971, pp. 1488–96.

16. Werbach, op. cit., p. 68.

17. *University of California at Berkeley Wellness Letter,* v. 12, n. 12, 9/96, p. 1.

18. Varma, SD, et al., "Light-induced damage to ocular lens cation pump: prevention by vitamin C," *Proceedings of the National Acadamy of Sciences,* v. 76, 1979, pp. 3504–6.

19. Atkinson, D, "Malnutrition as an etiological factor in senile cataract," *Eye, Ear, Nose and Throat Monthly*, v. 31, 1952, pp. 79–83.

20. Werbach, op. cit., p. 69.

21. Ross, WM, "Modeling cortical cataractogenesis—III: in vivo effects of vitamin E on cataractogenesis in diabetic rats," *Canadian Journal of Ophthalmology*, v. 17, n. 2, 1982, pp. 61–66; and Varma, SD, et al., *Photochemistry and Photobiology*, v. 36, n. 6, 1982.

22. Ketola, HG, *Journal of Nutrition*, v. 109, 1979, pp. 965–69.

23. Fujihira, K, "Treatment of cataract with ba-wei-ren (*hachimijiogan*)," *Journal of the Society of Oriental Medicine in Japan*, v. 24, 1974, pp. 465–79.

24. Christen, WG, et al., "Smoking cessation and risk of age-related cataract in men," *Journal of the American Medical Association*, v. 284, n. 6, 6/00.

25. American College of Ophthalmology web site: www.eyenet.org.

26. Robertson, W, et al., "Prevalence of urinary stone disease in vegetarians," *European Urology*, v. 8, 1982, pp. 334–39.

27. Griffith, H, et al., "A control study of dietary factors in renal stone formation," *British Journal of Urology*, v. 53, 1981, pp. 416–20.

28. Shaw, P, et al., "Idiopathic hypercalcemia: its control with unprocessed bran," *British Journal of Urology*, v. 52, 1980, pp. 426–69.

29. Rose, G, et al., "The influence of calcium content of water, intake of vegetables and fruit and of other food factors upon the incidence of renal calculi," *Urological Research*, v. 3, 1975, pp. 61–66.

30. Ulmann, A, et al., "Effects of weight and glucose ingestion on urinary calcium and phosphate excretion: implications for calcium urolithiasis," *Journal of Clinical Endocrinology and Metabolism*, v. 54, 1982, pp. 1063–67.

31. Zechner, O, et al., "Nutritional risk factors in urinary stone disease," *Journal of Urology*, v. 125, 1981, pp. 51–55.

32. Curhan, GC, et al., "Comparison of dietary calcium with supplemental calcium and other nutrients as factors affecting the risk of kidney stones in women," *Annals of Internal Medicine*, v. 126, n. 7, 4/97, pp. 553–55.

33. "Calcium treatment may prevent formation of kidney stones," *American Family Practice*, v. 2, n. 7, 7/76, p. 4; and Brockis, JG, et al., "The effects of vegetable and animal protein diets on calcium, urate and oxalate excretion," *British Journal of Urology*, v. 54, n. 6, 1982, pp. 590–93.

34. Johansson, et al., "Magnesium metabolism in renal stone formers: effects of therapy with magnesium hydroxide," *Scandinavian Journal of Urology and Nephrology*, v. 53, 1980, pp. 125–30.

35. Pac, CYC, and Fuller, C, "Idiopathic hypocitraturic calcium-oxalate nephrolithiasis successfully treated with potassium oxalate," *Annals of Internal Medicine*, v. 104, 1986, pp. 33–37.

36. Curhan, GC, et al., "A prospective study of the intake of vitamins C and B_6, and the risk of kidney stones in men," *Journal of Urology*, v. 155, n. 6, 6/96, pp. 1847–51.

37. Ulman, et al., op. cit.

Chapter 24

1. Oz, M, et al., "Complementary medicine in the surgical wards," *Journal of the American Medical Association*, v. 279, 1998, pp. 710–11.

2. Lemole, Gerald W, An *Integrative Approach to Cardiac Care*, Medtronic, Inc., 2000.

3. Norred, Carol, et al., "Use of complementary and alternative medicines by surgical patients," *American Association of Nurse Anesthetists Journal*, v. 68, n. 1, 2000, pp 13–18.

4. Ibid.

5. Sieron, A, et al., "Use of magnetic field in treatment of trophic leg ulcers, *Polski Tygodnik Lekarski,* v. 46, n. 37–39, pp. 717–19; Krag, C, et al., "The effect of pulsed electromagnetic energy (Diapulse) on the survival of experimental skin flaps: a study on rats," *Scandinavian Journal of Plastic and Reconstructive Surgery,* 1979: v. 13, n. 3, pp. 377–80; additional unpublished Magnatherm research, Jeff Lipsky, Kansas City, MO, 800–432–8003.

6. McGarey, W, *Physician's Reference Notebook,* A.R.E. Press, 1968, pp. 315–16.

7. "Vitamin E may delay healing," *Family Practice News,* 3/15–31/97.

8. Menard, M, "The effect of therapeutic massage on post-surgical outcomes," doctoral thesis, University of Virginia, 1995.

Index

A Surgeon Under the Knife (Nolen), 107
abdominal aortic aneurysm, 307–9
abdominal artery bypass operations, 300–302, 302(fig.)
abdominal perineal resection with colostomy, 441; and proctocolectomy with ileostomy, 444, 446
abdominoplasty ("tummy tuck"), 670–72, 671(fig.)
Abel, Robert, 693
abortion, 209, 210
abscess drainage, 422, 456, 479
acetaminophen, 126, 646, 653
acid blockers, 346
Acterberg, Jeanne, 47, 207
Actigal, 387
acupressure, 674
acupuncture, 25, 30; after surgery, 716; as alternative anesthesia, 119–20; for back problems, 620; for benign prostate enlargement, 561; for breast cancer, 208; for carpal tunnel syndrome, 661; and Chinese medicine, 73–74; for facial cosmetic problems, 674; for heartburn, 345; for hernia, 485, 491, 494; for hip joint damage, 653; for hyperthyroidism, 595; for inflammatory colitis, 428; for knee injuries, 641, 646; for lung cancer, 231; for malignant melanoma, 166; for neck problems, 630; in self-healing process, 17; for skin cancer, 161; for smoking cessation, 85; for stroke recovery, 318–19
acute cholecystitis, 382, 388
acute colitis, 425
acute pancreatitis, 397–400
Adalat, 273
Adams, Patch, 23, 60
adenocarcinoma, 240
adenoids, tonsils and, 684–90, 685(fig.)
adenoma polyps, 431, 432
adenomyosis, 520
adjuvant chemotherapy, 226, 227
adjuvant hormonal therapy, 226
adjuvant radiotherapy, 227

adjuvant treatment of breast cancer, 226–28
Advance Directive form, 108
Advanced Breast Biopsy Instrument, 188
Advil, 126, 127, 513, 621, 631, 634, 638, 646, 654
Air Force/Texas Coronary Atherosclerosis Prevention Study, 274
alcohol, 68, 69, 86, 174, 204–5, 268, 318, 350, 361, 375, 398, 400, 403, 432, 438, 581
Alcoholics Anonymous, 59, 400
Aldara, 477
Aleve, 126, 513
Alexander Technique, 51, 619
alkaline phosphatase, 106
alkaline reflux gastritis, 371
allergic diseases, fasting and, 84
Alleve, 622, 631, 634, 638, 646, 654
aloe vera, 79
alprostadil, 584
alternative healing methods, 25, 34, 73–83
alternative medicine, 13–14; alternative/complementary/integrative health centers, 30–31; avoiding blaming the victim, 27–28; choosing from among the alternatives, 26–27; death, 28–30; fundamentals of, 18–25; life support considerations, 28; most common alternatives, 25–26; operating room of the future, 30; pain relief, methods of, 127–29; protecting yourself from unreliable alternatives, 27; scientific research on, 26; self-healing, 17–18; special benefits of the alternative medicine approach, 104; third surgical opinion option, 94–95; why "alternative" medicine, 14–17
alternative medicine approaches, specific, 33–34; alternative approaches in addition to surgery, 89; alternative approaches instead of surgery, 87–88; alternative healing methods, 73–83; designing an alternative program, 34–35; diet, 64–73; fasting, 83–84; physician, heal myself, 88–89; quitting smoking, 84–85; sleep, 86–87; stress management techniques, 35–64; summary, 89–90

alternative medicine approaches to: abdominal aortic aneurysm, 308–9; anal fissures, 473–74; anal infection, 478; anal warts, 476–77; aneurysms, 308–9; appendicitis, 454–55; artery disease, 291–94; back problems, 613–21; benign prostate enlargement, 559–63, 563(fig.); breast cancer, 201–12; breast enlargement, 175–76; breast reduction, 179; carpal tunnel syndrome, 660–61; cataracts, 692–94; cervical cancer, 529–31; collapsed lung, 237; colon health, 414–15; colon polyps, 431–32; colorectal cancer, 435–39; convalescence, 137–39; coronary artery disease, 261–72; diverticular disease, 419–21; dysfunctional uterine bleeding, 509–13; endometriosis, 516–17; erectile dysfunction, 581–82; esophageal cancer, 350–51; excess body fat, 666–68; facial cosmetic problems, 673–74; fibrocystic disease and benign lumps, 191–92, 193; gallbladder disease, 384–87; goiter, 598–99; hemorrhoids, 463–67; hernias, 484–86, 489–91, 493–94, 496, 497–98; hiatal hernia and gastroesophageal reflux, 342–45; hip joint damage, 651–53; hyperthyroidism, 594–95; infections, 715; inflammatory colitis, 426–48; kidney stones, 17, 44, 701–4; knee injuries, 636–37, 640–41, 645–46; lipomas and sebaceous cysts, 147; lung cancer, 231, 241; lymph gland enlargement, 150; malignant melanoma, 165–67; moles, 145; nasal disorders, 678; nausea and vomiting relief, 125; neck problems, 630; nonpeptic stomach ulcer disease, 372–73; ovarian cancer, 546–47, 549–50; ovarian cysts and benign tumors, 542–43; pancreatic cancer, 404–5; pancreatitis, 397–98, 400–401; peptic ulcer disease, 360–67; pilonidal cysts, 156; preoperative preparation, 113–14; prostate cancer, 570–73; skin cancer, 158–59; skin infections, 152; stomach cancer, 356, 374–75; stroke prevention, 315–19; thinning hair and baldness, 680–82; thyroid cancer, 601–2; tonsil and adenoid disorders, 686–87; umbilical hernias, 489–91; uterine cancer, 534–35; uterine fibroids, 521–23; varicose veins, 329–31
Alzheimer's disease, antacids and, 365
American Academy of Neurology Practice Committee, 178
American Academy of Orthopedic Surgeons, 623
American Association for Cancer Research, 375, 438
American Board of Surgery, 93
American Cancer Society (ACS), 185; colon and rectum diseases, 434–35; lung cancer, 239, 240; organizations for postmastectomy patients, 221; PSA testing, 569; screening for colorectal cancer, 418
American College of Cardiology, 278
American College of Obstetrics and Gynecology, 4, 185
American College of Radiology, 186
American College of Surgeons, 185, 222
American Health, 95
American Heart Association, 203, 264, 278, 323
American Horticultural Association, 62
American Medical Association (AMA), 26, 120, 185
American Neurological Association, 623
American Society for Therapeutic Radiology and Oncology, 578
American Society of Clinical Hypnosis, 120
American Urological Association, 569
Amphogel, 345–46
amputation, due to vascular disease, 305–6
anal fissures, 472–76, 475(fig.)

anal fistulotomy, 480
anal infections, 478–80
anal/rectal abscess, incision and drainage of an, 479
anal warts, 82, 476–78
Anderson, J. W., 266
anesthesia, 114–15; acupuncture as alternative, 119–20; anesthetic choice considerations, 115–16; general, 116–17, 118–19; hypnosis as alternative, 120–21; intravenous medication, 126–27; local, 116–17; and preparation before surgery, 712–13; regional, 117–18
aneurysms, 307–11; abdominal aortic aneurysm, 307–8; surgical approaches to, 309–11, 310(fig.)
angina, 257–58
angiogram, 249, 290–91
angioplasty, 249, 250, 251, 276, 277(fig.), 278, 295–96, 296(fig.), 297(fig.), 320
ankylosing spondylitis, 60
anoscope, 461
antacids, 345–46, 355, 356, 365
anterior cruciate ligament (ACL) repair, 642, 643(fig.)
antibiotics, 19. *See also* drugs
antidepressants, 136, 631
antioxidants, 68, 148, 204, 267
antrectomy, 369, 370(fig.)
anus and rectum, 459–80, 460(fig.), 470(fig.), 475(fig.)
aortic aneurysm repair, 309–11, 310(fig.)
aortoiliac and aortofemoral bypass, 301, 302(fig.), 310 (fig.)
aphasia, 314
apomorphine, 584
appendectomy, 457–58, 457(fig.)
appendicitis, 66, 452–58, 452(fig.), 457(fig.)
appendix, 451–52
Archives of Dermatology, 330
arm block, 117
armpit lymph node biopsy, 217–18, 220
arnica, 81, 128
aromatherapy, 25, 30, 52–53, 86–87, 125, 582
Arsenicum album, 30
art, 55
arteries, 285–324, 287(fig.), 296(fig.), 297(fig.), 302(fig.), 303(fig.), 310(fig.), 313(fig.), 321(fig.)
arthritis: fasting and, 84; of the hip, 650; magnet therapy use for treatment of, 83; *qi gong* for treatment of, 49
arthrogram, 635
arthroscopy, 636
aspartame, 69, 71
aspiration biopsy, 143
aspirin, 126, 136, 295, 319, 362, 439, 621, 631, 646
asymptomatic bruits, 315; surgery and, 322–23
At Peace in the Light (Brinkley), 29, 31, 711
atelectasis, 134
atenolol, 273
atherectomy, 297, 297(fig.)
atherosclerosis, 254–57, 255(fig.), 282, 288, 292, 298, 307, 315–16
Atkins diet, 70, 251
Atkins, Robert, 251
atorvastatin, 257, 274
atypical ductal hyperplasia, 188
augmentation mammoplasty, 177–78, 179
Austin, S., 212
autoimmune diseases, fasting and, 84
automatic compression stockings, 135–36

Axid, 366
ayurveda, 74–75

Bach Flower Remedies, 81
back problems, 74, 78, 102, 607–27, 609(fig.), 611(fig.), 624(fig.)
baldness, thinning hair and, 680–84
balloon dilation, 564–65
Banov, Leon, 459
barium enema test, 417–18
basal cell skin cancer, 158–59, 161
Basmajian, John, 608, 620
BCG, 165
Beating Cancer with Nutrition (Quillin), 166, 206, 405, 572
beating heart bypass, 282
Beaumont, William, 363
beauty, 55
belladonna, 148
benign prostate enlargement (hypertrophy), 66, 558–67, 563(fig.)
benign prostate hypertrophy (BPH), 559
benign tumors, ovarian cysts and, 542–45
Benson, Herbert, 44, 45
Bergen, Candice, 674
Bergen, Edger, 270
Bernard, Claude, 22
beta-blockers, 273
beta-carotene, 204, 242, 267
Bett, Bari, 120
betulinic acid, 167
Beyondananda, Swami, 61
Bihari, Bernard, 405
bilateral sapingo-oophorectomy (TAH-BSO), 538–39, 538(fig.)
bilateral trunkal vagotomy, 369
bile duct and stomach bypass, 408–9
biliary colic, 382, 388, 391
biofeedback, 21, 48, 75–77, 271, 363, 620
biopsies, 171, 183, 185, 505; armpit lymph node biopsy, 217–18, 220; breast, 183, 185, 186–87; cone biopsy, 506; directed biopsy, 506; endometrial biopsy, 506; for male reproductive system disorders, 558; needle breast biopsy, 183, 187–88, 192, 217; open breast biopsy, 187, 189–90; pancreas needle biopsy, 396–97; punch biopsy, 505–6; sentinel lymph node biopsy, 215–16; skin surface, 143; thyroid needle biopsy, 592; transthoracic biopsy, 235–36
birth control pills, 210, 386, 523, 529–30, 543–44
bismuth, 365
bladder, cancer of the, 69
Blankenhorn, Neal, 292
bleeding ulcers, 367–69, 368(fig.)
blepharoplasty (eyelid surgery), 676–77, 677(fig.)
blood circulation of the brain, 312–13, 313(fig.)
blood clots, 135–36, 257, 275, 288
blood gases, 106, 235
blood pressure, 37, 308
blood tests, 106, 258, 382, 395, 416, 556, 580, 592, 701
blood thinners, 136, 319
blood urea nitrogen (BUN), 106
BlueCross BlueShield, 500
Board-Certified surgeons, 5, 93
body brace, 616

bodymind, 22
Boitano, Brian, 47
bone marrow transplant, 228, 229
bone scans, 558, 612
botulinum toxin injection, 474
bowel and bladder function, postoperative, 132–33
bowel cancer, 411
bowel habits, maintaining good, 466
bowel movements, 66
bowel obstruction, 424
bowel surgery, complications of, 449–50
Bowman-Birk protease, 204
Bowman Gray School of Medicine, 342
bra, wearing and not wearing a, breast cancer risk and, 210–11
Bradley, Craig, 13, 716
Braid, James, 120
brain angiography, 315
brain artery disease, 313–15
brain, blood circulation of the, 312–13, 313(fig.)
Brand, Stewart, 80
BRCA genes, 186, 195
breast, 171–72; appearance of your breasts, 174; breast biopsy, 186–87; breast enlargement, 174–78, 177(fig.); breast reduction, 179–81; breast specialist evaluation, 183; CAT, MRI, and PET scans, 186; development, structure, and function, 172–74, 173(fig.); diagnosis of breast disease, 181–90; fibrocystic disease and benign lumps, 190–93; mammography, 181, 183–86; needle breast biopsy, 183, 187–88, 192; open breast biopsy, 189–90; other cosmetic breast problems, 180–81; ultrasound scan, 186 breast cancer, 66, 171, 181, 184, 193–95, 197(fig.); adjuvant treatment of, 226–28; alternative medicine approaches to, 201–12; considerations in choosing your treatment program, 223–24; follow–up, 229; local treatment of the tumor, 224–26; locally advanced and inflammatory, 228; questions to ask your surgeon, 195–99, 200(table), 201(table); recurrent or metastatic, 228–29; risk factors for, 196(table); summary, 230; surgical approaches to, 212–23, 217(fig.), 219(fig.)
Breast Cancer (Austin), 212
breast conservation therapy (BCT), 213, 228; with follow-up radiation, 217–18, 217(fig.); vs. mastectomy, 224–26
breast-feeding, 209
breast self-examination (BSE), 181–82
breathing exercises, yoga, 42–44, 135, 208, 237
Brett, George, 459
Bricklin, Mark, 451, 485
Brinkley, Dannion, 29, 30, 50, 711
bromelain, 330
bruits, 322–23
Bryant, Paul "Bear", 270
budesonide, 428
bulking agents, 468, 474
Burkitt, Denis, 38, 325, 343, 385, 414, 420, 455, 462
Bush, George, 595
Byers, Tim, 205
bypass: abdominal artery bypass operations, 300–302, 302(fig.); bile duct and stomach bypass, 408–9; bypass graft, 300; coronary artery bypass grafting (CARB or "cabbage"), 278–82, 281(fig.); coronary bypass surgery, 37, 102, 249, 250, 251, 261–62, 280; failure

bypass: abdominal artery bypass operations (*cont.*) of vascular reconstruction, 305; internal stent bypass, 405; laparoscopic and endovascular bypass surgery, 304; leg artery bypass operations, 302–4, 303(fig.)

C-reactive protein (CRP), 257
cabbage juice, 362
Cabot-Zinn, Jon, 24
Cady, Blake, 603
caffeine, 68, 69–70, 86, 191, 204–5, 404, 704
Calan, 273
calcium, 106, 432
calcium channel blockers, 273–74
calendula, 81, 148
Canadian National Breast Screening Study, 202, 205
cancer: alternative treatment of, 17; bladder, 69; cervical, 500, 527–33, 528(table); cigarette smoking and, 69; coffee use and risk of, 69; colon, 38, 66; colorectal cancer screening, 418; dietary factors and, 65; esophageal, 349–53, 349(table), 352(fig.); hypnosis and pain relief in terminal cancer patients, 82; kidney, 69; lung, 69, 231, 239–48, 241(table), 245(fig.); ovarian, 545–50, 546(table), 548(fig.); pancreas, 69; pancreatic, 69, 402–9, 403(table), 406(fig.), 408(fig.); prostate, 66, 69, 567–75, 569(table); risks for cancer surgery, 103; skin, 141, 157–63; stomach, 374–77; thyroid, 600–604, 601(table); uterine, 533–36, 534(table). *See also* breast cancer
Cancer Prevention Program (Gaynor), 405
Cannigliaro, Tony, 270
capsaicin, 647
capsular contracture, 177
CarcinoEmbryonic Antigen (CEA), 442
cardiac catheterization, 260–61
cardiac problems, postoperative, 135
cardiopulmonary bypass machine, 280
cardiovascular disease: diabetes and, 37–38; role of hypnosis in, 82; yoga in prevention of, 37. See also heart disease
Cardizem, 273
caring, medical value and healing powers of, 19, 20
Carnegie-Mellon University, 110
Carofate, 366
carotid endarterectomy, 321–23, 321(fig.)
carpal tunnel syndrome (CTS), 83, 659–64, 663(fig.)
Carter, Jimmy, 459
Casey, Kenneth, 613
Castell, Donald, 342
Castelli, William, 264
castor oil, 145, 473
CAT scan: for aneurysms, 308; for appendicitis diagnosis, 454, 456; for arterial vascular disease diagnosis, 290; for back problems, 612; for breast cancer diagnosis, 186; for colon disease diagnosis, 418; for hernias, 484; for hip joint damage, 651; for kidney stones diagnosis, 701; for lung disease diagnosis, 234–35, 240; for male reproductive system disorders, 558; for neck problems, 629; for pancreatic disease diagnosis, 395; pelvic CAT, 504
cataracts, 690–98, 691(fig.), 696(fig.)
catecholamine, 192
catheter abscess drainage, 422
catheter techniques, radiologic, 295–98, 296(fig.)
caudal block, 117

Caverjet, 584
CCK-HIDA scan, 383, 388
Celebrex, 647
celecoxib, 647
cell patterns in tumors, 198
cellulite, 668
centella asiatica, 330
Center for Complementary and Alternative Medicine, 26
Centers for Disease Control (CDC), 25, 205
central IVs, 129–30
cerebral vascular accident (CVA), 311–12
cervical cancer, 500, 527–33, 528(table)
cervical dysplasia, 528
cervical intraepithelial neoplasia (CIN), 527
Cesarean section, 499; acupuncture for avoidance of a, 74; hypnosis as anesthesia for, 121
chamomile, 52, 125
Chandra, P., 150
chelation, 272, 293–94
chemotherapy: for cervical cancer, 532; for colorectal cancer, 440; hypnosis and side effects of, 82; for lung cancer, 231, 243; for ovarian cancer, 547; for pancreatic cancer, 405–6; for prostate cancer, 574; self-healing techniques and, 74; for treatment of breast cancer, 226, 228, 229, 230; for uterine cancer, 535
chest X-rays, 107, 234, 258
chewing gum and toothpicks, for quitting smoking, 85
children: disease-prevention education for, 25; groin hernias in, 496–97; massage therapy for premature infants, 50–51; response to alternative medicine techniques, 34; umbilical hernias in, 497–98
Chinese medicine, 26, 73–74, 120
chiropractic interventions, 25, 77–78, 345, 619, 641, 646, 653, 661, 716
chlorothiazide, 705
chocolate, eating, 18
Choices in Healing (Lerner), 17, 166, 206, 405, 572
cholecystectomies, 388–90, 389(fig.)
cholecystokinin (CCK), 383
cholesterol: atherosclerosis and, 255–57; cholesterol-lowering drugs, 274–75, 319–20; coronary artery disease and, 264–65; fatty diet and cholesterol levels, 66; high-density lipoprotein (HDL), 256, 266, 268, 269, 274, 275, 292, 293, 318; low-density lipoprotein (LDL), 256, 265, 266, 269, 274, 275; and risk of stroke, 316; yoga practice in lowering, 37
cholestyramine, 274
choline, 385
chronic back pain, 78
chronic inflammatory colitis, 425
chronic pancreatitis, 400–402
chronic pelvic pain, 527
cigarettes, alcohol, and caffeine, 68–70
cilostazol, 295
cimetidine, 346, 356, 365–66
cinnamon, 125
ciprofloxacin, 428
Circulation (journal), 278
claudication, 288, 295
claudication distance, 288
Clinoril, 646, 654
clopidogrel, 275, 319
codeine, 126
coenzyme A reductase inhibitors, 319–20

coffee, drinking, 69
Coggin, Joan, 60
colectomy, 433
Colestid, 274
colestipol, 274
colitis, 66
collapsed lung, 236–39
Collins, Robert, 49
colon, 411–50, 412(fig.), 420(fig.), 434(table), 445(fig.)
colon cancer, 38, 66, 416
colon polyps, 431–33
colonoscopy, 417
color therapy, 23, 24, 55–56
colorectal cancer, 418, 432, 433–43, 434(table)
colostomy, 446–47
colotomy with polyp excision, 433
Columbia-Presbyterian Medical Center, NYC, 39, 709
comfrey, 78–79
Compassion in Action (organization), 29, 30
complementary health centers, 30–31
complete blood count (CBC), 106
complete large bowel obstruction, 424
Condyline, 477
Condylomata accuminata, 476
Condylox, 477
cone biopsy, 506
constipation: associated with appendicitis, 455; following surgery, 108; laxatives causing, 464; yoga practice in relief of, 38
Consumer's Guide to Coronary Artery Bypass Graft Surgery, 102
continent ileostomy, 448
contraceptives, oral, 174, 210, 318, 386, 523, 529–30, 543–44
conventional medicine approaches to: anal fissures, 474; anal infections, 478–79; anal warts, 477; appendicitis, 455–56; artery disease, 294–98, 296(fig.), 297(fig.); for back problems, 621–22; benign prostate enlargement, 564; carpal tunnel syndrome, 564; cataracts, 694–95; cervical cancer, 531–32; colon polyps, 432–33; colorectal cancer, 439–40; coronary artery disease, 272–78, 277(fig.); diverticular disease, 421–22; dysfunctional uterine bleeding, 513–14; endometriosis, 517–18; erectile dysfunction, 582–85; esophageal cancer, 351; fibrocystic disease and benign lumps, 192; gallbladder disease, 387; goiter, 599; hemorrhoids, 468; hernia, 486, 494; hiatal hernia and gastroesophageal reflux, 345–46; hip joint damage, 653–54; hyperthyroidism, 595–96; inflammatory colitis, 428; kidney stones, 704–6; knee injuries, 637–38, 641, 646–47; lung cancer, 243; lymph gland enlargement, 150–51; malignant melanoma, 167; neck problems, 630–31; ovarian cancer, 547, 550; ovarian cysts and benign tumors, 543–44; pancreatic cancer, 405–6, 406(fig.); peptic ulcer disease, 365–67; preoperative preparation, 112–13; prostate cancer, 573; skin cancer, 161–62; skin infections, 154; stomach cancer, 375; stroke, 319–20; thinning hair and baldness, 681–82; thyroid cancer, 602; tonsil and adenoid disorders, 687; uterine cancer, 535; uterine fibroids, 523–24; varicose veins, 332–33
Coppen, A., 541
core needle biopsy, 143, 592
coronary angiography, 260–61

coronary artery bypass grafting (CARB or "cabbage"), 278–82, 281(fig.)
coronary artery disease, 66, 254–76, 255(fig.), 277(fig.), 278–84, 281(fig.)
coronary bypass surgery, 37, 102, 249, 250, 251, 261–62, 280
corset/body brace, 616
cortisone, 362
cortisone injections, 662
Coumadin, 319
Couric, Katie, 411, 417
Cousins, Norman, 23, 33, 47, 60, 61, 63
Covera, 273
COX-1 and COX-2 inhibitors, 646–47, 654
Crawford, Jane Todd, 5
Crile, George, 1
Crohn's disease, 132, 424–31
cryosurgery, 574
cryotherapy, 471, 477
culdoscopy, 505
culposcopy, 504
cystometrics, 557
cystoscopy, 557, 706
cystourethrogram, 557
cysts: cyst aspiration, 544; cyst excision, 544; ovarian cysts and benign tumors, 542–45

Danazol, 514, 518
Danocrine, 514, 518
Dartmouth protocol, 167, 169
Darvon, 126, 127
Daypro, 646, 654
Dean Ornish Lifestyle Program, 21, 92–93, 262–63
death, 28–30
decongestants, 562
deep relaxation, yoga, 40–42, 86, 92
dehydroepiandrosterone (DHEA), 128
DeKalb General Hospital, Decatur, GA, 61
Deltasone, 428
Demerol, 116, 126, 127, 128, 134
deodorants and antiperspirants, 210, 211
Depocar, 564
depression, 513; after surgery, 136
dermis, 142
dermoid cysts, 542
dermoid tumors, 542
diabetes: artery problems in, 286, 298; and atherosclerosis, 269; in cardiovascular and renal disease, 37–38; cholesterol levels, 275; foot care for diabetics, 294; high-fiber diet and, 66; the pancreas and malfunction of insulin production, 394; refined sugar intake, 67–68, 267; and risk of stroke, 316–17, 320; yoga program for type I and type II, 38 diabetic ulcers, magnet therapy use in treating, 83
diarrhea, 370, 371
diet, 25, 34, 64–65; acid-stimulating foods, 362; after surgery, 714; for appendicitis, 454–55; arterial disease and, 292–93, 308–9; before surgery, 710–11; for benign prostate enlargement, 560; for breast cancer, 202–5; for breast care, 179, 191; for cataracts, 693; for cervical cancer, 530; choosing whole foods, 70–71; cigarettes, alcohol, and caffeine, 68–70, 86; and circulatory disorders, 65; for colon polyps, 431–32; for colorectal cancer, 436–38; coronary artery disease

diet(*cont.*)
  and, 264–67; for diverticular disease, 420–21; for dysfunctional uterine bleeding, 500–501, 510; for endometriosis, 516; for erectile dysfunction, 581; for esophageal cancer, 350–51; for excess body fat, 667; for facial cosmetic problems, 673; fats, 66–67, 242, 264–66, 292–93, 361–62; fiber, 66, 203, 266, 343, 361, 463–64; for gallbladder disease, 384–85; for goiter, 598–99; good news in foods, 65; for hemorrhoids, 463–64; for hernias, 484, 490, 493, 496; for hiatal hernia and gastroesophageal reflux, 343, 344; for hip joint damage, 652; for hyperthyroidism, 595; for inflammatory colitis, 426–27; for kidney stones, 702–3, 705; for knee injuries, 645; for lung cancer, 242; lung diseases and role of, 135; for nasal disorders, 678; for ovarian cancer, 546; for ovarian cysts and benign tumors, 543; for pancreatic cancer, 402–3, 404; for pancreatitis, 398; phytochemicals, 68; postoperative nutrition, 130–32; for prostate cancer, 571–72; proteins, 67; red grape juice, 268; refined sugar, 67–68, 86, 204–5, 267, 426, 437; salt, 266–67; skin care and, 146, 147–48, 150, 153, 156, 159–60, 165–66; special nutritional formulas, 71–72; for stomach cancer, 375; for stomach ulcer disease, 361–62, 373; for stroke prevention, 316; Super Drinks, 71–72; for thinning hair and baldness, 681; for tonsil and adenoid disorders, 687; for uterine cancer, 534; for uterine fibroids, 522; for varicose veins, 329–30; vitamin and mineral supplements for your surgery, 72–73; vitamins and minerals, 68
digestive enzymes, 398
digital exam, 461
digitalis, 273
dihydrotestosterone (DHT), 559
Dilacor, 273
dilation and curettage (D&C), 99, 506–7, 514
Dilaudid, 126, 127
Diltia, 273
diltiazem, 273
dipyrimidol, 275
direct hernias, 482(fig.), 483
directed biopsy, 506
Directory of Board Certified Medical Specialists, 93
disease, preventing and treating disease by lifestyle choices, 25
diuretics, 273–74
Diuril, 705
diverticular disease, 419–24, 420(fig.)
diverticulitis, 66, 418, 422
diverticulosis, 38, 66, 414, 420–21
dobutamine, 260
Dole, Bob, 553, 573
dolphin swim programs, 62
Donaldson, William, 613
Doppler exam, 289
Doppler flow, 289
Dossey, Larry, 64
Downey, Morton, Jr., 239, 241
Dr. Ornish's Program for Reversing Heart Disease, 59
dreams, interpreting, 24
Dressed to Kill (Singer and Grismaijer), 210
drugs: affecting blood clotting, 275; alpha–blocking, 564; antibiotics and bowel rest for diverticular disease, 422; antibiotics for anal infections, 478–79; antibiotics for appendicitis, 456; antibiotics for skin infections, 152, 154; antiinflammatory, 126, 127, 621–22, 634; for arterial disease, 295; to avoid for peptic ulcer disease, 362; for back problems, 621–22; for carpal tunnel syndrome, 662; for coronary artery disease, 272–75; for endometriosis, 518; for erectile dysfunction, 579, 583–84; for gallbladder disease, 387; for hyperthyroidism, 596; and its effects on esophageal reflux, 344; for knee injuries, 638, 641; for neck problems, 631; nonsteroidal antiinflammatory drugs (NSAIDs), 126, 367, 631, 638, 646–47, 654; over-the-counter, 126, 345–46, 355, 362, 365–66, 462, 474, 646, 654; for prostate cancer, 574; to reduce risk of stroke, 319–20; stress testing with, 260; for ulcer disorders, 365–66; for uterine fibroids, 523 ductal carcinoma in situ (DCIS), 197, 198, 199, 213, 214, 219, 220
Duke, Jim, 18
dumping syndrome, 370, 371
duplex Doppler exam, 290, 314–15, 329
dysfunctional uterine bleeding (DUB), 507–15
dyspepsia, 355
dysplasia, 430

Eat More, Weigh Less (Ornish), 70, 293, 317
Echinacea, 19, 79, 141, 148, 153, 166
echocardiogram, 259
echocardiogram exercise stress test, 259–60
Ecotrin, 126
Edencare (nursing home project), 61
Edison, Thomas, 13
Efudex, 477
Einstein, Albert, 16
electric blankets, breast cancer risk and use of, 212
electrical stimulation, for pain relief, 128
electrocardiogram (EKG or ECG), 107, 258–59; EKG exercise stress test, 259
electrodessication and curettage, 162
electromyelogram (EMG), 76, 612, 620, 629
electron beam CT Scan, 260
Ellis, Steve, 278
emboli, 257
embolus, 307
Emory Medical Center, 608, 620
emotional support, 35, 57–58; group support, 58–59; laughter and play, 59–61; pets and plant therapy, 62–63
empathy, healing powers of, 19
Emperin, 126
endarterectomy, 299–300, 321–23, 321(fig.)
endometrial ablation, 514
endometrial biopsy, 506
endometrial hyperplasia, 526–27
endometriomas, 515, 542
endometriosis, 500, 515–20, 542
endorphins: and effects of meditation on endorphin levels, 45; endorphin levels and eating chocolate, 18; exercise and its effects on, 617; laughter and its effects on, 60; positive mental images and increase in, 46–47
Endoscopic Retrograde Cholangiopancreatography (ERCP), 390, 395–96
endoscopic ultrasound, 397
endoscopy, 359
endotracheal tube, 118

endovaginal ultrasound (EVUS), 504
endovascular bypass surgery, 304
endovascular stent grafts, 311
enkephalins, 45, 46
enterocoel IV, 129
environment, breast cancer and environmental factors, 195
ephedra, 115
epidermis, 142
epidermoid lung cancer, 240
epidural block, 117
epidural catheters, 126
epigastric hernia, 492
epithelial cancer, 546
erectile dysfunction (ED), 579–88
Ernst, Edward, 330
Esalen Institute, Big Sur, CA, 50
escin, 330
esophageal cancer, 349–53, 349(table), 352(fig.)
esophageal disease, 339–40
esophageal manometry, 340
esophageal pH testing, 340
esophageal reflux, 337, 341–46
esophagitis, 341, 371
esophagogram, 340
esophagoscopy, 340
esophagus, 337–53, 339(fig.), 349(table), 352(fig.)
essential fatty acids, 66
estrogen, 173, 174, 191, 194, 203, 209, 212, 500, 507–8
estrogen replacement therapy, 174, 192, 210, 275–76
ethylene-diamine-tetraacetic-acid (EDTA), 272
eucalyptus, 52, 53
evening primrose oil, 192
Evista, 227
excess body fat, 666–72, 669(fig.), 671(fig.)
excisional biopsy, 143, 189
exercise, 25, 56–57; for arterial disease, 293; for back problems, 616–17; for benign prostate enlargement, 562; for breast cancer, 208–9; for carpal tunnel syndrome, 660; for colorectal cancer, 438–39; for constipation, 455; for coronary artery disease, 268–69; for diverticular disease, 421; for dysfunctional uterine bleeding, 512; for erectile dysfunction, 582; for excess body fat, 667; for gallbladder disease, 386; for hemorrhoids, 465; for hernia, 485, 490, 494; for hiatal hernia and gastroesophageal reflux, 344; for hip joint damage, 653; for knee injuries, 637, 640–41, 645; for neck problems, 630; for prostate cancer, 572; for restful sleep, 87; for stroke prevention, 318; for thyroid cancer, 601; for uterine fibroids, 522; for vein disorders, 327, 330–31; yoga in your exercise program, 38
exopthalmus, 593
exploratory thoracotomy, 236
expressive-supportive groups, 59
extensive intraductal component (EIC), 198
external beam radiation, 573
external hemorrhoids, 468–69
extracorporeal shock wave lithotripsy (ESWL), 705–6
eye, the, cataracts, 690–98, 691(fig.), 696(fig.)
eyelid surgery, 676–77, 677(fig.)

face-lift, 672, 675–76, 675(fig.)
facial cosmetic problems, 672–77, 675(fig.), 677(fig.), 679–80

famotidine, 346, 365–66
fasting, 83–84
fat: dietary, 66–67, 242, 264–66, 292–93, 361–62; excess body fat, 666–72, 669(fig.), 671(fig.)
Fawzy, F., 59
Federal Drug Administration, 167, 169
feeding tubes, 131–32
Feldene, 646, 654
Fellow American College of Surgeons (FAC), 93
female reproductive system, 499–501; cervical cancer, 527–33, 528(table); diagnosis of female disorders, 502–7; dysfunctional uterine bleeding (DUB), 507–15; endometriosis, 515–20; ovarian cancer, 545–50, 546(table), 548(fig.); ovarian cysts and benign tumors, 542–45; structure and function, 501–2, 501(fig.); uterine cancer, 533–36, 534(table); uterine fibroids, 520–26, 521(fig.)
feminine healing modalities, 20
femoral angiography, 41
femoral hernias, 482(fig.), 483
fever, postoperative, 133
feverfew, 115
fibrin glue injection, 480
fibroadenomas, 190–91, 193
fibrocystic disease and benign lumps, 190–93
fibroid embolization, 523–24
fight-or-flight syndrome, 36, 51, 61
finasteride, 564, 681
fine needle aspiration biopsy (FNA), 187, 592
Fink, John, 16–17
"First Aid" and "Second Aid", concepts of, 20
fistulotomy, anal, 480
5 alpha-dihydrotestosterone (DHT), 681
5-fluorouracil (5-FU), 162, 477
5-hydroxy-L-tryptophan (5-HTP), 128
Flagyl, 428
Fleischauer, Aaron, 375
Flexeril, 621, 631
flexible fiberoptic bronchoscopy, 235
Foley catheter, 113
follicular stimulating hormone (FSH), 507–8
food allergies, 385, 427
Food and Drug Administration, U.S., 178, 227, 583
foot care, arterial disease and, 294–95
four-vessel brain angiography, 315
fragmin, 136
Framingham Study, 264–65, 318
free radicals, 68, 146
fresh air, breathing, 52
Fresno Recovery Care Center, CA, 111
fulguration, 449
functional cysts, 542

gallbladder, 379–91, 380(fig.), 383(fig.), 389(fig.), 396
gallstones, 66, 74, 380–81, 383–84, 383(fig.), 387, 397, 398
garlic, 79, 141, 148, 153, 166, 206, 267–68, 438
gastrin, 342, 357
gastroesophageal reflux (GERD), 341–49
gated radioisotope ejection fraction test, 260
Gaviscon, 346
gemfibrozil, 274
Gestrinone, 518
ginger, 125

ginkgo biloba, 115
ginseng, 115
Giuliani, Rudolf, 567
Gleason Score, 569
glucose levels, 106
gluteus maximus free flap, 223
goiter, 598–600
goldenseal, 79, 141
Goldman, Louis, 355
Gonzales, Nicholas, 405
Gonzales program, 405
goserelin, 518
Gracie, William, 384
Grave's disease, 275, 593–97
Gray's Anatomy, 50
Green, Elmer and Alyce, 271
green tea, 69–70
Greenway, Hubert, 161
Greer, Steven, 208
groin hernias, 482–89, 482(fig.), 496–97
Groshong catheter, 130
Group Health Cooperative, 542–43
group support, 21, 25, 58–59
Guy's Hospital, London, 212

H-2 acid-reducing drugs, 365–66
hair: hair removal before surgery, 113–14; hairpieces, 682; thinning hair and baldness, 680–84
Hair Club for Men, 681
Hannan, E. L., 281–82
Hart, Bruce, 2–3, 717–18
Harvard Medical School, 204
Harvard Nurses' Study, 386
Harvard University, 208, 266, 267
Hashimoto's thyroiditis, 598
Healing Diet, The (Lemole), 67
Healing from the Heart (Oz), 39
healing ridge, 133, 488
Healing Through Nutrition: A Natural Approach to Treating 50 Common Illnesses with Diet and Nutrition (Abel), 693–94
Healing Words (Dossey), 64
Health and Human Services, U.S. Department of, 4, 194
Health Care Financing Administration, U.S., 263
Health Professionals Follow-up Study, 421, 432
hearing tests, 686
heart, 249–51, 252(fig.), 253; angioplasty and stent treatment, 276, 277(fig.), 278; coronary artery disease and atherosclerosis, 254–76, 255(fig.), 277(fig.), 278–84, 281(fig.); how your heart works, 253–54, 253(fig.); and lung tests, 107
Heart and Estrogen/Progesterone Replacement Study, 275
heart disease, 26, 250, 513; Dean Ornish Heart Disease Reversal Program, 102, 249, 250, 269, 271, 292; Dean Ornish heart research support groups, 21; diet and, 65; heart attack, 109–10; use of massage for heart attack, 13–14. *See also* cardiovascular disease
heartburn, 337, 342, 343, 344, 345, 347
heat coagulation therapy, 471
Helicobacter pylori (H. pylori), 356, 359, 360, 365; *H. pylori* infection, 346, 366–67, 370, 372, 374
hematoma, 133
hemorrhoidectomy, 470–71
hemorrhoids, 65, 66, 91, 331, 459, 460, 462–72, 470(fig.)

hepar sulph, 148
heparin, 136
heparin-lock IV, 129
hepatic iminodiacetic acid (HIDA), 383
herbal shotgun, 18
herbal sling, 18
herbs, 25, 78–79; for anal fissures, 473; as antidepressant alternatives to drug therapy, 136; for back problems, 620; to be discontinued before surgery, 115; for benign prostate enlargement, 561; for breast cancer, 206; for cataracts, 694; for cervical cancer, 530–31;Chinese, 74; for dysfunctional uterine bleeding, 511; for endometriosis, 517; herbal remedies for smoking cessation, 85; for hernia, 485, 491, 494; immune-enhancing herbals, 148, 150; for inflammatory colitis, 427; for nausea following surgery, 125; for ovarian cysts and benign tumors, 543; for peptic ulcer disease, 364–65; for prostate cancer, 572; for restful sleep, 86–87; for uterine fibroids, 522; for varicose veins, 330
Hering-Breuer Reflex, 43
hernias, 65, 66, 481–98, 482(fig.), 488(fig.), 492(fig.)
heterocyclic amines, 204
hiatal hernia, 65, 341–48
Hickman catheter, 130
high blood pressure, 269, 293, 307, 308, 316, 318
high-density lipoprotein (HDL). *See* cholesterol
highly selective (parietal cell) vagotomy, 369–70, 370(fig.)
hip, 83, 649–58, 650(fig.), 656(fig.)
Hippocrates, 91, 111, 139
HMOs, 18, 102
Hodgkin's disease, 212
Holter monitor, 259, 314
homeopathy, 25, 30, 79–81, 137; after surgery, 715; for anal warts, 477; for back problems, 620; before surgery, 712; for benign prostate enlargement, 561–62; for goiter, 599; for heartburn, 345; for hemorrhoids, 465; for hernia, 485, 491, 494; for hyperthyroidism, 595; for lipomas and sebaceous cysts, 148; for peptic ulcer disease, 365; for skin cancer, 160; for skin infections, 153
Hong, M. K., 275
hormone blockers, 535
hormone replacement therapy (HRT), 194, 439, 513, 549
hormone therapy, for prostate cancer, 573
hormones, 173, 174, 194
hospice care, 30
hospital: checking into the, 107–8; hospital discharge, 136–37; hospital environment, 111–14; hospital history and physical examination, 108–9; origin of, 31
hot flashes, 513
Hoxey Formula, 206
Hudson, Tori, 531
human papilloma virus (HPV) infection, 476
humor therapy programs, 61
Hunter, David, 202, 204
hydrocele, 137
hydrochlorothiazide, 705
HydroDiuril, 705
hydromorphone, 126
hyperalimentation, 132
Hypericum, 81, 128, 136
hyperplastic polyps, 431
hypertension, 269, 293, 307, 308, 316

hyperthyroidism, 275, 593–97
hypnosis, 25, 29–30, 81–82; as alternative anesthesia, 120–21; for benign prostate enlargement, 561–62; for breast enlargement, 175; for breast reduction, 179; for goiter, 599; for heartburn, 345; for lipomas and sebaceous cysts, 148; for lung cancer, 231; for moles, 146; for pain relief, 128; for peptic ulcer disease, 364; for removing moles, 146; for skin cancer, 160; for skin infections, 153; for smoking cessation, 82, 85
Hypnosis in Obstetrics, 121
Hypnotic Induction Profile, 82
hysterectomy, 499, 500, 514, 519, 525, 536; avoiding, 536–37; complications of, 540–41; operations, 537–40, 538(fig.), 540(fig.)
hysterosalpingogram, 504
hysteroscopy, 504
Hytrin, 564

ibuprofen, 126, 127, 362, 513, 621, 634, 646, 654
ileoanal pouch, 430, 448
ileostomy, 444, 446, 447–48
illness-care system, 20
imagery: hypnosis and guided, 81–82; visualization and, 46–49
immune modulators, 206
immune stimulators, 153, 165
immunological theory, modern, 22
immunotherapy, 161, 167, 574
implants: breast, 176–78; for postmastectomy reconstruction, 222; prosthetic, 586–87
incentive spirometer, 135
incision problems, 133–34
incisional biopsy, 143, 189
incisional hernia, 491–95, 492(fig.)
Inderal, 273
Index Medicus, 95
indigestion, 355
indirect hernias, 482–83, 482(fig.)
Indocin, 646, 654
induction chemotherapy, 228
infections: alternative medicine for, 715; anal, 478–80; incision, 134; magnet therapy use for chronic, 83; skin, 149, 151–55
inflammation, atherosclerosis and, 257
inflammatory bowel disease (IBD), 425, 426, 427, 428, 429
inflammatory breast cancer, 228
inflammatory colitis (ulcerative colitis and Crohn's disease), 424–31
infliximab, 428
injection therapy for hemorrhoids, 469–70
inner jogging, 60
inositol, 141
insecticides, 205
insomnia, 513
Institute of Medicine, 178
Integral Health Center, VA, 95
integrated approach to surgery, 709–10; after surgery, 713–16; beyond the scalpel, 718; during surgery, 713; examples of integrative surgery, 717–18; getting ready for surgery, 710–13; preventing future recurrence, 716–17
integrative health centers, 30–31
intercostal nerve block, 117
interferon, 165

interferon alfa–2b, 167, 168, 169
interleukins, 60, 165
internal hemorrhoids, 469
internal stent bypass, 405, 406(fig.)
International Medical Electronics, Ltd., 83
Internet, as information source for surgery decision, 95
intimal hyperplasia, 297
intracavernosal injections, 584–85
intramuscular injection, 127
intraurethral pellets, 585
intravenous lines, 129; central IVs, 129–30; peripheral IVs, 129; problems with IVs, 130
intravenous medication, 126–27
intravenous pyelogram, 557
intubation, 118
intuitive healing, 23–24
iodine-131 uptake test, 592
Isoptin, 273

Jacobs, Marion, 59
Johnson, Ernest, 616–17, 618
Johnson, Lyndon, 24, 379
Joint Commission on Accreditation of Healthcare Organizations, 101–2
joint injections, 638, 647
Jollis, James, 278
Journal of Clinical Pharmacology, 87
Journal of the American Cancer Society, 207
Journal of the American Medical Association (JAMA), 53, 101, 102, 210, 262, 263, 265, 266–67, 276, 316, 318, 439, 541, 561, 661
juvenile hypertrophy, 179

Kadian, 127
Kaiser-Permanente Hospital, Walnut Creek, CA, 49
Kaiser-Permanente Medical Center, Los Angeles, 49
Kansas State University, 62
Katz, Ronald, 119
Kervorkian, Jack, 28
ketorolac, 126
kidney cancer, 69
kidney disease, 65
kidney stones, 17, 44, 698–708, 699(fig.)
Kirlian photography, 73
Kleinke, Chris, 175
Kloss, Jethro, 345
knee, 83, 634–49, 635(fig.), 639(fig.), 643(fig.), 648(fig.)
knee joint cartilage and bone damage, 644–49, 648(fig.)
knee ligament injury, 639–44, 643(fig.)
knee meniscus injury, 636–39, 639(fig.), 644
Koch pouch, 448
Kocher, Theodor, 604
Kübler-Ross, Elisabeth, 29
Kusserow, Richard, 94

lactate dehydrogenase (LDH), 106
Lahey Clinic, Boston, 614
laminectomy, 623, 624(fig.), 626
laminoforaminotomy, 632
laminotomy, 623–24, 624(fig.)
Lancet, 49, 120, 122, 240, 541
lansoprazole, 366
laparoscopic and endovascular bypass surgery, 304
laparoscopic appendectomy, 457–58, 457(fig.)

laparoscopic-assisted hysterectomy, 538(fig.), 539
laparoscopic colon surgery, 449
laparoscopic hernia repair, 487–88
laparoscopy, 505
laparotomy, 505
Lapinsky, Tara, 47
laryngeal mask airway (LMA), 118
laser hemorrhoidectomy, 471
laser scalpels, 30
lateral collateral ligament (LCL) repair, 642–44
latissimus dorsi flap, 223
laughter: healing powers of, 23; and play, 59–61
lavender, 30, 52, 53, 206
lecithin, 385
leg artery bypass operations, 302–4, 303(fig.)
Lemole, Gerald, 33–34, 67
lemon scent, 52
Lerner, Alan, 499
Lerner, Michael, 16–17, 38, 166, 206, 405, 572
Letterman, David, 251
leuprolide, 518
Levamisole, 169
Lewis, Carson, 99
Life Care Health Associates, 36
life support considerations, 28
lifestyle choices: lifestyle changes for heart patients,
    263–72; lifestyle habits in designing an alternative
    program, 34–35; and making an informed decision
    about surgeon, 91; preventing and treating disease by,
    25; preventing illness and changing lifestyle, 716
ligation and stripping, vein, 334–35, 334(fig.)
light, benefits of, 23
Lipitor, 257, 274
lipomas and sebaceous cysts, 146–49
liposuction, 149, 180, 665, 668–70, 669(fig.)
Lipsky, Jeffrey, 83
lithotripsy, 17, 705–6
liver disease, 275
liver-gallbladder flush, 331, 386–87
lobectomy, 245, 245(fig.), 246
lobectomy with isthmusectomy, 604–5, 605(fig.)
lobular cancers, 197–98
lobular carcinoma in situ (LCIS), 196, 197(fig.)
local excision, 441–42, 448–49
locally advanced breast cancer, 228
Locke, Steven, 58
Loma Linda University School of Medicine, 60
loop electrocautery excision procedure (LEEP), 506
Lopid, 274
Lopressor, 273
Love and Survival (Ornish), 59
love, healing powers of, 19, 23, 31
lovenox, 136
low anterior resection, 441, 444
low-density lipoprotein (LDL). See cholesterol
lower back pain, acupuncture for relief of, 74
lumpectomy, 171, 189, 217(fig.)
lung, 69, 231–48, 233(fig.), 245(fig.); postoperative lung
    problems, 134–35
lung cancer, 69, 231, 239–48, 241(table), 245(fig.)
lung disease: diagnosis of, 233–36; yoga breathing exercises
    for patients with chronic, 43
lung function tests, 107, 234–35
Lupron, 518, 523

lycopene, 68
lymph gland enlargement, 149–51
lymph node biopsy, 215–16
lymphocytes, 149

Maalox, 345–46
Macmillan, Harold, 558
magnesium, 106, 386
magnet therapy, 23, 24, 83, 153, 331, 620
magnetic resonance angiogram (MRA) scan, 291
magnetic resonance angiography, 315
magnetic resonance imaging (MRI), 186, 441, 504, 558,
    612, 629, 635–36, 651
male medical voice, 20
male reproductive system, 553–54; benign prostate enlarge-
    ment (hypertrophy), 558–67, 563(fig.); diagnosis of
    male disorders, 556–58; erectile dysfunction, 579–88;
    prostate cancer, 567–75, 569(table); structure and
    function, 554–55, 555(fig.)
malignant melanoma, 163–70, 165(table)
mammography, 181, 183–86
managed care, and choice of healthcare providers, 102
Mann, Horace, 25
Maracaine, 116
Marcus Welby, M.D. (TV program), 18
Marshall, Jan, 46, 60
marsupialization, 157
Maryland's Women's Health Study, 541
Massachusetts General Hospital, 311
massage therapy, 13–14, 25, 30, 50–51; after surgery,
    715–16; for back problems, 619; for breast cancer,
    211–12; for carpal tunnel syndrome, 661; for erectile
    dysfunction, 582; for facial cosmetic problems, 674;
    and getting ready for surgery, 711; for hip joint dam-
    age, 653; for knee injuries, 646; massage bars, 51; for
    restful sleep, 87; for smoking cessation, 85
mastectomies, 214; modified radical mastectomy, 219(fig.),
    220; simple mastectomy, 219–20, 219(fig.); skin-spar-
    ing mastectomy, 220, 222; total mastectomy, 218–21,
    219(fig.)
Mayo Clinic, 603
McDowell, Ephraim, 5
McLanahan, David, 4, 11–12
McLanahan, Jack, 58, 270, 654–55
McLanahan, Sandra, 3–4, 7–11
mechanical bowel obstruction, 424
medial collateral ligament (MCL) repair, 642–44, 643(fig.)
mediastinoscopy, 236, 240
Medicaid and Medicare: mastectomy coverage by, 222;
    Medicare carotid endarterectomy patients, 323;
    Medicare reimbursement for hospital stays, 136; vol-
    untary second surgical opinion programs, 94
Medical Journal of Australia, 87
Medical Self Care, 95
medications: anticancer, 161; diuretics, 705; female hor-
    mone medications, 513–14, 535; hemorrhoid, 468;
    intravenous, 126–27; for kidney stones, 705; pain,
    126–27, 134, 622, 631, 638, 646, 653–54; pain pills,
    127; for smoking cessation, 85; steroid, 694; ulcer
    causing, 362. See also drugs
medicine and surgery, integrating a new paradigm for,
    21–23
meditation, 24, 25; for breast cancer, 206–7; yoga, 44–46
medullary cancer, 601

Megace, 535
melanocytes, 142–43, 144
melanomas, 163–70, 165(table)
melatonin, 166
Melling, Andrew, 122
Menninger Clinic, 47, 271
Menninger Foundation, 75–76
menopause, 174, 209, 500, 536, 666
Menopause: How You Can Benefit from Diet, Vitamins, Minerals, Herbs, Exercise, and Other Natural Methods (Murray), 276
menorrhagia, 508
menstruation, 173, 212, 500, 507–8
Meperidine, 126
metastatic breast cancer, 228–29
methimazole, 596
methylxanthines, 191
Meticorten, 428
metoclopramide, 346
metoprolol, 273
metranidazole, 428
metrorrhagia, 508
Meyshens, Frank L., Jr., 436
microcalcifications, 184
microdiscectomy, 624, 624(fig.)
microwave thermotherapy, 565
Milken, Michael, 567
mind-body connection/mind-body research, 21, 22, 27, 111, 500
Mind Over Back Pain (Sarno), 617–18
mindfulness training, 24
minerals. *See* supplements
minimally invasive coronary artery bypass (MIDCAB), 283
Minipress, 564
Minnesota Multiphasic Personality Inventory (MMPI), 613
minoxidil, 682
mint, 52
modified radical mastectomy, 219(fig.), 220
moles, 144–46
Mondeville, Henri de, 61
Monitored Atherosclerosis Regression Study, 292
Monro, Robin, 37
Montana, Joe, 622, 625–26
Mooney, Vert, 621
morphine, 126, 127
Motrin, 126, 127, 367, 513, 621, 631, 634, 638, 646, 654
MsContin, 127
Multicenter Lifestyle Demonstration Project, 263
Murray, Michael, 276
muscle or pendulum testing, 24
muscle relaxants, 621, 622, 631
Muse system, 585
music therapy, 23, 24, 53–55, 87, 712, 713, 717, 718
Mutual of Omaha, 263
myelogram, 612–13
Mylanta, 345–46
myomectomy, 524–25

Nader, Ralph, 4
nafarelin, 518
Naltrexone, 405
Naprosyn, 126, 646, 654
naproxen, 126, 646, 654
nasal disorders, 677–79

nasogastric (NG) tubes, 113, 134
National Academy of Sciences, 178
National Cancer Institute (NCI): breast cancer surgery and premenopausal women, 212; determining risk factors for breast cancer, 195, 196(table); lung cancer, 240, 242;
National Cancer Advisory Board, 185; prostate examinations, 569
National Center for Health Statistics, 183–84
National Cholesterol Education Project, 66
National Commission on Cancer, U.S., 407
National Health and Nutrition Examination Survey Study, 652
National Institutes of Health (NIH), 26, 80, 224, 227; alternative medicine description, 6; and carotid endarterectomy surgery, 323; Center for Complementary and Alternative Medicine, 6; Cholesterol Education Project, 274–75; Dietary Reference Intake guidelines, 652; and erectile dysfunction, 579; Office of Alternative Medicine, 6
National Polyp Study, 432, 435
National Stroke Association: Consensus Statement, 318; drugs to reduce risk of stroke, 319, 320; Stroke Prevention Advisory Board, 312
National Surgical Adjuvant Breast and Bowel Project, 227
natural childbirth, 19
Natural Health, 95
natural killer (NK) activity, 47, 206–7
natural medicine, U.S. shift towards, 19
nazatadine, 366
neck fusion, 632–33
neck problems, 74, 627–33
needle ablation, transurethral, 565
needle aspiration, 187
needle biopsy: pancreas, 396–97; for thyroid disease, 592
needle breast biopsy, 183, 187–88, 192, 217
neoadjuvant chemotherapy, 228
nerve block, 612
nerve conduction tests, 612, 629, 660
nerve injections, 622
New Age Journal, 95
New Beauty: the Acupressure Face Lift (Wagner), 674
New England Deaconess Hospital, Boston, 603
New England Journal of Medicine, 6, 29, 178, 202, 208–9, 214, 251, 265, 266, 267, 274, 318, 361, 386, 456, 583, 585
New York Times, 81, 119
New York University, 221
Nieper, Hans, 405
nifedipine, 273
Nissen fundoplication, 347–48
nitrate drugs, 273
nitroglycerin, 273
nitroglycerin ointment, 474
Nolen, William, 33, 105, 107
Nolvadex, 227
nonmalignant skin growths, 143–44
nonpeptic stomach ulcer disease, 372–73
Norris, Pat, 47–48
Novocain, 116
Nuprin, 126
nurse-anesthetists, 114
Nurses' Health Study, 178, 210, 267, 269, 275, 316, 318, 436
nutrition. *See* diet

oat cell lung cancer, 241
obesity, 269
obstetrics, use of hypnosis in, 121
Ohio State University, 616, 618
omega-3 and omega-6 fatty acids, 66–67, 148, 265–66
omeprazole, 346, 347, 366
One Surgeon's Experience with Hypnosis (Werbel), 121
oophorectomy, 519, 538–39, 538(fig.), 544, 550–51
open appendectomy, 457–58, 457(fig.)
open breast biopsy, 187, 189–90
open nephrolithotomy, 707
open prostatectomy, 566
operating room of the future, 30
operative period, the, 114–23; adjusting to a new lifestyle,
        139; alternative medicine approaches to
        convalescence, 137–39; alternative methods of nausea
        and vomiting relief, 125; anesthesia, 114–21; blood
        clots in the veins, 135–36; blood tests, 106; cardiac
        problems, 135; checking into the hospital, 107–8;
        chest X–ray, 107; consultations from specialists, 109;
        early postoperative period, 123–25; heart and lung
        tests, 107; hospital discharge, 136–37; hospital envi-
        ronment, 111–12; hospital history and physical exam-
        ination, 108–9; immediate preoperative tests and
        preparations, 109; incision problems, 133–34; inten-
        sive care unit (ICU), 124–25; intravenous lines,
        129–30; late postoperative period, 125–36; lung prob-
        lems, 134–35; operating room, 121–23; patient advo-
        cate or ombudsman, 110; "postop blues", 136;
        postoperative activity, 133; postoperative fever, 133;
        postoperative nutrition, 130–32; postoperative pain
        control, 125–29, 134; postsurgical problems, 133; the
        preoperative period, 105–14; preoperative period,
        106; preoperative preparation, 112–14; reading your
        chart, 109–10; recovery room, 123–24; return of
        bowel and bladder function, 132–33; surgical consent
        forms, 110
orchiectomy, 574
Ornish, Dean, 6, 14, 15, 16, 21, 23, 26, 38, 59, 65, 66, 70,
        92–93, 251, 262–63, 293, 317, 570
Ornish Heart Disease Reversal Program, 102, 249, 250,
        269, 271, 292, 319
osteoarthritis, 650
osteopathic manipulation therapy (OMT), 77
osteopathy, 25, 77–78, 345, 619, 641, 646, 653, 661, 716
osteoporosis, 69, 227, 513, 616
ovarian cancer, 545–50, 546(table), 548(fig.)
ovarian cysts and benign tumors, 542–45
oxaprozin, 646, 654
oxicam piroxicam, 646, 654
OxyContin, 127
Oz, Mehmet, 39, 709, 718

Pacific Medical Center, San Francisco, Planetree Hospital
        Program at, 51, 110, 111, 112
pain control, postoperative, 125–26; alternative medicine
        methods of pain relief, 127–29; epidural catheters,
        126; intramuscular injection, 127; intravenous med-
        ication, 126–27; local measures, 127; methods of pain
        control administration, 126; pain pills, 127; types of
        pain medication, 126, 134
painkillers: for kidney stone pain, 17, 44; local anesthesia,
        116
painkilling substances, natural, 45, 46–47, 60

Painter, Robert L., 101
palliative surgery, 103
Palmer, Daniel David, 77
pancreas, 393–409, 394(fig.), 403(table), 406(fig.), 408(fig.)
pancreas needle biopsy, 396–97
pancreatectomy, total, 407–8
pancreatic abscess, 399
pancreatic cancer, 69, 402–9, 403(table), 406(fig.),
        408(fig.)
pancreatitis, 390; acute pancreatitis, 397–400; chronic pan-
        creatitis, 400–402
pantoprazole, 346
Pap smear, 503–5
papaverine, 584
papillary cancer, 601
papillotomy, 396
Paracelsus, 46
paracervical block, 117
Parafon Forte, 621, 631
Parham, Vistara, 411
partial colectomy, 423, 430, 441; and low anterior resec-
        tion, 444; with temporary colostomy, 423
partial mastectomy, 217
partial thromboplastin time (PTT), 106
Pasteur, Louis, 22
Patient Bill of Rights, 110
patient-controlled anesthesia (PCA), 126–27
Pediapred, 428
pelvic exenteration, 540
pelvic inflammatory disease (PID), 526
pelvic lymph node dissection, 578
pendulum testing, 2
pentazocine, 126
Pentoxifyline, 295
Pepcid, 346, 366
peppermint, 125
peptic ulcer disease (PUD), 359–72, 368(fig.), 370(fig.)
Percocet, 127, 622, 631, 638
percussion, 135
percutaneous discectomy, 624–25
percutaneous endoscopic gastrostomy (PEG tube), 132
percutaneous nephrolithotomy, 706–7
Percutaneous Transhepatic Cholangiography (PTC), 396
perianal abscess, 478
perianal fistula, 478
perineal prostatectomy, 576, 577(fig.), 578
peripheral IVs, 129
peripheral vascular disorders, diabetes and, 38
peripheral vascular surgery, 286
perirectal abscess, 478
Perocet, 126
persantine, 260, 275
pesticides, 205
PET scan, 186, 260, 263, 418
pet therapy, 23, 61–62
phentolamine, 584
Philbin, Regis, 250
phosphates, 69
physical exam: for appendicitis, 454; for arterial vascular
        disease diagnosis, 289; for back problems, 611; for
        brain artery disease diagnosis, 314; for carpal tunnel
        syndrome diagnosis, 660; for colon disease diagnosis,
        416; for coronary artery disease, 258; for diagnosis of
        female disorders, 502–7; for erectile dysfunction, 580;

for esophageal disease diagnosis, 339–40; for gallbladder disease, 382; for hernias, 484; for hip joint damage, 651; for kidney stones diagnosis, 701; for knee injuries, 635; for lung disease diagnosis, 234; for male reproductive system disorders, 556; for neck problems, 629; for pancreatic disease diagnosis, 395; for stomach disease diagnosis, 358–59; for thyroid disease diagnosis, 591; for tonsils and adenoids, 686; for varicose veins diagnosis, 329

physical therapy: for back problems, 621; for carpal tunnel syndrome, 661; for hip joint damage, 653; for knee injuries, 638, 641, 645

physicians: alternative medicine use for personal health problems, 19; average patient visits to, 18; of the future, 20; moving from doctor care to self-care, 21

Physician's Health Study, 275, 318, 694

physics, the human body and modern concepts of, 22

phytochemicals, 68, 191

phytoestrogens, 203–4, 500–501, 510, 516

Pierce, Ellison, 118–19

pigment stones, 381

pilonidal cysts, 155–57

Pittler, Max, 330

placebo effect, 42

Planetree Hospital Program, Pacific Medical Center, San Francisco, 51, 110, 111, 112

Planetree Project, University of Arizona Medical Center, 30

plant therapy, 23, 61–63

plaque, 250, 256

plastic surgery, 665–66

Plavex, 275, 304

Plavix, 319

play, laughter and, 59–61

Pletal, 295

pneumonectomy, 245, 245(fig.), 246, 247

pneumothorax, 236–39

Podocon-25, 477

podofilox, 477

podophyllin, 477

podophyllotoxin, 477

poetry, healing powers of, 23, 55

polycystic ovarian syndrome, 542

port-access coronary artery bypass (PAC-CAR or PORT-CAB), 283

Portacath catheter, 130

posterior cruciate ligament (PCL) repair, 642

postmastectomy reconstruction, 221–23

posture, 614–15

practitioners, alternative, and time spent with patients, 18

Pravachol, 274

pravastatin, 274

prazosin, 564

prednisolone, 428

prednisone, 362, 428

pregnancy: breast cancer and early, 209–10; breast enlargement during, 174; endometriosis and, 517; hemorrhoids during, 462; pseudopregnancy, 517–18; varicose veins during, 329

Prelone, 428

premenstrual syndrome (PMS), 173, 179

Preparation H, 462, 468

Prevacid, 366

Prevention magazine, 451, 485

Preventive Medicine Research Institute, 263

Preventive Services Task Force, U.S., 275

Prilosec, 346, 347, 366

Pritikin Hospital Plan, 111

Procardia, 273

proctocolectomy: with ileoanal pouch, 430; with ileostomy, 444, 446

progesterone, 173, 174, 194, 508, 517–18

prolactin, 174

prolapse of the uterus, 526

Propecia, 681–82

propoxyphene, 126

propranolol, 273

propylthiouracil (PTU), 596

Proscar, 564

prostaglandin, 584

prostate alkaline phosphatase (PAP) test, 556, 568

prostate cancer, 66, 69, 567–75, 569(table)

prostate disorders, 558–67, 563(fig.)

prostate specific antigen (PSA) test, 554, 556, 567, 568, 569

prostate stents, 565

prostatectomies, 566, 574, 576, 577(fig.), 578

prostheses, breast, 223

prosthetic implants, 586–87

proteins: dietary, 67; measuring, 106; for wound healing, 84

prothrombin time (PT), 106

proton pump inhibitors, 366

Protonix, 346

Provera, 535

psychological testing, 613

psychoneurocardiology, 58

psychoneuroendocrinology, 590

psychoneuroimmunology, 58, 206

Public Citizen's Health Research Group, 4

pulmonary embolus, 134

punch biopsy, 143, 505–6

Pycnogenol, 330

pyloroplasty, 369, 370–71

qi gong, 49–50, 161, 166, 208, 619

Questran, 274

Quillin, Patrick, 166, 206, 405, 572

Quinlan, Kathleen, 28

radiation treatment: for breast cancer, 212, 218; for cervical cancer, 531–32; for ovarian cancer, 547; for uterine cancer, 535

radical hysterectomy, 539, 540(fig.)

radical prostatectomy, 574, 578

radioactive iodine treatment, for hyperthyroidism, 596

radioactive isotope thyroid scan, 592

radioactive thallium stress test, 259

radiotherapy, 161, 243, 405, 439–40, 573

Raloxifene, 227

Ram Das, 16

Ranitidine, 346, 365–66

Reach-to-Recovery, 139, 221

Reagan, Ronald, 141, 411, 558

rectal cancer, 440

rectum, anus and, 459–80, 460(fig.), 470(fig.), 475(fig.)

rectus diastasis, 492(fig.), 493

recurrent breast cancer, 228–29

reduction mammoplasty, 180
reflexology, 51
reflux, 337, 341–49
regional neck nerve block, 117
Reglan, 346
Reiki, 51
Reladin, 646, 654
relaxation techniques. *See* stress management techniques
religion, science and, 15, 16
Remicade, 428
renal disease, diabetes and, 37–38
residual urine, 557
rest pain, 288
Reston, James, 119
Retin-A, 145, 160, 161
Retinoic acid, 145
retropubic prostatectomy, 576, 577(fig.), 578
reversible ischemic neurologic deficits (RINDs), 314
Rimm, Eric, 267, 268
Robaxin, 621, 631
rofecoxib, 647
Rogaine, 682
Rolaids, 345–46
rolfing, 51, 102, 619, 661
rose scent, 52
Ross, John, 4
Roto-Rooter, 297
Rowesa, 428
Roxicet, 126, 127
rubberbanding technique for hemorrhoids, 469, 470(fig.)
Rumi, 20
ruptured disk, 622
ruscus aculeatus, 330
Rush-Presbyterian-St. Luke's Medical Center, Chicago, 242

Sachs, Frank, 266
Said, Bob, 47
saline implants, 178
salpingectomy, 550–51
salt intake, 266–67
sand tray therapy, 61
sarcoma, 533
Sarno, John, 617–18, 621
Saved by the Light (Brinkley), 29, 50, 711
saw palmetto, 564
Scherwitz, Lawrence, 272
Scholz, Kenneth, 622
Schwarzkopf, Norman, 553
sciatica, 608
science: religion and, 15, 16; scientific research of alternatives, 26
Science journal, 271
scientists, 14–15
sclerotherapy, 333
scoliosis, 102
Scottish Cancer Trial, 227
Scripps Medical Center, La Jolla, CA, 161
sebaceous cysts. *See* lipomas and sebaceous cysts
segmental mastectomy, 217
segmentectomy, 245, 245(fig.)
self-care: moving from doctor care to, 21; self-care education, 25
self-healing capacity, alternative medicine and body's, 17–18

self-hypnosis, 82
Selzer, Richard, 1, 122
sentinel lymph node biopsy, 215–16
septoplasty, 679
septorhinoplasty, 679
seroma, 133
serotonin, 18, 45
serum electrolytes, 106
serum glutamine oxalate pyruvate transferase (SGPT), 106
serum glutamine oxalate transferase (SGOT), 106
Setterberg, Fred, 608
sexual transmitted disease (STD), 529
sharing, medical value of, 20
Sharp Recovery Center, San Diego, 111
shave biopsy, 143
shaving before surgery, 113–14
shiatsu, 51, 716
shock wave lithotripsy, 387
sickle cell anemia, 106
Sickles, Edward, 186
Siegal, Bernie, 23–24, 48, 123, 207
sigmoidoscope, 461
sigmoidoscopy, 417
sildenafil, 583
silicea, 148
silicone gel implants, 178
Simonton, Carl, 47
simple hysterectomy, 537–38
simple mastectomy, 219–20, 219(fig.)
simvastatin, 274
sitz baths, 467, 468, 471, 474, 478
skin, 141–70, 142(fig.), 165(table)
skin cancer, 141, 157–63
skin infections, 82, 149, 151–55
skin-sparing mastectomy, 220, 222
skin tags, anal, 468
sleep, 86–87, 129, 364, 686
sliding hiatal hernias, 341
slipped disk, 610
smoking: aneurysms and, 307, 308; arterial vascular disease and, 292, 298; back problems and, 615–16; breast cancer and, 206; cataracts and, 694; cervical cancer and, 530; children and, 25; cigarettes, 68–69; colon polyps and, 432; colorectal cancer and, 438; coronary artery disease and, 264; dietary factors and, 65; dysfunctional uterine bleeding and, 510; effects on breast milk, 174; erectile dysfunction and, 581; esophageal disease and, 344, 350; facial cosmetic problems and, 673; fibrocystic disease and, 191; hernia risk and, 485, 490, 493; hyperthyroidism and, 595; hypnosis in helping people to quit, 82; inflammatory colitis and, 427–28; lung cancer and, 231, 232, 239, 241–42; ovarian cysts, benign tumors and, 542–43; pancreatic cancer and, 403, 404; peptic ulcer disease and, 361; postoperative lung problems for smokers, 134–35; quitting, 84–85; stomach cancer and, 375; and stroke prevention, 318
Sneed, Catherine, 62–63
Society for Office-Based Surgery, 99
soft drinks, 69
soft science, 16
solid core needle biopsy, 187, 188
Soma, 621, 631
sonogram, 259, 289–90, 382–83, 395, 504, 557–58

soybean products, 191, 203–4
spa treatments, 52
sperm tests, 557
sphincterotomy, 396
Spiegel, David, 58, 59
spinal block, 117
spinal fusion, 625–26
spinal stenosis, 610
spiritual aspects of health and healing, 18, 19, 22, 23, 24, 25; accessing spiritual side before surgery, 711; stress management and innermost and spiritual connection, 35, 63–64
spirometry, 235
spondylosis, 628
sputum tests, 234
squamous cell lung cancer, 240
squamous cell skin cancer, 158–59, 161
St. John's Hospital, Los Angeles, 61
St. John's wort, 81, 115, 136
staging pelvic lymph node evaluation, 574
Staphylococcus, 152
staphysagria, 81
State University of New York, Buffalo, 53
steam and sauna treatments, 52, 687
Steele-Rosornoff, Renee, 621
Stein-Leventhal Syndrome, 509
Steiner, Charles, 608
Steiner, Rudolph, 55
stem cell transplant, 228
stent treatment, 276, 277(fig.), 278, 296, 297(fig.), 320, 405
stents, prostate, 565
stereotactic needle biopsy, 187–88
steroid injections, 631
stimulants, scents as, 52–53
"Stoke Belt", 317
stomach, 355–77, 357(fig.), 368(fig.), 370(fig.)
stomach bypass, 408–9
stomach cancer, 374–77
stool occult blood test, 416
stool softeners, 468, 474
Strawberry, Darryl, 411
Streptococcus, 152
stress exercise test, 107
stress management techniques, 25, 34, 35–36; for aneurysms, 309; aromatherapy, 52–53; art, poetry, beauty, and color, 55–56; for arterial disease, 293; before surgery, 711; for benign prostate enlargement, 562; for breast cancer, 206–7; for carpal tunnel syndrome, 661; for cervical cancer, 531; for collapsed lung, 237; for constipation, 455; for coronary artery disease, 268, 270–71; for dysfunctional uterine bleeding, 512; emotional support, 35, 57–63; for erectile dysfunction, 582; for excess body fat, 667; exercise, 56–57; for fibrocystic disease, 192; for gallbladder disease, 386; for goiter, 598; for heartburn, 345; for hemorrhoids, 466; for hernia, 498; for hyperthyroidism, 594–95; for inflammatory colitis, 427; innermost or spiritual connection, 35, 63–64; for lung cancer, 243; for malignant melanoma, 166; massage, therapeutic touch, reflexology, Reiiki, rolfing, shiatsu, and Alexander Technique, 50–51; music, 53–55; for pancreatitis, 398; for peptic ulcer disease, 362–64; relaxation techniques, 35, 36–46; for skin

cancer, 161; for skin infections, 153–54; *tai chi* and *qi gong*, 49–50; for thinning hair and baldness, 681; for tonsil and adenoid disorders, 687; for uterine cancer, 535; for uterine fibroids, 522; visualization and imagery, 46–49; water therapy, spa treatments, sunlight and fresh air, 52
stress testing with drugs, 260
stripping, vein, 334–35, 334(fig.)
stroke, 311–24, 313(fig.), 321(fig.)
subluxations, 77
subtotal gastrectomy, 376
subtotal hysterectomy, 537
subtotal thyroidectomy, 599, 604, 605(fig.)
sucralfate, 366
sulindac, 646, 654
Sullivan, Michael, 95
sunlight/sun exposure, 52, 212, 673
superficial basal cell cancer, 158
supplements: after surgery, 714; for aneurysms, 309; for back problems, 620; before surgery, 710–11; for benign prostate enlargement, 560–61; for breast cancer, 204, 205–6; for breast care, 179, 191–92; for carpal tunnel syndrome, 661; for cataracts, 693–94; for cervical cancer, 530; for colon polyps, 432; for colorectal cancer, 438; for constipation, 455; for coronary artery disease, 267–68; in the diet, 68; for dysfunctional uterine bleeding, 510–11; for endometriosis, 516–17; for erectile dysfunction, 581–82; for facial cosmetic problems, 673–74; for gallbladder disease, 385–86; for goiter, 599; for hemorrhoids, 465; for hip joint damage, 652; for inflammatory colitis, 427; for kidney stones, 703; for knee injuries, 637, 640, 645; for lung cancer, 242; minerals for restful sleep, 86; for nasal disorders, 678; for ovarian cancer, 546; for ovarian cysts and benign tumors, 543; for pancreatic cancer, 405; for prostate cancer, 572; for skin care, 146, 147–48, 150, 153, 156, 159–60, 165–66; for stomach ulcer disease, 364, 373; for stroke prevention, 317; for thinning hair and baldness, 681; for tonsil and adenoid disorders, 687; for uterine cancer, 534–35; for uterine fibroids, 522; for varicose veins, 330; vitamin and mineral supplements for your surgery, 72–73
support groups, 58–59, 668, 716–17; for back problems, 620–21; breast cancer, 207; changing from individual care to group support, 21; coronary artery disease, 271–72; for melanoma patients, 166; ovarian cancer, 547; prostate cancer, 573
support stockings, 332, 333
Suramin, 169
Surgeon General, U.S., *Physical Activity and Health* report, 208
surgery: for abdominal aortic aneurysm, 309–11, 310(fig.); for anal fissures, 474–75; for anal infections, 479–80; for anal warts, 477–78; for appendicitis, 456–58, 457(fig.); for arterial vascular disease, 292, 298–306, 302(fig.), 303(fig.); for back problems, 622–26, 624(fig.); for benign prostate enlargement, 564–66; for breast cancer, 212–23, 217(fig.), 219(fig.); for breast enlargement, 176–78, 177(fig.); for breast reduction, 179–80; for carpal tunnel syndrome, 662–63, 663(fig.); for cataracts, 695–97, 696(fig.); for cervical cancer, 532; for collapsed lung, 237–39; colon operations, 443–44, 445(fig.), 446–50; for colon polyps, 433; for colorectal cancer, 440–42; for coronary

surgery (*cont.*)

artery disease, 278–83, 281(fig.); cosmetic and reconstructive plastic surgery, 665, 666; for diverticular disease, 422–23; for dysfunctional uterine bleeding, 514; for endometriosis, 518–19; for erectile dysfunction, 585–87; for esophageal cancer, 351–52, 352(fig.); for excess body fat, 668–72, 669(fig.), 671(fig.); for facial cosmetic problems, 674–77, 675(fig.), 677(fig.); for fibrocystic disease and benign lumps, 192–93; for for dysfunctional uterine bleeding, 514–15; for for malignant melanoma, 167–69; future of, 30; for gallbladder disease, 388–91, 398(fig.); for goiter, 599; for hemorrhoids, 468–71, 470(fig.); hernia, 485, 486–89, 488(fig.), 491, 494–95, 496–97, 498; for hiatal hernia and gastroesophageal reflux, 346–48; for hip joint damage, 654–57, 656(fig.); for hyperthyroidism, 596–97; hysterectomy operations, 537–40, 538(fig.), 540(fig.); for inflammatory colitis, 429–30; integrating a new paradigm for medicine and, 21–23; for kidney stones, 706–7; for knee injuries, 83, 638–39, 639(fig.), 641–44, 643(fig.), 647–49, 648(fig.); for lipomas and sebaceous cysts, 148–49; for lung cancer, 243–47, 245(fig.); for lymph gland enlargement, 151; for malignant melanoma, 167–69; for moles, 146; for nasal disorders, 678–79; for neck problems, 631–33; and the new nonsurgical choices, 5–6; for ovarian cancer, 547–48, 548(fig.), 550–51, 551(fig.); for ovarian cysts and benign tumors, 544; for pancreatic cancer, 406–9, 408(fig.); for pancreatitis, 398–400, 401–2; for pilonidal cysts, 156–57; for prostate cancer, 574, 575–76, 577(fig.), 578–79; for skin cancer, 162–63; for skin infections, 154–55; for stomach cancer, 375–76; for stomach ulcer disease, 367–72, 368(fig.), 370(fig.), 373; for stroke prevention, 320–23, 321(fig.); for thinning hair and baldness, 682–83; for thyroid cancer, 602–6, 605(fig.); for tonsil and adenoid disorders, 688–89; for uterine cancer, 535–36; for uterine fibroids, 524–25; for varicose veins, 333–35, 334(fig.).

surgery, making a decision about: the alternative medicine third opinion, 94–95; choosing your hospital, 101–2; choosing your opinions, 92–93; choosing your surgeon, 93–94; cure, quality of life, and life extension, 103; educating yourself, 6–7; finalizing your choice of surgeon, 101; making an informed decision, 91–92; other sources of information, 95; philosophy of risk taking, 103; questions to ask at your initial doctor visits, 95–101; restrictions in choice of doctor or hospital, 102; the second surgical opinion, 94; should you have the operation?, 104; special benefits of the alternative medicine approach, 104; special benefits of the surgical approach, 103–4. *See also* integrated approach to surgery

surgical care, support groups and, 21

surgical consent forms, 110

sweat glands, 142, 143

Swedish massage, 51

Synarel, 518, 523

Synthroid, 594, 599

Tagamet, 346, 356, 365–66

tai chi, 49–50, 319, 619

talc, 547

talking, medical value of, 20

Talwin, 126

Tamoxifen, 169, 227, 535

Tapazol, 596

Tarlov, Edward, 614

Taylor, Andrew, 77

Taylor, Ronald, 615

tea: drinking, 69–70, 267, 317, 427; tea bags for hemorrhoid pain relief, 467

temper, controlling your, 318

temporary colostomy, 423

Tenormin, 273

terazosin, 564

Texas Tech University School of Medicine, 622

thallium exercise stress test, 259

therapeutic touch, 51

Thierot, Angelica, 111

thinning hair and baldness, 680–84

Third Opinion (Fink), 17

Thomas, Sue A., 36

thoracoscopy, 236

thrombolysis, 276, 297, 297(fig.)

thrombosis, 257, 288, 307

thyroid, 512, 522–23, 589–606, 590(fig.), 605(fig.)

thyroid cancer, 600–604, 601(table)

thyroid hormone level blood test, 592

thyroid sonogram, 592

thyroid stimulating hormone (TSH), 591, 598

Ticlid, 275, 304

ticlopidine, 275

tissue plasminogen activator, 276

tonsil and adenoid disorders, 684–90, 685(fig.)

toothaches, magnet therapy use for, 83

topical applications, 145–46, 148, 160–61, 166, 654

Topral, 273

Torudol, 126, 127

total abdominal hysterectomy (TAH), 537–38, 538(fig.); and bilateral sapingo-oophorectomy (TAH-BSO), 538–39, 538(fig.)

total gastrectomy, 376

total mastectomy, 218–21, 219(fig.)

total pancreatectomy, 407–8

total parenteral nutrition (TPN), 132

total proctocolectomy, 446; with permanent ileostomy, 430

total thyroidectomy, 599, 604, 605(fig.)

touch: medical value and healing powers of, 19, 20, 50; therapeutic touch, 51

tourniquet/intravenous Bier block, 117

traction devices, 630

TRAM flap procedure, 223

trans-fatty acids, 67

transabdominal sonogram, 504

transcient ischemic attacks (TIAs), 314, 320–21

transcutaneous nerve stimulation (TENS), 622

transformation, using your illness as a chance for, 24

transmyocardial revascularization (TMR), 282–83

transthoracic biopsy, 235–36

transurethral electrovaporization of the prostate (TVP), 566

transurethral incision of the prostate (TUIP), 565

transurethral needle ablation, 565

transurethral resection of the prostate (TURP), 564, 565–66, 574, 575–76, 577(fig.)

transvaginal hysterectomy, 538(fig.), 539

Trental, 295

tretinoin, 160
trigger-point therapy, 622
triglycerides, 256
trusses, hernia, 482, 486
tryptophan, 128
tubal ligation, 551(fig.)
tumescent liposuction, 669
"tummy tuck", abdominoplasty, 670–72, 671(fig.)
tumorectomy, 217
Tums, 345–46
Tylenol, 126, 646, 653
Tylenol #3, 126, 127, 622, 631, 638
Type A and B lifestyles/personalities, 36, 62
tyrosinase, 167

Udupa, K. N., 594
ulcerative colitis, 424–31
ulcers, 355, 356; nonpeptic stomach ulcer disease, 372–73;
    peptic ulcer disease, 359–72, 368(fig.), 370(fig.); stom-
    ach ulcer disease summary, 373–74
ultrasound-assisted liposuction, 670
ultrasound-guided needle biopsy, 188
ultrasound scan, 186, 484, 692
ultrasound (sonogram) exam, 289–90, 382–83, 418, 504
Ultrazyme, 398, 401
umbilical hernia, 489–91, 497–98
undifferentiated small cell and large cell lung cancer, 241
University of Alabama, 204
University of Arizona Medical Center, Planetree Project, 30
University of California, Irvine, 436
University of California, Los Angeles, 59, 84, 119
University of California, San Francisco, Medical Center,
    572
University of Massachusetts, 363
University of Miami, 621
University of Michigan, 384
University of Pennsylvania, 62, 119, 229
University of Southern California, 208
University of Texas, 47, 621
University of Texas Medical Center, 207
University of Virginia Medical Center, 128, 715–16
Unna boots, 332–33
upper GI (gastrointestinal) series, 359, 383
Uprima, 584
urethra culture, 556
urinalysis, 556, 701
urinary infection, 705
ursodiol, 387
uterine cancer, 533–36, 534(table)
uterine fibroids, 500, 520–26, 521(fig.)
uterine removal, 500

vacuum/constriction devices, 584
vaginal dryness, 513
vaginal pack, 530–31
vagotomy, 369–71, 370(fig.)
Valium, 621, 631
Van Nostrand, Randy, 52, 89, 141
varicose veins, 65, 66, 325, 327–36, 327(fig.), 334(fig.)
vascular disease, 286
vascular surgery, 292; for erectile dysfunction, 585–86
vasectomy, 572–73
vegetarian diet, 66–67, 266
veins, 325–36, 326(fig.), 327(fig.)

venogram, 329
ventral and incisional hernias, 491–95, 492(fig.)
verapamil, 273
Viagra, 579, 583–84
vibrational medicine, 23, 24
Vicodan, 126, 622, 631, 638
villous adenoma polyps, 431
Vioxx, 647
virginal hypertrophy, 179
visual laser ablation of the prostate (VLAP), 565–66
visualization and imagery, 46–49; for anal fissures, 473–74;
    for anal infections, 478; for anal warts, 477; for arter-
    ial disease, 294; for back problems, 621; before
    surgery, 712; for benign prostate enlargement, 562;
    for breast cancer, 206–7; for breast enlargement, 176;
    for breast reduction, 179; for carpal tunnel syndrome,
    661; for cervical cancer, 531; for collapsed lung, 237;
    for colorectal cancer, 439; for coronary heart disease,
    272; for diverticular disease, 421; for dysfunctional
    uterine bleeding, 512–13; for endometriosis, 517; for
    erectile dysfunction, 582; for excess body fat, 667; for
    fibrocystic disease, 192; for gallbladder disease, 387;
    for goiter, 599; for heartburn, 345; for hemorrhoids,
    466; for hernia, 485, 490, 494; for hip joint damage,
    653; for hyperthyroidism, 595; hypnosis and, 81–82;
    for inflammatory colitis, 428; for kidney stones, 704;
    for lipomas and sebaceous cysts, 148; for lung cancer,
    243; for malignant melanoma, 167; for ovarian can-
    cer, 547; for ovarian cysts and benign tumors, 543;
    for pancreatic cancer, 405; for pancreatitis, 398, 401;
    for peptic ulcer disease, 363–64; for pilonidal cysts,
    156; for prostate cancer, 573; for removing moles,
    146; for skin cancer, 161; for stroke recovery, 319; for
    thinning hair and baldness, 681; for thyroid cancer,
    602; using visualization to quit smoking, 85; for uter-
    ine cancer, 535; for uterine fibroids, 522; for varicose
    veins, 331
vitamins. See supplements
Volteren, 646, 654
voluntary second opinion programs, 94
volvulus, 424

Wagner, Lindsay, 674
Waldorf Schools, 55
Walford, Roy, 84
walking, 269; after surgery, 135, 138
warfarin, 319
Warhol, Andy, 380
warts, anal, 82, 476–78
water therapy, 52, 85
wave theory, 22
wedge resection, 245, 245(fig.)
weight, maintaining your, 209, 269, 293, 317, 330, 345,
    386, 465, 484, 490, 493, 496, 498, 512, 517, 522,
    572, 615, 645, 652, 693, 704
weight training, 57
Weil, Andrew, 30, 71
Werbach, Melvin, 694
Werbel, Ernest, 121
West, Stanley, 499
Whipple procedure, 407–8, 408(fig.)
White, Betty, 61
"Why Me?" (organization), 221
Williams, Robin, 60

Winfrey, Oprah, 26, 83
Wolff, M. S., 205
wrist, 658–64, 663(fig.)

X-rays: for appendicitis diagnosis, 454; for back problems, 612; chest, 107, 234, 258; chest X-ray for lung disease diagnosis, 234, 240; for coronary artery disease diagnosis, 258; for hip joint damage, 651; for kidney stones diagnosis, 701; for knee injuries, 635; limiting exposure to, 602; for neck problems, 629; for tonsils and adenoids, 686
Xylocaine, 116, 149, 162

Yale-New Haven Hospital, NY, 48
yoga, 24, 25, 30, 36–39; after surgery, 39–40, 40(fig.), 714; for aneurysms, 309; for back problems, 617–18; before surgery, 711; for benign prostate enlargement, 562, 563(fig.); breathing exercises, 42–44, 135, 208, 237; for carpal tunnel syndrome, 661; for cataracts, 694; for constipation, 455; for coronary artery disease, 268, 270–71; deep relaxation, 40–42, 86, 92; for dysfunctional uterine bleeding, 512; for erectile dys-function, 582; for excess body fat, 667; for facial cosmetic problems, 674; for goiter, 598; for hemorrhoids, 465–66; for hernia, 485, 490, 494, 498; for hip joint damage, 653; for hyperthyroidism, 594–95; for knee injuries, 637, 641, 645–46; for malignant melanoma, 166–67; meditation, 44–46; for nasal disorders, 678; for pain relief, 128; for peptic ulcer disease, 364; for pilonidal cysts, 156; postures, 37, 38–39; practicing yoga to quit smoking, 85; for prostate cancer, 572; for skin cancer, 161; for stroke prevention, 319; for thinning hair and baldness, 681; for vein disorders, 327, 330–31; yoga postures daily program, 39; yoga stretches after your operation, 39–40, 40(fig.); yoga stretches for breast cancer, 208

Zantac, 346, 365–66
Zappa, Frank, 567
zinc, 427, 511
Zocor, 274
Zolodex, 518, 523
Zone diet, 70
Zostrix, 647